ENCYCLOPEDIA OF
BIOETHICS

3RD EDITION

EDITORIAL BOARD

ENCYCLOPEDIA OF
BIOETHICS

3 RD EDITION

EDITED BY

STEPHEN G. POST

VOLUME

4

N – S

**MACMILLAN
REFERENCE
USA™**

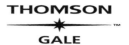

GALE

New York • Detroit • San Diego • San Francisco • Cleveland • New Haven, Conn. • Waterville, Maine • London • Munich

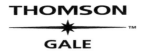

Encyclopedia of Bioethics, 3rd edition

Stephen G. Post

Editor in Chief

©2004 by Macmillan Reference USA.
Macmillan Reference USA is an imprint of The
Gale Group, Inc., a division of Thomson
Learning, Inc.

Macmillan Reference USA™ and Thomson
Learning™ are trademarks used herein under
license.

For more information, contact
Macmillan Reference USA
300 Park Avenue South, 9th Floor
New York, NY 10010
Or you can visit our Internet site at
http://www.gale.com

While every effort has been made to
ensure the reliability of the information
presented in this publication, The Gale Group,
Inc. does not guarantee the accuracy of
the data contained herein. The Gale Group,
Inc. accepts no payment for listing; and
inclusion in the publication of any
organization, agency, institution, publication,
service, or individual does not imply
endorsement of the editors or publisher.
Errors brought to the attention of the
publisher and verified to the satisfaction of
the publisher will be corrected in future
editions.

Library of Congress Cataloging-in-Publication Data

Encyclopedia of bioethics / Stephen G. Post, editor in chief.— 3rd ed.
    p. cm.
Includes bibliographical references and index.
    ISBN 0-02-865774-8 (set : hardcover : alk. paper) — ISBN
0-02-865775-6 (vol. 1) — ISBN 0-02-865776-4 (vol. 2) — ISBN
0-02-865777-2 (vol. 3) — ISBN 0-02-865778-0 (vol. 4) — ISBN
0-02-865779-9 (vol. 5)
    1. Bioethics—Encyclopedias. 2. Medical ethics—Encyclopedias. I.
Post, Stephen Garrard, 1951-
QH332.E52 2003
174'.957'03—dc22

2003015694

This title is also available as an e-book.
ISBN 0-02-865916-3 (set)
Contact your Gale sales representative for ordering information.

Printed in the United States of America
10 9 8 7 6 5 4 3 2

Front cover photos (from left to right): Custom Medical Stock;
Photo Researchers; Photodisc; Photodisc; AP/Worldwide Photos.

N

NANOTECHNOLOGY

• • •

Imagine a world in which manufacturing and medical treatments take place solely at a molecular level, a world in which human bodies are reengineered to include more durable tissues or to reverse past injuries. These are some of the dreams motivating scientists and engineers pursuing the field of nanotechnology. As the name implies, nanotechnology involves the engineering or manipulation of matter, and life, at nanometer scale, that is, one-billionth of a meter. (Ten hydrogen atoms side by side span 1 nanometer; the DNA molecule is 2.3 nanometers across). If feats such as those mentioned above were possible, then the structures of the human body and the current tools of humankind could be significantly altered. In recent years many governments around the world, including the United States with its National Nanotechnology Initiative, and scores of academic centers and corporations have committed increasing support for developing nanotechnology programs (Glapa).

The Birth of an Idea

The idea behind nanotechnology originated with Nobel laureate Richard Feynman in a speech he gave to the American Physical Society in 1959. He described the development of tools for molecular engineering, whereby things would be built molecule by molecule. He proposed, as a challenge to his colleagues, the writing of the entire *Encyclopedia Britannica* on the head of a pin. His startling claim was that this sort of task would not require a new understanding of physics and was completely compatible with what scientists already understood about the nature of force and

matter. Little was done in response to the Feynman challenge until the publication of works by K. Eric Drexler in the 1980s and 1990s. Drexler demonstrated the feasibility of such manipulation from an engineering perspective and provided a vision for the possible benefits of such technologies.

What Could Nanotechnology Do?

The list of potential uses of nanotechnology continues to expand. The primary focus of research at this point concerns miniaturization of electronic components (Bachtold et al.; Hornbaker et al.), but nanoscale materials may dramatically improve the durability of materials used in machinery and could result in less polluting and more efficient production methods. The U.S. military has a significant interest in nanotechnology and has created the Institute for Soldier Nanotechnologies (ISN). Among the initial aims of the ISN is to create stealth garments (and coatings) that are difficult to see or detect, are highly durable, and provide increased protection from penetrating objects. The institute aims to develop devices to rapidly and accurately detect biological or chemical weapon attacks. The ISN is also interested in using nanotechnology to help seamlessly integrate electronic devices into the human nervous system—creating the cyborg soldier.

There are many possible medical uses of microscopic, subcellular machines. Medical applications of nanotechnology include rational drug design; devices specifically targeting and destroying tumor cells (McDevitt et al.) or infectious agents; in vivo devices for the manufacture and release of drugs and for tissue engineering or reengineering at the site of need; early detection or monitoring devices; in vitro diagnostic tools amounting to a laboratory on a chip (Park, Taton, and Mirkin); devices to clear atherosclerotic lesions in coronary or cerebral arteries; and biomimetic nanostructures to repair or replace DNA or other organelles. Nanotechnology might be used to provide artificial replacements for red blood cells and platelets (Freitas, 1996), to augment or repair interaction between neurons in the brain, to improve biocompatibility and the interface between brain tissue and cybernetic devices, and to develop more durable prosthetic devices or implants (Drexler, 1986; Drexler and Peterson; Freitas, 1999; Crandell; BECON). Such tools have also been envisioned to provide new means of cosmetic enhancement, such as controlling weight, changing hair or skin color, removing unwanted hair, or producing new hair simulations (Crawford). Also, some of the potential therapeutic uses previously listed would lead to more effective treatment of life's greatest killers, such as cancer, infectious disease, and vascular disease, leading in turn to greatly enhanced human lifespans.

One other possible project to arise from nanotechnology has become the focus of a rigorous debate among members of the nanocognoscenti. This controversial device is the self-replicating assembler, which was first envisioned by Drexler in 1986. The assembler is in essence a form of artificial life, for not only would it manipulate its environment on a molecular or atomic level, as other nanomachines would, but it would also be coded and designed to replicate itself, potentially making endless copies of itself. Alternatively, nanomachines could be designed to function more as viruses, using the mechanisms in other living cells to help duplicate constituent parts and assemble them into a new machine. While it is beyond the scope of this entry to detail the elements of the debate between those who contend such devices can and will be developed and those who adamantly claim that Drexlerian assemblers are a physical impossibility, the assembler is an excellent starting point for the discussion of the ethical aspects of nanotechnology.

Ethical Issues

The ethical issues of nanotechnology can be grouped into five categories:

1. the challenges of prospective technology assessment and regulation;
2. environmental impact of nanotechnologies;
3. issues of justice and access to the goods and services that might accrue from nanotechnology;
4. the ethical and social implications of increased longevity that might result from medical nanotechnology; and
5. the issues of augmentation or enhancement of human attributes and function.

Accidents, Abuses, and Regulation

The vision for medical uses of nanotechnology is exciting, and if only a portion of the proposed devices prove possible, nanotechnology may benefit many thousands of patients. Any device that can operate on the subcellular level, however, can just as easily be designed to destroy as to repair or heal. In fact, it will be far easier to develop devices that kill. One of the first applications of medical nanotechnology involves a device that can target and destroy cancer cells. Despite the arguments over the feasibility of creating assemblers, it is not a far stretch to envision nanoscale weapons that could be borne on the winds or delivered through the water or food supply. Even if not self-replicating, such devices, with appropriate targeting or with the ability to synthesize toxic substances once inside the host could prove to be quite lethal or disabling. If assemblers were ever created, with the ability to self-replicate like bacteria, then the level of personal or environmental harm could be substantial.

Concern over the potential military or terrorist use of such technology, which could ultimately be fairly cheap to produce, and thus impossible to sufficiently regulate once in existence, has led some (even within the technology community) to contend that the only safe way to proceed is to choose not to develop the tools and methods of nanotechnology at all (Joy). In this view, the only way to prevent the potential devastating harms of a technology, or the consequences of malicious use of knowledge and technology, is to not develop the technology, or acquire the knowledge, in the first place. Arguments of this type, however, assume the burden of proving:

1. that the projected abilities of the device in question are possible to achieve;
2. that the feared harms cannot be prevented, controlled, or mitigated to an acceptable degree;
3. that it is feasible to achieve universal consensus that the area of technology and/or knowledge in question should not be pursued; and
4. that such a prohibition can be sufficiently policed.

In the case of the first issue, it seems very likely that biological nanodevices will be developed, most likely using a so-called bottom-up approach. That is, existing biological molecules and organelles will be used as models for creating tools to achieve the desired function, or these "natural" materials will be used in new ways. An example of this is a project that involved the conversion of the ATPase molecule, ubiquitous in living cells, into a molecular motor (Soong et al.). Therefore, because the development of functioning biomechanical nanodevices is highly probable, it is morally imperative to prospectively evaluate the possible impact of these technologies as they are being developed, so that appropriate safeguards can be implemented to protect against accidents, unanticipated consequences, or inappropriate uses of the technology.

While many disagree with Joy's conclusions, his concerns for the potential harms that autonomous technology could produce are legitimate. It is his response to the second issue, the likely ability or inability to control or protect against foreseeable or unforeseeable harms, that has led to the most dissent. Concerns have been raised that autonomous, self-replicating assemblers could escape control, and/or mutate, in such a way as to destroy life and the environment on a massive, cataclysmic scale. This is Drexler's (1986) so-called "gray goo scenario." In a 2000 article, however, Robert A. Freitas Jr. calculated that this nightmarish scenario is unlikely because of the ability to detect the activity of such biovorous devices early on and to neutralize them. In the early days of recombinant DNA research, there were many concerns about releasing lethal plagues into the environment, quite similar to a number of the concerns being voiced about nanotechnology. Yet the scientific community responded strongly and wisely to the challenges of DNA research, establishing procedural safeguards that remain in use (Krimsky; Fredrickson) and that serve as a model for developing and containing potentially harmful technologies.

Pursuing a similar course of prospective risk assessment and guideline development, the Foresight Institute published the "Foresight Guidelines on Molecular Nanotechnology" in 2000. The guidelines remain voluntary recommendations, but they could be used as a framework for formal regulation and licensing of biologically active nanodevices. Some of the recommended design principles include: (1) dependence on a single fuel source or cofactor that does not exist in the natural environment; (2) requiring constant signaling from an external source for the device to continue functioning; and/or (3) programming termination times (similar to apoptosis in living cells). While it is hopeful that all responsible researchers and engineers would embrace suggestions such as these, there will need to be formal regulation with serious economic, licensure, and punitive penalties for failure to comply. Additionally, the granting of licenses to perform research in nonlaboratory settings or to market nanodevices, as well as the awarding of patents, should be contingent upon proof of the ability to detect and destroy the devices in both in vitro and in vivo settings.

The idea that humankind could reach universal agreement to limit or forbid certain areas of research is naive, and very unlikely to happen, particularly when the field of knowledge in question may lead to vast improvements in health, lifespan, productivity, and so on. Even if consensus could be achieved, policing such restrictions will be essentially impossible. The force of curiosity, as well as the stubborn human heart's universal propensity to rebel against restriction, will ensure that the research will indeed take place, just not as rapidly as it might have otherwise. Rather it is wiser to direct the development of the technology in such a way as to prepare defenses concurrently along with the devices themselves. It is only in this way that humankind and individual societies can be prepared to meet the threats of terrorism, accidents, and other calamities resulting from the creation and/or abuse of a particular technology.

The Nano-Improved Human

As mentioned above, medical nanotechnology may provide exciting tools for healing injured tissue, repairing DNA, and treating neoplastic and infectious diseases, as well as for cosmetic applications. It is conceivable that some nanodevices may also be used to strengthen normal tissue; to manipulate certain DNA strands to alter traits; or to augment mental function, either via enhanced electronic interfaces at the cellular level or by direct stimulation of certain neural pathways. These latter possibilities immediately bring up difficult questions.

Should such uses of bionanotechnology be permitted? If they should, should the medical profession be involved with nonhealing, elective augmentation, and if not, then who should? Should people be allowed to use health insurance to cover the cost of such interventions? How can just access be ensured otherwise? Such augmentations, if successful, would create significant differentials in performance in the workplace, physical abilities, and so on. Consequently, the wealthy would get stronger and wealthier, further increasing their advantage over those who might not be able to afford the technology in question.

In his 1999 book *Nanomedicine,* Freitas suggested that nanotechnology, and by implication other potentially augmenting technologies, requires a new concept of disease that transcends the classic model of disordered function. He calls this new model the volitional normative model of disease, and he described it as follows:

> Disease is characterized not just as the failure of "optimal" functioning, but rather as the failure of either (a) "optimal" functioning or (b) "desired" functioning. Thus disease may result from:
>
> 1. failure to correctly specify desired bodily function (specification error by the patient),

2. flawed biological program design that doesn't meet the specifications (programming design error),

3. flawed execution of the biological program (execution error),

4. external interference by disease agents with the design or execution of the biological program (exogenous error), or

5. traumatic injury or accident (structural failure). (Freitas, 1999, p. 20)

While encompassing traditional understandings of disease, this model additionally takes disease out of the context of an objective pathophysiological assessment and turns disease into whatever the patient defines it to be. Any limitation or undesired trait may now be declared disease. Though ostensibly continuing the contemporary trend of patient self-determination to a new level, this approach is fraught with both danger and injustice. To declare that a condition is disease imposes a moral claim that services ought to be rendered for its modification, elimination, or amelioration. The balance between beneficence (the obligation to do good) and nonmaleficence (the obligation to prevent harm) may be inappropriately tipped to what the patient desires, rather than needs. Physicians would be reduced to agents of wish fulfillment and to technicians, rather than remaining healers. These issues already exist to some degree in the area of cosmetic surgery but will expand to involve most other areas of medicine as well. Further, claims to "treatment" would unjustly deplete healthcare resources and funds, potentially depriving those in real need of legitimate healing.

Conclusion

Nanotechnology offers exciting new tools for materials processing, more powerful and integrated electronic devices, and new medical therapies. Nanodevices, however, may also become instruments of harm, and they require prospective regulation and engineering to prevent both foreseeable and unforeseeable negative consequences. Nanodevices join a number of other developing technologies that offer the potential to alter or augment the human body. A prospective, widespread discussion of the implications of these technologies for the human species, the profession of medicine, and the world's communities should occur as soon as possible.

C. CHRISTOPHER HOOK

SEE ALSO: *Biomedical Engineering; Cybernetics; Enhancement Uses of Medical Technology; Human Dignity; Transhumanism and Posthumanism*

BIBLIOGRAPHY

Antón, Philip S.; Silberglitt, Richard; and Schneider, James. 2001. *The Global Technology Revolution: Bio/Nano/Materials Trends and Their Synergies with Information Technology by 2015.* Santa Monica, CA: RAND.

Bachtold, Adrian; Hadley, Peter; Nankanishi, Takeshi; et al. 2001. "Logic Circuits with Carbon Nanotube Transistors." *Science* 294: 1317–1320.

Crandell, B. C., ed. 1996. *Nanotechnology: Molecular Speculations on Global Abundance.* Cambridge, MA: MIT Press.

Crawford, Richard. 1996. "Cosmetic Nanosurgery." In *Nanotechnology: Molecular Speculations on Global Abundance,* ed. B. C. Crandell. Cambridge, MA: MIT Press.

Drexler, K. Eric. 1986. *Engines of Creation.* New York: Anchor.

Drexler, K. Eric. 1992. *Nanosystems: Molecular Machinery, Manufacturing, and Computation.* New York: Wiley.

Drexler, K. Eric, and Peterson, Christine. 1991. *Unbounding the Future: The Nanotechnology Revolution.* New York: Morrow.

Fredrickson, Donald S. 2001. *The Recombinant DNA Controversy: A Memoir.* Washington, D.C.: ASM Press.

Freitas, Robert A., Jr. 1999. *Nanomedicine,* vol. 1: *Basic Capabilities.* Austin, TX: Landes Bioscience.

Grethlein, Christian E., ed. 2002. "DoD Researchers Provide a Look Inside Nanotechnology." Special issue of *AMPTIAC Quarterly* 6(1).

Hornbaker, D. J.; Kahng, S.-J.; Misra, S., et al. 2002. "Mapping the One-Dimensional Electronic States of Nanotube Peapod Structures." *Science* 295: 828–831.

Joy, Bill. 2000. "Why the Future Doesn't Need Us." *Wired,* April, pp. 238–262.

Krimsky, Sheldon. 1982. *Genetic Alchemy: The Social History of the Recombinant DNA Controversy.* Cambridge, MA: MIT Press.

McDevitt, Michael R.; Ma, Dangshe; Lai, Lawrence T.; et al. 2001. "Tumor Therapy with Targeted Atomic Nanogenerators." *Science* 294: 1537–1540.

Mulhall, Douglas. 2002. *Our Molecular Future: How Nanotechnology, Robotics, Genetics, and Artificial Intelligence Will Transform Our World.* Amherst, NY: Prometheus.

Park, So-Jung; Taton, T. Andrew; and Mirkin, Chad A. 2002. "Array-Based Electrical Detection of DNA with Nanoparticle Probes." *Science* 295: 1503–1506.

Roco, Mihail, and Bainbridge, William Sims, eds. 2001. *Societal Implications of Nanoscience and Nanotechnology.* Arlington, VA: National Science Foundation.

Soong, Ricky; Bachand, George; Neves, Hercules; et al. 2000. "Powering an Inorganic Nanodevice with a Biomolecular Motor." *Science* 290: 1555–1558.

INTERNET RESOURCES

BECON (NIH Bioengineering Consortium). 2000. "Nanoscience and Nanotechnology: Shaping Biomedical Technology: Symposium Report, June 2000." Available from <http://www.becon.nih.gov/poster_abstracts_exhibits.pdf>.

Feynman, Richard. 1959. "There's Plenty of Room at the Bottom." Available from <http://www.zyvex.com/nanotech/feynman.html>.

Foresight Institute. 2000. "Foresight Guidelines on Molecular Nanotechnology." Available from <http://www.foresight.org/guidelines/>.

Freitas, Robert A., Jr. 1996. *Respirocytes: A Mechanical Artificial Red Cell: Exploratory Design in Medical Nanotechnology.* Foresight Institute. Available from <http://www.foresight.org/Nanomedicine/Respirocytes.html>.

Freitas, Robert A., Jr. 2000. "Some Limits to Global Ecophagy by Biovorous Nanoreplicators, with Public Policy Recommendations." Foresight Institute. Available from <http://www.foresight.org/NanoRev/Ecophagy.html>.

Glapa, Steven. 2002. "A Critical Investor's Guide to Nanotechnology." In Realis. Available from <http://www.inrealis.com/nano.htm>.

Institute for Soldier Nanotechnologies. 2003. Available from <http://www.aro.army.mil/soldiernano/>.

National Nanotechnology Initiative. 2003. Available from <http://www.nano.gov/>.

National Science and Technology Council. 2003. "Nanotechnology: Shaping the World Atom by Atom." Available from <http://itri.loyola.edu/nano/>.

NARRATIVE

• • •

Human beings are a narrative species. We tell stories incessantly; we read and listen to them, watch them unfold on screen and stage. In making and absorbing narrative—news, gossip, fiction, drama, anecdotes, and history—we spin and untangle explanatory accounts of the way the world works and how we and our fellow human beings act in every conceivable circumstance. Memories of the past and ideas of the future are expressed in narrative accounts of how the world was and how it will, or should, become. Individual identities and self-conceptions are packaged in life stories, part (and heirs) of larger family, community, and national stories that shape the life events and choices to become the chapters that follow. There is even evidence that narrative, rather than simply a creative use human beings have found for language, is instead the motive for its acquisition: Young children learn to talk in order to give some account of occurrences in their daily lives (Bruner).

For the most part, the word *narrative* is used interchangeably with *story* to designate a more or less coherent written, spoken, or (by extension) enacted account of occurrences, either historical or fictional. *Story,* however, is used more often, especially informally, to denote spoken and fictional accounts, while *narrative* emphasizes the inclusion of nonfiction or indicates a contrast with visual or numerical data, as in historiography or book production or computer science. *Narrative* tends to be used generically in literary theory, perhaps following the Russian formalist and French structuralist distinction between *story* and *plot,* where *story* designates the events, and *plot,* the ordering of those events in the literary or historical account. Thus, the story of Oedipus begins with the prophecy his parents receive before his birth; the plot of Sophocles' play begins when, years later, he learns from the same oracle that the plague that afflicts his city is punishment for the unavenged death of the old king. Narrative refers to the whole and implies, for any particular telling, the inseparability of plot and story.

As it orders events, narrative asserts or connotes some causal relation among those events and imputes character and motives to the actors (Forster). Yet, despite this linearity, conclusions are never foregone. As narrative depicts events embedded in the lives and concerns of its protagonists, circumstances unfold through time in all their contingency and complexity (Ricoeur). Whether it is the life story essential to moral understanding (Burrell and Hauerwas; MacIntyre) or the political history of a nation (White), narrative explores the way cause and effect are entangled with the variables of human character and motivation, with luck and happenstance. When moral principles or political generalizations are abstracted from events without the use of narrative, those details are left behind as inessential, even though for those involved such particulars may represent what is most valued in a life or a history. Narrative remains mired in the particulars of human experience. From its designation of certain details as relevant "facts" and certain occurrences as "events" to the use of rhetorical strategies in the representation and description of those facts and events, narrative is concerned with the construction and interpretation of meaning.

Narrative and Medical Knowledge

Because narrative is the primary way of organizing and communicating the sense human beings make of the world, the interpretive process integral to shaping and understanding a story is at the heart of human knowing. Thus, the investigation of narrative forms and practices is a fruitful way of understanding how knowledge is acquired and transmitted. To understand medical knowledge—whether the patient's illness, the physician's practice, ideas of causality, issues of medical ethics, or activities of clinical research—it is helpful to look at the historical and explanatory narratives patients and practitioners tell themselves and each other (Charon, 1986, 1994; Hunter, 1991; Miles and Hunter).

Clinical medicine is a radically uncertain field of knowledge. Based on human biology, a science more complicated and multileveled than physics or chemistry, medicine has the task of applying scientific knowledge to the care of individual human beings. Not only does the living matter of biology change—the influenza virus mutates annually, tuberculosis and gonorrhea become drug-resistant, HIV gains purchase in the human community—but even more reliably, illness, that is, the manifestation of disease in human beings, varies unpredictably from person to person. Despite the triumph of the germ theory, "disease" remains a label given to a complicated interaction of physiological phenomena—none of which need be a necessary or sufficient cause—in circumstances identified and construed culturally, socially, and personally. Much about disease can be known scientifically, if not entirely predictably; but both the patient's illness and his or her response to treatment remain complex events with multiple causes occurring in circumstances that are impossible or immoral to replicate.

Given such uncertainty, narrative in its various guises is essential to the scientific practice of medicine. Patients relate the history of their illness when they present themselves for medical attention; disease plots make up the clinical taxonomy found in textbooks; their variant subplots are stored in physicians' memories; written accounts of medical care preserved in charts fill hospital basements; case reports contribute, one by one, to clinical research. In the physician's office where patients are well known and practice is solitary, narration may dwindle to a nearly invisible minimum. But in academic medical centers where medicine is taught and research carried out—just where one might expect to find narratives banished by the ever-present concern for scientific objectivity—narrative flourishes. The clinical case is not only the record of care but the mainstay of clinical education and academic discourse. Cases are presented at morning report, at teaching rounds, patient-care conferences, grand rounds, ethics conferences, informally in halls and locker rooms, and around lunch tables. The case record is compiled in the hospital chart by several hands. When anomalies occur, the case becomes the vehicle for communication and further investigation that may lead to sustained clinical or laboratory research. As the translation and interpretation of the patient's account of illness, augmented by further investigation, the medical narrative enables clinicians to apply scientific knowledge and therapeutic judgment to the understanding and relief of illness in particular human beings.

The case thus constitutes the scientific data in the investigation and treatment of a patient's malady. Confronted with the signs and symptoms, guided by the patient's story, the physician asks questions, sorts the information into a list of possible diagnostic plots, and then sets to work to eliminate from consideration the least probable and most life-threatening and to confirm the most likely. The goals of this medical retelling of the patient's story are representational: fidelity to the clinical observation of the patient and minimalization of the observer's (and the patient's) subjectivity. To this end the conventions of the medical case are strict and almost inviolable. The narrator is all but effaced, appearing only as a signature authorizing the passive voice, while the patient's experience is subordinated to the medical retelling of illness events and physical signs, a version that resolutely ignores the fear and bewilderment, the loss of control, and the suffering that may attend the experience of illness. This is not meant to be cruel; it is meant to provide the patient with an objective gaze that is capable of establishing with some certainty what the matter is so that treatment may begin and, with luck, health may be restored.

The physician's familiarity with other cases grounds the investigation and, indeed, the whole interpretive, diagnostic circle. Whether read and heard about or, better, observed and directly experienced, these cases make up an intellectual storehouse backed by the myriad of information accumulated in publications and through consultation. Well understood and ready to hand, this body of practical knowledge enables physicians to apply physiological principles, textbook summaries, and clinical wisdom to signs and symptoms presented by individual patients, testing each particular case against those established, more abstract patterns. There are no all-encompassing laws of disease, and physicians must learn not only operative rules and their variants, but also the habits of perception that narrative enforces, habits that will stand them in good stead for a lifetime of practice in a field where knowledge and practice constantly change—and new diseases appear. The case narrative is the means by which such a store of exemplars is assembled both in formal education and in practice (Dreyfus and Dreyfus), and is the medium for the consultation, further investigation, and publication that are the hallmarks of modern academic medicine.

Narrative and Bioethics

The centrality of narrative characteristic of clinical medicine is shared with other case-based disciplines of knowledge, such as law, moral theology, and criminal detection. In these domains, knowledge is not simply a "top-down," theory-driven activity. Research must be conducted retrospectively, and knowing is interpretive, accumulated from the experienced scrutiny of many individual instances in the light of general rules. The case—a term common to them all—functions as both exemplar and test of more general formulations: legislation, ethics, criminology, and biological science. In everyday practice, "in the trenches," these generalizations are extended or refined as they are applied, and practical expertise is developed in the continual search for more nearly adequate rules.

Narrative is also central to bioethics. Not only does it provide an opportunity for imaginative moral reflection for its audience, it is equally the proving ground of moral argument. Although the contemporary study of bioethics, especially medical ethics, until recently has focused almost exclusively on principles (Beauchamp and Childress; Pellegrino), the applicability of moral principles is inevitably gauged against the particular case, and cases regularly provoke the careful study and refinement of the rules. Indeed, the rehabilitation of casuistry—dealing with questions of right and wrong—has been the work of philosophers in bioethics (Toulmin; Jonsen and Toulmin; Jonsen).

The role of narrative in moral life is well established with regard to literature (Horace; Coles; Banks). Along with history, which is also strongly narrative, fictional narrative has long been regarded as a moral teacher—especially in that most narrative of eras, the nineteenth century. Both literary theory and historiography have struggled against this assumption of moral didacticism in the twentieth century. French historians of the *Annales* school and American cliometricians (mathematical and statistical analysts) have attempted to reduce the narrative element in history writing in favor of numerical data—the records of glacially slow and macroscopic social change for the former, and a microanalysis of economic statistics for the latter. In literature, from the "art-for-art's-sake" movement at the turn of the last century through Dadaist experimentation to the frequently reported "death" of the novel, twentieth-century writers defied critics to draw morals from their stories. For much of the century, literary critics, too, eschewed moralism in favor of the aesthetics of "the work itself," relegating morals to a matter of folk tales. Thus, it was oddly fitting that when structuralists reanimated a critical concern with narrative it was necessary to turn to Vladimir Propp's *The Morphology of the Folktale* (1968; Todorov; Brooks). More recently, literary theorist Wayne Booth and philosopher Martha Nussbaum have made strong cases for literature as the medium of moral knowledge.

Literature's usefulness for moral reasoning lies not only in its themes and characters—those elements the McGuffey

Readers drew upon for the "morals" that concluded their tales—but also in the interpretive reasoning it requires. As in clinical reasoning, narrative negotiates the application of general truths about human experience to the individual case. Readers know that murder is evil, but they turn to *Macbeth, Crime and Punishment,* or *Native Son* to reflect on precisely why and how. At the same time, narrative also tests such moral truths. Its representation of the particular instance asks implicitly whether circumstances can ever be extenuating; it negotiates on behalf of ethical inquiry, as it does for medical diagnostics, the imprecise and uncertain fit between general rule and particular instance.

The narrative that constitutes the bioethics case likewise plays a role in moral reasoning. The purpose of constructing and presenting a case in bioethics should not be limited to the illustration of a rule or principle any more than in medicine (Arras; Donnelly). It is rather to set out accounts of events in order to explore imaginatively their meaning for the people they affect and to determine what action should be taken. Because narrative's representation of subjective experience gives its audience access to the perception and judgment of other human beings, good ethics cases offer a means of thinking about the meaning of illness in the life of the patient, and about the role of the physician and the meaning of a patient–doctor interaction in the life of the physician. These are traditional themes of literature, and beyond literature—the themes of the unwritten stories, the gossip, and the self-revelation—that convey and test social values and give texture both to individual lives and to culture. To read and listen to stories and to watch them enacted on screen and stage is to open the understanding to the experience of other people, and to the meaning that experience has for them. Physicians do the former all the time, asking their patients about pain or the history of an illness, talking about the effects of disability or the likelihood of death. But imagining the meaning of experience for other people is very difficult and rarely undertaken (Kleinman; Waitzkin); for physicians, traditional, professional reticence and self-protection are obstacles (Katz). The desire for just this sort of understanding from another person, especially one pledged to a certain disinterested concern, informs both nostalgia for the legendary general practitioner and Anatole Broyard's request that his physician "spend five minutes thinking about my case" (1992). A longing for an interpreter who will both hear our stories in all their physical starkness and nevertheless see in us human subjects, people who create meaning in the story of our lives, may underlie the burgeoning interest in medical ethics. The public discussion of troubling cases—in the mass media, in the courts, in drama and film and autobiography, and in ethics courses—reveals a narrative hunger for meaning in the face of death. Indeed,

Walter Benjamin (1936) has located in death's certainty the closure that narrative meaning requires.

As in clinical medicine, the use of narrative in bioethics is necessitated by the limits of human knowledge, and an attention to narrative enforces an awareness of these limits for both narrator and audience. Not only does the audience understand that the narrator's knowledge is limited, but, in addition, both narrator and audience know—or soon learn—that the knowability of the narrated is limited (Hunter, 1993). What happens next? Then? And then? The unfolding of narrative through time captures the contingencies of causation, the radical uncertainty of the most ordinary life, the uncontrolled variables that resist attempts to regularize and codify social knowledge. More questions may yield more information, yet uncertainty is best met not by the pursuit of every elusive clue, but by a sense of the balance of knowledge and tolerable ignorance sufficient for action. Although always accountable to social and cultural norms—indeed, these norms are operating in the framing and interpretation of narratives—moral knowledge is inevitably subjective, always open to question, discussion, elaboration, retelling, and reinterpretation.

In bioethics as in clinical medicine, narrative knowledge is always situated knowledge. Just as every malady has its patient, every tale has a teller—either the voice of an omniscient author or a character who has been witness to the events—and every narrator has an audience, imagined or real, to whom the story is addressed. Narratives are enmeshed in the circumstances of their telling, even when, as with clinical cases, the form is specially designed to extricate itself from those circumstances. Cases do not drop pure and untouched from the sky, nor do they contain a truth or essence that could be revealed if only the circumstances of their telling were stripped away. Instead, they are narratives constructed and presented by human beings who are making an effort to be understood—or to deceive, to impress an audience, or to reinterpret an event. Even stories meant to be perfectly transparent—medical cases, news reports, ethics cases—are framed by their all-but-invisible tellers and interpreted by their audience. Though the narrator may be a disinterested and impartial observer, there is nevertheless a standpoint from which the story is told (Chambers). Some things will be emphasized or privileged, others will be out of the narrator's view. While norms exist and exert their force, they do so variously and unpredictably, and determining how they do so is one of the tasks that readers and listeners undertake. Narrators are revealed to their audience, in part, by the stands they take in relation to both the norms of society and the conventions of the narrative genre. This tension between tale and teller (or tale and the untold) is always a part of the narrative.

Where the sense of events offered by a narrative is contested or where its interpretation is in doubt, the narrative itself comes under scrutiny. The reader or listener begins to ask about the narrator and the narrative frame. Who is telling the story—the physician, the patient, a family member, an ethicist? Why is it told? In what circumstances? How does the teller frame the story to include or ignore culture, history, life stories, power relations, economic conditions, the history of the present question? Because an understanding of the problem turns upon the answers to these questions, this is where the study of ethical discourse must begin (Chambers, 1994). Cases may be narratively impoverished and morally inadequate even when bioethical principles are followed and apparently right conclusions are reached.

Through narrative, bioethics partakes of an ongoing dialogue among human beings perceiving and acting in the world. This is not a theoretical but a practical activity with strong resemblances to the clinical epistemology of which medical-case narrative is a part. As in medicine, the "facts" are sometimes of uncertain relevance and the circumstances may not be replicable, but the representation of experience through time acknowledges and puts to use the inevitable subjectivity of human understanding (Ricoeur). The subjectivity and apparent relativism unavoidable in narrative openly represents one of the conditions of moral discourse. There is no neutral position or Archimedean platform beyond nature from which a narrator, cleansed of bias, may see "truth" or "reality" in all its uncluttered purity. Indeed, narrative may be most valuable as a guarantee against this positivist assumption, for an awareness of narrative and its workings is a constant reminder that there is no absolute truth, no certainty. For the most part, stories are relatively straightforward about the conditions of their acquisition and telling. They make no pretense to objectivity—or when they do, the pretense is readily apparent as yet another storytelling genre. Narratives can be questioned: The potential prejudices of the narrator's situation beg to be understood. The interpretation of narrative may be one of the few ways human beings have of seeing our customary blind spots as both narrators and interpreters. As Ernst Hans Gombrich (1960) observed about the perception of art, there is no innocent, no "naked eye." And if there is no sight without a lens, it can become second nature to inquire into the character and quality of the lens in any particular instance—and to adjust it as needed.

Narrative exists in dialogue with other narratives, other interpretations—including the principles that, distilled from accounts of good and evil, have come to represent those accounts. Stories are not a substitute for norms and principles, just as clinical medicine does not replace medical research and case law does not render legislation irrelevant. Historians know well that every story implies an answering account, one that will surely—at last!—set the record straight. If the physician tells the patient's story, no one truly believes that it is the only story that matters; nor is the patient's story sufficient; otherwise the patient would not have sought medical help. The two are in dialogue. The goal is not a synthesis or a determination of a "truth" that will swallow up other accounts, but a sustainable representation of incommensurability, a consensus that may be acted upon. Ethics is practical knowledge, forged experientially and honed on circumstance. It is practiced in the negotiation of story and teller, story and listener, story and answering story. Because, in narrative, inquiry is inseparable from explanation, narrators and audiences must test the sources of our stories, compare versions, and sustain a healthy skepticism about answers. Thus, narrative represents the conditions of moral discourse, even as it is the principal medium of that discourse.

KATHRYN MONTGOMERY HUNTER (1995)
BIBLIOGRAPHY REVISED

SEE ALSO: *Ethics: Moral Epistemology; Health and Disease: The Experience of Health and Illness; Literature and Healthcare; Metaphor and Analogy; Value and Valuation*

BIBLIOGRAPHY

Arras, John D. 1991. "Getting Down to Cases: The Revival of Casuistry in Bioethics." *Journal of Medicine and Philosophy* 16(1): 29–51.

Bakhtin, Mikhail M. 1981. *The Dialogic Imagination: Four Essays.* tr. Michael Holquist. Austin: University of Texas Press.

Beauchamp, Tom L., and Childress, James F. 1989. *The Principles of Bioethics.* 3rd edition. New York: Oxford University Press.

Benjamin, Walter. 1968 (1936). "The Storyteller: Reflections on the Works of Nikolai Leskov." *Illuminations: Essays and Reflections,* pp. 83–109, tr. Harry Zohn. New York: Schocken.

Booth, Wayne C. 1987. *The Company We Keep: An Ethics of Fiction.* Berkeley: University of California Press.

Brody, Howard. 1987. *Stories of Sickness.* New Haven, CT: Yale University Press.

Brody, Howard. 2002. *Stories of Sickness.* New York: Oxford University Press.

Brooks, Peter. 1984. *Reading for the Plot: Design and Intention in Narrative.* New York: Alfred A. Knopf.

Broyard, Anatole. 1992. *Intoxicated by My Illness: And Other Writings on Life and Death.* New York: Clarkson Potter.

Bruner, Jerome S. 1990. *Acts of Meaning.* Cambridge, MA: Harvard University Press.

Burrell, David, and Hauerwas, Stanley. 1977. "From System to Story: An Alternative Pattern for Rationality in Ethics." In *Knowledge, Value and Belief,* pp. 111–152, Vol. 2 of *The Foundation of Ethics and Its Relationship to Science,* ed. H. Tristram Engelhardt, Jr., and Daniel Callahan. Hastings-on-Hudson, NY: Hastings Center.

Carson, A. M. 2001. "That's Another Story: Narrative Methods and Ethical Practice." *Journal of Medical Ethics* 27(3): 198–202.

Chambers, Tod S. 1994. "The Bioethicist as Author: The Medical Ethics Case as Rhetorical Device." *Literature and Medicine* 13(1): 60–78.

Chambers, Tod S. "From the Ethicist's Point of View: The Literary Nature of Ethical Inquiry." In manuscript.

Charon, Rita. 1986. "To Render the Lives of Patients." *Literature and Medicine* 5: 58–74.

Charon, Rita. 1994. "Narrative Contributions to Medical Ethics: Recognition, Formulation, Interpretation, and Validation in the Practice of the Ethicist." In *A Matter of Principles? Ferment in U.S. Bioethics,* pp. 260–283, ed. Edwin R. DuBose, Ronald Hamel, and Laurence J. O'Connell. Valley Forge, PA: Trinity Press International.

Charon, R. Alta. 2001. "The Patient-Physician Relationship. Narrative Medicine: A Model for Empathy, Reflection, Profession, and Trust." *Journal of the American Medical Association* 286(15): 1897–1902.

Charon, Rita, and Montello, Martha, eds. 2002. *Stories Matter: The Role of Narrative in Medical Ethics.* London: Routledge.

Coles, Robert. 1979. "Medical Ethics and Living a Life." *New England Journal of Medicine* 301(8): 444–446.

Donnelly, William J. 1992. "Hypothetical Case Histories: Stories Neither Fact Nor Fiction." Presented at a meeting of the Society for Health and Human Values, Tampa, Fla., May 1.

Dreyfus, Hubert L., and Dreyfus, Stuart E. 1987. "From Socrates to Expert Systems: The Limits of Calculative Rationality." In *Interpretive Social Science: A Second Look,* pp. 327–350, ed. Paul Rabinow and William M. Sullivan. Berkeley: University of California Press.

Ellos, W. J. 1998. "Some Narrative Methodologies for Clinical Ethics." *Cambridge Quarterly of Healthcare Ethics* 7(3): 315–322.

Forster, E. M. 1927. *Aspects of the Novel.* New York: Harcourt, Brace.

Glaser, Barney G., and Strauss, Anselm L. 1967. *The Discovery of Grounded Theory: Strategies for Qualitative Research.* Chicago: Aldine.

Gombrich, Ernst Hans. 1960. *Art and Illusion: A Study in the Psychology of Pictorial Representation.* Bollingen Series, no. 35. New York: Pantheon.

Hester, D. Micah. 2002. "Narrative as Bioethics: The 'Fact' of Social Selves and the Function of Consensus." *Cambridge Quarterly of Healthcare Ethics* 11(1): 17–26.

Horace. 1960. *The Ars Poetica of Horace,* ed. Augustus S. Wilkins. New York: Macmillan.

Hunter, Kathryn Montgomery. 1991. *Doctors' Stories: The Narrative Structure of Medical Knowledge.* Princeton, NJ: Princeton University Press.

Hunter, Kathryn Montgomery. 1993. "The Whole Story." *Second Opinion* 19: 97–103.

Hunter, K. M. 1996. "Narrative, Literature, and the Clinical Exercise of Practical Reason." *Journal of Medicine and Philosophy* 21(3): 303–320.

Jones, A. H. 1997. "Literature and Medicine: Narrative Ethics." *Lancet* 349(9060): 1243–1246.

Jonsen, Albert R. 1991. "Of Balloons and Bicycles—or—The Relationship Between Ethical Theory and Practical Judgment." *Hastings Center Report* 21(5): 14–16.

Jonsen, Albert R., and Toulmin, Stephen. 1988. *The Abuse of Casuistry: A History of Moral Reasoning.* Berkeley: University of California Press.

Katz, Jay. 1984. *The Silent World of Doctor and Patient.* New York: Free Press.

Kleinman, Arthur. 1988. *The Illness Narratives: Suffering, Healing, and the Human Condition.* New York: Basic Books.

Kuczewski, Mark G. 1999. "Commentary: Narrative Views of Personal Identity and Substituted Judgment in Surrogate Decision Making." *Journal of Law, Medicine and Ethics* 27(1): 32–36.

Levine, Peter. 1998. *Living Without Philosophy: On Narrative, Rhetoric, and Morality.* Albany: State University of New York Press.

MacIntyre, Alasdair C. 1981. *After Virtue: A Study in Moral Theory.* Notre Dame, IN: University of Notre Dame Press.

Mattingly, Cheryl, and Garro, Linda C., eds. 2000. *Narrative and the Cultural Construction of Illness and Healing.* Berkeley: University of California Press.

Miles, Steven, and Hunter, Kathryn Montgomery. 1990. "Case Stories." *Second Opinion* 15: 60–69.

Nelson, Hilde Lindemann, ed. 1997. *Stories and Their Limits: Narrative Approaches to Bioethics (Reflective Bioethics).* London: Routledge.

Newton, Adam Zachary. 1995. *Narrative Ethics.* Cambridge, MA: Harvard University Press.

Nicholas, B., and Gillett, Grant. 1997. "Doctors' Stories, Patients' Stories: a Narrative Approach to Teaching Medical Ethics." *Journal of Medical Ethics* 23(5): 295–299.

Nussbaum, Martha C. 1986. *The Fragility of Goodness: Luck and Ethics in Greek Tragedy and Philosophy.* Cambridge, Eng.: Cambridge University Press.

O'Toole, J. 1995. "The Story of Ethics: Narrative as a Means for Ethical Understanding and Action." *Journal of the American Medical Association* 273(17): 1387, 1390.

Pellegrino, Edmund D. 1993. "The Metamorphosis of Medical Ethics: A Thirty-Year Retrospective." *Journal of the American Medical Association* 269(9): 1158–1162.

Propp, Vladimir. 1968. *The Morphology of the Folktale,* 2nd edition, rev. tr. Laurence Scott. Austin: University of Texas Press.

Ricoeur, Paul. 1988. *Time and Narrative,* 3 vols. tr. Kathleen McLaughlin Blamey and David Pellauer. Chicago: University of Chicago Press.

Spike, J. 2000. "Narrative Unity and the Unraveling of Personal Identity: Dialysis, Dementia, Stroke, and Advance Directives." *Journal of Clinical Ethics* 11(4): 367–372.

Todorov, Tzvetan. 1977. *The Poetics of Prose,* tr. Richard Howard. Ithaca, NY: Cornell University Press.

Tong, Rosemary. 1998. "The Ethics of Care: A Feminist Virtue Ethics of Care for Healthcare Practitioners." *Journal of Medicine and Philosophy* 23(2): 131–152.

Toulmin, Stephen. 1982. "How Medicine Saved the Life of Ethics." *Perspectives in Biology and Medicine* 25(4): 736–750.

Tovey, P. 1998. "Narrative and Knowledge Development in Medical Ethics." *Journal of Medical Ethics* 24(3): 176–181.

Turner, L. 2001. "Narrative, Thick Description, and Bioethics: Cases, Stories, and Simone de Beauvoir's 'A Very Easy Death'." *Journal of Clinical Ethics* 12(2): 122–130.

Waitzkin, Howard. 1991. "The Politics of Medical Encounters: How Patients and Doctors Deal with Social Problems." New Haven, CT: Yale University Press.

White, Hayden. 1981. "The Value of Narrativity in the Representation of Reality." In *On Narrative,* pp. 7–23, ed. W. J. Thomas Mitchell. Chicago: University of Chicago Press.

NATIVE AMERICAN RELIGIONS, BIOETHICS IN

• • •

Using the phrase "Native American" signals a recognition that there are indigenous peoples on the North American continent who retain distinct ethical perspectives within the mainstream cultures of the United States and Canada. Terms such as "First Peoples," "American Indian," and "Amerindian" are also used to refer to the indigenous peoples of the Americas. Each term has a history of use and limitations in its reference. For example, there are no actual people who call themselves Native Americans in their traditional language; rather, there are distinct ethnic groups who were on the North American continent prior to the arrival of Europeans, Africans, and Asians. Prior to contact with European settlers in the fifteenth century, it is believed, there were over 2,000 different native communities on the continent. Over 700 of these ethnic groups have survived repeated invasions, epidemic diseases, cultural genocide, and ideological exploitation. Thus, when we use the term "Native American," it is at a general level of understanding and reference that is fictional and conceptual. A deeper understanding of Native Americans must move to another level of reference, beginning with the names by which indigenous peoples know themselves.

In this entry the following system will be used. The indigenous name will be followed by the popular name in Canada and the United States. The peoples who call themselves Anishinabe are also known as Chippewa/Ojibwe, Ottawa, and Pottawatomi. In some instances, there are historical and sociological reasons for differentiating specific tribal names among a larger nation such as the Anishinabe. So also, the term Haudenosaunee, or "Long-House People," is the name of the northeastern North American peoples whom the French called Iroquois. Either term is often used to indicate individual nations within the Haudenosaunee political confederation, or "long house": Seneca, Cayuga, Onondaga, Oneida, Tuscarora, and Mohawk. Other examples can be listed: Apsaalooke/Crow; Tsistsistas/Cheyenne; Muskogee and Miccosukkee/Creek; Dine/Navajo; Ashiwi/Zuni; Tohono O'odham/Papago; and Skittagetan/Haida. This usage recognizes the right of a people to be known by the name by which they describe themselves.

The term *religion* raises a similar ethical concern; it carries associated references that can mislead an inquiry into Native American ways. The term *religion* derives from the Latin *religio,* "to bind fast." Traditionally this has carried associations from its Mediterranean-Atlantic heritage, namely, to be reunited, after a pilgrimage through life, with the personal, monotheistic, creator God who transcends earthly existence. The connotations of monotheism, the one deity as personal and transcendent, and a pilgrimage orientation to life are embedded in the term *religion* for many Euro-American Christians.

In contrast, the term *lifeway* emphasizes the road of life as indigenous people see it. Such a perspective can be associated with the concept "worldview," a distinct way of thinking about the cosmos and of evaluating life's actions in terms of those views. The Dakota/Sioux lawyer and professor of history Vine Deloria, Jr., speaks thus of an Indian ethical view of the universe: "In the moral universe all activities, events, and entities are related, and consequently it does not matter what kind of existence an entity enjoys, for the responsibility is always there for it to participate in the continuing creation of reality" (Deloria, p. 63). This view understands all life forms as having purpose, as being related, and as being cocreators of the world they occupy. The religious structure that flows from these views gives rise to a moral imagination in which the sacred is immanent, within the earth, and revealed in one's contemplation of natural occurrences. All life in one's local bioregion is both interdependent and participating in the act of creation evident, for example, in the changing seasons. The term *bioregion,* is used here to suggest the Native American reverence and respect for all life forms in the local region. Indians have traditionally understood their local bioregion as filled with moral purpose, interrelated, and alive.

Cosmic Interdependence

Moral actions in Native American lifeways are acts in harmony with a sacred power that is believed to pervade the world and is experienced most immediately in the local bioregion. While moral actors are not limited to the human community, any particular human is seen as integrated into the larger harmony by means of his or her community. Someone who has committed a crime is not made into an outsider by virtue of an isolated act. Rather, the one who is out of balance must be brought back, if possible, into the community by ritual treatment with that power believed to pervade the cosmos.

Native peoples in North America have articulated terms such as Wakan Tanka (Lakota), Kitche Manitou (Anishinabe), or Akbatatdia (Apsaalooke), which convey an understanding of the mysterious presence and fullness of pervasive cosmic power. These terms have often been used by nonnative missionary traditions to communicate ideas regarding the sacred, especially belief in a personal God. While such usage may be sanctioned by Christian native peoples, some traditional practitioners object to this interpretation as misleading. Sacred power, and the native terms used to evoke that mystery, do not indicate a patriarchal deity but emphasize the web of cocreative relationships throughout the spiritual realms and the ecological terrain, or bioregion. This pervasive power is experienced in a plurality of manifestations, or spirits, that relate to the presence of transformative power in distinct spiritual realms of the cosmos but especially to the local bioregion. Thus, Native American lifeways may be described as manifesting an "ethical naturalism" in which moral choices flow from the desires of individuals and communities to flourish within the limits and opportunities of nature as understood by the people and as typically observed within the particular bioregional conditions of a people (Lovin and Reynolds).

Synthetic Ethics

Questions of the relation of ethics to ritual and myth are also analytical themes in the study of religion, but in Native American traditions these questions are inextricably linked. This article will attempt to communicate this ethical wholeness by describing practices related to both ritual and the daily life of native North American peoples. One term used throughout this entry, *synthetic ethics,* refers to the Native American effort to bring people into the most immediate and profound encounter with resources for thought and for food: the bioregion, the animals hunted, the human community, the seasons, and the spiritual realm.

Synthetic ethics signifies the seamless whole of the Native American world in which personal actions affirm mythic values and in which ritual actions reflect relationships established with the surrounding bioregion. Rather than abstract principles, these ethical relationships correspond to moral metaphors transmitted in the myth stories. Such generative metaphors as the living earth and purposeful animals cause a person to contemplate, as ethical experiences, the seasons, or the hunt, or the eating of local foods at their harvest time. American Indian moral imagination arises from formal structures that are believed to govern personal and community life as well as the bioregion and the larger cosmos. Such a worldview implies integration of a situational ethic, which guides one in daily life, and a cosmological ethic, which flows from the harmonious rhythms of nature. Thus, the terms *lifeway, synthetic ethics,* and *bioethics* are used in this entry to suggest the wholeness or totality of a good life that is lived in thoughtful relationship to the seasons and the living bioregion.

Each particular native people has its own terms for such concepts as synthetic ethics and lifeway. For example, Winona LaDuke writes:

> The ethical code of my own Anishinabeg community of the White Earth Reservation in northern Minnesota keeps communities and individuals in line with natural law. *"Minobimaatisiiwin"*—it means both the "good life" and "continuous rebirth"—is central to our value system. In *minobimaatisiiwin,* we honor women as the givers of lives, we honor our *Chi Anishinabeg,* our old people and ancestors who hold the knowledge. We honor our children as the continuity from generations, and we honor ourselves as a part of creation. Implicit in *minobimaatisiiwin* is a continuous habitation of place, an intimate understanding of the relationship between humans and the ecosystem and of the need to maintain this balance. (p. 70)

It is possible to find similar expressions by elders from indigenous communities in North America that articulate the relationship between social justice and ecojustice in their lifeway. The range of indigenous terms need not be discussed here but, where appropriate, such terms will be introduced.

Land and the Human Presence

Three features of Winona LaDuke's description of Anishinabe/Ojibwe ethical naturalism—enduring habitation (land), cosmological understanding (lifeway), and ecological balance (synthetic ethics)—can be used to frame the Native American appreciation of land and the human presence. The Winter Dance among the Okanagan/Salish/Colville peoples of Washington State provides a unique insight into the relationships of land, lifeway, and synthetic ethics. The Winter Dance introduces us to a developed native North American lifeway in which ritual participation is believed to transform individuals, communities, and bioregions. Moreover, the Salish understand the relationships established during the ritual as historical, that is, they deepen as an individual matures in the ethical path.

While this ritual, from the interior Salish-speaking peoples of the Columbia River plateau, has been selected for discussion here, it should be emphasized that the themes discussed have parallels in many distinct native North American rituals. The Green Corn, or Busk, ceremony of the Muskogee in the Southeast, the Shalako and Winter Solstice rituals of the Ashiwi in the Southwest, the Ashkisshe, or Sun Dance, of the Northern Plains Apsaaloke and many more rituals throughout Indian country continue to be performed in sacred settings by traditional practitioners.

OKANAGAN/SALISH/COLVILLE WINTER DANCE. Among many Salish people the Winter Dance begins the annual ritual calendar. Rituals performed during the calendar year include individual and communal activities, such as sweatlodge ceremonies, vision questing, stick gambling, curing rituals, and first fruits and harvest festivals for deer, salmon, and root crops. However, the major ritual, which draws together all of the old subsistence and healing rituals, is the Winter Dance. This dance is a complex renewal ritual convened by individual sponsors from late December through February. An abbreviated form of the ceremony can be performed at any time for someone in need. Simply by ritually establishing the center pole, the most significant symbol of the bioregion, in the middle of the dance house the curative and transformative powers of the Winter Dance can be evoked.

The Winter Dance ritual complex is especially focused on the singing of guardian spirit songs over the successive days of the ceremonial (Grim, 1992). Singing begins in the evening of each day and continues until dawn. "Ceremonial" also refers to the accompanying ritual activity that occurs during the day, such as feasting, sweat-lodge rituals (healings, purifications, petitions), giveaways, stick-game gambling, and storytelling. At the ritual heart of the Winter Dance, however, is the individual-guardian spirit relationship. Most important, this spirit-human exchange generates and reenacts the time of the traditional mythic stories, or cosmogony, in which the universe was created. The Salish moral imagination is established in this cosmogonic symbolism that is believed to renew community life and to regenerate plants and animals. Thus, individual-guardian spirit relationships form the core of the Salish synthetic ethics in which stories, songs, and symbolic actions bind individual, community, and bioregion together to generate a sacred cohesiveness and a spiritual empathy. This Native American ritual, then, provides an excellent example of the close relationship between land, lifeway, and synthetic ethics.

Prior to contact with mainstream America and the establishment of the reservation system in the nineteenth century, the Winter Dance provided the major impetus for independent villages to undertake ritual diplomacy with other villages. The ritual was the locus of interaction that smoothed individual conflicts and encouraged group cohesion. Thus, the multifaceted Winter Dance diminished aggressive rivalry between villages and brought them together for the shared task of world renewal. Just as the Winter Dance was the locus for negotiation between fiercely independent and self-governed villages, so this ritual continues to be the central place for negotiation between the human and spirit realms.

As a world renewal ceremony the Winter Dance calls the spirit powers of the bioregion into reciprocal relationship with the human communities. This ceremonial makes explicit the interdependence of minerals, plants, animals, and humans through the songs that are sung by those who have had visionary experiences of these spirits in special places of the bioregion. There is no explicit recitation of a cosmogony during the Winter Dance; however, during the days between the evening and all-night ritual activity, individuals are encouraged to tell stories. Coyote stories are especially popular on these occasions. While there is no single cosmogony among the Salish people, the cycle of Coyote stories has cosmogonic features that describe the formative activities in the time of mythic beginnings (Mourning Dove, 1933). The often humorous Coyote stories are ensembles of generative moral metaphors in which the ambiguous and mistaken actions of Coyote are narrated as examples of inharmonious behavior. Thus, the formal activities of singing vision songs and the giving of gifts, as well as the informal storytelling, serve to activate a ritual logic that informs participants of both the sources of motivation for a moral life and the purposive world around them.

The most significant symbol of land and the human presence is the center pole, a lodgepole pine ninety or so inches high. The center pole, symbolic of the bioregion, is set up in the middle of the dance hall. It is the most significant place for contact with, and communication from, guardian spirits. Songs and giveaways are the mode of the moral imagination during this ritual, and the singers are said to experience a spirit sickness because of their proximity to the cosmogonic powers. The singers go to that center pole to sing, speak in moral exhortation to the assembled community, and give gifts just as the ancient mythic spirits gave to humans. While dancing around the pole to the songs of the visionaries, the participants are said to be like the animals who "are moving around" during the snows of the Winter Dance season. The very structure of the Winter Dance as animals moving about the land is presented as having moral force in Salish thought. More than simply isolated ritual acts or symbolic gestures, it is understood as bringing a person and a community into the moral order established during the time of the cosmogonic events when the mythic plants, minerals, and animals decided to give their bodies to humans for food.

In the traditional Winter Dance singers renewed themselves in the centering experience of the ceremony, and by doing so re-created their village communities. Much has been lost due to the intrusion of the dominant Euro-American worldview, which has devalued the sacredness of the community of all life forms and has often misunderstood the visionary experiences of guardian spirits. Still, the Salish Winter Dance retains striking continuity with a traditional ethics of giving, evident in the giveaway features of the ritual, and of empathy, apparent in the spirit sickness. This is because of the evocation in the Winter Dance ritual of the ancient cosmogonic knowledge transmitted in the sacred power (*sumix*) of the mineral, plant, and animal persons, in the spirit sickness of the singers, and in the cosmic symbolism of the centering tree. This relationship between ritual and ethics can be labeled "synthetic" to signal the holistic character of the traditional lifeway of these people.

Health, Sickness, and Healing

Knowledge of health, reproduction, and death among particular native North American peoples developed in relation to their investigative exchange with bioregions, and in historical contacts among indigenous peoples long before the arrival of Europeans. One ancient religious practice, that of the healer, or shaman, still embodies traditional knowledge of bioregions accumulated over centuries of historical change. Comparative studies in shamanism suggest that Native American peoples brought healing practices with them in their transcontinental passages from Siberia as long as 40,000 years ago. The shaman, as a specialist in psychological and spiritual healing, can be contrasted in some native North American traditions with herbalists, who also sought to cure ills. Among the Winnebago of the western Great Lakes region of Wisconsin the following advice was given to young men who were about to seek a vision experience:

> There are individuals who know [the virtues and powers]. It is sad enough that you could not obtain [blessings from the more powerful spirits] during fasting; but at least ask those who possess plants to take pity on you. If they take pity on you, they will give you one of the good plants that give life [to man] and thus you can use them to encourage you in life. However, one plant will not be enough for you to possess. All [the plants] that are to be found on grandmother's hair, all those that give life, you should try to find out about, until you have a medicine chest [full]. Then you will indeed have great reason for being encouraged. (Blowsnake, p. 75)

Such advice not only emphasizes the disciplined attention given to the plant world and to those who know the healing properties of plants but also suggests the broad connections between religion, ethics, and bioregion.

The last 500 years of historical contacts with Eurasia have brought "virgin soil epidemics," diseases against which native peoples had no natural defense (Crosby), resulting in demographic devastation among Native American populations (Dobyns). The initial challenge to and decline in the ritual authority of Native American shamans due to disease during the seventeenth, eighteenth, and nineteenth centuries did not lead to the disappearance of these ritual practitioners. Rather, as epidemics subsided, traditional practices were often given full credit for effecting cures (Trigger). Currently, traditional healers are often found working with scientific medical practitioners on many reserves and reservations.

Mainstream American popularizations of surviving Native American healing practices resulted, during the nineteenth century, in misunderstandings of herbal healers or medicine persons (Albanese). This has led to romantic fictional accounts of shamans as creative individualists. One characteristic that courses through all of this interest in Native American health systems is the close connection between medicine and religion. As we have emphasized in the use of the term *lifeway,* religion is a relational practice, and an indigenous shaman always stands in close connection with his or her bioregional community.

Ritual specialists capable of diagnosing disease, treating ailments, and guiding the dead are found in all traditional native North American settings (Hultkrantz). In many agricultural communities these specialists organized in priesthoods that transmitted traditional lore and ritual experiences that addressed specific sicknesses. Among the Ashiwi/Zuni in the Southwest, research on the human body was extensive and, during healing rituals, patterns symbolic of the somatic knowledge of Zuni healers were drawn on the patient (Hultkrantz). The physiology and anthropology informing this ritual, however, were not necessarily drawn from cadaver experiments or empirical observations of social structure. These healing societies typically abhorred cutting a dead body, for it still embodied ancestral animating principles in the process of release or dying. Often specialists in dreams, visions, and spiritual travel to other-than-human realms were believed to have acquired knowledge of the human body that could not have been obtained by observational means (Deloria).

The gathering-and-hunting societies of the period before the late nineteenth century, as well as many of these extant native communities, generally sanction individual shamans. Different from priests, who may be inducted into a healing cult through a personal healing or clan privilege to learn a traditional body of lore (Ortiz), shamans are usually called by vivid experiences of spirits that "adopt" them and enable them to respond to specific needs of their people (Grim, 1983). Myths among diverse native North American peoples, such as the Apsaalooke/Crow and the Dine/Navajo, often described a hero or heroine as someone who had been abandoned by the people and consequently, "adopted" by a spirit power (Eliade; Grim, 1983; Sandner; Sullivan).

Disease in a traditional Native American setting is usually attributed to transgression of a cosmological principle, performance of prohibited behavior, intrusion of an object "shot" into a diseased individual by witchcraft, or loss of a vital soul. Prohibitions in a native context often constitute a major ethical system involving hundreds of rules for the treatment of living organisms, handling the remains of organisms, and strategies for living with the spiritual powers in the bioregion. The Koyukon people of Alaska, for example, have an elaborate system of rules and regulations called *hutlanee* (Nelson). Disease and death can result from breaking these rules and disrupting the natural balance of *sinh taala,* "the power of the earth." Koyukon shamans, *diyinyoo,* know the spiritual powers that reside in the bioregion and use their power to diagnose disease, to treat illness, and to restore *sinh taala,* the foundation of their medicine. Shamans and elders teach the wisdom needed to restore the power of the earth and to meet death with knowledge of the paths to those places in the bioregion where the dead one will live. These teachings are found in the stories from the Distant Time, or *Kk'adonts'idnee,* in which the origin, design, and functioning of nature were established. Instituted in Distant Time, the *hutlanee,* moral codes for conserving game animals and the environment, are not simply superstitions but the Koyukon synthetic ethics that governs life.

Disease that results from "object intrusion," or witchcraft, often implies a worldview in which balance or harmony between one's body and the local bioregion has been purposely broken by a malicious individual. Among the Dine/Navajo, the health of an individual is not an isolated case but a matter of the whole community of life. The "beauty," or *hozho,* inherent in the world can be put out of harmony by the malicious act of witchcraft. Cosmological ceremonies of great beauty, called chantways, are conducted by ritual specialists, or singers, to reestablish the diseased person's bodily harmony by removing the intruded object or retrieving lost vitality. The key relationship in Dine/Navajo rituals is that between the Holy People, *Diyin Dine'e,* who are potentially malevolent as numinous forces in the landscape, and the Dine themselves, as earth-surface people. To reestablish health, the ritual evokes the Holy People, who are the inner forms of the elements of nature. Through the narrative power of language, especially in a form of the chantway called Enemyway, which exorcises evil, the chaos of witchcraft can be transformed into order and beauty (Witherspoon). The synthetic ethics of the Dine/Navajo people does not expel malicious people from the community, where there would be no opportunity to undo their evil. Rather the hope is that they also can be restored to "beauty" and cosmic harmony.

In the Dine/Navajo Emergence Myth, the basic narrative source for the chantway stories, the beauty of the earth is evoked in the following chant to restore health: "Then go on as one who has long life, Go on as one who is happy, Go with blessing before you, Go with blessing behind you, Go with blessing below you, Go with blessing above you, Go with blessing around you, Go with blessing in your speech, Go with happiness and long life, Go mysteriously" (Sandner, p. vii). Through this repetitive language, the chanters amplify sacred power and control the inner forms of themselves, of their patients, and of the spiritual powers in the landscape that have been evoked into the sandpainting ritual. The chanter restores the blessedness of the one sung over by bringing the patient into the healing environment.

Current Ethical Perspectives

Major ethical issues involving native North American peoples have coalesced around the following three areas: ancestral bones, religious freedom, and sovereignty. The passage of the Grave Protection and Repatriation Act of 1990 has helped to slow the pillage of ancestral Native American gravesites. So also the itemization of Native American holdings in major museums will enhance the possibility of the return of sensitive religious material to native peoples from whom it was often improperly obtained.

Serious questions of trust and sovereignty between the American government and Native American peoples have arisen in the late twentieth century in a series of court cases in which indigenous religious freedom has been curtailed. The history of mainstream American cultural and legislative antagonism toward Native American lifeways had been momentarily reversed in the passage in 1978 of the American Indian Religious Freedom Act. However, a sequence of Supreme Court cases (especially *Lying v. Northwest Indian Cemetery Protection Association* and *Employment Division v. Smith*) has challenged the sovereignty of Native American lifeways and demonstrated an unwillingness to recognize their sacred relationships to land.

The emergence at the end of the twentieth century of a global voice of indigenous people comes as a result of such negative factors as the environmental crisis and the proximity of indigenous peoples to undeveloped areas on the globe. In the United States and Canada, native North American peoples, having been pushed onto reservations and reserves away from the majority populations of mainstream culture, now manage resources and undeveloped land. Native American peoples have increased their close contact with other indigenous peoples around the globe in an effort to protect themselves from environmental racism, the imposition of projects such as hydroelectric dams and toxic dump sites that destroy the environments of minority peoples. Gatherings such as the United Nations Earth Summit in Rio de Janeiro in 1992 and the meetings titled "Changing Ecological Values in the 21st Century" in Kyoto, Japan, in 1993 have included native North American representatives. Meetings have also brought together representatives from the world's religions to talk with elders from Native American lifeways about their traditional environmental ethics.

The remarkable resurgence of native North American peoples in the late twentieth century, after 500 years of suppression, derives from a complex process, but undoubtedly the knowledge transmitted in traditional ethics is a singular component of their endurance. Often dismissed as superstitious or derogatively labeled as primitive, the affective and holistic insights of native peoples are now recognized as ways of knowing grounded in close relationship with local bioregions. Those native teachers who still know this ethical system present their insights as a gift, a giveaway, to dominant America, which for so long juxtaposed the "nobility" of Enlightenment reason with the "contemptible character" of native thought. For traditional native North American peoples, the world is alive and, far from being a random collection of objects, is seen by some as our Mother and by many as a community of knowing subjects. Rather than a branch of knowledge, bioethics, in a native North American context, brings one to the heart of a way through life.

JOHN A. GRIM (1995)

SEE ALSO: *Abortion; Alternative Therapies; Animal Welfare and Rights; Body; Bioethics, African-American Perspectives; Conscience, Rights of; Environmental Ethics; Ethics: Religion And Morality*

BIBLIOGRAPHY

Albanese, Catherine L. 1990. *Nature Religion in America: From the Algonkian Indians to the New Age.* Chicago: University of Chicago Press.

Blowsnake, Sam. 1963 (1923). *The Autobiography of a Winnebago Indian,* ed. and tr. Paul Radin. University of California Publications in American Archaeology and Ethnology, 16(7). New York: Dover.

Crosby, Alfred W. 1986. *Ecological Imperialism: The Biological Expansion of Europe, 900–1900.* Cambridge: Cambridge University Press.

Deloria, Vine, Jr. 1993. "If You Think About It, You Will See That It Is True." *Noetic Sciences Review* no. 27 (Autumn): 62–71.

Dobyns, Henry F. 1983. *Their Number Become Thinned: Native American Population Dynamics in Eastern North America.* Knoxville: University of Tennessee Press.

Eliade, Mircea. 1964. *Shamanism: Archaic Techniques of Ecstasy.* New York: Bollingen Foundation.

Grim, John A. 1983. *The Shaman: Patterns of Siberian and Ojibway Healing.* Norman: University of Oklahoma Press.

Grim, John A. 1992. "Cosmogony and the Winter Dance: Native American Ethics in Transition." *Journal of Religious Ethics* 20(2): 389–413.

Hoppal, Mihaly, and Von Sadovszky, Otto, eds. 1989. *Shamanism: Past and Present.* 2 vols. Budapest: International Society for Trans-Oceanic Research.

Hultkrantz, Ake. 1992. *Shamanic Healing and Ritual Drama: Health and Medicine in Native North American Religious Traditions.* New York: Crossroads.

Jilek, Wolfgang G. 1982. *Indian Healing: Shamanic Ceremonialism in the Pacific Northwest Today.* Surrey, B.C.: Hancock House.

Kunitz, Stephen J. 1983. *Disease, Change, and the Role of Medicine: The Navajo Experience.* Berkeley: University of California Press.

LaDuke, Winona. 1992. "Minobimaatisiiwin: The Good Life." *Cultural Survival Quarterly* 16(4): 69–71.

Lovin, Robin W., and Reynolds, Frank E., eds. 1985. *Cosmogony and Ethical Order: New Studies in Comparative Ethics.* Chicago: University of Chicago Press.

Lyons, Oren. 1987. "Communiqué No. 11." *Traditional Circle of Elders* (Denver), September 11.

Mourning Dove. 1990 (1933). *Mourning Dove: A Salishan Autobiography,* ed. Jay Miller. Lincoln: University of Nebraska Press.

Nelson, Richard K. 1983. *Make Prayers to the Raven: A Koyukon View of the Northern Forest.* Chicago: University of Chicago Press.

Ortiz, Alfonso. 1969. *The Tewa World: Space, Time, Being, and Becoming in a Pueblo Society.* Chicago: University of Chicago Press.

Sandner, Donald. 1979. *Navaho Symbols of Healing.* New York: Harcourt Brace Jovanovich.

Sturtevant, William C., ed. 1978–. *Handbook of North American Indians.* 20 vols. to date. Washington, D.C.: Smithsonian Institution.

Sullivan, Lawrence E., ed. 1989. *Native American Religions.* New York: Macmillan.

Thornton, Russell. 1987. *American Indian Holocaust and Survival: A Population History since 1492.* Norman: University of Oklahoma Press.

Trigger, Bruce G. 1985. *Natives and Newcomers: Canada's "Heroic Age" Reconsidered.* Montreal: McGill-Queen's University Press.

Vogel, Virgil J. 1970. *American Indian Medicine.* Norman: University of Oklahoma Press.

Witherspoon, Gary. 1977. *Language and Art in the Navaho Universe.* Ann Arbor: University of Michigan Press.

NATURAL LAW

• • •

Natural law is perhaps the most ancient and historically persistent concept in Western ethics. Philosophers like Aristotle regarded nature as a ground of justice. Theologians like Thomas Aquinas distinguished between natural and supernatural sources of morality and law. By it Thomas Jefferson sanctioned a revolution. With it political reformers like Martin Luther King, Jr., justified civil disobedience. Upon it political philosophers like John Locke have built theories of the origin and limits of the civil state; and international lawyers, such as Hugo Grotius and Samuel Pufendorf, the order of justice between states. Despite disagreements about the theory of natural law, international bodies appeal to unwritten sources of rights to healthcare.

U.S. constitutional law has used natural law to clarify and sometimes amend the written law. Natural law undergirds the Thirteenth (1865) and Fourteenth Amendments (1868), which outlawed slavery and secured rights of U.S. citizens against state jurisdictions. Natural law also serves as a method of judicial interpretation, from which the judge looks beyond the written text of the Constitution in order to identify and vindicate rights of citizens. Today, constitutional debates have become the most public and controversial forum of natural-law discussion (Dworkin, 1985; Ely). Inasmuch as natural law is widely regarded as the moral basis for rights of privacy or personal autonomy, it is implicated in some of the most difficult biomedical issues, including abortion, reproductive technologies, and euthanasia.

The question of natural law emerges when we consider human laws and customs (Sokolowski). None is perfect, and some appear to be wicked. We then ask: What is the norm of reason in matters of morality and justice? Are moral norms merely the artifacts of human reason, devised to serve the circumstances of a particular culture? Or is there a ground that transcends cultures and histories? On what basis can laws be morally criticized and rectified?

Since these questions are fundamental to all ethical inquiry, what makes natural law different from other normative theories? There is no tidy answer. An array of moral theorists, using different theories, agree (1) that there are objective, though unwritten, moral grounds for right reason in the legislation and adjudication of human law; and (2) that moral reason must be guided by, and respect, certain values inherent in human nature (e.g., rationality and the capacity for free choice). If natural law means that moral and legal norms are grounded in reason, and that right exercise of human reason requires respect for goods inherent in human nature, then it would be exceedingly difficult not to hold a natural-law theory of one sort or another.

The healthcare professional exploring natural-law issues will face a debate often abstract and bewildering. First, what starts as a debate over particular issues in law, politics, or healthcare often becomes a debate over the concept of natural law itself. Second, what distinguishes one natural-law theory from another is not always clear; there seem to be as many different theories of natural law as there are theorists. In any case, one must remember that the rubric "natural law" often hides important disagreements among its proponents, as well as significant agreements among those who dispute its particular formulations and applications. Third, until recently natural-law thinking for the most part has not directly addressed biomedical issues. A well-developed body of natural-law literature, as found in legal, moral, and political theory, does not yet exist for biomedical issues. Thus, it will be helpful to summarize some of the main historical and philosophical themes of natural law.

Ancient Themes

Ancient Greek philosophers asked whether law and morality are due principally to nature or to convention. Aristotle, who is sometimes credited as the father of natural law, contended that "[w]hat is just in the political sense can be subdivided into what is just by nature and what is just by convention. What is by nature just has the same force everywhere and does not depend on what we regard or do not regard as just" (*Nicomachean Ethics,* 1134b18). While Aristotle certainly held that there are standards for judging whether a law is "in accord with nature" (*Rhetoric,* 1373b6), whether he had a doctrine of "natural law" is much debated (Miller). The proposition that moral judgment is rooted in the soil of nature, and not merely in human artifice, does not necessarily mean that nature is a "law."

The form of natural-law theory that came to influence Western culture arose from the confluence of Stoic, biblical, and Christian Scholastic ideas. Cicero, the ancient authority most often cited by Christians, wrote:

> True law is right reason in agreement with nature; it is of universal application, unchanging and everlasting; it summons to duty by its commands, and averts from wrongdoing by its prohibitions.... It is a sin to try to alter this law, nor is it allowable to attempt to repeal any part of it, and it is impossible to abolish it entirely.... [there is] one master and ruler, that is, God, over us all, for he is author of this law, its promulgator, and its enforcing judge. (*De Re Publica,* 3.22.33)

Similarly, Thomas Aquinas said that "the participation in the eternal law by rational creatures is called the law of nature" (*Summa theologica,* 1947, I-II, q. 91, a. 2). Nature *as law* requires the notion that natural standards are promulgated by God. The human intelligence finds itself not merely in a natural order but under a divine commonwealth, which is a rule of law in the exemplary sense.

Aquinas and Natural Law

Since the theory of natural law as developed by Thomas Aquinas is widely regarded as the epitome of the premodern position, let us summarize his view. In the *Summa theologica,* Aquinas maintains that for something to be called law, it must be: (1) reasonable, in the sense of directing action; (2) ordained to the common good; (3) legislated by the proper authority; and (4) duly promulgated (I-II, q. 90). The eternal law, whereby the world is ruled by divine providence, satisfies these criteria in an exemplary way (q. 91, a. 1). Natural law, however, is principally that part of divine reason accessible to the human intelligence. It is not to be confused with the order of the physical or biological world. Law is predicated only by a kind of similitude with the order found in nonrational entities (q. 91, a. 2 ad 3).

The first principle of the natural law is that "Good is to be done and pursued and evil avoided" (q. 94, a. 2). By nature, the human agent is inclined toward certain intelligible goods. Though Aquinas never claimed to provide an exhaustive list, these goods include life, procreation and care of offspring, entering into society, and knowing the truth about God. The first precepts of natural law take the form that something is to be done and pursued with respect to these goods, or resisted if contrary to them. Why call the precepts "natural"? Because the objectives of action are grounded in human nature antecedent to our deliberation and choice. In this sense, nature signifies the (human) essence directed to its specific operation. The term *natural* also indicates that the first precepts stand as the basic axioms of action, and are known naturally (*naturaliter*) rather than learned by study or by inference. Why call the objects of these inclinations "precepts" or "law"? Aquinas maintains that human agents are capable of seeing that certain goods are worthy of pursuit; they also grasp, in an elementary way, that in choices one is morally bound to act in accord with these goods.

The first precepts, however, are not a complete moral code. Aquinas holds that human reason must develop and apply them. First precepts are developed in terms of "secondary precepts," which spell out further implications for human action. For example, from the precept that one must act in accord with the good of life and resist what is contrary to it, we reason that murder is wrong. The first precepts also require "determinations," supplied by custom and positive laws. The "determinations" are ways that the natural law is made effective in the human community. Thus, while the care and education of offspring are enjoined upon humankind by a first precept of the natural law, how, where, and when the duty is discharged are determined by custom or positive law. Here, the virtue of prudence is paramount.

In the Thomistic scheme, the moral order in human law and politics is a kind of ecosystem, requiring for its proper function not only the universally binding precepts of natural law but also good customs, intelligently framed and emended positive laws, and acquired virtues, by which the laws are obeyed not just externally but also in the interior act of the will. It is therefore not advisable to isolate the doctrine of natural law in Aquinas from the rest of his account of

moral agency. First, Aquinas flatly rejects the idea that human beings ever existed in a pure state of nature (I, q. 95, a. 1), unlike the ahistorical "state of nature" models of the modern era. Created in grace and wounded by sin, the concrete human condition, according to Aquinas, is in need of tutoring and, ultimately, of transformation by divine grace. Aquinas insists, for example, that the two great ends of the natural law—the love of God and of neighbor—obscured by sin and evil customs, require repromulgation by divine positive law (q. 100, aa. 5, 11). Second, the greater part of his *Treatise on Law* (I-II, qq. 90–108) puts the natural law in the double context of the divine positive law of the Old Testament (*lex vetus*) and the New Testament Law of Grace (*lex nova*). Biblical history shapes Aquinas's fully considered judgment and exposition of the natural law.

Aquinas can be absolved of the charge that he confuses moral and physical meanings of nature, as well as the charge that his account is ahistorical. Yet his theory of natural law does rely on a teleological conception of providence, and the historical cast of his thought is informed by the biblical narrative. These features are not accidental. To the extent that modern theorists reject the credibility of the teleological science of nature, and aim to provide an account of natural law that is neutral with respect to theological suppositions, the Thomist theory will be of more historical than systematic interest.

Modern Theories

In modern times, the concept of natural law has undergone considerable doctrinal and institutional development. Although the theological framework of natural law was maintained as part of public rhetoric well into the nineteenth century, it was no longer the main interest of natural lawyers. As Lloyd Weinreb notes: "The puzzles with which Aquinas and others grappled when they tried to understand the place of humankind in nature appear in [modern] guise as part of the effort to describe the relationship of the individual to the state" (p. 67). This shift of perspective and emphasis, from cosmological and theological themes to the more narrow political and legal issues of natural law, is complicated. Leo Strauss has argued that the ancient and modern theories are so radically different that they ought not to be confounded. Whether there is continuity or discontinuity between premodern and modern versions of natural law remains a disputed subject in the scholarly literature. While we cannot discuss this in detail, we can cite at least two problems that have shaped the modern approach.

NATURAL LAW AND MODERN SCIENCE. By the seventeenth century, the phrase "natural law" was expropriated by the modern sciences to denote purely descriptive or predictive aspects of natural bodies. In optics, astronomy, and physics, the relation between nature and law no longer expressed the *human* participation in divine providence but, rather, the intelligible, measurable, and predictable regularities in physical nature (Ruby). Teleological understanding was abandoned in favor of mechanistic explanations that relied exclusively upon material and efficient causes. The success and prestige of the physical sciences made it difficult thenceforth to interrelate the moral and physical meanings of natural law without falling into equivocation. How, for example, can law be predicated on nature without conflating physical and moral necessities? In the physical sciences, law denotes the measurable and predictable properties of things that have no freedom. But in the practical or moral sphere, law denotes principles that govern human freedom. These two meanings of natural law—nature as amenable to description and prediction, and nature as a prescriptive norm of freedom—present an ongoing theoretical difficulty in modern thought about the subject.

NATURAL LAW AND THE PUBLIC ORDER OF RIGHTS. The humane focus of natural law concerns legal and political problems of the relationship between the individual and the state. In the seventeenth and eighteenth centuries, human nature rather than authority allegedly vested in churches or kings came to represent the legitimate origin of the state and its rule of law. Philosophers and jurists wrested natural law from the controversial settings of religion and custom, and attempted to reduce it to self-evident laws of reason sufficient to ground a public order of law and rights. While the well-known dictum by Hugo Grotius that the natural law would have validity even if God did not exist captures something of the modern temper, even more pertinent is his assertion that "[j]ust as mathematicians treat their figures as abstracted from bodies, so in treating law I have withdrawn my mind from every particular fact" (Grotius, Prolegomena nos. 11, 58). Modern natural-law theorists emphasize apodictic, nongainsayable propositions, and filter out anything dependent upon the mediation of culture and religion. These theories are expected to cut through religious and political controversy in order to secure that minimum of rational consensus needed for public purposes (Gewirth). In contrast with the ancients and medievals, the minimalistic bent of modern theories is not designed to mesh with the virtue of prudence.

Natural Social Necessities

Given the new scientific meanings of nature and law, as well as the practical need to devise principles of justice sufficient

to limit the modern state, two approaches to natural law dominate the modern period. One tradition keys natural law to what is needed for survival and societal peace. By nature, human beings are vulnerable, and need a certain minimal protection of their interests. Thomas Hobbes set the pattern of this tradition. Other examples of this approach are David Hume's "circumstances of justice," Oliver Wendell Holmes's "can't helps," and H. L. A. Hart's "minimum natural law." Natural law sets a background for customs and laws prohibiting violations of life, limb, and property. The advantages of this approach are at least threefold. First, the desire to protect one's life and property, insofar as it can be described and predicted, comports with the physicalist model of nature and law favored by the modern sciences. Second, it picks out elementary goods and bads that are apt to win consensus. These basic needs do not seem to depend upon the idiosyncrasies of particular individuals and their private life plans. Third, at least in the Anglo-American world, issues of life, limb, and property are easily recognized and adjudicated within a system of positive law.

However, natural necessities provide little or no reason to recognize absolute moral norms or rights that might resist the utilitarian calculations of a political majority acting for its alleged interests in peace and security. As Oliver Wendell Holmes said in his famous essay on natural law: "The most fundamental of the supposed preexisting rights—the right to life—is sacrificed without a scruple not only in war, but whenever the interest of society, that is, of the predominant power in the community, is thought to demand it" (p. 314). It is one thing to say that any system of positive law must work against the background of natural human necessities; it is quite another to hold that these pervasive natural facts about the human condition carry any prescriptive or moral force.

Natural Right of Autonomy

Another tradition, typified by Kant's dictum that one "[m]ust act as if the maxim of your action were to become through your will a universal law of nature" (Kant, no. 421, p. 30), emphasizes the autonomy of moral agents. This natural law can be expressed in the categorical imperative that humanity in one's person and in the person of others must be respected as an end in itself. As developed by many modern theorists, autonomy is a concept variously described as "moral independence" (Dworkin, 1985, p. 353), "the free choice of goals and relations as an essential ingredient of individual well-being" (Raz, p. 369), and "personal sovereignty" (Reiman, p. 43). Is autonomy a fact about human nature, or is it a moral ideal? There is disagreement about this (Schneewind). Reiman, for example, maintains that

"Personal sovereignty [indicates] a natural fact about human beings, consideration of which will lead us to the natural ground of equality between human beings" (p. 43). Put thus, autonomy embraces both a natural fact and a moral principle.

Some version of the autonomist theory is the preferred approach in much of contemporary natural-law theory, for the autonomist position emphasizes specifically moral principles of law rather than mere natural necessities. It seeks to tell us not what agents typically want or need, but how and why human beings must be respected. Moreover, it comports with the humanistic premise that human beings have a native dignity based upon a rational capacity to determine their conduct. It is the rational capacity that sets (at least some) human beings apart from other entities of nature, and constitutes the axioms of the moral world.

Despite its wide appeal, three problems routinely crop up in connection with the autonomist position. First, it is not always clear whether we are enjoined to respect the capacity for autonomy or the rightful exercise of that capacity. If we are enjoined to respect the capacity itself, are we thereby duty bound to respect the agent when he or she uses the capacity in a wicked way? In short, do agents have a moral right to do moral wrong? Second, the rights and obligations that flow from this "natural" fact of autonomy are difficult to formulate except in very general terms. What can a right to autonomy mean, except that persons ought not to be treated as mere objects; and what can this mean, except that a person ought to be treated according to sound moral considerations (Raz)? Hence, while autonomists emphasize a natural right to be treated equally, it is a humanist premise rather than the conclusion of moral reasoning (Raz). Third, we can ask whether the natural capacity for self-determination is adequate for moral reasoning about the status of other nonhuman species, prehuman entities (genetic material), incipient human life (embryos), and human beings whose autonomy is diminished.

Catholic Natural-Law Theory

The Roman Catholic Church is the only international institution to hold a natural-law doctrine in both the premodern and modern phases of the theory. Conciliar decrees, papal encyclicals, and canon law both reaffirm the natural law and have applied it across a range of moral issues (Fuchs; Finnis, 1980b). The encyclical *Veritatis splendor* (1993) gives considerable attention to natural law. Drawn chiefly from the work of Augustine and Aquinas, the papal formulation of natural law in *Veritatis* is traditional, emphasizing the status of natural law as real law, promulgated by God. Although there is only passing reference to biomedical

issues, the encyclical represents perhaps the clearest exposition of the theoretical underpinnings of natural law by a modern pope. The concept of natural law has also recently been applied to natural rights. The new Code of Canon Law (1983) asserts the right of the church to address secular affairs insofar as such affairs pertain to "fundamental rights of the human person" (canon 747/2).

Over the past three decades natural-law debate has focused upon the encyclical *Humanae vitae* (1968), which condemned contraception as a violation of the natural law, not because it is artificial but because it is contrary to nature. The encyclical's premise is that marriage (apart from considerations of sacramental theology) naturally contains both a procreative and a unitive good. The moral question is whether these goods can be deliberately separated in the particular conjugal act. The natural-law reasoning of *Humanae vitae* has been interpreted in quite different, and sometimes contradictory, ways by moral theologians. A 1991 study finds that at least six natural-law positions have emerged in the debate (Smith). This is because the encyclical is terse, and does not spell out its argument in the fashion of an academic exercise. But it is also due to the fact that the encyclical outlines an argument at three levels, each of which is open to debate: (1) that the conjugal act must preserve the intrinsic order toward the procreative end; (2) that the unitive and procreative goods of marriage must not be separated; (3) that the integrity of marriage cannot be maintained in its totality unless it is maintained in each and every conjugal act. Hence, its analysis of nature concerns not only the natural order of the sexual function but also the natural goods of marriage as well as the nature of the human sexual act itself. Whatever might be said about the document, it does not present a simple natural-law argument.

Critics like Charles Curran have charged that *Humanae vitae* confuses the physical and moral structures of human acts. Curran also charges the encyclical with adopting a "classicist worldview and methodology" that comports with neither the methods of the sciences nor the relativizing of nature by the history of salvation. Bernard Häring raises objections similar to Curran's. Not only in matters of reproduction, but also more generally in biomedical issues, Häring notes that the physician no longer defines himself as a servant of "ordered potentialities and powers of nature." Rather, he "increasingly considers himself an architect and sculptor of the given stuff of nature" (Häring). So, too, the moral theologian, he argues, must emphasize the divine mandate to creatively mold and intervene in nature. As so often happens in debates about natural law, the practical issue at hand (in this case, contraception) quickly opens onto the more abstract philosophical and theological questions about the meaning of nature and how it relates to norms of conduct.

In 1987, Joseph Cardinal Ratzinger, prefect of the Congregation for the Doctrine of the Faith, issued *Instruction on Respect for Human Life (Donum vitae)*. The *Instruction* addressed a number of biomedical issues, including experimentation upon human embryos; methods of prenatal diagnosis; and in vitro fertilization, both homologous (the meeting in vitro of the gametes of married spouses) and heterologous (the use of gametes coming from at least one donor other than the spouses). Whereas *Humanae vitae* contended that the procreative good cannot deliberately be suppressed in favor of the unitive good, Cardinal Ratzinger argued that the natural law also prohibits separating procreation from the unity and love of the spousal act. While the argument is similar to *Humanae vitae,* Cardinal Ratzinger makes it clearer that natural law is a moral law, not to be confused with a "set of norms on the biological level." By nature, the conjugal act is a "personal" act of love between spouses. This guarantees that the transmission of life is an act of procreativity rather than mere reproduction. The *Instruction,* therefore, maintains that in vitro fertilization, whether homologous or heterologous, is contrary to the personal and unitive meaning of the marital act.

With respect to human rights, Cardinal Ratzinger argues that in vitro fertilization violates not only the natural structure of the marital act but also the "inalienable rights" of the child. The child cannot be treated as an object serving the interests of the parents but, rather, must be treated as an end in itself. Parents have only the right to perform those acts that are per se ordered to procreation. Were parents to have a right to reproduce, by whatever means, then the child would be an object to which one has a right of ownership. At least on matters of bioethics, the *Instruction* represents an important development in the linkage between a traditional natural-law conception of the marital act with distinctively modern arguments concerning natural rights.

Natural-law theory is in a period of transition among Catholic scholars. Some scholars working in the Thomistic tradition now emphasize the role of the virtues rather than the juridical themes of natural law (Bourke; MacIntyre). Others, notably John Finnis (1980a) and Germain Grisez (1983), have developed a theory of the relationship between practical reason and "basic human goods" (e.g., life, knowledge, play, aesthetic experience, sociability, practical reasonableness, and religion). The aim of the theory is to identify moral norms governing how basic goods ought to be chosen. It was first undertaken by Germain Grisez (1964; 1983); John Finnis (1980a) has systematically applied Grisez's work to the whole field of jurisprudence. The natural-law component of the theory is much criticized. Some argue that

it has no clear connection to the Thomistic doctrine of natural theology (Hittinger, 1987); others, particularly proportionalists, argue that absolute moral norms are not easily generated by such generalized forms of human well-being (McCormick). Although there is considerable agreement among Catholic philosophers and theologians that natural law is important, there is less agreement about how to deal systematically with the subject.

Natural Law in Law and Bioethics

Constitutional and legal issues have occupied recent secular debates over natural law. It is noteworthy that the philosophical ground of the debate between natural lawyers and legal positivists continues to be revisited (see essays in George, 1992). At a more concrete level, however, discussion has focused upon civil liberties, particularly the right of privacy. Since this area of the law is the bellwether for many important biomedical questions, we will briefly outline the state of this discussion.

In *Griswold v. Connecticut* (1965), the Supreme Court invalidated a Connecticut statute forbidding the sale to and use of contraceptives by married people. The Court held that a zone of privacy protects marriage from intrusive governmental actions. Since the Constitution and its amendments do not mention the right of privacy, the Court was widely regarded as using natural law in constitutional interpretation. Indeed, the use of natural law was more controversial than the result in this particular case. In *Eisenstadt v. Baird* (1972), which invalidated a Massachusetts statute prohibiting the sale of contraceptives to unmarried people, Justice William Brennan reasoned that the right of privacy generally covers the decision of individuals, married or single, to make decisions about whether to "bear or beget" children. In *Roe v. Wade* (1973), the right to privacy was extended to abortion. Since then, it has been cited by lower courts as precedent for paternal refusal to allow the implantation of embryos. Other biomedical issues have also surfaced in the courts in terms of natural rights: "There is a fundamental natural right expressed in our Constitution as the 'right to liberty,' which permits an individual to refuse or direct the withholding or withdrawal of artificial death-prolonging procedures …" (*Cruzan v. Harmon,* 760 S.W.2nd 408, 434 [Mo. banc 1988] [Higgins, J., dissenting]).

It is unfortunate that some of the thorniest biomedical questions have been formulated legally in terms of a right to privacy. The moral substance of the right is often moved to the periphery in favor of the controverted issue of natural law as a tool of constitutional interpretation. Setting aside the legal questions, we can ask what are the ground and scope of a right to privacy. It is widely held that the moral basis of the right rests upon the natural autonomy of individuals to make decisions about their bodies, with respect not only to sexual conduct but also to many life-and-death concerns. The notion of the body as property has a long philosophical pedigree in the Anglo-American world (e.g., John Locke); the notion that there exists a field of private or self-regarding actions is traceable to a number of different moral theorists (e.g., John Stuart Mill). Moral and legal theorists generally have attempted to unite these themes under a right of autonomy or moral independence (surveyed in Hittinger, 1990). In *Planned Parenthood v. Casey* (1992), the U.S. Supreme Court reaffirmed its holding in *Roe v. Wade*. It is significant, however, that the Court discussed the right in the language of autonomy, and brought this language under the legal rubric of "liberty" (in section one of the Fourteenth Amendment), rather than "privacy." Because privacy has such disputable grounds in the positive law, this move from privacy to liberty in *Casey* can be read as an effort to find more secure grounds in the positive law for the moral right to autonomy.

Two problems attend the formulation of a right to autonomy. First, it is not clear that a natural right to autonomy can be applied with analytic precision. Even if we narrow the scope of autonomous actions to those that relate to use of the body, it would seem that contraception, abortion, and euthanasia are very different kinds of acts—not only materially but also morally. Hence, it can be objected that although autonomy is a necessary element in our consideration of these issues, it is not a sufficient condition for how they ought to be settled. Second, in Western history, the great tradition of natural rights has concerned the limitation of the coercive power of the state. In legislation and in public policy, a natural rights argument can be expected to shed light upon the principles that ought to govern the ends and the means of public force. But the right of autonomy provides only the most inchoate ground for distinguishing between legitimate and wrongful actions on the part of the state. Why, for example, should the state be prevented from intruding upon decisions about reproduction but not those concerning suicide or euthanasia? All these acts concern the body, and are plausible instances of the individual's interest in his or her autonomy. If the difference consists in the moral specifications of the acts (if, for example, abortion is adjudged morally licit or at least indifferent, while suicide and assisted euthanasia are deemed morally wicked), then autonomy needs to be augmented with other principles in order to draw a line between what belongs to the individual and what belongs to the state. If, on the other hand, one has a natural moral right to act autonomously regardless of the moral specifications of the acts, then one would seem to have a natural right to do

wrong. While a government might have other reasons to tolerate wicked acts, it is unclear how a government can be bound to respect a right to do a moral wrong.

Since bioethics encompasses matters of physiological well-being, moral choice, and justice, some version of natural law might seem indispensable to how we should frame and resolve the issues. Despite theoretical problems and disagreements, nature stubbornly remains a standard for health (Kass). Until nature is exorcised, it will continue to invite natural law reflection on norms of medical practice. Modern technology urgently bids us to investigate the moral relevance of the contrast between nature and art. Furthermore, it would be hard to imagine a future in which citizens stop making claims about rights in the area of healthcare and the allocation of its resources. Natural law has become part of our repertoire of moral discourse about rights. Yet, as one critic of natural law has stated the problem: "Either the allegedly universal ends [of natural law] are too few and abstract to give content to the idea of the good, or they are too numerous and concrete to be truly universal. One has to choose between triviality and implausibility" (Ely, p. 51). The same can be said of any of the standard normative theories of ethics, whether deontological or utilitarian. With respect to any abstract theory, especially one as prodigious as natural law, one must look carefully at its different versions, and also take the applications of the theories on a case-by-case basis.

RUSSELL HITTINGER (1995)
BIBLIOGRAPHY REVISED

SEE ALSO: *Abortion, Religious Traditions: Roman Catholic Perspectives; Christianity, Bioethics in; Embryo and Fetus: Religious Perspectives; Enhancement Uses of Medical Technology; Ethics: Normative Ethical Theories; Ethics: Religion and Morality; Eugenics and Religious Law: Christianity; Fertility Control: Social and Ethical Issues; Law and Morality; Reproductive Technologies: Ethical Issues; Transhumanism and Posthumanism; Virtue and Character*

BIBLIOGRAPHY

Aquinas, Thomas. 1947. *Summa theologica,* tr. Fathers of the English Dominican Province. New York: Benzinger Brothers.

Arkes, Hadley. 2001. "The 'Laws of Reason' and the Surprise of the Natural Law." *Social Philosophy and Policy* 18(1): 146–175.

Bourke, Vernon. 1974. "Is Thomas Aquinas a Natural Law Ethicist?" *Monist* 58(1): 52–66.

Code of Canon Law. 1983. Latin-English ed. Tr. Canon Law Society of America. Washington, D.C.: Canon Law Society of America.

Congregation for the Doctrine of the Faith. 1987. *Instruction on Respect for Human Life in Its Origin and on the Dignity of Procreation: Replies to Certain Questions of the Day (Donum vitae),* tr. Vatican. Boston: St. Paul Publications.

Curran, Charles E. 1985. "Natural Law." Ch. 5 In *Directions in Fundamental Moral Theology.* Notre Dame, IN: University of Notre Dame Press.

Devine, Philip E. 2000. *Natural Law Ethics (Contributions in Philosophy, No. 72).* Westport, CT: Greenwood Publishers.

Dworkin, Ronald A. 1982. "'Natural' Law Revisited." *University of Florida Law Review* 34: 165–188.

Dworkin, Ronald A. 1985. "A Matter of Principle." Cambridge, MA: Harvard University Press.

Ely, John H. 1980. *Democracy and Distrust: A Theory of Judicial Review.* Cambridge, MA: Harvard University Press.

Finnis, John. 1980a. *Natural Law and Natural Rights.* Oxford: Clarendon Press.

Finnis, John. 1980b. "The Natural Law, Objective Morality, and Vatican II." In *Principles of Catholic Moral Life,* ed. William E. May and William E. Baum. Chicago: Franciscan Herald Press.

Fuchs, Josef. 1965. *Natural Law: A Theological Investigation,* tr. Helmut Reckter and John A. Dowling. New York: Sheed and Ward.

Gahl Jr., Robert A. 1997. "From the Virtue of a Fragile Good to a Narrative Account of Natural Law." *International Philosophical Quarterly* 37(4): 457–472.

George, Robert P. 1998. *Natural Law and Moral Inquiry: Ethics, Metaphysics, and Politics in the Work of Germain Grisez.* Washington, D.C.: Georgetown University Press.

George, Robert P., ed. 1992. *Natural Law Theory: Contemporary Essays.* Oxford: Clarendon Press.

George, Robert P., ed. 2001. *Natural Law, Liberalism, and Morality: Contemporary Essays.* New York: Oxford University Press.

Gewirth, Alan. 1984. "Law, Action, and Morality." In *The Georgetown Symposium on Ethics: Essays in Honor of Henry Babcock Veatch,* pp. 67–90, ed. Henry Veatch and Rocco Porreco. Lanham, MD: University Press of America.

Grisez, Germain. 1964. *Contraception and the Natural Law.* Milwaukee, WI: Bruce.

Grisez, Germain. 1983. *Christian Moral Principles, The Way of the Lord Jesus,* vol. 1. Chicago: Franciscan Herald Press.

Grotius, Hugo. 1925. *On the Law of War and Peace,* tr. Francis W. Kelsey. Oxford: Clarendon Press.

Gomez-Lobo, Alfonso. 2002. *Morality and the Human Goods: An Introduction to Natural Law Ethics.* Washington, D.C.: Georgetown University Press.

Häring, Bernard. 1973. *Medical Ethics.* Notre Dame, IN: Fides.

Hall, Pamela M. 1999. *Narrative and the Natural Law: An Interpretation of Thomistic Ethics.* Notre Dame, IN: Notre Dame University Press.

Hart, Herbert L. A. 1961. "The Minimum Content of Natural Law." In *The Concept of Law,* pp. 189–195. Oxford: Clarendon Press.

Hittinger, Russell. 1987. *A Critique of the New Natural Law Theory.* Notre Dame, IN: University of Notre Dame Press.

Hittinger, Russell. 1990. "Liberalism and the American Natural Law Tradition." *Wake Forest Law Review* 25: 429–499.

Holmes, Oliver Wendell. 1918. "Natural Law." *Harvard Law Review* 32. In *Holmes's Collected Legal Papers,* pp. 310–316. New York: Harcourt, Brace and Howe, 1920.

Kant, Immanuel. 1981. *Grounding for the Metaphysics of Morals,* tr. James W. Ellington. Indianapolis: Hackett.

Kass, Leon R. 1985. *Toward a More Natural Science: Biology and Human Affairs.* New York: Free Press.

Lisska, Anthony J. 1996. *Aquinas's Theory of Natural Law: An Analytic Reconstruction.* New York: Clarendon Oxford Press.

MacIntyre, Alasdair C. 1988. *Whose Justice? Which Rationality?* Notre Dame, IN: University of Notre Dame Press.

McCormick, Richard A. 1981. "Bioethics and Method: Where Do We Start?" *Theology Digest* 29(4): 303–318.

Miller, Fred D. 1991. "Aristotle on Natural Law and Justice." In *A Companion to Aristotle's Politics,* pp. 279–306, ed. David Keyt and Fred D. Miller. Oxford: Basil Blackwell.

Murphy, Mark C. 1995. "Self-Evidence, Human Nature, and Natural Law." *American Catholic Philosophical-Quarterly* 69(3): 471–484.

Passerin d'Entrèves, Alessandro. 1970. *Natural Law: An Introduction to Legal Philosophy,* 2nd edition. London: Hutchinson University Library.

Paul, Ellen Frankel; Miller, Fred Dycus; and Paul, Jeffrey, eds. 2001. *Natural Law and Modern Moral Philosophy (Social Philosophy and Policy).* New York: Cambridge University Press.

Raz, Joseph. 1986. *The Morality of Freedom.* Oxford: Clarendon Press.

Reiman, Jeffrey. 1990. *Justice & Modern Moral Philosophy.* New Haven, CT: Yale University Press.

Ruby, Jane E. 1986. "The Origins of Scientific 'Law.'" *Journal of the History of Ideas* 47: 341–359.

Schneewind, Jerome B. 1986. "The Use of Autonomy in Ethical Theory." In *Reconstructing Individualism,* pp. 64–75, ed. Thomas C. Heller, Morton Sosna, and David E. Wellbery. Stanford, CA: Stanford University Press.

Smith, Janet E. 1991. *Humanae Vitae: A Generation Later.* Washington, D.C.: Catholic University of America Press.

Sokolowski, Robert. 1992. "Knowing Natural Law." In *Pictures, Quotations, and Distinctions: Fourteen Essays in Phenomenology,* pp. 277–291. Notre Dame, IN: University of Notre Dame Press.

Strauss, Leo. 1953. *Natural Right and History.* Chicago: University of Chicago Press.

Sullivan, Denis. 2000. "Disagreement and Objectivity in Ethics: Aquinas on the Common Precepts of the Natural Law." *American Catholic Philosophical Quarterly* 74(Suppl.): 231–244.

Traina, Cristina L. H. 1999. *Feminist Ethics and Natural Law: The End of the Anathemas (Moral Traditions and Moral Arguments Series).* Washington, D.C.: Georgetown University Press.

Weinreb, Lloyd L. 1987. *Natural Law and Justice.* Cambridge, MA: Harvard University Press.

NEUROETHICS

• • •

Neuroethics involves the analysis of ethical challenges posed by chemical, organic, and electromechanical interventions in the brain. The term *neuroethics* is used by European neurologists to refer to ethical issues in brain disorders, such as strokes or epilepsy, and it has also been used at times for ethical concerns in psychiatry, child development, and brain injury rehabilitation. In 2001, however, the language expert William Safire reinvigorated the term, applying it to the ethical challenges of emerging neurotechnologies.

Neuroethics encompasses both research and clinical applications of neurotechnology, as well as social and policy issues attendant to their use. The literature predominantly focuses on psychopharmaceuticals and their proper clinical and social uses; brain scanning (especially its use for jurisprudence); regenerative neurology, such as fetal-cell transplants in the brain (e.g., for Parkinson's disease); implantable information-processing devices that interface with the brain (such as cochlear implants); and electrical stimulation of the brain, both externally (through transcranial magnetic stimulation) and internally (through deep brain stimulation).

Neuroethics is a content field, defined by the technologies it examines rather than any particular philosophical approach. The field's distinctiveness derives from novel questions posed by applying advanced technology to the brain, the seat of personal identity and executive function in the human organism. Advances in the understanding of brain function pose challenges to certain philosophical suppositions about human nature, exposing fallacies in people's self-conceptions, revealing disparities between social or biological groups in brain function, and tying together traits and states in novel ways. Intervention technologies raise questions about the proper limits of therapeutics, the desirability of human enhancement, and the right to access information directly from a person's brain that may even be hidden from his or her own conscious mind.

Neuroscientific Advances

Until the last few decades of the twentieth century, few ethical procedures were available that could directly reveal the details of brain functioning. Neurological and psychiatric interventions were crude. Scientists generally tried to understand the brain by correlating pathologies to loss of function, stimulating areas of the brain during surgery, or using electroencephalographs (EEGs) to glean how brain waves correspond to function. In contrast, technologies such as brain scans now provide less invasive access to brain activities. At the same time, new classes of psychopharmaceuticals and innovative neurotechnologies have increased medicine's ability to directly influence brain function.

Psychopharmaceuticals

Pharmaceutical advances are changing the way mental illness is conceptualized, defined, diagnosed, and treated. Medications that manipulate the major neurotransmitter systems (i.e., catecholamines, cholinergic and serotonergic systems), show great specificity and few side effects compared to older drugs. Psychopharmaceuticals pose two ethical challenges: (1) how to best utilize these tools in treating neurological and mental illnesses; and (2) how to assess the widespread use of these drugs outside medical settings.

MEDICAL USES. The proper role of drugs in treating mental illness has been a topic of ethical concern at least since the second half of the nineteenth century, and the issue periodically captures public attention. In the late 1980s, fluoxetine (Prozac), a drug classed as a *selective serotonin reuptake inhibitor* (SSRI), hit the market, and within three years it became the most highly prescribed antidepressant in the world. In his widely-read *Listening to Prozac* (1993), Peter Kramer described how patients on Prozac reported enhanced self-worth and confidence, less sensitivity to social rejection, and more risk-taking in their lives. However, as patients underwent these transformations, they began to wonder which was their "real self"—the pre-Prozac personality, or the personality improved by the drug?

What are the implications of a pill that seems to alter personality, not just cure illness? Will Prozac replace self-examination as the treatment of choice for life's challenges? Pharmaceutical research continues to produce drugs that can alter cognition (cogniceuticals) and mood, and the temptation will be to consider traits like shyness, irritability, or forgetfulness medically relevant simply because drugs that can alter these mental states are available. What are the social implications of drug choices—is it significant that when American society wanted women at home the drug of choice was Valium (a tranquilizer), and now that workplace assertiveness is valued it is Prozac?

Some have similarly criticized the widespread use of Ritalin to treat attention deficit disorders in children, suggesting that what is being treated is a normal variation in children's attentional capacities that would not be labeled pathological in other societies or other historical periods. The pressure for early diagnosis and treatment has resulted in calls for large-scale testing of children (Rowland et al., 2001; Shea et al., 1996) and claims of the overuse of psychiatric medication (Diller; Miller et al., 2001).

"LIFESTYLE" DRUGS. Inducing desired mental states through ingestion is at least as old as the discovery of fermentation. However, the growing power of modern psychopharmaceuticals to specifically alter mood or cognition, or to enhance traits such as memory or attentiveness is one of the most promising and challenging developments of the twenty-first century.

Pharmaceuticals developed for identified pathologies such as depression, erectile dysfunction, and narcolepsy also have the potential to improve or augment otherwise average or typical functioning. Drugs are often prescribed to help people moderate shyness, stage fright, occasional erectile difficulties, mild depression, or distractibility. Through such "cosmetic psychopharmacology" people will increasingly be able to chemically micromanage their mood states and cognitive skills. The demand for "lifestyle" drugs will alter the role of the clinician and strengthen the role of direct-to-consumer marketing of drugs. Drugs that can alter mood, attention, or cognitive functioning may also have social policy implications, such as their use to control prison populations or to enhance employee performance.

Brain Imaging

Brain imaging technologies generally look at blood flow to areas of the brain during mental activities. The technology began with the development in the 1970s of computerized axial tomography (CAT scans, which use X-rays), functional magnetic resonance imaging (fMRI, which uses magnets and radio waves), and positron emission tomography (PET scans, which use an injected radioactive isotope). By examining areas of metabolic activity in the brain during a specific cognitive or affective process, scientists can map that process to brain structure (morphometry), or identify irregularities. The use of imaging technology raises three general kinds of ethical issues: (1) our understanding of brain processes—and therefore of who we are; (2) proper medical uses of imaging; and (3) the desirable social uses of imaging.

UNDERSTANDING MENTAL PROCESSES. Neuroscientists suggest that, in principle, virtually all human states, from love to laziness to empathy to irritability, have brain correlates that may be detectable through brain mapping. J. F. Pujol and colleagues, for example, showed that the size of the cingulate gyrus (which coordinates sensory input with emotions) is significantly correlated with levels of emotions such as worry, fearfulness in the face of uncertainty, and shyness with strangers. If claims that imaging can identify emotional tendencies, musical talent, aggressiveness, or spatial acuity are true, this could alter ways of understanding people. Schools, employers, or the military could potentially use such technologies to categorize and track their students or workers.

Imaging research is exploring even complex activities such as moral judgments. For example, a 2001 study by Joshua Greene and colleagues used fMRI to study 100 subjects presented with a classic ethics vignette: given the choice, most people would redirect a train onto a track where one person would be killed rather than keep it on a track where five would be killed. However, they would not physically push a single person in front of the train to stop it from killing five others, even though both cases involve killing one to save five. The researchers found that emotional centers of the brain were much more active when considering physically pushing someone onto the track (a *moral-personal* scenario) than when simply pulling a switch (a *moral-impersonal* scenario). Such systematic differences in brain patterns may give us insight into hidden aspects of moral decision making.

MEDICAL USES OF IMAGING. Imaging studies have already challenged medical nosologies (classifications), discovering new pathological processes and revealing specific disease susceptibilities or risks. For example, the finding that psychiatric syndromes affect multiple brain structures has challenged the view that mental illness reflected particular abnormalities in discrete areas of the brain.

Familiar ethical concerns of medical procedures such as imaging include the risks of radiation and obtaining informed consent from the cognitively impaired. Imaging also raises novel concerns, however. A history of depression, drug abuse, or other brain pathologies, as well as certain behavioral traits, can leave lasting morphological traces that can be seen on certain types of scans. In 1977, Wayne Drevets and colleagues reported that people with a history of depression had 48 percent less gray matter in their left subgenual prefrontal cortex than those without such a history, while those with bipolar illness were 39 percent smaller. Scanning done for other purposes can be used to detect these morphological signatures, raising significant privacy concerns.

SOCIAL USES OF IMAGING. Imaging technology will pose significant challenges to policymaking and jurisprudence. The ability to detect neurological signs of alcoholism, aggression, sexual inclinations, and other behaviors would be a tempting target for law enforcement personnel and other agents of social control. Scans can already detect identifiable responses in some people with phobias when they are presented with a feared stimulus (Birbaumer et al.), or former drug addicts when presented with drugs (Childress, et al.)—even if they try to suppress the response, and even if the stimulus is presented to them subliminally. In a controversial study, Phelps and colleagues showed white males pictures of unfamiliar black faces, and showed a correlation between their levels of racism and levels of activity in the amygdala (the seat of emotions such as fear). Other imaging studies have shown that some false memories can be distinguished from true memories (Schacter et al.), and that lies can be distinguished from truth-telling (Langleben et al.). The use to which such devices might be put raise significant privacy and justice concerns.

Brain-Computer Interfaces

Brain-computer interfaces (BCIs) are defined as systems in which commands from the brain to the external world are communicated technologically rather than passing through the brain's normal output pathways of peripheral nerves and muscles (Wolpaw et al.). BCIs include using EEGs to translate brain waves into actions and using neurologically implanted chips and electrodes that can communicate with external computers.

The most common BCI is the cochlear implant, used by over 30,000 people worldwide. The technology, which allows deaf people and those severely hard of hearing to perceive sound, is controversial, in part because it is imperfect and can thus trap users between hearing and deaf cultures. Much of the deaf community has also been opposed to the device, believing that deafness represents a culture rather than a disability, and that there is no need to try and "fix" it. In contrast, visual prostheses for persons with degenerative retinal disease have generated no such reaction from the blind.

Investigational BCIs include implanted extracellular electrode arrays that allow those with spinal chord injuries to control their environments by being able to manipulate mechanical devices with brain waves (Nicolelis). Integrating computer technology into human physiology is beginning to create cyborgs—organisms that are partly organic and partly machine. In the case of brain prostheses, which impact one's sense of identity and enhance basic human activity such as communication or cognition, questions of informed consent, privacy, and autonomy become important (Maguire and McGee).

Cell Transplants

Neural cells from fetuses have been transplanted (with mixed results) into patients with syndromes such as Parkinson's disease (Kordower et al.), raising ethical questions of informed consent, the appropriateness of implanting foreign tissue in the brain, and the potential destruction of a fetus or embryo for therapeutic purposes. In addition, integrating cells from one person into another's brain raises issues of identity and autonomy, which will become even more trenchant if proposals to attempt full or partial brain transplants are ever realized.

External and Internal Stimulation of the Brain

Transcranial magnetic stimulation (TMS) disrupts normal functioning of the brain using a pulse from a magnetic coil held over the skull. It "turns off" an area of the brain by creating a transient functional lesion, and certain kinds of TMS may even improve performance in memory and reasoning tasks. Researchers are also now using direct electrical stimulation of the brain to treat tremors associated with Parkinson's disease and severe chronic pain. The technology also seems to improve major depression, obsessive-compulsive disorder, and other psychiatric conditions. However, the long-term effects of these technologies are unknown, raising questions of safety and of obtaining informed consent when risks are difficult to define.

General Ethical and Social Concerns

Neurotechnologies have specific characteristics that raise unique concerns. However, the overall development of such powerful tools also has general implications for ethics and social policy.

SELFHOOD. The working assumption of most neuroscientists is that all human properties—personality, mind, and even soul—are emergent properties of the brain, and that no change in thought or sense of selfhood could occur without corresponding changes in neurophysiology. Neuroscience has already laid claim to the location of a sense of selfhood in the frontal lobes, for example. Frontotemporal dementia can result in significant changes in political social or religious values (Miller et al.), and frontal lobe trauma can cause personality change (Mataro et al.).

The attempts to trace human cognitive activity to brain structures raise important philosophical and religious questions. What would be the implications of discovering that traits like loving or moral reasoning have neurological (i.e., electrochemical) correlates? Does it reduce love to a biological artifact or epiphenomenon, or erode people's sense of free will? Further, if selfhood is embodied in specific areas of the brain, what are the implications of manipulating those areas pharmaceutically? Can neuroscience demonstrate that a beloved parent with Alzheimer's disease is no longer the person he or she was because the seat of selfhood in the brain has been damaged? And whether or not selfhood is actually an emergent property of the brain, what is the impact of neuroscientific materialism and determinism (the concepts that personhood is fundamentally rooted in brain substance and that it determines the shape and scope of our personhood) on the progress of neuroscience itself, or on the public's view of things like selfhood and the soul?

ENHANCEMENT. Human beings use many strategies and technologies to enhance their cognitive and affective functioning, from mnemonics (memory aids) to ingesting coffee or amphetamines. The enhancement debate centers primarily on the attempt to bypass mechanisms such as learning or behavioral reinforcement and directly moderate brain electrochemistry or structure (Wolpe). Drawing on the body's own resources, or manipulating the external environment to effect change, does not raise the same ethical challenges.

Enhancement, which refers to attempts to improve "normal" cognitive and affective functioning, poses two basic questions. The first, and more philosophical, question is about categorization: what do terms such as *average* or *normal* functioning, or even *disease* mean, when we can improve functioning across the entire range of human capability? If Prozac can lift everyone's mood, what then is "normal" affect? Will sadness or inner struggle be pathologized? If we can all be happy and well-adjusted through a drug such as Prozac, should insurance pay to reach that state of bliss? The second question addresses a broader social concern: should people be encouraged to, or discouraged from, ingesting pharmaceuticals to enhance behaviors, skills, and traits? What are the personal and social implications of using drugs or other neurotechnologies to micromanage mood, improve memory, maintain attentiveness, or improve sexuality?

Neurotechnologies ask one to explicitly consider the kind of "self" one wants to have or, perhaps, to be. For some, the astounding ability to manipulate human biology is an integral part of being human. For others, it is an affront to humanity. This is an argument for which there are no right or wrong answers, emerging as it does from two philosophically different visions of human life. Yet therein lies the tension of the enhancement debate, and there is little doubt that the debate will involve the ancient desire to control the workings of the mind.

Social Policy

PRIVACY AND CONFIDENTIALITY. Some brain-imaging technologies progressively image the skull as well as the brain, and computer programs can thus reconstruct the face of the person being scanned. Unlike other technologies, such as genetic analysis, imaging often cannot be done anonymously. Yet scientists have already founded brain-imaging data banks and made thousands of scans available to researchers (Van Horn et al.). Brain waves may also soon be as identifiable as fingerprints, and they may have social uses such as surveillance, raising serious questions about invasion of privacy.

JURISPRUDENCE. Imaging studies have often looked for structural differences in the brains of criminals and murderers, especially those diagnosed with antisocial personality. More recently, research has identified some functional signatures of lie detection, and now *brain fingerprinting,* a type of brain wave analysis, is being used to determine if people have ever seen particular faces, pictures, or crime scenes before (Farwell and Smith). Attorneys have tried to enter brain scans as evidence in criminal proceedings in a number of states, with mixed results. There is no doubt, however, that the use of brain scans in criminal justice venues will increase.

POLITICS AND POLICY. The quest to locate human traits in the brain also has political implications. Morphological attempts have been made to support or refute claims of racial intelligence hierarchies, and to attempt to demonstrate that sexual orientation has structural brain correlates. As the technology develops, society will have to answer questions such as: Should imaging be used in insurance profiling for life insurance or health insurance? Will it replace testimony or other clinical measures in determining competence or mental illness? Will employers be allowed to use imaging to screen employees or look for special aptitudes? Will pharmaceutical solutions to social problems become increasingly acceptable, as in the case of some uses of Ritalin in the classroom? The answers to these and other questions of neuroethics will have a powerful effect on the nature of American society in the coming decades.

PAUL ROOT WOLPE

BIBLIOGRAPHY

Birbaumer, N.; Grodd, W.; Diedrich, O.; et al. 1998. "fMRI Reveals Amygdala Activation to Human Faces in Social Phobics." *NeuroReport* 9(6): 1223–1226.

Blank, Robert H. 1999. *Brain Policy: How the New Neuroscience Will Change Our Lives and Our Politics.* Washington, D.C.: Georgetown University Press.

Childress, A. R.; Mozley, P. D.; McElgin, W.; et al. 1999. "Limbic Activation During Cue-Induced Cocaine Craving." *American Journal of Psychiatry* 156(1): 11–8.

Diller, L.H. 1996. "The Run on Ritalin: Attention Deficit Disorder and Stimulant Treatment in the 1990s." *Hastings Center Report* 26(2): 12–14.

Drevets, W. C.; Price, J. L.; Simpson, J. R., Jr.; et al. 1997. "Subgenual Prefrontal Cortex Abnormalities in Mood Disorders." *Nature* 386(6627): 824–827.

Farah, Martha. 2002. "Emerging Ethical Issues in Neuroscience." *Nature Neuroscience* 5: 1123–1129.

Farwell, L. A., and Smith, S. S. 2001. "Using Brain MERMER Testing to Detect Concealed Knowledge Despite Efforts to Conceal." *Journal of Forensic Sciences* 46(1): 1–9.

Greene, Joshua D.; Sommerville, R. Brian; Nystrom, Leigh E.; et al. 2001. "An fMRI Investigation of Emotional Engagement in Moral Judgment." *Science* 293(5537): 2105–2108.

Illes, Judy, ed. 2002. "Brain and Cognition: Ethical Challenges in Advanced Neuroimaging." *Brain and Cognition,* Special Issue, 50(3).

Kordower, J. H.; Freeman, T. B.; Chen, E. Y.; et al. 1998. "Fetal Nigral Grafts Survive and Mediate Clinical Benefit in a Patient with Parkinson's Disease." *Movement Disorders* 13(3): 383–393.

Kramer, Peter. 1993. *Listening to Prozac.* New York: Viking Press.

Langleben, D. D.; Schroeder, L.; Maldjian, J. A.; et al. 2002. "Brain Activity during Simulated Deception: An Event-Related Functional Magnetic Resonance Study." *Neuroimage* 15(3): 727.

Maguire, G. Q., Jr., and McGee, E. M. 1999. "Implantable Brain Chips? Time for Debate." *Hastings Center Report* 29(1): 7–13.

Mataro, M.; Jurado, M.A.; Garcia-Sanchez, C.; et al. 2001. "Long-term Effects of Bilateral Frontal Brain Lesion: Sixty Years after Injury with an Iron Bar." *Archives of Neurology* 58(7): 1139–1142.

Miller, A.R.; Lalonde, C.E.; McGrail, K.M.; and Armstrong, R.W. 2001. "Prescription of Methylphenidate to Children and Youth, 1990–1996." *Canadian Medical Association Journal.* 165(11): 1489–94.

Miller, M.D., Seeley, W. W., Mychack, P.; et al. 2001. "Neuroanatomy of the Self." *Neurology* 57: 817–821.

Nicolelis, M. A. 2001. "Actions from Thoughts." *Nature* 409(6818): 403–407.

Phelps, E. A.; O'Connor, K. J.; Cunningham,W.A.; et al. 2000. "Performance on Indirect Measures of Race Evaluation Predicts Amygdala Activation." *Journal of Cognitive Neuroscience* 12(5): 729–738.

Pujol, J., A.; Lopez, J. Deus; et al. 2002. "Anatomical Variability of the Anterior Cingulate Gyrus and Basic Dimensions of Human Personality." *Neuroimage* 15(4): 847–55.

Rowland, A.S.; Umbach, D.M.; Catoe, K.E.; et al. 2001. "Studying the Epidemiology of Attention-deficit Hyperactivity Disorder: Screening Method and Pilot Results." *Canadian Journal of Psychiatry (Revue Canadienne de Psychiatrie)* 46(10): 931–40.

Safire, William. 2001. "Stem Cell Hard Sell." *New York Times,* July 5: 17A.

Schacter, D. L.; Reiman, E.; Curran, T.; et al. 1996. "Neuroanatomical Correlates of Veridical and Illusory Recognition Memory: Evidence from Positron Emission Tomography." *Neuron* 17(2): 267–274.

Shea, K.M.; Rahmani, C.H.; and Morris, P.J. 1996. "Diagnosing Children with Attention Deficit Disorders through a Health Department-Public School Partnership." *American Journal of Public Health* 86(8 Pt 1): 1168–1169.

Van Horn, J. D.; Grethe, J. S.; Kostelec, P.; et al. 2001. "The Functional Magnetic Resonance Imaging Data Center (fMRIDC): The Challenges and Rewards of Large-scale Databasing of Neuroimaging Studies." *Philosophical Transactions of the Royal Society of London: Biological Sciences* 356(1412): 1323–1339.

Wolpaw, J. R.; Birbaumer, N.; McFarland, D. J.; et al. 2002. "Brain-Computer Interfaces for Communication and Control." *Clinical Neurophysiology* 113(6): 767–791.

Wolpe, Paul Root. 2002. "Treatment, Enhancement, and the Ethics of Neurotherapeutics." *Brain and Cognition* 50(3): 387–395.

NURSING ETHICS

• • •

The development of nursing ethics has paralleled the development of nursing as a profession. As nursing has evolved from the use of the rules of hygiene in caring for the sick (Nightingale) to a profession that defines its practice realm as the promotion of health, the prevention of illness, the restoration of health, and the alleviation of suffering (International Council of Nurses), so has nursing ethics evolved from following rules of conduct in attending the sick (Robb) to an identified field of inquiry within bioethics (Fry and Veatch).

Early Interpretations of Nursing Ethics

During the first half of the 20th century, interpretations of nursing ethics tended to view the nurse as a chaste, good woman in Christian service to others, and as an obedient, dutiful servant. To Florence Nightingale (1820–1910), who had responded to a religious calling to nursing, a good nurse was committed to the ideal of doing what was right. Being of the highest character, the good nurse was disciplined by moral training and could be relied upon to do her Christian duty in service to others.

This view of the good nurse as a good woman pervaded early textbooks on nursing ethics. Isabel Hampton Robb 1860–1910), the first president of the American Nurses Association (ANA), thought that the nurse must be a dignified, cultured, courteous, well-educated, and reserved woman of good breeding. Like Nightingale, she considered the nurse's work as ministry, as "a consecrated service, performed in the Spirit of Christ" (Robb, p. 38). Thus, moral virtue, moral duty, and service to others were established as important foundations upon which later interpretations of nursing ethics would be built.

At one time, nursing ethics was virtually indistinguishable from nursing etiquette and the performance of duty. Nursing etiquette included forms of polite behavior, such as neatness, punctuality, courtesy, and quiet attendance to the physician. The nurse demonstrated her acceptance of her moral duties by following rules of etiquette and being loyal and obedient to the physician (Robb). Early textbooks on the subject describe nursing ethics as the ideals, customs, and habits associated with the general characteristics of a nurse, and as doing one's duty with skill and moral perfection.

Some important distinctions were made between etiquette and ethics, however. Nurses learned proper ward etiquette in order to promote professional harmony in patient care, and this etiquette became the foundation for all other nursing behaviors. Ethics, however, was taught to promote moral excellence and technical competence on the part of the nurse. Ethics was viewed as a science, the knowledge of which would enable the nurse to carry out prescribed duties with moral skill and technical perfection.

Following World War II, the nurse's role in patient care slowly shifted from that of the physician's obedient helper to that of an independent practitioner who could be held accountable for what had been done or not done in providing patient care. A shift in the understanding of nursing ethics accompanied this shift in roles. The nurse's moral responsibilities were no longer couched solely in terms of obedience to authority and institutional loyalty. Instead, the nurse now claimed authority for independent clinical decisions in patient care, including ethical decisions.

In the second half of the twentieth century, contemporary nursing ethics began to develop in several directions. First, recently developed codes of nursing ethics were revised. Second, dramatic changes occurred in the teaching of nursing ethics. Third, nurses' attitudes and values, moral development, moral-reasoning abilities, and ethical practice or behavior were empirically studied. Fourth, the moral concepts of nursing practice were philosophically analyzed. Finally, consideration was given to the development of theories of nursing ethics.

The Development and Revision of Nursing Codes of Ethics

As professional nursing developed, nursing organizations began to discuss the need for a code of ethics for nursing practice. In the United States, the 1897 meeting of the newly constituted ANA was the first occasion for members of the profession to discuss such a code. The ANA House of Delegates, however, did not accept a code of ethics until 1950. Revised in 1960, 1968, 1976, 1985 and 2001, the ANA Code of Ethics for Nurses with Interpretive Statements "provides a framework for nurses to use in ethical analyses and decision-making" (p. 6). While the development of the ANA Code of Ethics for Nurses was in process, the International Council of Nurses (ICN), established in 1900, was developing an international code of nursing ethics. A draft of this code was presented and accepted at the 1953 ICN Congress held in Sao Paulo, Brazil. The ICN Code for Nurses was revised in 1965, 1973, and 2000 and has been translated into several languages. The ICN published guidelines on the use of the Code for Nurses in 1977, 1994, and 2002.

A significant number of national nurses' associations throughout the world have also developed codes of ethics. Among the areas of agreement are nursing responsibility for practice competence; the need for good relations with coworkers; respect for the life and dignity of the patient; protection of patient confidentiality; and the ethical responsibility not to discriminate against patients on the basis of race, religious beliefs, cultural practices, or economic status (Sawyer). Like other professional codes of ethics, nursing codes provide important ethical standards that nurses can refer to when faced with questions of ethics or unethical practices on the part of coworkers and institutions. They are also an important historical record of the ethical concepts and principles considered important to nursing practice over time. Their periodic revisions have thus helped to shape the development of modern nursing ethics.

Like all professional codes of ethics, nursing codes are hard to apply to patient care. Since such codes represent moral ideals rather than specific action guides, professional nursing organizations have developed lengthy interpretations of nursing codes of ethics, or produced guidebooks with case applications of a code (Fry and Johnstone). In the United Kingdom, the Nursing and Wifery Council has published advisory documents to supplement its Code of Professional Conduct.

Teaching Ethics in Nursing Education

During the 1970s, the models of nurses' ethical decision making used in nursing-education programs were critically examined. A study of ethics teaching in 209 accredited baccalaureate nursing programs in the United States revealed that general ethics content was integrated into the curricula of two-thirds of the programs surveyed (Aroskar). The majority of the programs also expressed a need for the teaching of more specific nursing ethics content. Several textbooks on nursing ethics have helped to define this content (e.g., Benjamin and Curtis; Bishop and Scudder; Fry and Veatch; Yeo and Morehouse). According to these textbooks, both the teaching of ethics in nursing curricula and the analysis of ethical conflicts as they occur in nursing practice can enhance nurses' ethical decision-making abilities. They also agree that the ethical problems nurses most often experience involve: (1) balancing harms and benefits in patient care; (2) protecting patients' autonomy; and (3) distributing nursing-care resources.

As various approaches to teaching ethics in nursing education developed, a consensus emerged that the overall goal of teaching ethics to nurses is to produce an ethically accountable practitioner who is skilled in ethical decision making. Intermediate goals of ethics teaching are to: (1) examine personal commitments and values in relation to the care of patients; (2) engage in ethical reflection; (3) develop skill in moral reasoning and moral judgment; and (4) develop the ability to use ethics for reflection on broader issues that have policy implications and for research on the moral foundations of practice. These goals focus on the fact that ethics is a form of inquiry used by every nurse in clinical practice. Broad general acceptance of these goals in nursing education prompted research into nurses' ethical decisions and the types of ethical issues nurses confront in patient care.

Nursing-Ethics Research

The earliest recorded nursing-ethics research project was Rose Helene Vaughan's 1935 study of the diaries of ninety-five student and graduate nurses who recorded the ethical problems they encountered in nursing practice over a three-month period. Vaughan's analysis identified 2,265 moral problems, 67 problems of etiquette, and 110 questions about ethical behavior. The ethical problem the nurses faced most often was the lack of cooperation between nurses and physicians, and among nurses in general. Other ethical problems noted were: duties to the nursing school, lying

(including dishonest charting), duties to patients, lust, and problems of temperance. Vaughan concluded that the problem of lack of cooperation her subjects experienced signaled nurses' growing awareness of their responsibilities to society and the role they were playing in patient care. She recommended more emphasis on ethics education in nursing to ensure a high standard of individual morality, which she believed would "raise the nursing professional above and beyond the slightest suggestion of social disapproval" (p. 105).

Despite this early interest in nurses' ethical problems, nursing-ethics research did not begin in earnest until the 1980s. Research efforts initially focused on the ethical reasoning abilities and ethical behaviors and judgments among practicing nurses (Ketefian and Ormond). These studies focused on the ability of the nurse to make moral judgments, on the hypothetical ethical behavior of the nurse, and on nurses' perceptions of ethical problems. Methodologically, the studies were designed to document the cognitive abilities of nurses to make moral judgments.

A few studies in nursing ethics have measured nurses' ethical decision-making styles, factors influencing nurses' ethical decisions, and the consistency of the way nurses make ethical decisions (Ketefian and Ormond). Nursing-ethics research has also looked at the attitudes and values of nurses concerning ethical issues (Davis and Slater). Other topics studied include: how frequently nurses in different practice environments encounter specific ethical issues in their practices; how disturbed they are by ethical problems; and the influence of demographic and work-related variables on the frequency and the disturbance levels of ethical issues (Berger, Severson, and Chvatal; Fry and Damrosch; Fry and Duffy; Omery et al.; Scanlon).

The problems most frequently encountered by the nurse subjects in these studies are: (1) staffing patterns that limit patient access to nursing care, (2) pain relief and management, (3) inappropriate allocation of resources, (4) prolonging life with inappropriate measures, and (5) working with incompetent and irresponsible colleagues. However, it is still not known how nurses respond to particular issues when they experience them, or how nurses use resources in the workplace to handle specific issues. Furthermore, it is not clear which workplace factors influence the abilities of nurses to handle issues and which ethics resources in the workplace are most helpful to the ethical practice of nurses. Further research is clearly needed, particularly as changes occur in healthcare delivery and nurses are presented with new and more difficult etical issues that may affect patient outcomes.

The theoretical frameworks used to interpret study results in nursing-ethics research also need evaluation. Since nursing is largely practiced by women, theoretical structures should include the process of ethical decision making by women as well as men. Furthermore, researchers should use structures that can account for the nature and process of ethical decisions made by nurses—and how they contrast with those of other healthcare workers, such as physicians (Fry). This means that theoretical structures that are developed from the study of one gender alone, or that consider ethical decisions as decisions made by physicians, might not be appropriate for the study of nurses' ethical decisions. In considering appropriate theoretical frameworks, clarity about the moral concepts of nursing is very important.

Moral Concepts of Nursing Ethics

Advocacy, accountability, collaboration, and caring are foundational moral concepts for nurses' principled, ethical decision making (Fry and Johnstone). They are important because they enjoy a firm place in nursing standards and ethical statements throughout the history of the nursing profession and help define the ethical dimensions of the nurse–patient relationship.

ADVOCACY. Advocacy may be defined as the active support of an important cause (Fry and Johnstone). In nursing, it describes the nature of the nurse–patient relationship and has been interpreted as a legal metaphor for the nurse's role in relation to a patient's human and moral rights within the healthcare system (Winslow). Others have interpreted advocacy as the moral concept that defines how nurses view their responsibilities to the patient (Gaylord and Grace; Sellin; Snowball).

Advocacy has been associated with courage and heroism. It may also be understood as the means by which the nurse participates with the patient in determining the meaning that the experience of illness, suffering, or dying has for that individual (Gadow). Francesca Lumpp, a nurse educator, has even argued that two general ethical principles—respect for human dignity and fidelity—are rooted in the advocacy concept. Some nurse-ethicists have interpreted advocacy as the ethical principle that justifies what nurses do to protect the human dignity, privacy, choice (when applicable), and well-being of the patient (Fry and Johnstone). This last view of advocacy seems most consistent with the values expressed in nursing codes of ethics and the primary ethical responsibilities of the nurse.

ACCOUNTABILITY. The concept of accountability seems to have two major attributes: answerability and responsibility. Nurses are assumed to carry personal responsibility for nursing practice and are expected to justify, or "give an account" of, their nursing judgments and actions according to the profession's ethical standards or norms. Terms of legal accountability for nursing practice are contained in licensing procedures and state-regulated nursing practice acts, while terms of moral accountability appear as norms in codes of nursing ethics and other standards of nursing practice. By virtue of agreeing to perform nursing care, the nurse accepts accountability for performing such care according to these standards and norms.

While accountability is a basic moral value in nursing practice, mechanisms for evaluating the accountability levels of nurses need to be developed. A few codes of nursing ethics have focused on accountability as a central moral concept (ANA; Australian Nursing Council; United Kingdom Central Council, 2002), and at least one national nursing organization has provided documentation on the extent of nursing accountability in professional practice (United Kingdom Central Council, 1996).

COOPERATION. Cooperation is active participation with others to obtain quality care for patients, collaboration in designing nursing care, and reciprocity to those with whom nurses professionally identify, such as physicians and other healthcare workers. It implies consideration for the values and goals of those with whom one works. The concept of cooperation encourages nurses to work with others toward shared goals, to make mutual concerns a priority, and to sacrifice personal interests to maintain the professional relationship over time.

Cooperation has been included in several codes of nursing ethics as a moral concept of nursing practice (ANA; Australian Nursing Council, ICN; Irish Nursing Board). While early views on nursing ethics linked cooperation to a special loyalty shared by members of the professional group (Robb), later views linked cooperation to the need to compromise individual goals and interests in order to achieve a mutually determined and higher level of patient care (Benjamin and Curtis; Fry and Johnstone).

CARING. The moral concept of caring has long been valued in the nurse–patient relationship. Caring behavior is considered essential to the nursing role and is presumed to affect how humans experience health—as well as life itself. For nurses, caring is directed toward the protection of the health and welfare of patients, and it indicates a commitment to the protection of human dignity and the preservation of human health (Fry and Johnstone).

Recent feminist interpretations of human caring relate caring to the protection, welfare, or maintenance of another person (Noddings). Others have defined caring as a moral obligation or duty among health professionals (Pellegrino), or as a form of involvement with others that engenders concern for how they experience their world (Benner and Wrubel). These views indicate two attributes of the concept. First, caring is a natural human sentiment, the way all humans relate to their world and to each other (Noddings). It exists as a structural feature of human growth and development before caring behaviors actually commence. Second, caring is linked to moral or social ideals, such as the human need to be protected from the elements or the need for love. Caring, in this sense, might be interpreted as a commitment toward certain patient outcomes, especially the protection of human dignity and the preservation of human health (Shiber and Larson; Valentine).

It has been suggested that caring is really a therapeutic "presence" that includes both an attitude of personal concern and skill and knowledge about caring (Bishop and Scudder). Caring, in this view, is not emotion or sentimental, but is a way of being with others that assures them of personal concern for their well-being. Such a presence fosters the well-being of individuals by transforming how they experience their world, and it ultimately fosters the healing process. Patients know that they are not only being cared for, but that the one providing care really does care about them.

Theories of Nursing Ethics

Progress in the development of a theory of nursing ethics has been slow, partly because of disputes about the relationship of nursing ethics to medical ethics—and to the discipline of ethics itself. Some ethicists claim that there is little that is morally unique to nursing practice (Veatch). The same moral issues confront everyone in the healthcare setting, regardless of whether one is a physician, nurse, or patient. This means that *nursing ethics* is a legitimate term only insofar as it refers to a subcategory of medical ethics. Since medical ethics is the ethics of all judgments made within the biomedical sciences, nursing ethics is simply the ethical analysis of those judgments made by nurses, in much the same way that physician ethics is the ethical analysis of those judgments made by physicians. Any theory of nursing ethics will, therefore, be exactly like medical-ethics theory. According to this view, a theory of nursing ethics may not even be necessary.

Others argue that nursing ethics is not just another form of applied ethics or medical ethics (Gamete). If the moral concepts and obligations inherent in nursing practice are different from (yet compatible with) those of other health professions, then nursing ethics may have a distinct voice in healthcare. If so, nursing ethics will use traditional and contemporary forms of philosophical analysis to describe the moral phenomena of nursing practice, to critically assess the language and conceptual foundations of nursing practice, and to raise normative claims about the aims of nursing practice within the healthcare sphere. It will provide a perspective on what is good and bad, or right and wrong, in nursing practice, and will thus lead to ethical principles that can be used to guide nursing judgments and actions. It will be nursing-ethics theory and not medical-ethics theory.

Regardless of its form, any theory of nursing ethics will need to address the relevance of the moral concepts of nursing practice in the years ahead. As the twenty-first century reveals new moral challenges in healthcare, nursing ethics must respond with conviction about the integrity of its moral concepts and develop practice-based theories of nursing ethics. If it is to claim its promise as a form of philosophical inquiry for the field of bioethics, it must also continue to move ahead on the expansion of nursing-ethics research and identify what is known and not known about nurses' ethical practices in a changing healthcare environment.

SARA T. FRY (1995)
REVISED BY AUTHOR

SEE ALSO: *Autonomy; Beneficence; Care: Contemporary Ethics of; Compassionate Love; Feminism; Medical Codes and Oaths; Narrative; Nursing, Profession of; Nursing, Theories and Philosophy of; Palliative Care and Hospice; Professional-Patient Relationship: Ethical Issues; Profession and Professional Ethics; Teams, Healthcare; Trust; Women as Health Professionals*

BIBLIOGRAPHY

American Nurses Association (ANA). 2001. *Code of Ethics for Nurses with Interpretative Statements.* Washington, D.C.: Author.

Aroskar, Mila A. 1977. "Ethics in the Nursing Curriculum." *Nursing Outlook* 25(4): 260–264.

Australian Nursing Council, Royal College of Nursing. 2002. Code of Ethics for Nurses in Australia. Dickson, ACT: Author.

Benjamin, Martin, and Curtis, Joy. 1992. *Ethics in Nursing,* 3rd edition. New York: Oxford University Press.

Benner, Patricia E., and Wrubel, Judith. 1989. *The Primacy of Caring: Stress and Coping in Health and Illness.* Menlo Park, CA: Addison-Wesley.

Berger, M. C.; Severson, A.; and Chvatal, R. 1991. "Ethical Issues in Nursing." *Western Journal of Nursing Research* 13: 514–521.

Bishop, Anne H., and Scudder, John R. 2001. *Nursing Ethics: Holistic Caring Practice,* 2nd edition. Boston: Jones and Bartlett.

Davis, Anne J., and Slater, Patricia V. 1989. "U.S. and Australian Nurses' Attitudes and Beliefs About the Good Death." *Image* 21(1): 34–39.

Fry, Sara T. 1989. "Toward a Theory of Nursing Ethics." *Advances in Nursing Science* 11(4): 9–22.

Fry, Sara T., and Damrosch, Shirley. 1994. "Ethics and Human Rights Issues in Nursing Practice: A Survey of Maryland Nurses." *The Maryland Nurse* 13: 11–12.

Fry, Sara T., and Johnstone, Megan-Jane. 2002. *Ethics in Nursing Practice: A Guide to Ethical Decision Making,* 2nd edition. Geneva: International Council of Nurses.

Fry, Sara T., and Veatch, Robert M. 2000. *Case Studies in Nursing Ethics,* 2nd edition. Boston: Jones and Bartlett.

Gadow, Sally. 1980. "Existential Advocacy: Philosophical Foundations of Nursing." In *Nursing: Images and Ideals,* ed. Stuart F. Spicker and Sally Gadow. New York: Springer.

Gaylord, Nancy, and Grace, Pamela. 1995. "Nursing Advocacy: An Ethics of Practice." *Nursing Ethics* 2: 11–18.

International Council of Nurses (ICN). 2000. *Code of Ethics for Nurses: Ethical Concepts Applied to Nursing.* Geneva: Author.

Irish Nursing Board (An Bord Altranais). 2000. Code of Conduct. Dublin: Author.

Jameton, Andrew. 1984. *Nursing Practice: The Ethical Issues.* Englewood Cliffs, NJ: Prentice Hall.

Ketefian, Shake, and Ormond, Ingrid. 1988. *Moral Reasoning and Ethical Practice in Nursing: An Integrative Review.* New York: National League for Nursing.

Lanara, Vassiliki A. 1981. *Heroism as a Nursing Value: A Philosophical Perspective.* Athens: Sisterhood Evniki.

Lumpp, Francesca. 1979. "The Role of the Nurse in the Bioethical Decision-Making Process." *Nursing Clinics of North America* 14(1): 13–21.

New Zealand Nurses Organization, Professional Services Committee. 1995. *Code of Ethics.* Wellington, New Zealand: Author.

Nightingale, Florence. 1859. *Notes on Nursing: What It Is, and What It Is Not.* London: Harrison and Sons.

Noddings, Nel. 1984. *Caring: A Feminine Approach to Ethics and Moral Education.* Berkeley: University of California Press.

Omery, Anna; Henneman, E.; Billet, B.; et al. 1995. "Ethical Issues in Hospital-Based Nursing Practice." *Journal of Cardiovascular Nursing* 9: 42–53.

Pellegrino, Edmund D. 1985. "The Caring Ethic: The Relation of Physician to Patient." In *Caring, Curing, Coping: Nurse, Physician, Patient Relationships,* ed. Anne H. Bishop and John R. Scudder. Tuscaloosa: University of Alabama Press.

Robb, Isabel Hampton. 1921. *Nursing Ethics: For Hospital and Private Use.* Cleveland, OH: E. C. Koeckert.

Sawyer, Linda M. 1989. "Nursing Codes of Ethics: An International Comparison." *International Nursing Review* 36(5): 145–148.

Scanlon, Colleen. 1994. "Ethics Survey Looks at Nurses Experiences." *The American Nurse* (November–December): 22.

Sellin, S. C. 1994. "Out on a Limb: A Qualitative Study of Patient Advocacy in Institutional Nursing." *Nursing Ethics* 2: 19–29.

Shiber, Stella, and Larson, Elaine. 1991. "Evaluating the Quality of Caring: Structure, Process, and Outcome." *Holistic Nursing Practice* 5: 57–66.

Snowball, Jane. 1996. "Asking Nurses About Advocating for Patients: Reactive and Proactive Accounts." *Journal of Advanced Nursing* 24: 67–75.

United Kingdom Central Council, Nursing and Midwifery Council. 1996. *Guidelines for Professional Practice.* London: Author.

United Kingdom Central Council, Nursing and Midwifery Council. 2002. *Code of Professional Conduct.* London: Author.

Valentine, Kathleen. 1991. "Comprehensive Assessment of Caring and Its Relationship to Outcome Measures." *Journal of Nursing Quality Assessment* 6: 59–68.

Vaughan, Rose Helene. 1935. "The Actual Incidence of Moral Problems in Nursing: A Preliminary Study in Empirical Ethics." Ph.D. diss. Washington, D.C.: Catholic University of America.

Veatch, Robert M. 1981. "Nursing Ethics, Physician Ethics, and Medical Ethics." *Law, Medicine, and Health Care* 9(5): 17–19.

Winslow, Gerald R. 1984. "From Loyalty to Advocacy: A New Metaphor for Nursing." *Hastings Center Report* 14(3): 32–40.

Yeo, Michael, and Moorhouse, Anne, eds. 1996. *Concepts and Cases in Nursing Ethics,* 2nd edition. Peterborough, ON: Broadview Press.

INTERNET RESOURCE

Fry, Sara T., and Duffy, Mary E. 2000. "Ethical Issues in Nursing Practice: How They Are Experienced and Handled by New England RNs" (abstract). Chestnut Hill, MA: Boston College School of Nursing. Available from <http://www.bc.edu/nursing/ethics>.

NURSING, PROFESSION OF

• • •

Care for the ill or injured has existed since the beginning of recorded history, but modern nursing, as it is now known, had its beginnings in the nineteenth century with Florence Nightingale, who viewed nursing as a self-defining moral practice focused on caring. Nevertheless, for decades after Nightingale established the school of nursing at St. Thomas's Hospital in London, nursing made accommodations to other established institutions, especially medicine and hospitals—accommodations that dimmed Nightingale's original vision. Only after the nursing profession accomplished the tedious but necessary task of developing its craft and the institutions that any new venture must have in order to establish itself within a society did it engage in a concerted effort to establish its identity. Beginning in the 1960s, nursing attempted to gain recognition as a profession by applying science to nursing. Then in the 1980s, it began to identify itself as a caring practice, using qualitative methods of the human sciences to articulate the meaning of nursing practice.

Nightingale's Vision

"A new art and a new science has been created since and within the last forty years. And with it a new profession—so they say; we say, *calling*," wrote Florence Nightingale in 1893 to the meeting of the International Congress of Charities, Correction and Philanthropy in Chicago (Nightingale, 1949 [1893], p. 24). This congress initiated the organization of the nursing profession in the United States and Canada. Nightingale considered her "calling" a moral imperative from God (Woodham-Smith).

Nightingale preferred to designate nursing a "calling" rather than a "profession" to underscore its identity as a self-defining practice with a dominant moral sense. Nightingale regarded nursing as a way for women to make positive contributions to society. She recruited only women of the highest moral character, thus attempting to overcome the public impression that most nurses were alcoholics or prostitutes. In the male-dominated society of Nightingale's time, "refined" women did not work outside the home.

As medical science advanced, nurses increasingly came to be considered handmaidens of physicians, as Nightingale had feared. One reason she rejected the germ theory was that she feared it would lead to what eventually came to be called intervention medicine. She foresaw that intervention medicine would lessen the centrality of nursing care in healthcare (Rosenberg). Intervention medicine led to the belief that physicians cure by intervening in the development of disease, whereas nurses merely care for those being cured. Furthermore, science and applied science were regarded as masculine activities, whereas caring was believed to be a feminine activity.

The primary focus of caring was one's own family. Thus, in the early part of the twentieth century, much nursing care was given by young women who, for the most part, were waiting to fulfill what was seen as their primary calling: to care for family. While they were students, these young women were a cheap source of labor for hospitals.

The few career nurses in hospitals directed these novice nurses, who gave most of the direct nursing care. Most nursing care in hospitals, then, was not given by nurses who could be called professionals in any sense of the word.

World War II (1939–1945) required that large numbers of women enter the industrial workforce for the first time, and nurses serving in the armed forces attracted greater attention to the importance of nursing. This apparent advance in women's professionalism, however, merely implied that it was permissible for women to work outside the home when unusual circumstances demanded it. During the 1950s, nursing seemed not to progress as a profession except that married women were accepted into schools of nursing and allowed to practice in hospitals; the traditional view of women's vocation continued to prevail. In her 1976 book, *Hospitals, Paternalism, and the Role of the Nurse,* Jo Ann Ashley argued that hospital paternalism and sexist attitudes of physicians contributed to the exploitation of nurses, who were kept subservient. Susan M. Reverby concluded in her 1987 book titled *Ordered to Care* that nurses were "so divided by class that their common oppression based on gender could not unite them" (p. 6), and that nurses saw caring for patients as a duty that "constrained nursing's effort to control its own practice and occupational future" (p. 199).

Throughout history, men, particularly in religious orders and in military service, provided nursing care for the ill and wounded. But since the development of modern nursing, few men have entered nursing as a vocation. Even with the encouragement of men to enter nursing in the last decades of the twentieth century, the percentage of male nurses in the United States remained fairly constant at approximately 3 to 5 percent (HRSA).

Nursing is mainly a woman's vocation throughout the world. According to Constance Holleran, writing in a 1992 issue of *Nursing Administration Quarterly,* one reason that few men enter nursing is that "the problems of nursing and nurses truly are universal: few well-prepared nurses, poor career structures, and lack of resources. It is only a question of degree" (p. 3). Holleran also observed that hospitals in many countries have no budget for nursing and that in some countries there are many nursing administrators but few nurses who give direct care.

Gaining Recognition as a Profession

The question of whether nursing is a profession has concerned nursing organizations and scholars since the 1960s. Early attempts to gain recognition as a profession were based primarily on criteria drawn from disciplines outside of nursing. Using sociological criteria, Amitai Etzioni contended in the 1969 book, *The Semi-professions and Their Organization,* that although nursing had some of the characteristics of a profession, it could not be classified as a profession. In a major study to assess how far nursing had advanced in its attempt to become a profession between 1970 and 1980, researchers used six sociological criteria to determine its progress: a long and disciplined educational process; discretionary authority and judgment; an active and cohesive professional organization; acknowledged social worth; significant commitment and contribution to human well-being; and a unique body of knowledge and skill (Lysaught). These sociological criteria are helpful in understanding the controversy surrounding nursing's claim to be a profession.

A LONG AND DISCIPLINED EDUCATIONAL PROCESS. The first criterion has been one of the most difficult for nursing to meet because of the tension between hospital and collegiate programs. In the United States, nurses are prepared to be registered nurses in multiple ways: by diploma programs in hospitals; by associate degree programs, usually in community colleges; and by baccalaureate degree and graduate degree programs in colleges and universities. Every major study of nursing in the twentieth century, however, recommended that nursing education should be placed in the mainstream of collegiate education (Committee for the Study of Nursing; National Commission for the Study of Nursing; National Commission on Nursing). As early as 1965, the American Nurses Association (ANA) recommended that all those licensed to practice nursing should be educated in institutions of higher education and that the baccalaureate degree in nursing should be the minimum preparation for beginning professional nursing practice. While many hospital diploma programs have closed because of falling enrollment and financial constraints on hospitals, associate degree programs have proliferated and now represent the largest proportion (57%) of basic nursing programs (HRSA). Baccalaureate programs have also steadily increased in number, as have accelerated programs for individuals who have undergraduate degrees in another field and wish to pursue a career in nursing.

As was true of the early history of nursing in the United States, other countries have traditionally prepared nurses for practice in hospital schools of nursing. In many countries there continues to be no university-level basic or graduate (postbasic) programs for nurses (Holleran), although the general trend is toward more formal, university education. Progress toward collegiate education as the basic entry level has, however, been varied. In Canada, for example, nursing education is well established in the university system, with more than eighty-five schools offering the bachelor of science degree. Prince Edward Island has had the baccalaureate degree as the required entry level for nurses since 1992 (Thomas and Arseneault). The baccalaureate degree is the basic preparation in Denmark, which has twenty-four schools of nursing and has offered graduate degrees since 1991. In Asia, many countries have nursing education models similar to the United States. Japan, for example, has baccalaureate degree programs in nursing as well as associate degree and diploma programs (Anders and Kanai-Pak). Korea has over 100 colleges offering a nursing degree, while China offers an associate degree in eighty-nine colleges and a baccalaureate degree in forty-nine universities, in addition to graduate programs.

Progress in nursing education in lesser-developed countries has been slow but encouraged by the support of the World Health Organization (WHO). Established in 1948 by the United Nations as its specialized agency for health, WHO supports advances in nursing education by designating "WHO Collaborating Centers" in universities in the United States and elsewhere. The WHO Centers then serve as resources for nursing schools and organizations in countries needing assistance, such as Uganda, Mexico, and some smaller European nations.

Graduate education in nursing in the United States began to develop in the 1960s. Master's degree programs were established primarily in the clinical specialties of nursing practice, such as adult health, maternal and child health, and psychiatric/mental health. Although doctoral programs in nursing in the United States originally developed slowly, they more than doubled, from twelve to twenty-seven, between 1974 and 1984 (Brodie), and by 1993 had doubled again. Other countries have followed a similar pattern, and doctorates in nursing can now be pursued in many countries.

DISCRETIONARY AUTHORITY AND JUDGMENT. In the United States, regulation of nursing practice and enforcement of standards for practice and education first occurred at the turn of the twentieth century through the establishment of state boards of nursing. These boards, composed of members of the nursing profession, set criteria for the practice of nursing and established evaluation procedures to ensure that nurses are capable of practicing safely and effectively. The state boards in the 1950s created standardized testing for licensure to practice at the basic level, and they also regulate advanced nursing practice (e.g., nurse practitioners, nurse midwives) in most states.

The National League for Nursing (NLN), an organization of nurses and citizens concerned with improving nursing, has significantly influenced the standards of nursing through the development of voluntary accreditation of educational programs. The NLN has established criteria to determine the quality of nursing education and formulated procedures for accreditation of all types of educational programs that meet their criteria.

State and national nursing associations have exercised their influence in the political arena since they first supported legislation to create state boards of nursing. In the 1980s and 1990s, they concentrated on developing a political agenda that sought a greater influence on state and national legislation affecting nursing practice, nursing education, and health issues. Prior to this time, nurses had little influence in developing healthcare policy. In 1992, however, two significant events demonstrated nursing's increased influence on healthcare policy. First, the Community Health Accreditation Program (CHAP) of the NLN won "deemed status" from the federal government; this means that community health agencies that have met the standards of accreditation by CHAP are considered to have met the federal government's conditions for participating in the Medicare program and can receive Medicare reimbursement. Second, the Joint Commission on Accreditation of Healthcare Organizations created an at-large nursing seat on its board of commissioners. This body is the official accrediting agency of hospitals and other healthcare organizations, and it consequently has a great influence on the standards of healthcare in hospitals.

As nursing education has advanced to the graduate level, specialized fields of practice have been established and formal organizations, such as the Oncology Nursing Society and the American Association of Critical Care Nurses, have been formed to establish standards of practice for these specialties. In order to ensure a high standard of practice, certification examinations for specialty practice are now available and are considered a necessary additional credential for professional advancement in some areas.

In 1965 a new level of nursing practice was created with the establishment of the first nurse practitioner program at the University of Colorado. Nurse practitioners are nurses who have completed an additional specialized educational program that extends practice into areas of responsibility traditionally thought to be part of medical practice, such as diagnosis and the prescribing of medications. Nurse practitioners focus primarily on the prevention of illness, maintenance of wellness, and management of chronic health problems. More recently, nurse practitioners have been employed by both hospitals and physician practice organizations to assist with the care of acutely ill, hospitalized patients. Other types of advanced practice nurses include clinical nurse specialists, nurse anesthetists, and nurse midwives.

Regulation and credentialing for the four types of advanced practice nurses are done through a variety of arrangements between boards of nursing and boards of medicine. Legislation has been passed in many states that authorizes nurse practitioners to write prescriptions. Many states permit nurses in advanced practice to receive direct payment for services from third-party payers such as Medicare, Medicaid, and private insurance. Because medical diagnoses are not always appropriate indexes for nursing practice, the North American Nursing Diagnosis Association was created in the 1980s to develop nursing diagnoses that would further standardize nursing practice and could serve as a basis for establishing a system of reimbursement for nurses.

In the 1980s and early 1990s, many nurses in the United States began to focus on providing primary healthcare. Nurse-managed centers for primary care were established across the country, often located in homeless shelters, housing projects, and other settings, expressly to meet the needs of the poor, who have limited access to healthcare.

ACTIVE AND COHESIVE PROFESSIONAL ORGANIZATION. The lack of a cohesive professional organization in 1981 was evident in the following statement made by Jerome P. Lysaught in a book published that year, titled *Action in Affirmation:* "What is needed for the professionalization of nursing is a new birth of leadership, individual and organizational, that can conceive of ways to unite the more than 20 associations that currently draw their membership from nurses" (p. 24). Activities in the international arena promoted by the International Council of Nurses (ICN) and the World Health Organization would eventually bring nursing in the United States to a more cohesive union.

The ICN, established in 1899 as an independent, nongovernmental federation of national nursing associations worldwide, is the only representative international body of the whole nursing profession. Nursing's involvement in the projects of WHO, an intergovernmental, interdisciplinary agency representing more than 160 countries, is administered by the chief nurse scientist, who maintains communications with the six regional offices of WHO and other international organizations related to nursing. There is a close working relationship between WHO and ICN, both of which are headquartered in Geneva, Switzerland.

In 1977 WHO set the year 2000 as the target date for the attainment of the highest possible level of health for all people and specified primary healthcare as the key to attaining optimal health. In keeping with WHO's goal, the ICN has encouraged its member associations around the world to prepare nurses to participate more fully in a primary healthcare system.

Nursing in the United States has been moving toward a greater role in primary care since the development of the nurse practitioner role. It has, however, needed political influence to achieve this and other reforms. Nurses gained greater political power in 1991 when the American Nurses Association, the National League for Nursing, and the American Association of Colleges of Nursing joined to form the Tri-Council for Nursing; the council was later joined by the American Organization of Nurse Executives. The increasing influence of nursing in the political arena is evident in a document titled "Nursing's Agenda for Health Care Reform" (ANA), developed by the Tri-Council and formally supported by sixty-four nursing organizations in early 1993 ("Additional Endorsements"). The Tri-Council has led the effort to gain acceptance by the U.S. Congress of measures that would increase primary healthcare in community-based settings; foster community responsibility for personal health, self-care, and informed decision making in selecting healthcare services; and facilitate the use of the most cost-effective providers in the most appropriate settings ("Fifty-eight Organizations").

ACKNOWLEDGED SOCIAL WORTH AND STRONG LEVEL OF COMMITMENT. The 1981 Lysaught study reported that the public had a high appreciation of nurses' social worth but that nurses ranked low in commitment because only 40 percent of licensed registered nurses were employed full-time. This was clearly an inappropriate use of quantitative criteria to measure commitment, which cannot be measured in this manner. Commitment in nursing refers to the nurse's determination to foster the well-being of patients/clients. Using qualitative methods, Patricia E. Benner found that commitment to the patient's well-being was present to a high degree in those who were considered excellent nurses. Anne H. Bishop and John R. Scudder Jr. (1990) also found such commitment evident in narratives in which nurses described their most fulfilling experiences as nurses.

The recognition of the "worth" of nursing as a profession has been greatly improved by research findings that have demonstrated the link between levels of nurse staffing in hospitals and adverse patient outcomes, including infections and increased mortality rates (Aiken, Smith, and Lake; Kovner and Gergen; Blegen, Goode, and Reed). This evidence, coupled with widespread shortages of nurses in almost every country, has brought enormous attention to the essential nature of nurses' contribution to healthcare. As has been true historically when shortages reached severe levels, these forces have also begun to prompt improved salary levels, better working conditions, and increased access to education through government subsidies (Buerhaus, Staiger, and Auerbach).

UNIQUE BODY OF KNOWLEDGE AND SKILL. The development of a unique body of knowledge and skill depends in significant measure on funding for research. During the 1970s, the federal Division of Nursing, which is within the U.S. Public Health Service, focused its priorities for research on clinical studies that would determine the health problems needing nursing intervention, the effectiveness of nursing practice, and the means of appropriating research findings into practice for the improvement of patient care. Funding for nursing research was enhanced with the establishment in 1986 of the National Center for Nursing Research within the National Institutes of Health (NIH). The later conversion of the center to an institute—the National Institute of Nursing Research—with the same status as other institutes within NIH, has further established the importance of continued development of nursing knowledge.

The majority of nursing research in the United States in the 1960s and 1970s tended to use scientific models and to approach nursing knowledge as an applied science. Often theories were imported into nursing from the natural and behavioral sciences in an effort to create a credible body of knowledge concerning nursing that would enhance nurses' status in the academic community. This applied approach was perhaps predictable, given that only one-third of nursing educators and scholars took their initial graduate degrees in nursing (Moses). Since the mid-1980s, however, a growing number of nursing scholars have used the qualitative methodology of the human sciences to conduct research in the practice of nursing. The significant increase in nursing scholars holding doctorates continues to broaden the approaches to research in nursing, and the different approaches can be seen in the increasing number of nursing journals, including many devoted specifically to nursing research.

Enhancing the Status of Nursing

A review of the nursing literature demonstrates that nursing continues to seek its identity in almost all parts of the world. Everywhere, nurses face difficulties in establishing the authority of their own practice because of the elevated status of men and the lowered status of women. In a 2001 report from WHO titled *Strengthening Nursing and Midwifery,* low salaries and poor working conditions, often stemming from the status of nursing as a women's profession, was identified as a major cause of persistent nursing shortages in many countries.

Nurses are increasingly attempting to enhance their legitimate authority to direct nursing care by establishing the worth of their own practice. For example, in her 1982 book, *On Nursing: Toward a New Endowment,* Margretta Styles contended that nursing would be "better served by a set of internal beliefs about nursing than a set of external criteria about professions." She proposed the "bare necessities" (p. 121) for professionhood: (1) nurses recognize the social significance of nursing by being certain about the nature and importance of their work; (2) nurses respond to the moral imperative of their work and perform to the utmost of their ability by being well prepared in knowledge, skill, and attitude; and (3) nurses realize that responsibility and authority are shared through collegiality and collectivity in order to preserve the wholeness of the profession.

Benner, author of the 1984 book, *From Novice to Expert: Excellence and Power in Clinical Nursing Practice,* attempted to learn about nursing by studying its actual practice rather than applying theories from outside of nursing. Working with a team of nursing scholars, she used the qualitative research methods of narrative and interpretative phenomenology to describe the experiences of nurses in practice. She identified seven domains of nursing: the helping role, teaching/coaching, patient diagnosing and monitoring, effectively managing rapidly changing situations, administering and monitoring therapeutic interventions and regimens, monitoring and ensuring the quality of healthcare practices, and organizational and work-role competencies. Furthermore, she identified the progression of nurses through five stages, from novice to expert, illustrating each stage with exemplars that reflect clinical knowledge. Benner's study is significant to the advancement of nursing knowledge because it illustrates, in part, that knowledge can be developed from nursing practice itself, as opposed to studies that attempt to reveal knowledge through the application of theories.

Like Benner, Bishop and Scudder Jr. (1990, 1991) showed that phenomenological interpretation of nursing practice is appropriate to the study of nursing. They concluded that nursing is a practice with an inherent moral sense and is appropriately studied as a practical human science. Benner, Bishop, and Scudder are part of a growing number of scholars who are attempting to define nursing by using the concept of caring. They employ qualitative research methodology to clarify the meaning of nursing and to improve nursing.

Conclusion

Those who are interpreting nursing from the inside of nursing approach the meaning of the term *profession* in a different way than those who follow the applied approach. The latter attempt to show that nursing is a profession by applying criteria for any profession to nursing. Using these criteria has helped to establish nursing as a profession; the criteria, however, often function as norms to be achieved, and thus actually form, rather than merely assess, nursing. Those who interpret nursing from the inside are not primarily interested in demonstrating that nursing is a profession, although they are confident that it is when its identity is disclosed. They are attempting to articulate the meaning of nursing as it is practiced and are focused on improving that practice. The nursing practice they describe has advanced in ways that Nightingale could not have foreseen. It is nevertheless the same self-defining moral practice focused on caring envisioned by her.

ANNE H. BISHOP (1995)
REVISED BY BARBARA J. DALY

SEE ALSO: *Autonomy; Beneficence; Care: Contemporary Ethics of; Compassionate Love; Feminism; Medical Codes and Oaths; Narrative; Nursing Ethics; Nursing, Theories and Philosophy of; Palliative Care and Hospice; Professional-Patient Relationship: Ethical Issues; Profession and Professional Ethics; Teams, Healthcare; Trust; Women as Health Professionals*

BIBLIOGRAPHY

"Additional Endorsements for Nursing's Agenda." 1993. *American Nurse* 25(March): 8.

Aiken, Linda H.; Smith, Herbert L.; and Lake, Eileen T. 1994. "Lower Medicare Mortality among a Set of Hospitals Known for Good Nursing Care." *Medical Care* 32(8): 771–787.

American Nurses Association (ANA). 1991. *Nursing's Agenda for Health Care Reform.* Washington, D.C.: American Nurses Publishing.

Anders, Robert L., and Kanai-Pak, Masako. 1992. "Karoshi: Death from Overwork … A Nursing Problem in Japan?" *Nursing and Health Care* 13(4): 186–191.

Ashley, Jo Ann. 1976. *Hospitals, Paternalism, and the Role of the Nurse.* New York: Teachers College Press.

Benner, Patricia E. 1984. *From Novice to Expert: Excellence and Power in Clinical Nursing Practice.* Menlo Park, CA: Addison-Wesley.

Bishop, Anne H., and Scudder, John R., Jr. 1990. *The Practical, Moral, and Personal Sense of Nursing: A Phenomenological Philosophy of Practice.* Albany: State University of New York Press.

Bishop, Anne H., and Scudder, John R., Jr. 1991. *Nursing: The Practice of Caring.* New York: National League for Nursing.

Blegen, Mary A.; Goode, Colleen J.; and Reed, Laura. 1998. "Nurse Staffing and Patient Outcomes." *Nursing Research* 47(1): 43–50.

Brodie, Barbara. 1986. "Impact of Doctoral Programs on Nursing Education." *Journal of Professional Nursing* 2(6): 350–357.

Buerhaus, Peter I.; Staiger, Douglas O.; and Auerbach, David I. 2000. "Implications of an Aging Registered Nurse Workforce." *Journal of the American Medical Association* 283(22): 2948–2954.

Chick, Norma P. 1987. "Nursing Research in New Zealand." *Western Journal of Nursing Research* 9(3): 317–334.

Committee for the Study of Nursing. 1923. *Nursing and Nursing Education in the United States,* ed. Josephine C. Goldmark. New York: Macmillan.

Etzioni, Amitai, ed. 1969. *The Semi-professions and Their Organization: Teachers, Nurses, Social Workers.* New York: Free Press.

"Fifty-eight Organizations Support Nursing's Reform Agenda." 1992. *American Nurse* 24(February): 24.

Gortner, Susan R., and Lorensen, Margarethe. 1989. "Development of Nursing Science in Scandinavia." *Nursing Outlook* 37(3): 123–126.

Health Resources and Services Administration (HRSA). National Center for Health Workforce Information and Analysis. 2001. *U.S. Health Workforce Personnel Factbook.* Washington, D.C.: U.S. Department of Health and Human Services.

Holleran, Constance. 1992. "Perspective of the International Council of Nurses." *Nursing Administration Quarterly* 16(2): 2–3.

Kovner, Christine, and Gergen, Peter J. 1998. "Nurse Staffing Levels and Adverse Events following Surgery in U.S. Hospitals." *Image: Journal of Nursing Scholarship* 30(4): 315–321.

Lysaught, Jerome P. 1981. *Action in Affirmation: Toward an Unambiguous Profession of Nursing.* New York: McGraw-Hill.

Moses, Evelyn B. 1990. *The Registered Nurse Population: Findings from the National Sample Survey of Registered Nurses, March 1988.* Washington, D.C.: U.S. Department of Health and Human Services, Public Health Service, Health Resources and Services Administration, Bureau of Health Professions, Division of Nursing.

National Commission for the Study of Nursing and Nursing Education. 1970. *An Abstract for Action,* ed. Jerome P. Lysaught. New York: McGraw-Hill.

National Commission on Nursing. 1983. *Summary Report and Recommendations.* Chicago: Author.

Nightingale, Florence. 1860 (reprint 1946). *Notes on Nursing: What It Is, and What It Is Not.* Philadelphia: J. B. Lippincott.

Nightingale, Florence. 1893 (reprint 1949). "Sick Nursing and Health Nursing." In *Nursing of the Sick,* ed. Isabel A. Hampton Robb. New York: McGraw-Hill.

Reverby, Susan M. 1987. *Ordered to Care: The Dilemma of American Nursing, 1850–1945.* Cambridge, UK: Cambridge University Press.

Rosenberg, Charles E. 1979. "Florence Nightingale on Contagion: The Hospital as Moral Universe." In *Healing and History: Essays for George Rosen,* ed. Charles E. Rosenberg. New York: Dawson Science History.

Styles, Margretta. 1982. *On Nursing: Toward a New Endowment.* St. Louis, MO: C. V. Mosby.

Thomas, Barbara, and Arseneault, Anne-Marie. 1993. "Accreditation of University Schools of Nursing: The Canadian Experience." *International Nursing Review* 40(3): 81–84.

Woodham-Smith, Cecil. 1951 (reprint 1983). *Florence Nightingale, 1820–1910.* New York: Atheneum.

World Health Organization (WHO). 2001. *Strengthening Nursing and Midwifery: Progress and Future Directions.* Geneva: Author.

INTERNET RESOURCES

American Nurses Association. 2003. Available from <http://www.nursingworld.org>.

Canadian Nurses Association. 2003. Available from <http://www.cna-nurses.ca>.

National Institute of Nursing Research. 2003. Available from <http://www.nih.gov/ninr/>.

National League of Nursing. 2003. Available from <http://www.nln.org>.

World Health Organization Collaborating Centres. 2003. Available from <http://whqlily.who.int/general_infos.asp>.

NURSING, THEORIES AND PHILOSOPHY OF

• • •

Any theory or philosophy of nursing involves a quest for nursing identity. The quest that began in the last quarter of the twentieth century has been fostered by several factors, including nursing education's move from the hospital to the academy, changes within nursing itself, and the feminist movement. Although there were nursing schools in a few universities before the 1950s, the movement to place nursing education and research in universities has accelerated since then. This move required nursing to establish its place in an academic setting. Usually nursing schools were placed in the natural or applied sciences, and consequently, nursing initially attempted to establish its identity as a science. The attempt to identify nursing with natural science led to scientific studies of nursing, but these studies, while important, did not show that nursing itself was a science. Recognition that nursing was a human practical activity led to the use of the behavioral sciences to give a scientific account of nursing. In both cases, nursing itself could, at best, be called an applied science. It was hoped that scientific studies of nursing would lead to a theory of nursing and that theory would prescribe nursing practice. But attempts to use theory to prescribe nursing practice were far removed from the way nursing was practiced.

Involvement in an academic setting eventually broadened the meaning of nursing beyond that of applied science. The applied approach had been fostered by nurses taking graduate degrees in other fields and applying their methods and concepts to nursing. The development of master's and doctoral degree programs in nursing fostered a movement away from this applied approach.

Graduate study in nursing developed as nursing became more complex and required nurses to make their own decisions concerning patient care. The development of intensive care units in hospitals initiated the expansion of specialization and technical knowledge into nursing care. As this trend grew, care for patients increasingly required nurses to make decisions without specific directives from physicians. As nurses became more responsible for patient care, they began to question the traditional control of nursing care by physicians and hospital administrators. Critical examination of their dependence on others encouraged nurses to seek an independent identity for nursing.

The feminist movement enhanced the desire of nurses to be independent from control of physicians and hospital administrators. Feminist theorists pointed out that society, including healthcare institutions, undervalued care and nurturing and overvalued command, technology, and hierarchical structure. Feminists enhanced the determination of nurses to become self-directing professionals rather than workers who followed the directions of physicians and administrators.

The Primacy of Caring

As nurses articulated their own practice, they became aware that nursing was focused on care rather than on science or applied science. Beginning in 1978, a series of annual conferences turned to the task of interpreting the meaning of caring as it related to nursing. The significance of this approach to nursing is evident in the following comment by a nurse who attended one such conference: "This is the first time I have ever heard nurses talk about caring or care as related to nursing care. I had nothing like these concepts in my nursing program, and yet they make sense and seem so logical and essential to nursing. In our classes, we were taught about curing medical diseases, understanding medical diagnostic techniques, and everything but caring" (National Caring Conference, p. vi). Published regularly, the proceedings of these conferences constitute a developing interpretation of caring as the source of identity for nursing. Philosophical interpretation of caring has been fostered

by the International Association for Human Caring, initiated by Madeleine M. Leininger, and the Center for Human Caring at the University of Colorado, initiated by Jean Watson.

The Phenomenology of Nursing

In her phenomenological interpretation of nursing, Patricia E. Benner articulated the meaning of nursing by drawing exemplars of excellent nursing from concrete nursing practice. In sharp contrast to using theories to prescribe the meaning of nursing, Benner disclosed the meaning of nursing excellence through descriptions of care for patients/clients in specific situations. These exemplars of excellence were interpreted to clarify and enhance the meaning evident in nursing practice. From the study of these exemplars, she identified seven domains of nursing practice with thirty-one distinct nursing competencies. For example, one of the domains is the helping role, and two of the competencies of the helping role are: (1) providing comfort measures and preserving personhood in the face of pain and extreme breakdown; and (2) maximizing the patient's participation and control in his or her own recovery (Benner). Rather than following the tradition in nursing of using definitions of good nursing to prescribe practice, Benner conveyed the meaning of excellence through the work of excellent practitioners. Her study showed that knowledge of excellence gained from practice is essential to any adequate definition of nursing. Benner's work illustrated the use of hermeneutic phenomenological methodology in nursing in that she disclosed the meaning of nursing excellence through exemplars in actual practice and interpreted their significance for the identity of nursing.

Nursing is the practice of caring, according to Anne H. Bishop, a nurse, and John R. Scudder Jr., a philosopher. Like Benner, Bishop and Scudder employed hermeneutic phenomenology to articulate the meaning of nursing (Bishop and Scudder, 1990, 1991). Nursing is a practice in that it is a traditional way of caring for patients that fosters the patient's well-being. The moral sense of nursing inherent in the caring relationship between nurse and patient is disclosed by phenomenological interpretation.

Confused thought has been fostered in nursing by the tendency to use the term *nursing* to mean both care for patients and the study of that care. Bishop and Scudder called the study of nursing the "discipline" of nursing to distinguish it from the practice. They maintained that the discipline of nursing should be a human science because it studies how nurses care for patients. Furthermore, it is a practical human science because the discipline attempts to improve nursing practice as well as to study it. Practices, such as nursing, are expanded and enhanced by the realization of possibilities that are inherent in the practice.

Bishop and Scudder affirmed the tendency to find the identity of nursing in caring. Although they articulated the meaning of care primarily from nursing practice, they found the interpretations of care by feminists Carol Gilligan and Nel Noddings particularly helpful in their articulation. Gilligan's "web of connection" forms a context for an interpretation of nursing as the bringing together of patient, nurse, physician, hospital administration, and family into "wholistic care" (Bishop and Scudder, 2001). Noddings's interpretation of care as engrossment in the situation of the other and shift of concern to the well-being of the other enhances Bishop and Scudder's interpretation of nursing care as fulfillment of the moral sense of fostering the well-being of patients. Bishop and Scudder also argued that the integral relationship between the moral sense and nursing practice is clearly evident in Benner's description of nursing excellence (1984). Nursing practice, as they interpret it, consists of two fundamental stances: first, wholistic care that focuses on cooperative care, articulated by Bishop and Scudder; second, the stance of recognized nursing competence in which nurses are free to direct care, described by Benner. Nursing's purpose, however, is not to become autonomous, as is often stressed by nursing reformers, but instead to foster the patient's well-being. Because nursing has this fundamental moral sense, the primary purpose of ethical considerations of nursing should be to foster excellent care—a care that promotes wellness while respecting the dignity and rights of each person.

Unlike Benner and Bishop and Scudder, who seek the identity of nursing in nursing practice, Sally Gadow (1980) attempted to give nursing a new identity with her interpretation of nursing as "existential advocacy." She drew her conception of existential advocacy from the stress on authenticity that is central to existential phenomenology. "Being authentic," in existentialist phenomenology, entails choosing oneself. Because the primary meaning of being human, for the existentialist, is self-direction, it follows that nurses should become existential advocates who foster authentic human being for those facing illness, treatment, and possible death. The nurse becomes an existential advocate by "participating with the patient in determining the personal meaning which the experience of illness, suffering, or dying is to have for that individual" (Gadow, p. 97).

Nursing Ethics

Pursuit of nursing ethics began in earnest in 1979 when a series of meetings in New York and New England brought together philosophers and nurses to begin development of a specific nursing ethic. Since then, many books and articles on nursing ethics have applied philosophical understanding to the moral dilemmas faced by nurses. Most nursing ethicists have applied philosophical inquiry and/or systems to moral problems that nurses encounter, especially those originating in advances in medical science. A different approach to nursing ethics begins not with philosophical ethics but with the moral imperative inherent in nursing practice. When the moral sense of nursing is given its due, according to Benner (1984) and Bishop and Scudder (1990, 1991), the primary concern of nursing ethics becomes fulfillment of its moral sense. Hence, the primary thrust of nursing ethics becomes fulfilling the moral sense of nursing practice rather than resolving moral problems that, although arising out of practice, are treated as adjuncts to practice.

The philosophers who took part in the aforementioned conferences that brought nurses and philosophers together in search of a nursing ethic also asserted that "the long-standing concern of philosophy to assist in the process of emancipation" should be brought to bear on the "long subjugation of the nurse" by helping nursing move "away from its position of political and intellectual subordination" (Spicker and Gadow, p. xiv). Nurses, who had long been impatient with being under the control of physicians and hospital administrators, were seeking greater individual and professional autonomy. The demand for greater autonomy was supported by feminist philosophy and by critical theory. Critical theory was used to disclose the hidden power structures in healthcare that denied nurses self-direction (Allen; Thompson).

Nurses also became interested in philosophy from their attempt to challenge the dominant scientific methodology and criteria for knowledge that prevailed when nursing first entered the academy. Recognition that nursing was primarily a human activity concerned with caring relationships between nurse and patient led nursing scholars to become involved in qualitative research and to use the methodology of the human sciences. A significant number of nurses became regular participants in the Society for Phenomenology and Human Sciences and the International Human Science Research Conference. Nursing scholars who found the stress on empirical rational science too restrictive welcomed Barbara Carper's expanded conception of knowledge. She contended that nursing knowledge should include not only scientific empirical knowledge but also three other ways of knowing in nursing—knowledge of how to make morally right choices, knowledge gained from personal experience, and knowledge of how to practice the art of nursing. Carper's patterns of knowing generated much interest among nurses who had long recognized that scientific knowledge alone was not adequate for nursing practice.

Attempts to Develop an Explicit Philosophy of Nursing

Initial interest in investigating nursing philosophically came from the quest for an independent identity for nursing and from encountering issues concerning ethics, knowledge, and justice within nursing itself. These first attempts could be called philosophical interpretations of nursing. An early attempt to foster the development of the philosophy of nursing was the establishment of the Institute for Philosophical Nursing Research at the University of Alberta, Canada. The institute invites nursing scholars with philosophical interests and talents to biannual conferences to discuss issues involved in developing a philosophy of nursing. The institute, through its conferences and publications, seeks to "establish common ground in nursing philosophy, accommodate diversity of thought in nursing philosophy, and articulate a sound philosophy of nursing" (Kikuchi and Simmons, p. 4).

Starting in the late 1990s and continuing into the early 2000s, the pace at which the philosophy of nursing was developing quickened. There is now a journal, *Nursing Philosophy*, that is broadening the philosophy of nursing beyond its former stress on hermeneutic and existential phenomenology to include the analytic, pragmatic, and postmodern traditions. The International Philosophy of Nursing Conference has met several times in Great Britain and Ireland, providing a forum for philosophical consideration. Discussion of the philosophy of nursing is being fostered on an Internet service called Nurse-Philosophy, which was initiated by Scottish scholars who also conduct a series of seminars on the same subject. An entire issue of *Scholarly Inquiry for Nursing Practice: An International Journal* has been devoted to the philosophy of nursing. Jan Reed and Ian Ground wrote an introduction to analytic philosophy, specifically for nurses, that uses nursing examples and considers nursing issues. New philosophies of nursing have expanded philosophical interpretations of nursing to include process and analytic philosophy. Janice M. Brencick and Glenn A. Webster, interpreting nursing from a process perspective, applied philosophical considerations of the universal and particular to nursing practice in their 2000 book, *Philosophy of Nursing*. Unfortunately, they disregarded previous studies of the philosophy of nursing with the exception of the work of Jean Watson. In contrast, Steven D. Edwards, in his 2001 book of the same name, developed an analytic philosophy of nursing in interaction with most of the extant works on the philosophy of nursing and developed a unified philosophy of nursing, thinking as an insider with degrees and standing in both nursing and philosophy.

Future Considerations

As the philosophy of nursing develops and matures, it may become a more integral part of the discipline of nursing. At present, however, many questions remain. Will the philosophy of nursing maintain its initial focus on the meaning of nursing, or will it refocus on philosophical issues and concerns? Will it bring nursing concerns into interaction with understandings, issues, and methods of philosophical traditions, or will it concentrate on philosophical issues and concerns that are to be applied to nursing? Furthermore, will philosophers of nursing become specialists who talk primarily to each other, or will the philosophy of nursing become an integral part of the development of a nursing discipline dedicated to the articulation and improvement of nursing practice?

JOHN R. SCUDDER, JR.
ANNE H. BISHOP (1995)
REVISED BY AUTHORS

SEE ALSO: *Autonomy; Beneficence; Care, Contemporary Ethics of; Compassionate Love; Feminism; Medical Codes and Oaths; Narrative; Nursing Ethics; Nursing, Profession of; Palliative Care and Hospice; Professional-Patient Relationship: Ethical Issues; Profession and Professional Ethics; Teams, Healthcare; Trust; Women as Health Professionals*

BIBLIOGRAPHY

Allen, David G. 1987. "The Social Policy Statement: A Reappraisal." *Advances in Nursing Science* 10(1): 39–48.

Benner, Patricia E. 1984. *From Novice to Expert: Excellence and Power in Clinical Nursing Practice.* Menlo Park, CA: Addison-Wesley.

Benner, Patricia E., and Wrubel, Judith. 1989. *The Primacy of Caring: Stress and Coping in Health and Illness.* Menlo Park, CA: Addison-Wesley.

Bishop, Anne H., and Scudder, John R., Jr. 1990. *The Practical, Moral, and Personal Sense of Nursing: A Phenomenological Philosophy of Practice.* Albany: State University of New York Press.

Bishop, Anne H., and Scudder, John R., Jr. 1991. *Nursing: The Practice of Caring.* New York: National League for Nursing.

Bishop, Anne H., and Scudder, John R., Jr. 2001. *Nursing Ethics: Holistic Caring Practice,* 2nd edition. Boston: Jones and Bartlett.

Brencick, Janice M., and Webster, Glenn A. 2000. *Philosophy of Nursing: A New Vision for Health Care.* Albany: State University of New York Press.

Carper, Barbara. 1978. "Fundamental Patterns of Knowing in Nursing." *Advances in Nursing Science* 1(1): 13–23.

Edwards, Steven D. 2001. *Philosophy of Nursing: An Introduction.* Basingstoke, UK: Palgrave Macmillan.

Fry, Sara T. 1989. "Toward a Theory of Nursing Ethics." *Advances in Nursing Science* 11(4): 9–22.

Gadow, Sally. 1980. "Existential Advocacy: Philosophical Foundation of Nursing." In *Nursing: Images and Ideals: Opening Dialogue with the Humanities,* ed. Stuart F. Spicker and Sally Gadow. New York: Springer.

Gilligan, Carol. 1982. *In a Different Voice: Psychological Theory and Women's Development.* Cambridge, MA: Harvard University Press.

Kikuchi, June F., and Simmons, Helen, eds. 1994. *Developing a Philosophy of Nursing.* Thousand Oaks, CA: Sage.

National Caring Conference. 1981. *Caring: An Essential Human Need: Proceedings of Three National Caring Conferences,* ed. Madeleine M. Leininger. Thorofare, NJ: Charles B. Slack.

Noddings, Nel. 1984. *Caring: A Feminine Approach to Ethics and Moral Education.* Berkeley: University of California Press.

Reed, Jan, and Ground, Ian. 1997. *Philosophy for Nursing.* London: Arnold.

Scholarly Inquiry for Nursing Practice: An International Journal. 1999. 13(1).

Spicker, Stuart F., and Gadow, Sally, eds. 1980. *Nursing: Images and Ideals: Opening Dialogue with the Humanities.* New York: Springer.

Thompson, Janice L. 1987. "Critical Scholarship: The Critique of Domination in Nursing." *Advances in Nursing Science* 10(1): 27–38.

Watson, Jean. 1985. *Nursing: Human Science and Human Care: A Theory of Nursing.* Norwalk, CT: Appleton-Century-Crofts.

INTERNET RESOURCE

"Nurse-Philosophy Listserv." JISCmail. 2003. Available from <http://www.jiscmail.ac.uk/lists/nurse-philosophy.html>.

O

OBLIGATION AND SUPEREROGATION

• • •

Much human behavior in the biomedical sphere is governed by moral principles. Due to their particular importance, medical relationships, in the wide sense of the term, have always been considered to be subject to evaluation in terms of justice, duty, obligation, and rights. Thus, the allocation of medical resources is weighed in terms of justice and fairness; the physician's professional role and powerful status define his or her professional duties; the contractual agreement and the special trust of patients places the doctor under a wide variety of obligations toward them; and the particularly urgent needs and interests of human beings (fetuses, handicapped persons, people in coma, and all sickly people included) grant them the right to be medically treated and respected. The regulation of medical practice under these terms of rights and duties has been acknowledged throughout history and formulated in a series of doctors' oaths. More recently there has been a growing trend to safeguard morally required behavior in medical practice under legal rules, on the one hand, and political (state) control, on the other. This institutionalization of medical relations has led to the effective enforcement of the moral rights and duties of patients and physicians, but also to the depersonalization, even dehumanization, of these relations.

Some forms of heroic sacrifice, volunteering, and beneficence have been traditionally treated as situated beyond the call of duty. This article seeks to establish the important (though limited) role of such behavior in the medical domain, especially against the background of the growing legislation, politicization, and commercialization of medical

life. Eager to safeguard universal compliance, impartial distribution, and equal treatment, medical ethicists have tended to ignore the unique virtues of the morality of supererogation as a complement to the morality of duty.

The Theological Sources of Supererogation

The term *supererogation* derives from the Latin verb meaning "to pay out more than is required." The first source for its use as an ethical concept goes back to the Latin version of the New Testament. In the famous parable, the Good Samaritan offers money to an innkeeper to care for a wounded man found on the road, and promises to repay the innkeeper "over and above" for any extra expenses (Luke 10:35). Consequently, Good Samaritanism has been closely associated with supererogatory behavior.

Yet the parable of the Good Samaritan does not distinguish explicitly between the obligatory and the supererogatory, but rather between the merely legally binding (to which the priest and the Levite in the biblical story seem to be exclusively committed) and moral or truly virtuous behavior (manifest in the deeds of the Good Samaritan). The explicit distinction between two types of moral norms, the commanded and the recommended, is better formulated in the contrast between keeping one's lawful riches and leading a life of total poverty (Matthew 19:16–24), or between lawful marriage and self-imposed chastity (1 Corinthians 7:25–28), or between ordinary religious faith and total commitment to a religious way of life.

Perpetual poverty, perfect chastity, and perfect obedience thus became the paradigm cases of evangelical counsels (*consilia*), which, in contrast with the religious commandments (*praecepta*), were considered by the church fathers and medieval theologians (from Augustine to Thomas Aquinas) to be truly meritorious. Other acts, by which one could freely choose to go beyond the religious precepts, included penance, patience, fasting, and martyrdom, as well as mercy (as opposed to justice) and beneficence (as in the bestowal of gifts). Living by the commandments guaranteed salvation, but following the counsels exemplified perfection.

Both the ideal of monastic life and the institution of sainthood were based on the gradually evolving two-level morality of duty and supererogation. Accordingly, two separate systems of norms applied to two categories of believers, ordinary people and those who had a special vocation or a particular moral capacity. In a later stage in the development of the idea of supererogation, it was claimed that the superabundant merit of the acts of those who belonged to the second category of believers (Jesus and the saints) was bequeathed to the spiritual treasury of the church, and could be dispensed by the pope to help sinners achieve salvation. Thus, the two systems of religious morality were linked by a mystical principle of transference of merit, from those who have a surplus to those who are in debt. The system of indulgences was based on the idea that the supererogatory merit of saintly people could compensate for the sins of ordinary folk. But the papal distribution of indulgences, gradually commercialized in the late Middle Ages, became one of the central targets of the reformers' attacks on the Roman Catholic Church.

Martin Luther, John Calvin, and the Anglican Church questioned the theological foundations of the very idea of supererogation. If mortal human beings could not hope ever to carry out the religious precepts or commandments, how could they hope to do more than was required of them? The reformers' belief that salvation could be achieved only through God's grace, rather than through "good works," made the idea of supererogation absurd and blasphemous, a "superabomination." The denial of a two-tier religious morality directly challenged the ideas of sainthood, monasticism, and indulgences. The metaphysical rejection of freedom of the will undermined the Catholic idea of *licentia*, that playroom for the virtuous exercise of free choice to do more than is required, which served as the condition and moral justification of supererogation conduct. The theological debate over the concept of supererogation not only is the historical source for the parallel philosophical discussion in secular ethics, but also may serve as the model for this discussion. For despite the obvious differences between the two arenas (particularly on the objects of supererogatory acts, God and human beings, respectively), they share the basic features of the issue: the relation between goodness and duty, the limits of duty, the nature of free will, the place of virtue and perfection in a deontological theory, and the question of whether there are two categories of moral agents who are subject to moral requirements of different scope and stringency.

Supererogation in Ethical Theory

The subject of supererogation, rather surprisingly, did not receive much philosophical attention in ethical theory until the 1950s. In his pioneering article, James Urmson challenges the traditional tripartite classification of moral actions into the permissible (what one may do), the obligatory (what one ought to do), and the forbidden (what one ought not to do). Saintly and heroic acts are adduced as typical examples of actions that do not fall into any of these categories but still have a distinct moral value. However, breaking the neat framework of the threefold division of moral action turns out to be a controversial enterprise. For example, it has to overcome the resistance of logicians, who try to draw a systematic analogy between the permissible and the possible, the forbidden and the impossible, and the obligatory and the necessary, thus creating a unified system of logic. If an act is morally good, how can it not be obligatory? And if there are good reasons for leaving it *non*obligatory, cannot supererogation be analyzed in terms of the permissible? And finally, should supererogatory behavior not be considered forbidden, as a dangerous illusion of conceited and morally self-indulgent agents, who violate self-regarding duties and the principles of impartiality and fairness?

There are three kinds of answers to these questions regarding the seemingly paradoxical nature of supererogation: anti-supererogationism, qualified supererogationism, and unqualified supererogationism. Anti-supererogationism denies the existence of actions that go beyond the call of duty. Pure deontological theory, such as Kant's doctrine of the categorical imperative, is a typical example of this view. Obligatoriness (moral necessity) exhausts the moral sphere; duty is the only legitimate motive in morality; and universalizability is the ultimate test for the morality of actions. Hence there is no room for the nonobligatory, charity-based personal action that is typical of supererogation. Acts of beneficence or heroic self-sacrifice are either "imperfect duties" (which for Kant are no less binding than their "perfect" counterparts) or cases of moral fanaticism motivated by self-love.

Some forms of utilitarianism are no less anti-supererogationist. Thus, for the eighteenth-century utilitarian William Godwin, promoting the overall good (including the agent's) is the absolute and only moral duty. This view leaves no room for supererogatory action (e.g., doing a favor), since either its beneficiary has a "complete right" over it or it is wrong ("unjust") to do it because of other people's rights (including the agent's). The derivation of "ought" statements from statements about the good (utility, happiness) leads George Edward Moore, too, to a straightforward denial of supererogation.

Modern utilitarian theorists point to the logical difficulty in distinguishing between utility-promoting actions that are obligatory and utility-promoting actions that are not obligatory, since such a distinction requires an appeal to a nonutilitarian principle. The common ground on which deontological and consequentialist anti-supererogationists rest their case seems to be the purely impersonal conception of morality, a conception typically expressed by the universalization principle or the classical utility principle of an agent-independent promotion of overall goodness "in the world." Impersonalism of this kind leaves no room for altruism, personal sacrifice, or the expression of individual preference.

Qualified supererogationism tries to do more justice to our common belief in the value of supererogatory conduct. It concedes that in some abstract or ideal sense every good action is obligatory, but highlights the circumstances that make such a morality too demanding, even absurd. Some utilitarians, like John Stuart Mill, distinguish between the prevention of harm (which is obligatory) and the altruistic promotion of the good (which deserves gratitude, honor, and moral praise). Henry Sidgwick is willing to distinguish between what a person ought to do and what people are justified in blaming him or her for not doing. Thomas Aquinas states that while the commandments apply to everyone, the counsels are directed only to the few who are capable of following them or who have made the life of perfection their special vocation. Rule utilitarians, as well as contract theorists like David Richards, point to the possible decrease in overall happiness through the adoption of a general rule enforcing supererogatory action as a duty, and at the same time to the general social benefit derived from leaving it to individual discretion. Even Kant, in his later ethical writings, acknowledges the existence of "duties of virtue" that "others cannot compel us (by natural means) to fulfill," as they are concerned with the adoption of ends, are binding only in the "internal" sense, and create no corresponding rights in the recipient. Finally, John Rawls and Joseph Raz analyze supererogation in terms of exemption: the exemption that "natural duty" allows in cases of high risk or loss to the agent (Rawls), or that granted by the second-order "exclusionary permission" not to act on the best balance of first-order reasons (Raz).

Qualified supererogationism is reductive in nature: it insists on accommodating supererogatory acts within a deontic framework (i.e., the language of duties and obligations). Every moral action is in principle required, though considerations of exemption, risk, disutility of enforcement, personal (in)capacity, excuses, difficult psychological circumstances, and rights define a supererogatory subcategory. Unqualified supererogationism, on the other hand, insists on placing the supererogatory "beyond duty" in the absolute, nonreductive sense (Urmson; Feinberg; Heyd). Supererogatory behavior is fully optional, that is, it lies beyond any kind of duty, under any condition, and for any moral subject. No excuse is needed for not acting heroically.

Definition and Justification of Supererogation

Most definitions of supererogation display the same general form, pointing to the asymmetry of commission and omission of actions. Thus supererogatory acts are said to be those acts that are good to do but not bad not to do, or right (just, virtuous, praiseworthy) to do but not wrong (unjust, vicious, blameworthy) to refrain from doing. These definitions, however, fail to capture either the special merit of supererogatory acts or their particular optional character. More sophisticated attempts retain the asymmetry but mix the contrasted pairs (e.g., "non-obligatory well doings," according to Roderick Chisholm, or "meritorious non-duties," according to Joel Feinberg). Still, the definition of supererogation, at least of the unqualified version, must refer explicitly to the normative status of the acts in question, to their particular value, and to the person-relative features of these acts (the agent as well as the recipient).

A possible definition contains the following four conditions for an act to be supererogatory:

1. It is neither obligatory nor forbidden.
2. Its omission is not wrong and does not deserve sanction or criticism, either formal or informal.
3. It is morally good, both by virtue of its intended consequences and by virtue of its intrinsic value (being beyond duty).
4. It is done voluntarily for the sake of someone else's good, and is thus meritorious.

The first condition characterizes supererogatory acts in negative terms (being nonobligatory), but the second emphasizes their purely optional nature. This distinction between the permissible and the optional points to the specific double value of the latter as opposed to the moral neutrality of the former: it is not only the good effect of supererogatory action that makes it praiseworthy; it is its motive, which is completely "free," that is, not even an "ought." This combination of desirable consequences and virtuous motive is the source of the moral merit ascribed to the agent of supererogatory acts.

It should be noted that the goodness of supererogation lies in its leading to consequences that are of moral value, that is, of the same type or on the same scale as those of obligatory action. This is clearly manifest in supererogatory transcendence of duty, such as "going the second mile" or doing more than one's job requires. In that respect, supererogation is continuous with the morality of duty. But the fact that the source of the value of a supererogatory act lies no less in the voluntariness of its motive points to its conceptual dependence on the idea of duty, that is, its being correlative to duty. It should be noted that there are ethical theories that are not based on the concept of duty at all (but rather on the idea of virtue, as in Aristotle). Such theories do not leave room for supererogation as it is defined here.

The general justification of supererogation is twofold: on the one (negative) hand, it has to do with the basic autonomy of individuals to lead their lives in ways not always subordinated to moral principles such as the overall good. On the other (positive) hand, it is associated with the supplementation of the impersonal and universal core of ethical theory with a personal dimension. This is expressed both by the agent's discretion and by the choice of the particular recipient of the beneficent act. Supererogation in that respect is highly important for social cohesion, trust, and friendship in society—values that cannot be fully achieved even in an ideally just society in which every person performs his or her duties and obligations. This justification for unqualified supererogationism is reminiscent of the debate about the legal enforcement of morality: In the same way that there are moral reasons for leaving some moral duties beyond the reach of the law, so there are moral reasons for leaving some morally good acts out of the system of moral duties and obligations. The Good Samaritan first took care of the wounded man (which was not his legal duty but certainly his moral duty); then he offered to pay the innkeeper "over and above," that is, for the expenses involved in housing and feeding the man (which was not even his moral duty).

Typical examples of supererogatory acts are saintly and heroic acts, which involve great sacrifice and risk for the agent and a great benefit to the recipient. However, more ordinary acts of charity, beneficence, and generosity are equally supererogatory. Small favors are a limiting case, because of their minor consequential value. Volunteering is an interesting case of supererogation, because it refers to the procedure by which the agent of an obligatory act is selected. That is to say, someone ought to do the act, but due to its particular difficulty or risk, it is hard to decide who. Finally, there are supererogatory forbearances, in which the agent refrains from taking a morally justified action that would have a negative impact on another. Forgiveness, pardon, and mercy are typical examples: we would have been justified in punishing a criminal, but we decided to exercise mercy or pardon.

Supererogation in Medical Ethics

The place of supererogation in medical ethics has been almost completely ignored, both in the theoretical discussions of supererogation and in the vast literature on medical ethics. This might be explained by the fact that both fields are relatively new, and by the tendency to bind the vital aspects of medical practice and relationship in a firm system of well-defined rights, duties, and obligations. The issues of confidentiality, informed consent, abortion, euthanasia, and allocation of scarce resources revolve around the debate on the rights of patients and the duties of doctors, the principles of justice, or the responsibilities of state and society to their members. However, there are some areas of medical practice in which supererogation has a central role to play, cases that could also help in understanding and justifying the theoretical distinction between obligation and supererogation: the collection and allocation of blood, organ donation, surrogate motherhood, and medical experimentation.

Anti-supererogationists would tend to deny that some medical matters lie beyond the sphere of moral duty and social justice. In their attempt to reduce allegedly supererogatory conduct to one of three categories—the obligatory, the permissible, and the forbidden—they may, for instance, claim that blood donation is a moral duty, that surrogacy arrangements should be completely forbidden, or that participation in medical experiments should be left to the morally neutral (permissible) regulation of the free market. Grounding vital medical relationships in supererogatory altruistic motives offends our moral sense of equality, both in the access to treatment and in the undertaking of risks. Legislation and the market are two powerful alternatives that safeguard impartiality and personal neutrality, which are principal values in the ethics of duty and justice.

Qualified supererogationists would admit that ideally all medical practice should be subjected to universal deontic principles, especially since it deals with matters of life and death in which we want people to have equal chances, rights, and duties. But they point to the limit of what can be expected of individuals by way of giving and taking risks, particularly when the sacrifices required are of the same kind as the health needs of others that create the call for sacrifice. Therefore, when the health of a sick person requires an organ donation that would expose the donor to serious health hazards, one must leave the decision to the personal discretion of the donor. Institutional control or regulation under impersonal rules (such as legislation) is immoral, either because most people cannot make the required sacrifice ("ought" implies "can"), or because it could be counterproductive in utilitarian terms (the sacrifice of the donor being greater than the potential benefit to the recipient). Furthermore, the market mechanism, which is so efficient in much of our economic life, may lead to the exploitation of the poor by the rich or to other morally repugnant consequences related to the commercialization of human life and health.

The unqualified supererogationist shares many of these apprehensions but adds a positive justification for a "moral free zone" in medical life. Beyond the realm of relations of duties and rights, there is in medical practice some room for a totally free exercise of giving. It is a reflection of personal autonomy; it is grounded in a personal interest in another individual, and it creates personal relations; it strengthens social ties and cohesion. Blood donation is a typical example. Collection of blood for medical use in modern society can be based on a free-market system in which blood is freely bought and sold, or on a legally enforced system of duties (e.g., of young people to donate blood once a year), or on a fully voluntary system, as in Great Britain, in which people volunteer to give blood and patients get it free. Economists like Kenneth Arrow favor "the economy of charity," and believe that the market can better handle the needed balance of supply and demand of blood. Furthermore, they claim that altruism is itself a scarce resource, and therefore should be used only when necessary. Richard Titmuss and Peter Singer, on the other hand, argue that the commercialization of blood donation is potentially destructive to society, especially because it concerns a "commodity" that has no price, that is, it is extremely valuable to the recipient and of almost no value to the donor. They add that altruism is not a scarce resource but, rather, a good that grows the more it is exercised. The supererogatory model is thus considered as superior both to the market mechanism and to the political (legal) arrangement of collection and allocation.

The donation of organs (like kidneys) is different in that it is much more costly to the donor than the donation of blood (particularly in the case of living donors). It is also more personal than the anonymous donation of a blood bank, as it usually involves someone personally close to the donor. Unlike blood donation (which may be considered morally obligatory though not legally enforceable), giving away a nonrenewable part of one's body is typically supererogatory, in the "saintly and heroic" sense. Ideals of personal responsibility, family ties, friendship, and particular emotional commitments make personal sacrifices like organ donation valuable beyond their sheer utility (which sometimes is tragically doubtful).

Surrogate motherhood can also be regulated by market mechanisms or left to voluntary, altruistic agreements. Beyond the controversial aspects of surrogacy (having to do with the interests of a third party, the child, and with the possibility of a change of mind by the surrogate mother), we may note that most legal systems prefer to leave it as a supererogatory matter. Thus, agreements on surrogacy are not considered criminal (forbidden) in many countries but are not enforced by the courts (in contrast with ordinary contracts). Commercialization is often treated as undesirable, even patently immoral and illegal.

Finally, medical experimentation on human subjects in most countries is now allowed only on the basis of volunteering. No person, sick or healthy, is required (legally or even morally) to take part in any experiment. On the other hand, participating in the enterprise of medical research and progress is definitely of great moral value. By altruistically giving our share to medical research, we express our gratitude to those in the past who made us beneficiaries of medical progress (Jonas). The supererogatory nature of participation in medical experimentation is typically connected to the case of volunteering, in which it is a moral "ought" that someone (in a group) do the job but no particular individual can be identified as having to do it. As opposed to any selection procedure based on substantive criteria (like merit), or formal criteria (like random devices, which are particularly attractive as a fair means of imposing burdens in risky situations), volunteering is completely supererogatory.

We may conclude, then, by pointing to the special status of supererogation in some aspects of medical ethics as combining the advantages of both morality and the market, as well as avoiding some of the dangers of both. A supererogatory system of blood collection is on the one hand of moral worth (no less, and even more, than its alternative regulation according to principles of duty fairness in a politically centralized system of collection and allocation), yet fully optional (as in the case of buying and selling in the market). On the other hand, it avoids the danger of exploitation, typical of the market mechanism, as well as the danger of compulsion, typical of often-abused political power or of social pressure. Supererogation can partly counter the undesirable trends of both commercialization and politicization of modern medical life by leaving an outlet for the autonomous and spontaneous exercise of supererogatory beneficence.

DAVID HEYD (1995)
BIBLIOGRAPHY REVISED

SEE ALSO: *Beneficence; Care; Compassionate Love; Epidemics; Ethics: Normative Ethical Theories; Family and Family*

Medicine; Long-Term Care: Home Care; Maternal-Fetal Relationship; Medicine, Profession of; Nursing Ethics; Organ and Tissue Procurement; Professional-Patient Relationship

BIBLIOGRAPHY

Aquinas, Thomas. *Summa theologica,* esp. I, q. 21; I, II, q. 108; II, II, q. 31, q. 32, q. 106, q. 184; and suppl., q. 25.

Arrow, Kenneth J. 1972. "Gifts and Exchanges." *Philosophy and Public Affairs* 1(4): 343–362.

Chisholm, Roderick M. 1963. "Supererogation and Offence: A Conceptual Scheme for Ethics." *Ratio* 5 (1): 1–14.

Feinberg, Joel. 1968. "Supererogation and Rules." In *Ethics,* pp. 391–411, comp. Judith J. Thomson and Gerald Dworkin. New York: Harper & Row.

Fishkin, James S. 1999. *The Limits of Obligation.* New Haven, CT: Yale University Press.

Godwin, William. 1971 (1793). *Enquiry concerning Political Justice.* 3rd edition. Oxford: Clarendon Press.

Heyd, David. 1982. *Supererogation: Its Status in Ethical Theory.* Cambridge, Eng.: Cambridge University Press.

Jonas, Hans. 1969. "Philosophical Reflections on Experimenting with Human Subjects." *Daedalus* 98, pp. 219–247.

Kamm, Frances Myrna. 1985. "Supererogation and Obligation." *Journal of Philosophy* 82: 118–138.

Kant, Immanuel. 1948 (1785). *The Moral Law; or, Kant's Groundwork of the Metaphysic of Morals,* ed. and tr. John Paton. London: Hutchinson.

Kant, Immanuel. 1964 (1797). *The Metaphysic of Morals,* Part II, tr. Mary Gregor. New York: Cambridge University Press.

McKay, A. C. 2002. "Supererogation and the Profession of Medicine." *Journal of Medical Ethics* 28(2): 70–73.

McNamara, Paul. 1996. "Making Room for Going beyond the Call." *Mind* 105(419): 415–450.

Mellema, Gregory. 1991. *Beyond the Call of Duty: Supererogation, Obligation, and Offence (SUNY Series in Ethical Theory).* Albany: State University of New York Press.

Mill, John Stuart. 1969 (1865). "Auguste Comte and Positivism." In *The Collected Works of J. S. Mill,* vol. 10, pp. 261–368. Toronto: University of Toronto Press.

New, Christopher. 1974. "Saints, Heroes and Utilitarians." *Philosophy* 49: 179–189.

Prichard, Harold A. 1990. *Moral Obligation, Duty & Interest.* New York: Oxford University Press.

Rawls, John. 1971. *A Theory of Justice.* Cambridge, MA: Harvard University Press/Belknap Press.

Raz, Joseph. 1975. "Permissions and Supererogation." *American Philosophical Quarterly* 12(2): 161–168.

Richards, David A. J. 1971. *A Theory of Reasons for Action.* Oxford: Clarendon Press.

Schumaker, Millard. 1977. *Supererogation: An Analysis and Bibliography.* Edmonton, Alta.: St. Stephen's College.

Singer, Peter. 1972. "Famine, Affluence, and Morality." *Philosophy and Public Affairs* 1(3): 229–243.

Thomasma, David C., and Kushner, Thomasine. 1995. "A Dialogue on Compassion and Supererogation in Medicine." *Cambridge Quarterly of Healthcare Ethics* 4(4): 415–425.

Titmuss, Richard M. 1973. *The Gift Relationship: From Human Blood to Social Policy.* Harmondsworth, U.K.: Penguin.

Urmson, James O. 1958. "Saints and Heroes." In *Essays in Moral Philosophy,* pp. 198–216, ed. Abraham I. Melden. Seattle: University of Washington Press.

Wellman, Carl, ed. 2002. *Rights and Duties: Six Volume Set (Ethical Investigations).* London: Routledge.

Wolfe, Alan. 1991. *Whose Keeper?: Social Science and Moral Obligation.* Berkeley: University of California Press.

OCCUPATIONAL SAFETY AND HEALTH

• • •

I. Ethical Issues

II. Occupational Healthcare Providers

I. ETHICAL ISSUES

The workplace setting presents unique problems for public health because, on the one hand, virtually all its hazards are environmental and can be prevented or controlled, while, on the other hand, it is a setting for social conflict with large economic stakes. Occupational injury and disease are economic phenomena resulting from social decisions about technology and the use of labor in the production of goods and services. The rights of property owners, even in state socialist systems; the economic obligations of managers to owners of enterprises; and the imbalance of power between labor and management present particular problems for occupational health. The position of health and safety professionals in industry is frequently problematic because of tensions between their responsibilities to employers and the ethical codes of their professions. The imperatives of production and profit frequently override other responsibilities for the health and welfare of employees.

Industrial hygiene is the principal profession applying scientific and engineering methods to the protection of workers from toxic chemicals, dust, other air contaminants, and job hazards. The basic industrial-hygiene approach to the work environment places engineering controls at the top of a hierarchy of methods for workers' health protection. This approach is enshrined in the ethical codes of the profession. A typical listing of industrial-hygiene approaches places substitution, process change, and isolation or enclosure at the top of the list. Methods that rely on personal protective equipment are considered less effective and are to be resorted to only when engineering controls are not feasible. The professional emphasis is on management's responsibility to provide a safe work environment rather than on workers' self-protection or adaptation to hazardous conditions.

Equity, or fairness in the distribution of society's material benefits, is not a primary concern in the economic theory or operation of the modern market. Public policy is predicated on the assumption that market mechanisms promote and reward efficiency. Policymakers presume that tax and/or subsidy policy will be used to cushion the effects on individuals or groups damaged in socially unacceptable ways, such as utter impoverishment. The market model minimizes the costs of factors of production, including labor, through entrepreneurial pursuit of profit. The role of government is restricted severely. Since consumer choice rules in the model, firms are guided in the production of goods and services by the willingness of consumers to pay, and resources are directed to consumers' financially expressed desires. Selfish motives are presumed of everybody, yet the model claims efficient results.

Even the strongest advocate of the market economy understands the limits of market efficiency. In the market model, collective consumption of goods and services, such as national defense, malaria control, road building, and the like, may be handled legitimately by the government. Further, where there are monopolistic imperfections in markets, where information is restricted or the mobility of labor and capital is impaired, the government may intervene. In addition, where costs or benefits are not internalized by the firm, air, water, wild animals, and the like are "free goods"; they cannot be considered in entrepreneurial calculations and "inefficient" solutions may result. For instance, a firm may use a process hazardous to human health if it will not bear the cost of worker illness that occurs years later. The existence of externalities is an argument for government intervention to force private parties to internalize these costs.

On what grounds does the government intervene to protect workers' health? Some would argue that imperfect information, imbalances in bargaining power, and other deviations from the perfect market model require that the state intervene on behalf of workers' health and safety. Others would argue that even if markets were working perfectly, the society has an overriding interest in the health of its members, including workers, and that it has a longer time frame than any of the market participants is willing to consider. Thus, market failure to deliver socially desirable ends, because of either imperfections or externalities, justifies state intervention.

Historical Overview

Occupational health has rarely received much attention from the public. Historically, the commitment of the United States to economic advancement through technology has made its society myopic about its toll on workers' health. Through much of U.S. history, workers themselves have been too engaged in the pressing task of making a living for their families to pay much attention to widespread occupational safety and health problems. The labor movement has not been strong enough to force public attention to these issues on a continual basis.

In Europe, the tradition of occupational medicine is much greater. In the sixteenth century, the occupational health problems of miners and foundry and smelter workers were studied by Paracelsus. Bernardino Ramazzini (1633–1714) wrote a classic text on the occupational diseases of workers.

The industrial revolution brought a host of new health and safety problems to European workers. The social reform movements in England, for instance, sought protection for child labor and to restrict the working day to ten hours. Protective labor legislation was passed in 1833 (the Factory Act) and in 1842 (the Mines Act). Both occupational medicine and the trade union movement in Great Britain were launched in the nineteenth century as responses to awful conditions in many workplaces.

In the nineteenth century, the industrial revolution brought to the United States a host of safety problems and some public concern. Massachusetts created the first factory inspection department in 1867 and in subsequent years enacted the first job safety laws in the textile industry. The Knights of Labor, an early trade union, agitated for safety laws in the 1870s and 1880s, and by 1900 minimal legislation had been passed in the most heavily industrialized states.

After 1900, the rising tide of industrial accidents resulted in passage of workers' compensation laws; by 1920 virtually all states had adopted this no-fault insurance program. Previously, workers seeking financial compensation and medical care for industrial accidents had to sue their employers—and their employers had three extremely effective defenses. First, the courts accepted the notion that in a free market, workers assumed the responsibility for established occupational risks. Second, employers were absolved from responsibility for accidents to the extent that a worker's own actions contributed to the mishap. Third, in the eyes of the courts, employers were not financially responsible for injuries caused by fellow employees of the injured worker. In an economy of highly skilled artisans in which the labor process was controlled by the workers themselves, this defensive troika might have been reasonable; in an economy of mass production, high-speed assembly lines, and detailed division of labor, the illusion of worker autonomy fell of its own political weight. No-fault industrial accident insurance was the solution adopted by the states.

Throughout the 1920s, the rise of company paternalism was accompanied by the development of occupational medicine programs. Much attention was paid to preemployment physicals rather than industrial hygiene and accident prevention. Occasional scandals, like cancer in young painters of radium watch dials, reached the public attention, but until the resurgence of the labor movement in the 1930s, Congress did not pass important national legislation. The Walsh-Healey Public Contracts Act of 1936 required federal contractors to comply with health and safety standards, and the Social Security Act of 1935 provided funds for state industrial-hygiene programs. The Bureau of Mines was authorized to inspect mines.

After World War II, occupational health and safety again receded from public attention, as sympathy for the labor movement declined and the nation took a turn to the right. An exception to the general neglect of the field was passage of the Atomic Energy Act of 1954, which included provision for radiation safety standards. Not until the 1960s, when labor regained some political influence, did the issue reemerge. Injury rates rose 29 percent during the 1960s. A major mine disaster in 1968 at Farmington, West Virginia, in which seventy-eight miners were killed, captured public sympathy. In 1969, the Coal Mine Health and Safety Act was passed, and in 1970, the broader Occupational Safety and Health Act became law.

Regulatory Effects

A fundamental aspect of the new law was the unambiguous statement of employer responsibility for occupational health and safety. A new regulatory agency, the Occupational Safety and Health Administration (OSHA), was created in the U.S. Department of Labor. OSHA could require employers to provide safe and healthy workplaces and to promulgate and enforce safety standards. In addition, the OSHA Act established the National Institute for Occupational Safety and Health (NIOSH) as part of the U.S. Public Health Service, to do research and evaluate health hazards in the work environment.

Initially, OSHA adopted a host of so-called consensus standards. In addition to extending the Walsh-Healey regulations for government contractors to the rest of industry, the new agency adopted many of the voluntary guidelines developed by the American National Standards Institute and the American Conference of Government Industrial Hygienists. While this enabled OSHA to enter the field running, with standards to enforce, many of the guidelines were inappropriate as legal standards. Some were contradictory; others were overly detailed or anachronistic. For instance, OSHA adopted a requirement that toilet seats be split in the front, an idea that persisted from the day when people believed syphilis was caught from contaminated toilets. When Eula Bingham became head of OSHA in 1977, one of her earliest and most important tasks was standards simplification: throwing out inappropriate, ineffectual, or silly standards.

The process of developing new standards, however, was slow and cumbersome, involving substantial litigation before any new worker protection was extended. Perhaps the most tortuous path was that of the field sanitation standard for farm workers, which required that farmers provide clean water and toilet facilities for workers in the field. The standard took fourteen years to develop and ultimately was issued only because the courts required OSHA to do so. However, when OSHA, in a heroic effort to update its standards, adopted hundreds of new permissible exposure limits for air contaminants in the late 1980s, this wholesale revision was rejected by the federal courts as failing to meet the procedure required for standard development. In any case, since OSHA's inception, enforcement of standards has left much to be desired, largely because of understaffing.

While the OSHA Act covered most workers in the private sector, the Coal Mine Health and Safety Act established a special regulatory body to deal with the high-risk mining industry. Authority to regulate pesticide exposure of agricultural workers was assigned to the U.S. Environmental Protection Agency (EPA); OSHA bears responsibility for other aspects of farm employment, such as migrant-labor camp conditions and field sanitation.

The most important extensions of worker protection in recent years have been linked to growing public concern with general environmental issues. For instance, amendments to federal environmental laws in 1987 required both OSHA and the EPA to adopt safety and training requirements for a broad range of hazardous-waste workers and emergency personnel dealing with hazardous materials.

Federal government policy during the 1980s was characterized by a neoconservative, antiregulatory stance. Public-health advocates complained of the slow pace of OSHA standards promulgation, the federal ceding of enforcement authority to states, the failure to protect worker-complainants from employer discrimination, and the decimation of NIOSH's budget. The decline of the U.S. trade union movement has further weakened the political impetus for OSHA enforcement activity. In the early 1990s, efforts at legislative reform stressed streamlining OSHA procedures for developing standards and enhancing workers' right to act.

Perhaps the most pressing problems in occupational health arise from the increasing integration of the world economy. In North America, the development of a continental free-trade agreement may threaten the work environment standards of Canada and the United States while bringing a host of new hazards to Mexico. The export of hazardous technologies, products, and waste represents increasing challenges for public health worldwide. On the one hand, our understanding of the nature of health hazards to workers has been improving; on the other hand, the restructuring of the world economy may undercut the political will to control these hazards.

The Rights to Know, to Refuse, to Act

Until the 1980s, workers in the United States did not have a legal right to know the names of hazardous materials to which they were exposed. This seems odd, since even market economists argue that good information is necessary if markets are to reflect working conditions correctly. Nevertheless, it was not until 1980, in the final days of the Carter administration, that OSHA promulgated a "right to know" regulation. The Reagan administration withdrew the proposed rule in 1981, and a political fight for this right ensued on state and local levels. Time and again, coalitions of workers' organizations and community environmental groups won state and local laws mandating the right to know. Finally, OSHA came forth with the Hazard Communication Standard, which, although not as rigorous as some of the local ordinances, nevertheless extended a fundamental right to a wide range of workers across the country. This public-health regulation had to contend with competing property rights of corporations, such as the protection of trade secrets. Proposed legislation that would have required notification of workers discovered in NIOSH studies to be at high risk of occupational disease failed to pass Congress for such economic reasons. In addition, conservatives discovered that providing information involved economic costs to employers and sometimes to government. Companies argued that they should not be required to reveal essential substances or aspects of production processes because business competitors might obtain this information. OSHA was required to balance the protection of worker health with the protection of business's intellectual property rights.

Soon after the Hazard Communication Standard became law, labor advocates argued that the right to know was of little use as long as workers could not use such information to change hazardous working conditions. The OSHA Act made the violation of safety regulations an offense punishable by the government but gave workers only a very limited right to refuse hazardous work, and then only when there was objective evidence (not just fear) of imminent life-threatening danger. Moreover, the OSHA Act focused on the rights of individuals, not on collective worker action for health and safety. Health and safety advocates demanded an expanded right to refuse hazardous work, as well as the mandating of workplace health and safety committees with the right to act. Such committees, which already exist in countries other than the United States (Sweden, for instance), would mark a major departure in the regulatory approach in the United States. Worker empowerment is a substantially different approach from state regulation of the work environment.

Medical Monitoring, Reproductive Hazards, and Hazards to Minority Workers

Even though there is a long history of the use of preemployment examinations by occupational physicians in the United States, medical testing and monitoring remains a controversial area. Key ethical issues include confidentiality of medical records; inappropriate discrimination against minorities, women, and disabled or hypersusceptible employees; and "blaming the victim" vs. reducing exposures. Some OSHA standards require medical monitoring; perhaps one of the most distressing issues is the failure of OSHA and employers to analyze accumulated data systematically.

Because job segregation by gender continues to exist in the United States, women and men sometimes experience different health hazards. Perhaps the most controversial now concern reproduction. Some employers have sought to bar fertile women from jobs in which exposures to hazardous chemicals are within legal limits but may pose risks to a fetus. In some instances, where removal from such work involved serious income and/or opportunity loss, some women have agreed to sterilization in order to meet employer "fetal protection" requirements. Women's organizations and trade unions argue that such policies constitute unfair discrimination against women. The U.S. Supreme Court prohibited such policies in its decision in the case *Johnson Controls, Inc. v. UAW* in the spring of 1991 (110 S.Ct. 1522, 111 S.Ct. 1196).

Similarly, discrimination against and segregation of workers of color in the United States results in their having some of the most hazardous jobs. The situation of illegal immigrants exacerbates the problem, since they are fearful of turning to government for protection. Minority workers frequently have no union representation and are at the mercy of particularly exploitative employers. Migrant farm workers experience some of the most difficult conditions, in part because responsibility for their protection is split between the EPA, which regulates pesticides and related chemicals, and OSHA, which regulates labor camps. Domestic workers are another group largely composed of people of color who have little protection.

Workers' Compensation, Cost-Benefit Analysis, and the Value of Life

When workers are injured or killed on the job in the United States, workers' compensation programs at the state level are supposed to provide quick income support and medical care or a death benefit. These programs may provide a maximum of two-thirds of the average wage in the state, the rationale being that workers must have a financial incentive to return to work. No payment for pain or suffering is allowed. Workers are barred from suing their employers in this "no-fault" insurance scheme. There is no question that many workers suffer severe economic, as well as physical, hardship as a result of industrial injuries. Nevertheless, many employers complain about "cheaters" and fraud in the system, as well as about rising insurance premiums.

There is much debate about whether workers' compensation provides adequate compensation to workers who are injured on the job, and about the efficacy of the system for preventing injury; however, it seems evident that the system does not deal effectively with occupational diseases such as cancer and respiratory diseases. Workers have the burden of demonstrating that their illness is job-related. Diseases of long latency and that may have multiple causes are rarely diagnosed as occupational and workers suffering from them are rarely compensated. Because the workers' compensation system failed to deal with asbestos-related disease, workers' attorneys initiated third-party liability suits in the 1970s and thereafter against asbestos suppliers, who, although they were not direct employers of the sick workers, had failed to warn asbestos product users about the hazards of the material. In this way, the inadequacies of the workers' compensation system have driven the occupational disease problem into the civil courts. Essentially, both the workers' compensation system and the civil courts place dollar values on worker health or life by making employers or suppliers pay monetary compensation for occupational disease or injury.

Massachusetts, for instance, publishes a chart indicating the amount of money a worker will receive, under its workers' compensation regulations, for loss of different parts of the body. This system is not a satisfactory way to provide equitable compensation to sick workers because of the lengthy proceedings, the legal expenses, and the high probability that suits will fail.

Workers' compensation programs are not the only situations in which dollar values are placed on workers' health or life. Under the Reagan administration, all regulatory agencies had to calculate the costs and benefits of proposed government regulations. Thus OSHA was forced not only to estimate the costs to industry of compliance with new standards but also was required to place a dollar value on the lives and/or health saved. Economists have devised a variety of ways to estimate the value of a life through surveys of "willingness to pay" to save a life, analyses of apparent risk premiums (higher wages for higher risk jobs) in labor markets, and other techniques for evaluating human capital. Estimates range from as little as $28,000 to several million dollars per life saved. Perhaps the most common approach is to imagine that a worker is a bond or security that will yield a return for some years in the future and that the stream of earnings a worker would receive is a reasonable measure of the worker's productivity. How much such a bond (or worker) would be worth now depends on the size of the earnings stream and on the interest rate that an investor could obtain on alternative bonds or securities. Thus, the present value of human capital can be calculated, and the value of lives saved or lost can be compared with the cost to industry of improvements in the work environment. It is important to note that economists always discount the future: Economists believe that the gain or loss of a dollar ten years from now counts less than a gain or loss of a dollar now. Another approach is to compare the wages of risky jobs with those that are less risky. Then the risk premium is considered to be the amount that workers themselves assign to their health. In a manner similar to the human capital approach, such calculations require us to assume that the markets work well and that wages are adequate measures of the value of labor and reflect the preferences of workers.

Some public-health advocates have argued that there is an inherent antiregulatory bias in such cost–benefit analysis because of the difficulties of placing dollar values on nonquantifiables such as pain, suffering, loss of loved ones, and the like. In addition, cost–benefit analysis attempts to equate economic losses of employers with health and life losses of workers, which critics argue is inappropriate. Another serious difficulty is the problem of discounting the future. What is the appropriate interest rate to use in calculating the present value of a stream of costs or benefits that extends into the distant future? Who should decide the worth of a health benefit twenty years from now? Proponents of such economic approaches claim that there is really little choice in the matter, that public policy requires such calculation. People balance costs and benefits in an ongoing, practical way, even if exact calculations are not made. Certainly, companies must do such balancing. Thus, cost–benefit analysis utilizes market-based evaluation in situations brought about by the failure of the market to treat worker well-being adequately.

Society, by enacting laws and regulations through the political process, has decided to try to override the market. In the United States, as in other nations, worker health and safety appear to be attended to inadequately by employers and managers in charge of production. Even when workers have this information about occupational hazards, they frequently seem to lack the economic power to act to protect themselves. When government intervenes to protect workers, business interests have reasserted their belief in the primacy of economic concerns. Worker health and safety is an important arena in which the values of the market and the values of health and society are in conflict.

CHARLES LEVENSTEIN (1995)
BIBLIOGRAPHY REVISED

SEE ALSO: *Environmental Health; Hazardous Wastes and Toxic Substances; Harm; Public Health Law; Injury and Injury Control;* and other *Occupational Safety and Health* subentries

BIBLIOGRAPHY

Bayer, Ronald, ed. 1988. *The Health and Safety of Workers: Case Studies in the Politics of Professional Responsibility.* New York: Oxford University Press.

Bayer, Ronald, ed. 1996. *The Health and Safety of Workers: Case Studies in the Politics of Professional Responsibility.* New York: Oxford University Press.

Franco, G. 2001. "The Future of Occupational Health Practice: Reconciling Customer Expectation and Evidence-Based Practice." *Occupational Medicine* 51(8): 482–484.

Hansson, Sven Ove. 1998. *Setting the Limit: Occupational Health Standards and the Limits of Science.* New York: Oxford University Press.

Harms-Ringdahl, Lars. 2002. *Safety Analysis: Principles and Practice in Occupational Safety.* New York: Taylor & Francis.

Howard, G. 1996. "Disability Discrimination Act 1995: An Occupational Health Nightmare?" *Occupational Health* 48(4): 135–138.

Institute of Medicine, Committee to Assess Training Needs for Occupational Safety, Health Personnel Safety in the United States. 2000. *Safe Work in the Twenty-First Century.* Washington, D.C.: National Academy Press.

Kloss, Diana M. 1999. *Occupational Health Law.* Boston, MA: Blackwell Science.

LaMontagne, A. D., and Needleman, C. 1996. "Overcoming Practical Challenges in Intervention Research in Occupational Health and Safety." *American Journal of Industrial Medicine* 29(4): 367–372.

Levy, Barry S., and Wegman, David H., eds. 1988. *Occupational Health: Recognizing and Preventing Work-Related Disease,* 2nd edition. Boston: Little, Brown.

Marson, G. K. 2001. "The 'Value Case' for Investment in Occupational Health." *Occupational Medicine* 51(8): 496–500.

Mendeloff, John M. 1988. *The Dilemma of Toxic Substance Regulation: How Overregulation Causes Underregulation at OSHA.* Cambridge, MA: MIT Press.

New Solutions: A Journal of Environmental and Occupational Health Policy. 1990–. Denver, CO: Alice Hamilton Memorial Library.

Raffle, P. A. B.; Lee, W. R.; McCallum, R. I.; and Murray, R. 1987. *Hunter's Diseases of Occupations,* rev. edition. London: Hodder & Stoughton.

Robinson, James C. 1991. *Toil and Toxics: Workplace Struggles and Political Strategies for Occupational Health.* Berkeley: University of California Press.

Rosner, David, and Markowitz, Gerald E., eds. 1987. *Dying for Work: Workers' Safety and Health in Twentieth-Century America.* Bloomington: Indiana University Press.

Wald, Peter H., and Stave, Gregg M., eds. 2001. *Physical and Biological Hazards of the Workplace.* Hoboken, NJ: John Wiley and Sons.

Westerholm, Peter, and Menckel, Ewa. 1999. *Evaluation in Occupational Health Practice.* New York: Oxford University Press.

II. OCCUPATIONAL HEALTHCARE PROVIDERS

Occupational-health services—the focus of professional personnel, their healthcare and equipment, the programs offered for the prevention of disease and promotion of wellness—have become an increasingly important field in preventive medicine and public health during the twentieth century. The goal of these services is to develop and implement interventions that improve the health and safety of the workplace. They have advanced not only as a result of general developments in preventive medicine and public health but also because of increasing emphasis on the rights of employees and their overall welfare.

The occupational-health profession faces challenges represented by global economic competition, changes in labor force demographics, expanding markets, and new and different occupational and nonoccupational hazards to which workers are exposed. Occupational epidemiology is flourishing, and detailed studies of groups at risk are demonstrating previously unrecognized associations between work exposure and certain adverse health effects. Striking advances in molecular biology are bringing new tools and new insights into cellular aberrations induced by occupational exposure to physical and chemical agents, potentially offering the possibility of very early detection of occupational disease or risk, including risks to the fetuses or offspring of workers. New rules and regulations are helping workers gain information on the toxicity of materials with which they are working and the precautions that must be taken to prevent excess exposure. Good translations of the technical literature into appropriate language ensure that previously guarded information becomes available to work groups. At the same time, the consumer movement has demanded and spread available data, and the Freedom of Information Act has brought disclosures of data not previously available. All these developments have significant ethical implications for the practice of occupational health, and therefore for those who engage in that practice: occupational-health professionals in occupational-health surveillance, specifically, screening programs. The ultimate goal of these services is to develop and implement interventions that improve some aspect or modify determinants of the health and well-being of people who work. Before embarking on an overview of these ethical issues, it is well to consider the relationships of occupational-health professionals to industrial management, relationships that may have ethical implications. Occupational health services may be provided through: (1) a complete in-plant health program with a full-time physician; (2) a partial in-plant health program with a physician in attendance for a portion of the day; (3) an out-of-plant medical program executed almost exclusively in the offices of private physicians; or (4) contract health programs.

In the complete in-plant health program, organizational placement of occupational-health professionals in the managerial structure may suggest to employees that the surveillance activities operate exclusively to protect the company. And although this situation has markedly improved, too often in the past many occupational-health professionals took the position that the company was always right. Such professionals ignored their responsibility to advise management on all matters pertaining to the health of employees, including deficiencies that required resolution or correction. The economic interest of the company may prompt management to pressure occupational-health professionals into a position of unilateral loyalty. This may lead to the expectation by managers that because the occupational-health physician is "one of them," some or all risk-assessment data,

including information regarding chemical or other hazardous exposures for certain employees, will be shared irrespective of its confidential content. Unquestionably, the goal of a healthy company and the goal of healthy workers can collide, and when they do come into conflict, occupational-health personnel must be aware of their ethical responsibility to the health of the workers and to the principles of occupational medicine.

As industries seek to reduce the cost of health services, and as the social and scientific context of the workplace changes, less than full-time on-site occupational-health services may become more common. These arrangements can raise ethical issues of another kind, including questions about active advertising or direct solicitation of contracts for such services and about "self-referral"—the physician's referral of patients to an outside facility in which he or she has a financial interest. Growing evidence suggests that more and more physicians own healthcare facilities to which they refer patients for services but at which they do not practice. The danger in occupational medicine is that part-time physicians may be strongly tempted to see their work as a golden opportunity to generate patients for off-site, private treatment facilities in which they own an interest, including services covered by workmen's compensation (Swedlow et al.).

The principle that guides these relationships of service is that physicians and other occupational-health personnel cannot use their relationship with industry as a means to build their private practice. The American Medical Association's Council on Ethical and Judicial Affairs affirmed:

> However others may see the professional, the physicians are not simply business people with high standards. Physicians are engaged in the special calling of healing, and in that calling they are fiduciaries of their patients. They have different and higher duties than even the most ethical business purpose. There are some activities involving their patients that physicians should avoid whether or not there is evidence of abuse. (Council on Ethical and Judicial Affairs)

The Code of Ethical Conduct for Physicians Providing Occupational Medical Service emphasizes this principle in the following way: "Physicians should … avoid allowing their medical judgement to be influenced by any conflict of interest." Addressing the same issue, the *Guide to Developing Small Plan Occupational Health Programs* states:

> The plant physician should never use his industrial affiliation improperly as a means of gaining or enlarging his private practice. If he observes these ethical relationships, the plant physician should experience no difficulty in establishing cordial

relationships with other physicians in the community and gaining mutual cooperation on the problem. (1983, p. 13)

Surveillance Screening

Issues of privacy, confidentiality, and informed consent pervade almost every program activity for the assessment, preservation, restoration, and improvement of the health of workers at the place of employment. In screening programs especially, these issues are brought into bold relief. They may relate to the screening program itself or to the use of the results, which are designed to determine if the worker's health remains compatible with the job assignment and to detect any evidence of impaired health that may be attributed to employment.

Many such programs are ill-conceived from both a scientific and an ethical point of view. Problems of test validity and predictive values may weaken any appeal of beneficence. For example, some employers may insist on genetic testing even though the science of identifying genetic factors that may contribute to the occurrence of job-related illness is still in its infancy. The correlation of a genetic risk presumed to pose dangers (i.e., chromosomal damage) for the later occurrence of disease may not mean that all or most with the risk factor will become ill. Also, other genetic factors or environmental factors (such as smoking) may be necessary for the development of the disease. Thus, the use of genetic screening to identify and protect workers who might be at increased risk of disease in a workplace cannot be justified by the ethical principle of beneficence where there are low correlations between risk factors like genetic markers and disease. Just as there is uncertainty about who, or how many, could be harmed, so there is uncertainty about how industry should respond. There would be some physical risks associated with medical testing procedures.

Second, there would be risks to the worker from use of the screening information. These include the loss of a job or reassignment to a lower-paying or less desirable job, loss of self-esteem, and, possibly, stigmatization as "genetically inferior." Such a label conceivably could result in the person's exclusion from certain jobs in an entire industry. Historically disadvantaged groups—women and/or ethnic or racial minority workers—would be further disadvantaged. The use of such tests, in short, may provide no real benefit to the company and may cause harm to the worker.

The rapid growth of new molecular and biochemical tools in occupational medicine has resulted in the development of biological indexes or markers for predicting occupational diseases. Scientists hope that these biological indexes or markers will stand as early warnings of the occurrence of occupational risk and disease. Occupational medicine may use biological markers to enhance early detection and treatment of disease; occupational epidemiology may use them as indicators of internal exposure at the workplace or of potential health risks and the need for workplace monitoring. The use of these tools in workplace screening touches on areas of basic concern to most people: opportunity for employment, job security, health, self-esteem, and privacy. In the case of a biological marker known to reflect susceptibility, for example, should a worker who tests positive or has a higher measurement be removed from the workplace? If so, should the occupational-health professional recommend that the worker be offered an equivalent job in the same industry? Or should the occupational-health professional recommend that management clean up the workplace to protect the most sensitive worker? To complicate matters, most biological markers of occupational disease are presumed to predict group risks (increased rates of disease among workers), and these levels of risk are still sufficiently low as to not be reliable guides to which individuals are threatened. Therefore, it is important that workers be informed in advance that the results are interpretable only on the group level. Test results given to workers should be presented and discussed on the basis and in the context of the information that is available on the variability within groups of workers and between individuals (National Research Council).

Of equal importance is the treatment of the data generated by biological-marker testing. One concern of employees who have been screened would be to prevent the spread of embarrassing, damaging, or false information about themselves, particularly to potential employers. The Code of Ethical Conduct for Physicians Providing Occupational Medical Service provides that employers are entitled to receive counsel about the medical fitness of an individual in relation to work but are not entitled to diagnoses or specific details. No one in healthcare challenges the fact that the medical record is a confidential document. But many managers believe they should have access to it when there is interest in an individual employee. However, diagnostic information is not needed for placement of an employee or for changes in his or her workstation because of change in health status. The occupational-health physician can state that an individual is physically or emotionally capable for all work or that an employee should not work in areas where there are high concentrations of certain organic vapors. This information meets the needs of management and does not change the privilege of the medical information under the control of the occupational-health physician. The Code of Ethical Conduct of the American Occupational Medicine Association is clear on this issue:

Treat as confidential whatever is learned about individuals served, releasing information only when required by law or by overriding public health considerations or to other physicians at the request of the individual according to traditional medical ethical practice and recognize that employers are entitled to counsel about the medical fitness of an individual in relation to work but are not entitled to diagnoses or details of a specific nature.

Medical records usually need to be kept for a long time because of linkages between occupational exposure and disease or dysfunction with long latency periods. These are usually the kinds of disease (cancer, for example) that are most sensitive in terms of workers' feelings about privacy. Records become part of large data systems to which government regulatory agencies, courts, and law enforcement officials may have relatively easy access. Workers are concerned that leakage of sensitive information will affect their mobility and employability.

Confidentiality is seldom an absolute value. Information about patients may be revealed under certain circumstances, including those in which workers themselves give consent to provide it to insurance companies or other physicians. Because they are concerned about possible misuse of information from screening programs, or because they wish to know of risks to their health, employees may want access to their medical records. The ethical principle of autonomy implies a duty to provide employees with information about their health, even when it is not clear what the information means. The duty would be even stronger when the information is highly predictive of a risk of disease.

Autonomy would also appear to require that the workers be fully informed of the nature of any screening procedure to which they will be subjected. While the concept of informed consent would be most crucial in occupational-health research, it is also applicable to medical screening. In the latter case, even though the procedures are clearly beneficial, their application to work without informed consent is a paternalistic action.

Epidemiologic Investigations

The results of screening programs may suggest the need for epidemiologic studies to provide additional information on adverse health effects from occupational exposure. These studies may be conducted by occupational epidemiologists. Even prior to the U.S. Occupational Safety and Health Act of 1970, companies involved in formulating and synthesizing chemicals had hired epidemiologists to conduct in-house studies. Such research is an important aspect of an employer's obligation to employees, consumers, and the public in general.

In conducting epidemiologic studies, occupational-health professionals have obligations to workers who are the study subjects as well as to the company's management, who ordered the study and will pay for it. Sometimes these obligations conflict, and the occupational-health professional must sort out ethical as well as scientific priorities. Depending on where the request for the study originates, for example, there may be conflict even in the initial decision as to whether the study should be undertaken. The analysis and interpretation of the data the study generates may be affected by its expected implications. Economic implications may be intertwined with political ones. Epidemiologic studies of workers who are occupationally exposed to neurotoxins or reproductive toxins, for example, may lead to political conflict between labor and management, with government as a possible third party. The dispute is essentially about the occupational environment rather than economic issues with political factors as a secondary concern. Here the company's epidemiologist may be under pressure to respond more fully to his or her responsibilities to the employer than to any professional obligation to the workers (Gordis).

As the research project proceeds, the subjects should be kept informed of its progress, subjects' privacy should be respected, and confidentiality of data should be maintained. This is an important task because the concept of research can be disquieting to workers and to management as well. When, in the course of the study, management and other investigators who are not part of the study ask that investigators share data on an individual basis, investigators face conflict between professional obligations and legal ones. Under the provisions of the Toxic Substances Control Act, for example, epidemiologists are required to communicate substantial risk to the U.S. Environmental Protection Agency within fifteen days after learning of such risk. This information is then made available to the public. Here the professional obligation is to make the best interpretation of the facts, perhaps even to the extent of realizing that the best interpretation cannot be made without additional facts. When there is no time for the investigator to gather additional data, he or she has an obligation to make the best interpretation of the data that is available (Bond, 1991).

Ethical guides for communicating potential health risk have not been defined. In this context, occupational-health personnel are often called on to distinguish between the significant and the trivial. The problem does not lie where real risk can be identified and effective action by the company can result in real benefit to the worker. The technical and ethical conflicts arise when the occupational-health specialist must decide whether a given risk is acceptable, or whether it must be disclosed when not enough is known to be able to measure the presumed risk, and when there are acceptable alternatives. In such cases the occupational-health investigator must act judiciously, in the best interest of the health and well-being of the workers. Withholding pertinent information or providing unqualified, incomplete, or uncertain data may be detrimental to the worker and/or the company.

Conclusion

Economic performance is not the only responsibility of industry any more than educational performance is the only responsibility of a college or university. Unless economic performance is balanced with broader responsibilities for the health and safety of workers, industry will ultimately fail. The public's interest in health and safety, and its broader interest in the rights of workers, including the right to know of risks they face, seem a permanent feature of modern American capitalism. The demand for socially responsible industries and for workers' health and safety will not go away. These responsibilities involve concern about all factors that influence the health of employees, including assuring the availability of health services that are preventive and constructive. These services are not the work of any one group but depend on the cooperative activities of medicine, chemistry, toxicology, engineering, and many others. In this setting industry must recognize and respect the unique position of occupational-health-service providers and assist them in providing impartial, professional counsel to both management and employees. The occupational-health-service providers must be honest, consistent, courageous, and defenders of confidentiality.

Albert Jonsen states the case well:

In a general way, the environment of modern industry comes about through investments from employer and employee alike, each making certain sorts of contributions. In our modern concept of relationship of those diverse contributions, we attribute right of ownership to employers and a variety of rights regarding wages and working conditions to employees. It is now common to consider that among these employees' rights is the right to know about hazards of the work environment.

They also have the right to know about interrelated elements of occupational safety and health. Ensuring those rights involves a great diversity and complexity of ethical responsibilities—interlocked with privacy, confidentiality,

and professional and legal obligations—of the occupational-health-service provider.

Anticipating these complex ethical issues and developing sound approaches for resolving them are significant challenges to those healthcare professionals who have the responsibility to promote the health and well-being of people who work. Specifically, however, their responsibility is played out in the context of the workplace where many other healthcare professionals have the responsibility to promote workers' health.

BAILUS WALKER, JR. (1995)
BIBLIOGRAPHY REVISED

SEE ALSO: *Conflict of Interest; Corporate Compliance; Divided Loyalties in Mental Healthcare; Environmental Health; Hazardous Wastes and Toxic Substances; Harm; Public Health Law; Injury and Injury Control;* and other *Occupational Safety and Health* subentries

BIBLIOGRAPHY

Ashton, Indira, and Gill, Frank S. 2000. *Monitoring for Health Hazards at Work.* Boston, MA: Blackwell Science Inc.

Bohle, Philip, and Quinlan, Michael. 2000. *Managing Occupational Health and Safety: A Multidisciplinary Approach,* 2nd edition. Victoria: MacMillan Co. of Australia.

Bond, Gregory G. 1991. "Ethical Issues Relating to Conduct and Interpretation of Epidemiologic Research in Private Industry." In *Industrial Epidemiology Forum's Conference on Ethics in Epidemiology,* pp. 295–345, ed. William E. Fayerweather, John Higgenson, and Tom L. Beauchamp. New York: Pergamon.

Bond, M. B. 1971. "Occupational Medical Services for Small Employee Units." *Rocky Mountain Medical Journal* 68(11): 31–36.

Council on Ethical and Judicial Affairs. American Medical Association. 1992. "Conflict of Interest: Physician Ownership of Medical Facilities." *Journal of the American Medical Association* 267(17): 2366–2369.

Cullen, M. R. 1999. "Personal Reflections on Occupational Health in the Twentieth Century: Spiraling to the Future." *Annual Review of Public Health* 20: 1–13.

Erickson, Paul A. 1996. *Practical Guide to Occupational Health and Safety.* Burlington, MA: Academic Press.

Feldstein, A. 1997. "Quality in Occupational Health Services." *Journal of Occupational and Environmental Medicine* 39(6): 501–503.

Felton, J. S. 2000. "Occupational Health in the USA in the Twenty-First Century." *Occupational Medicine* 50(7): 523–531.

Feyer, Anne Marie, and Williamson, Ann, eds. 1998. *Occupational Injury: Risk, Prevention and Intervention.* New York: Taylor & Francis.

Frick, Kaj; Jensen, P. L.; Quinlan, Michael; and Wilthagen, T., eds. 2000. *Systematic Occupational Health and Safety Management.* Oxford: Pergamon Press.

Gordis, Leon. 1991. "Ethical and Professional Issues in the Changing Practice of Epidemiology." In *Industrial Epidemiology Forum's Conference on Ethics in Epidemiology,* pp. 95–155, ed. William E. Fayerweather, John Higgenson, and Tom L. Beauchamp. New York: Pergamon.

Higgenson, John, and Chu, Flora. 1991. "Ethical Considerations and Responsibilities in Communicating Health Risk Information." In *Industrial Epidemiology Forum's Conference on Ethics in Epidemiology,* pp. 515–565, ed. William E. Fayerweather, John Higgenson, and Tom L. Beauchamp. New York: Pergamon.

"International Code of Conduct (Ethics) for Occupational Health and Safety Professionals." 2001. *International Journal of Occupational and Environmental Health* 7(3): 230–232.

Jonsen, Albert R. 1991. "Ethical Considerations and Responsibilities When Communicating Health Risk Information." In *Industrial Epidemiology Forum's Conference on Ethics in Epidemiology,* pp. 695–725, ed. William E. Fayerweather, John Higgenson, and Tom L. Beauchamp. New York: Pergamon.

National Research Council. 1992. "Biological Markers in Immunotoxicology." Washington, D.C.: Author.

Nielsen, Ronald P. 1999. *OSHA Regulations and Guidelines: A Guide for Health Care Providers.* Clifton Park, NY: Delmar Learning.

Plomp, H. N. 1999. "Evaluation of Doctor-Worker Encounters in Occupational Health: An Explanatory Study." *Occupational Medcine* 49(3): 183–188.

Rosenstock, Linda, and Hagopian, Amy. 1987. "Ethical Dilemmas in Providing Health Care to Workers." *Annals of Internal Medicine* 107(4): 575–580.

Sadhra, Steven S., and Rampal, Krishna G., eds. 1999. *Occupational Health: Risk Assessment and Management.* Boston, MA: Blackwell Science.

Swedlow, Alex; Johnson, Gregory; Smithline, Neil; and Millstein, Arnold. 1992. "Increased Costs and Rates in the California Workers' Compensation System as a Result of Self-Referral by Physicians." *New England Journal of Medicine* 327(21): 1502–1506.

Westerholm, Peter. 1999. "Challenges Facing Occupational Health Services in the Twenty-First Century." *Scandinavian Journal of Work, Health, and Environment* 25(6): 625–632.

Westerholm, Peter, and Menckel, Ewa, eds. 1999. *Evaluation in Occupational Health Practice.* New York: Oxford University Press.

Ziegler, J. 1997. "The Worker's Health: Whose Business is it?" *Business and Health,* suppl. A, 15(12): 26–30.

ONCOLOGY

SEE *Cancer, Ethical Issues Related to Diagnosis and Treatment*

ORGAN AND TISSUE PROCUREMENT

• • •

I. Medical and Organizational Aspects

II. Ethical and Legal Issues Regarding Living Donors

I. MEDICAL AND ORGANIZATIONAL ASPECTS

Organ transplantation is high-technology medicine in one of its most extreme forms. It is very expensive, employs advanced biotechnologies, and requires large teams of highly trained specialists. It is used to intervene when the final stage of an illness is reached, and although it can save lives, it does not provide a "cure" or a return to a preexisting condition of health. Patients with transplants require constant, ongoing treatment with highly sophisticated and often quite dangerous medications.

But unlike most other advanced medical technologies, organ and tissue transplantation also depends on people. The only source of human organs and tissues is donations. In most instances these donations must be obtained from a young person who has died under sudden and tragic circumstances: by automobile accident, suicide, murder, and so forth. The organ procurement system's role is to provide a bridge between human tragedy and high technology.

The Supply of Organ Donors

During the first half of the 1980s the supply of cadaveric organ donors grew continually and rapidly. In 1982, there were 3,681 cadaveric kidney transplants. In 1986, there were 7,089, an increase of almost 100 percent (or almost 25% a year). Since 1986, the rate of increase has slowed. In 1992, 7,202 cadaveric kidney transplants were performed, representing donations from about 4,500 donors. In 2000, 8,089 cadaveric kidney transplants were done, representing 5,986 donors. According to the United Network for Organ Sharing (UNOS), the number of donors increased to 6,081 in 2001 and the number of transplants to 8,203. Although this was one of the largest number of organ donors in any year in U.S. history, the leveling out of the donor supply in the United States continues to cause disquiet and debate over the efficacy of the organ procurement system and the adequacy of the principles underlying it.

While organs have been transplanted in most nations of Western Europe, in Japan, and in some places in the Middle East, the infrastructure necessary to obtain organ donors routinely exists only in North America and Western Europe. (While Japan certainly has the necessary resources and expertise, cultural factors, including discomfort with brain death and a strong commitment to intact burial, have militated against the development of such a system there.) The Eurotransplant International Foundation, serving Germany, Austria, the Benelux nations, and Slovenia, is the second-largest organ procurement system in the world and the largest in Europe. In 2000, 3,099 cadaveric kidneys were transplanted in the Eurotransplant region, as well as more than 642 hearts and 1,285 livers. France and the United Kingdom have both operated national organ procurement systems since the 1980s, and 1,486 cadaveric kidneys were transplanted in the United Kingdom and Ireland in 2000 and 1,840 in France. Scandia Transplant (serving Scandinavia) is an organization of long standing; it provided kidneys for 630 transplants in 2000. Since the early 1990s, both Italy and Spain have developed transplantation and organ procurement systems. Spain's program now provides about 1,350 donors a year—the highest rate of donation in Europe. Over 1,900 cadaveric kidney transplants were done in Spain in 2000. Italy has been less successful, but 1,308 kidneys were transplanted there in 2000. About 19,000 kidney transplants were done in Western Europe in 2000, considerably more than in the United States. But the U.S. system remains the largest single system in the world, with almost 17,600 cadaveric kidney transplants completed in 2000 (UK Transplant; UNOS).

Of course kidneys are not the only organs being transplanted. In 1990 over 4,700 livers and over 4,100 hearts were transplanted worldwide, along with more than 1,000 pancreases and 250 lungs or heart–lung combinations. By 2000, 2,202 hearts and 4,664 livers were transplanted in the United States alone. In Europe an additional 1,991 hearts and 4,733 livers were transplanted. Since 1990 others organs have joined the list: intestines, lungs, and pancreases in particular. During the late 1980s, the total number of heart and liver transplants grew very rapidly, although the number of donors did not. This reflected an increase in multiple-organ donation. Donors who previously donated only kidneys were increasingly providing hearts, livers, and/or pancreases. In the United States, by 1992, 72 percent of all organ donors provided more than one organ (UNOS). In 2001 the percentage certainly exceeded 76 percent and was, perhaps, higher still. While trustworthy data are difficult to

obtain, it is probable that in 1982 the percentage was less than 25 percent.

The number of actual donations must be understood in relation to the number of potential donors. A groundbreaking study headed by Kenneth J. Bart and conducted for the Centers for Disease Control estimated that in 1975 between 54.5 and 115.8 donors per million persons—about 25,000 to 26,000 potential donors—were available that year in the United States (Bart et al., 1981b). More recent work has applied more restrictive criteria to the examination of hospital death records, with one study finding an estimated national donor pool of between 10,000 and 12,500 (Nathan et al). Although divergent, these estimates both show that actual donation rates are not close to exhausting the potential supply of donors. They also indicate that the size of the donor pool is very sensitive to donor criteria, especially age. Medical criteria for acceptable donors are not fixed by immutable laws but change as transplant experience changes, and perhaps as the need for organs changes. The donor pool is itself a somewhat flexible and changing concept.

CRITERIA FOR DONATION. The one immutable medical criterion for organ donation has been brain death, or more exactly, the determination of death by brain-death criteria. Once the circulation of blood ceases, an organ very rapidly becomes useless for transplantation unless it is cooled. For this reason organ donors must be kept on machines that maintain respiration and heartbeat after death. Because the heart must be kept pumping, death must be declared on the basis of total and irreversible cessation of brain function—brain death. The causes of death that are consistent with organ donation are therefore sharply limited to those involving damage to the central nervous system. Trauma is the most common cause of such damage. Almost 43 percent of all donors in 2000 died of head trauma (about 25 percent died in auto accidents) and over 41 percent of kidney donors died of strokes (OPTN).

The need for organs is believed to be so severe that even the brain-death criterion is being questioned. Efforts are under way in a number of locations to test the feasibility of employing donors whose hearts are not beating for organ donation (i.e., donors who suffer cardiac arrest before organ retrieval). Professional support for this approach is reflected in the Institute of Medicine's 2000 report on non-heart-beating organ transplantation. This report cites studies estimating that up to a 20 percent increase in kidney donation could result from organ procurement organizations (OPOs) actively seeking non-heart-beating donors. Actual change, however, has been slow. As of 1998 only half of all OPOs had a protocol for obtaining donations from non-heart-beating donors. No more than a dozen OPOs are actively engaged in such efforts and less than 3 percent of all donors fall into that category.

Other medical criteria also limit the potential supply of organs. Cancer, systemic infections, HIV, hepatitis, and other diseases can exclude a donor because of the possible transmission of the disease to the organ recipient. High blood pressure, diabetes, and many other conditions can damage an organ and thereby render it unsuitable for transplantation.

The most general limiting factor is the age of the donor. There is little unanimity among transplant centers on acceptable donor age. In general the criteria for kidney donors is the least exclusive, and that for heart donors the most exclusive. Young donors are preferred; in the 1980s kidney donors over fifty-five were considered unsuitable, as were male heart donors older than forty. Over time, age criteria have loosened noticeably. From 1978 to 1987 the percentage of kidney donors over fifty went from 5 percent to 10 percent, and the percentage over thirty grew from about 30 percent to 40 percent (Takemoto and Terasaki). According to UNOS, in 2000 about 31 percent of cadaveric organ donors were fifty years old or older; almost 8 percent were over sixty-five. Eurotransplant protocols now consider kidney and liver donors up to age seventy-five as suitable—subject to individual evaluation. Increases in acceptable donor age can enlarge the donor pool substantially, especially when combined with an increasing percentage of donors dying from causes other than trauma.

The Procurement Systems

Organ donation requires an institutional structure to identify willing donors, obtain consent, procure the organ, and distribute it to the transplant team. These are the tasks of the organ procurement system.

LOCAL CONTEXT. The earliest organ procurement organizations in the United States were founded around 1970. They were purely local organizations that grew up around kidney transplantation teams and were meant to address those teams' needs for transplantable organs. By the mid-1980s, over ninety of these organizations had been formed; virtually no area of the nation was unserved.

While the organ procurement system has undergone many changes since the early 1980s, the local components of organ procurement success have not changed. The central factor in successful organ procurement is timely information about potentially suitable donors. Only a very small percentage of deaths can lead to an organ donation, and the window

of time available for action is short. Cooperation from hospital personnel, specifically doctors and nurses in intensive care units (ICUs), is essential. A referral from these professionals (i.e., notification that a potential donor is under treatment) is required for the donation process to begin. OPO personnel typically spend more of their time encouraging doctors and nurses to make referrals than they do on organ procurement itself. This persuasion takes the form of in-service training sessions, one-on-one visits, and visits to the ICU itself. Success in obtaining referrals is the key determinant of successful organ procurement (Prottas, 1989).

A second factor of great importance is targeting appropriate hospitals. Not all hospitals are equally good sources of potential donors: Some see little trauma, and some lack the capacity to make brain-death determinations. OPOs that target their professional education efforts where the return can be the greatest are likely to be more successful than those that work with every hospital in their area.

The final step in the procurement process is obtaining permission from families. This is a very delicate matter. Families of potential donors have suffered a terrible loss. Some OPOs prefer to have their own, experienced staff approach the family. Others depend more heavily on hospital staff. All depend on the physicians involved to inform the family that their relative has died. U.S. law forbids paying families to permit donation. All organ donation decisions are therefore voluntary and altruistic.

THE DONATION DECISION. The American public, indeed the publics of all Western nations, appear to be very supportive of organ donation (Gallup Organization; Bergström and Gäbel; Moores et al.). Support levels for organ donation of 90 percent are routinely found in large-scale surveys. In the United States these rates vary by race/ethnicity, education, and income. White Americans, middle-class Americans, and well-educated Americans are more supportive of organ donation than are nonwhites and poorer and less-educated citizens. The differences, however, are all within the context of very high levels of support. African-American levels of support approach 80 percent (Prottas, 1994).

Actual willingness to donate is lower but still large. Survey data indicate that 75 to 80 percent of the population is willing to give permission for organ donation by a relative when they know that the person has been declared dead, even if they never discussed this issue with the deceased (Batten and Prottas). Here, too, there are significant differences across social classes and ethnicities. Actual permission rates obtained are another measure of public willingness to donate—although they are somewhat obscured by who is asked and the skills of those requesting permission. Permission rates vary among OPOs but generally lie between 45 and 50 percent (Siminoff et al., 2001).

There are two general categories of reasons that the public gives for being willing to donate the organs of a deceased relative. The more important is a desire to help another person. Families that have actually allowed a donation and the general public both report that they support donation so that someone's life can be saved. The families of donors also assert that they permitted donation in order that something positive could come out of the death of their relative—a factor that is only slightly less likely to be mentioned than the desire to save a life. The general public is less likely to give the solace of donation as a reason for its support of donation, but it still is the second most commonly given reason. Indeed, families and the general public agree that organ donation can help the families of the donor in the grieving process (Prottas and Batten; Batten and Prottas).

The reasons people give for their unwillingness to donate seem to reflect a mistrust of the medical establishment and the donation process. Among the most commonly given reasons is a fear that permission will compromise the care received or prolong the suffering of the relative. The second reason, closely aligned to the first, assumes that donation-related activities are occurring while the patient is still alive. From 45 to 65 percent of those unwilling to give permission for donation give answers of this sort as the explanation for their unwillingness. Of this group, 60 percent also say that they would not give permission because the donation process is too complicated. Finally, about a third attribute their unwillingness to expected resistance from other family members (Prottas and Batten).

Some of these reservations relate directly to the donation process itself and to communication between OPOs and the public. Others may reflect more basic mistrustful or alienated attitudes toward medical institutions. In this regard the greater unwillingness to donate found among ethnic minorities and among poorer citizens becomes more comprehensible.

The donation process itself seems to have important effects on willingness to donate. The core process of asking to donate is the same for all OPOs and hospitals, but differences in details can matter. Once the medical suitability of a patient has been determined, the family must be approached with the patient's terminal prognosis and—then or somewhat later—with a request for donation. A physician must present the fact of brain death, but the request for donation can be made by a doctor, a nurse, or a member of the local OPO. In different places the patterns vary. In some cases the organ procurement specialists carry the main burden of talking with the families because they are trained and experienced in this kind of encounter. In other locales, nurses will assume the responsibility because they often have the best rapport with the family, developed while the patient was being treated. A well-managed process, based on good communications and good relationships between families and the clinicians caring for the patients, can influence the permission rate (Siminoff et al., 2001).

The most common cause of death for an organ donor is accident trauma, and most donors are young; as a result, most family decision makers are parents. In recent years the age of donors has increased, and a larger percentage have died from cerebrovascular accidents. This has led to an increase in the percentage of decision makers who are spouses—most generally wives, because male donors outnumber female donors.

Donor families generally feel that the donation process was well handled, and almost 90 percent would make the same decision over again. The criticisms that do emerge usually regard the timing of the request and the clarity of the brain-death explanation (Batten and Prottas). Some of these criticism can be met by improved permission-seeking behavior (Siminoff et al., 2001), but others may reflect reactions to the loss of a loved one itself.

SYSTEM CONTEXT. Prior to 1986 the Southeastern Organ Procurement Foundation was the only regional OPO in the United States. It operated the United Network for Organ Sharing, a computer system listing most of the patients in the United States awaiting an organ. This computer list was simply a compilation of individual OPO lists, was readily accessible, and made inter-OPO organ sharing possible. However, the disposition of kidneys (few other organs were procured at that time) remained solely in the hands of the procuring agency.

Some OPOs were far more effective than others. Some procured forty kidneys per million population served; others, only eight. Cost per kidney also varied tremendously, from lows of $6,000 to $7,000 to highs of over $20,000. The percentage of organs not actually transplanted—in effect, wasted—was also very high and variable. In Europe 4 to 5 percent of the kidneys procured were discarded; the U.S. rate was almost 20 percent (a difference now virtually eliminated by improvements in the United States). Organ distribution criteria were different in different areas; often they were unwritten and inconsistently applied. Some transplant hospitals believed that when donor and recipient had similar immunological characteristics, the probability of successful transplantation was much higher. Others felt such matching was of little importance. Those who believed in matching offered to share organs more frequently than those who did not, and this tended to decrease access to transplants for their patients.

PUBLIC INVOLVEMENT. The dual issues of system efficacy in organ procurement and equity in organ allocation induced the U.S. Congress to become directly involved in organ procurement and transplantation matters. In 1972, Congress established the End Stage Renal Disease (ESRD) Program through an amendment to the Social Security Act. Under this program, people suffering from renal failure automatically became eligible for Medicare coverage. Although most of the budget of this several-billion-dollar program pays for renal dialysis, renal transplantation and organ procurement costs are also covered. Under the ESRD Program, the federal government began paying the expenses of the nation's ninety OPOs. This financial involvement of the government, coupled with public concerns about efficacy and equity, led to major changes in the organ procurement system in the late 1980s.

Starting in 1984 with the Organ Transplantation Act, Congress moved to restructure two key aspects of the organ procurement system by supporting the formation of a national organization to oversee the sharing of organs and by reforming the governance of OPOs themselves. By 1986 certain principles and structures were agreed upon that have come to define the U.S. organ procurement system. The most basic principle was that human organs are a public resource and that the organ procurement system was a steward of the public in its handling of organs. Each OPO and each transplant surgeon could be held accountable for organ allocation decisions. OPOs were now required to have public representatives on their boards.

A federally funded agency, the Organ Procurement and Transplantation Network (OPTN), was established to act as the public's agent in matters of organ allocation. This organization was given the authority to set rules controlling organ allocation at both the local and the interagency level and to enforce those rules on all OPOs. Only member agencies of OPTN could procure organs; only member hospitals could transplant organs, on pain of losing Medicare reimbursement. OPTN was also given the authority to set membership standards, including those regarding personnel training and transplant outcomes. These standards had to be met if an OPO or a hospital was to be involved in organ procurement or transplantation. While OPTN has been very conservative in the use of its powers, deferring to local practices and preferences whenever possible, the federal government now essentially has final say on how human organs are to be allocated to patients.

In the late 1980s, the Health Care Financing Administration (HCFA) exercised its right to set standards for the certification of OPOs, which included the definition of a service area for each OPO that was, to a large degree, the grant of a monopoly to procure organs in that area. Because HCFA rules precluded multiple OPOs in a single service area, there was a significant decrease in the number of OPOs in operation. As of 2000, the United States had some sixty-seven certified OPOs.

The next major increase in government involvement was the passage of "required request" laws at both the federal and the state level. The philosophical underpinning of these laws is the belief that organ donation is a right that families have and that medical institutions have an obligation to facilitate the exercise of that right. While there are differences among the various required request laws, they all share the same basic elements. Each requires that hospitals have a system in place to ensure that the family of every medically appropriate donor is asked if they wish to permit an organ or tissue donation. Reimbursement under Medicare can be denied to any hospital without such a system. These laws appear to have been reasonably successful in ensuring that families are given the option of donation (Siminoff et al., 1995). It is less clear that they have increased actual donation rates (Anderson and Fox; Viring).

In 1998 an additional step was taken when "routine referral" rules were promulgated. These rules require that hospitals inform OPOs of all imminent deaths. The goal of this regulation was to ensure that organ donation professionals are involved in the process from its earliest stages. It was predicated on a concern that not all suitable donors were being identified and that in-hospital personnel lacked the skills necessary to effectively request donation (OPTN). No systematic evaluation of the effect of this approach has been done but there is little indication of a system-wide increase in donation.

Finally, in the last years of the 1990s, the federal government became more actively involved in issues of organ allocation. There is a long-standing dispute over whether the queue for a transplant should reflect only patient characteristics or whether the OPO or the region procuring the donation ought to be given some form of preferred position. The dispute is complex and until recently the federal government took little active part. In the last half of the 1990s, however, the Department of Health and Human Services became actively involved in the debate and finally promulgated rules designed to minimize all allocation factors that did not pertain to the individual patient's characteristics. This appears to be the last in a decade-long series of changes that increased the influence of public bodies over professional ones in structuring the transplantation system.

DONATION RULES. Federal law defines the terms of exchange in organ donation. It is against federal law to buy or sell human organs and tissues. Organ and tissue donation requires explicit consent from the donor's family or a signed donor card. An alternative system exists called "presumed consent." This system reverses the burden of proof regarding family permission. Under it, if a family does not express an objection to organ donation, their permission is presumed. Austria, Belgium, Finland, France, Greece, Norway, Portugal, and Spain have presumed-consent laws (Eurotransplant), but it is unclear how often they are implemented. Certainly some nations do not actually procure organs under these laws but insist on obtaining explicit permission from families. Spain may be the only general exception, although even there detailed hospital-level data is hard to find.

In the United States, about half the states have some form of presumed-consent laws with regard to cornea donations. According to these laws, corneas can be removed from cadavers under the jurisdiction of the medical examiner, based on permission from the medical examiner's office. Some states require a minimal effort to contact families, but others do not.

ORGAN TRANSPLANTATION AND TISSUE PROCUREMENT SYSTEMS. The laws regarding organ procurement apply to tissue procurement in most ways. Tissue donation, too, must be voluntary and uncompensated, and families have the right to be given the option to donate when the medical circumstances are appropriate. However, the organizational structure of the tissue banking system is different from that of organ banking. Organ procurement is a closely regulated, federally financed system; tissue procurement is neither.

The system for procurement of musculoskeletal tissue (bone, tendons, fascia, ligaments) is virtually unregulated, except insofar as it falls under laws forbidding payments, certain Food and Drug Administration quality regulations, and required-request laws. Shared professional and technical concerns have begun to translate into discussion of procurement and distribution practices. Few rules have been agreed to, and there are no enforcement mechanisms. Government involvement in tissue banking is very recent and has occurred in response to public health concerns about the spread of AIDS and hepatitis via transplanted tissue.

The organ and tissue procurement systems, however, increasingly overlap at the operational level. Cooperation of hospitals and their medical staffs is central to the success of both, and there is overlap in terms of donor families as well.

Because of this, OPOs and tissue banks have found themselves in conflict regarding access to hospital staff and to families. In response, most OPOs have expanded their activities to include tissue banking. Over 80 percent of OPOs report being involved in tissue procurement. Detailed data on the exact nature of those involvements is not available, but it appears that most OPOs now have some permanent organizational relationship within the tissue procurement field. This may take the form of having a tissue division or being within a larger organizational umbrella with a tissue procurement agency. In other cases, local agreements, especially with eye banks, have generated cooperation. The large size and unregulated nature of tissue banking, however, has left the relationships between the two systems diverse and complex.

JEFFREY M. PROTTAS (1995)
REVISED BY AUTHOR

SEE ALSO: *Cybernetics; Death, Definition and Determination of; Dialysis, Kidney; Healthcare Resources, Allocation of; Medical Futility; Medicare; Mistakes, Medical; Organ and Tissue Procurement; Organ Transplants, Medical Overview of; Organ Transplants, Sociocultural Aspects of; Technology; Xenografts;* and other *Organ and Tissue Procurement* subentries

BIBLIOGRAPHY

Anderson, K. S., and Fox, D. M. 1988. "The Impact of Routine Inquiry Laws on Organ Donation." *Health Affairs* 7:65–78.

Bart, Kenneth J.; Macon, Edwin J.; Humphries, Arthur L., Jr.; et al. 1981a. "Increasing the Supply of Cadaveric Kidneys for Transplantation." *Transplantation* 31(5): 383–387.

Bart, Kenneth J.; Macon, Edwin J.; Whittier, Frederick C.; et al. 1981b. "Cadaveric Kidneys for Transplantation: A Paradox of Shortage in the Face of Plenty." *Transplantation* 31(5): 379–382.

Batten, Helen Levine, and Prottas, Jeffrey M. 1987. "Kind Strangers: The Families of Organ Donors." *Health Affairs* 6(2): 35–37.

Bergström, Christina, and Gäbel, Hakan. 1991. "Organ Donation and Organ Retrieval Programs in Sweden, 1990." *Journal of Transplant Coordination* 1(1): 47–51.

Eurotransplant International Foundation. 1992. *Eurotransplant Newsletter 91.* Leiden, Netherlands: Author

Evans, Roger W.; Orians, Carlyn E.; and Ascher, Nancy L. 1992. "The Potential Supply of Organ Donors: An Assessment of the Efficacy of Organ Procurement Efforts in the United States." *Journal of the American Medical Association* 267(2): 239–246.

Eye Bank Association of America. 1991. *Eye Banking Statistics.* Washington, D.C.: Author.

Health Care Financing Administration. 1990. *ESRD Program Highlights.* Washington, D.C.: Author.

Moores, B.; Clarke, G.; Lewis, B. R.; et al. 1976. "Public Attitudes towards Kidney Transplantation." *British Medical Journal* 1(6010): 629–631.

Nathan, Howard, et al. 1991. "Estimation and Characterization of the Potential Organ Donor Pool in Pennsylvania." *Transplantation* 51(1): 112–149.

Organ Procurement and Transplantation Network (OPTN). 2000. *Annual Report 2000.* Richmond, VA: Author.

Prottas, Jeffrey M. 1989. "The Organization of Organ Procurement." *Journal of Health Politics, Policy, and Law* 14(1): 41–55.

Prottas, Jeffrey M. 1994. *The Most Useful Gift: Altruism and the Public Policy of Organ Transplants.* San Francisco: Jossey-Bass.

Prottas, Jeffrey M., and Batten, Helen Levine. 1991. "The Willingness to Give: The Public and the Supply of Transplantable Organs." *Journal of Health Politics, Policy, and Law* 16(1): 121–134.

Siminoff, Laura A.; Arnold, R. M.; Caplan A. L.; Virnig, B. A.; and Seltzer, D. L. 1995. "Public Policy Governing Organ and Tissue Procurement in the United States; Results from the National Organ and Tissue Procurement Study." *Annal of Internal Medicine* 123(1) 10–17.

Siminoff, Laura A.; Gordon, Nahida; Hewlett, Joan; et al. 2001. "Factors Influencing Families' Consent for Donation of Solid Organs for Transplantation." *Journal of the American Medical Association* 286(1): 71–77.

Takemoto, Steven, and Terasaki, Paul I. 1988. "Donor and Recipient Age." In *Clinical Transplants,* ed. Paul I. Terasaki. Los Angeles: UCLA Tissue Typing Laboratory.

U.S. Institute of Medicine. Division of Health Care Services. 2000. *Non-Heart-Beating Organ Transplantation: Practice and Protocols.* Washington, D.C.: National Academy Press.

Virnig, B. A., and Caplan, A. L. 1992. "Required Request: What Difference Has It Made?" *Transplant Proceedings* 24: 2155–2158.

INTERNET RESOURCES

Gallup Organization. 1993. "The American Public's Attitude toward Organ Donation and Transplantation." Questionnaire conducted for the Partnership for Organ Donation. Available from <http://www.transweb.org/reference/articles.htm>.

Organ Procurement and Transplantation Network (OPTN), Annual Report, Chapter 3, 6/2003. Available from <http://optn.org/data/annualReport.asp>.

UK Transplant. 2003. "Statistics." Available from <http://www.uktransplant.org.uk/statistics/statistics.htm>.

II. ETHICAL AND LEGAL ISSUES REGARDING LIVING DONORS

History and Background

As the number of suitable cadaver organs available for transplantation has leveled off in the last decade, the use of living donors has become increasingly important. However, the history of living donors goes back to the earliest successes in transplantation. In 1954 Dr. Joseph E. Murray performed the first successful organ transplantation at Peter Bent Brigham Hospital in Boston by transplanting a healthy kidney from twenty-three year-old Ronald Herrick into his identical twin brother Richard—thus proving the viability of soild organ transplantation. While the histories of other types of transplantation primarily consist of cadaver donors, a shortage of organs as well as improved results have led to the use of living donors for kidney, lung, liver, pancreas, and small-bowel transplantations.

The first kidney transplantation surgeries were successful because there were no immunological barriers—the organs came from identical twins. Once transplantation was proven possible, research increasingly focused on overcoming immunological barriers that cause organ rejection. Success came in the early 1960s with the immunosuppressive agent azathioprine. "Its use in combination with chronic corticosteroid therapy provided the first effective means for preventing immune-mediated destruction of allografts in clinical transplantation" (Woodle, p. 902). Improved results throughout the 1970s led to an increasing shift to cadaver sources. Living donors were still used in this period, but until the early 1980s surgeons restricted living organ donations to kidneys and usually required the donor to be a parent, sibling, or child of the recipient (Fox and Swazey). Further success came in 1979 when results from trials at Peter Bent Brigham Hospital and the University of Colorado showed that cyclosporine combined with steroids controlled rejection better than any past drug therapy. By 1983 the FDA released cyclosporine for general use, increasing graft survival by 30 percent or more. Due to increasing public education throughout the 1980s, the number of cadaver organs available for transplantation continued to grow. This in conjunction with the increasing success of immunosuppressive agents led to an increased use of cadaveric kidneys; due to advances in immunosuppression there was no need for a genetic match. Outcome data were still better for living transplants than cadaver, but many speculated that the need for living organ donors would continue to diminish. In 1985 Thomas Starzl, a pioneering transplant surgeon, argued that advances in cadaver transplant would challenge the morality of living organ donations.

By the early 1990s the number of suitable cadaver donor organs leveled off and waiting lists grew, leading to a renewed interest in living organs. Other types of living organ transplantation became increasingly more successful. The first successful living related liver transplantation in the United States took place in 1989. At first the recipients were typically infants receiving a lobe from a parent. But transplantation between adults has been increasingly successful;

the first successful adult living liver transplantation was reported in Japan in 1994 and the first in the United States occurred in 1998. Adult to adult transplantation is technically more difficult than the pediatric procedure and the risk to the donor is far greater than a kidney donation. The death in January 2002 of Mike Hurewitz, who donated a portion of his liver to his brother at Mt. Sinai Hospital in New York, has increased safety concerns. The New York State Department of Health shut down the hospital's transplant program, one of the largest in the country, for six months. An investigation found no fault with the surgery, only with post-surgical care. Living donors for liver transplantation are almost always genetically or emotionally related to the recipient; so-called Good Samaritan or nondirected donations are very rare. UNOS reports that out of 5,327 liver transplants in 2002 only 359 were from living donors.

The first successful living lung transplantation took place at Stanford University in October 1990. In living lung donation a pair of adult donors each donate one lobe (left or right) to one recipient. The number of such transplantations is still quite low. In 2002 only 13 living donor lung transplants were reported in the United States (UNOS). Other living donor transplantations also include the pancreas and small-bowel. Because there is no shortage of cadaveric sources for either organ, living donor transplants are rare, but increasing due to better patient outcomes (Margrieter). Living donor pancreas transplantation is increasingly being supplanted by islet cell transplants.

Drug therapies continue to improve, and since the number of cadaveric organs remains fixed and there is a growing gap between the available supply and demand of organs and tissue, living donation increases. New technologies such as laparoscopic live-donor nephrectomy first performed in 1995 have made it less burdensome to be a living kidney donor. According to UNOS data, between 1999 and 2000 living donor kidney transplants increased 16.5 percent. In 2001, of the 24,076 organ transplantations performed in the United States, more than 6,507 were living donor transplantations. In 2000 UNOS began pilot testing "paired exchange" and "list-paired exchange" programs that provide further incentives for living donations. Transplant centers increasingly accept Good Samaritan or nondirected living kidney donors (Matas et al.).

Ethical, Legal and Policy Issues

ETHICAL ISSUES. While living organ donors were initially limited to blood relatives to reduce the risk of immune rejection, improved immunotherapy has expanded the pool of potential donors far outside of those related by blood, to those who are emotionally related to each other. This has resulted in expanding the notion of "relatedness" to include people related by marriage (spouses and in-laws) as well as those who are not traditionally considered relatives—friends, co-workers, members of the same church or other community group, and even those with very limited emotional ties, such as so-called Good Samaritans. With this extension of the concept of living donation, it became a logical and relatively short step from tangentially related directed living organ donors to organ donations from altruistic strangers.

How far should living donation be allowed to go? Is informed consent sufficient to justify any living donation to which a prospective donor would voluntarily consent? In other areas of medicine, and clinical research, there are limits to the risk to which healthy people—related or not—should be allowed to consent. For many, increasing risk to the donor tilts the balance away from being acceptable, meaning that at very high levels of risk, no living donor should be allowed to undertake organ donation.

One of the concerns in nondirected or Good Samaritan living donation is that strangers should not be allowed to accept the same level of risk as related donors. The argument is that relatedness matters, such that related donors have more to gain from the donation and so can be allowed to accept greater risk. The justification is that seeing a loved one's life saved or health improved is a greater benefit than the psychological benefit to a stranger of performing an altruistic act. But one can also argue that both types of donors stand to realize substantial benefits, albeit of different varieties, and that it should be up the individuals to determine whether the benefits are sufficient to justify taking the associated risks.

Some thinkers have argued that intimates may actually have an obligation to be a living organ donor (Ross), but this would seem to create a duty of heroism. There is a history of courts refusing to require beneficent acts on the part of individuals, even if they would be lifesaving (*McFall v. Shimp*, 1978). In moral philosophy, this is the distinction between actions that are obligatory and those that are supererogatory. We laud people to perform acts that are "above and beyond the call of duty," but do not require such acts of them—to do so would create a duty of heroism, demanding too much of individuals in the process and undermining the value of what it means to be truly heroic. That being said, we may think it is more understandable, and even expected, for relatives to donate an organ to someone within their family, which raises its own ethical concerns. The most important problem is pressure within the family to donate and the effect it can have on decision making—undermining effective informed consent, which must be a mainstay of any living organ donation (The Authors for the Live Organ Donor Consensus Group).

Many transplant centers go so far as to offer prospective donors false medical excuses so they do not need to tell their family member that they are unwilling to donate (ibid).

LAW AND POLICY. Specific laws covering living organ and tissue donors vary greatly between countries. In the United States the chief law addressing organ donation is the National Organ Transplant Act of 1984 (NOTA). NOTA established the Organ Procurement and Transplantation Network (OPTN), which is responsible for maintaining a national registry for organ matching, increasing the "effectiveness and efficiency of organ sharing and equity in the national system of organ allocation," and increasing the "supply of donated organs available for transplantation." The United Network for Organ Sharing (UNOS) administers the OPTN under government contract. The OPTN does not oversee living donor transplantation. However, UNOS collects data about living donor transplants in the United States and develops and recommends policies covering a range of issues including living donors. Living donation is handled by the center or hospital performing the transplantation and Medicare dictates the only organ transplantation regulations. A hospital or transplant center can opt to ignore these regulations, but will be ineligible for Medicare reimbursements.

A number of international organizations have adopted policies on human organ transplantation that include specific guidelines for living donors. For example, the World Health Organization's (WHO) "Guiding Principles on Human Organ Transplantation" states:

> Organs for transplantation should be removed preferably from the bodies of deceased persons. However, adult living persons may donate organs, but in general such donors should be genetically related to the recipients. Exceptions may be made in the case of transplantation of bone marrow and other acceptable regenerative tissues. An organ may be removed from the body of an adult living donor for the purpose of transplantation if the donor gives free consent. The donor should be free of any undue influence and pressure and sufficiently informed to be able to understand and weigh the risks, benefits and consequences of consent.

In addition, "The human body and its parts cannot be the subject of commercial transactions. Accordingly, giving or receiving payment (including any other compensation or reward) for organs should be prohibited" (WHO). The World Medical Association's "Statement on Human Organ and Tissue Donation and Transplantation" also states that

"In the case of living donors, special efforts should be made to ensure that the choice about donation is free of coercion" and persons incapable of making informed decisions should be donors in only "very limited circumstances." The Live Organ Donor Consensus Group argues that a living donor should be competent, willing, and free of coercion as well as medically suitable and psycho socially suitable (The Authors for the Live Organ Donor Consensus Group). Living donor qualifications usually include good general health, physically fit, free from high blood pressure, diabetes, cancer, kidney, and heart disease.

Donation by Minors

The early case law in the United States focuses on minors or persons incapable of consenting to being living kidney donors. In 1957 the Massachusetts Supreme Court ruled in *Masden v. Harrison* that the 19-year-old twin brother Leonard Masden could be a living kidney donor to his brother Leon. Based on the testimony of a psychiatrist who had interviewed both brothers, the court recognized that although the operation had no therapeutic value to Leonard, it had a compelling psychological value. The death of his brother would have "grave emotional impact" on Leonard. While the NOTA does not specifically address the use of minors as donors, many countries have legislation specifically addressing this issue. For example, Spain, Greece, and the Russian Federation prohibit the removal of organs from minors, although many make exceptions for bone marrow donation to a family member. In France donation is restricted to first-degree relatives. The Live Organ Donor Consensus Group was generally opposed to the use of a minor, but recognized that there may be exceptional circumstances. When the donor is mentally retarded or ill, courts have often concluded that the donor would benefit emotionally or psychologically.

Financial Incentives

Title III of the NOTA prohibits the purchase of organs: "It shall be unlawful for any person to knowingly acquire, receive, or otherwise transfer any human organ for *valuable consideration* for use in human transplantation if the transfer affects interstate commerce" (NOTA Sec. 301 [a]; emphasis added). Violators are subject to a fine up to $50,000 and/or up to five years in prison. According to the statute, "The term 'valuable consideration' does not include the reasonable payments associated with the removal, transportation, implantation, processing, preservation, quality control, and storage of a human organ or the expenses of travel, housing, and lost wages incurred by the donor of a human organ donor in connection with the donation of the organ" (NOTA Sec. 301 [a]). The Department of Justice is responsible for enforcing this prohibition, but there have been few public cases. There remains great confusion over how valuable consideration should be interpreted and understood. For example, a Pennsylvania plan to offer donor families $300 towards funeral expenses was replaced out of fear that it came to close to violating NOTA. Its replacement, the Expense Benefit Plan for Organ Donors and Their Families offers a $300 benefit per organ donor to pay for food and lodging costs.

There are reports of an increasing worldwide black market in human organs and there are few policy approaches to addressing it. For example, federal law does not prevent people from re-entering the United States after transplantation.

Health insurance coverage varies. If the recipient is covered by Medicare's end-stage renal disease program, Medicare covers the donor's expenses. The Organ Donor Leave Act of 1999 provides 30 days of paid leave for federal employees who are living donors for transplantations. A handful of states have passed similar laws. There have been some movements to provide donor insurance to cover the medical risk of donation.

Exchange Programs

The goal of exchange programs is to increase the supply of kidneys available for transplant to overcome problems of ABO and cross-match incompatibilities. In paired exchange, two living donors, who are mismatched donors for their intended recipient, effectively swap kidneys. In list-paired exchanges, a living donor donates a kidney to the general pool. In return, the intended (but mismatched) recipient advances on the waiting list for a cadaveric kidney. In 2001 Tufts-New England Medical Center launched the first exchange program, indicating it was approved by UNOS. But it is unclear what authority UNOS has over such programs. UNOS' general counsel argues that Section 301 does not apply to exchange programs, but others have expressed concerns over the meaning of "valuable consideration."

Distribution of Nondirected Donations

In recent years transplant centers have begun considering nondirected kidney donations by community members. A National Conference on the Nondirected Live Organ Donor advocates caution and suggest a framework for institutions that are considering accepting nondirected kidney donations. The conference document recommends ethical and practice guidelines. Some question how nondirected donations should be distributed. Should they remain at the transplant center first solicited, or should they enter the general pool? There is general agreement that donors cannot request that certain demographic groups do or do not receive their donation. There have been recent calls for a national system to be developed so that organs from nondirected donors can go to the first patient on a national list rather than to the first patient at the center where the organ is donated. Such an approach has been developed on a local basis by the consortium of transplant centers in the Washington, D.C. area, and may serve as a model for national expansion.

Conclusion

The growing gap between the available supply and the demand for solid organs means that the search will continue for new sources of organs. We can all agree that living donation is a growing source of solid organs, as evidenced by the fact that the number of transplanted kidneys from living donors has surpassed the number from cadaveric donors at some of the leading transplant centers in the United States. The question is not whether living organ donation will continue, but rather what conditions and policies ought to apply to make it ethically acceptable.

JEFFREY KAHN
SUSAN PARRY

SEE ALSO: *Beneficence; Bioethics, African-American Perspectives; Cybernetics; Death, Definition and Determination of; Dialysis, Kidney; Healthcare Resources, Allocation of; Informed Consent; Medical Futility; Medicare; Mistakes, Medical; Obligation and Supererogation; Organ Transplants, Medical Overview of; Organ Transplants, Sociocultural Aspects of; Technology; Xenografts;* and other *Organ and Tissue Procurement* subentries

BIBLIOGRAPHY

The Authors for the Live Organ Donor Consensus Group. 2000. "Consensus Statement on the Live Organ Donor." *Journal of the American Medical Association* 284: 2919–2926.

Fox, Renée C., and Swazey, Judith P. 1992. *Spare Parts: Organ Replacement in American Society.* New York: Oxford University Press.

Margreiter, Raimund. 1999. "Living-Donor Pancreas and Small-Bowel Transplantation." *Langenbeck's Archives of Surgery* 384: 544–549.

Matas, Arthur J.; Garvey, Catherine A.; Jacobs, Cheryl L.; Kahn, Jeffrey P. 2000. "Nondirected Donation of Kidneys from Living Donors." *New England Journal of Medicine* 343: 433–436.

McFall v. Shimp. 10 Pa. D. & C.3d 90. Allegheny County Ct. (1978).

National Organ Transplant Act. Public Law No. 98–507 (1984).

Organ Donor Leave Act. H.R. 457, Pub Law No. 106–56 (Sept. 24, 1999).

Ross, Lainie F.; Rubin, David T.; Siegler, Mark; et al. 1997. "Ethics of a Paired-Kidney-Exchange Program." *New England Journal of Medicine* 336: 1752–1755.

World Health Organization. 1991. "Guiding Principles on Human Organ Transplantation." Geneva, World Health Organization.

World Medical Organization. 2000. "Statement on Human Organ and Tissue Donation and Transplantation." Adopted by the 52nd WMA General Assembly in Edinburgh, Scotland.

Woodle, E. Steve. 2003. "A History of Living Donor Transplantation: From Twins to Trades." *Transplantation Proceedings* 35: 901–902.

INTERNET RESOURCES

Ritsch, Malcolm E., Jr. 2003. "Intended Recipient Exchanges, Paired Exchanges and NOTA § 301." Available from <http://www.unos.org/news/newsDetail.asp?id=265>.

United Network for Organ Sharing. 2003. "Transplants by Donor Type." Available from <http://www.optn.org/latestData/rptData.asp>.

ORGANIZATIONAL ETHICS IN HEALTHCARE

• • •

Organizational ethics in healthcare, which sometimes is referred to as institutional ethics, can be defined as the ethical analysis of decisions and actions taken by healthcare organizations, that is, institutional boards or committees and individuals acting as agents of those organizations. This entry begins with background observations about organizational ethics as a subfield and then addresses the history of concern about this topic, the major issues in the field, ethical perspectives and strategies for addressing those issues, the relationship of organizational ethics to clinical ethics committees, institutional review boards and compliance programs, the development of organizational ethics programs in healthcare institutions, and some of the current issues in the field.

Background

There has been much discussion of whether organizational ethics should be considered a subcategory of the clinical issues that normally are addressed by institutional ethics committees or is more closely related to business ethics. This issue is significant inasmuch as it affects the scope of the problems involved in the field, the perspective adopted to address those issues, and the question of who should have responsibility for dealing with these matters (for example, clinical medical ethics committees or administrative units). Organizational ethics clearly is related both to clinical medical ethics in that institutional policies and actions affect patient care and to business ethics in that many institutional issues are primarily business concerns involving financial matters, strategic planning, and compliance with legal regulations—issues that do not affect patient care directly. Healthcare organizations, of course, also have business relations with patients with respect to the payment of bills and insurance matters.

As in the field of business ethics generally, there has been some discussion in the published literature on healthcare organizational ethics of whether institutions and organizations can be considered moral agents in a meaningful sense in light of the fact that they are not individuals with moral sensitivities, motives, or consciences. Organizations do, however, set goals and take actions in pursuit of those goals, although their actions often result from collective rather than individual decisions. Also, organizations normally are evaluated and judged as to whether their goals and actions are morally acceptable, and they often are held accountable for harm done or are praised for morally worthy policies and actions. Although organizations may be thought to have a moral status slightly different from that of individuals, it cannot be doubted that they are responsible agents in an ethically meaningful sense.

History

In the United States ethical problems in relation to organizations have been recognized since bioethics as a field began to take shape. The issue of research involving human subjects was raised in the 1960s and came to public attention in the 1970s with the revelation of the disregard of informed consent and the misinformation given to African-American males in the Tuskegee Study. Although this was an issue with clear organizational implications, research ethics came to be treated as a special concern.

This led to the establishment of the institutional review board system rather than to consideration of other issues in organizational ethics. The distribution of scarce medical equipment for renal dialysis (as a matter of triage) was debated in the 1970s, raising procedural issues concerning who was to make such decisions on behalf of healthcare organizations and on what basis. The ethical propriety of for-profit healthcare institutions was the subject of conferences held by the National Institute of Medicine in the early 1980s and editorials in the *New England Journal of Medicine*.

It was not until the 1990s that healthcare organizational ethics began to be identified as a separate field. The American Hospital Association issued a management advisory in 1992 and later instituted its Organizational Ethics Initiative, an ethics education program for hospital administrators. The Woodstock Theological Center convened a seminar on organizational ethics in healthcare in 1994, although the framework that was adopted for consideration of the topics addressed was one of "professional" ethics. Almost simultaneously with the publication of the Woodstock report in 1995, the American College of Healthcare Executives issued a major revision of its 1970 Code of Ethics for healthcare management professionals, a document with lasting merit that spells out definite standards of conduct.

A major step in the development of the field came in 1995 when the Joint Commission for Accreditation of Healthcare Organizations unexpectedly added requirements for "Organization Ethics" to its accreditation standards for all healthcare organizations. Those standards required that hospitals have a code of ethical behavior addressing marketing, admissions, transfer, discharge and billing practices (issues related to patients), and "the relationship of the hospital and its staff members to other healthcare providers, educational institutions and payers." The required hospital code also must protect "the integrity of clinical decision making, regardless of how the hospital compensates or shares financial risk with its leaders, managers, clinical staff, and licensed independent practitioners" (Joint Commission on Accreditation of Healthcare Organizations). Although the full implications of these standards have not yet been determined, this action effectively established the field as an area of administrative responsibility and a discipline worthy of separate attention.

Organizational ethics in healthcare has been recognized as a concern in other countries, although these issues are more likely to be considered matters of health regulation and planning in public health systems. Numerous publications on the subject have appeared since the mid-1990s in Europe, and the Comisión Nacional de Bioética of Mexico held its first conference on organizational ethics in healthcare institutions in 2002.

Major Issues in Organizational Ethics

Concerns normally associated with organizational ethics in the United States include a wide variety of issues. Among the most common are the following.

Charity and uncompensated care pose financial problems for most institutions. From an ethical perspective, however, healthcare institutions must consider ways to provide a level of care consistent with their mission and the needs of the community. Not-for-profit institutions have an obligation to provide public benefits in return for their tax-exempt status; some states in the United States have begun to require community assessments to determine the nature and level of the services needed.

Ethical issues in managed care have been discussed widely under the heading of organizational ethics. These issues include conflict of interest problems, reasonable benefit and exclusion regulations, and the provision of fair hearings of appeals if treatment is denied.

After the promulgation of government regulations in 1999, confidentiality of patient information became more of an organizational issue than a matter of professional responsibility. This is appropriate in light of the multiplicity of providers involved in patient care and the maintenance and transfer of patient records electronically.

Consideration of employee wages and benefits involves judgments about a "living" or "just" wage at the lower end of the scale and merit at the higher end. The fairness of wages for employees relative to other employees, or the "comparable worth" of positions and responsibilities, is another factor. Hiring and promotion practices along with downsizing raise ethical issues for healthcare organizations, as do relations with labor unions.

Organizations that provide human services also face problems of discrimination either by employees or by clients on the basis of race, ethnicity, gender, disability, and religion. Diversity training that is based on a firm institutional commitment to equal and sensitive treatment often is considered necessary.

Advertising and marketing concerns require special attention to the needs of vulnerable populations as well as the common standards of fairness in advertising. Pharmaceutical companies, some of whose practices have been criticized for decades, should be considered healthcare providers. Professional associations and healthcare institutions can have a significant influence on the practices of pharmaceutical companies and other suppliers.

Environmental concerns of healthcare organizations constitute a serious issue. These concerns include not only proper disposal of medical and toxic waste but comprehensive plans for the reduction of waste and solid waste management.

Other ethical issues for healthcare organizations that have been discussed include governmental relations (including lobbying) and community relations, externally, and socially responsible investing and professional relations, internally.

Perspectives and Strategies

Traditional Western ethical perspectives have been applied to organizational ethics issues. Those perspectives include utilitarianism (which has a certain affinity with the stakeholder strategy noted below), rationalism (which has provided support for organizational policy development and codes of ethical behavior), virtues theory and idealism (which has been supportive of mission statement analysis), and various contextual theories, including feminist ethics (which have drawn attention to historical institutional responsibilities and relations). Leonard Weber has proposed a priority list of principles for decision making that takes into account patients' interests along with organizational interests and community benefit. In addition to the application of normative ethical perspectives to institutional ethics issues, the following organizational strategies have been proposed.

PROFESSIONAL APPROACHES. The American Medical Association has addressed organizational ethics issues from the perspective of the historical responsibilities and obligations of healthcare professionals. This approach has been expanded to include the obligations of professionals other than physicians: The Code of Ethics of the American College of Healthcare Executives (2000) established standards for healthcare administrators. The professional codes of lawyers, accountants, and engineers, along with those of clergypersons and social workers, also should be included in this approach inasmuch as professionals from those fields work in healthcare institutions.

Professional approaches to organizational ethics have been especially successful in addressing conflict of interest problems. Conflicts of interest occur whenever a decision maker has an interest in making a particular decision on the basis of factors other than the interest of the patient (if it is a professional decision) or the interest of the organization (if it is a decision made as an agent of an institution). The conflict can be a matter of personal gain from the decision in question or can be a conflict between responsibility to a patient and responsibility to an institution. Conflicts of interest also can occur when there is institutional pressure on an individual to depart from the spirit or letter of a professional code. Professional codes of accountants, social workers, clergypersons, lawyers, and administrators must be considered along with those of physicians and nurses.

THE STAKEHOLDER STRATEGY. This perspective, which has been borrowed from business ethics, focuses on the consequences of institutional decisions for the many stakeholders and stakeholder groups that are affected (Evans and Freeman). Stakeholders in healthcare organizations include professionals, employees, business partners, and the community, in addition to patients. Spencer et al. (2000) have proposed the adaptation of a stakeholder strategy that involves a specific priority list of stakeholder interests for healthcare institutions: patient populations, professional excellence, organizational viability, community access, and public health.

THE MISSION STATEMENT STRATEGY. This perspective derives a critical examination of organizational decisions and actions directly from the mission and goals adopted by an institution. Those goals can be subjected to ethical evaluation (Hall) and often have to be elaborated and applied through high-level institutional decision making.

CORPORATE CULTURE ANALYSIS. This approach represents an application of the organizational theory common in business ethics to the analysis of healthcare institutions (Boyle et al.). As collective entities, healthcare organizations generate patterns of behavior, both formal and informal, that can be analyzed with respect to their ethical dimensions and implications.

Although specific strategies may differ, there is general agreement among commentators that organizational ethics issues involve many dimensions besides ethical considerations and that a multidisciplinary approach is needed. The purpose of the organizational ethics perspectives and strategies described in this entry is to highlight the ethical dimension of institutional decision making at all levels.

Relationships with Clinical Ethics Committees, Institutional Review Boards, and Compliance Programs

Organizational ethics is closely related to clinical medical ethics in that many clinical ethical problems have organizational implications. Difficulties with nursing, pharmacy, and other professional services may result from staffing decisions. The availability, adequacy, and confidentiality of medical records are organizational matters. Institutional policies often govern clinical issues such as orders not to resuscitate and palliative care. The organization and availability of social services, including ethics consultation, also is an organizational responsibility. Healthcare organizations also have direct relations with patients with respect to admissions, discharge, and transfer as well as billing and other financial matters. Inasmuch as any of these issues involve organizational decisions and actions, they may move out of the jurisdiction of clinical ethics committees and into the wider realm of organizational ethics.

The relationship of organizational ethics to institutional review boards for the protection of human subjects in medical research involves less of an overlap of responsibilities. Healthcare organizations need to provide resources and staff for institutional review boards, but the activities of those boards is subject to specific federal guidelines. It is appropriate, however, for healthcare organizations to decide whether research projects are consistent with the mission of the institution and/or interfere with other staff responsibilities.

Organizational ethics also is closely related to compliance programs. Although organizational compliance programs have a responsibility for bringing institutional activities into conformity with federal and state regulations, such programs also may be considered to have responsibility for the conformity of activities to institutional mission statements or ethical goals. Although this responsibility is mentioned specifically in the Federal Sentencing Guidelines under which compliance programs are established, those programs have tended to focus on legal compliance and ignore ethical goals and objectives that go beyond the law.

Some authors have suggested that organizational ethics should be conceived of as a comprehensive perspective or program that would include clinical ethics, compliance, and institutional review board functions in a single organizational unit or division. These activities, however, are generally well-established institutional programs, and it may make little sense to attempt to include them organizationally under a new unit that has its own problems and issues to address.

Organizational Ethics Programs in Healthcare Institutions

Healthcare institutions have considered various methods for addressing organizational ethical issues and bringing ethical perspectives into organizational cultures. Because concern for these issues has been raised in discussions of clinical ethics, some commentators think that the mandate of clinical ethics committees could be expanded to include

institutional issues. It generally is recognized, however, that organizational issues can be quite different from clinical matters and that clinical ethics committees normally do not include the administrators who have responsibility for these issues or individuals with relevant administrative competencies and experience. If organizational ethics concerns are to be addressed within the scope of a clinical ethics program, therefore, a separate track or process may be necessary.

A few healthcare organizations have formed separate organizational ethics committees, but considerable time probably will be needed for those new units to acquire the perspective, the sense of role, and the credibility within the organization necessary to be effective. Other suggestions for organizational ethics programs in healthcare institutions involve the use of consultants and governing board subcommittees and the assignment of the function to compliance programs. Although there has been general agreement that as a result of the nature of the issues involved, organizational ethics programs must involve top administrative and governing board representatives, the issue of the involvement of employees and professionals from all levels within the organization and outside community members is more problematic.

Current and Future Issues in Healthcare Organizational Ethics

Although the organizational ethics issues mentioned above are areas of organizational activity that will require attention well into the future, it is worth mentioning three issues that have not been addressed adequately to date.

First, providing access to basic healthcare for all people remains the foremost challenge for healthcare organizations. In countries with national health systems the challenge takes the form of finding adequate funding, educating skilled personnel and professionals, and eliminating bureaucratic problems. In countries with largely privatized healthcare systems, such as the United States, the problem entails providing care for those who, because they are unemployed, underemployed, or working poor, lack access to care for financial reasons. This may be considered a social or political issue with a scope wider than that of any individual healthcare organization, but in countries where healthcare is provided by nonprofit corporations it is an organizational problem as well.

Nonprofit organizations generally are thought to have a public obligation to provide healthcare to people who cannot afford to pay. Competitive pressures on organizations, however, in many cases have moved this mission off the corporate agenda. Many nonprofit healthcare organizations view charity care as a business loss rather than an essential organizational goal, and many investor-owned healthcare corporations refuse to accept the provision of charity care as either a mission goal or a public obligation. Serious attention to this problem would require community needs assessments and regular social audits of institutional performance.

Second, there is the question of how healthcare institutions can develop and promote ethical perspectives within the organization. Ethical concern for the issues mentioned above is still for the most part a matter of informal discussion among administrators, members of clinical ethics committees, and academic and social commentators. Including top administrators and governing board members in organizational processes for addressing ethical issues is essential but often difficult. Few organizations have formal mechanisms for an ethical consideration of organizational issues, and even fewer involve top administrators or governing board members in that process. Many administrators seem to believe that compliance programs can take care of ethical concerns adequately or that ethical concerns are a matter of community perspectives that should be left to the governing board.

Third, the excessively aggressive practices of pharmaceutical companies must be addressed. This issue has become more than just a matter of professional marketing practices. It is a social issue in that society is becoming increasingly dependent on prescription drugs. Healthcare organizations have a significant role to play in educating the public about the dangers of overmedication and in curbing the aggressive advertising practices of pharmaceutical companies.

ROBERT T. HALL

SEE ALSO: *Corporate Compliance; Healthcare Management Ethics; Just Wages and Salaries; Managed Care*

BIBLIOGRAPHY

Boyle, Philip; Dubose, Edwin R.; Ellingson, Stephen J.; et al. 2001. *Organizational Ethics in Health Care: Principles, Cases, and Practical Solutions.* San Francisco: Jossey-Bass.

Evans, William M., and Freeman, R. Edward. 1996. "A Stakeholder Theory of the Modern Corporation: Kantian Capitalism." In *Ethical Issues in Business: A Philosophical Approach,* 5th edition, ed. Thomas Donaldson and Patricia Werhane. Upper Saddle Ridge, NJ: Prentice-Hall.

Hall, Robert T. 2000. *An Introduction to Healthcare Organizational Ethics.* Oxford, Eng.: Oxford University Press.

Joint Commission on Accreditation of Healthcare Organizations. 1988. *HAS: 1998 Hospital Accreditation Standards.* Oakbrook Terrace, IL: Joint Commission on Accreditation of Healthcare Organizations.

Khushf, George. 1997. "Administrative and Organizational Ethics." *HealthCare Ethics Committee Forum* 9(4): 299–309.

Spencer, Edward M.; Mills, Ann E.; Rorty, Mary V.; and Werhane, Patricia H. 2000. *Organization Ethics in Health Care.* Oxford, Eng.: Oxford University Press.

Weber, Leonard J. 2001. *Business Ethics in Healthcare: Beyond Compliance.* Bloomington: Indiana University Press.

Woodstock Theological Center. 1995. *Ethical Considerations in the Business Aspects of Health Care.* Washington, D.C.: Georgetown University Press.

INTERNET RESOURCE

"American College of Healthcare Executives Code of Ethics: As Amended by the Council of Regents at its Annual Meeting on March 25, 2000." <http://www.ache.org/abt_ache/code.cfm>.

ORGAN TRANSPLANTS, MEDICAL OVERVIEW OF

• • •

The first successful kidney transplant, performed by Dr. Joseph Murray at Boston's Peter Bent Brigham Hospital, took place in 1954. Since then, remarkable advances have occurred in transplantation. Antirejection drugs have dramatically improved success rates, and the vast majority of recipients are restored to well-being and enjoy productive and active lives. Better preservation of organs allows longer storage times, so organs can be transported over greater distances. In addition to kidneys, numerous other organs, including livers, hearts, lungs, and pancreases, are commonly transplanted today. Certain areas remain problematic, however. The control of rejection of transplanted organs is not yet perfect, and post-transplant complications, such as infection and cancer, can still threaten the health of recipients. But the major obstacle remains the inadequate number of organs available to meet the need of potential recipients on the waiting list.

Development of Transplantation

Attempts to transplant a kidney from one person to another began in the 1930s. These attempts were based on laboratory experiments by Alexis Carrel, a researcher who had developed a technique for suturing blood vessels in 1902. These early transplants all failed because the recipient's immune system recognized that the transplanted organ (often called a *graft*) was a foreign substance. The immune system then attacked and destroyed the organ, a process known as *rejection*. Success was finally achieved in 1954 because the donor and recipient were identical twins. Identical twins have the same tissue type, so the recipient's immune system perceives the transplant organ as a part of its own body, and rejection does not occur. Because every healthy person has two kidneys, one kidney can be donated from a living person to another person.

An organ or tissue that is transplanted between genetically identical twins is called an *isograft. Allografts* are organs or tissues that are transplanted between genetically nonidentical people, which occurs when organs or tissues are donated from a deceased person (cadaver donor). An *autograft* is a tissue transplanted from one part of a person's body to another part, such as when a burn victim has healthy skin grafted from one area of the body to the burned area. A *xenograft* is an organ or tissue transplanted from a different species, for example, a pig liver transplanted into a human.

During the 1950s, antirejection drugs had not yet been developed, so transplants were limited to kidneys from identical-twin donors. In 1959, however, Murray and his colleagues at Brigham Hospital again achieved a historic feat. They transplanted a kidney from a nonidentical twin to his brother, who had undergone total body X-ray treatment (irradiation). This treatment suppressed the patient's immune response so that his body accepted the new organ, and he lived for twenty-six years after the transplant. Irradiation was also tried with kidney transplants from cadaver donors. For most patients, however, the outcome was fatal because the irradiation weakened their immune systems too much. Although they accepted the transplanted organ, patients died from infection because their natural defenses against bacteria and viruses were reduced. It seemed evident that irradiation for transplantation "was too dangerous to be practical" (Starzl).

During this time, chemical immunosuppression (drug therapy) was being studied. In 1960 the French surgeon René Küss achieved successful nonrelated kidney transplantation using a combination of total-body irradiation, steroids, and 6-mercaptopurine. Azathioprine (also called Imuran) was later derived from 6-mercaptopurine. The combination of azathioprine and prednisone (a type of steroid) to prevent organ rejection, suggested by Sir Roy Calne, was a clinical milestone in 1962, as kidney transplant results improved and fewer side effects occurred.

In 1967 a heart and a liver were each successfully transplanted—the heart by Dr. Christiaan Barnard in Capetown, South Africa, and the liver by Dr. Thomas Starzl in Denver, Colorado. These successful transplants were followed by a flurry of activity as hospitals worldwide rushed to perform transplant surgery. Lung, bowel, and pancreas transplants were all attempted during the 1960s. Most of these attempts failed, however, and many transplant programs were abruptly stopped. Methods of suppressing the immune system were too crude to achieve the fine balance needed to control rejection but avoid fatal infection. By 1975 there were only two liver transplant programs in the world. Starzl was continuing to transplant in Denver, Colorado, and Calne was leading a program in Cambridge, England.

The modern era of transplantation began in the late 1970s and the early 1980s, when drugs to prevent rejection were discovered that were vastly superior to existing ones. The first of these was cyclosporine, a drug that acted much more specifically on the patient's immune system. It primarily affected those cells that were responsible for initiating the rejection process. Other drugs followed, including FK506 and OKT3, which quickly found their place in patient management. The decade of the 1980s witnessed a proliferation of transplant centers worldwide.

Refinements in surgical techniques and better methods to preserve donor organs also contributed to improved patient outcome, and successful kidney, liver, and heart transplants became routine. Lung transplantation was developed at the Toronto General Hospital in Canada, where single-lung transplantation was established in 1983 and double-lung transplantation in 1986. By the year 2000 more than 600,000 organ transplants had been performed worldwide, and transplant centers with special interests accumulated huge experiences that benefited not only their own patients, but those in other centers as well. At the University of Minnesota alone, more than 1,000 pancreas transplants had been performed by 2000 (Sutherland et al.).

Success with bowel transplantation was more difficult to achieve compared to other organs. The intestine has a large number of cells called *lymphocytes,* which help trigger rejection and also react against the recipient (graft-versus-host disease). Bowel transplantation was not successfully performed until the late 1980s when a patient in Kiel, Germany, and another in Paris, France, had prolonged survival. The first successful combined small-bowel and liver transplant took place at University Hospital (London, Canada) in 1988. Experience from these centers and from Pittsburgh showed that bowel transplants could be worthwhile for selected patients who either had part of their bowel removed or had inadequate bowel function. The antirejection drug FK506 improved the success rate of bowel transplantation, and patients could resume eating a normal diet after their transplant without the need for special intravenous feeding solutions.

Transplantation of islet cells from the pancreas first occurred in the mid-1970s. Rather than transplanting the donor's whole pancreas, the insulin-producing islet cells were removed from the donor pancreas. The cells, injected into the portal vein of the recipient's liver, adhered to the liver. The cells then began producing insulin. For diabetic patients who had to take insulin to stabilize their blood-sugar levels, islet-cell transplantation eliminated or reduced the need for daily insulin injections. Although reports began to emerge of short-term and prolonged insulin independence in 1990 (Scharp et al.), it was not until ten years later that the most significant progress to date was made. The transplant team at the University of Alberta, in Edmonton, Canada, developed a specific protocol of antirejection drugs combined with the transplantation of fresh islets from more than one donor to supply a critical mass of insulin-producing cells (Shapiro et al.). That success has led the National Institutes of Health to sponsor an international trial of islet transplantation using the Edmonton protocol. Because of the inadequate number of cadaver donors, however, animal islet cells, probably from pigs, may be required in the future.

The Cadaver Organ Donor

Traditionally, death has been declared on the basis of cardiopulmonary criteria: The heart stops beating and the patient can no longer breathe. Once the heart stops, oxygen-rich blood is no longer pumped to the body's organs, and the organs' cell functions begin to deteriorate. During the 1960s, organs came either from living donors (for kidneys) or from cadaver donors who were declared dead by the traditional cardiopulmonary criteria (non-heart-beating donors). The first successful liver transplants in 1967 used organs from donors who were removed from ventilators (artificial breathing machines) and pronounced dead after the heart had stopped.

As medical technology progressed and it became possible to maintain bodies after death using mechanical support, doctors needed to determine when a patient could be declared dead. Accordingly, in 1968, an ad hoc committee comprising medical doctors, a lawyer, a philosopher, and a theologian convened at the Harvard Medical School to define acceptable criteria for brain death. They decided that death could be declared by neurologic criteria as well as

traditional cardiac criteria. Brain-dead donors, with the assistance of a ventilator, have oxygen circulating in their blood, which maintains the usefulness of organs for transplant. Brain death is declared after a series of tests have been performed. The cause of death, such as trauma, intracerebral hemorrhage, hypoxia, or primary brain tumor, must be known. Patients with potentially reversible conditions, such as hypothermia or drug-induced coma, are not considered potential donors. To be declared brain dead, therefore, a patient must be in an irreversible coma and not respond to pain. There are no brain-stem reflexes, so the patient does not breathe, swallow, or blink. Apnea testing shows that the patient cannot breathe when taken off the ventilator. After death, tests ensure that the deceased patient is a suitable donor, without disease or infection that could possibly be transmitted to the transplant recipient. In 1971 Finland became the first nation to accept the legality of brain-death criteria. Most countries recognize the legal status of brain death and accept brain death as a medical basis to declare death.

Brain-dead donors are preferred for transplant, rather than non-heart-beating donors, because they almost invariably provide better quality organs. When non-heart-beating donors are used, transplants are usually limited to tissues and kidneys, and sometimes the liver. By the time the heart has stopped beating and death is declared through the absence of pulse and respiration, other organs, such as the heart and lungs, are too damaged for transplant. Because of the worldwide shortage of organ donors, however, many countries have explored the possibility of using non-heart-beating donors in addition to brain-dead donors.

Non-heart-beating donors fall into two categories: uncontrolled and controlled. Uncontrolled non-heart-beating donors are those in whom death is sudden and unexpected, without any preparatory time to plan for organ removal. Examples are victims of accidents or heart attacks who arrive in hospital emergency rooms *in extremis* (at the point of death), perhaps after the heart has already stopped beating. They do not respond to resuscitative measures, their lives cannot be saved despite all medical efforts, and they are pronounced dead. Consent for donation has to be obtained urgently, and organ removal is a hasty event, usually performed under far less than ideal circumstances. Still, the organs may have been deprived of blood flow and oxygen for so long that they are irreparably damaged and would not function if transplanted.

Controlled non-heart-beating donors are those in whom death is a planned event. The patient, with a hopeless prognosis, is going to have life support withdrawn because the patient and next of kin wish to forgo any measures or interventions that would prolong life. The patient has previously expressed the wish to donate after death, and consent for donation is obtained prior to death. Surgical removal of organs is timed to occur within minutes of cardiac arrest. In this situation, the organs are generally less damaged than they are with uncontrolled non-heart-beating donors.

Non-heart-beating donors have been used in Spain, the Netherlands, and the United States, although these countries have predominantly used brain-dead donors. Before 1988, when Sweden adopted its brain-death laws, transplant programs retrieved and transplanted livers from donors whose hearts had stopped beating. In 1995 an international workshop on non-heart-beating donors was held in Maastricht, Netherlands, and recommendations were put forward to guide transplant specialists on the use of nonheartbeating donors (Koostra).

The Living Organ Donor

Normal, healthy individuals can donate one of their kidneys or a part of another organ for transplantation. Because of the limited number of cadaver donors and the increasing population of patients developing kidney failure each year, greater use is being made of kidneys from living donors. The best long-term results of kidney transplantation are those achieved with living donors. In countries that typically use cadaver donors, the rate of living donors varies. In the United States, approximately 35 percent of all kidney transplants are from living donors; in Canada, 48 percent; and in the United Kingdom, only 6 percent. Japan has brain death-criteria, but acceptance of the concept for purposes of organ donation has been slow. Consequently, 78 percent of kidney transplants are from living donors.

Advances in minimally invasive surgery now allow kidneys to be removed from living donors through much smaller incisions, allowing for earlier discharge (as early as 48 hours), and shortening the overall recovery period for the donor. The procedure is referred to as *laparoscopic* kidney removal. Rather than making a long and painful incision over the flank with removal of a rib to retrieve the kidney, slender instruments the diameter of a pencil are inserted into the abdominal cavity through tiny incisions. Carbon dioxide is used to fill the abdominal cavity, which allows the organs to separate from one another. With the use of fiber optics, a camera sees the inside of the abdomen and projects the picture onto a screen for the surgeon. Then the kidney is dissected from its attachments and removed through an incision just large enough for the kidney to fit through the muscles and skin (2 to 3 inches). The donors experience much less pain after the surgery, they recover more quickly, and return to normal activity and employment sooner.

A portion of the liver, lung, pancreas, or bowel can be removed from a living adult and transplanted into a suitably sized recipient, either a child or an adult who is smaller than the donor. Blood-group matching and size matching of the donor and recipient are very important. In most instances, living donors are either genetically related to the recipients or "emotionally related," such as a spouse or close friend. Parent-to-child living-donor liver donation began in the early 1990s, and it has become common in major pediatric transplant centers. A small segment (one-quarter) of the liver is removed from the donor. The use of living liver donors has significantly reduced the number of children dying while on transplant waiting lists. Adult-to-child lung donation is also possible, by removing a lobe of a donor's lung and transplanting it into the chest cavity of a child whose diseased lung has been removed. Living liver donation can also be performed between two adults. Rather than using a small part of the donor liver, as in a parent-to-child transplant, the largest lobe of the liver, which makes up about two-thirds of the organ, is removed and transplanted into a size-matched adult recipient.

Given the severe shortage of donated cadaver organs, relatives, especially parents, may feel compelled to donate. The donor must understand the risks and benefits of donation. Although living donors place themselves at risk, they may experience a psychological benefit from saving, or attempting to save, their loved one's life. In addition, the recipient does not have to wait as long for the transplant and will likely be healthier. This factor, combined with a reduced ischemic time (the length of time the organ has no blood supply) may provide greater success than transplants from cadaver donors. Because the donor and recipient operations can take place simultaneously, the organ does not have to be stored and transported, and ischemia is reduced and organ function is not compromised.

The operative risk of a kidney donor dying is approximately 3 in 10,000 (Najarian et al.). There is general acceptance that the risk is considered low enough to justify the procedure. The risk for a person donating the major portion of the liver is estimated to be much higher, perhaps ten times as high. The exact percentage is not known because no national or international registry has accumulated all the donor data to document the risk. However, deaths have occurred, and some have been widely published in the press (Strong). Experience from individual centers indicates that the chance of a postoperative complication that may interfere with the recovery of the liver donor is as high as one in five patients. Some physicians and surgeons have questioned the justification for living donation that could potentially harm the donor. On the other hand, living donations are an important avenue to reduce the organ shortage. Without living donors, many patients would be denied transplantation.

Organ Retrieval and Preservation

After patients are declared dead and consent has been obtained, they are transferred to an operating room where organs and tissues are removed. Local surgeons may remove organs and send them to a transplant center, or often the transplant team travels to the donor hospital to remove and transport the organs. Surgical teams from different centers may be involved, and each team may remove a different organ before returning by air or ground travel (depending on the distance) to its own transplant center. Organ and tissue recovery is a delicate surgical procedure. Transplant staff are careful to prevent visible disfigurement so that usual funeral arrangements for the donor, including an open casket, are possible.

In the operating room, an incision is made on the donor that extends from the sternal notch (breastbone) to the pelvis. The rib cage and abdomen are retracted so the organs can be seen easily, and the organs are examined for damage or disease that may not have been detected by earlier tests. If the organ appears normal, the surgeon begins to carefully dissect, or cut away, the tissue surrounding the organ. The aorta (the blood vessel through which blood flows from the heart to the rest of the body) is then clamped, and a tube is inserted into it. Through that tube a specially prepared, cold solution (4°C) is infused to flush blood out of each organ and lower the organ's temperature. Cold acts as a metabolic brake, reducing the oxygen requirements of the organ to near zero, thereby helping to preserve the organ. If several organs are to be removed, the procedure takes approximately two to three hours. The heart or lungs are removed first, the liver and small bowel next, followed by the pancreas and kidneys. The kidneys are removed together and then separated—the kidneys are preserved and stored separately so that they can be transplanted into two patients.

Each organ is immersed in cold preservation solution and stored in a sterile container, which is surrounded by ice, and transported in an insulated cooler. Because storage times are limited, recipient surgery has to be timed in relation to the donor procedure. When the donor and recipient are at the same transplant center, the surgeries can be done simultaneously so that organs do not have to be cold-stored for long periods. When the ischemic time is shortened, initial organ function is better after transplant.

Various solutions have been developed to preserve organs, including Collins, Euro-Collins, HTK, and UW solutions. Different solutions can be used for different organs removed from the same donor. There are limits to the time that organs can be stored ("cold ischemic time") before permanent cell damage occurs and the organ cannot be used for transplant. Typically, kidneys are transplanted within 24 hours and livers are transplanted within 12 hours. Heart and lung preservation times remain limited to between 4 to 6 hours.

Whereas most organs are flushed and stored in a cold solution for transport, kidneys can be preserved by two methods: cold storage or machine perfusion. Most often, kidneys are immersed in a cold solution and stored in a sterile container (cold storage). With perfusion, the kidney is attached to a machine that periodically flushes a cold solution through the kidneys until they are transplanted. Long-term results show that kidney transplants are equally successful whether they are cold-stored or machine-perfused.

Organ Distribution

Potential recipients are assessed by transplant teams that evaluate each patient's disease to determine if a transplant is needed, and how quickly it is needed. General criteria are that the potential recipient has a disease for which transplantation is good treatment, and that there are no other health issues that would make a transplant too risky. Transplant centers define their own specific criteria for patient acceptance on waiting lists, such as age and rehabilitation potential. Once on the list, each patient should have an equitable chance of receiving an organ, because policy guidelines have been formulated to ensure appropriate and fair distribution of organs.

Several factors may be considered in selecting the recipient once an organ has been donated: blood group; tissue type (for kidneys); body size of donor and recipient; amount of time the patient has been waiting; proximity to the transplant center; and the patient's current health and "status rating." When their names are added to waiting lists, potential recipients are assigned a status code rating that describes their medical condition. For example, a rating of "1" is given to a patient whose health is stable and who is waiting at home. The highest number, "4," is given to a patient who is on life support in an intensive care unit and may die within days without a transplant. This number or rating changes as the patient's health changes so that the most urgent patients can receive transplants first.

When an organ becomes available, the most suitable recipient on the waiting list is identified through computer and telephone communication between transplant centers and organ procurement agencies. The role of the agencies is to facilitate the procurement of organs after a donor is identified, and assist in the distribution of organs to appropriate recipients according to allocation guidelines. In some countries, such as Canada and the United Kingdom, the agencies are run and funded by governments. In the United States, they are independent organizations that act as arms of the transplant centers. They cover specific geographic regions and charge the transplant centers for the costs they incur. The transplant centers pass on the costs to the recipients' medical insurance. Transplant centers maintain waiting lists of potential recipients for matching with donors in their own region. National waiting lists are also maintained for sharing donor organs between regions, depending on the priority of sick patients. In the United States, the United Network for Organ Sharing (UNOS) maintains a national, computerized list of potential recipients.

In Scandinavia (Norway, Sweden, Finland, and Denmark), Scandiatransplant organizes the exchange of transplant organs. Exchange rules have evolved over time, but transplant organs generally cross international boundaries easily. The UK Transplant Service serves all of Britain and is linked with other agencies in western Europe. In Europe, organ-matching agencies in Italy, France, Spain, and other countries arrange organ distribution according to agreed-upon rules. Eurotransplant, located in the Netherlands, registers potential recipients and distributes organs among the Netherlands, Belgium, Luxembourg, Germany, and Austria.

Rejection and Immunosuppression

After the transplant, the body's attempt to reject the organ is normal, since the function of the immune system is to recognize and attack foreign substances, including a transplanted organ. There are three types of organ rejection: hyperacute rejection; acute rejection; and chronic, long-term rejection. Hyperacute rejection occurs when the recipient's immune system, pre-sensitized by antibodies, immediately recognizes the transplant as foreign. The organ is rejected within minutes to hours. This type of rejection can be avoided if "crossmatch" tests using the donor's and the recipient's blood are performed before the transplant. Although hyperacute rejection can be avoided, acute or chronic rejection may still occur. Acute rejection is characterized by rapid onset, usually several days after the transplant. The closer the match between donor and recipient

tissue, the less likely an acute rejection episode will occur. This is particularly important in kidney transplantation. Chronic rejection develops more slowly, occurring many months or years after transplantation, and it gradually compromises function of the graft.

Transplant patients take drugs to suppress the immune response and prevent rejection. Drug therapy (immunosuppression) is usually started during the transplant surgery, and continues after the transplant. Larger doses of drugs are given in the first few weeks after transplantation, when the risk of acute rejection is the greatest. The doses are tapered over time, and most patients need relatively small doses years after their transplant. If acute rejection occurs, the dosage of the patient's regular antirejection drugs may be increased temporarily. Alternatively, other immunosuppressants, such as OKT3, antilymphocyte globulin, or antithymocyte globulin, may be added temporarily to reverse rejection episodes. New immunosuppressants continue to be investigated in clinical trials and animal studies to assess their effectiveness and side effects.

The antirejection drug cyclosporine was first used in transplant patients in 1978. The first clinical studies showed improved patient and organ survival. Until the 1990s, cyclosporine was the mainstay of immunosuppression. Another drug, FK506 (tacrolimus) is a valuable alternative to cyclosporine. Although it is a completely different molecule from cyclosporine, it has a similar effect on the immune system. Either cyclosporine or FK506 is used as baseline immunosuppression in most organ recipients. Prednisone (a steroid) is commonly used as well, but much smaller doses are required because of the effectiveness of cyclosporine and FK506. There are other immunosuppressive drugs that may be added, depending upon specific patient characteristics, the organ transplanted, and the doses of the other drugs being given. Immunosuppression protocols vary among transplant centers, but, as a general principle, drug doses are reduced over time to low levels to minimize the risk of side effects.

Immunosuppression requires a careful balance so that organ rejection is prevented and side effects are minimized. All immunosuppressive drugs have some side effects. Because they affect the body's immune response, white blood cells may be less effective in fighting bacteria and infections. Infections may occur more frequently and be more difficult to treat. The more severe effects may include impaired kidney function, hypertension, or the development of cancer. In some patients, adverse side effects can be minimized or prevented when a combination of drugs is used and a large amount of a single drug is avoided. When large amounts of a

TABLE 1

Patient and Graft Survival Rates after Transplantation

Transplant	1 year patient	1 year graft	5 year patient	5 year graft
living kidney	98%	95%	91%	78%
cadaver kidney	95%	89%	82%	65%
liver	88%	81%	74%	66%
heart	86%	85%	70%	69%
lung	77%	76%	44%	42%
heart-lung	60%	58%	42%	41%
pancreas	93%	76%	84%	42%
bowel	79%	64%	50%	37%

SOURCE: UNOS Scientific Registry Data, 2001 OPTN & SRTR Annual Report.

drug are given, negative side effects, such as impaired kidney function from cyclosporine or weight gain and hypertension from prednisone, may be more likely to occur.

Success of Transplantation

Table 1 shows the survival rates after various organ transplants—success is highest with the kidney and lowest with the bowel. Usually, both patient and graft survival rates are measured. Patient survival rates may be higher because patients may survive even though the transplant fails. This is true especially for kidney recipients who can return to kidney dialysis machines if the graft fails, and pancreas or islet-cell transplant patients, who may resume insulin injections. For other organs, such as the liver, the patient can have a repeat transplant if the first graft fails, and thus patient survival is higher than graft survival. Success rates for a second or third transplant, if a patient is fortunate enough to receive one, are lower, however. When a patient has rejected a kidney transplant, it is often more difficult to find a "match" for a second kidney. The patient's immune system has memory cells and antibodies that persist and would aggressively attack a second transplant if it shared tissue proteins with the first graft.

While the most objective evidence of the success of transplantation is survival, more and more emphasis is appropriately being given to the patient's quality of life. With increasing numbers of recipients entering the second decade after their transplant, long-term goals should be aimed at restoring patients to their pre-illness level of health and social functioning. A major transplant study in the United States reported that 80 to 90 percent of kidney, heart, liver, and pancreas recipients are physically active (Evans). This study also asked transplant recipients to rate their quality of life—their "life satisfaction," "well-being," and "psychological affect." The average scores reported by kidney, heart, liver, and pancreas recipients are similar to scores reported by the general public, indicating a comparable quality of life (see Table 2). Many other studies have also shown that the majority of transplant recipients enjoy a good quality of life and complete rehabilitation (Pinson et al.; Bravata et al.; Ostrowski et al.). Transplantation produces improvement in their physical health, social functioning, and ability to perform daily activities. The sense of well-being and satisfaction with life of most recipients is similar to the general public—they are able to return to work, and they enjoy their families without any restriction on their physical activity. Before modern immunosuppression and all of the advances that have occurred in transplantation since the 1980s, recipients led precarious existences. Today, they are encouraged to live lives that are as close to normal as possible. Indeed, every second year the Transplant Olympic Games are held, and hundreds of organ recipients from around the globe compete at a high level.

Transplant recipients are expected to follow good health habits, including regular exercise and appropriate attention to diet and weight. Transplant patients take immunosuppressive drugs to prevent organ rejection for the rest of their lives, although there are occasional patients who have been able to be weaned completely from their immunosuppressive drugs. However, lack of compliance regarding medication is one of the causes for graft loss in the long term. Despite this need for continued medication, patients report remarkable life satisfaction and well-being.

Transplantation Costs and Reimbursement

Transplantation is expensive, as are many other medical therapies and surgical treatments. In view of limited healthcare resources, society must determine the extent of its willingness to fund transplantation. An important consideration, however, is the number of years and quality of life obtained from transplantation. Numerous studies have documented the cost savings of kidney transplantation when compared to its alternative, dialysis. It is widely recognized that transplantation is the most cost-effective treatment for end-stage kidney disease. Although transplantation initially costs more than dialysis, the costs are fully recouped within three years after surgery (Loubeau et al.). Other studies report that liver and heart transplantation are also cost effective. The cost effectiveness of lung transplantation is limited by its lower survival rates and high costs (Anyanwu et al.).

In the United States, funding through Medicare and Medicaid has provided coverage for many kinds of transplants at approved transplant centers. Approved centers must have performed at least a specified number of transplants with a certain level of success to receive these funds. Medicare has been the primary provider of kidney transplant coverage, although coverage has also been provided for certain patients requiring bone marrow, cornea, heart, or liver transplants. Medicaid coverage has varied from state to state, but usually bone marrow, cornea, kidney, and liver transplants have been covered. Heart transplants have been widely available, but coverage for heart-lung, lung, and pancreas transplants has been limited. Most states have covered the cost of organ retrieval, and every state has paid for antirejection drugs for the first year after the transplant. During the 1990s, drug coverage increased, and new transplant patients now have coverage for three years.

In the United States, private insurance and the patient's own financial resources are often necessary. Even when public and private insurance covers transplantation, patients may only be partially reimbursed. The total costs for organ retrieval, surgery, and follow-up healthcare may not be reimbursed, so the patient may have substantial medical bills to pay.

In Canada, provincial health programs cover the costs of organ retrieval, transplant surgery, and medical care. The major cost for recipients is transportation to the transplant center, which may be located in another province. The antirejection drug cyclosporine is paid for for all transplant recipients by a government-sponsored program. Costs are paid as long as patients take the drug, regardless of the socioeconomic status of patients. If patients take other immunosuppressive drugs, these costs may be completely or partially reimbursed by work benefits, private insurance, or special plans for patients with limited finances. Long-term follow-up care is covered by the patient's provincial healthcare plan.

TABLE 2

Quality of Life Assessment

Population	Life Satisfaction[1]	Well-Being[2]	Psychological Affect[3]
Kidney recipient	5.25	11.01	5.23
Heart recipient	5.11	11.11	5.49
Liver recipient	6.70	n/a	6.40
Pancreas recipient	5.40	11.03	5.35
General population	5.55	11.77	5.68

1. Range of values, 1.0 to 7.0, where 7.0 = positive satisfaction;
2. Range of values, 2.1 to 14.7, where high score = positive well-being;
3. Range of values, 1.0 to 7.0, where 7.0 = positive affect.

SOURCE: Evans, Roger W., 1991.

In Europe, according to European Economic Community (EEC) agreements, patients may be eligible for transplant in other countries, with their own governments paying the costs. Patients from countries outside the EEC may also receive transplants, but they have to pay the costs themselves. As more programs have developed, however, fewer patients need to travel to other countries for their transplants.

Expanding the Pool of Cadaveric Organs

Given the success of transplants, and the prevalence of diseases that result in organ failure, more patients are being referred for transplant surgery. The inadequate supply of organs, however, limits the number of transplants, so waiting lists continue to grow (see Figure 1). Transplant programs, therefore, continue to expand their criteria for acceptable organs and are trying innovative ways to procure more organs. One prime example is the use of organs from donors who are older than ideal. As a person ages, hardening of the arteries occurs to greater or lesser degrees in almost everyone, accompanied by deterioration in the function of various organs. Less-than-perfect donor organs have been used, and studies have shown that they can function adequately when certain criteria are met (Wall et al.; Loebe et al.). For example, both kidneys from an older cadaver donor can be transplanted into one patient, and this can provide the recipient with an adequate mass of functioning kidney tissue. The liver is affected by aging much less than other organs, and livers from donors in their seventies, and even eighties, can be successfully transplanted when other variables are satisfactory. For unknown reasons, the blood vessels that feed the liver are rarely affected by hardening of the arteries. Unsuitable hearts, which would not usually be used, have been transplanted as "biological bridges" in urgent situations until a suitable heart has been found.

FIGURE 1

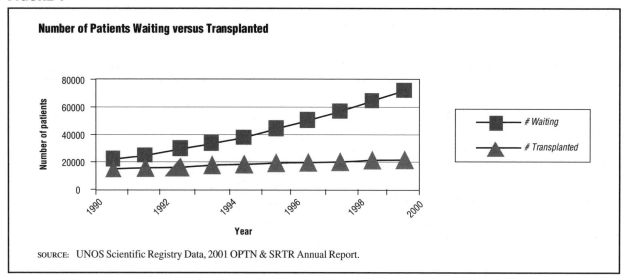

Number of Patients Waiting versus Transplanted

SOURCE: UNOS Scientific Registry Data, 2001 OPTN & SRTR Annual Report.

The liver from a cadaver donor can be split in two for transplant into two suitably sized patients. The procedures are technically complex, however, and there is a greater risk of complications. The applicability of this procedure is also limited by the need for multiple surgical teams operating simultaneously. Additional constraints are those imposed by limited preservation times, especially if the intended recipients are located in different transplant centers. Nevertheless, good results are obtainable. The practice of *domino transplantation* allows a recipient's healthy organ to be removed and transplanted into another patient. For example, when a patient needs a double-lung transplant, he or she may receive a combined heart-lung transplant because it is easier technically to include the donor heart with the transplant as opposed to just the lungs. In this situation, the healthy heart of the recipient can be transplanted into another recipient rather than being discarded. So the recipient of the lungs is both a donor (heart) and a recipient (lungs and heart).

Transplant specialists face dilemmas when less-than-optimal donor organs are offered for transplantation. Obviously, they want the best outcome for their recipients, but the lack of donor organs may force them to make compromises. And while doctors must do what they can to make effective use of donated organs, society must also do its part to maximize organ donation rates. Even if organs were donated from every potential cadaveric donor, however, the supply would still not satisfy the need. Thus, other alternatives such as mechanical hearts and animals as sources for organs have to be explored.

CALVIN R. STILLER (1995)
REVISED BY CALVIN R. STILLER
WILLIAM J. WALL

SEE ALSO: *Artificial Hearts and Cardiac Assist Devices; Body: Cultural and Religious Perspectives; Cybernetics; Death, Definition and Determination of; Dialysis, Kidney; Healthcare Resources, Allocation of; Informed Consent; Life, Quality of; Organ and Tissue Procurement; Organ Transplants, Sociocultural Aspects of; Technology*

BIBLIOGRAPHY

Anyanwu, A.C.; McGuire, A.; Rogers, C. A.; et al. 2002. "An Economic Evaluation of Lung Transplantation." *Journal of Thoracic and Cardiovascular Surgery* 123(3): 411–418.

Azoulay, D.; Castaing, D.; Adam, R.; et al. 2001. "Split-Liver Transplantation for Two Adult Recipients: Feasibility and Long-Term Outcomes." *Annals of Surgery* 233(4): 565–574.

Bravata, D. M.; Olkin, I.; Barnato, A. E.; et al. 1999. "Health-Related Quality of Life after Liver Transplantation: a Meta-analysis." *Liver Transplantation Surgery* 5(4): 318–331.

Cronin, D. C.; Millis, M.; Siegler, M.; et al. 2001. "Transplantation of Liver Grafts from Living Donors into Adults—Too Much, Too Soon." *New England Journal of Medicine* 344(21): 1633–1637.

Evans, R. W. 1991. *The National Cooperative Transplantation Study.* Seattle, WA: Battelle-Seattle Research Center.

Evans, R. W., and Kitzmann, D. J. 1998. "An Economic Analysis of Kidney Transplantation." *Surgical Clinics of North America* 78(1): 149–174.

Grewal, H. P.; Thistlethwaite, J. R.; Loss, G. E.; et al. 1998. "Complications in 100 Living-Liver Donors." *Annals of Surgery* 228(2): 214–219.

Hauptman, P. J., and O'Connor, K. J. 1997. "Procurement and Allocation of Solid Organs for Transplantation." *New England Journal of Medicine* 336(6): 422–431.

Hummel, M; Michauk, I.; Hetzer, R.; et al. 2001. "Quality of Life after Heart and Heart-Lung Transplantation." *Transplantation Proceedings* 33: 3546–3548.

Kizilisik, A. T.; Grewal, H. P.; Shokouh-Amiri, M. H.; et al. 2001. "Ten Years of Chronic Immunosuppressive Therapy following Orthotopic Liver Transplantation: Impact on Health and Quality of Life." *Transplantation Proceedings* 33: 3448–3449.

Koostra, G. 1995. "Statement on Nonheartbeating Donor Programs." *Transplantation Proceedings* 27(5): 2965.

Loebe, M; Potapov, E. V.; Hummel, M.; et al. 2000. "Medium-Term Results of Heart Transplantation Using Older Donor Organs." *Journal of Heart and Lung Transplantation* 19(10): 957–963.

Loubeau, P. R.; Loubeau, J. M.; Jantzen, R.; et al. 2001. "The Economics of Kidney Transplantation versus Hemodialysis." *Progress in Transplantation* 11(4): 291–297.

Najarian, J. S.; Chavers, B. M.; McHugh, L. E.; et al. 1992. "Twenty Years or More of Follow-Up of Living Kidney Donors." *Lancet* 340: 807–810.

Ostrowski, M.; Wesolowski, T.; Makar, D.; et al. 2000. "Changes in Patients' Quality of Life after Renal Transplantation." *Transplantation Proceedings* 32: 1371–1374.

Pinson, C.W.; Feurer, I. D.; Payne, J. L.; et al. 2000. "Health-Related Quality of Life after Different Types of Solid Organ Transplantation." *Annals of Surgery* 232(4): 597–607.

Pomfret, E. A.; Pomposelli, J. J.; Lewis, W. D.; et al. 2001. "Live Donor Adult Liver Transplantation Using Right Lobe Grafts: Donor Evaluation and Surgical Outcome." *Archives of Surgery* 136: 425–433.

Sagmeister, M.; Mullhaupt, B.; Kadry, Z, et al. 2002. "Cost-Effectiveness of Cadaveric and Living-Donor Liver Transplantation." *Transplantation* 73(4): 616–622.

Scharp, David W.; Lacy, Paul E.; Santiago, Julio V.; et al. 1990. "Insulin Independence after Islet Transplantation into Type 1 Diabetic Patient." *Diabetes* 39: 515–518.

Seiler, C. A.; Muller, M.; Fisch, H. U.; et al. 1998. "Quality of Life after Liver Transplantation." *Transplantation Proceedings* 30: 4330–4333.

Shapiro, A. M.; Lakey, J. R.; Ryan, E. A.; et al. 2000. "Islet Transplantation in Seven Patients with Type I Diabetes Mellitus Using a Glucocorticoid-Free Immunosuppressive Regimen." *New England Journal of Medicine* 343(4): 230–238.

Starzl, Thomas E. 1992. *The Puzzle People: Memoirs of a Transplant Surgeon.* Pittsburgh, PA: University of Pittsburgh Press.

Stiller, Calvin. 1990. *Lifegifts: The Real Story of Organ Transplants.* Toronto: Stoddart.

Strong, R. W. 1999. "Whither Living Donor Liver Transplantation?" *Liver Transplantation and Surgery* 5: 536–538.

Sutherland, D. E.; Gruessner, R. W.; Dunn, D. L.; et al. 2001. "Lessons Learned from More Than 1,000 Pancreas Transplants at a Single Institution." *Annals of Surgery* 233(4): 463–501.

Tousignant, P.; Guttmann, R. D.; and Hollomby, D. J. 1985. "Transplantation and Home Hemodialysis: Their Cost-Effectiveness." *Journal of Chronic Disease* 38(7): 589–601.

Trotter, J. F.; Wachs, M.; Everson, G. T.; et al. 2002. "Adult-to-Adult Transplantation of the Right Hepatic Lobe from a Living Donor." *New England Journal of Medicine* 346(14): 1074–1082.

Wall, William; Mimeault, Richard; Grant, David; et al. 1990. "The Use of Older Donor Livers for Hepatic Transplantation." *Transplantation* 49: 377–381.

Weber M.; Dindo, D.; Demartines, N.; et al. 2002. "Kidney Transplantation from Donors without a Heartbeat." *New England Journal of Medicine* 347(4): 248–255.

ORGAN TRANSPLANTS, SOCIOCULTURAL ASPECTS OF

• • •

Transplantation has been defined by the American medical profession and by U.S. society at large as a "gift of life" since the first human organ grafts were performed in the mid-1950s. This conception has its roots in the Judeo-Christian tradition of American society, which defines the life of an individual as a gift that comes directly or indirectly from God and that creates an obligation to reciprocate (Parsons, Fox, and Lidz). The notion of organ transplantation as a gift is not institutionalized, or even invoked, in societies with other religious traditions (such as Japan with its Buddhist, Shinto, and Confucian background; or Pakistan, with its Islamic worldview). Initially in the United States, the idea of a gift was used metaphorically, with little awareness or analysis of its implications. Only gradually, through clinical experience and interpretive input from psychiatrists, social workers, and social scientists, did the psychological, social, and cultural meanings and repercussions of the gift-exchange aspects of transplantation become more apparent and better understood (Fox and Swazey, 1978).

Despite all the biomedical and social changes that have ensued within and around the field of organ replacement, the "gift of life" aspects of seeking, giving, and receiving a human organ have remained central to the dynamics and meaning of transplantation in U.S. society. The increased frequency of organ transplants, and their greater routinization in certain regards, have not eliminated the gift elements from these surgical and medical acts or reduced their effects on donors, recipients, and their families (Fox and Swazey, 1992).

Marcel Mauss's Gift-Exchange Paradigm

"The theme of the gift, of freedom and obligation in the gift, of generosity and self-interest in giving reappear in our society like the resurrection of a dominant motif long forgotten," wrote the renowned French sociologist Marcel Mauss in his classic 1925 essay *The Gift* (p. 66). To a remarkable degree, organ transplantation has been shaped by the triple set of "symmetrical and reciprocal" obligations that, according to Mauss, govern all gift exchange, no matter how spontaneous and expressive it may appear to be. These are the entwined obligations to offer and give, to receive and accept, and to seek and find an appropriate way to repay. Failure to live up to any of these obligations, Mauss pointed out, produces major social strains that affect the giver, the receiver, and those associated with them.

Mauss also emphasized that gifts have "emotional" and symbolic as well as "material" value and meaning. In this sense, he said, the gift and the obligations attached to it are "not inert." Rather, "the spirit of the thing given" and received is "alive and often personified." It "pertains to a person," and because it does, it creates a "sort of spiritual bond" between donor and recipient (pp. 10–11). Anthropomorphic and magical connotations of the gift have proved to be as characteristic of the modern medical, scientific, and technological milieus in which the giving and receiving of organs through transplantation take place, as of the settings in "primitive" and "archaic" societies that were the contexts of Mauss's study.

Obligations to Give Organs

The gift-exchange paradigm illuminates many of the distinctive psychological and social phenomena that donors, recipients, their families, and the transplant team encounter. To begin with, even though the U.S. organ donation system has been organized around the cardinal societal principles of voluntarism and freedom of choice, the situations in which transplants are performed subject prospective donors and their families to strong inner and outer pressures to make such a gift. This is most apparent in the case of live organ transplants, which usually involve the donation of a kidney to a parent, sibling, or child who is gravely ill with end-stage disease. Most transplant teams scrupulously try to avoid urging close biological kin to offer themselves as donors. Nevertheless, they do inform patients and their families that a live kidney transplant from a relative who is a "good tissue match" is likely to have a better prognosis than a cadaver transplant from a nonrelated donor. In addition to the biomedical reasons that favor a live kidney donation, its

symbolic meaning virtually obliges every family member at least to consider making such a gift. The integrity, intimacy, and generosity of the family and each of its members are involved in their individual and collective willingness to give of themselves to a terminally ill relative in this supreme, life-sustaining way (Simmons, Klein, and Simmons).

It would be easy to assume that because cadaver organs come from persons who are unrelated and unknown to recipients, such donations are relatively free from inner and outer gift-giving pressures. Nevertheless, under the circumstances in which the option of donating cadaver organs arises, families may feel emotionally and spiritually constrained to make such a gift of life when this prospect is presented to them by an organ procurement team. Most cadaver organs are obtained from young, healthy persons who have been fatally injured in a vehicular accident or a homicide or who have taken their own lives. These sudden and unexpected deaths are especially tragic and fraught with problems of meaning. In the face of this sort of death, the grief-stricken family may be motivated to donate their young relative's organs by their intense need to make redeeming sense out of what they would otherwise experience as morally and existentially absurd.

Obligations to Receive Organs

The candidate-recipient who is offered a live or cadaver organ is subject to strong, complementary pressures to receive it. Whatever the potential recipient's reservations may be about a transplant, great reluctance or outright refusal to accept the lifesaving gift that is offered symbolically implies a rejection of the donor and of the donor's relationship to the recipient.

There are several recurrent sets of reasons why recipients may be reluctant to accept the kind of gift of life that a donated organ represents. First, the recipient may not want a living, related donor exposed to the degree of discomfort, danger, or sacrifice that a transplant entails. Second, the recipient may feel that receiving an organ from this individual would make the relationship between them too emotionally complicated and difficult. Third, whether the proffered organ comes from a live relative or a deceased stranger, the recipient may be heavily burdened by the realization that it is such an extraordinary gift that he or she will never be able to repay it. Fourth, the recipient may have great concern or apprehension about absorbing a donated part of another known or unknown individual into his or her body, person, and life.

Receiving a donor's organ summons up buried, often animistic feelings that people have about their vital organs and the integrity of their body, along with the sort of anthropomorphic reactions to such a gift that Mauss identified. Many recipients of cadaveric organ transplants grapple with the haunting sense that psychic and social as well as physical qualities of the unknown donor have been transferred into their body, personhood, and life. Writing about his experiences as a liver transplant recipient, Richard McCann vividly expressed such feelings—depicting the donor organ as a "bearer of its own cellular memories" and describing the long nights when he thought of the donor, always "with great tenderness," sometimes perceiving the donor as a male and sometimes as a female. The strong interest that many recipients of cadaver organs and their kin have in knowing what kind of person the donor was and what the donor's family is like is related to this phenomenon. So, too, is the eagerness of donor families to learn something about the persons to whom living parts of their deceased relatives have been given, and about their families.

In the early years of human organ transplants, during the 1950s to mid-1960s, medical teams were inclined to reveal the identities of the donors of cadaver organs, their recipients, and their families, and to provide details of their backgrounds and lives. Physicians believed that these intimate participants in the acts of transplantation giving and receiving were entitled to such knowledge. They also thought it would enhance the meaning of the transplant experience for the recipient and recipient's family and afford consolation and a sense of completeness to the donor's family.

With the passage of time and increased clinical experience, however, transplant teams became more wary about the information they conveyed. They were discomfited by the way in which recipients, their kin, and donor families personified cadaver organs, and by how many of them not only arranged to meet but also tried to become involved in each other's lives, as if they were indebted and related to one another. These interactions were major factors that led most transplant units to establish the normative practices of guarding the anonymity of cadaveric donors and of exercising great restraint in divulging any information about the donor to the recipient or about the recipient to the donor's family. Although transplanters developed this policy out of their desire to reduce some of the stress that the symbolically charged gift of an organ entails for all who are involved in it, they express some ambivalence about its merits and uncertainty about its consequences. The policy of anonymity has been challenged as paternalistic by donor families and recipients, in the "National Communication Guidelines" developed by the National Donor Family (NNF) council in collaboration with a number of transplant organizations including the United Network for Organ Sharing (UNOS)

and the U.S. Department of Health and Human Service's Division of Organ Transplants (Corr et al., p. 625).

Obligations to Repay the "Gift of Life" and the "Tyranny of the Gift"

At the center of organ transplantation is a gift of surpassing significance—in the words of philosopher Hans Jonas, a "supererogatory gift … beyond duty and claim" (p. 16). Paradoxically, it is an offering that so perfectly epitomizes an ultimate Judeo-Christian value—the injunction to give of one's self to others in ways that include strangers as well as kin—that it transcends what is ordinarily asked or expected of people. The sublime meaning of what is exchanged, along with the literal and figurative sense in which a living part of the giver comes to reside and function inside the recipient, usually creates a very strong bond between the donor, the recipient, and their families. The sense of oneness and ennoblement that a donor or donor's family and a recipient often experience as a result of the life-giving and life-receiving acts in which they have participated can greatly enrich them, emotionally and spiritually.

But as Mauss could have foretold, what recipients believe they owe to donors, and the sense of obligation they feel about repaying "their" donor for what has been given, weigh heavily upon them. This psychological and moral burden is especially onerous because the gift the recipient has received from the donor is so extraordinary that it is inherently nonreciprocal. It has no physical or symbolic equivalent. As a consequence, the giver, the receiver, and their families may find themselves locked in a creditor–debtor vise. Because of their feelings of great indebtedness, recipients of live organs may have difficulty in maintaining psychic distance and independence from donors and in asserting their own separate identity and being. In some instances, their struggle to do so may cause a serious rupture in the relationship between recipient and donor. Renée C. Fox and Judith P. Swazey have called these aspects of the gift-exchange dimensions of transplantation "the tyranny of the gift" (1978, chap. 1).

Alterations in the Theme of the Gift: Efforts to Procure More Organs

The 1980s and 1990s brought a number of significant changes in the ways the U.S. medical community and public thought about the gift of a transplantable organ, and in how they acted in relation to their conception of it. The primary precipitants of these changes were the growing preoccupation with the shortage of organs and the increasing efforts that were made to augment the supply of both living and cadaver donors.

The 1980s were marked by a substantial expansion in the number and types of transplants and retransplants, in the number of hospitals doing these procedures, and in the number of patients on waiting lists. The discovery and pervasive use of cyclosporine, a more effective immunosuppressive drug for managing the rejection reaction triggered by transplanted organs, was a key biomedical factor that contributed to this transplant "boom." To the distress of organ procurement agencies and transplanters, these increases occurred in the face of a plateauing of cadaveric donors and a slight decline in living donors. The "alarming number of patients who die waiting" for a transplant (Peters, p. 1302) led members of the transplant community and their advocates to define the organ shortage as a "public health crisis" (Randall, p. 1223). In the context of various policy strategies that were deployed to combat this growing "crisis," the concept and theme of transplantation as a gift of life underwent a number of alterations.

GREATER USE OF LIVING DONORS. Efforts to enlarge the supply of organs included a greater interest in the use of living donors. This resulted in an expansion of the kinds of live-donor transplants that surgeons were willing to perform, and significant redefinitions by the transplant community of how, for purposes of giving and receiving an organ, donors and recipients can be nonbiologically "related" to each other. Increasingly active and large-scale campaigns to recruit future donors were also mounted, urging people to "make a miracle" by giving a gift of life through the provisions of the Uniform Anatomical Gift Act. (Promulgated in 1968 and adopted in some form by every state by 1973, the act enables individuals to legally signify their willingness to have their bodily parts used for transplantation after their death; if the deceased's wishes are unknown, the act grants the next of kin the right to make this decision.)

Beginning in the 1980s, the fact that the supply of cadaveric kidneys was not large enough to meet the growing demand for them, along with advances in immunosuppression, emboldened a number of medical centers to undertake kidney transplants from unrelated live donors. In effect, something akin to a collective taboo against performing this type of graft had previously existed among transplant physicians. A new term appeared in the medical literature: "emotionally related donors," meaning persons whose relationship to recipients, though not biological, was analogously close (including spouses, in-laws, adopted children, and kinlike friends). In 1985 the Council of the Transplantation Society (CTS) issued a set of "guidelines for the donation of kidneys by unrelated living donors" that legitimated their use in exceptional circumstances "when a satisfactory cadaver or living related donor cannot be found." These normative recommendations expressed continuing concern about the motives of such donors, about the recognition and protection to which they were entitled for such "a gift of extraordinary magnitude," and about the ever-present danger "in the current climate of commercialization" that, particularly in the case of "living stranger donors," the covert buying and selling of organs might be involved (CTS, p. 716). Because living donations have become a "burgeoning source of organs," some concern also has been expressed about the risk of "trading [the donor's] health or even life for that of [the recipient]" (Kahn, p. 4).

In the atmosphere produced by the acceleration in the number and range of transplants performed, the mounting sense of crisis over the organ shortage, and the increased support given to live-donor kidney transplants, liver and lung transplantation from living donors was tried for the first time in the United States. The initial liver recipients, in 1989, were two infants with biliary atresia, a congenital, usually fatal condition, each of whom received a liver lobe from a parent. In 1991 a nine-year-old girl received two successive live-donor lung-lobe transplants: first from her father and then, when this did not provide enough lung capacity, another transplant from her mother. During the second procedure, the child died of heart failure. Partly because the liver has the mysteriously unique ability to regenerate itself, live liver-lobe transplants have since included donations from friends and, in one instance, a "stranger"; but like lung-lobe transplants, they are still relatively uncommon and done only at a few highly sophisticated transplant centers.

Another form of live donation, employed since 1984, has generated even greater uncertainty and debate about "the permissible limits of one of our most powerful instincts, the one that leads us to fight for the life of our children" (Quindlen). These cases involve conceiving and giving birth to a baby in order to provide a bone marrow donor for one's dying child when no donor with a compatible tissue type can be located. In 1990 the case that received the most attention, because of the decision to go public, was that of the Ayala family, whose nineteen-year-old daughter, Anissa, was slowly dying of chronic myelogenous leukemia. Her parents announced that they had conceived a child on the one-in-four chance that the baby's tissue type would be compatible with Anissa's. There was a tissue match, and at age fourteen months the baby had her bone marrow withdrawn and infused into her sister. The Ayalas' story was viewed by many as an act of love as well as of science—all the more so because the parents made it clear that they never would have considered aborting the fetus if its tissue type did not match Anissa's. Pervading all the discussion surrounding this case, however, was disquietude about how morally acceptable it was to bring a baby into the world to provide life-sustaining treatment for another child; about the baby's inability to consent to this role; about the psychological impact that the condition of the donor child's birth could have on her sense of identity and of her reason for being; and about how blameworthy she might feel, or be made to feel, if in the end her transplanted tissue failed to help her sister (Kearney and Caplan).

By 2002 all these issues had been extended to an analogous situation, one in which hematopoietic stem cells from umbilical cord blood or bone marrow might cure or alleviate a disease affecting the blood or immune system of a child. Conceiving a baby to serve as a stem cell donor was a possibility for the parents of such a child, and using in vitro fertilization followed by selective abortion, or preimplantation genetic diagnosis and selective embryo transfer had become viable biomedical options (Robertson, Kahn, and Wagner).

NON-HEART-BEATING DONORS. Another effort to increase the supply of organs has been the use of what are termed planned or controlled *non-heart-beating donors,* an effort that was initiated by a 1991 protocol at the University of Pittsburgh. In such cases, a family agrees to have life-sustaining treatment withdrawn from a close relative who is terminally ill but not brain dead, so that the person's organs can be retrieved for transplants. In effect, this constitutes a return to the cardiopulmonary criteria that were used to pronounce donors of cadaver organs dead before the concept of brain death was adopted in the United States in the late 1960s and progressively took its place alongside the more traditional means for declaring a person dead on the basis of irreversible cessation of circulatory and respiratory functions. The use of non-heart-beating donors helped bring to the surface and intensify pervasive conceptual confusion and unease about the relationship between these dual means of determining and declaring death. It also raised troubling questions about the exact borderline between life and death; how long an interval should be observed after the complete cessation of cardiac and pulmonary function before death is pronounced; whether giving drugs to non-heart-beating donors to minimize the effects of warm ischemic time on the viability of their organs could hasten or cause their death; and the compatibility of procuring organs in this manner with the humane and respectful treatment of dying patients and their families (Fox; IOM, 1997; Arnold and Youngner; Youngner, Arnold, and DeVita).

BROADER STANDARDS FOR CADAVERIC ORGANS. Criteria for what are deemed to be acceptable cadaveric organs have also been "liberalized and expanded" in the drive to perform more transplants. These broadened, less stringent standards include using organs from donors of increasing age; from persons with medical conditions such as diabetes and hypertension and certain infections; and from persons with some hemodynamic instability or chemical imbalances, or whose organs have undergone increased preservation time (IOM, 1997). While transplant experts have hopefully predicted that using what are sometimes called such "marginal" organs could markedly increase the donor supply, they have acknowledged that the concomitant financial and human costs, and lower graft and recipient survival, should be seriously considered (IOM, 1997).

XENOTRANSPLANTATION. Along with the measures taken to increase the number of human donor organs, the 1990s brought a surge of renewed interest in xenotransplantation—grafting animal organs, tissues, and cells into human beings—accompanied by strong appeals to end the informal moratorium that had been called on interspecies organ transplants in the United States and numerous European countries because of the immediate postoperative deaths of all but one of the patients on whom the procedure had been previously tried. The reignited interest in xenotransplantation has been deliberated by bodies such as the U.S. Food and Drug Administration, the Centers for Disease Control and Prevention, the National Institutes of Health, and the National Academy of Sciences' Institute of Medicine. All these groups have focused special attention on the "greater than zero" risk that xenotransplants could trigger zoonosis, the transmission of known and unknown animal pathogens into the human population (IOM, 1996). In a historical era when the most daunting problems of world health emanate from the "emergence" and "reemergence" of infectious diseases in epidemic and pandemic proportions, this consideration has had a sobering and restraining effect on the intrepidness with which the prospect of providing animal organs for the long lines of people awaiting transplants has moved forward.

"REQUIRED REQUEST" AND "PRESUMED CONSENT." Seeking remedies for the shortfall of organs has also involved identifying and attempting to alter attitudes and role behavior of physicians and nurses. In this connection, in the mid-1980s bioethicist Arthur L. Caplan proposed the establishment of "required-request" procedures in hospitals to ensure that the next of kin or the legal guardian of every potential donor was notified of the transplantation option and was asked to make a donation of their relative's organs for this purpose (Caplan, 1984a, 1984b). Although required request had been drafted into state and federal legislation and incorporated into hospital accreditation standards by the end of the 1980s, studies suggest that its influence has been minor (Annas; Caplan, 1988).

In Western Europe, serious attention has been given to the use of "presumed consent" or "opting out" as a way to increase the number of cadaveric organs. This is a system that legally allows the use of a deceased patient's organs for transplantation, unless the patient had formally registered the desire not to be a donor. This system has resulted in notable increases in organ procurement rates in a number of European countries. There is evidence, however, that if the "opting out" system requires the next of kin to be informed about organ removal from their dead relative before it is done, physicians may be less inclined to initiate the procurement process and families more likely to object to the donation. Opinion polls have shown that there is a strongly held and wide-ranging resistance to its establishment as a basis for organ and tissue procurement in the United States, as well as in Great Britain and the Netherlands (Kokkedee). It has been suggested, but not systematically investigated, that "opting out"—rather than "opting in"—may run counter to the social expectations and cultural values of individuals, families, and health professionals in these societies.

From "Gifts of Life" to Market Commodities?

Throughout its history in the United States, human organ transplantation has been steadfastly defined and ardently promoted as a gift of life, and the National Organ Transplant Act of 1984 made it illegal for "any person to knowingly acquire, receive, or otherwise transfer any human organ for valuable consideration for use in human transplantation." Nonetheless, recurrent proposals have been made to provide some sort of financial recompense for this act of giving. These proposals have had a dual purpose: to recognize what donors and their families have contributed and to provide an additional incentive for organ donation. None of the proposals has involved the outright buying and selling of organs. Rather, they have entailed various forms of so-called regulated compensation, or what has euphemistically been termed "rewarded gifting," such as granting a paid medical leave to living donors (the Organ Donor Leave Act, enacted in 1999) or advocating the partial reimbursement of funeral expenses for cadaveric donors. Among the most pecuniary of these suggested measures has been a Congressional proposal to give tax credits or refunds for an organ donation (the Gift of Life Tax Credit Act of 2001). The most market-oriented notion, espoused by some jurists, economists, and health policy analysts and managers, is that of a "futures market" in

cadaveric organs that would allow healthy persons to contract for the sale of their organs for transplantation, to be retrieved and used after their death (Cohen; Hansmann). Neither the tax credits nor the futures market plan has been implemented.

The search to devise monetarily expressed incentives and rewards for organ donation that will help alleviate the organ shortage, without violating the prohibition against buying or selling organs, has been occurring in the larger context of the existence of a global black market for organs from living donors (Scheper-Hughes). In the United States, the search has been characterized by a continuous veering toward financial incentives and a continuous veering away from them. This ambivalence is exemplified by the outcome of a bill, originally signed into law in Pennsylvania in 1994, that created an Organ Donation Awareness Trust Fund, part of which was intended to pay up to $3,000 to a cadaver donor's family to defray funeral expenses, and to study the impact of this arrangement. After nearly eight years of debate and delay, state health officials abandoned the program on the grounds that it came too close to offering cash for organs. Instead, in 2002 they created a program to offer a modest $300 benefit to pay directly for food and lodging costs incurred by a donor's family (Wiggins). Another proposal, which "released a torrent of protest" during a committee hearing, was introduced in June 2002 by the Council on Ethical and Judicial Affairs of the American Medical Association (AMA); it involved offering a $300 to $500 payment to families of cadaveric donors and was coupled with a study to determine the effects of such payments. If the AMA House of Delegates approved the council's recommendations, however, a pilot study would require changes in the federal law that prohibits such financial incentives (Peck). To date, at least in American society, every such attempt to institute compensatory measures for organ donation has elicited as much concern and opposition as support; and it has called forth strong affirmations about the "symbolic" association of organ transplantation with "altruism" and "social good" and the importance of not subverting its meaning by monetarizing the gift that it constitutes (Delmonico et al.).

RENÉE C. FOX
JUDITH P. SWAZEY (1995)
REVISED BY AUTHORS

SEE ALSO: *Body: Cultural and Religious Perspectives; Cybernetics; Death, Definition and Determination of; Life, Quality of; Medicine, Anthropology of; Medicine, Sociology of; Organ and Tissue Procurement; Organ Transplants, Sociocultural Aspects of*

BIBLIOGRAPHY

Annas, George J. 1988. "The Paradoxes of Organ Transplantation." *American Journal of Public Health* 78(6): 621–622.

Arnold, Robert M., and Youngner, Stuart J., eds. 1993. "Ethical, Psychosocial, and Public Policy Implications of Procuring Organs from Non-Heart-Beating Cadavers." Special issue of *Kennedy Institute of Ethics Journal* 3(2)

Caplan, Arthur L. 1984a. "Ethical and Policy Issues in the Procurement of Cadaver Organs for Transplantation." *New England Journal of Medicine* 311(15): 981–983.

Caplan, Arthur L. 1984b. "Organ Procurement: It's Not in the Cards." *Hastings Center Report* 14(5): 9–12.

Caplan, Arthur L. 1988. "Professional Arrogance and Public Misunderstanding." *Hastings Center Report* 18(2): 34–37.

Cohen, Lloyd R. 1989. "Increasing the Supply of Transplantable Organs: The Virtues of a Futures Market." *George Washington Law Review* 58(11): 1–51.

Council of the Transplantation Society (CTS). 1985. "Commercialisation in Transplantation: The Problems and Some Guidelines for Practice." *Lancet* 2(8457): 715–716.

Corr, Charles A.; Coolican, Margaret B.; Nile, Lucy G.; Noedel, Nancy. 1994. "What is the Rationale for or against Contacts between Donor Families and Transplant Recipients?" *Critical Care Nursing Clinics of North America* 6(3): 625–632.

Delmonico, Francis L.; Arnold, Robert; Scheper-Hughes, Nancy; et al. 2002. "Ethical Incentives—Not Payment—for Organ Donation." *New England Journal of Medicine* 346(25): 2002–2005.

Fox, Renée C. 1993. "An Ignoble Form of Cannibalism: Reflections on the Pittsburgh Protocol for Procuring Organs from Non-Heart-Beating Cadavers." *Kennedy Institute of Ethics Journal* 23(2): 231–239.

Fox, Renée C., and Swazey, Judith P. 1978. *The Courage to Fail: A Social View of Organ Transplants and Dialysis,* 2nd edition. Chicago: University of Chicago Press. Reprint, with a new introduction by the authors. New Brunswick, NJ: Transaction Publishers, 2002.

Fox, Renée C., and Swazey, Judith P. 1992. *Spare Parts: Organ Replacement in American Society.* New York: Oxford University Press.

Hansmann, Henry. 1989. "The Economics and Ethics of Markets for Human Organs." In *Organ Transplantation Policy: Issues and Prospects,* ed. James F. Blumstein and Frank A. Sloan. Durham, NC: Duke University Press.

Jonas, Hans. 1970. "Philosophical Reflections on Experimenting with Subjects." In *Experimentation with Human Subjects,* ed. Paul A. Freund. New York: George Braziller.

Kahn, Jeffrey. 2000. "Giving 'til It Hurts: How Far to Go in Living Organ Donation?" *Bioethics Examiner* 3(4): 1, 4.

Kearney, Warren, and Caplan, Arthur L. 1992. "Parity for the Donation of Bone Marrow." In *Emerging Issues in Biomedical Policy: An Annual Review,* vol. 1, ed. Robert H. Blank and Andrea L. Bonnicksen. New York: Columbia University Press.

Kokkedee, William. 1992. "Kidney Procurement Policies in the Eurotransplant Region: 'Opting In' versus 'Opting Out.'" *Social Science and Medicine* 35(2): 177–182.

Mauss, Marcel. 1925 (reprint 1954). *The Gift: Forms and Foundations of Exchange in Archaic Societies,* tr. Ian Cunnison. Glencoe, IL: Free Press.

McCann, Richard. 1999. "The Resurrectionist." In *Body,* ed. Sharon Sloan Fiffer and Steve Fiffer. New York: Avon.

Parsons, Talcott; Fox, Renée C.; Lidz, Victor. 1972. "The Gift of Life and Its Reciprocation." *Social Research* 39(3): 367–414.

Peters, Thomas G. 1991. "Life or Death: The Issue of Payment in Cadaveric Organ Donation." *Journal of the American Medical Association* 265(10): 1302–1305.

Quindlen, Anna. 1991. "The Heart's Reasons." *New York Times,* June 6.

Randall, Terri. 1991. "Too Few Human Organs for Transplantation, Too Many in Need ... and the Gap Widens." *Journal of the American Medical Association* 265(10): 1223, 1227.

Robertson, John A.; Kahn, Jeffrey P.; and Wagner, John E. 2002. "Conception to Obtain Hematopoietic Stem Cells." *Hastings Center Report* 32(3): 34–40.

Scheper-Hughes, Nancy. 2000. "The Global Traffic in Organs." *Current Anthropology* 41(2): 191–224.

Simmons, Roberta G.; Klein, Susan D.; and Simmons, Richard L. 1977. *Gift of Life: The Social and Psychological Impact of Organ Transplantation.* New York: Wiley. Reprint, published with new introduction as *Gift of Life: The Effect of Organ Transplantation on Individual, Family, and Societal Dynamics,* by Roberta G. Simmons, Susan Klein Marine, and Richard L. Simmons. New Brunswick, NJ: Transaction Books, 1987.

U.S. Institute of Medicine (IOM). Division of Health Care Services. 1996. *Xenotransplantation: Science, Ethics, and Public Policy.* Washington, D.C.: National Academy Press.

U.S. Institute of Medicine (IOM). Division of Health Care Services. 1997. *Non-Heart-Beating Organ Transplantation: Medical and Ethical Issues in Procurement.* Washington, D.C.: National Academy Press.

Wiggins, Ovetta. 2002. "PA Donors Get $300 Boost." *Philadelphia Inquirer,* May 27.

Youngner, Stuart J.; Arnold, Robert M.; and DeVita, Michael A. 1999. "When Is 'Dead'?" *Hastings Center Report* 29(6): 14–21.

INTERNET RESOURCE

Peck, Peggy. 2002. "AMA Ethics Group Considers Financial Incentives for Donor Organs." *Reuters Medical News.* Available from <http://www.medscape.com>.

P

PAIN AND SUFFERING

• • •

Suffering demands explanation and relief. Some appear to suffer in excess of their actions, the innocent suffer as the evil do, and the best suffer with the worst. Theologies and theodicies attempt to cope with the paradox of a holy, omnipotent, omniscient, just god and the presence of suffering. Healers and systems of medicine arise in every culture in response to suffering. Yet what suffering is, where in the human condition it originates, and in what direction its solution is, remain poorly understood.

Pain is the most commonly considered source of suffering, so much so that the two terms are commonly linked—as in "pain and suffering." They are, however, distinctly different forms of distress. Understanding what pain is, and how it is related to but different from suffering, provides an introduction to the topic.

How the Nervous System is Involved in Pain: The Nociceptive Apparatus

The nervous system pathways—the nociceptive apparatus—involved in the transmission of noxious stimuli do not simply transfer information from an injured part to the central nervous system. They are part of a system in which the information can be either enhanced, diminished, or suppressed. The modulation of the noxious sensation occurs as part of the process of perception where meaning influences the original message.

Skin, muscles, and internal organs are supplied with nerve endings that come from several types of nerve fibers.

Some are specifically responsive to mechanical, thermal, and chemical stimuli that give rise to the noxious physical sensation called nociception. These nociceptive nerve fibers enter the spinal cord and make complex connections with the spinal nerves that ascend to the thalamus and from there to areas of the cortex of the brain. Neural pathways from the higher centers, in what is called the endogenous pain control system, descend to make connections in the dorsal horn of the spinal cord in the area where the pain fibers make their initial central connections. These descending tracts are able to modulate the nociceptive signal by exerting an inhibitory effect specifically on pain-transmission neurons.

In addition to neural pathways, which do not merely transmit noxious sensations but change their character, chemical messengers and their receptors within the nervous system also have an influence on the message. Naturally occurring brain peptides such as enkephalin and beta-endorphin, collectively known as endorphins, exert analgesic effects in different areas of the nervous system by binding to specialized receptors. These same receptors also bind drugs such as morphine or meperidine, allowing them to provide pain relief. Other neurotransmitters, such as serotonin and dopamine, also have effects that temper the transmission of nociceptive messages.

Pain as Perception

Historically, knowledge about nociception as neural transmission of noxious stimuli predated knowledge about the modulation of the nociceptive process. This simplified view of nociception fits the mechanical understanding of the nervous system that has held until recent times. This view accounts for the fact that the noxious sensation that is nociception is so commonly confused with pain and that the two terms, although distinct, are often used interchangeably. Nociception provides the noxious sensation resulting from extremes of mechanical pressure or temperature that is interpreted by the organism as pain.

Because pain is a perception based on sensory information from the nociceptive apparatus—just as seeing something is a perception based on information from the visual apparatus—it involves a cognitive effort that requires judgment. The place of cognition in the process may be questioned in acute, severe, or momentary pain, but most pain is longer lasting and more ambiguous in source and meaning.

Nociception is usually followed by aversive action. The reflexive withdrawal of a burned hand, however, has little applicability to understanding human pain. The actions of humans in response to pain generally take into account the location, severity, cause, and anticipated course of the pain. Knowledge and judgment are required. Reactions to pain range from the momentary to well-laid future plans. While the former may depend on reflexes, the latter do not. *Pain is the entire process of sensing, interpreting, and modulating the nociceptive process, assigning cause, anticipating course, and determining response.* As a consequence, it is obvious why it is a source of confusion that human pain does not exist without sentience. Unconscious or comatose persons may demonstrate nociceptive reactions such as reflex withdrawal from noxious stimuli or elevations in pulse and blood pressure. Consciousness, however, is required for the full experience of pain. This is why a useful working definition of pain is experience reported in the statement "it hurts."

Attempts to refute the subjective nature of pain may take the form of statements that pain is usually accompanied by physiologic changes in, for example, pulse and blood pressure, but the body and its physiology are part of the person and nothing happens to one part that does not happen to all. Confusions such as this are residua of the mind–body dichotomy that has ruled medical science for centuries and still disorders understanding. The fact that pain cannot be measured has been a source of great frustration to investigators. Noxious stimuli and nociceptive responses can be quantified, but pain cannot. The difficulty of understanding pain is part of the age-old conundrum of how a physiological event becomes a feeling or a thought and how thoughts and feelings are translated into physiology.

Chronic Pain

Chronic pain—by definition, pain lasting more than six months—represents a greater challenge to understanding than acute pain. What is known about the nociceptive system does not explain the phenomenon of chronic pain.

There is evidence that the reparative response that occurs after damage to peripheral nerves may alter their function in a manner that perpetuates or exaggerates their response to noxious stimuli. Similar modifications of the whole nociceptive apparatus, including the function of its neuroendocrine component (for example, endorphins), may provide some basis for pain that continues after the initial stage of tissue damage. Nonetheless, paucity of solid evidence to resolve the enigma of chronic pain has led to speculation and hypothesis based more on belief than on knowledge. For example, various schemata have been developed that explain chronic pain in many ways: as a result of continued tissue damage (e.g., rheumatoid arthritis); because of psychic perpetuation of organic pain (e.g., phantom limb pain); or from emotional factors believed to precipitate the organic (e.g., duodenal ulcer); as well as to hypothesized states of psychogenic pain arising from psychic conflicts experienced in a somatic manner (Whitehead and Kuhn).

The problem has also been framed as a conflict between peripheralists and centralists. The peripheralist believes that there must be continued nociceptive input and that treatment should be directed toward blocking the presumed nociceptive process with analgesics or nerve blocks and by other means. Centralists believe that although some peripheral pathology with nociceptive consequences initiated the pain, under some circumstances it can be continued "as a self-perpetuating physiological generator mechanism within the central nervous system" (Crue).

The Role of Meaning

Human pain, acute or chronic, involves the constant and interactive contribution of both psychic and physical determinants. The most important psychological component of pain is its meaning, that is, its significance and its importance. Significance denotes the event as a this or a that: "Chest pain (of this type) signifies a heart attack." Importance evaluates the event: "A heart attack will be the end of my active life." These two functions of meaning are always intertwined and arise from the concepts (e.g., heart attacks) to which they refer. The interpretation of a pain as arising from, for example, cancer, contains within it ideas of process: "Cancer comes from ... and goes on to become ..." as well as to ideas of the impact on the person: "Cancer pain is terrible and heralds death." Things have affective, physical, and spiritual as well as cognitive meanings. People act on their interpretation of the consequences of the distress, doing what is necessary on their part for it to improve. For example, a person who develops unexpected chest pain while walking may stop because it is impossible to continue. But the person may also walk more slowly in the future, deny the pain's significance, go to an emergency room, worry, panic, take nitroglycerin, or any of a variety of actions, in response to what the person believes the symptom means.

The Distinction between Pain and Suffering

Suffering is closely related to pain because pain is a common cause of suffering, but they are distinct forms of distress. People may report suffering when a pain, such as that caused by a dissecting aortic aneurysm, is overwhelming. Or they may tolerate even extremely severe pain if they know what it is, know that it can be relieved, or know that it will soon end. Less intense pain may be a source of suffering if the person does not know its source or believes that it has a dire cause (e.g., cancer), cannot be controlled, or will be "never-ending." Suffering can sometimes be controlled merely by changing the meaning of the pain. Clinicians working with terminally ill patients frequently see suffering patients grunting with pain who cannot be comforted. When their pain has been adequately relieved and it has been demonstrated that such relief will be forthcoming if the pain should return, they will frequently tolerate the same level of pain (by their report) without requesting medication. Once assured that relief is possible, suffering often subsides although the pain remains. It is difficult to relieve the suffering of patients who are frightened without also relieving their fear.

People may suffer from pain even when the pain is not present. Some who have had severe pain will suffer from the fear of the pain's return even when they are pain-free. People with severe and frequent migraine may suffer from their fear of a return of the headache. These headaches have repeatedly ruined what would otherwise have been pleasurable or important experiences: Family relationships, jobs, sports, and virtually everything that is dear to the person may have been negatively influenced by the headaches. Not surprisingly, such patients may be obsessed with their headaches and their attempts at relief virtually to the exclusion of other aspects of life. They suffer when they do have the actual pain and also when they do not.

The distinction between pain and suffering is clarified by the case of the pain of childbirth. Different kinds of pain relief, some more effective than others, are popular in different parts of the United States. The more important issue seems to be the degree to which the woman is in control of her own labor and delivery, rather than the absolute control of pain. Control of the process of childbirth does not relieve pain, but appears to prevent suffering. In other cases, symptoms such as dyspnea (labored respiration), choking, or even diarrhea may be sources not of pain but of suffering if

they are sufficiently severe. In fact, suffering may be present in the absence of any symptoms. Parents, particularly if they are helpless in the situation, commonly suffer at the sight of their children in pain. Grinding poverty may be a source of suffering, as well as betrayal or the loss of one's life work.

The Role of the Future

The role of the future in these situations of suffering is crucial. In cases of overwhelming pain, in long-continued ("never-ending") pain accompanied by fear of the inability to continue to "take it," and in the situation where the pain is suspected of having terrible meaning, a sense of future is necessary in order to suffer. In each of these instances—when at the moment the pain is not overwhelming, the person is "taking it," and the fact of a dreadful disease does not yet exist—the body cannot worry; it knows no future. The body cannot supply information about the future because at any moment, for the body, the future does not yet exist. Only imagination, beliefs, memories, or ideas can supply the information necessary to provide a "future." In other words, in order to suffer, there must be a source of thoughts about possible futures.

To summarize thus far: Although suffering may attend pain, they are distinct. There may be pain without suffering. There may be suffering without pain. There seems to be no suffering without an idea of the future. Bodies do not have the beliefs, concepts, ideas, or fantasies necessary to create a future—only persons do. One can conclude that although bodies may experience nociception, bodies do not suffer. Only persons suffer.

Suffering Defined

Suffering is a specific state of severe distress induced by the loss of integrity, intactness, cohesiveness, or wholeness of the person, or by a threat that the person believes will result in the dissolution of his or her integrity. Suffering continues until integrity is restored or the threat is gone. The whole person does not mean solely the whole biological organism or the solid-bounded object, although it may be the object of the threat. Persons, while they may be identified with their bodies, cannot be whole in body alone. Nor should the threat to the whole person be understood as solely a quantitative matter (i.e., that persons subjected to more than X amount of pain or Y amount of tissue destruction suffer, even if this amount of pain or tissue destruction may virtually always cause suffering), since one individual may suffer from pain considered unimportant by another. Suffering may occur in relationship to any part of a person.

Wholeness, Self, and Person Defined

Suffering helps define the concept of person. Person is not mind, body, or self, although persons have all of these things. The word *self,* as employed here, denotes that aspect of the person that is an object of the consciousness of a person—the person's own consciousness or that of another. It has cohesive characteristics and it exists over time. Persons cannot be known in their entirety and they cannot be known by reducing them to their parts. As one does that, the person disappears. A topography, however, is possible. A person is the composite entity made up of its body, its selves, its history, its collected beliefs, its believed-in future, unconscious, incorporated society and culture, associations with others including the family, the family's history, its political dimension, secret life, and transcendent dimension.

Persons are also constructed by their ideas and beliefs, by the past, the present, and a sense of the future, as well as by a sense of some level of stability in the environment. Suffering may thus be initiated by profound changes in the person's physical, political, or social world. Clinical observation suggests that the suffering of some patients is initiated by their inability to explain what has happened to them. "What did I do that made this happen to me?" is not merely a question but a metaphysical statement about how the world works. If the person's beliefs and demand for explanations are too rigid and the person cannot accept fate or uncertainty, then the integrity of the person is violated by the unexplained injury.

If physicians focus on the sick person, as necessitated by suffering, they will require knowledge of persons in the way that they presently have knowledge of the body. Persons, however, are different from other objects of science and so they pose difficulties for twentieth-century understanding. Considering persons as ahistorical, atomistic individuals, in which the body is separate from the mind—largely the stance of the sciences, the law, and some schools of philosophy—is not supported by a knowledge of suffering. The sciences of humankind, including psychology and the social sciences, have followed the lead of the physical sciences in employing reductive methodologies, but these lead to a distorted understanding. Similarly, division of the sciences of humankind into the physical, psychological, and social leads away from an understanding of persons and therefore of suffering. Virtually everything that is social is also ultimately physical and psychological. A person is not an object with physical or temporal boundaries, but rather he or she is a process in a trajectory through time. The challenge to a scientific understanding of persons lies in accepting these characteristics.

Suffering is Unique and Individual

Suffering is always individual because it can arise in relation to any aspect of a person, and persons are necessarily unique and particular. If the suffering of two people is initiated by an identical physical insult (e.g., the same kind of severe burn or similar overwhelming pain), the suffering of each will be unique and particular because it becomes suffering by virtue of its effect on a particular dimension or characteristic of the suffering person. No one can know with certainty why another person suffers. One can know that someone is suffering, but not what it is about this specific person that leads to the suffering. Sufferers themselves may not know. What threatens the loss of wholeness of one person is not necessarily the same as that which jeopardizes another. In chronic illness this distinctiveness is more easily seen. Here, suffering can arise because the sick person may not be accepted by, feel at home in, or be able to meet the expectations of others. The way these feelings affect the person will be unique to that person. These difficulties may evoke loneliness, anger, or feelings of unfairness, abandonment, or hurt. The suffering person will be focused on the feeling and the external source that is seen as its cause, not on suffering per se. This is because the same feelings may cause suffering in one person but not in another, and the suffering itself is the result of the disruption of the person arising from the discomfort. Even when suffering is caused by physical pain, the person feels pain, not suffering.

Purpose

To be whole and able to suffer is to have aims or purposes. One of these purposes, central purpose, is the preservation and continued evolution of myself as I know myself. Purposes entail actions. When suffering exists, the identity that the sufferer fears will disintegrate is an identity expressed in purposeful action—legs walk, hands grasp, eyes see, minds have ideas. Purposes and their enabling actions may not require anything from consciousness, but they are nonetheless self-defining. Illness and other sources of suffering interfere with actions that may be conscious, below awareness, or habitual, and thus contribute to damaging the integrity of the person and lead to suffering.

The suffering of the chronically ill may start with the inability to accomplish their previously important purposes. It may actually begin when it finally dawns on the chronically ill person that the life of illness that has been held off for so long and with such effort and determination is now truly imminent. Again, notice that suffering begins not merely when persons cannot do something but when they become aware of what the future holds, even though at the time of recognition their function has not yet worsened. The task of the person, of identity, indeed of wholeness, is the centralization of purpose, while disease, pain, and suffering may contribute to the defeat of such purpose. Pain or other symptoms may focus the person's attention on the distressed body part so completely that central purpose is lost (Bakan). This is probably always true of suffering, which arises with the loss of the ability to pursue purpose and also defeats purpose. It is one of the wonders of humanity, on the other hand, to see how a central purpose, exemplified in the biblical story of Job, may overcome suffering as well as disease and pain.

Suffering Always Involves Self-conflict

The source of suffering is usually seen as outside the sufferer. What is usually identified as the origin of the suffering is the thing that causes the pain, or the pain itself, the life circumstances, or the stroke of fate. In fact, however, suffering always involves self-conflict. Thinking about acute pain, one wonders how this can be. The clue lies in the fact that meaning is essential to suffering. The threat to the person's intactness or integrity resides in the meaning of the pain or beliefs about its consequences. The book of Job provides an illustration of the place of self-conflict in suffering. That there is a God and that God is just are not merely facts for Job; they are part of his self-understanding. Job is a righteous man, but his friends taunt him: If Job is righteous as he says, God would not punish him. Job responds, "Yet does not God see my ways and count my every step?" (31: 4). On the other hand, he wants to defend himself before God: "I would plead the whole record of my life and present that in court as my defense" (31: 37). If God knows his every step and God is just, why would he have to defend himself? The suffering of Job, generally identified with the awful things that happen to him, has as its deeper source the conflict between that part of him that knows that God is aware of his every step and is a just God, and that part of him that believes (with his friends) that only the wicked are punished. Either he is wicked when he knows he is not, or God is not just.

The saints offer a contrary example. Reaching toward Christ by sharing the bodily suffering of others or through punishments imposed on the body are familiar aspects of early Christianity. Denial of bodily needs, tolerance of awful afflictions, and self-inflicted torture are commonplace in the histories of the saints. Adversities and pains are seen as allowing the holy person to identify with the suffering of Christ. Conflict with the body and the tolerance of the pain

do not cause conflict within the person because they permit reaching a desired goal. If there were no Christ with whom to identify, then suffering would follow.

The sick, especially the chronically ill, are often unable to do what they need to do to ensure their self-esteem and their ability to be like others and be admired by others, to excel. But they do not stop wanting to meet these standards, which they usually picture as existing outside of themselves. The resulting internalized conflict of the sick person with the external world becomes self-conflict.

Confrontations between the person and his or her body, as well as dissension within the various aspects of the individual, can threaten to destroy the integrity of the person. This is most easily seen when the demands of the body conflict with the needs of the person. Pain or other symptoms, disabilities, medical care, or other needs may require attention to the body that deters the person from pursuits or purposes considered vital, or they may require attention to the body that the person finds extremely onerous. The body may become an untrustworthy "other" that fails the sick person when it is most needed. It may be a source of humiliation because of, for example, loss of bowel or bladder control. The body's needs, sexual or otherwise, may force the person to engage in behaviors that lead to social failures. Conflicts between the person and the body may cause suffering when no illness is present. The internal struggle that may occur in regard to sexual desire is notorious. Even in acute pain, self-conflict is present. If the person did not care about the pain or its consequences, did not resist its overwhelming force, and instead became completely passive or resigned to the injury, suffering would not occur. This represents extreme self-discipline. People want to live, to resist the pain, to fight back, and therein is the genesis of the suffering.

Suffering is a Lonely State

Because the individual is ultimately unknowable and suffering is unique and individual, involving a withdrawal of purpose from the social world and marked by self-conflict, suffering is inevitably a lonely condition. The inability to know with certainty why someone is suffering, and thus to identify truly with the sufferer, creates difficulties for its treatment. The treatment and relief of suffering, *even when pain cannot be relieved,* is often best accomplished by attempting to overcome its loneliness. This is illustrated in Tolstoy's superb story about sickness and suffering, *The Death of Ivan Ilych.* Virtually the only relief from his suffering that Ilych experiences late in his illness is the constancy and compassion of the servant, Gerasim, who stays with him when all others have effectively abandoned him (Reich).

Persons are communal in origin and by nature. They cannot be known or understood apart from their social being. As a consequence, the sufferer's inherent loneliness furthers the suffering. Because the sufferer's loss of connection with the group is one of the most important aspects of suffering both from the standpoint of its origins and its opportunities for relief, the loneliness of the sufferer is not only the feeling of being alone but an absence from the general "we-ness" of the world, from a shared participation in spirit. The idea of spirit reaches back into the history of both philosophy and religion. The word has many meanings in different traditions, but fundamentally, spirit has to do with the relationship of individuals to the group and to an overriding belief in the existence of God, Nature, or other transcendency. For the purposes of understanding suffering, spirit in a Hegelian sense is useful: some sort of general consciousness that unites all persons (Solomon).

Pain or Suffering in Special Groups

Until recently, minor surgical procedures were performed on newborns and very young infants without anesthesia in the belief that they did not feel pain. Whether their perception is of pain in the manner of fully functioning adults, where other psychological factors such as meaning play a part, is not as important as the understanding that newborns and very young infants (as known from neuroanatomic criteria, psychophysiologic measures, and their behaviors) experience nociception and resulting sensory pain and thus require anesthesia and analgesia. The situation is not as clear for fetuses, but they also exhibit aversive responses to nociceptive stimuli, suggesting the need for analgesia (Anand and Carr).

Depending on the depth of coma, patients in coma may or may not experience nociception as shown by whether they react to nociceptive stimuli. Reaction to painful stimuli is employed as a measure of the depth of coma and is often the first sign of recovery of central nervous system function. Nociception does not appear to be present in persons in a persistent vegetative state (Katayama et al.).

By definition, comatose patients and patients in a persistent vegetative state cannot suffer. Since suffering involves persons and their appreciation of their own intactness or threats to it, and requires a sense of identity, of the past, and of the future, these features must be present for suffering to occur. The applicability of these criteria to fetuses and neonates is unknown, but young children have the capacity to suffer.

Philosophical Issues

The history of medicine, like much of philosophy, has been marked by the dichotomy between empiricism and rationalism. In medicine, empiricism has also been identified with vitalism, the belief that there exist forces for health within the patient—the *physis* of the Hippocrates. For more than 150 years, medicine has been dominated by rationalist thought that has focused on disease as known by the objective criteria of pathoanatomic or pathophysiologic alterations. Diagnostic and therapeutic interventions and the actions of physicians have been based on the science of medicine and its conviction that all illness and pathophysiology would be explained by the laws of physics and chemistry. Symptoms and the reactions of sick persons to their diseases have been treated as epiphenomena, matters of less importance than science, and given over to the art of medicine, which was ranked lower than that of science.

In recent decades, however, the sick person has become more important. This is largely the result of vitalist-empiricist beliefs expressing themselves as a desire for a more "holistic" medicine, as well as changes in the social context of medicine since the 1960s. During the period of the civil-rights movement and the women's movement in the United States, patients (and more recently persons with disabilities) have achieved the social status of full personhood. The rise of bioethics in the United States during this period has played an important part in this social transformation. Recent interest in pain and suffering can be attributed both to the fact that they defy explanation on purely physicochemical grounds and to the increased attention being given to the experience of the sick person.

The concept of patient autonomy has been of central importance in bioethics, but suffering can put the sufferer's autonomy in question, creating ethical dilemmas. Autonomy implies a self-directed individual with consistent goals and intentions springing from a rational evaluation of situations and norms. Reasoning about choices is coupled here with coherence of purpose—central purpose. The ability to remain autonomous requires that things over which one has no control do not remove all of one's choices or the ability to choose. For the suffering person, autonomy is removed when purposes are directed by the immediate needs of the sick body or by the compulsion to address what is perceived to be the source of suffering. This creates difficulties for an ethics that relies heavily on the principle of autonomy. The exercise of authentic choice in this circumstance requires the help of others, individuals who can represent suffering persons to others and, perhaps, to themselves. The difficult task in these situations is to help the sufferer make choices and act as if suffering were absent. But suffering is marked by loneliness that can deny the help of others. The loss of autonomy following severe illness is usually obvious, while the fact that autonomy is no longer present because of suffering may not be apparent. Actions that are beneficent or even nonmaleficent in relation to the suffering person, in contrast to the ill person, may not be obvious. Thus, what is known about suffering casts doubt on the usefulness of an ethics of principle such as that advocated by Tom Beauchamp and James Childress. In contrast, the nature of suffering suggests the importance of a communitarian view of ethics where the relations of individuals to each other as members of a community guide notions of the right and the good. Stanley Hauerwas has raised questions about the obligations of physicians to relieve suffering—if, in fact, medicine could remove all suffering—in view of the importance often placed on the benefit of suffering. Rather, the duty to alleviate suffering highlights the physician's classical responsibility to have compassion for the suffering person, as in the story of the Good Samaritan, even in the absence of the ability to lift the burden of the sufferer (Hauerwas).

Theological Perspectives on Suffering

SUFFERING AS A RESULT OF HUMAN SIN.
A commonly employed explanation of suffering is to see it as the fault of human beings, as punishment or retribution for individual or group actions or sins. The idea that God keeps tabs on individual actions and punishes sinners is widespread. This corresponds to the conviction of one of Job's friends: "As I have seen, those who plow iniquity and sow trouble reap the same" (Job 4: 8). Yet, it is obvious that the innocent as well as the evil are made to suffer. In the New Testament (Luke 13: 1 and John 9), Jesus indicates the mistake of interpreting each evidence of suffering as the consequence of someone's sins. A recent Apostolic Letter of Pope John Paul II (1984) on the Christian meaning of suffering acknowledges the Old Testament writings that show suffering as punishment inflicted by God for human sins, but goes on to disavow such a simple understanding.

SUFFERING AS EDUCATIONAL AND EVIDENTIARY.
Where would we be without suffering to tell us what is important, make us better, to lead us back into the paths of righteousness? Suffering, in this view, offers the opportunity to learn humility.

> My son, do not spurn the Lord's correction
> or take offence at his reproof;
> For those whom he loves the Lord reproves,
> and he punishes a favorite son. (Proverbs 3: 11, 12)

But it could not provide such opportunities in the absence of a God of grace and love. The prophets provide many examples of this view of the importance of human suffering. But suffering also reveals to the sufferer a greater depth of human experience and meaning. After the experience of suffering, the person is led to a richer understanding of the meaning of being human, a greater concern for the suffering of others, and away from the superficialities that too often characterize daily existence.

SUFFERING AS SACRIFICIAL AND LEADING TO SOME GREATER GOOD.
Both on a religious and a secular basis, it is not unusual for suffering persons to believe that their suffering is a form of selfless service to others. Through the acquisition of meaning in this fashion, the suffering is alleviated. It should be remembered that suffering occurs when the intactness or integrity of the person is threatened or disrupted, and it can be relieved when the person is reconstituted even if the agency of its occurrence continues. Giving meaning to the distress, which is what occurs in sacrificial suffering, is one way the person can be made whole again. The suffering of one may benefit many. The suffering of the prophets in the service of Israel is such an example. Another is the crucifixion of Jesus, an evil done by others, turned by God into Christianity's central saving act and a demonstration of the power of love over suffering.

SUFFERING RESULTING FROM THE FORCES OF EVIL OR CHAOS.
This view suggests that God is not the only supernatural force and that there exist powers that are specifically evil. Satan is such an example, although he is specifically mentioned only three times in the Old Testament; the best known of these mentions appears in Job. In the New Testament, the Devil, Satan, demons, or evil spirits are frequently mentioned as sources of suffering. Modern peoples are frequently uncomfortable with such images, yet suffering on a huge scale has occurred so often in recent times that it seems necessary to draw on some other source of evil while keeping God a positive, loving, and just force. Another variant, nondemoniac, implies that there is a limit to the power of God and that he is just one force in the universe. God, in this view, should be called on for what he can do, but one should realize his limitations. A popular book employs this explanation for the problem raised in its title, *When Bad Things Happen to Good People* (Kushner). The mystical tradition of Judaism denies these limitations, insisting that to speak of God as one ("Hear, O Israel, the Lord is God, the Lord is One" [Deut. 6: 4]) is to speak of the unity of all. Everything is God, good and evil, joy and suffering. "And know today and bring it home to your heart

that the Lord, He is God, in the heavens above and on the earth below—there is none other" (Deut. 4: 39) (Luzzatto).

SUFFERING AS MYSTERIOUS OR MEANINGLESS. For the classical Greeks, fate and the actions of the gods are indifferent to humankind's ideas of good or justice. Unconcerned fate has, however, a beginning, a middle, and an end and what starts must ultimately be realized. In the Greek tragedies, the terrible end is foretold in the beginning, the middle is the attempt of the hero to live the heroic existence, while in the end the suffering and tragedy that had been foretold must necessarily occur. Suffering and tragedy, then, have their origins in meaningless fate, but they follow from initial actions of humans. A somewhat similar conclusion is reached in the reincarnation religions such as Buddhism and Hinduism: Suffering in this life is inherent in existence, following, in part, from desire in a previous existence that determines the current behavior that leads to suffering. Since one cannot know what transpired in the previous animation, suffering in this life appears to be the result of capricious fate. Deliverance can only come by escape from individual personality, and ultimately, by giving up desire.

The Old Testament, particularly in Job and Ecclesiastes, explores the problem of suffering in depth, ultimately concluding that it is beyond the ability of ordinary mortals to explain. Explanation itself, and the reasoning on which it is based, may be the problem. In their early speeches, Job's counselors know that he must have transgressed, otherwise he would not be punished. Simple explanation—the connection of logically related, but largely unexamined, premises leading to a conclusion—particularly of the facile type presented by Job's counselors, prevents any deeper understanding. If, for example, Job's privations are not punishment directed at him, but occur as part of the natural order of God's universe, then the search for the explanation itself prevents an acceptance of the mystery. Yet the acceptance of mystery, of the fundamentally unsolvable, points the way to changes in fundamental presuppositions and to the relief of suffering. Religion for the Preacher of Ecclesiastes and for Job represents the general, not simple, truths, including the goodness of God, that have the capacity for transforming character and relieving suffering when they are sincerely held and vividly apprehended, even in the painful void of evidence for their truth. It belongs to the depth of religious spirit to have felt forsaken by God (Whitehead).

A consideration of the nature of suffering opens possibilities for reflection and study about the nature of persons, the relation of persons to their bodies, the goals of medicine, relationships between persons and within communities, and the place of spirit in the lives of individuals. It is little wonder that consideration of suffering and its place in the human condition and in the relationship of God to humankind has occupied human thought throughout the ages—and still the questions remain.

ERIC J. CASSELL (1995)

SEE ALSO: *Authority in Religious Traditions; Autonomy; Chronic Illness and Chronic Care; Care; Compassionate Love; Health and Disease: The Experience of Health and Illness; Life, Quality of; Life Sustaining Treatment and Euthanasia; Medicine, Anthropology of; Palliative Care and Hospice; Pastoral Care and Healthcare Chaplaincy; Rehabilitative Medicine; Suicide*

BIBLIOGRAPHY

Anand, K. J. S., and Carr, D. B. 1989. "The Neuroanatomy, Neurophysiology, and Neurochemistry of Pain, Stress, and Analgesia in Newborns and Children." *Pediatric Clinics of North America* 36(4): 795–822.

Bakan, David. 1968. *Disease, Pain, and Sacrifice: Toward a Psychology of Suffering.* Chicago: University of Chicago Press.

Beauchamp, Tom L., and Childress, James F. 1994. *Principles of Biomedical Ethics,* 4th edition. New York: Oxford University Press.

Cassell, Eric J. 1982. "The Nature of Suffering and the Goals of Medicine." *New England Journal of Medicine* 306(11): 639–645.

Cassell, Eric J. 1991. *The Nature of Suffering and the Goals of Medicine.* New York: Oxford University Press.

Cleary, Francis X. 1974. "Biblical Perspectives on Suffering." *Hospital Progress* (December): 54–58.

Crue, Benjamin L. 1985. *Chapter in Evaluation and Treatment of Chronic Pain,* ed. Gerald M. Aronoff. Baltimore: Urban and Schwarzenberg.

Frankl, Viktor E. 1962. *Man's Search for Meaning: An Introduction to Logotherapy,* tr. Ilse Lasch. Boston: Beacon Press.

Hauerwas, Stanley. 1979. "Reflections on Suffering, Death, and Medicine." *Ethics in Science and Medicine* 6: 229–237.

John Paul II. 1984. "Salvifici doloris." *Acta Apostolica Sedis* 76 (March 1): 201–250, tr. under the title "Salvifici doloris: On the Meaning of Christian Suffering." *The Pope Speaks* 29 (Summer): 105–139.

Katamaya, Yoichi; Tsubokawa, Takashi; Yamamoto, Takamitsu; Hirayama, Teruyasu; Miyazaki, Shuhei; and Koyama, Seigon. 1991. "Characterization and Modification of Brain Activity with Deep Brain Stimulation in Patients in a Persistent Vegetative State: Pain-Related Late Positive Component of Cerebral Evoked Potential." *Pacing and Clinical Electrophysiology* 14, no. 1: 116–121.

Kushner, Harold S. 1981. *When Bad Things Happen to Good People.* New York: Schocken.

Loewy, Erich H. 1991. *Suffering and the Beneficent Community: Beyond Libertarianism.* Albany, NY: State University of New York Press.

Lovejoy, Arthur O. 1961. *Reflections on Human Nature.* Baltimore: Johns Hopkins University Press.

Luzzatto, Moshe Hayyim. 1982. *The Knowing Heart: The Philosophy of God's Oneness,* tr. Shraga Silverstein. Jerusalem: Feldheim.

Reich, Warren T. 1989. "Speaking of Suffering: A Moral Account of Compassion." *Soundings* 72(1): 83–108.

Scarry, Elaine. 1985. *The Body in Pain: The Making and Unmaking of the World.* New York: Oxford University Press.

Simundson, Daniel J. 1980. *Faith under Fire: Biblical Interpretations of Suffering.* Minneapolis, MN: Augsburg.

Solomon, R. C. 1972. "Hegel's Concept of 'Geist.'" In *Hegel: A Collection of Critical Essays,* ed. Alasdair C. MacIntyre. Notre Dame, IN: University of Notre Dame Press.

Whitehead, Alfred North. 1974. *Religion in the Making.* New York: New American Library.

Whitehead, Willard, III, and Kuhn, Wolfgang F. 1990. "Chronic Pain: An Overview." In vol. 1 of *Chronic Pain,* pp. 5–48, ed. Thomas W. Miller. Madison, CT: International Universities Press.

PALLIATIVE CARE AND HOSPICE

• • •

The terms *palliative care* and *hospice* are frequently used interchangeably to describe an approach to the care of individuals who are likely to die in the relatively near future from serious, incurable disease, for whom the principal focus of care is quality of life and support for the patient's family. The terms gained currency in the last third of the twentieth century as a result of significant changes in the leading causes of death in the developed countries of the industrialized world. In these countries prior to 1900, most people died relatively quickly, usually from acute, infectious diseases. They typically died at home, attended by family and friends. Because little in the way of medical technology was available to prevent or delay death, the costs of care were low, and the dying person and her caregivers could emphasize the interpersonal and spiritual aspects of dying.

By contrast, at the beginning of the twenty-first century most people in the developed world die from chronic, degenerative diseases such as cancer, cardiovascular disease, lung disease, and degenerative neurological disease. Death usually follows a prolonged period of progressive loss of function and numerous distressing symptoms, of which pain and shortness of breath are the most feared by patients, along with fear of the unknown. Because considerable medical technology now exists that can postpone death, costs are often high and most people die in hospitals or nursing homes, attended by strangers. For patients who die at home, the financial, physical, and emotional burdens of caregiving fall heavily on isolated nuclear families, and predominantly on women.

The Early Days of the Hospice Movement

The "hospice movement," as it is popularly known, is generally agreed to have started in 1967 with the opening of St. Christopher's Hospice in London under the charismatic leadership of Dr. Cicely Saunders. Hospices were a feature of the Middle Ages in Europe, usually run by religious orders, and offered safety, healing, and rest to weary and often wounded travelers. It was therefore an obvious name to give to institutions founded in France, Ireland, and England around the turn of the nineteenth century to care for the dying. What made St. Christopher's and those that followed different was Saunders's insistence on scientific rigor and professional education and training.

Few people were likely to return home from these pioneer hospices, but they would get skilled relief of their pain and suffering, whatever its nature or origin, in a sensitively nourished environment of love, safety, and peace for them and their relatives. That better care of the dying was needed was attested to by many comments of the dying themselves, grieving relatives who looked back in horror and sadness at what patients had had to suffer, and by an increasing number of papers published in reputable medical journals detailing this suffering. At what most must have felt the loneliest time of their life, the dying described themselves as having no attention paid to their suffering and getting no answers to their questions. They not only experienced a spectrum of physical suffering, but endured fear, depression, loneliness, and a sense of being undervalued by society. They often felt deserted by their doctors, whom they found difficult to trust when so rarely were they told the true nature of their mortal illness and what lay ahead. The dying either lived with relatives who, hoping to protect them, conspired with the doctors to keep them in ignorance, or in hospitals where the focus of attention was sophisticated investigations and aggressive treatments designed to cure.

Palliative Care

It was soon recognized that the word hospice, though widely understood and accepted by the English-speaking world, would never be universally acceptable because it had a different meaning in French and Spanish. Balfour Mount, who established a specialized unit at the Royal Victoria Hospital in Montreal in 1974 based on the principles he had learned at St. Christopher's, coined the term *palliative care* to circumvent the language problem. Because it was already in medical parlance, the healthcare professions accepted this term. Today physicians working in this field describe themselves as palliative medicine physicians and nurses as palliative care nurses, while the services where they work (the original hospices) are called specialist palliative care services.

The acceptance and adoption of palliative care by other healthcare professionals has not always been straightforward, however. Many claimed they were already providing it, in spite of the many reports of uncontrolled suffering. A few suspected it was euthanasia under another name. Some were convinced it was not based on well-proven therapeutic regimens but was simply complementary or alternative medicine applied to the dying. Others questioned why it seemed to focus on the care of people with malignant disease when patients suffering end-stage cardiac, neurological, and respiratory disease, or AIDS, had similar and often unmet needs (Addington-Hall).

Definition and Scope

It was easy to define hospice care when it focused on the final days of life. It soon became apparent, however, that better care was needed long before this terminal phase. Hospital-based teams were created to provide care for patients in the hospital units where they were still receiving treatments intended to cure or slow the progress of their underlying disease. Things could also be improved when people were being cared for at home, where most wanted to remain as long as possible, though, contrary to what has always been said, not necessarily to die there (Hinton; Ward). A range of services was developed to assist primary physicians caring for people at home, including home visits by nurses and other professionals and day-care units for patients who could be brought into a center for clinical assessment and creative occupational therapy.

Palliative care was no longer synonymous with "care of the dying." Yet, as the field has developed, it has struggled to define itself in a way that captures its broader scope— reflecting its appropriateness for patients earlier in their disease process, who are not imminently dying—without resorting to euphemisms chosen to disguise the fact that the care is for people who, sooner rather than later, will die of their illness. The most commonly used definition is that devised by the World Health Organization. It emphasizes that the principles of palliation—the relief of physical, psychosocial, and spiritual distress, and respect for the needs

of relatives—are appropriate from the time of diagnosis. In an attempt to produce a more succinct definition, called for when palliative medicine was recognized as a medical specialty in the United Kingdom in 1987, palliative care was defined as the study and care of patients with active, progressive, far-advanced disease and a limited life expectancy, for whom the focus of care is the quality of life.

This definition does not limit palliative care to people with malignant disease, nor does it state a prognosis in terms of months or weeks. It is worded so as not to be confused with care of the elderly, care of the chronically ill, or care of the incurable (which would embrace many of the conditions seen daily by physicians). Unfortunately, it omits mention of relatives, or the fact that palliative care can be provided only by an interdisciplinary team. Its strength lies in its unequivocal focus on quality of life rather than on cure or prolongation of life, the declared objectives of much of modern medical care.

J. Andrew Billings, who in 1998 reviewed many of the competing definitions, concluded that the following definition achieves the best balance of completeness and concision:

> Palliative care is comprehensive, interdisciplinary care, focusing primarily on promoting quality of life for patients living with a terminal illness and for their families. Key elements for helping the patient and family live as well as possible in the face of life-threatening illness include assuring physical comfort, psychosocial and spiritual support, and provision of coordinated services across various sites of care. (p. 80)

Two further statements, endorsed by the government of the United Kingdom, have been found challenging and helpful:

- It is the right of every person who needs it to receive high quality palliative care, irrespective of his or her diagnosis.
- It is the responsibility of every clinician to provide high quality palliative care. (Doyle, p. 6)

In applying these principles in the complex, highly differentiated world of the health professions, it is helpful to note that palliative care can be provided at three levels: principles, techniques, and specialist care.

Palliative care principles are integral to all good clinical care, and they are applicable at every stage of a patient's care, whatever the nature of the illness. Every doctor and nurse should be applying these principles, even when they are still defining the nature and cause of an illness or its symptoms.

Palliative techniques are usually the responsibility of professionals such as surgeons and interventional radiologists, who, for example, create ostomies, insert stents, and provide palliative radiation. None of these procedures is intended to cure, but each can bring about relief in suffering.

Specialist palliative care is provided by those who have undergone specialist training as stipulated by their accrediting professional body. In such countries and regions as the United Kingdom, Australasia, and Hong Kong, specialist palliative care units are those where all senior doctors and nurses are accredited specialists and where members of professions allied to medicine (physiotherapists, occupational therapists, clinical pharmacists, clinical psychologists, and music, art, and stoma therapists) have all had additional training pertinent to palliative care. Such services are usually affiliated with local medical and nursing colleges.

Quality, Value, and Meaning of Life

As palliative care continues to develop, it is being recognized that with the drugs and techniques currently available, and the increasing skills to use them, it is relatively easy to achieve physical comfort, but that even when that has been achieved a person may still feel frightened, lonely, unwanted, or undervalued. Those working in the field now realize that, beyond the management of physical symptoms, palliative care is primarily concerned with three things.

First is quality of life. Many quality-of-life assessment tools specific to palliative care are now available to healthcare professionals (Clinch, Dudgeon, and Schipper; Higginson). Each attempts to measure quality as perceived by the patient or relative and not by the attending professionals. Robust research is now confirming what has long been suspected, that patients not given the information they seek experience more physical and psychosocial suffering and describe a lower quality of life than those kept informed according to their wishes. To many people's surprise, this has proven to be the case not only in the West but also in diverse cultures and among peoples of various faiths in the Middle and Far East.

The second concern is value of life. As people approach death they increasingly wonder whether their lives have been of any value to others and to the community, and whether they still have any value as persons when they are incapacitated by a fatal illness, dependent on others, and, as they are often reminded, expensive to care for. Surveys in the United States have shown that patients' loss of independence and fears of being a burden to others are more often the primary motivations in requesting assisted suicide or euthanasia than is physical pain (Emanuel et al.; Sullivan, Hedberg, and Fleming). Respecting the individual patient's assessment of

the value of her life, while remaining vigilant for the effects of depression or social isolation, presents one of the most profound clinical and ethical challenges in palliative care. Yet, the skills for eliciting and responding to this form of suffering are seldom addressed in medical and nursing schools.

The third concern is meaning of life. When, and only when, their physical suffering has been relieved and their families cared for, do dying people begin to ask existential questions. Though a diminishing proportion of people in the West now claim to have a meaningful religious faith, more than 75 percent of dying people want to discuss the meaning of life, suffering, and death, and they may be disappointed if no one is interested in helping them. Once again, in the absence of some training in the humanities, doctors and nurses in the increasingly secularized Western society find themselves ill-equipped to help with this issue.

The Development of Palliative Care Worldwide

From the handful in operation in 1967, there are now more than 6,200 palliative care programs in over 100 countries. In its birthplace, the United Kingdom, palliative care services are readily and freely accessible to all. The National Health Service runs one-fifth of these services, and 25 percent of the operating costs of the others are met by government, the balance being met from voluntary funding of more than US$450 million annually. A typical palliative care in-patient unit in the United Kingdom, with 10 to 100 beds, admits annually twenty to twenty-five patients per bed, where each will stay for an average of eleven to fourteen days. The portion of patients able to return home varies between 40 and 60 percent, higher if there is an effective community palliative care service and a day unit. Seldom do more than 15 percent of patients who have conditions other than cancer receive palliative care in the United Kingdom, a considerably smaller percentage than in the United States.

Though palliative care services are being developed in many countries, most are modeled on those of the United Kingdom and the United States, rather than being designed to meet local needs and cultures. Palliative care is still not available to the 75 percent of the world's population, for whom curative treatment of life-threatening disease is either unavailable or inaccessible. There are still only a relative handful of medical schools worldwide that include palliative care in the curriculum, and fewer still where a specialist teaches it. Even when it is mentioned in undergraduate medical courses it is rarely included in the training of subspecialists who—in the West—provide the bulk of the care to critically ill patients. Only in those countries where there are doctors working full time in the field is palliative care rapidly gaining credibility and acceptance.

Palliative Care in the United States

The first hospice program in the United States opened in Connecticut in 1974. Most early programs relied heavily for financial support on private, local philanthropy and grants. Beginning in 1983, patients over the age of sixty-five could elect to receive a "hospice benefit" under the Medicare program. A patient certified by his physician as "terminally ill" (defined as having a life expectancy of six months or less) may waive access to Medicare coverage of curative treatments for the terminal illness, in return for a package of services aimed at symptom control and improved quality of life. These services would otherwise not be covered or would be provided in an uncoordinated manner. The Medicare hospice benefit (payable as a per diem reimbursement to Medicare-certified hospice providers) includes nursing care in the home (up to sixteen to twenty hours per week, with temporary twenty-four-hour care available under limited "crisis" circumstances); medical appliances and drugs; home-makers, home health aides, and volunteers for personal and respite care; physician services; short-term hospitalization; physical and occupational therapy; psychological and spiritual support; social services; and bereavement counseling (Center for Medicare Education).

Medicare requires hospices to conform to several procedural and staffing requirements in order to receive federal funds. Among the most significant requirements are that the hospice must have a core, interdisciplinary team made up of at least a physician, a registered nurse, a social worker, and a chaplain or other counselor; that patients must have an identified primary-care provider in the home (usually a family member or someone else who is available on a twenty-four-hour-per-day basis); and that no more than 20 percent of the total aggregate number of days of care provided by the hospice may be in inpatient settings.

Since Medicare funding became available, the number of hospice programs in the United States has increased dramatically. From 1982 to 2000, the estimated number of providers grew from 500 to 3,100. The number of patients served increased from approximately 1,000 to approximately 700,000 between 1975 and 2000. Cancer patients made up 57 percent of hospice admissions in the United States in 2000, followed by patients with heart disease (10%), dementia (6%), lung disease (6%), end-stage kidney disease (3%), and end-stage liver disease (2%) (NHPCO).

In contrast to community- and home-based hospice care, hospital-based palliative care programs are a much more recent development in the United States. As recently as 1998, only 15 percent of U.S. hospitals reported having any services devoted to end-of-life care (Pan et al.). In a survey of 5,810 member hospitals by the American Hospital Association in 2000, 13.8 percent of the 4,856 respondents reported having a palliative medicine service, while 22.7 percent reported a hospital-based hospice program, and 42 percent reported a pain management service.

Inpatient palliative care units on the British or Canadian model are still relatively rare in the United States. Hospital-based palliative care teams primarily provide consultation for symptom management, patient and family counseling, and conversations designed to determine appropriate goals of care (Pan et al.). Financial pressures on acute-care hospitals in the United States usually dictate the swift discharge (to home or nursing facility) of any patient for whom acute hospital interventions are no longer indicated. This restricts the ability of the hospital palliative care team to assist in the course of the patient's dying. The role of the team at that point is most often to assure as smooth a transfer as possible to another setting, which may or may not include ongoing palliative care by specialist professionals.

Unlike in Great Britain, where there are now more specialist palliative medicine physicians than oncologists, palliative medicine has not been recognized as a medical subspecialty in the United States. Beginning in 1996, however, the American Board of Hospice and Palliative Medicine began to administer a certifying examination for physicians who wished to be known for special competence in the field. A separate organization, the Hospice and Palliative Nurses Association, administers a certifying examination for nurses and began a certification program for palliative care nursing assistants in 2002.

Ethical and Policy Issues in Palliative Care and Hospice

Many of the ethical issues that arise in the care of the dying are similar to issues that arise in many other areas of healthcare, such as truthfulness and confidentiality, decision-making authority in the professional–patient relationship, the appropriate use and allocation of technology and other healthcare resources, the conduct of research, and the locus of ethical responsibility when care is provided by a team (Randall and Downie). Other issues are more commonly associated with the care of the terminally ill, though not absent from other arenas, such as decision making for patients who have lost the capacity to make or communicate their own decisions, withholding or withdrawing life-sustaining treatment, and hastening death by assisting in suicide or through active euthanasia.

The latter issue tends to receive the greatest attention from bioethics scholars and policymakers. Moral distinctions between various actions or choices that can hasten the time of death can be exquisitely fine (Quill, Lo, and Brock). Yet, for all the persistent and intense debate surrounding the issues of suicide and euthanasia (Battin, Rhodes, and Silvers), "terminal sedation" and the doctrine of double effect (Fohr), or the differences, if any, between "allowing to die" and "causing to die" (Brock; Clouser), another set of issues are no less vexing and affect far more people. These are the questions of access to and quality of palliative care services.

The dimensions of the problem of access to palliative care are suggested by the following data from the United States. According to the National Hospice and Palliative Care Organization (NHPCO), of the 2.4 million people who died in the United States in 2000, approximately one-fourth died while receiving hospice care. Approximately half died in hospitals, 25 percent died in a nursing facility, and another 25 percent died at home; the percentage of home deaths has remained relatively stable for several decades, despite Gallup polls that consistently indicate that over 85 percent of Americans would prefer to die at home.

It is true that dying at home is an imperfect marker for the adequacy of palliative care. In fact, in most developed countries, the better the palliative care provision in hospitals and the community, the fewer the number of people who die at home, with home deaths now approaching 20 percent in most European countries. A more telling statistic is that of patients who received hospice care in 2000, one-third died within seven days of admission, despite the six months of benefits allowed under the Medicare hospice program. The median length of stay for hospice patients in the United States has been dropping steadily for several years; the NHPCO reports that it was only twenty-five days in 2000. Although the reasons for these trends are still being investigated, the following are likely to be significant contributing factors: the difficulty of making precise estimates of life expectancy—as is required for Medicare hospice eligibility—especially for diseases other than cancer (Teno et al.); patients' reluctance to accept the label "terminally ill"; the requirement that patients forgo Medicare reimbursement for treatments with curative intent; and many physicians' identification of a hospice referral with "giving up."

In the United States, hospice and palliative care have not yet fully overcome the legacy of opposition to mainstream scientific medicine that characterized their beginnings in the 1970s. The growth of rigorous scientific research in palliative care, the publication of textbooks, and the growth of a cadre of palliative medicine specialists with a base in academic medical centers should ameliorate this problem in the years to come. For the present, however,

hospice and palliative care remain near the margins of the American healthcare system. In the realm of education, a 1997 survey of fourth-year medical students and third-year medical residents found that both groups rated their preparation in end-of-life care worse than for many other common clinical tasks (Block and Sullivan), and analyses of leading medical textbooks reveal that, on average, end-of-life issues are addressed on only 1.6 percent of the pages (Block). In the realm of financing of services or research, the desire to forestall or prevent death overwhelms support for hospice and palliative care. Precise data are difficult to obtain, but one indicator of the relative lack of support for palliative as opposed to curative medicine is presented in a 1997 report from the Institute of Medicine of the National Academy of Sciences. The report cites a personal communication from an official from the National Institutes of Health (NIH), who estimated that in fiscal year 1996, NIH spent about $70 million on pain research out of an overall budget of $12 billion.

From the policy perspective, the greatest challenge facing palliative care in the United States at the beginning of the twenty-first century is to fashion a system of financing and delivery of care that is flexible enough to provide services as they are needed along the complete continuum from diagnosis of life-threatening illness through the (often unpredictable) period of disability and functional decline, into the last phases of active dying and family bereavement (Lynn). The system would, at a minimum, encourage the open acknowledgment by physicians and patients of the possibility of dying, advance planning to anticipate complications and likely needs for care, meticulous attention to physical symptoms and to psychological and spiritual suffering, support for the family, and the creation of settings for care that respect the personal and spiritual significance of death and loss.

Worldwide, the challenge of access to competent palliative care is no less daunting. Among the principal causes for alarm are the number of people living with HIV/AIDS—estimated by the United Nations at 40 million at the end of 2001—and the large projected increase in deaths from tobacco products, which the World Health Organization predicts could triple by 2020 from the 2000 level of 3.5 million (Brundtland). In both cases, almost all of the increase is expected to occur in the developing world. Global efforts to teach the principles of modern palliative care, and to incorporate them in healthcare systems, are lagging far behind the manifest need, despite curative technologies and medications remaining unavailable or unaffordable for most of the world's poor.

Where palliative care is available, there is the challenge of providing care in ways that respect different cultural and religious views. Most professionals who enter the field do so because they want to help people die well. But what does it mean to "die well"? What is a "good death"? There is no single, universal answer to either of these questions. That the modern hospice movement was first promulgated largely by Christians may have hindered its development among people of other faiths for whom the "hospice philosophy" may have been hard to separate from theological commitments that they did not share. Even with respect to elements of a "good death" on which most people could probably agree—freedom from pain, resolution of personal affairs, the supportive presence of loved ones—there is room for considerable personal variation. People differ in their willingness to face the reality of their imminent death; in their desire to talk about their feelings to friends, family, or caregivers; in how they balance pain relief against alertness; and in their willingness to tolerate increasing weakness, dependency, and uncertainty rather than trying to control the timing and manner of their death through an act of suicide or euthanasia. This variability requires health professionals to approach patients and families as individuals, in an effort to provide care that is consistent both with patient and family values and with their own conscience.

DEREK DOYLE

DAVID BARNARD

SEE ALSO: *AIDS: Healthcare and Research Issues; Cancer, Ethical Issues Related to Diagnosis and Treatment; Care; Compassionate Love; Death; Dementia; Healthcare Resources, Allocation of; Informed Consent; Life, Quality of; Life Sustaining Treatment and Euthanasia; Long-Term Care; Nursing, Profession of; Pastoral Care and Healthcare Chaplaincy; Social Work in Healthcare; Teams, Healthcare*

BIBLIOGRAPHY

Addington-Hall, Julia. 1998. *Reaching Out: Specialist Palliative Care for Adults with Non-Malignant Diseases.* London: National Council for Hospice and Specialist Palliative Care Services.

Battin, Margaret; Rhodes, Rosamond; and Silvers, Anita; eds. 1998. *Physician-Assisted Suicide: Expanding the Debate.* New York: Routledge.

Billings, J. Andrew. 1998. "What Is Palliative Care?" *Journal of Palliative Medicine* 1(1): 73–81.

Block, Susan. 2002. "Medical Education in End-of-Life Care: The Status of Reform." *Journal of Palliative Medicine* 5(2): 243–248.

Block, Susan, and Sullivan, Amy. 1998. "Attitudes about End-of-Life Care: A National Cross-Sectional Study." *Journal of Palliative Medicine* 1(4): 347–355.

Brock, Dan. 1992. "Voluntary Active Euthanasia." *Hastings Center Report* 22(2): 10–22.

Brundtland, Gro. 2001. "The Future of the World's Health." In *Critical Issues in Global Health,* ed. C. Everett Koop, Clarence Peterson, and M. Roy Schwartz. San Francisco: Jossey-Bass.

Center for Medicare Education. 2001. *The Medicare Hospice Benefit.* Washington, D.C.: Author.

Clinch, Jennifer; Dudgeon, Deborah; and Schipper, Harvey. 1998. "Quality of Life Assessment in Palliative Care." In *Oxford Textbook of Palliative Medicine,* ed. Derek Doyle, Geoffrey Hanks, and Neil MacDonald. New York: Oxford University Press.

Clouser, K. Danner. 1977. "Allowing or Causing: Another Look." *Annals of Internal Medicine* 87: 622–624.

Doyle, Derek. 1997. *Dilemmas and Directions: The Future of Specialist Palliative Care: A Discussion Paper.* London: National Council for Hospice and Specialist Palliative Care Services.

Doyle, Derek; Hanks, Geoffrey; and MacDonald, Neil, eds. 1998. *Oxford Textbook of Palliative Medicine.* New York: Oxford University Press.

Emanuel, Ezekiel; Fairclough, Diane; Daniels, Elisabeth; et al. 1996. "Euthanasia and Physician-Assisted Suicide: Attitudes and Experiences of Oncology Patients, Oncologists, and the Public." *Lancet* 347: 1805–1810.

Fohr, S. Anderson. 1998. "The Double Effect of Pain Medication: Separating Myth from Reality." *Journal of Palliative Medicine* 1(4): 315–328.

Higginson, Irene. 1992. *Quality, Standards, Organizational, and Clinical Audit for Hospice and Palliative Care Services.* London: National Council for Hospice and Specialist Palliative Care Services.

Hinton, John. 1994. "Can Home Care Maintain an Acceptable Quality of Life for Patients with Terminal Cancer and Their Relatives?" *Palliative Medicine* 8(3): 183–196.

Joint United Nations Programme on HIV/AIDS. 2002. *Report on the Global HIV/AIDS Epidemic 2002.*

Lynn, Joanne. 2001. "Serving Patients Who May Die Soon and Their Families: The Role of Hospice and Other Services." *Journal of the American Medical Association* 285(7): 925–932.

Mount, Balfour. 1997. "The Royal Victoria Hospital Palliative Care Service: A Canadian Experience." In *Hospice Care on the International Scene,* ed. Cicely Saunders and Robert Kastenbaum. New York: Springer.

National Hospice and Palliative Care Organization (NHPCO). 2001. *Facts and Figures.* Alexandria, VA: Author.

Pan, Cynthia; Morrison, R. Sean; Meier, D.; et al. 2001. "How Prevalent Are Hospital-Based Palliative Care Programs? Status Report and Future Directions." *Journal of Palliative Medicine* 4(3): 315–324.

Quill, Timothy E.; Lo, Bernard; and Brock, Dan W. 1997. "Palliative Options of Last Resort: A Comparison of Voluntarily Stopping Eating and Drinking, Terminal Sedation, Physician-Assisted Suicide, and Voluntary Active Euthanasia." *Journal of the American Medical Association* 278(23): 2099–2104.

Randall, Fiona, and Downie, R. S. 1996. *Palliative Care Ethics: A Good Companion.* Oxford: Oxford University Press.

Saunders, Cicely. 1998. "Foreword." In *Oxford Textbook of Palliative Medicine,* ed. Derek Doyle, Geoffrey Hanks, and Neil MacDonald. New York: Oxford University Press.

Sullivan, Amy; Hedberg, Katrina; and Fleming, David. 2000. "Legalized Physician-Assisted Suicide in Oregon—The Second Year." *New England Journal of Medicine* 342(8): 598–604.

Teno, Joan; Weitzen, Sherry; Fennell, Mary; et al. 2001. "Dying Trajectory in the Last Year of Life: Does Cancer Trajectory Fit Other Diseases?" *Journal of Palliative Medicine* 4(4): 457–464.

U.S. Institute of Medicine. Division of Health Care Services. Committee on Care at the End of Life. 1997. *Approaching Death: Improving Care at the End of Life,* ed. Marilyn Field and Christine Cassel. Washington, D.C.: National Academy Press.

Ward, Audrey. 1985. "Home Care Services for the Terminally Ill." Sheffield, UK: University of Sheffield, Medical Care Research Unit.

World Health Organization. 1990. *Cancer Pain Relief and Palliative Care.* Geneva, Switzerland: Author.

INTERNET RESOURCE

Joint United Nations Programme on HIV/AIDS. 2002. *Report on the Global HIV/AIDS Epidemic 2002.* Available from <http://www.unaids.org/publications/>.

PASTORAL CARE AND HEALTHCARE CHAPLAINCY

• • •

Pastoral care normally refers to the help given by ordained ministers, priests, and other persons with designated religious roles (such as deacons and members of Roman Catholic religious orders) to suffering, troubled, or perplexed persons. In the simplest and most profound sense, *pastoral care* has been defined from a Christian perspective as "the attempt to help others, through words, acts, and relationships, to experience as fully as possible the reality of God's presence and love in their lives" (Holst, p. 46). The term is primarily Christian but it is sometimes used analogously in other faith traditions (e.g., the rabbi's care in Judaism). Recently the term *spiritual care* has been introduced into secular healthcare settings as a less specifically Christian alternative term. In any case, when pastoral or spiritual care is provided in healthcare facilities by pastors or rabbis sponsored by the institution, it is known as *healthcare chaplaincy.* This article largely focuses on healthcare chaplaincy because it is the primary way in which contemporary pastoral care becomes involved with the issues of bioethics.

Historically, pastors have extended their care to a wide range of personal needs and concerns, from struggles of faith, doubt, moral failure, and problems of conscience to marriage and family conflict and the suffering involved in illness, tragedy, and death. In Christian care, the historic, ritualized "means of grace"—sacrament, scripture, prayer—continue to be important resources of pastoral care, especially in situations of crisis (e.g., dying). But in many situations conversational methods predominate. Pastoral conversation emphasizes the caregiver's psychological understanding and ability to foster a therapeutic or healing mode of relationship and style of conversation with the person receiving care. This includes empathic listening, the ability to form emotionally honest, trusting relationships, and the care receiver's active participation with the pastor in the search for healing and wholeness. At the root of their care, pastoral caregivers help persons find the kind of faith and value commitments that can sustain, enrich, and give redemptive meaning to their lives, and "to experience as fully as possible the reality of God's presence and love in their lives" (Holst, p. 46).

Pastoral care and healthcare chaplaincy are often distinguished from another ministerial specialization—pastoral counseling. When this distinction is made, pastoral counseling is commonly defined as a specialized form of ministry characterized by an intentional contract between the pastoral caregiver and the person or family seeking help, usually involving a series of prearranged counseling sessions. This structured form of care contrasts with the more casual and varied forms of caring relationships that parish pastors and healthcare chaplains typically form. Though many ministers, priests, rabbis, and healthcare chaplains provide short-term counseling of the more formal kind, pastoral counseling as a specialized ministry is devoted entirely to this work. To a large extent it is a form of psychotherapy or family therapy (and is often called "pastoral psychotherapy"), and usually involves a number of sessions and the payment of a fee. Pastoral counselors, like healthcare chaplains, have specialized training requirements, professional organizations (principally, the American Association of Pastoral Counselors), and standards of certification. They serve on the staffs of larger churches, in pastoral counseling centers, and in other professional settings, and are often licensed by state governments as pastoral (or other) counselors, psychologists, or marriage and family therapists.

Pastoral Care in Healthcare Settings: The Healthcare Chaplain

FUNCTIONS AND ROLE. Much of what healthcare chaplains do involves helping persons and families (of all faiths) with the emotional and spiritual dimensions of the healing process, offering support and therapeutic care in situations of crisis and grief, helping to resolve conflicts and communication difficulties, and consulting in situations of bioethical and other decision making. Most chaplains also develop an extensive ministry with nurses, physicians, aides, administrators, and others in medical settings who carry significant emotional burdens and moral concerns. Chaplains promote communication between patients, families, and staff concerning religious and cultural traditions that may bear upon medical decisions (e.g., concerning blood transfusion, abortion, and the use of life-support technologies). They often become involved in discussions with all parties involved in healthcare decisions. In addition, healthcare chaplains form educational relationships with local clergy and congregations, function as liaisons between the healthcare institution and the community, and serve on the boards of related community organizations. As more and more medical care is provided on an outpatient basis, and as more congregations develop healthcare emphases and programs, these aspects of their work are expected to increase.

Chaplains often play a significant role in hospital ethics committees; in many instances, they helped to organize these committees in the late 1970s and 1980s. The chaplains' role in ethics committees, as in their consulting with patients and families on bioethical decisions, consists largely in promoting good communication and mutual understanding, interpreting religious and cultural traditions, resolving conflicts, clarifying moral issues, and facilitating free and responsible moral decision-making. It is a basic principle of the Association of Professional Chaplains, the National Association of Catholic Chaplains, and similar national certifying organizations that healthcare chaplains respect the belief and value systems of others and refrain from proselytizing or trying to impose their own convictions on them.

Many healthcare institutions sponsor professional training programs in pastoral care called "clinical pastoral education" (C.P.E.). These programs train not only future chaplains in pastoral care, but also large numbers of theological students, pastors, and members of religious orders not seeking specialized ministry certification. C.P.E. students minister under the supervision of a highly trained and certified chaplain supervisor with whom they meet individually and as a group to analyze and reflect on their work. Such reflection involves intense examination of detailed case reports, personal reflection on the trainees' ways of caring for other persons, and consideration of the psychological, social, cultural, theological, and ethical questions involved in their experiences. Pastoral supervision evolved in the second half of the twentieth century into a distinct and important specialization within healthcare chaplaincy.

RELATION OF HEALTHCARE CHAPLAINCY TO OTHER HEALTHCARE PROFESSIONS. Most pastors who serve in healthcare settings hold a broad, liberal understanding of themselves and their ministries that enables them to cooperate easily with the medical profession and to work pastorally with a wide range of persons. They do not limit their ministries to persons with problems that are explicitly defined in religious or moral terms, but seek to become related to persons in supportive and therapeutic ways whatever the immediate, presenting needs or issues may be.

Thus their work often closely resembles, in certain respects, that of psychiatrists, psychologists, psychiatric nurses, social workers, and patient representatives. The chaplain functions as an integral member of the healthcare team. He or she is "cross trained" in a variety of institutionally valuable skills usefully integrated into a single profession: "psychosocial and spiritual counselor, clinical ethicist, patient representative and ombudsperson, cultural anthropologist and religious scholar, gatekeeper of community resources and public relations expert, and health promoter" (Burton, p. 2). But the chaplain's range of competencies also raises questions of vocational distinctiveness and identity for other professionals and sometimes for themselves. The situation is made more challenging by the fact that pastoral identity in healthcare facilities is usually not expressed solely or principally through the performance of religious rituals or conversation confined to overtly religious problems.

What then gives the chaplain's wide-ranging work comprehensive definition and focus? The answer to this question is much debated within the profession. In general, however, pastoral identity in healthcare settings has two intimately related poles of concern: healing and health, and religion (Burton). Chaplains are significantly identified with each. The distinctiveness of the profession lies in the way these two poles interrelate in an ambiguous but creative unity in the performance of the chaplain's professional function.

At one pole there is a concern for and participation in the processes of health and healing. While healthcare chaplains do not practice medicine or psychiatry, they believe that the meanings and values by which people live, and the quality of their personal relationships, play an important role in the organic processes of illness and health. They also believe that a comprehensive concern for human well-being, including health and healing, is integral to the faith traditions they represent. Thus chaplains believe that religion supports the fundamental aims of medicine and healthcare. And they see their ministries as essentially involved in the process of healing, which they understand in comprehensive terms as healing of the whole person—body, mind, and spirit. Consequently, they view themselves as significant members of the healthcare team, and increasingly they are being viewed in that way by the medical professions.

At the other pole, healthcare chaplains are committed to representing religious meanings and values that include but transcend the values of health and healing. They seek to enable people to find and experience, which ultimately can fulfill their lives and redeem them from the threats of meaningless shame, guilt, and death that pervade all of life, in illness as well as in health. And they set health and healing as values into an encompassing faith perspective that affirms the meaningfulness of life whether or not healing occurs. For the healthcare chaplain, this larger context is ultimately rooted in the reality and loving power of God, who makes health possible, but who also makes meaning, hope, and love possible in every circumstance of life, in illness and adversity as well as in health and wholeness.

Thus pastoral identity is bipolar, committed to both healing and religious faith and to their essential interrelationship. It is the ambiguous but disciplined interplay of these polar commitments that constitutes the distinctive orientation of healthcare chaplaincy.

EDUCATION, CERTIFICATION, AND LICENSURE. Nearly all specialized healthcare chaplains today hold college and seminary degrees or have other appropriate theological education, and have been ordained or otherwise endorsed by their religious denominations. Healthcare chaplains are not licensed by state governments, though some who also practice specialized pastoral counseling are licensed as pastoral counselors, psychologists, or marriage and family therapists.

Most full-time, professional healthcare chaplains have trained for their ministries through clinical pastoral education as described above. The C.P.E. certification is sponsored mainly by the Association for Clinical Pastoral Education, the National Association of Catholic Chaplains, the Canadian Association for Pastoral Education, and similar bodies in other countries. In 2002 the Association for Clinical Pastoral Education listed 350 accredited C.P.E. training centers and 600 certified C.P.E. supervisors. Similar organizations and C.P.E. programs exist in Canada and a number of other countries. An international organization closely related to the movement, the International Council for Pastoral Care and Counselling, meets quadrennially.

Various national professional associations also exist for specialized healthcare chaplains, principally the Association of Professional Chaplains, the National Association of Catholic Chaplains, and the National Association of Jewish Chaplains. These organizations set high standards for professional practice that are enforced through rigorous certification and review procedures. A consortium of these and related organizations publishes the *Journal of Pastoral Care*. There is also a large umbrella organization in the United States and Canada, the Congress on Ministry in Specialized Settings (COMISS), that sponsors joint meetings of pastoral-care organizations.

HISTORY OF HEALTHCARE CHAPLAINCY IN THE UNITED STATES. Hospital chaplaincy, like the hospital itself, had its origin in the ancient and medieval Christian church. The rise of the modern secular hospital in the late nineteenth century, however, was not immediately accompanied by the presence of chaplains as members of hospital staffs. Such pastoral ministry as occurred in secular hospitals was usually provided by retired clergy with no special training for the work beyond general parish experience, often on a voluntary and/or part-time basis. This pattern has continued in some smaller institutions, but today healthcare chaplaincy is fully established as a specialized ministerial profession, and chaplains are employed as regular staff members by most large healthcare institutions.

The turn toward specialized, highly trained, professional healthcare chaplaincy had its roots in the "religion and health" movement early in the twentieth century, in which a positive relation between religion and modern medicine was first seriously explored (Holifield). In the 1920s, this led to the first attempts to train theological students in clinical settings (Thornton). Notable was the groundbreaking work of a physician, William S. Keller, who placed theological students in a general hospital in Cincinnati in 1923, and Anton T. Boisen, a Congregational minister who began what became the "clinical pastoral training movement" with his pioneering program relating religion to mental disorders at Worcester State Hospital in Massachusetts in 1925. Boisen had the key support of two physicians, the distinguished Boston medical educator, Richard C. Cabot, and the progressive superintendent of Worcester State Hospital, William A. Bryan. Soon thereafter another physician, Flanders Dunbar, noted for her research in psychosomatic medicine, became a major leader of the movement. These and other early innovators were convinced that not books but intensive clinical experience—learning to interpret the experience of real human beings, to read the "living human documents" through clinical encounters—held the key to developing a realistic and profound theological understanding of human nature and the art of effective pastoral care (Boisen). The movement developed rapidly in the postwar period, when many training centers were organized, chaplain supervisors certified, and staff chaplaincy positions created in mental and general hospitals.

Clinical pastoral education was seldom undertaken in congregational settings, partly for pedagogical and practical reasons related to the abundance of pastoral opportunities in hospitals, and partly for financial reasons—hospitals were better able to pay for these programs than churches or seminaries. Most programs were sponsored by hospitals, and C.P.E. programs remained largely unrelated to the formal curricula of the theological seminaries until the late 1950s and 1960s. C.P.E. thus acquired a somewhat nonecclesiastical, "secular" style and appearance, and there has always been a concern that C.P.E. students would develop a confused professional identity as a result of C.P.E.'s close ties to the medical establishment.

Medical institutions still comprise the vast majority of C.P.E. training centers. Today, however, C.P.E. is widely embraced by the "mainline" Protestant and Catholic churches, and C.P.E. programs are a common, and often required, component of Protestant, Catholic, and some Jewish theological education. Healthcare chaplaincy itself is similarly established as a highly specialized, professionally trained and certified form of ministerial practice. Most hospital administrations require staff chaplains to have completed a year or more of C.P.E. or its equivalent. The Association of Professional Chaplains, the National Association of Catholic Chaplains, and similar organizations require C.P.E. in their certification standards.

Philosophical and Cultural Orientations

RELATION OF RELIGION AND HEALTH. The high degree of professional cooperation existing today between pastoral caregivers and medical professionals represents a remarkable and relatively recent development in both medicine and religion. In ancient and medieval times medicine and religion often enjoyed a close relationship; healing rites, exorcisms, pilgrimages, and health cults flourished. But with the Protestant Reformation and the later rise of modern science and scientific medicine, Christian ministry began a long retreat from its tradition of involvement in healing, and theology grew increasingly wary of making scientific, empirical claims about the natural world. An intellectual and professional schism between religion and medicine resulted. As medicine became scientific and ministry became confined to matters of God and the soul, corresponding spheres of professional influence were delineated: physicians cared (scientifically) for the body; clergy cared (spiritually) for the soul. Medical science assigned mental and emotional disorders, traditionally considered problems of the soul, to the body as organically caused, and regarded them as at least potentially treatable by physical (i.e., medical) means.

With the development of dynamic psychiatry and the religion and health movement in the early twentieth century, such distinctions began to blur. Psychoanalysis and related developments in psychiatry revealed psychogenic factors in many psychiatric disorders, while empirical studies in psychosomatic medicine demonstrated the profound effects of emotional and spiritual attitudes on physical health and healing. At the same time, theology began to recover biblical, holistic conceptions of human personhood, salvation, and the healing potential of religious ministry. In this theology the welfare of the whole person, physical, mental, and spiritual, was regarded as a profound unity. The result was a gradual closing of the theoretical gap between medicine and religion and the emergence of a more collaborative style of work between physicians and pastoral caregivers.

INFLUENCE OF THERAPEUTIC PSYCHOLOGY. Prior to the twentieth century, pastoral care was dominantly concerned with problems that could be clearly or outwardly identified as religious and moral in nature or as having religious significance, such as faith, doubt, sin, repentance, and the mysteries of suffering, illness, death, and dying. Contemporary pastoral care, however, at least as practiced in the larger Christian denominations (sectarian churches being the usual exception), holds to broader conceptions of Christian ministry, human welfare, and the meaning of salvation. In these traditions, physical welfare and emotional health play prominent parts in the overall meaning of salvation; ministry's sphere of concern includes the total health and welfare of persons and families in *this* world. Often this understanding gives prominence to psychology as an adjunctive discipline, and ministry acquires a distinctly psychotherapeutic style and orientation. This has been especially evident in the mainline Protestant denominations, but it is increasingly true of Roman Catholic and some conservative Protestant traditions. Judaism has historically emphasized the values of human health and welfare.

This therapeutic style of ministry has important ethical and professional consequences. Typically, it seeks to broaden moral discussion in healthcare settings from a focus on the content of moral decisions—what to do—to a focus on the process and quality of the decision making itself. Healthcare chaplains try to foster the psychological conditions that will facilitate free and responsible moral judgment and decision. These conditions include relationships of trust that permit open, honest communication among all parties concerning feelings as well as ideas and opinions. Though facilitating such conditions is not usually thought of as a form of moral guidance, it obviously has important moral value. Some pastoral authorities, however, while affirming this approach, have also urged pastoral caregivers to engage the substantive questions of ethics more directly in their caring ministries (Browning, 1976, 1983; Carnes).

AFFINITIES WITH SITUATION ETHICS AND CHARACTER ETHICS. Pastoral care, including healthcare chaplaincy, has not been highly articulate concerning the traditions of philosophical and theological ethics out of which it has operated (Carnes). Most pastoral theologians have concentrated instead on theological questions of human nature and the relation of religion to health (Browning, 1983; Holifield). However, much of the informal ethical reflection in the field has probably been influenced chiefly by some form of situation ethics. Situation ethics holds that fixed laws and rules are inadequate for moral decision making; decisions must be reached through a careful assessment of the particulars of each situation, guided by very general principles such as love, justice, and responsibility. Pastors with therapeutic training often exemplify this orientation since they tend to be concerned more about the specifics of situations than the application of abstract moral rules and principles (Poling, 1984b). Their typical ethical question is likely to be: "What is the appropriate, responsible, loving, or just thing to do in this situation, given its many complexities and dynamics?"

Pastoral care also has a close affinity with what is called the "ethics of character and virtue," though this connection is seldom recognized (Poling, 1984a). Conceptions of personality implicit in therapeutic psychology often function as secular character ideals within pastoral care. For example, healthcare chaplains commonly assume that psychological self-knowledge and the ability to experience oneself and others fully, without the distorting effects of emotional defensiveness, is desirable not only as an aspect of mental health but as a moral good—as a basis for free and responsible moral action. In many situations, as a matter of principle, healthcare chaplains are therefore likely to be as concerned about the emotional health and maturity of the persons exercising moral judgment as about the decisions they reach. This commitment to an ethic of character and virtue thus easily complements the field's general tendency to support situational or contextual forms of ethical reasoning.

RELATION OF THEORY AND PRACTICE. Many of the ways pastors have ministered to troubled and suffering persons over the centuries may be regarded as a practical implementation of the ethical principles of the pastors' religious communities and traditions. Practice has tended to follow theory, "applying" it.

But human needs and problems do not always fit neatly into prescribed categories and practices, and social and cultural forces change over time; contemporary problems of bioethics provide many cases in point. In such situations, pastoral care cannot operate as a straightforward application of established moral theories and principles. Conscientious improvising becomes necessary, especially in times of rapid social, cultural, and technological change.

Thus moral theory does not always easily or clearly guide practice; in fact, to some degree it reflects practice and is changed by practice. To this extent pastoral care, over time and in concert with other social and cultural factors, gradually helps moral theory to evolve. The Jewish *responsa* literature, representing the accumulated moral debates and evolving traditions of Judaism's encounter with novel problems over many centuries, provides massive evidence of this process in one tradition (Meier). A similar process, though often less explicit and legally constructed, has occurred in Christian pastoral care (Browning, 1976). This can be seen in changing contemporary pastoral attitudes in the mainstream Protestant churches on issues like divorce, remarriage, abortion, and artificial life support. Pastoral caregiving is thus culturally innovative as well as conservative, and represents (as Browning argues) a practical form of "moral inquiry."

Issues in Healthcare Chaplaincy

Like other health-oriented professions, healthcare chaplaincy faces a number of challenges as the technology and institutional forms of healthcare undergo rapid and extensive developments. Four major contemporary challenges may be noted:

1. Multiculturalism and minority concerns constitute an increasingly visible and important feature of the social landscape in which healthcare chaplaincy functions. This fact presents novel professional issues for healthcare chaplaincy. Today's hospital chaplains must understand a growing range of religious and ethnic cultures and find ways of relating their ministries with appropriateness and integrity to persons with religious faiths and social customs different from their own. They must also be able to help persons of non-Western cultural and religious traditions relate to the social values and practices of advanced Western healthcare facilities.

2. The overlap of professional roles in contemporary healthcare settings intensifies the problem of defining the healthcare chaplain's pastoral identity. This question is becoming urgent. As institutional budget pressures increase, many healthcare chaplains and pastoral departments have been forced to define their identities and defend the value of their ministries to healthcare administrators, often in quantifiable, cost-benefit terms alien to the traditional meanings and purposes of ministry.

3. How (in theory or practice) can chaplains maintain an institutionally appropriate neutrality yet remain significantly committed to their traditions of faith? Focusing on *process* rather than *content* in moral decision making, and maintaining an institutionally proper value-neutral stance on specific questions, are clearly helpful in this regard. But such public neutrality may beg important questions. Is there any way for ethical commitments and insights of particular religious traditions to contribute to contemporary moral reflection in institutional decision-making and policy formation? How can healthcare chaplains represent their traditions without imposing themselves inappropriately on others or abusing their institutional positions?

4. Healthcare chaplains are being drawn into *discussions* of healthcare policy in their institutions and in the larger society. This expanded arena offers new opportunities to witness to their moral and spiritual commitments, by questioning unjust policies and practices and advocating the rights of the poor, for example. But it also raises difficult questions. How far and in what way—if at all—should healthcare chaplains develop this expression of their ethical integrity in place of, or in addition to, their work of holistic healing, care and compassion?

RODNEY J. HUNTER (1995)
REVISED BY AUTHOR

SEE ALSO: *Beneficence; Care; Compassionate Love; Death: Western Religious Thought; Grief and Bereavement; Mental Health: Meaning of Mental Health; Teams, Healthcare; Trust; Value and Valuation*

BIBLIOGRAPHY

Boisen, Anton T. 1971 (1936). *The Exploration of the Inner World.* Philadelphia: University of Pennsylvania Press.

Browning, Don S. 1976. *The Moral Context of Pastoral Care.* Philadelphia: Westminster Press.

Browning, Don S. 1983. *Religious Ethics and Pastoral Care.* Philadelphia: Fortress Press.

Burck, J. Russell. 1983. "The Chaplain amid Dilemmas of Health-Care Ethics." *American Protestant Hospital Association Bulletin* 47(3): 69–76.

Burton, Laurel Arthur, ed. 1992. *Chaplaincy Services in Contemporary Health Care.* Schaumburg, IL: College of Chaplains.

Carnes, Ralph L. 1995. "Ruminations on Some Approaches to Bioethics." *Journal of Pastoral Care* 49: 125–128.

Hayes, Helen; Van der Poel, Cornelius J.; and National Association of Catholic Chaplains. 1990. *Health-Care Ministry: A Handbook for Chaplains.* New York: Paulist Press.

Holifield, E. Brooks. 1983. *A History of Pastoral Care in America: From Salvation to Self-Realization.* Nashville, TN: Abingdon Press.

Holst, Lawrence E., ed. 1985. *Hospital Ministry: The Role of the Chaplain Today.* New York: Crossroad.

Hunter, Rodney J.; Malony, H. Newton; Mills, Liston O.; and Patton, John; eds. 1990. *Dictionary of Pastoral Care and Counseling.* Nashville, TN: Abingdon Press.

Journal of Health-Care Chaplaincy. 1987–. New York: Haworth Press.

Lapsley, James N. 1990. "Moral Dilemmas in Pastoral Perspective." In *Dictionary of Pastoral Care and Counseling,* ed. Rodney J. Hunter. Nashville, TN: Abingdon Press.

Marty, Martin E., and Vaux, Kenneth L., eds. 1982. *Health/ Medicine and the Faith Traditions: An Inquiry into Religion and Medicine.* Philadelphia: Fortress Press.

Meier, Levi. 1990. "Medical-Ethical Dilemmas, Jewish Care and Counseling In." In *Dictionary of Pastoral Care and Counseling,* ed. Rodney J. Hunter. Nashville, TN: Abingdon Press.

Mitchell, Kenneth R. 1972. *Hospital Chaplain.* Philadelphia: Westminster Press.

Poling, James N. 1984a. "Ethical Reflection and Pastoral Care: Part I." *Pastoral Psychology* 32(2): 106–114.

Poling, James N. 1984b. "Ethical Reflection and Pastoral Care: Part II." *Pastoral Psychology* 32(3): 160–170.

Second Opinion. 1986–. Park Ridge, IL: Park Ridge Center.

Thornton, Edward E. 1970. *Professional Education for Ministry: A History of Clinical Pastoral Education.* Nashville, TN: Abingdon Press.

INTERNET RESOURCES

VandeCreek, Larry, and Burton, Laurel, eds. "Professional Chaplaincy: Its Role and Importance in Healthcare." Hospital Chaplaincy Gateway. Available from <http://www.healthcarechaplaincy.org/publications/white_paper_05.22.01>.

PATENTING ORGANISMS AND BASIC RESEARCH

• • •

Patents give inventors the right to prevent others from making, using, or selling their inventions for a limited time. The U.S. Constitution justifies the patent system as a way to promote technological progress (U.S. Constitution, Article I, Section 8, Clause 8). The U.S. patent system promotes technological progress through the financial incentives it creates for innovation and through its disclosure requirement. In exchange for exclusive rights patent applicants must disclose their inventions in terms that enable others who are skilled in the field to make and use them (U.S. Patent Act, Section 112). When a patent is issued, that broad disclosure becomes available to the public, and when the patent term expires, the public is free to make, use, and sell the patented invention.

Background and History

As commercial interest in biological products and processes has grown, inventors have turned to the patent laws, seeking rights to inventions that involve living materials. Under traditional patent doctrine, patents on living materials raise a number of concerns. For example, products and phenomena of nature are not patentable under U.S. law even when they are newly discovered (*Funk Brothers Seed Co. v. Kalo Inoculant Co.*).

Even before the explosion of modern commercial biotechnology, however, judicial decisions reduced the significance of that obstacle to patent protection by permitting patents on materials derived from natural sources through human intervention, such as purifications of naturally occurring products, as long as the patent claims did not cover the products in their natural state. Under that interpretation of the law, courts upheld the validity of patents on purified prostaglandins (*Bergstrom*), purified acetylsalicylic acid (*Kuehmsted v. Farbenfabriken*), and a purified adrenaline composition (*Parke-Davis & Co. v. H. K. Mulford & Co.*). Nonetheless, before 1980 it was not entirely clear that living materials were patentable. (*Funk Brothers Seed Co. v. Kalo Inoculant Co.*).

The 1980 decision of the U.S. Supreme Court in *Diamond v. Chakrabarty* stated unequivocally for the first time that living materials are patentable. In that case the Court held that a living single-celled bacterium that was transformed with DNA plasmids (small circles of bacterial DNA) through human intervention to give it the capacity to break down multiple components of crude oil could be patented as a "manufacture" or "composition of matter." In arriving at that decision the Court stated that the patent statute allows patents to be issued on "anything under the sun that is made by man" (*Diamond v. Chakrabarty*, p. 309).

With that broad directive from the Supreme Court the Patent and Trademark Office (PTO) quickly expanded the categories of living organisms it considered eligible for patent protection. In 1985 the PTO held that corn plants were eligible for standard utility patents, as opposed to the more limited plant variety protection (*Hibberd*), and two years later it held that polyploid oysters fell within the range of patentable subject matter (*Allen*). Shortly afterward the commissioner of patents issued a notice stating that the PTO "now considers nonnaturally occurring nonhuman multicellular living organisms, including animals, to be patentable subject matter" (U.S. Patent and Trademark Office 1077:24). Any claim covering a human being would not be considered patentable, however, because "the grant of a limited, but exclusive property right in a human being is prohibited by the Constitution."

The first patent on a genetically altered animal (U.S. Patent No. 4,736,866) was issued in April 1988 to Harvard University for the development of a mouse harboring a human oncogene that makes it susceptible to cancer (HARVARD/Onco-Mouse Application). The decision to extend patent protection to animals generated considerable public controversy and was the focus of numerous hearings in the U.S. Congress (Dresser).

In 1998 the PTO's policy of refusing to grant patents on human beings was tested by a patent application on "chimeric embryos" (embryos containing human and nonhuman cells) filed by Jeremy Rifkin. In rejecting the application the PTO argued that Congress did not intend product patents on human organisms to fall within the scope of patentable subject matter (Ho). The widespread adoption of cloning techniques has tested the PTO's policy once again. By 2001 the PTO had granted patents on cloning *processes* that produce mammalian embryos, both human and nonhuman (U.S. Patent Nos. 6,211,429 and 6,235,970).

Although national patent laws vary somewhat, as a general rule the range of biotechnology inventions that can be patented outside the United States is somewhat more restricted than it is under U.S. law. Two provisions of the European Patent Convention have presented obstacles to the issuance of standard utility patents covering plants and animals in Europe (Dickson). Article 53(b) of the European Patent Convention states that European patents will not be issued for plant or animal varieties and essentially biological processes for the production of plants or animals with the exception of microbiological processes and the products of those processes. Article 53(a) of the European Patent Convention bars the issuance of a patent on an invention if its publication or exploitation would be contrary to public order or morality. The European Patent Office (EPO) concluded, however, that neither of those provisions barred the issuance of a European patent to Harvard University for its transgenic mouse (HARVARD/Onco-Mouse Application).

The recently issued European Biotechnology Directive generally follows the European Patent Convention and the case law of the EPO but suggests that slight human interference is sufficient to make a process for the production of plants and animals patentable (European Community Directive 98/44, 1998). In addition, Article 6 of the directive specifically prohibits, among other things, patents on processes for cloning human beings and processes for modifying the germline identity of human beings.

Objections to Patenting Organisms

Some of the objections to patenting living organisms, including humans, that have emerged in the wake of these legal developments are better understood as objections to the underlying technology rather than to its protection under patent law (Dresser; Merges). Objections of this character include concerns about the hazards of genetic engineering to public health and to the environment and concerns that transgenic animal research involves cruelty to animals. With respect to humans many people believe that creating humans through cloning processes violates principles of freedom, equality, and human dignity (President's Council on Bioethics).

One might question whether these kinds of objections are the concern of the patent laws or whether they might be met better through other types of regulation or outright prohibition of the research. However, withholding commercial rewards may be an effective way to slow the pace of such research without prohibiting it altogether (Kass). Some have argued that the patenting of life forms promotes an unwholesome or irreverent materialistic conception of life (Hoffmaster). A strong version of this argument holds that characterizing a life form as a patentable manufacture or composition of matter reduces a patented organism to a material object (Kass). A more attenuated version of that argument would stress the potential for commercial interests to debase people's attitudes toward life when life forms are treated as commodities to be bought and sold in the market (Murray). However, because patents do not provide an affirmative right to use an invention (they provide only a right to bar others from using it), the extent to which patents contribute to commodification is not clear. Allowing the creation of particular life forms, as well as patents on those life forms, patents would be consistent, for example, with a regime in which sales of life forms were banned (Rai).

Ownership of Other Living Materials

Moral objections have been voiced to the ownership of living materials such as the human genome sequence and single-nucleotide polymorphisms (SNPs), which are single-base variations in the genetic code. In both of those cases, however, preemptive actions to put genetic information into the public domain largely have prevented such ownership. In the case of the human genome sequence the public

Human Genome Project instituted a policy of putting large-scale genomic sequence information immediately into the public domain (National Human Genome Research Institute). As a consequence the private company Celera, which had undertaken its own sequencing project, could not patent raw genome data. Moreover, although Celera maintains its genome database as a trade secret, the value of that database is diminished by the fact that genome data are publicly available. In the case of SNP data a consortium of pharmaceutical companies that were worried about the effects of patents on those upstream research inputs came together to fund an effort to put SNPs into the public domain (SNP Consortium Website). The public domain also has been enhanced to some extent by the recent decision of the PTO to require that those who seek to patent DNA sequences show the functional significance of those sequences (Patent and Trademark Office).

A major arena in which the ownership of living materials continues to raise moral concerns pertains to the ownership of human genes. Companies that own those genes often require universities and other institutions that perform genetic tests to pay large licensing fees. In some cases the size of the fee has led institutions to stop performing such tests (Merz).

REBECCA S. EISENBERG (1995)
REVISED BY ARTI K. RAI

SEE ALSO: *Agriculture and Biotechnology; Animal Research; Commercialism in Scientific Research; Environmental Ethics; Law and Bioethics; Pharmaceutical Industry; Private Ownership of Inventions; Technology*

BIBLIOGRAPHY

Allen, Ex parte. 1987. 2 U.S.P.Q.2d 1425 (PTO B.d Pat. App. & Interf. 1987).

Armitage, Robert A. 1989. "The Emerging U.S. Patent Law for the Protection of Biotechnology Research Results." *European Intellectual Property Review* 11(2): 47–57.

Bergstrom, In re. 1970. 427 F.2d 1394, 57 (C.C.P.A.) 1240, 166 U.S.P.Q. (BNA) 256.

Diamond v. Chakrabarty. 447 U.S. 303, 65 L. Ed. 2d 144, 100 S. Ct. 2204 (1980).

Dickson, David. 1989. "Europe Tries to Untangle Laws on Patenting Life." *Science* 243(4894): 1002–1003.

Dresser, Rebecca. 1988. "Ethical and Legal Issues in Patenting New Animal Life." *Jurimetrics Journal* 28(4): 399–435.

European Community Directive 98/44/EC. 1998. *Official Journal of the European Communities,* July 30, pp. 213/13–213/21.

Funk Brothers Seed Co. v. Kalo Inoculant Co. 333 U.S. 127, 192 L. Ed. 588, 68 S. Ct. 440 (1948).

HARVARD/Onco-Mouse Application No. 85 304 490.7. 1991. *European Patent Office Reports* 525.

Hibberd, Ex parte. 1985. 227 U.S.P.Q. 473 (PTO Bd Pat. App. & Interf.).

Ho, Cynthia. 2000. "Splicing Morality and Patent Law: Issues Arising from Mixing Mice and Men." *Washington University Journal of Law & Policy* 2: 247–286.

Hoffmaster, Barry. 1989. "The Ethics of Patenting Higher Life Forms." *Intellectual Property Journal* 4: 1–24.

Kass, Leon R. 1981. "Patenting Life." *Commentary* 72(6): 45–57.

Kuehmsted v. Farbenfabriken. 179 F. 701 (7th Cir.), cert. denied, 220 U.S. 622, 55 L. Ed. 613, 31 S. Ct. 724 (1910).

MacKenzie, Debora. 1992. "Europe Debates the Ownership of Life." *New Scientist* 133(1802): 9–10.

Merges, Robert P. 1988. "Intellectual Property in Higher Life Forms: The Patent System and Controversial Technologies." *Maryland Law Review* 47: 1051–1075.

Merz, Jon; Kirss, Antigone G.; Leonard, Debra G. B.; and Cho, Mildred K. 2002. "Diagnostic Testing Fails the Test." *Nature* 415: 577–579.

Murray, Thomas H. 1987. "On the Human Body as Property: The Meaning of Embodiment, Markets, and the Meaning of Strangers." *University of Michigan Journal of Law Reform* 20(4): 1055–1088.

Parke-Davis & Co. v. H. K. Mulford & Co. 189 F. 95 (S.D.N.Y. 1911), aff'd, 196 F. 496 (2d Cir. 1912).

Patent and Trademark Office. 2001. "Utility Examination Guidelines." *Federal Register* 66: 1092.

President's Council on Bioethics. 2002. *Human Cloning and Human Dignity: An Ethical Inquiry.* Washington, D.C.: Author.

Rai, Arti K. 2002. "Patenting Human Organisms: An Ethical and Legal Analysis" (working paper prepared for President's Council on Bioethics).

U.S. Congress, House Committee on the Judiciary. 1988. *Patents and the Constitution: Transgenic Animals: Hearings before the Subcommittee on Courts, Civil Liberties and the Administration of Justice.* 100th Cong., 1st Sess.

U.S. Constitution, Article 1, Section 8, Clause 8. *United States Code Annotated* (St. Paul, West, 1987).

U.S. Patent Act. 35 United States Code Annotated §§101, 112, 161–164 (St. Paul, West, 1984, and Supp. 1992).

U.S. Patent and Trademark Office. 1987. "Commissioner's Notice, Animal Patentability." *Official Gazette of the Patent and Trademark Office* 1077: 24.

World Council of Churches. Church and Society. 1982. *Manipulating Life: Ethical Issues in Genetic Engineering.* Geneva: Author.

INTERNET RESOURCES

National Human Genome Research Institute. 1996. Policy Regarding Intellectual Property of Human Genome Sequence. Available from <http://www.nhgri.nih.gov/Grant_info/Funding/Statements/RFA/intellectual_property.html>.

SNP Consortium. 2003. Available from <http://www.snp.cshl.org>.

PATERNALISM

. . .

Paternalists maintain that restricting the autonomy of persons is justified if these persons would be likely to cause serious harm to themselves or fail to secure an important benefit for themselves. The main ethical issue is whether paternalistic interventions are morally justified, and if so, under what conditions. In bioethics, rightful authority in the patient–physician relationship and public-health interventions have been the focus of the discussion. For health policy, paternalism is central to questions concerning the government's role in promoting healthy lifestyles and preventing self-caused injury and illness.

Many actions, rules, and laws are commonly justified by appeal to some paternalistic principle. Examples include laws that protect drivers by requiring seat belts; restrictions on the availability of drugs; rules prohibiting a healthy subject of biomedical research from voluntarily undergoing a high-risk procedure; overriding adult refusals of treatment; disclosing confidential information about a patient to protect the patient's health; involuntary commitment to hospitals; interventions to prevent suicides; and denial of an innovative therapy to someone who wishes to receive it. Laws are the usual vehicle for translating paternalistic beliefs into public policy, but individual actions and institutional policies can also have paternalistic roots.

Early History in Ethical Theory

In an eighteenth-century discussion, the philosopher Immanuel Kant denounced paternalistic government ("imperium paternale") for its benevolent cancellations of the freedoms of its subjects (pp. 58–59). However, it was the nineteenth-century English philosopher John Stuart Mill who presented the first systematic attack on paternalism, a term he avoided, in his 1859 monograph *On Liberty*:

> The only purpose for which power can be rightfully exercised over any member of a civilized community, against his will, is to prevent harm to others. His own good, either physical or moral, is not a sufficient warrant. He cannot rightfully be compelled to do or forbear because it will be better for him to do so, because it will make him happier,

because in the opinions of others, to do so would be wise, or even right. These are good reasons for remonstrating with him, or reasoning with him, or persuading him, or entreating him, but not for compelling him .... In the part which merely concerns himself his independence is, of right, absolute. (p. 223)

Mill thus articulated a principle that properly restricted social control over individual liberty, regardless of whether such control is political, religious, or of some other type. He defended his principle with the utilitarian argument that granting people liberty rather than subjecting them to paternalism produces the best possible conditions for social progress and for the development of individual character and talent. Independent of his commitment to utilitarianism, Mill's *On Liberty* has played a more important role in discussion of paternalism than any treatise in ethical theory.

Neither Mill nor Kant anticipated that a paternal model of justified intervention into the affairs of competent adults might be extended to interventions with adult persons who, like children, have only a restricted or compromised capacity to choose autonomously. Yet this latter and broader model has become the most widely defended account of paternalism.

Definitions of Paternalism

The word *paternalism* refers loosely to acts of treating adults as a benevolent father treats his children, but the term has been given both a narrow and a broad meaning in ethical theory. In the narrow sense, paternalism refers to acts or practices that restrict the autonomy or liberty of individuals without their explicit consent; justification for such actions is either the prevention of some harm they stand to do to themselves, or the production of some benefit for them that they would not otherwise secure. This conception of paternalism leads to the following definition: Paternalism is the intentional limitation of the autonomy of one person by another, where the person who limits autonomy justifies the action exclusively by the goal of helping the person whose autonomy is limited (Dworkin, 1992; Beauchamp and McCullough). Following this definition, an act of paternalism overrides the value of respect for autonomy on some grounds of beneficence. Paternalism seizes decision-making authority by preventing persons from making or implementing their own decisions.

Many writers object to this analysis of paternalism because it does not comprehend the meaning of the term as it has descended from common usage and venerable legal precedent, where the notion is linked to guardianship, surrogate decision making, and government intervention to protect the vulnerable. The root sense of paternalism in ordinary language ("government as by a benevolent father") is joined with the law's wide-ranging use of terms such as *parens patriae* to produce a broad meaning that includes interventions into both autonomous and nonautonomous actions. Those who follow this broad vision recommend the following definition: Paternalism is the intentional overriding of one person's known preferences by another person, where the person who overrides justifies the action by the goal of benefiting the person whose will is overridden. Under this second definition, if a person's stated preferences do not derive from a substantially autonomous choice, overriding his or her preferences can still be paternalistic. The only essential condition of paternalism is beneficent treatment that overrides a known preference; a condition of substantial autonomy is not essential (VanDeVeer; Kleinig).

Defenders of the first definition argue that there are compelling reasons for resisting this second definition. First, paternalism originates in ethical theory as an issue about the valid limitation of freedom and autonomy. To include cases involving persons who lack substantial autonomy, such as drug addicts or the mentally disabled, broadens the term in a way that obscures the central issue, which is how, whether, and when liberty or autonomy can be justifiably limited. Second, the legal concept of *parens patriae* powers has its own subtleties and complexities. Courts do not apply this notion across the same range of thought and conduct that paternalistic literature treats as problematic. To incorporate a marginal legal doctrine together with the vagueness of ordinary language might prove more confusing than instructive in the end.

These two definitions are currently contested in literature. However, defenders of these two definitions need not disagree on all controversies about the meaning of paternalism. For example, it has sometimes been said that the term *paternalism* is inherently pejorative because it implies that authorities may treat adults such as hospital patients as if they were children lacking considered preferences of their own; therefore, they reason, the term is tainted by illegitimate authoritarianism or repressive dominance (Feinberg, 1980, 1986; Sherwin). Proponents of the above two definitions are free either to accept or to resist this interpretation. For example, they can both resist this pejorative meaning by arguing that paternalism suggests nothing beyond an analogy to respectable parental benevolence, in which parents act in the best interests of their children for good reason.

Weak (Soft) Paternalism and Strong (Hard) Paternalism

Joel Feinberg's distinction between weak and strong paternalism has profoundly affected literature on the subject.

Although he switched to the language of "soft" and "hard" paternalism in his later work (1986), the terms "weak" and "strong" seem to have more deeply influenced the bioethics literature and will be used here.

In weak paternalism, one "has the right to prevent self-regarding harmful conduct only when it is substantially nonvoluntary or when temporary intervention is necessary to establish whether it is voluntary or not" (Feinberg, 1971, p. 113). This type of paternalism confines permissible limitations of autonomy to substantially nonautonomous (or nonvoluntary) behaviors. For example, it is permissible to pick up injured, partially incoherent victims of automobile accidents who refuse ambulance service and to admit against their will mentally ill persons who are dangerous to themselves. In strong paternalism, however, it is proper to protect or benefit a person by autonomy-limiting measures even if the person's contrary choices are autonomous. This paternalism supports interventions that protect competent adults against their will; that is, it controls or restricts substantially autonomous behaviors. For example, refusing to release a competent hospital patient who will die outside the hospital but requests the release knowing the consequences is an act of strong paternalism.

Weak paternalism is built on conditions of compromised ability or dysfunctional incompetence. When conduct that affects only the actor is restricted, some degree of autonomy may be present in the restricted actor, but the action must be substantially nonautonomous. Conditions that can significantly compromise the ability to act autonomously include the influence of psychotropic drugs, painful labor while delivering a child, and a blow to the head that affects memory and judgment. In medical situations, a patient's illness can be so devastating that it affects decision-making capacity. As the patient becomes weaker, less aware, or less alert, his or her dependence on the physician increases. A member of the medical profession who overturns the preferences of a substantially nonautonomous patient in the interests of the person's medical welfare acts paternalistically and justifiably by the standards of weak paternalism. For this reason, weak paternalism has been widely accepted in law, medicine, and moral philosophy as an appropriate basis for intervention.

Strong paternalism, by contrast, supports some interventions intended to benefit a person whose choices and actions are informed and autonomous. Strong paternalism usurps autonomy by either restricting the information available to a person or overriding the person's informed and voluntary choices. These choices may not be fully autonomous or voluntary, but in order to qualify as strong paternalism the choices of the beneficiary of paternalistic intervention must be substantially autonomous or voluntary. For

example, a strong paternalist would prevent a patient capable of autonomous choice from receiving diagnostic information that might lead to suicide. Unlike weak paternalism, strong paternalism does not require any conditions of compromised ability, dysfunctional incompetence, or encumbrance as the basis of intervention (although strong paternalists of course accept the justifiability of weak paternalistic interventions as well).

Justification of Paternalism and Antipaternalism

Defenders of paternalism in ethical theory have paid more attention to the justifying grounds for paternalism than to the type of paternalism justified. Some justifications range widely and defend both strong and weak paternalism. Typically, however, a condition in the argument states or hints that only weak paternalism is justified, although strong paternalism is the most controversial and interesting type of paternalism and may be the only type worth the effort of justification.

JUSTIFIED PATERNALISM. Defenders of paternalism often appeal to either a principle of rational consent or a principle of welfare or beneficence in order to justify their position. In one prominent justification, Gerald Dworkin argues that paternalism should be regarded as a form of "social insurance policy" that fully rational persons would take out for their protection (1972, p. 65). That is, paternalism is justified under conditions to which an impartial rational agent would consent if he or she were to appreciate the possibility of being tempted at times to make decisions to commit acts that are potentially dangerous and irreversible. The agent might at other times be driven to do something that would be considered too risky if he or she could objectively assess the situation—for example, smoking or drinking so heavily that health and life are endangered. A paternalistic health policy would remove or severely restrict the availability of tobacco and alcohol. In other cases, persons might not sufficiently understand or appreciate the dangers of their conduct, or might distort information about their circumstances. Seat-belt laws and motorcycle-helmet laws have often been enacted on this paternalistic basis.

Dworkin argues that a paternalistic act that denies a person an immediate liberty may paradoxically protect deep autonomy (i.e., the person's deeper values and preferences about the principles and standards on which he or she ought to act). A physician might lie to a patient, for example, in order to prevent a suicide, if the physician knows that the patient really wants to live and will later calm down and not commit suicide, although the patient is presently in no position to appreciate this fact. Dworkin argues that rational consent (consent that would be given) is the only acceptable way to express the conditions of justified paternalism. Many philosophers subsequently agreed with this thesis and made some form of consent a necessary condition of justified paternalism. However, justifications on bases other than consent have also been attempted (Dworkin, 1972; see VanDeVeer; and Kleinig).

A justification based on consent may do more to obscure than to clarify the issues. If the paternalist's objective is to protect or improve the welfare of another, then intervention can be justified by harm-avoidance or benefit-production, as is the case in the justification of parental actions that override the wishes of their children. Children are treated paternalistically not because they will subsequently consent or would have consented were they rational, but because they will have better lives. This justification rests on providing for their welfare, not on respecting their autonomy.

THE JUSTIFICATION OF ANTIPATERNALISM. Some believe that paternalism is never justified. Mill supported this position, but with the important qualification that we are justified in restricting a person's liberty temporarily in order to ensure that the person is acting intentionally with adequate knowledge of the consequences of the action; once warned and informed, the person must be allowed to choose whatever course he or she desires. One need not be a follower of Mill's utilitarianism to defend this antipaternalism. For example, it can be defended by appeal to principles of respect for autonomy and privacy. Perhaps the most widely shared reason antipaternalists oppose (strong) paternalism is that it interferes with the authority of the individual, insults autonomous agents, and fails to treat them as moral equals (Childress).

The antipaternalist permits an initial, temporary infringement of liberty and privacy in the belief that persons who have a well-formed, autonomous resolution to do something harmful to themselves will have ample opportunity to perform the action after the temporary intervention has occurred. Intervention, in this limited respect, need not be a deep moral offense. Defenders of weak paternalism, however, view this qualified antipaternalism as insufficient because it disallows some highly desirable forms of intervention, such as long-term involuntary hospitalization for those in need of medical attention. Who, they reason, would not support altruistic beneficence directed at confused cardiac patients, ignorant consumers, frightened clients, and young persons who know little about the dangers of alcohol, smoking, drugs, and motorcycles? No caring and decent person would leave these individuals unprotected, and no reasonable philosopher would defend a normative thesis that permits such outcomes.

Weak paternalists thus project the appearance of steering a moderate and reasonable course between two radical and excessive extremes, strong paternalism and antipaternalism. The solution to the problem of paternalism, from their perspective, is to present the most defensible form of weak paternalism. But a severe stumbling block lies in the path of this tempting resolution of the issues: Weak paternalism has no clear substantive moral disagreement with antipaternalism, and therefore there is no reason to choose one over the other. Protection from harm caused to an individual by conditions beyond his or her knowledge and voluntary control—for example, by conditions beyond his or her self—is not an intervention that antipaternalists either criticize or disallow; they deny only the acceptability of intervention with substantially autonomous, self-caused harm. Weak paternalists too condemn such actions as an unjustifiable form of strong paternalism.

Weak paternalism, then, seems to be a defensible but noncontroversial position that virtually everyone accepts in some form. As Feinberg notes, it is "severely misleading to think of [weak paternalism] as any kind of paternalism," because weak paternalism is not "'paternalistic' at all, in any clear sense" (1986, pp. 12–14). Both weak paternalism and antipaternalism agree on the following critical claims:

(a) It is justifiable to interfere in order to protect persons against harm from their own substantially nonautonomous decisions; and

(b) it is unjustifiable to interfere in order to protect persons against harm from their own substantially autonomous decisions.

Weak paternalism is thus not a form of paternalism that can be distinguished in any morally important respect from antipaternalism. Weak paternalism does not seem to rest on a liberty- or autonomy-limiting principle independent of some moral principle of beneficence that supports prevention of harm to others (see Feinberg, 1971, pp. 107f., 124, and Feinberg, 1986, p. 13). Feinberg sarcastically suggests that the label "soft antipaternalism" seems to mean the same as "soft paternalism" (1986, p. 15).

The weak paternalist and the antipaternalist also join hands in opposition to the strong paternalist, who alone allows interventions that override and violate substantially autonomous actions.

THE JUSTIFICATION OF STRONG PATERNALISM. Although substantial autonomy is necessarily overridden in strong paternalism, conditions can be specified by a strong paternalist to restrict severely the range of justifiable interventions. For example, the strong paternalist might maintain that interventions are justified only if: no acceptable alternative to the paternalistic action exists; a person is at risk of serious harm; risks to the person that are introduced by the paternalistic action itself are not substantial; projected benefits to the person outweigh risks to the person; and any infringement of the principle of respect for autonomy is minimal.

Strong paternalism, so interpreted, will stand or fall on the strength of the argument that major welfare interests under some specifiable conditions legitimately override relatively minor autonomy interests. Many cases can be found that fit this model. For example, when healthy persons with no heart disease volunteered as subjects in a research study to have an artificial heart transplanted at the University of Utah, it was entirely reasonable that a review committee declared that the risk relative to benefit for a healthy subject is morally unacceptable and that they should not be allowed to undergo the procedure (Beauchamp and Childress).

Issues of Paternalism in Bioethics

Many examples of controversial paternalistic justifications are found in bioethics. Only a few general topics are treated here.

OVERRIDING REFUSALS OF TREATMENT. It is sometimes controversial whether procedures should be withheld or withdrawn even when the patient refuses the procedures. Justifications for overruling a patient's refusal of therapy need not be paternalistic, but they often are paternalistic because their objective is to prevent harm that would be caused by the patient's refusal. The issue is not whether a physician actually knows what is best for the patient, but whether the patient has a right to refuse treatment even if the refusal is harmful and the treatment beneficial.

Persons of questionable competence who refuse therapy present delicate moral problems and difficult conceptual issues about whether interventions are paternalistic. For example, do schizophrenic patients have a right to refuse a therapy for dehydration if a physician determines it to be safe and efficacious, and would an intervention after a refusal be paternalistic? Similarly, do children who understand what is being done to them have a right to refuse therapies when their parents and physicians judge these therapies to be essential, and are such interventions paternalistic?

OVERRIDING REQUESTS FOR TREATMENT. Patients or their legal representatives occasionally request medical procedures that physicians believe are harmful, ineffective, or futile. The physician may then refuse to act on these requests for paternalistic reasons. If the requests by patients are incompatible with accepted standards of care or conflict with the physician's conscientious beliefs about standards of care, a physician's refusal to comply may be justified for these apparently nonpaternalistic reasons of appropriate physician conduct. Nonetheless, the interventions are paternalistic whenever the primary ground of noncompliance with the request is that the treatment is not in the patient's best interests. Moreover, setting professional standards of practice is itself often a paternalistic attempt to protect patients' interests, and as such may be either justified or unjustified paternalism (Childress; Brett and McCullough). The same argument can be applied to drug policies of a government agency that refuses to accept requests for experimental therapies on grounds of risk to patients.

PARTIAL DISCLOSURES TO PREVENT HARM. Physicians and families often argue that a particularly devastating diagnosis or prognosis should not be disclosed to a patient. The concern is that bad news might adversely affect the patient's health or lead the patient to commit suicide. If the patient asks for the information or expects a truthful disclosure, it is paternalistic to withhold the truth. Physicians also occasionally make difficult medical decisions without consulting the parents of seriously ill newborns. These actions too are paternalistic if the objective is to prevent anguish to the parents. Other examples extend beyond serious patient illness. For example, genetic counselors sometimes use potential marital conflict for a patient as a reason not to disclose a condition such as nonpaternity, thereby depriving a patient of information generated in part by materials the patient provided.

In a much-quoted article on medical ethics, L. J. Henderson claimed that "the best physicians" use the following as their primary guide: "So far as possible, 'Do No Harm.' You can do harm by the process that is quaintly called telling the truth. You can do harm by lying…. But try to do as little harm as possible, not only in treatment with drugs, or with the knife, but also in treatment with words" (p. 823). The premise that some information may legitimately be withheld or disclosed only to the family for the patient's good is a clear instance of this rule and an equally clear case of paternalism. Why the family, rather than the competent patient, is given the information without the patient's prior permission is itself an important issue concerning paternalistic medical practices.

INVOKING THE THERAPEUTIC PRIVILEGE. Therapeutic privilege is a legally recognized privilege of the physician to withhold information from a patient if disclosure would cause serious deterioration in the physical, psychological, or emotional condition of the patient. This privilege has long been used in clinical settings to justify not obtaining consent and has elicited a particularly furious exchange over whether autonomy rights can be validly overridden for paternalistic reasons.

The courts have yet to develop a standard for appropriate use of the therapeutic privilege that renders it coherent with requirements of informed consent. If stated broadly, physicians can withhold information when disclosure would cause any countertherapeutic deterioration, however slight, in the physical, psychological, or emotional condition of the patient. If stated narrowly, physicians can withhold information if and only if the patient's knowledge of the information would have serious health-related consequences—for example, by jeopardizing the success of the treatment or harming the patient by critically impairing relevant decision-making processes. Confusion has also surrounded appropriate measures of rationality, psychological damage, and emotional stability under the standard of therapeutic privilege. Loose standards can permit physicians to climb to safety over a straw bridge of speculation about the psychological consequences of information, and this threat of abuse has made the therapeutic privilege highly controversial.

HEALTH POLICY FOR EXCESSIVE RISK. Antipaternalists argue that paternalistic standards for policy would authorize too much intervention. Paternalism could in principle prohibit smoking, drinking, and hazardous recreational activities such as hang gliding, mountain climbing, and white-water rafting, making such activities subject to criminal sanctions. Careful defenses of paternalism would disallow these extreme interventions, and at best antipaternalist arguments establish only a rebuttable presumption against paternalistic intervention. Nonetheless, antipaternalists are convinced that an unacceptable latitude of judgment would remain in contexts in which power is subject to abuse. Strong paternalism suggests that it would be permissible and perhaps obligatory to restrain and punish those who violate paternalistic rules. If so, antipaternalists argue, the state would be permitted to coerce morally heroic or valiant citizens if they act in a manner "harmful" to themselves. More generally, the state would be empowered to take away from persons the right to make decisions about their lives whenever officials view risks as excessive.

GOVERNMENT AGENCY RESTRICTIONS. Some government bureaus can be viewed, at least in part, as paternalistic guardians. For example, the Food and Drug Administration (FDA) in the United States is chartered to restrict persons from purchasing foods, drugs, and medical devices that are unsafe or inefficacious. A controversial decision by the FDA in 1992 to severely restrict the use of silicone-gel breast implants exemplifies paternalistic controversies that have beset the FDA. Women had elected implants for over thirty years, either to augment their breast size or to reconstruct their breasts following mastectomies. Over two million women in the United States had had these implants (three million worldwide) when, in April 1992, the FDA restricted the use of silicone-gel breast implants until additional studies could be conducted to establish their safety. Concerns centered on the implants' longevity, rate of rupture, and link with various diseases. Those who defended complete prohibition contended that no woman should be allowed to take a risk of unknown but potentially serious magnitude because her consent could not be informed. The FDA defended a restrictive policy, rather than prohibition, holding that patients with breast cancer and others have a legitimate need for breast reconstruction. The FDA distinguished sharply between reconstruction candidates and augmentation candidates, arguing that the favorable risk–benefit ratio is confined to reconstruction candidates (Kessler).

Critics of this decision charge that the government's decision is inappropriately paternalistic, especially in contrast to the more permissive public decisions reached in European countries. These critics argue that subjective benefits for many women outweigh the identified risks, and opinion surveys indicate that 90 percent of women receiving the implants are satisfied with the results (see Parker). Critics argue that the only defensible policy is to permit the continuing use of silicone-gel breast implants while requiring adequate disclosure of information about risks. Raising the level of disclosure standards is, from this perspective, more appropriate than raising the level of paternalistic restraints on choice.

THE MODEL OF PATERNAL AUTHORITY. The term *paternalism* has often been criticized as sexist and in need of correction to *parentalism*. However, some feminists in bioethics as well as some critics of paternalistic medical practices have argued that this usage is a rare case in which gendered language should be retained on grounds that an appropriate link is made between the privileges of a father in a patriarchical family and the privileges of physicians in an authoritarian medical system. The thesis is that just as hierarchical arrangements have long been the norm in the family, so paternalism has been the norm in medicine; to appreciate the need to revise authority structures in the family should similarly point to the need to revise the model of rightful authority in medicine (see Sherwin).

This criticism extends beyond analysis of the meaning of paternalism. It assumes the persistence among physicians, male and female, of the belief that a paternal model of authority is requisite in clinical practice because of compromised reasoning abilities in patients, the essential need for technical information in medical decision making, and the needs many patients have for an authority figure as healer. Susan Sherwin (1992) and other writers in bioethics have argued for replacing this traditional paternalistic model with a radically different model of the physician–patient relationship, such as a model based on friendship or on contract.

However, those who support justified paternalism in medicine believe that paternalism, properly understood, fits coherently with our normal expectations of altruistic beneficence and fiduciary responsibility in professional healthcare relationships. Their model is that of a dedicated professional who possesses superior knowledge, experience, and skills and who seeks to further a patient's best interest. Whether pieces of these two starkly different models can be joined consistently is a matter of widespread controversy in bioethics.

SUICIDE INTERVENTION. Many views about reporting, preventing, or intervening in suicide are paternalistic. Because of the extreme and irreversible effects of suicide, some defenders of intervention believe that a principle of respect for life creates an obligation to prevent suicide that overrides obligations based on the principle of respect for autonomy. A weaker account relies on Mill's strategy: Intervention is justified to establish autonomy in the person; but after it is determined that the person's decisions are substantially autonomous, further intervention would be unjustified. (Kleinig discusses several other paternalistic arguments for suicide intervention.)

Both this weaker account and stronger accounts have been defended on grounds that others do sometimes know our best interests with more insight and foresight than we do. It is often difficult to know how much ability persons have to act autonomously or how much insight they have into their "best interests." The stronger account is also defended on grounds that many suicidal persons are under intense strain or the influence of drugs or alcohol, clinically depressed, destabilized by a crisis, or simply wish to end their pain, and that these persons can be helped with their problems by health professionals. Another defense is that failure to intervene symbolically communicates to potential suicides an absence of communal concern and diminishes a feeling of communal responsibility. Finally, some argue that

it is a justified form of paternalism for friends and healthcare professionals to infringe confidentiality by reporting suicide threats to those who may be in a position to help prevent the acts. Some even defend a paternalistic obligation to report suicide threats (Bloch).

INVOLUNTARY INSTITUTIONALIZATION. Finally, a vast literature surrounds the involuntary hospitalization of persons who have never harmed others or themselves but are thought to stand in danger of inflicting such harm or of being vulnerable to harm by others. A major part of the contemporary rationale for use of police powers for the emergency detention and civil commitment of those dangerous to themselves is a paternalism supported by the knowledge that treatment has often helped persons over a momentary crisis. These interventions can involve a double paternalism: a paternalistic justification for commitment and a paternalistic justification for forced therapy (e.g., psychotherapy) after commitment.

Conclusion

Bioethics in the 1970s and 1980s exhibited a strong tendency to reject paternalism as an unjustified tampering with autonomy. However, from the mid-1980s through the mid-1990s many voices began to be heard that were more sympathetic to various paternalistic appeals. Paternalism seems likely to continue to be a viewpoint that will gain or lose adherents as the issues and larger social context shift. We may never again see the concentrated flurry of scholarly interest in this subject that was exhibited from the mid-1970s to the mid-1980s, but paternalism is not likely to be an issue that will soon disappear.

TOM L. BEAUCHAMP (1995)

SEE ALSO: *Autonomy; Behavior Control; Beneficence; Coercion; Freedom and Free Will; Institutionalization and Deinstitutionalization; Professional-Patient Relationship; Public Health; Suicide*

BIBLIOGRAPHY

Beauchamp, Tom L., and Childress, James F. 1994. *Principles of Biomedical Ethics,* 4th edition. New York: Oxford University Press.

Beauchamp, Tom L., and McCullough, Laurence B. 1984. *Medical Ethics: The Moral Responsibilities of Physicians.* Englewood Cliffs, NJ: Prentice-Hall.

Bloch, Kate E. 1987. "The Role of Law in Suicide Prevention: Beyond Civil Commitment—a Bystander Duty to Report Suicide Threats." *Stanford Law Review* 39(4): 929–953.

Brett, Allan S., and McCullough, Laurence B. 1986. "When Patients Request Specific Interventions: Defining the Limits of the Physician's Obligation." *New England Journal of Medicine* 315(21): 1347–1351.

Buchanan, Allen. 1978. "Medical Paternalism." *Philosophy and Public Affairs* 7(4): 371–390.

Childress, James F. 1982. *Who Should Decide? Paternalism in Health Care.* New York: Oxford University Press.

Dworkin, Gerald. 1972. "Paternalism." *Monist* 56(1): 64–84.

Dworkin, Gerald. 1992. "Paternalism." In *Encyclopedia of Ethics,* pp. 939–942, ed. Lawrence C. Becker. New York: Garland.

Feinberg, Joel. 1971. "Legal Paternalism." *Canadian Journal of Philosophy* 1: 105–124, rev. in *Social Philosophy.* Englewood Cliffs, NJ: Prentice-Hall 1973. Recast in *Harm to Self* (below).

Feinberg, Joel. 1980. "The Child's Right to an Open Future." In *Whose Child? Children's Rights, Parental Authority, and State Power,* pp. 124–153. Edited by William Aiken and Hugh LaFollette. Totowa, NJ: Rowman and Littlefield.

Feinberg, Joel. 1986. *Harm to Self.* Vol. III, *The Moral Limits of the Criminal Law.* New York: Oxford University Press.

Henderson, L. J. 1935. "Physician and Patient as a Social System." *New England Journal of Medicine* 212(18): 819–823.

Kant, Immanuel. 1974. (1793). *On the Old Saw: That May Be Right in Theory But It Won't Work in Practice,* tr. E. B. Ashton. Philadelphia: University of Pennsylvania Press.

Kessler, David A. 1992. "Special Report: The Basis of the FDA's Decision on Breast Implants." *New England Journal of Medicine* 326(25): 1713–1715.

Kleinig, John. 1983. *Paternalism.* Totowa, NJ: Rowman & Allanheld.

Mill, John Stuart. 1977. (1859). *On Liberty.* In *Collected Works of John Stuart Mill,* vol. 18. Toronto: University of Toronto Press.

Parker, Lisa S. 1993. "Social Justice, Federal Paternalism, and Feminism: Breast Implants in the Cultural Context of Female Beauty." *Kennedy Institute of Ethics Journal* 3(1): 57–76.

Pellegrino, Edmund D., and Thomasma, David C. 1988. *For the Patient's Good: The Restoration of Beneficence in Health Care.* New York: Oxford University Press.

Purdy, Laura M. 1992. *In Their Best Interest: The Case against Equal Rights for Children.* Ithaca, NY: Cornell University Press.

Sartorius, Rolf, ed. 1983. *Paternalism.* Minneapolis: University of Minnesota Press.

Sherwin, Susan. 1992. *No Longer Patient: Feminist Ethics and Health Care.* Philadelphia: Temple University Press.

VanDeVeer, Donald. 1986. *Paternalistic Intervention: The Moral Bounds on Benevolence.* Princeton, NJ: Princeton University Press.

PATIENTS' RESPONSIBILITIES

• • •

I. Duties of Patients

II. Virtues of Patients

I. DUTIES OF PATIENTS

Today, popular culture in the United States seems to be stressing health promotion and disease prevention; it is easy to get the impression from many sources that if one does not exercise regularly, eat the proper foods, and avoid tobacco and other dangerous substances, one has failed in a fundamental duty. In medicine and nursing, a vast literature has accumulated on "patient compliance"; despite some reminders that patients ought to be viewed as autonomous agents—the wisdom of the term *compliance* has been called into question—much of this literature assumes that the patient has a duty to follow advice given by the health professional. By contrast, eighteenth- and nineteenth-century codes of medical ethics, which listed responsibilities that patients owed to their physicians in order to balance the responsibilities that physicians were said to owe to their patients, have been condemned by most modern authors as paternalistic and self-serving. Whether patients owe any duties to health professionals and to others, and the extent of those duties if they exist, remain problematic. The topic has been much less studied in bioethics than the duties owed by professionals to patients and to society.

Duties Owed to Health Professionals

Many helpful models of the professional–patient relationship are based on some variant of social contract or covenant; and those models would imply that patients owe at least some duties to the professionals. These models deny the assumption that underlies most eighteenth- and nineteenth-century codes of medical ethics, namely, that professional ethics is a matter to be decided solely by professionals themselves, with no necessary role for patients in determining the rights and responsibilities that constitute professional ethics. It is this exclusion of patients from defining professional ethics, and not the idea of patient responsibilities per se, that permits the criticism that the alleged responsibilities of patients are paternalistic.

Are there any duties patients themselves would agree they owe to health professionals? Duties that would reasonably fall under this heading are so closely linked to the adequate carrying out of the professional role that their violation would make it impossible for the professional to provide the patient with the care the patient expects and demands. Such duties, properly circumscribed, cannot pose a threat to any patients' rights, because all such rights exist within a relationship whose purpose is to provide the patient with healthcare from a professional. Indeed, Meyer argues that the very notions of patients' rights and autonomy presuppose such a relationship.

Martin Benjamin proposes two such patient responsibilities: (1) honoring commitments, including compliance with a treatment regimen one has consented to carry out; and (2) disclosing relevant information, especially data needed to reach an accurate diagnosis and management plan for the illness. He is careful to insist that no patient has a duty to adopt any treatment plan merely because a professional recommends it; otherwise, there would be no patient right to informed consent. However, once the patient has agreed to try a plan, the patient has an obligation either to continue with the treatment or to inform the professional in a timely manner if circumstances (such as medication side effects) have made it impossible to do so. In this way, we acknowledge both the patient's right to autonomous choice and the professional's need to rely on disclosure of information and honoring of commitments in carrying out the assigned role.

Duties Owed to Identified Others

In general, duties owed to identified others are justified by the nature of the relationship between the patient and that other party. For example, as an extension of the duty to protect the interests of and to avoid harm to members of one's family, patients could have a duty to disclose health information (such as information about communicable diseases and genetic conditions) that would otherwise be protected by the right of confidentiality.

Where it is difficult to specify the precise nature and scope of the relationship, there will be a corresponding disagreement about the duties one owes. For instance, there is controversy about the duties that a pregnant woman owes to the fetus or the unborn child, in avoiding behaviors that might pose a health risk to herself or to the fetus and, in some instances, in either seeking or failing to seek an abortion. Such controversy will be resolved at least in part by more satisfactory conceptions of the precise relationship between

the pregnant woman and the fetus or child. For instance, viewing the mother and fetus as two strangers with a conflict of basic interests hardly seems to do justice to the actual nature of their bond.

Duties owed because of specific contractual relationships are much easier to understand and to justify. For example, if an insurance policy does not cover a particular laboratory test unless it is required to diagnose a specific condition, the patient has a duty not to ask the physician to falsify the claim form and say that he or she suspects the condition, when in fact the patient merely wants to know the laboratory value as a screening measure.

Duties Owed to Other Patients Generally

A patient in a modern technological society receives many benefits because of sacrifices made by patients in the past. I could not receive a medication for an infection unless that drug had been tested in research subjects. I could not receive care from a highly qualified physician or nurse unless that professional, as a student, had practiced on other patients, under supervision. It would seem at first glance that I would have a corresponding duty to serve as a research subject or as "teaching material" when I could do so with relatively little risk and inconvenience. But the healthcare system generally regards such participation as fully voluntary, not as arising out of any duty. The difference between these two views may be a result of differences in the level of moral analysis—one may acknowledge that one owes a moral duty as an individual, even if as a policy matter the institution is unwilling or unable to enforce any such duty. A full analysis of the duties, if any, that patients owe in such circumstances may nonetheless hinge upon the general theory of justice one adopts.

Duties Owed to Society

An important debate centers upon whether one's entitlement to healthcare services, or the portion of the cost of care that one bears, should hinge on the extent to which one has adhered to a healthy, low-risk lifestyle—an increasingly difficult task, as science regularly uncovers previously unappreciated health risks.

One proposal to fund expanded healthcare coverage and benefits in the United States, for instance, includes a substantial increase in the tax on cigarettes. This could be justified purely as a matter of public health, since empirical evidence suggests that a number of people will stop smoking as a result of the tax. In turn, the public-health agenda could be justified in part by referring to a patient's duty to himself or herself to avoid serious health risks (though some analytic philosophers would claim that a duty to oneself is incoherent, since if someone owes a duty to me, I can always voluntarily release him or her from that duty), or to the duty that an individual owes to close family members not to abandon them or decrease one's ability to support them by running unnecessary and substantial health risks. Alternatively, the tax could be justified as a matter of justice, with those who voluntarily adopt unhealthy behaviors having some responsibility to pay for a larger share of the overall health costs. According to this latter line of analysis, the tax is therefore justified even if it fails to persuade any current smokers to stop.

Some of the debate about a duty to avoid health risks centers upon the addictive nature of some undesirable behaviors. Addiction implies a loss of voluntary control, suggesting that any duty not to engage in that behavior is correspondingly weakened, assuming that I cannot have a duty to do what I cannot do. On the other hand, a careful analysis of most addictive behavior patterns reveals certain actions that do appear to be under voluntary control, even if other aspects of the pattern seem to be characterized by loss of control. For instance, smokers may elect not to sign up for smoking-cessation counseling, and may socialize in settings where they know the temptation to smoke will be high.

To some extent, linking entitlement to care with a duty to remain healthy depends on where one stands on a spectrum between individualistic and communitarian conceptions of healthcare justice. On a purely individualistic approach, I have no responsibility to help pay for the health needs of anyone else; on a communitarian interpretation, we all have a shared responsibility to provide decent care for all, and that sense of shared responsibility is undermined by efforts to assign differential duties to pay to different citizens on the basis of their personal behaviors. Also, a duty to avoid health risks seems more justifiable when it is applied even-handedly rather than being used to condemn those whose lifestyles differ from one's own. Finally, a policy based on a duty to avoid health risks seems justifiable in inverse proportion to its personal intrusiveness. Thus a tax on the sale of cigarettes appears more justifiable than refusing healthcare to those whose diseases are caused by smoking, or spying on citizens in their homes to be sure that they really have stopped smoking.

HOWARD BRODY (1995)
BIBLIOGRAPHY REVISED

SEE ALSO: *AIDS; Autonomy; Behavior Control; Confidentiality; Epidemics; Family and Family Medicine; Harm;* *Maternal-Fetal Relationship; Paternalism; Patients' Rights; Professional-Patient Relationship; Profession and Professional Ethics; Public Health; Substance Abuse*

BIBLIOGRAPHY

Benjamin, Martin. 1985. "Lay Obligations in Professional Relations." *Journal of Medicine and Philosophy* 10(1): 85–103.

Gatens-Robinson, Eugenie. 1992. "A Defense of Women's Choice: Abortion and the Ethics of Care." *Southern Journal of Philosophy* 30(3): 39–66.

Gorovitz, Samuel. 1984. "Why You Don't Owe It to Yourself to Seek Health." *Journal of Medical Ethics* 10(3): 143–146.

Greiner, K. Allen. 2000. "Patient-Provider Relations—Understanding the Social and Cultural Circumstances of Difficult Patients." *Bioethics Forum* 16(3): 7–12.

Little, Miles, and Little, J. M. 1995. *Humane Medicine: A Leading Surgeon Examines What Doctors Do, What Their Patients Expect from Them, and How the Expectations of Both Are Not Being Met.* New York: Cambridge University Press.

May, William F., and Soens, A. L., eds. 2000. *The Ethics of Giving and Receiving: Am I My Foolish Brother's Keeper?* Dallas, TX: Southern Methodist University Press.

Meyer, Michael J. 1992. "Patients' Duties." *Journal of Medicine and Philosophy* 17(5): 541–555.

Sider, Roger C., and Clements, Colleen D. 1984. "Patients' Ethical Obligation for Their Health." *Journal of Medical Ethics* 10(3): 138–142.

Stimson, Gerry V. 1974. "Obeying Doctor's Orders: A View from the Other Side." *Social Science and Medicine* 8(2): 97–104.

Ulrich, Lawrence P. 2001. *The Patient Self-Determination Act: Meeting the Challenges in Patient Care (Clinical Medical Ethics).* Washington, D.C.: Georgetown University Press.

Wikler, Daniel. 1987. "Personal Responsibility for Illness." In *Health Care Ethics: An Introduction,* pp. 326–358, ed. Donald Van DeVeer and Tom Regan. Philadelphia: Temple University Press.

II. VIRTUES OF PATIENTS

Although considerable attention has been given to virtues in medicine (Drane; Pellegrino and Thomasma, 1993), most writings focus on the virtues of caregivers rather than on those of care receivers. Patients writing about their experiences of illness (Abram; Sacks; Scott-Maxwell) often struggle with questions of virtue and character, but they tend not to express those questions in systematic or theoretical form. Little has been written on patients' virtues per se.

Several commentators suggest that virtues of different people involved in medicine have to be correlated with the goals or purposes of the medical encounter (Drane; Pellegrino and Thomasma, 1993). For example, in *For the Patient's*

Good, Edmund Pellegrino and David Thomasma (1988) suggest that the virtues of a good patient include truthfulness, probity (or an effort to uphold one's end of the healing relationship), justice, tolerance, and trust (which includes some elements of gratitude and friendship). These virtues arise out of the model of obligations appropriate to the internal goods of the practice of medicine. In *The Virtues in Medical Practice,* Pellegrino and Thomasma add benevolence, humility, and courage. These virtues, which apply to practitioners as well as patients, "dispose both parties to act well in relation to the ends of medicine" (1993, p. 194).

However, Edmund Pincoffs argues that virtues cannot be reduced simply to qualities related to the internal goods of a practice. If virtues are correlative to role-specific duties, as Tom Beauchamp and James Childress suggest, then patients might be expected to exhibit the virtues correlative to their duties of truthfulness, compliance with treatment regimen, and respect. However, such a view would neglect important virtues, such as gratitude, that are not readily identified with action guides.

Both Karen Lebacqz and William F. May address the virtues of patients as qualities that emerge in response to the situation of illness or limitation, but not specifically as qualities having to do with the doctor–patient or caregiver–care receiver relationship and not specifically as correlated with duties. Drawing on both fictional (Solzhenitsyn) and real-life (Abram; Fox; Scott-Maxwell) stories of patients, Lebacqz addresses the virtues of patients generally. May treats the virtues of the elderly within the general context of their confrontation with limitation, adversity, and death.

In line with other commentators (Drane; Hauerwas; Pellegrino and Thomasma, 1988), Lebacqz argues that virtue, which can be defined as a unity of the self, is not the same as specific *virtues.* Virtues are qualities or traits of character judged to be excellent. They emerge as general stances toward the world or as responses to situations. The situation of patients is generally characterized by bodily change, threats to self-identity and understanding, and the assumption of a new social role—that of "patient," with all its indignities, loss of control, and powerlessness. The virtues of patients are "excellences" in response to these situational changes.

Using classical virtue theory (Pieper), Lebacqz proposes that two "cardinal" virtues and one "theological" virtue are particularly appropriate to the situation of patients. Fortitude, or courage in the face of fear, is the first virtue for patients, who often wonder whether they have the strength to do what is needed. Fortitude includes both endurance and attack: both accepting limits and railing against limitation.

Prudence, or acting in accord with the real, is crucial for patients, who must learn to deal with new realities in their lives. The first aspect of prudence is perception; the second aspect is the willingness to act on what is perceived. Perception includes both listening, or contemplation, and removing hardness from the heart in order to value the little things in life.

Finally, Lebacqz suggests that hope in the sense of trust in the attainment of ends is crucial for patients (cf. Hauerwas, who argues that hope forms every virtue). In the face of despair and even terror, hope keeps patients from falling into despair. Humor is a central component of such hope.

Lebacqz stresses that there is no single pattern of virtue for patients and no one way of expressing relevant virtues. While she follows the Aristotelian pattern of assuming virtue to be a mean between extremes, she notes that virtues are culturally conditioned and, hence, what is considered virtuous in one culture may not be in another. For example, patient waiting might be prized in some cultures while aggressive resistance would be in others. Whereas Pellegrino and Thomasma (1988) note that healthcare providers often consider the "good patient" to be the one who is willing to suffer, Lebacqz rejects long suffering as a central virtue for patients. Similarly, virtues might be assessed differently for men and women in different cultures.

May's treatment of virtues of the elderly stresses several of those noted by Lebacqz. May also puts courage at the head of the list, and includes in it both endurance and attack. He places the virtue of prudence into the broader category of wisdom, and uses traditional categories to propose that prudence includes *memoria,* or learning from the past; *docilitas,* or the capacity to be silent and thus to perceive; and *solertia,* a readiness for the unexpected and an openness to the future. He does not list hope per se, but does include humor or *hilaritas* ("celestial gaiety") as a virtue related to wisdom.

May also adds some virtues of the elderly in situations of illness. Since patients are "receivers," May argues that humility is a crucial virtue for them. It removes the sting from the humiliations that they must endure. While Lebacqz argues that patience is not always a virtue, May suggests that purposive waiting and taking control of one's own spirit under circumstances of adversity is a virtue. For the elderly, May adds the virtues of benignity, letting go of one's possessions in openhanded love, and simplicity, learning to travel unencumbered. Finally, he suggests that integrity is a virtue that expresses unity of character and implies both uprightness and wholeness. Although May does not list theological virtues per se, he does suggest that integrity points to the transcendent dimension.

These different treatments of patients' virtues suffice to indicate that there is no single list of virtues appropriate to patients and no agreed mechanism for deriving such a list. Nonetheless, using Pincoffs's sorting scheme, we might suggest that patients need both instrumental and noninstrumental virtues.

Instrumental virtues are geared toward the goal of restoring health. These fit best with the view that virtues are qualities intrinsic to the goods of an institution or practice such as medicine. In the case of patients, such instrumental virtues would include complying with appropriate treatment regimens (probity) and telling the truth about one's situation (honesty). These virtues support the goal of working toward the patient's health.

Patients also need noninstrumental virtues. In these, Pincoffs includes: (1) aesthetic qualities such as serenity, which comes close to May's virtue of simplicity; (2) meliorating qualities such as tolerance and tactfulness, which come close to notions of humor utilized by both Lebacqz and May; and (3) moral virtues such as fairness and honesty, akin to virtues urged by Pellegrino and Thomasma.

There is general agreement, then, that virtues are qualities of persons generally admired or praised in a culture, and that certain qualities are particularly important for patients: courage (or fortitude), wisdom (especially prudence), humor, hope, truthfulness, and faithfulness to the task of healing, whether through long-suffering endurance or through attack and resistance. In spite of this agreement, the assessment of what constitutes a virtue will be culturally conditioned and will likely reflect the biases of dominant groups in a culture.

KAREN LEBACQZ (1995)
BIBLIOGRAPHY REVISED

SEE ALSO: *Beneficence; Care; Conscience, Rights of; Death; Healing; Law and Morality; Maternal-Fetal Relationship; Narrative; Pain and Suffering; Patients' Responsibilities: Duties of Patients; Professional-Patient Relationship; Trust; Virtue and Character*

BIBLIOGRAPHY

Abram, Morris B. 1982. *The Day Is Short: An Autobiography.* New York: Harcourt Brace Jovanovich.

Beauchamp, Tom L., and Childress, James F. 1989. *Principles of Biomedical Ethics,* 3rd edition. New York: Oxford University Press.

Brody, Howard. 1994. "Patients' Responsibilities." In *Encyclopedia of Bioethics,* ed. Warren T. Reich. New York: Macmillan.

Drane, James F. 1988. *Becoming a Good Doctor: The Place of Virtue and Character in Medical Ethics.* Kansas City, MO: Sheed and Ward.

Fox, Renée C. 1959. *Experiment Perilous: Physicians and Patients Facing the Unknown.* Glencoe, IL: Free Press.

Greiner, K. Allen. 2000. "Patient-Provider Relations—Understanding the Social and Cultural Circumstances of Difficult Patients." *Bioethics Forum* 16(3): 7–12.

Hauerwas, Stanley. 1985. "Virtue." In *Powers That Make Us Human: The Foundations of Medical Ethics,* pp. 117–140, ed. Kenneth Vaux. Urbana: University of Illinois Press.

Lebacqz, Karen. 1985. "The Virtuous Patient." In *Philosophy and Medicine,* vol. 17: *Virtue and Medicine: Explorations in the Character of Medicine,* ed. Earl E. Shelp, pp. 275–288. Dordrecht, Netherlands: D. Reidel.

Loewy, Roberta Springer. 2000. *Integrity and Personhood: Looking at Patients from a Bio/Psycho/Social Perspective.* New York: Plenum Publishers.

May, William F. 1991. *The Patient's Ordeal.* Bloomington: Indiana University Press.

May, William F. and Soens, A. L., eds. 2000. *The Ethics of Giving and Receiving: Am I My Foolish Brother's Keeper?* Dallas, TX: Southern Methodist University Press.

Midwest Bioethics Center. 2000. "Guidelines for Providing Ethical Care in Difficult Provider-Patient Relationships." *Bioethics Forum* 16(3): SS1–SS8.

Pellegrino, Edmund D., and Thomasma, David C. 1988. *For the Patient's Good: The Restoration of Beneficence in Health Care.* New York: Oxford University Press.

Pellegrino, Edmund D., and Thomasma, David C. 1993. *The Virtues in Medical Practice.* New York: Oxford University Press.

Pieper, Josef. 1966. *The Four Cardinal Virtues: Prudence, Justice, Fortitude, and Temperance.* Notre Dame, IN: University of Notre Dame Press.

Pincoffs, Edmund L. 1985. "Two Cheers for Meno: The Definition of the Virtues." In *Philosophy and Medicine,* vol. 17: *Virtue and Medicine: Explorations in the Character of Medicine,* ed. Earl E. Shelp, pp. 111–131. Dordrecht, Netherlands: D. Reidel.

Sacks, Oliver W. 1984. *A Leg to Stand On.* New York: Summit.

Scott-Maxwell, Florida. 1968. *The Measure of My Days.* New York: Knopf.

Schaeffer, Marilyn. 2000. "The Impatient Patient—Reexamining Difficult Patient-Provider Relationships." *Bioethics Forum* 16(3): 13–16.

Solzhenitsyn, Aleksandr Isavich. 1969. *Cancer Ward,* tr. Nicholas Bethell and David Burg. New York: Bantam.

Ulrich, Lawrence P. 2001. *The Patient Self-Determination Act: Meeting the Challenges in Patient Care (Clinical Medical Ethics).* Washington, D.C.: Georgetown University Press.

provide for their protection or assertion, and frequently limit their exercise without recourse (Annas and Healey).

PATIENTS' RIGHTS

• • •

I. ORIGIN AND NATURE OF PATIENTS' RIGHTS

In most industrialized countries it is taken for granted that citizens have a right to medical care, but there is much less recognition of rights in medical care. In the United States, in contrast, concentration has historically been on rights that individuals may exercise in the medical-care context, whereas only in the mid-1990s has discussion begun to focus on rights to medical care (or at least the right to medical insurance). From "informed consent" to the "right to abortion" to the "right to die," patients' rights have become both a political slogan and a part of broader political agendas.

Although initially the trend toward recognizing patients' rights concentrated on the institutional setting in which medical care was delivered, and focused on issues such as natural childbirth and informed consent, by the 1990s the trend was visible throughout the healthcare system in the United States and was spreading internationally.

The doctor–patient relationship has historically been described as based on trust rather than on the monetary considerations evident in the more typical business transaction. Nevertheless, increased expectations and increased cost have contributed to patients' views of themselves as "consumers," and by the 1980s hospitals began considering themselves private businesses. U.S. courts and legislatures had previously moved to protect the weaker party from abuses of power in areas formerly unregulated, such as landlord–tenant, seller–buyer, creditor–debtor, employer–employee, police–suspect, and warden–prisoner relationships. The law has now also come to the aid of patients asserting their rights in medical situations.

The recognition of patients' rights flows from two fundamental premises: (1) The healthcare consumer possesses certain interests, many of which may properly be described as rights, that are not automatically forfeited by entering into a relationship with a physician or a healthcare facility; and (2) many physicians and healthcare facilities fail to recognize the existence of these interests and rights, fail to

History

In 1969, the Joint Commission on Accreditation of Hospitals (JCAH)—a private, voluntary accreditation organization composed of members from the American Hospital Association (AHA) and the American Medical College of Surgeons—issued its proposals for revisions in its standards. The National Welfare Rights Organization (NWRO), a grass-roots consumer organization spawned during the activist 1960s, responded in June 1970 by drafting a document containing twenty-six demands; this was the first comprehensive statement of "patients' rights" from the consumers' perspective. Included were provisions for such things as grievance procedures, community representation on hospital governing boards, nondiscrimination on the basis of source of payment, restrictions on transfers, provisions on privacy and confidentiality, and prompt attention to patients' requests for nursing assistance (Silver). After months of negotiation, a number of these items were specifically written into the revised standards of the JCAH. By the late 1980s, issues of access to care, of respect and dignity, privacy and confidentiality, consent, refusal of treatment, and patient transfer to another facility were specifically addressed in a new section of their accreditation manual called "Rights and Responsibilities of Patients" (Annas, 1989).

In late 1972, the American Hospital Association adopted a Patient Bill of Rights based on the premise that "[the] traditional physician–patient relationship takes on a new dimension when care is rendered within an organizational structure ... the institution itself also has a responsibility to the patient." The text of the AHA bill of patient rights called for acknowledgment of the rights to (1) respectful care; (2) current medical information; (3) information requisite for informed consent; (4) refusal of treatment; (5) privacy; (6) confidentiality; (7) response to requests for service; (8) information on other institutions touching on the patient's care; (9) refusal of participation in research projects; (10) continuity of care; (11) examination and explanation of financial charges; and (12) knowledge of hospital regulations. In 1992, items on access to medical records and use of advance directives were added. Although the listing remains vague and incomplete, and there is no enforcement mechanism, it moves in the direction of more adequately informing patients of their rights.

Between 1974 and 1988, many states, including Arizona, California, Illinois, Kentucky, Maryland, Massachusetts, Michigan, Minnesota, New Hampshire, New York,

Pennsylvania, Rhode Island, and Vermont, adopted a patients' bill of rights by regulation or statute (Annas, 1989). All fifty states have adopted some form of advance healthcare directive document, such as a living will or durable power of attorney, in which people can express their wishes regarding medical care should they become incompetent. Both former President Nixon and Jacqueline Kennedy Onassis used such documents in 1994.

The American Medical Association (AMA), probably because of its traditional paternalistic philosophy, did not seriously consider adopting its own version of the patients' bill of rights until 1989. Five of the six provisions of its proposal—the rights of patients to access information in the medical record and to make treatment decisions and the rights to respect, to confidentiality, and to continuity of care—seem to have been uncontroversial. The bill of rights was rejected by the AMA House of Delegates, however, because of its sixth provision: "The patient has the right to essential health [medical] care." In the absence of some national healthcare program, or unless the patient has a preexisting relationship with a physician or insurance program or is experiencing an emergency medical condition, there is no "right to medical care" in the United States (although opinion polls taken since 1948 show that most physicians and Americans believe this right either exists or should exist).

International Scope of the Movement

Although "rights talk" is uniquely American (as are the Bill of Rights and Declaration of Independence), the patients' rights movement should not be viewed as unique to any one country. In 1975, for example, the Parliamentary Assembly of the Council of Europe submitted a draft recommendation to its sixteen member-nations recommending that all necessary action be taken to ensure that the sick can receive relief from their suffering and that people can prepare adequately for death; that commissions be established to study the issue of euthanasia; and that physicians be impressed "that the sick have a right to full information, if they request it, on their illness and the proposed treatment, and to take action to see that special information is given when entering hospitals as regards the routine, procedures and medical equipment of the institution." By 1990, work on a European Declaration of the Rights of Patients was well under way (Westerhall and Phillips; Leenen et al.). In 1991, a national conference on patients' rights was held in Japan, and at the impetus of tort lawyers and some physicians, a trend toward recognizing patients' rights is developing in that country as well.

The worldwide trend toward recognizing human rights in health should be viewed in context of the worldwide trend toward recognizing human rights in general. Recognition of rights to bodily integrity in general, for example, translates into a right to refuse treatment in the medical context. In this regard documents such as the Nuremberg Code (1947), the United Nations Universal Declaration of Human Rights (1948), and the United Nations International Covenant on Civil and Political Rights (1966) should be viewed as foundational (Annas and Grodin; Sieghart).

Patients' Rights in Context

Historian Paul Starr discusses the patents' rights movement in the United States as part of the "generalization of rights," distinguishing the movement to recognize healthcare as a basic human right (still unfulfilled) from the movement to work for rights in healthcare. In his words, "The new health care rights movement went beyond traditional demands for more medical care and challenged the distribution of power and expertise" (p. 389). Grass-roots consumer organizations in some states, such as Oregon, have begun to influence health policy, as have activist groups such as ACT-UP. Courts, of course, have contributed greatly to this trend, especially through decisions defining the doctrine of informed consent and by upholding treatment refusals as an individual's right to the exercise of liberty. But no one should have to go to court to have rights vindicated. Some have suggested the establishment of ethics committees to help patients enforce their rights, but such committees usually represent institutional interests more than the rights of individual patients (Annas, 1993). There is a need for an effective enforcement mechanism and an efficient dispute-resolution mechanism. Institutional and professional interests have made agreement on these issues difficult, and legal requirements to adopt such mechanisms may be needed.

One effective method of protecting patients' rights would be the establishment, either by the government under a national healthcare system or by health-insurance plans, of a patients' rights advocate program. The advocate should have the authority, under the direction of the patient, to exercise the patient's rights and powers on behalf of the patient. Such individuals could operate at the institutional level, but they are more likely to be effective in health plans, multi-institutional settings, and, of course, under any national health plan (Annas and Healey).

GEORGE J. ANNAS (1995)
BIBLIOGRAPHY REVISED

SEE ALSO: *Abortion: Contemporary Ethical and Legal Aspects; Abortion: Legal and Regulatory Issues; Abuse, Interpersonal; Access to Healthcare; Autonomy; Confidentiality; Conscience, Rights of; Disability: Legal Issues; Ethics: Normative Ethical Theories; Feminism; Genetic Discrimination; Human Rights; Informed Consent; Law and Bioethics; Law and Morality; Privacy and Confidentiality in Research; Privacy in Healthcare; Race and Racism;* and other *Patients' Rights* subentries

BIBLIOGRAPHY

Annas, George J. 1989. *The Rights of Patients: The Basic ACLU Guide to Patient Rights,* 2nd edition. Carbondale, IL: Southern Illinois University Press.

Annas, George J. 1993. *Standard of Care: The Law of American Bioethics.* New York: Oxford University Press.

Annas, George J. 1998. *Some Choice: Law, Medicine, and the Market.* New York: Oxford University Press.

Annas, George J., and Grodin, Michael A., eds. 1992. *The Nazi Doctors and the Nuremberg Code: Human Rights in Human Experimentation.* New York: Oxford University Press.

Annas, George J., and Healey, Joseph M., Jr. 1974. "The Patient Rights Advocate: Redefining the Doctor-Patient Relationship in the Hospital Context." *Vanderbilt Law Review* 27(2): 243–269.

Baker, Robert; Emanuel, Linda L.; Caplan, Arthur; and Latham, Stephen R., eds. 1999. *The American Medical Ethics Revolution: How the AMA's Code of Ethics Has Transformed Physicians' Relationships to Patients, Professionals, and Society.* Baltimore: Johns Hopkins University Press.

Buetow, S. 1998. "The Scope for the Involvement of Patients in their Consultations with Health Professionals: Rights, Responsibilities and Preferences of Patients." *Journal of Medical Ethics* 24(4): 243–247.

Corsino, Bruce V. 1996. "Bioethics Committees and JCAHO Patients' Rights Standards: A Question of Balance." *Journal of Clinical Ethics* 7(2): 177–181.

D'Oronzio, Joseph C. 2001. "A Human Right to Healthcare Access: Returning to the Origins of the Patients' Rights Movement." *Cambridge Quarterly of Healthcare Ethics* 10(3): 285–298.

Gross, Michael L. 1999. "Autonomy and Paternalism in Communitarian Society: Patient Rights in Israel." *Hastings Center Report* 29(4): 13–20.

Inlander, Charles B., and Pavalon, Eugene I. 1990. *Your Medical Rights: How to Become an Empowered Consumer.* Boston: Little, Brown.

JCAHO (Joint Commission on Accredation of Healthcare Organizations). 1998. *Ethical Issues & Patient Rights across the Continuum of Care.* Washington, D.C.: Author.

Kinney, Eleanor Dearman. 2002. *Protecting American Health Care Consumers.* Durham, NC: Duke University Press.

Leenen, Henk; Gevers, Sjef; and Pinet, Genevieve. 1993. *The Rights of Patients in Europe: A Comparative Study.* Deventer, Netherlands: Kluwer.

Mann, Jonathan; Gruskin, Sofia; and Grodin, Michael A., eds. 1999. *Health and Human Rights.* London: Routledge.

Parker, Lisa S. 1995. "Incidental Findings: Patients' Knowledge, Rights, and Preferences." *Journal of Clinical Ethics* 6(2): 176–179.

Schneider, Carl E. 1998. *The Practice of Autonomy: Patients, Doctors, and Medical Decisions.* New York: Oxford University Press.

Sieghart, Paul. 1983. *The International Law of Human Rights.* Oxford, U.K.: Clarendon Press.

Silver, Laurens H. 1974. "The Legal Accountability of Nonprofit Hospitals." In *Regulating Health Facilities Construction,* pp. 183–200, ed. Clark C. Havighurst. Washington, D.C.: American Enterprise Institute.

Starr, Paul. 1982. *The Social Transformation of American Medicine.* New York: Basic Books.

Sweet, M. P., and Bernat, J. L. 1997. "A Study of the Ethical Duty of Physicians to Disclose Errors." *Journal of Clinical Ethics* 8(4): 341–348.

Westerhall, Lotta, and Phillips, Charles, eds. 1994. *Patient's Rights: Informed Consent, Access and Equality.* Stockholm: Nerenius & Santérus.

Worth-Staten, Patricia A., and Poniatowski, Larry. 1997. "Advance Directives and Patient Rights: A Joint Commission Perspective." *Bioethics Forum* 13(2): 47–50.

II. MENTAL PATIENTS' RIGHTS

The strength of a society's commitment to justice and humanity can often be assessed by examining its treatment of its most vulnerable and/or disliked citizens. Few individuals have been as disliked, feared, persecuted, or stigmatized as have the mentally ill. Briefly reviewing the treatment of the mentally ill can provide a useful perspective in addressing present issues in mental patients' rights.

This article will examine mental patients' rights, including legal rights (judicial decisions, legislative and administrative enactments); human wants (basic human rights and entitlements); and clinical needs (the mental-health view of the right of every citizen to be free of the pain and limitations of mental illness).

In the United States, the mentally ill have historically experienced deprivation of many rights enjoyed by other citizens. Since colonial times there has been essentially a two-tier system distinguishing the treatment of the rich from that of the poor. The insane rich were usually kept at home—or more recently, in private institutions—and concealed from society to protect the reputation of their families, while the insane poor were left to the care of local communities. If the insane poor were seen as harmlessly deranged, society's main fear was that they would become public charges and drain the community's resources. To prevent this from happening, the mentally ill were often subjected to whipping and banishment, forced to wander from village to village. If they refused to leave their home community, their "treatment" frequently was incarceration in the local jail or poorhouse (Deutsch).

During the nineteenth century "moral treatment" was brought to America by a Quaker clergyman, the Rev. Thomas Scattergood. Great success, as high as 90 percent improvement in conditions, was reported by its early practitioners. The treatment was accomplished by removing patients from their family and community and placing them in a peaceful rural retreat—the asylum—where, under the absolute control of the physician, they lived a highly disciplined existence and engaged in useful employment (Rothman). "Moral treatment" represented an improvement in the conditions under which the mentally ill were treated. While still deprived of the legal and civil rights enjoyed by other citizens, they were at least given humane and hopeful treatment. This improvement, however, did not last long. By the end of the nineteenth century, as the result of a large influx of immigrants and a growing population of chronic patients, the asylums became overcrowded and inadequately staffed. Overcrowding and disorder created justification for mechanical restraints and punishments that grew in usage and severity; hospitals became human warehouses instead of treatment centers.

The failings and increasing harshness of public asylums did not lead to their dismantlement. Loose commitment laws facilitated the expulsion of the mentally ill from an increasingly urban society less willing to tolerate them. Efforts to improve conditions were sporadic, and progress was slow and uneven. Despite numerous books and exposés, including Clifford Beers's *A Mind That Found Itself* (1930), Albert Deutsch's *The Shame of the States* (1948), and Mary Jane Ward's *The Snake Pit* (1946, later made into a movie), the period of incarceration without adequate treatment continued well into the first half of the twentieth century.

By the mid-1950s, the mental-health community began to express its discontent with the situation in state mental hospitals. The resident population soared to 550,000, and approximately 40 percent of hospital beds were in state and county mental hospitals. The president of the American Psychiatric Association declared in 1958, "I do not see how any reasonably objective view of our mental hospitals today can fail to conclude that they are bankrupt beyond remedy" (Solomon, p. 7).

Public concern about the plight of the nation's mentally ill led Congress to establish the Joint Commission on Mental Illness and Health in 1955. The commission advocated the goal of community-based mental-healthcare accessible and responsive to the needs of all citizens. Community

mental-health centers would provide the mentally ill with treatment close to their homes and jobs, and would reduce the need for prolonged or repeated hospitalization. As the result of the development of psychotropic medicine (medications that therapeutically affect an individual's mood or cognitive thoughts), expansion of community-based care, increased public concern about civil rights, and some greater tolerance of alternative behaviors, the population of the hospitalized mentally ill dropped to 220,000 during the 1960s and 1970s. This process of deinstitutionalization, however, did not always proceed smoothly. Frequently, patient discharges from hospitals occurred precipitously and without adequate aftercare. In addition, communities protested that they were becoming "dumping grounds" for patients unprepared for the demands of community living and for whom no adequate support system had been established (*Stone v. Miller,* 1974).

Despite the increased willingness of the public to support improved care for the mentally ill within their home communities, the plight of those treated in large state hospitals was still characterized by dehumanization, inadequate facilities, and insufficient staff. Such conditions provoked a flurry of lawsuits during the 1960s and 1970s, which led to increased attention to the rights of the mentally ill. These cases fit into three broad categories: the right to treatment; the right to refuse treatment; and the right to be placed in the least restrictive alternative. A fourth right, the right to liberty, represented by the U.S. Supreme Court's *O'Connor v. Donaldson* decision (1975), has aspects that encompass the three other categories.

Right to Treatment and Right to Liberty

During the 1960s, mental-health litigation reflected the increased activism of many civil-rights attorneys who turned their attention to mental patients' rights. In a parallel development, courts that had previously refused to rule on matters of medical treatment began, during the same period, to question whether conditions that would enable treatment to occur actually existed in facilities to which the mentally ill were committed. The concept of a right to treatment was first enunciated by Morton Birnbaum, who wrote the following in an *American Bar Association Journal* article:

> The fact that a person has a mental ailment is not a crime. Therefore, if anyone is voluntarily restrained of his liberty because of mental ailment, the state owes a duty to provide him reasonable medical attention. If medical attention reasonably adjusted to the needs is not given, the person is not a patient, but ... virtually a prisoner. (Birnbaum, p. 499)

As a result of such thinking, a number of lawsuits were filed under the rationale of a constitutional right to treatment. Facilities in which widespread abuses and violation of clinical and legal rights were common were excellent targets for such litigation. Such was the situation that existed in certain hospitals in 1971, when the *Wyatt v. Stickney* lawsuit was brought against the Alabama Mental Health System. It was established during the trial that the state legislature had seriously underfunded Parlow and Bryce hospitals, leading to severe understaffing, deterioration in services and facilities, and limitation on treatment and basic care for the patients there. As a result of the rights violations described in the trial, the judge promulgated minimum standards for nearly every aspect of institutional care and a detailed program for implementation.

The minimum standards promulgated by the court include the following: a provision against institutional peonage; a number of protections to ensure a humane psychological environment; minimum staffing standards; provision for a human-rights committee at each institution; detailed physical standards; minimum nutritional requirements; a provision for individualized evaluations of patients, habilitation plans, and programs; minimum staff/patient ratios; and a requirement that every mentally impaired person has a right to the least restrictive setting necessary for treatment (*Wyatt v. Stickney,* 1971).

The courts have felt justified in moving into the vacuum caused by a lack of national standards to assure the treatment rights of involuntarily committed psychiatric patients. In the *O'Connor* decision, for example, the Supreme Court dismissed as "unpersuasive" the argument that the court should not be involved, noting: "Where treatment is the sole asserted ground for depriving a person of liberty it is plainly unacceptable to suggest that courts are powerless to determine whether the asserted ground is present" (*O'Connor v. Donaldson,* 1975, p. 574, n. 10). In other cases, such as *Wyatt v. Stickney,* the judges have consulted with various professional organizations, taken expert testimony, and come up with what they considered minimum standards. These standards tend to be more of the mortar-and-brick and staff-to-patient-ratio variety than to pertain directly to the quality of treatment. The basis behind the right-to-treatment issues as reflected in *Wyatt* and other cases is the expectation that if a psychiatric patient is to be involuntarily confined in order to be treated, then the facility in which he or she is placed should at least have the minimum capacity to deliver such treatment as will assure the patient's recovery and release. To do other than this is to "warehouse" patients and thus violate their constitutional right to liberty. The limited holding of the Supreme Court's *O'Connor* decision emphasized this point: "A state cannot constitutionally confine without *more*

[emphasis added], a nondangerous individual who is capable of surviving safely in freedom by himself or with the help of willing and responsible family members or friends" (*O'Connor v. Donaldson,* 1975, p. 576).

Changing Perspectives on Patient-Physician Relationships

The Supreme Court's decision in *O'Connor v. Donaldson* reflects an evolving philosophy about the rights of the mentally ill in relation to society and to mental-health practitioners. For hundreds of years, many concerned with care and treatment of the mentally ill believed that their condition categorically prevents them from accurately perceiving reality and making reasoned judgments. Therefore it was considered the state's duty, according to the principle of *parens patria* (the state acting as a good parent to the nation's citizens) to take care of such afflicted individuals, and to prevent them under the state's police power from harming themselves or others, or disturbing the peace and safety of the community (Fowlkes).

Consistent with these commitment perspectives has been the psychiatric view that life and health or physical and emotional well-being are at the pinnacle of any hierarchy of values and should be maintained at any cost—even if the cost is a considerable loss of liberty for the individual whose health is at stake (Kopolow, 1976). A corollary to this position is the belief that mental illness is a disease of processes that impairs an individual's judgment and capacity for responsible action in relation to self and others. In refusing hospitalization and treatment, therefore, the patient's wishes might very well be discounted and viewed as symptoms of his or her mental illness (Sadoff and Kopolow).

A countervailing philosophy was reflected in the civil-liberties perspective and shared by a growing number of lawyers and mental-health professionals concerned with human rights. This view maintains that although a person's physical and mental health are important they are not necessarily of the highest value, and that freedom of the individual to place a higher value on other things should be respected. Those espousing this view maintain that what is called "mental illness" is not a process that necessarily interferes with or invalidates a person's will or lessens responsibility for his or her behavior (Szasz). Even psychotic individuals should have their wish to live at home rather than in a state mental hospital taken into consideration by the judges and psychiatrists who determine their fate.

Increasingly, states have abandoned the *parens patria* doctrine as being intrusive into the lives of individuals and have begun to utilize a more limited criterion of dangerousness as the justification for the use of "police power" for commitment. The *O'Connor* court seemed to sanction a definition of dangerousness as applied to civil commitment when it declared:

> Of course, even if there is no foreseeable risk of self injury or suicide, a person is literally dangerous to himself if for physical or other reasons he is helpless to avoid the hazards of freedom either through his own efforts or with the aid of willing family members or friends. (*O'Connor v. Donaldson*, 1975, p. 574, n. 9)

As a result of such court decisions, the test for commitment in many states now requires that the person be harmful to self or others by reason of mental illness and that no less restrictive alternative exists (Stone).

Initially, right-to-treatment decisions such as *Wyatt v. Stickney* and the right-to-liberty case of *O'Connor v. Donaldson* were welcomed by some mental-health professionals who viewed litigation as a potentially effective means for obtaining the release of patients who were receiving only custodial care or should not have been institutionalized in the first place. Others considered litigation as an intrusion into clinical practices that would produce great disruption in the mental-health system and no long-term benefit for patient care. While this debate continues, it does seem clear that litigation did focus public attention on the plight of the hospitalized mentally ill and, at least in the short term, resulted in pressure on legislatures to increase mental-health appropriations in order to avoid litigation or to avert increased court intervention.

Traditionally, the decisions about therapies and medical procedures have been within the domain of the treating professional responsible for the patient. In many states, patients who were hospitalized involuntarily were considered incompetent to make decisions on their own behalf. As a result of these medical and legal perspectives, patients frequently were denied the rights of other citizens when they were hospitalized. They were not permitted to vote; often they could not make phone calls or correspond without censorship of their mail. Additionally, they were not told what was happening to them or the consequences of the treatment imposed on them.

In the past, patients within an institution experienced a double limitation on their rights—one created by their disabilities and the other by the inherent organization of an institutional system. Even now, the prevailing atmosphere in many hospitals and especially psychiatric facilities perpetuates dependency and helplessness (Goffman).

While the actual disabilities that require institutional care limit a patient somewhat, the prejudging of his or her capacities by the staff may constitute an even greater obstacle. Even at the most enlightened institution, there will inevitably be a strain between the needs of the individual to live a life free of outside control and the institution's need to deliver care efficiently and effectively. Within a mental-health institution or any long-term-care facility, such organizational factors can be dehumanizing and promote frustration, regimentation, and despair. In addition, the stigmatization of mentally ill patients throughout history has seriously hampered attempts to protect their rights, meet their clinical needs, and advance their basic human wants.

Right to Refuse Treatment

The right to refuse treatment in many ways encompasses virtually all other rights of patients and raises fundamental questions as to the extent of control that can be exerted by a treater over a person who may not wish to participate in treatment. The issues raised by this right include the right to privacy, personal sovereignty, inviolability of one's thoughts, freedom from harm, freedom from cruel and unusual punishment, and the issue of the least restrictive alternatives to institutionalization (Perlin, 1979).

From the legal perspective, the right to refuse treatment arises from a composite of postulated constitutional sources including the constitutional right to freedom from harm and the constitutional right to privacy. While the courts and legislatures in recent years have been active in assuring patients the right to refuse such intervention as electroconvulsive therapy and psychosurgery, they have been slower to recognize the right to refuse psychotropic medication (Clayton).

Many individuals with mental illness wish to avoid psychotropic medication because of the potential side effects, which range from merely unpleasant (dry mouth, tiredness, blurry vision) to permanent and disfiguring (tardive dyskinesia, involuntary muscle movement). In addition, some mentally ill patients refuse medication not for the side effects but because the medication works well and therefore forces them to surrender the positive defensive adaptation of the psychotic state. Such adaptations may include an increased sense of importance and power, an ability to shut out problems that exist in the real world, and the support offered by hospitals and physicians (Appelbaum, 1988).

In various jurisdictions, including Massachusetts (*Rogers v. Okin*, 1979), New York (*Rivers v. Katz*, 1986), New Jersey (*Rennie v. Klein*, 1978), and the nation (*Washington v. Harper*, 1990), mental-health attorneys have sought to expand and clarify issues related to the right to refuse treatment, especially medication. Among the issues examined have been questions such as the right to protect all mental processes (thoughts, feelings, beliefs) from governmental interference; the right to protect autonomy over one's own body; the effectiveness of involuntary treatment versus voluntary treatment; and the questions of whether the potential benefits of drug treatment are worth the risks and who should be permitted to make this decision (Perlin, 1979).

The courts in the cases cited above sought to establish various procedures to protect patient autonomy and decision making in refusing antipsychotic medication. While these court decisions and subsequent legislative statutes have attempted to make the right to refuse treatment a legal and clinical reality, recent studies have revealed serious practical complications in applying these principles. One such study examined the assumption by the courts that patients' refusals of treatment are based on autonomous decision making. The study concluded that for most patients the decision to refuse psychotropic medication is a manifestation of their illness and does not reflect autonomous functioning or consistent beliefs about mental illness or its treatment (Schwartz et al.).

A study done by Paul Appelbaum noted that while refusal of treatment was not uncommon, ultimately most of the patients received treatment during their hospitalization (1988). Some clinicians have studied the cost of implementing court-mandated protection programs in the wake of the *Rogers* decision. On the basis of the studies' results, these clinicians have concluded that from the economic perspective, such programs are not cost-effective (Schouten and Gutheil). Furthermore, some authors have noted that the right to refuse treatment may infringe on the constitutionally based right to treatment for involuntarily committed mental patients (Blais). Thus the battle continues to be fought. On one side is concern for patients' autonomy and for protection from intrusive and potentially dangerous procedures. On the other side is concern for the clinical needs of patients and the necessity of interventions that can restore them to mental and physical freedom. The future evolution of this right will need to take into consideration not only legal and psychiatric perspectives but also the reality of the consequences of court intervention.

Right to the Least Restrictive Alternative to Hospitalization

A third important right that has received increasing judicial and psychiatric attention is the right to the least restrictive alternative to hospitalization. Many mental-health departments have seen deinstitutionalization as an effective way to reduce the cost of mental-healthcare; unfortunately, clinical services have not always followed patients to their communities.

The trend toward community-based services (least restrictive alternative to hospitalization) was initially heralded as the answer to improved quality and more responsive services. However, it has only partially addressed the need to protect mental patients' rights in the community. In place of the neglect by large institutions, many ex-patients now suffer from the despotic control of boardinghouse managers; in place of "voluntary work with token rewards," they now face long hours of inactivity; in place of even rudimentary treatment plans, they now receive larger doses of tranquilizers administered by untrained persons. These patients also face the continuing threat that unless they conform and follow the rules, they will be rehospitalized (Kopolow, 1979). While community-based services are less restrictive than institutional care, services are only as good as a community is willing to make them.

In the case of *Dixon v. Weinberger* (1974), Judge Aubrey Robinson ruled that patients in the District of Columbia have a statutory right to treatment in the least restrictive alternative to institutionalization. Responsibility was placed on the District of Columbia and the federal government to prepare a plan to identify and transfer patients to newly created community facilities. It is significant to note that twenty years later, the court's orders still have not been fully implemented. This case clearly shows the limitation of the courts in establishing rights when a community is resistant to, or incapable of, compliance. Another important judicial decision that has relevance to least restrictive treatment is *O'Connor v. Donaldson*. In this decision, the court acknowledged that states have a legitimate interest in providing care and assistance to patients, but it also declared that the patients' preferences should be recognized as well:

> The mere presence of mental illness does not disqualify a person from preferring his home to the comforts of an institution. Moreover, while the States may arguably confine a person to save him from harm, incarceration is rarely if ever a necessary condition for raising the standards of those capable of surviving safely in freedom. (*O'Connor v. Donaldson*, 1975, p. 575)

The court's movement toward a standard of ability to survive and the expectation that the least drastic means of treatment will have to be used put increased pressure on communities to develop an adequate range of services. To have such a range of services, however, requires commitment of resources that, as the *Dixon* case so clearly pointed out, may be slow in coming. The right to the least restrictive alternative will become meaningful only when communities invest adequate resources to develop such alternatives and provide mechanisms such as patient advocates to protect and advance patients' rights within the community or within an institution.

Advocacy

Advocacy has many meanings, depending on the interests and priorities of the various groups using it: mental-health professionals, consumers, attorneys, citizens' organizations. In its classic sense it means "to summon to one's assistance, defending, or calling to one's aid." The present-day connotation of conflict or antagonism is not inherent in the basic concept of advocacy, but results from the manner in which some advocates pursue their duties.

The mentally ill, as noted previously, suffer from prejudice and stigmatization that make it difficult for them to advocate their own causes. In addition to these factors, the complexity of the support and treatment programs and the need for change agents in what is essentially a conservative system make the need for advocates especially important. Advocacy, as related to patients' rights, is the responsibility of many individuals and professionals, including lawyers, psychiatrists, social workers, and concerned citizens. While it is obvious that it is the responsibility of the legal profession to advocate for legal rights of patients, the term also has other useful meanings within the mental-health service delivery system. After pure legal rights have been established and attorneys are available to patients to ensure their protection, other issues remain that cannot and should not be resolved through the legal system. Such issues, including staff attitudes, environmental conditions, and alternative treatment services, which influence the quality of the day-to-day life of mental patients, can be more effectively dealt with through administrative and legislative actions.

It is clear that no one approach or even one professional group can perform all the necessary tasks of mental-health advocacy. Advocacy functions can be divided into three broad categories:

1. Education and training of hospital staff regarding the nature of patients' rights and the best way to assure their protection.
2. Establishment of procedures to allow the speedy resolution of problems, questions, or disagreements that may or may not be legal rights. Such procedures would enable quick and efficient resolution outside the courtroom of legal and nonlegal rights issues.
3. While functions (1) and (2) can be properly handled by appropriate state agencies, a final category requires the use of independent outside lawyers and agencies: provision for independent and readily available legal support when it is necessary to litigate

for protection of patients' rights after internal procedures have failed.

A major controversy in advocacy is whether the predominant emphasis should be on internal or external rights-protection programs. An external advocacy program system would be implemented by individuals who are totally independent of the mental-health system. An internal advocacy program would be implemented by employees of the service system. Arguments for external programs relate to the concept that the advocate is ultimately loyal and responsible to the client. An advocate who is an employee of a department or agency of state government may have divided loyalty. An alternative perspective is that not all state employees are equally subject to that conflict—for example, someone working in an independent section or agency of the state government.

Internal rights-protection or advocacy programs, however, frequently tend to be highly efficient in solving complaints about daily living and in planning for future patients'-rights needs. They have easier access to patient records, can participate in program policy development, have a more collegial relationship with administrators that engenders trust and greater cooperation, and have the ability to identify problems to be corrected without outside pressures or publicity. Unfortunately, such programs suffer from the double danger of co-optation and replacement at the discretion of administrators.

An external advocacy program can use persuasion, and when persuasion fails, litigation is always a backup position. Such a program can bypass administrative changes for quick action; however, court cases may move slowly. Therefore, while external advocacy may have a limited range of action, it nonetheless can be powerful and decisive in producing change in a system now receptive to patients' rights protection. This analysis of internal and external advocacy programs clearly illustrates a patient's need for the availability of both programs. Such comprehensive advocacy programs can go far in assuring that patients'-rights concerns do not become mere rhetoric or window dressing, but are permitted to make substantive changes necessary to create a more responsible mental-health system.

Conclusion

In answering the question "What rights do mental patients have?" it is important to go beyond judicial decisions, administrative actions, or legislative statutes, and look at the status of the mentally ill in American society. The rights of mental patients have historically been disregarded and denied. The mentally ill were frequently viewed as incompetent to make decisions, and society's concern was to place them in institutions where they would cause neither themselves nor others harm and where they might receive treatment for their conditions.

The patients'-rights movement, made up of civil-rights attorneys, enlightened mental-health professionals, and former patients, has waged a struggle in courts, in legislatures, and in local communities to stop patient abuse, end stigmatization, increase needed community services, and empower patients to exert their full civil rights. Major patients'-rights litigation in the areas of right to treatment, right to refuse treatment, right to least restrictive alternatives, and right to liberty have led to increased recognition of the existence of these rights. But it is clear, when one examines the plight of the mentally ill down through history, that "something else" is needed if there is to be no recurrence of the cycle of abuse, exposé, improvement, neglect, and abuse again.

This "something else" that can safeguard patients' rights is the advocate. Mental patients already have extensive rights under the Constitution. The problem is not simply granting or recognizing rights but protecting them. Only through the continuing efforts of the advocates will the mentally ill truly have the rights enjoyed by other citizens. In the case of patients, as in the case of other citizens, "the price of freedom is eternal vigilance." The advocate provides the vigilance that helps assure that the legal rights, human wants, and clinical needs of the mentally ill are protected and promoted.

LOUIS E. KOPOLOW (1995)
BIBLIOGRAPHY REVISED

SEE ALSO: *Autonomy; Coercion; Competence; Informed Consent: Issues of Consent in Mental Healthcare; Institutionalization and Deinstitutionalization; Mental Health Services; Mental Illness: Conceptions of Mental Illness; Mental Institutions, Commitment to; Paternalism; Professional-Patient Relationship;* and other *Patients' Rights* subentries

BIBLIOGRAPHY

Appelbaum, Paul S. 1986. "The Rising Tide of Patients' Rights Advocacy." *Hospital and Community Psychiatry* 37(1): 9–10.

Appelbaum, Paul S. 1988. "The Right to Refuse Treatment with Antipsychotic Medications: Retrospect and Prospect." *American Journal of Psychiatry* 145(4): 413–419.

Appelbaum, Paul S. 1997. "Almost a Revolution: An International Perspective on the Law of Involuntary Commitment." *Journal of the American Academy of Psychiatry and the Law* 25(2): 135–147.

Beers, Clifford W. 1930. *A Mind That Found Itself: An Autobiography.* Garden City, NY: Doubleday.

Benn, Piers. 1999. "Freedom, Resentment, and the Psychopath." *Philosophy, Psychiatry, and Psychology* 6(1): 29–39.

Birnbaum, Morton. 1960. "The Right to Treatment." *American Bar Association Journal* 46(5): 499–505.

Blais, Norman N. 1975. "Forced Drug Medication of Involuntarily Committed Mental Patients." *Saint Louis University Law Journal* 20: 100–119.

Clayton, Ellen Wright. 1987. "From Rogers to Rivers: The Rights of the Mentally Ill to Refuse Medication." *American Journal of Law and Medicine* 13(1): 7–52.

Cournos, Francine; McKinnon, Karen; and Adams, Carole. 1988. "A Comparison of Clinical and Judicial Procedures for Reviewing Requests for Involuntary Medication in New York." *Hospital and Community Psychiatry* 39(8): 851–855.

Deutsch, Albert. 1948. *The Shame of the States.* New York: Harcourt, Brace.

Dixon v. Weinberger. No. 74285 (C.D.D.C. Feb. 14, 1974).

Failer, Judith Lynn. 2002. *Who Qualifies for Rights: Homelessness, Mental Illness, and Civil Commitment.* Ithaca, NY: Cornell University Press.

Falk, A. J. 1999. "Sex Offenders, Mental Illness and Criminal Responsibility: The Constitutional Boundaries of Civil Commitment after *Kansas v. Hendricks.*" *American Journal of Law and Medicine* 25(1): 117–147.

Fowlkes, E. Oliver. 1978. "Mental Patients Rights." In *Proceedings: Symposium on Safeguarding the Rights of Recipients of Mental Health Services.* Washington, D.C.: U. S. Government Printing Office.

Freddolino, Paul P., and Appelbaum, Paul S. 1984. "Rights Protection and Advocacy: The Need to Do More with Less." *Hospital and Community Psychiatry* 35(4): 319–320.

Freddolino, Paul P.; Moxley, David P.; and Fleishman, John A. 1989. "An Advocacy Model for People with Long-Term Psychiatric Disabilities." *Hospital and Community Psychiatry* 40(11): 1169–1174.

Goffman, Erving. 1961. *Asylums: Essays on the Social Situations of Mental Patients and Other Inmates.* Chicago: Aldine.

Gostin, Lawrence O. 2001. "Beyond Moral Claims: A Human Rights Approach in Mental Health." *Cambridge Quarterly of Healthcare Ethics* 10(3): 264–274.

Guimon, Jose, 2001. *Inequity and Madness: Psychosocial and Human Rights Issues.* New York: Kluwer Academic Publishers.

Harold, James, and Elliott, Carl. 1999. "Travelers, Mercenaries, and Psychopaths." *Philosophy, Psychiatry, and Psychology* 6(1): 45–48.

Kopolow, Louis E. 1976. "A Review of Major Implications of the *O'Connor v. Donaldson* Decision." *American Journal of Psychiatry* 133(4): 379–383.

Kopolow, Louis E. 1979. "The Challenge of Patients' Rights." *Advocacy Now* 1(1): 19–21.

Levy, Robert M., and Rubenstein, Leonard S. 1996. *The Rights of People with Mental Disabilities: The Authoritative ACLU Guide to the Rights of People with Mental Illness and Mental Retardation.* Carbondale, IL: Southern Illinois University Press.

Miller, Robert D.; Rachlin, Stephen; and Appelbaum, Paul S. 1987. "Patients' Rights: The Action Moves to State Courts." *Hospital and Community Psychiatry* 38(4): 343–344.

O'Connor v. Donaldson. 95 S.Ct. 2486. (1975).

Olsen, Douglas P. 1998. "Toward an Ethical Standard for Coerced Mental Health Treatment: Least Restrictive or Most Therapeutic?" *Journal of Clinical Ethics* 9(3): 235–246.

Perlin, Michael L. 1979. "The Right to Refuse Treatment: A New Right Emerges." *Advocacy Now* 1(1).

Perlin, Michael L. 1993. "Decoding Right to Refuse Treatment Law." *International Journal of Law & Psychiatry* 16(1–2): 151–177.

Rennie v. Klein. 653 F. 2d. 83 (3d Cir. 1981); vacated 458 U.S. 1119 (1982).

Rivers v. Katz. 67 N.Y. 2d. 485 N.E. 2d. 337, 504 N.Y.S. 2d. 74. (1986).

Rogers v. Okin. 478 F. Supp 1342. D.Mass. (1979).

Rothman, David J. 1971. *The Discovery of the Asylum: Social Order and Disorder in the New Republic.* Boston: Little, Brown.

Sadoff, Robert, and Kopolow, Louis E. 1977. "The Mental Health Professional's Role in Patient Advocacy." In *Mental Health Advocacy: An Emerging Force in Consumer Rights,* pp. 36–41, ed. Louis Kopolow and Helene Bloom. Washington, D.C.: U. S. Government Printing Office.

Saks, Elyn R. 2002. *Refusing Care: Forced Treatment and the Rights of the Mentally Ill.* Chicago: University of Chicago Press.

Schouten, Ronald, and Gutheil, Thomas G. 1990. "Aftermath of the Rogers Decision: Assessing the Costs." *American Journal of Psychiatry* 147(10): 1348–1352.

Schwartz, Harold I.; Vingiano, William; and Perez, Carol Bezirganian. 1988. "Autonomy and the Right to Refuse Treatment: Patients' Attitudes after Involuntary Medication." *Hospital and Community Psychiatry* 39(10): 1049–1054.

Solomon, Harry C. 1958. "Presidential Address: The American Psychiatric Association in Relation to American Psychiatry." *American Journal of Psychiatry* 115(1): 1–10.

Stefan, Susan. 2001. *Unequal Rights: Discrimination against People with Mental Disabilities and the Americans with Disabilities Act.* Washington, D.C.: American Psychological Association.

Stone, Alan A. 1975. *Mental Health and the Law: A System of Transition.* Washington, D.C.: U.S. Government Printing Office.

Stone v. Miller. 373 F. Supp. 177 (E.D.N.Y. 1974).

Szasz, Thomas S. 1961. *The Myth of Mental Illness: Foundations of a Theory of Personal Conduct.* New York: Hoeber-Harper.

Veatch, Robert M. 1981. *A Theory of Medical Ethics.* New York: Basic Books.

Ward, Mary Jane. 1946. *The Snake Pit.* New York: Random House.

Washington v. Harper. 494 U.S. 210 (1990).

Wyatt v. Stickney. 325 F. Supp. 781 (M.D. Ala. 1971).

Ziegenfuss, James T., Jr. 1986. "Conflict between Patients' Rights and Patients' Needs: An Organizational Systems Problem." *Hospital and Community Psychiatry* 37(11): 1086–1088.

PEDIATRICS, ADOLESCENTS

• • •

Adolescents, defined as young people between the ages of thirteen and eighteen, have much more autonomy and much more extensive rights to make their own choices about healthcare than their parents did when they were adolescents. Constitutional and other law on reproductive issues and the development of the rights of privacy and of confidentiality also affect adolescents' rights to seek or to refuse healthcare. Until the ratification in 1971 of the Twenty-Sixth Amendment to the U.S. Constitution, which gave eighteen-year-olds the right to vote in federal elections, a "minor" was anyone under the age of twenty-one. Almost all states then changed their laws to make eighteen the age of majority.

Consent to Medical Treatment

Under the common law of England, from which the American legal system evolved, children were, in effect, possessions of their fathers. Until 1772, a mother had no right to her eldest son's custody after his father's death if her husband had chosen to make a will, leaving the boy to another man. Because women could not own property, mothers had the right to custody only of their daughters and their noninheriting younger sons. Even into the twentieth century, fathers retained rights to control their children to the point of brutality. Before 1903 nowhere in the United States was child abuse a crime, because it interfered with the father's right to discipline his children in any way he saw fit. The reporting of child abuse was not mandated until the 1960s. In the context of medical care, the father's total authority was recognized by allowing him to sue a physician who had provided nonemergency medical treatment to a minor—even completely successful treatment—if the father's consent had not been obtained.

Beginning in the 1960s, however, epidemics of sexually transmitted infections (STIs) in adolescents were worsened because the teenagers would not seek medical care if their parents would find out they had been infected. Not only did they remain untreated, they spread the infections to sex partners. Physicians all over the country and the American Medical Association itself began to lobby state legislators to enact statutes permitting minors to receive treatment for STIs in confidence. By the end of the 1960s all states had such statutes and thereafter also added statutes permitting confidential treatment for drug or alcohol abuse problems.

At the same time, about half of the states also enacted general minor consent statutes. Although the ages vary from fourteen to sixteen, these statutes allow a minor who has attained that age to consent to general medical or surgical care, although since 1973 and the Supreme Court's decision in *Roe v. Wade,* many states have enacted exceptions to this consent related to abortion. Even in states that do not have general consent statutes, courts apply what is known as the "mature minor rule" and hold that a physician is not liable for failing to obtain parental consent to provide medical or surgical services to an adolescent as long as the adolescent is as capable of giving informed consent as an adult would have been.

Therefore, whether a particular minor can consent to a particular medical intervention depends not only on the age and maturity of the adolescent but also on the severity of the condition and the risks of the proposed treatment. Most physicians would be perfectly willing to treat an adolescent for an earache without involving parents, but most, if not all, would not consider treating the same teenager for leukemia without her parents' involvement.

These conflicts rarely involve illness sufficiently severe to require hospitalization, however, because minors are insured, if at all, as dependents in their parents' health insurance plans. A hospital will not permit a nonemergency admission unless the parent agrees to pay or to have their insurance do so. If the physician has not obtained parental consent to a nonemergency procedure, the parent does not have to pay the bill.

In an emergency, parental consent is not required, no matter how young the child, if the parent cannot immediately be found. If a four-year-old falls at preschool and is brought to the emergency department or to his physician's office, if his parents are called but cannot be located, and if the physician proceeds to suture the child's cut, parents cannot thereafter object. In fact, it might be regarded as malpractice to allow an injured child to be denied care because his parent could not be reached.

Parental consent is also not required if the minor is emancipated. Minors are emancipated if they are married or in the military, and in most (but not all) states they are considered emancipated if they do not live with their parents and are self-supporting. Most states also consider a teenage mother to be emancipated, and in some states a pregnant minor is emancipated.

Refusal of Medical Treatment

If an adolescent is able to consent to a particular medical intervention, she is equally able to refuse it even if her parents wish her to have it. These situations usually involve non-life-threatening illnesses.

In no state may a minor execute a legally binding living will (a directive that describes patient preferences in certain medical situations, such as the use of a respirator, to be invoked if the patient is not able to express his or her wishes at the time the decision must be made) or durable power of attorney (a directive that appoints a specific person as the patient's agent to make decisions on the patient's behalf when the patient cannot do so). This does not mean, however, that the young person's views should not be considered. When an adolescent, or even a younger child, has a terminal illness, and there is no realistic hope of improvement, even if parents want to try "one more thing," if the patient wants to change the goal to palliative care, the physician should support the patient's wishes. (Palliative care is that which seeks to alleviate symptoms produced by a life-threatening disease or its treatment and to maintain the patient' quality of life when the medical condition is not remediable.)

Where lifesaving treatment is likely to be successful, but the adolescent does not wish to have it, courts in most states will not allow the patient to refuse. Examples of this situation have involved adolescents who have expressed the desire to refuse blood transfusions for religious reasons. Although a few judges have determined that the teenager had realistically assessed the situation and could give an informed refusal (e.g., *In re E.G.* [1990]), most others, on essentially identical facts, have simply stated that minors may not refuse lifesaving treatment (e.g., *In re Application of Long Island Jewish Medical Center,* [1990], *Novak v. Cobb County-Kennestone Hospital Authority,* [1996]).

Parents, of course, may not refuse lifesaving therapies for their children on religious or other grounds. Furthermore, if a child dies when reasonable medical care more probably than not would have saved the child, the parents may be successfully prosecuted for manslaughter or even murder (*Commonwealth of Pennsylvania v. Nixon* [2000]).

The "refusal of treatment" may, of course, involve many issues other than legal ones. An adolescent can very easily be so uncooperative that treatment is, for all practical purposes, impossible and he may either threaten to or actually run away.

Confidentiality

If an adolescent is deemed by a physician to be capable of giving informed consent and the adolescent's parent is not involved, the patient is entitled to the same degree of confidentiality that an adult patient would have. If the physician does not involve a parent before the treatment is given, the patient will understandably assume that the care is confidential. If the physician then notifies a parent, the patient's trust in all medical personnel is likely to be destroyed. In some cases, particularly those involving sexual behavior, parents may reject and evict their child when they learn the information, and some of these young people have been driven to suicide (Remafedi, 1999).

In some situations, such as treatment for STIs or for alcohol or drug abuse problems, state statutes mandate confidentiality. Some, in fact, specifically forbid billing parents in these circumstances, lest the parent find out about the treatment from the bill.

The most difficult issue about intrafamily confidentiality in the care of adolescents today involves those who have HIV disease. Although in normal situations parents would be included in decision making when an adolescent has a very serious and perhaps fatal disease, AIDS is likely to engender parental reactions that may be adverse to the patient's medical care—the adolescent may be expelled from the family home and left to live on the streets or be subjected to emotional and physical abuse if remaining at home. While all authorities agree that the patient should be encouraged to include parents in decision making about the disease, there is increasing agreement that if the adolescent is able to consent to testing and counseling, she should be promised confidentiality. This assumes, of course, that medications can be provided free or at very low cost, because health insurance is usually in the parent's name and notice to parents would be given of payments to pharmacies.

AIDS clinics have ample evidence suggesting that adolescents will not come for testing, much less treatment, if they are not assured of confidentiality. Long-term follow-up studies indicate that teenagers whose parents do not know that they are HIV positive fare as well as those whose parents are involved (Kipke and Hein).

The reverse issue in confidentiality occurs when a parent knows the adolescent's diagnosis and does not wish the adolescent to know. The physician's duty is to the patient, not to the patient's parent, so the physician may disregard the parent's request if she deems it in the patient's best interest. In no case, even if the physician is willing to accede to the parent's request, may she lie to her patient, so questions must be answered truthfully even if this leads to the patient's discovery of the diagnosis.

Although this is usually a question of ethics, in some cases there may be legal consequences to the physician for failing to make sure the patient understands the implications of his disease, including the risk of transmission to others. For example, if an adolescent has HIV/AIDS, and the parent is in denial that the adolescent is sexually active, protection of others requires that the patient understands the disease, its ramifications for others, and how to prevent infection through safe-sex practices.

In situations where requests for information come from outsiders, the adolescent patient's rights to privacy and confidentiality are as extensive as those of an adult. A school principal without permission from a parent to obtain medical information about a student has no more right to that information than does the student's neighbor.

Contraception

Contrary to the belief that adolescents are more sexually active than they used to be, the American teenage childbearing rate was 96 per 1,000 girls aged fifteen to nineteen in the late 1950s but fell to 49 per 1,000 by 2000. American girls who are sexually active are much more likely to become pregnant than their European counterparts. The percentage who are sexually active is about the same, but the pregnancy rate is much higher—the U.S. rate is four times higher than Germany's, six times higher than France's, and eight times higher than that of the Netherlands. A study conducted in 2000 by Harold Leitenberg and Heidi Saltzman found that 77 percent of American females and 85 percent of males had had intercourse by age nineteen.

In the 1965 case *Griswold v. Connecticut,* the U.S. Supreme Court held that married couples have a right to privacy that encompasses their decisions about whether to have children. State laws that made dissemination of information about or prescription of birth control a crime were found to be unconstitutional. This right was expanded to unmarried adults in 1972 (*Eisenstat v. Baird*) and in 1977 to minors (*Carey v. Population Services*).

In 1970 Congress enacted Title X (Family Planning Services) of the Public Health Services Act. This established federally funded family planning services and required that they be provided without regard to religion, creed, age, marital status, or number of pre-existing pregnancies, regardless of outcome. In 1978 the act was amended specifically to include teenagers. Attempts during the administration of Ronald Reagan to require parental notification if a girl received services were held unconstitutional. By statute, in federally funded clinics, services are confidential. There is, however, no obligation on a physician in private practice or an institution that does not receive federal family planning funds to provide contraceptives to anyone of any age.

Many adolescents go directly to family planning clinics instead of their customary healthcare provider because they do not trust their physicians or nurse practitioners to keep their confidences. Thus if an unrelated illness arises where it may be important to know whether an adolescent is taking birth control pills, the physician whom she does not trust is most unlikely to get a truthful answer.

Sexual Abuse

If a very young adolescent (under age fourteen) seeks contraceptives, sexual abuse should be considered but not assumed. After all, asking for contraceptives in and of itself requires some degree of maturity. Many very young girls may well be involved in exploitive relationships with older men; this constitutes statutory rape as well as abuse. In most states the statutory rape statute provides an age differential beneath which the relationship is presumed consensual and above which it constitutes a crime. In most states the differential is five years, so if a fifteen-year-old girl is having a relationship with a nineteen-year-old boy, it is not a crime, but if he is twenty-five, it is. In the mid-1980s the California attorney general issued an order that all sexual activity by children under fourteen had to be reported as sex abuse, and reports were to be made by anyone who had knowledge that a child under fourteen had a sexually transmitted disease or had asked for birth control. In a 1986 case (*Planned Parenthood Affiliates of California v. Van de Kamp*), this order was struck down by the California Court of Appeals as invasive of the minor's rights of privacy.

Abortion

When the Supreme Court decided *Roe v. Wade* in January 1973, all the plaintiffs were adult women. Many state legislatures responded to the decision by enacting laws requiring consent to abortion by a married woman's husband and consent by a parent to a minor's abortion. The Supreme Court quickly declared unconstitutional any requirement of a husband's consent (*Planned Parenthood Association of Missouri v. Danforth*) but in subsequent decisions permitted states to restrict a minor's right to consent (*Planned Parenthood Association of Kansas City v. Ashcroft*. Since the Ashcroft case in 1983, a state may require parental consent as long as it also provides a "bypass" procedure whereby the young woman may apply to a judge to find her "sufficiently mature" to consent to the procedure. The judge's role is to determine the girl's maturity: The judge's personal opinion of abortion is supposed to be irrelevant. In

some states, almost no young women are found "too immature"; in others most girls, even those weeks from their eighteenth birthdays, are routinely turned down. In an article published in the *Minnesota Law Review* in 2001, Nicole A. Saharsky noted that of the twenty-three states allowing a juvenile to be sentenced to death when convicted of murder, eighteen are also among the most restrictive in limiting the decisions of young women of exactly the same age to have abortions on the grounds that they are too immature. (If there is no state statute, the young woman's right to consent to abortion is the same as her right to consent to any other medical procedure.)

Of course, if a young woman is "too immature" to make this decision, she is altogether likely to be too immature to care for the baby she will have in a few months. It should be remembered that an adolescent mother, no matter how young, has the authority to surrender her baby for adoption, even if her parents strenuously object. Her parents, conversely, have never been given the right to surrender the infant for adoption over her objections. A teenage mother, no matter how young, has the same responsibilities and decision-making authority for her baby as she would if she were thirty. With the exception of a very few states, the teenage mother's parents have no duty to provide for her baby and in some states, because she is emancipated by childbirth, they may refuse further support for her as well, and evict her and the baby from the household (*A.N. v. S.M., Sr.* [2000]).

Since 1998 there have been several cases in which a girl lied about her age to obtain an abortion, and her parents, upon discovering the situation later, sued the physician who performed it. All of the girls were sixteen or seventeen and claimed to be eighteen. In each case, the suit was unsuccessful, because the consent statutes do not impose a duty on abortion providers to verify the patient's age. The cases *Jackson v. A Woman's Choice* and *McGlothin v. Bristol Obstetrics* held that the girls were "mature minors."

If parents have the right to refuse to permit their daughter to have an abortion, do they have the right to require her to have one if they think she is too young to have a baby? Logically, if she is too immature to say yes, she is also too immature to say no. There are very few cases on the subject, but in all instances the courts held that a girl has the right to refuse. None of those cases, however, came from states with parental consent statutes. There is only one case that can be located in which a physician, without telling his minor patient that she was pregnant, performed an abortion at the behest of the patient's mother and lied to the girl about the procedure. Years later she found out the truth and sued the physician. In 1995 the Texas Supreme Court, in *Powers v. Floyd,* ruled that the physician had not violated the girl's rights. The court held that although the state law had changed by the time the girl discovered the truth, at the time of the abortion, the girl could not refuse abortion because she equally could not consent.

Mental Health Issues

Adolescence is a period during which many serious psychiatric disorders such as schizophrenia begin to surface. Parents, confronted with "normal" rebellious behavior by their teenager, may think he or she has suddenly become mentally ill.

CONSENT TO TREATMENT. The issue of the young person's right to seek mental health treatment is unlikely to involve private psychotherapy, because the parent can refuse to pay the bill and in most cases a young person cannot afford it. A more practical question involves an adolescent's right of access to a community mental-health facility, a drug treatment center, or a counseling center for troubled adolescents. Community mental-health centers are probably covered by the normal rules of minor consent that apply to other medical treatment, because those institutions, most of which receive federal funds, must be careful to comply with requirements of proper licenses and credentials for all staff.

In some cases, however, treatment may be offered by caregivers without formal medical credentials. In drug rehabilitation centers, for example, many of the personnel may be former drug addicts without formal mental health training. Although this may be a viable method of treating addiction, it complicates the issue of the legal right of the adolescent to seek care. All statutes granting adolescents specific authority to consent to medical treatment, and all cases in which these issues have been decided, have dealt with the rights of young people to receive treatment from physicians, nurses, and other healthcare providers who fall within the boundaries of "mainstream medicine." Minor treatment statutes quite specifically refer to treatment given by physicians. Although there are no cases on the point, it is unlikely that courts would extend these rights of consent to encompass an unemancipated minor's right to seek treatment from a chiropractor; it is even more unlikely that a court would hold that an adolescent's right to consent to care would apply to situations in which the minor would choose to consult an alternative healer such as a naturopath. Parents in many cases have been found guilty of child neglect if they refused treatment from physicians and took their children to alternative healers, so it is most improbable that young people have the right to go to the same practitioners on their own. Drug rehabilitation clinics not directed by physicians and nurses and places where therapy is provided

by persons outside the credentialed healthcare system undoubtedly would be held to fall into the same category.

REFUSAL OF TREATMENT. Many forms of behavior that may seem perfectly rational to an adolescent can be interpreted by a parent to be sufficiently abnormal to warrant psychiatric intervention, at least on an outpatient basis. By definition, this discussion involves those minors who would generally be considered "normal neurotics" in adult psychiatry. Such adolescents are functional and are not engaging in criminal or dangerous antisocial behavior. They have not engaged in definitive delinquent behavior and are not dangerous to themselves or others. They may be defiant at home, missing school for a few days but not becoming dropouts, refusing to dress as their parents think appropriate, or engaging in equally distressing but non-dangerous activities.

As discussed above, if minors have the right to consent to treatment, a court would probably hold that they have the right to refuse it. More to the point, however, as a fact of psychiatric practice, although it might be possible to subdue a teenager physically in order to remove his or her appendix, it is absolutely impossible to carry out any form of effective psychotherapy on an unwilling patient. The patient will simply refuse to discuss anything. At least one court has held that a school system violates the minor's right of privacy if it sets up a system of routine psychological evaluations in the absence of any behavior that indicates serious emotional disturbance that may require treatment.

CONFIDENTIALITY AND PSYCHIATRIC TREATMENT. What is the psychiatrist's obligation of confidentiality to the adolescent patient? When confidentiality issues arise because schools or other outside entities such as insurance companies or employers want information, the minor's confidentiality protection is as extensive as that of an adult patient. The conflicts arise when the patient's parent is the party who wants the information.

Because young children are almost never treated except in the context of family therapy, this problem rarely, if ever, arises, but it does arise often with adolescents. The parent–child relationship may be genuinely adversarial, the parent may be terrified that the adolescent will disclose family secrets or tell the mental health professional about abuse, or the parent may just want to know whether, for example, her daughter is sexually active. Increasingly, as well, when parents are divorced and a child is in therapy, there are attempts to "get" the other parent or to attempt to change custody based on what the adolescent has told the psychiatrist.

Several cases from the 1990s and early 2000s (including *Abrams v. Jones* [2000] and *In re Daniel C. H. v. Daniel O. H.* [1990]) have held that a parent does not have the right to access his child's psychiatric records over the objection of either the adolescent patient or the mental health professional who believes that such disclosures are not in the patient's best interests.

INPATIENT TREATMENT. There are two distinct standards for commitment of adult patients to psychiatric institutions. Involuntary commitment of adults is reserved for those persons who are "dangerous to themselves or others" or are considered "gravely mentally disabled." For the latter, the legal definition covers patients who, as the result of mental illness, cannot provide the necessities of life—food, clothing, shelter, and medical care—for themselves. Voluntary commitment occurs when the patient and the patient's physician agree that treatment would be beneficial.

Minors of any age fall into an altogether different category. By statute many states allow "voluntary" commitment of children by their parents. Minors who are committed as "voluntary" patients at their parents' behest have fewer legal protections than adult patients do. Adult voluntary patients in a psychiatric hospital can leave at will unless, after arrival at the hospital, they are deemed to fall within one of the categories applied to involuntary patients ("dangerous" or "disabled"), at which point a judge must hold a hearing and the patient must be civilly committed or allowed to leave. Involuntary patients, on the other hand, have a right to a judicial hearing at the time of admission to the hospital and the right to release when they are no longer dangerous to themselves or others. Most states, however, stipulate that minors may not leave a psychiatric hospital without the approval of their parents. If parents choose not to have their child released, the patient cannot legally leave the hospital. Thus, on a standard of reasonable due process of law, hospitalized minors are in a far more restricted legal position than adults.

The case law indicates that there are many situations in which abusive parents have sought to incarcerate their children in psychiatric hospitals for reasons having nothing to do with the children's condition. In the 1960s, for example, some male adolescents were confined to hospitals for months or years because they refused to cut their hair. In many cases, it has become clear that adolescents have been committed to psychiatric hospitals without any serious attempt by admitting psychiatrists to discover whether the young people are really mentally ill.

If a child or adolescent has conflicts with a parent, society apparently concludes that the young person, not the parent, is the one with the problem. This is not necessarily true. In particular, as many judicial decisions have indicated, a parent cannot be assumed to have the best interests of a child at heart when commitment proceedings are undertaken.

In the early 1970s, several cases held that children do have certain minimal rights of due process before being committed to a psychiatric institution, and a right to be released from a hospital or an institution for the mentally handicapped on constitutional grounds if they have been denied a fair hearing and representation by counsel. As a result of these decisions, many states enacted statutes stipulating that younger children (under the age of thirteen or fourteen) could be admitted "voluntarily" to psychiatric hospitals by their parents, but minors over the statutory age had a right to a hearing, counsel, and due process, either at the minor's request or automatically. Where those statutes exist, the rights conferred by them are enforceable in the state courts under state constitutional rights of due process.

In 1979, however, the U.S. Supreme Court in *Parham v. J. R.* held that if a state legislature did not choose to enact such a statute, a minor's federal constitutional rights were not violated by "voluntary" admission to a mental hospital by a parent, even if the minor was not free to leave the institution thereafter. The court held that to protect minors from abuses of parental authority, the decision to admit had to be reviewed by a "neutral fact finder," but the fact finder could be a staff physician, "so long as he or she is free to evaluate independently the child's mental and emotional condition and need for treatment." After that decision, no more states enacted due process statutes for minor mental patients. In those states that have not enacted statutes providing for judicial intervention in a minor's commitment, the young person has no right to be evaluated by an independent psychiatrist or to consult a lawyer and may even be denied the right to contact a grandparent or other relative for help.

As press reports in 1991 indicated, some profit-making psychiatric hospitals admitted any adolescent patient whose parents sought his or her admission. Some of these hospitals paid bounties to high school guidance counselors to persuade parents that their children needed hospitalization and then, after the unsuspecting parents admitted them, refused to release the patients for weeks or months. The possibility of abuse of this population is a very serious one, because once hospitalized, the patients can be totally isolated from outside contact. State legislators and judges have been unwilling to deal with the problems of bad-faith actions by either parents or physicians.

An increasingly important problem today involves the rights of young people whose parents have had them admitted to an alcohol or drug treatment facility. The courts in at least two states have held that because these institutions do not claim to be "mental (psychiatric) hospitals," any rights to judicial intervention the minor may have under state law if admitted to a psychiatric hospital do not apply, and that the courts will not question the parent's right to admit the adolescent, even in the absence of an institutional definition of "addiction" to which the adolescent presumably conforms (*R. J. D. v. The Vaughn Clinic* [1990], *Department of Health and Rehabilitative Services v. Straight* [1986]). Thus a minor unjustly confined in a psychiatric hospital or addiction facility may have no recourse to, or even a right to contact, outside help of any sort. By contrast, if the parent wishes to turn for help to the juvenile court system and have the child declared "unmanageable" for precisely the same behavior, the child has a presumption of innocence, the right to counsel, and the right to a full hearing.

Participation in Research

In 1974 Congress passed the National Research Act, establishing the National Commission for the Protection of Human Subjects of Biomedical and Behavioral Research. Congress mandated that the commission study the problems of biomedical research and report to the Secretary of Health, Education, and Welfare (now the Secretary of Health and Human Services) on what ethical principles should be applied in research funded by or performed under the direction of the federal government. The Commission was also specifically mandated to consider the ethical and regulatory issues involved in research on a variety of "special populations" deemed particularly vulnerable, including children. The Commission issued significant studies and regulatory recommendations on each of the groups. Most of the recommendations are now federal regulations.

In general, research on minors is permissible if it involves no greater than minimal risk (defined as "the probability and magnitude of physical or psychological harm that is normally encountered in the daily lives, or in the routine medical or psychological examination, of healthy children"); or, when greater risk is involved, if there is likely to be a direct benefit to the young person. Parental permission is required for research on most preadolescent children. The Commission's recommendations and the final regulations permit adolescents to participate in some research projects without parental consent. If the local institutional review board (IRB) determines that a research protocol is designed for a subject population for which parental or guardian permission is not a reasonable requirement, the researcher may include adolescents as subjects without parental involvement. Any waiver of parental permission must be accompanied by the IRB's acceptance of a substitute mechanism for the protection of adolescent subjects or a finding that they are not being placed at any risk. The

discretion afforded to the IRB by the regulations for protecting the rights and welfare of the human subjects of all ages in the institution of which it is a part make it extremely unlikely that research that could endanger an adolescent would ever be approved. It is most improbable that any IRB would waive parental permission for adolescent participation in any project that included a serious risk of even minimal harm.

The three following types of research normally involve adolescents who participate without parental consent:

1. Research in which adolescence is relevant. For example, a researcher might wish to question pregnant teenagers coming to a prenatal clinic about their knowledge of contraception at the time they became pregnant.
2. Research in which adolescence is irrelevant. For example, a researcher might wish to draw small amounts of blood from volunteers, and a sixteen-year-old, seeing the poster, volunteers.
3. Research that involves an attempt to recruit subjects from all age groups. For example, an epidemiologist might wish to do a community survey about knowledge of HIV infection, and some of the people she approaches in the local shopping mall are adolescents.

It is likely that an IRB would approve these studies as suitable for adolescent consent without parental involvement. There is a fourth type of research, however, that normally requires parental involvement:

(4) Research that is not related to the patient's age but that involves investigational therapy. If an adolescent patient has a disease for which the patient's physician-researcher wishes to administer such therapy, parental permission would almost certainly be sought. Investigational therapies that involve risk (and most do, at least to the same degree that comparable standard treatment does) are reserved for the treatment of serious illness.

It is most unlikely that a physician would be caring for an adolescent ill with the sort of serious condition on which this type of research is done without involvement of parents. It is most unlikely that an IRB would approve this even if the investigator wished to deal with the adolescent patient alone.

Research in schools involving "normal educational practices" is usually exempt from requirements of either IRB review or parental permission. This type of research might, for example, compare two methods of teaching multiplication and has been held to carry no risk of harm. Before passage of the Family Educational Rights and Privacy Act

(FERPA) in 1992 and the Protection of of Pupil Rights Amendment (PPRA) of 2002, school-based surveys of children or psychological research involving children were also considered to be of no risk as long as the children were not individually identifiable. Under the 2002 Protection of Pupil Rights Amendment; however, parents may inspect instructional materials to be used in any surveys or evaluations sponsored or funded by the U.S. Department of Education. Schools also are required to adopt policies in conjunction with parents about surveys sponsored by other entities. Under the amendment and regulations to carry it out (as published by the Department of Education), written parental consent is now mandatory before minor students are required to participate in any federally supported in-class survey that would reveal information concerning:

1. political affiliation;
2. mental and psychological problems potentially embarrassing to the student or the student's family;
3. sex behavior and attitudes;
4. illegal, antisocial, self-incriminating, and demeaning behavior;
5. critical appraisals of other individuals with whom respondents have close family relationships;
6. legally recognized privileged or analogous relationships such as those of lawyers, physicians, and ministers; or
7. income.

If a student may refuse to participate, parental consent is apparently not required. If any research is funded by or is to be submitted to any agency of the federal government or if the institution in which the research is being conducted has agreed to evaluate all research (regardless of funding source) by federal standards, the participants must be advised that they may refuse to participate without penalty or loss of benefits.

Although the National Commission's recommendations included a provision that even small children should have the right to refuse to participate in any studies from which they will not derive benefit, the final regulations on research on children did not include this provision. By the time adolescents can make a decision to participate in research, they can certainly can make a decision to refuse.

ANGELA RODDEY HOLDER (1995)
REVISED BY AUTHOR

SEE ALSO: *Abortion: Contemporary Ethical and Legal Aspects; Autonomy; Care; Children; Coercion; Competence; Confidentiality; Family and Family Medicine; Infanticide; Informed Consent; Paternalism; Pediatrics, Overview of Ethical Issues in; Sexual Behavior, Social Control of; Students as Research Subjects*

BIBLIOGRAPHY

Abrams v. Jones.. 43 Tex. Sup. Ct. J. 1064, 35 SW.3d 620 (2000).

American Academy of Pediatrics. Committee on Adolescence. 1999. "Contraception and Adolescents." *Pediatrics* 104: 1161–1166.

American Academy of Pediatrics. Committee on Pediatric AIDS. 1999. "Disclosure of Illness Status to Children and Adolescents with HIV Infection." *Pediatrics* 103: 164–166.

American Academy of Pediatrics. Committee on Pediatric AIDS and Committee on Adolescence. 2001. "Adolescents and Human Immunodeficiency Virus Infection: The Role of the Pediatrician in Prevention and Intervention." *Pediatrics* 107: 188–190.

American College of Physicians. 1989. "Health Care Needs of the Adolescent." *Annals of Internal Medicine* 110: 930–935.

American Medical Association. Council on Scientific Affairs. 1993. "Confidential Health Services for Adolescents." *Journal of the American Medical Association* 269: 1420–1424.

A. N. v. S. M., Sr. 333 NJ Super. 566, 756A.2d 625 (2000).

Application of Long Island Jewish Medical Center, In re. 147 Misc.2d 724, 557 NYS 2d 239. (1990).

Bellotti v. Baird. 443 U.S. 622 (1979).

Bertuglia, Jessica. 2001. "Preserving the Right to Choose: A Minor's Right to Confidential Reproductive Health Care." *Women's Rights Law Reporter* 23: 63.

Carey v. Population Services International. 431 U.S. 678 (1977).

Commonwealth of Pennsylvania v. Nixon. 761 A.2d 1151. Pa (2000).

Daniel C. H. v. Daniel O. H., In re 220 Cal. App. 3d 814, 269 Cal. Rptr. 624 (1990).

Davis, A. J. 2001. "Adolescent Contraception and the Clinician: An Emphasis on Counseling and Communication." *Clinical Obstetrics & Gynecology* 44: 114–121.

Department of Health and Rehabilitative Services v. Straight. 497 So 2d 692. Fla App (1986).

Doig, Christopher, and Burgess, Ellen. 2000. "Withholding Life-Sustaining Treatment: Are Adolescents Competent to Make These Decisions?" *Canadian Medical Association Journal—Journal de l'Association Médicale Canadienne* 162: 1585–1588.

Driggs, Ann Eileen. 2001. "The Minor Doctrine: Do Adolescents Have a Right to Die?" *Health Matrix* 11: 687.

E.G., In re. 133 Ill. 2d 98, 549 NE. 2d 322. (1990).

Eisenstadt v. Baird. 405 U.S. 438 (1972).

English, Abigail. 1990. "Treating Adolescents: Legal and Ethical Considerations." *Medical Clinics of North America* 74: 1097–1112.

English, Abigail. 2000. "Reproductive Health Services for Adolescents: Critical Legal Issues." *Obstetrics and Gynecology clinics of North America* 27: 195–211.

English, Abigail, and Morreale, Madlyn. 2001. "A Legal and Policy Framework for Adolescent Health Care: Past, Present, and Future." *Houston Journal of Health Law & Policy* 1: 63.

Ginsberg, Karyn, and Slap, Gail. 1995. "Adolescents' Perceptions of Factors Affecting Their Decisions to Seek Health Care." *Journal of the American Medical Association* 273: 1913–1918.

Griswold v. Connecticut. 381 U.S. 479 (1965).

Hartman, Rhonda G. 2001. "Adolescent Decisional Autonomy for Medical Care: Physician Perception and Practices." *University of Chicago Law School Roundtable* 8: 87.

Hawkins, Lisa Ann. 1992. "Living Will Statutes: A Minor Oversight." *University of Virginia Law Review* 78: 1581.

Holder, Angela R. 1985. "Minors' Rights to Consent to Medical Care." *Journal of the American Medical Association* 257: 3400–3402.

Jackson v. A Woman's Choice. 503 SE.2d 422, 130 NC App. 590 (1998).

Jackson, Shelley, and Hafemeister, Thomas L. 2001. "Impact of Parental Consent and Notification Policies on the Decisions of Adolescents to be Tested for HIV." *Journal of Adolescent Health* 29: 81–93.

Jacobstein, C. R., and Baren, J. M.. 1999. "Emergency Department Treatment of Minors." *Emergency Medical Clinics of North America* 17: 341–352.

Katerberg, Robert J. 1998. "Institutional Review Board, Research on Children, and Informed Consent of Parents: Walking the Tightrope between Encouraging Vital Experimentation and Protecting Children's Rights." *Journal of College and University Law* 24: 545.

Kipke, Michelle, and Hein, Karen. 1990. "Acquired Immunodeficiency Syndrome in Adolescents." *Adolescent Medicine: State of the Art Reviews* 1(3): 429–449.

Kun, Joan Margaret. 1996. "Rejecting the Adage 'Children Should Be Seen and Not Heard': The Mature Minor Doctrine." *Pace Law Review* 16: 423.

Lantos, John, and Miles, Steven. 1989. "Autonomy in Adolescent Medicine: A Framework for Decisions about Life-saving Treatment." *Journal of Adolescent Health Care* 10: 460–466.

Leiken, Sanford. 1993. "The Role of Adolescents in Decisions concerning Their Cancer Therapy." *Cancer* 71: 3342–3346.

Leitenberg, Harold, and Saltzman, Heidi. 2000. "A Statewide Survey of Age at First Intercourse for Adolescent Females and Age of Male Partners." *Archives of Sexual Behavior* 29: 203–215.

McGlothin v. Bristol Obstetrics. WL 65459. Tenn. App. (1998).

Novak v. Cobb County–Kennestone Hospital Authority. 74 F.3d 1173 (11th Cir. 1996).

Parham v. J.R. 442 U.S. 584 (1979).

Planned Parenthood Affiliates of California v. Van de Kamp. 181 Cal. App. 3d 245, 226 Cal. Rptr. 361 (1986).

Planned Parenthood Association of Kansas City v. Ashcroft. 462 U.S. 476 (1983).

Planned Parenthood Association of Missouri v. Danforth. 428 U.S. 52 (1976).

Powers v. Floyd. 904 SW.2d 713. Tex. App. (1995).

Protection of Pupil Rights Amendment. U.S. Code. Vol. 20, sec. 1232h34 CFR Part 98. (1978).

Public Health Service Act. U.S. Code. Vol. 42, secs. 300–300a(8). (1970 as amended 1988).

Remafedi, Gary. 1987. "Male Homosexuality: The Adolescent's Perspective." *Pediatrics* 79: 326–330.

Remafedi, Gary. 1999. "Sexual Orientation and Youth Suicide." *Journal of the American Medical Association* 282: 1291–1292.

Roe v. Wade. 410 U.S. 113 (1973).

R. J. D. v. Vaughn. 572 So 2d 1225. Ala (1990).

Saharsky, Nicole A. 2001. "Consistency as a Constitutional Value: A Comparative Look at Age in Abortion and Death Penalty Jurisdictions." *Minnesota Law Review* 85: 119.

Silverstein, Helena. 2002. "Inconceivable?" *Law and Inequality* 20: 141.

Society for Adolescent Medicine. 1997. "Confidential Health Care for Adolescents: Position Paper of the Society for Adolescent Medicine." *Journal of Adolescent Health* 21: 408–415.

Traugott, Isabel, and Alpers, Ann. 1997. "In Their Own Hands: Adolescents' Refusal of Medical Treatment." *Archives of Pediatrics & Adolescent Medicine* 51: 922–927.

PEDIATRICS, INTENSIVE CARE IN

• • •

While sickness and death are an inevitable part of the human condition, they are never expected in childhood. Even though the number of pediatric intensive care unit (ICU) beds is only a small fraction of the number of adult ICU beds, the practice of pediatric intensive care medicine raises a disproportionate number of complex and unresolved ethical issues, including those related to decision making for critically ill children as well as issues related to end-of-life care in this setting.

Informed Consent

Children in the intensive care unit often have diminished capacity to participate in decision making, either on the basis of their age, their illness, or a combination of both. Although these children are noncompetent in terms of their capacity to give informed consent, they differ from noncompetent adults in several important ways. For example, most of the important legal cases involving noncompetent adults have concerned patients who were never expected to regain competency, that is, adults with chronic and usually progressive medical problems. Children are different, because in most cases their competency and decision making-capacity is expected to recover and grow. Therefore, with adults the emphasis is on respecting their *former* autonomy; with children the challenge is to faithfully preserve options for their *future* autonomy.

CHILDREN NOT ABLE TO PARTICIPATE IN DECISION MAKING. Children in the intensive care unit are often very ill, and many require high levels of analgesia and sedation to tolerate life-sustaining treatments such as mechanical ventilation. In addition, from the newborn period through early childhood, even healthy children are not able to participate in decisions about their medical care. For all these patients, parents are generally viewed as their surrogate decision makers. Up until the nineteenth century or so, children were seen essentially as the "property" of their parents, and parents were seen as having a "right" to make these medical decisions. Although this is no longer the case, the presumption in favor of parental decision making is based upon several persuasive considerations:

1. Parents have strong emotional bonds to their children and are powerfully motivated to make decisions that are in the best interests of their children;

2. An assumption is made that children will grow up to espouse many of the same values as their parents, therefore parental decisions are more likely to resemble the kinds of decisions that children will make when they become competent;

3. Parents will usually have to shoulder and live with the consequences of the decisions that are made on behalf of their children (including financial obligations), so they should have some say in making those decisions; and

4. Parents are held responsible for most of the nonmedical decisions that need to be made on behalf of the child (housing, food, schooling, etc.), so they should have responsibility for the medical decisions as well.

An interesting and largely unresolved question is how to balance the interests of the child against the interests of the family as a whole when these are in conflict. Consider, for example, a child who has sustained severe brain injury following an accident, and the family is given the option of either withdrawing life support and allowing the child to die or continuing with treatment that will likely lead to survival of the child with severe disabilities. Is it legitimate for the parents to factor the interests of the family as a whole into their decision, and to consider the impact (psychological, financial, spiritual, etc.) that raising a severely disabled child will have on other members of the family? The traditional view has been that only the best interests of the child should be considered. Yet families with children are profoundly interdependent, and parents often have responsibility for fairly balancing the interests of one family member against another, such as in the way that financial resources are distributed for various needs, projects, and interests. Because parents are rarely required to fully account for the reasons behind their decisions about life-sustaining treatments, it is likely that these potential conflicts are operative but remain unarticulated and unexplored in many of these situations.

CHILDREN ABLE TO "ASSENT" TO MEDICAL TREATMENT. The concept of "assent" to treatment for pediatric patients was first proposed by the National Commission for the Protection of Human Subjects of Biomedical and Behavioral Research in the 1970s. Based upon knowledge of normal childhood development, this commission proposed that children between the ages of seven and fourteen should be asked for their assent to medical treatment. Above the age of fourteen, they suggested, children should generally be presumed to have full decision-making capacity. In an article published in 1998 in the *American Journal of Law and Medicine,* Leonard H. Glantz observed that this "rule of sevens" has also appeared in legal decisions, with the view that below the age of seven a child is irrebuttably decisionally incapacitated, from seven to fourteen years there is a rebuttable presumption of decisional incapacity, and for those between fourteen years and the age of majority there is a rebuttable presumption of decisional capacity.

The American Academy of Pediatrics (AAP) extended this concept in 1995, claiming that the entire "doctrine of 'informed consent' has only limited *direct* application in pediatrics. Only **patients** who have appropriate decisional capacity and legal empowerment can give their **informed consent** to medical care. In all other situations, parents or their surrogates provide **informed permission** for diagnosis and treatment of children with the **assent** of the child whenever appropriate" (bold and italics in original) (Kohrman et al., p. 314).

In its definition of the term, the AAP said that "assent" should include at least the following elements:

1. Helping the patient achieve a developmentally appropriate awareness of the nature of his or her condition;

2. Telling the patient what he or she can expect with tests and treatment(s);

3. Making a clinical assessment of the patient's understanding of the situation and the factors influencing how he or she is responding (including whether there is inappropriate pressure to accept testing or therapy);

4. Soliciting an expression of the patient's willingness to accept the proposed care. (Kohrman et al., p. 315)

Regarding this final point, the AAP added: "no one should solicit a patient's views without intending to weigh them seriously. In situations in which the patient will have to receive medical care despite his or her objection, the patient should be told that fact and should not be deceived" (Kohrman et al., p. 316).

"EMANCIPATED" AND "MATURE" MINORS. Two legal categories that give special status to patients under the age of majority also need to be mentioned (Holder). Emancipated minors fall into a legal category that grants certain individuals under the age of majority all of the rights of an adult to consent to medical care. State laws vary, but most states specify by statute the conditions under which a minor is considered emancipated. Generally, minors are emancipated when they are married, are parents, or are on active duty in the armed forces. In some jurisdictions minors are emancipated when they are above a certain age (e.g., sixteen years), are not financially supported by their parents, and are either not subject to parental control or their parents have consented to their emancipation (note that runaways would therefore not generally be considered emancipated).

Many states have either statutory or case law for the treatment of "mature minors." Mature minors are not emancipated, but they may nevertheless have the legal power to consent to some forms of medical treatment. Although the mature minor concept provides legal protection to physicians who treat adolescents, the patient's parents are not financially responsible for treatment rendered without their consent.

Conflicts among Clinicians, Patients, and Patients' Parents

Just as adolescents may have the capacity to participate in their decision making, they are also well known to have the capacity for (what most adults regard as) irrational behavior. Billy Best, for example, was a sixteen-year-old patient diagnosed with Hodgkin's disease in 1994. He and his parents were told he had an 80 to 90 percent chance of cure with chemotherapy and low-dose radiation. Although he reportedly had only "minor" side effects from the chemotherapy (including hair loss, nausea, and fatigue), after several months he refused treatment and ran away from home. This situation was resolved only when his clinical team chose to honor his refusal of treatment while still monitoring him for evidence of cancer.

Clinicians and parents have not always refrained from imposing standard treatment, however. In New York in 1991, for example, a fifteen-year-old was diagnosed with an anterior mediastinal tumor. The patient's father had died of carcinoma of the lung four months earlier. Based largely upon his phobia of needles, the patient refused to undergo diagnostic surgery. His mother asked the court for an order directing the child to submit to surgery. The court found that surgery was urgently required and ordered the sheriff's department to take him to the hospital, restrain him if necessary, and supervise him while he was in the hospital.

These two cases illustrate the kinds of problems that arise in the gray area of late adolescence, when patients do not yet have the nearly unqualified rights of adults to refuse medical therapy, yet parents no longer have the authority to mandate their children's treatment. The best recommendation that can be made is for clinicians to attempt to persuade adolescents regarding the optimal approach to their care. When these recommendations are refused, however, clinicians must decide whether this refusal is reasonable, all things considered, or whether it is in the patient's best interest to seek a court order imposing the standard therapy. When in doubt, the bias should be toward potentially life-prolonging treatment, because this is the path that is least likely to foreclose options for the patient as she matures into a fully functioning autonomous adult.

End-of-Life Care

Just as pediatric intensivists need to have coherent strategies and plans for managing patients with clinical syndromes such as acute respiratory or renal failure, so they need to have a systematic approach to caring for children who are dying. The most important components of this approach relate to the "mechanics" of withdrawing life support and to the provision of sedation and analgesia.

WITHDRAWAL OF LIFE-SUSTAINING TREATMENTS. Although pediatric ICUs have a much lower mortality rate than most adult ICUs, they are similar in that an increasing proportion of deaths follow the withdrawal of life-sustaining treatment. One survey of adult ICUs found that 90 percent of the deaths followed a decision to limit therapy (Prendergast and Luce). Similarly, a study of more than 100 consecutive deaths in three Boston pediatric ICUs found that about two-thirds of the deaths followed the withdrawal of life-sustaining treatment (Burns et al.). In the Boston study, the treatment withdrawn in all cases was mechanical ventilation, reflecting that the cause of death in children in the ICU is very often related to respiratory failure, in contrast to adults where the proximate causes of death are more diverse.

SEDATION AND ANALGESIA AT THE END OF LIFE. Current ethical and legal guidelines place importance upon the intentions of clinicians in administering analgesics and sedatives at the end of life. Specifically, clinicians should administer doses that are intended to relieve pain and suffering but that are not intended to directly cause death. Because intentions are essentially subjective and private, the only ways to infer the nature of an individual's intentions are by self-report and by an analysis of his or her actions. Accordingly, documentation of one's intentions in the patient's chart is an important part of providing end-of-life care. For example, when a clinician administers morphine in small doses every ten or twenty minutes, it is plausible to conclude that the clinician intends to make the patient comfortable and not to directly cause the patient's death. On the other hand, when a clinician administers a large dose of morphine to a patient who is not profoundly tolerant, it is difficult not to conclude that the clinician did in fact intend the death of the patient (Truog et al., 2001).

Although ethical and legal guidelines require that sedatives and analgesics be administered in doses based on the patient's comfort, they provide little advice about what to do when the clinician and the family disagree about whether or not the patient is comfortable. Consider a patient who is near death and having "agonal" respirations. The family may find these very distressing, despite reassurances from the clinicians that the patient is unconscious and not experiencing any pain or suffering. Should the physician administer additional opioid to the patient, with the intention of making the patient appear more peaceful for the benefit of the family? Although controversial, many pediatric intensivists would do so, on the ethical grounds that doing so may be of great benefit to the family members in terms of how they remember the child's death, while the potential for this action to harm the patient is small.

TERMINAL EXTUBATION VERSUS TERMINAL WEAN. A systematic approach to ventilator withdrawal at the end of life was first proposed in the early 1980s, with this approach involving a gradual reduction in the ventilator settings over several hours. Since then, there has been an ongoing debate regarding the best method of withdrawing mechanical ventilation.

One recommended approach, commonly referred to as "terminal extubation," involves the removal of the endotracheal tube, usually following the intravenous administration of sedatives and/or analgesics. The second technique, known as a "terminal wean," is performed by gradually reducing the amount of supplemental oxygen the patient is receiving and/or the rate at which the ventilator is providing breaths to the patient, leading to the progressive development of hypoxemia and hypercarbia. In the latter technique there is considerable variability in the pace of the process, with some completing the wean over several minutes and others stretching it over several days (Truog et al., 2001).

The preferred approach varies widely. A 1992 survey of critical-care physicians found that 33 percent preferred terminal weaning, 13 percent preferred extubation, and the remainder used both. These preferences were correlated with specialty: surgeons and anesthesiologists were more likely to use terminal weaning, whereas internists and pediatricians were more likely to use extubation (Faber-Langendoen).

The principle advantage of the terminal wean is that patients do not develop any signs of upper airway obstruction during the withdrawal of ventilation. They therefore do not develop distress from either stridor or oral secretions, and if the wean is performed slowly with the administration of sedatives and analgesics, they do not develop symptoms of acute air hunger. These advantages not only promote the comfort of the patient but also reduce the anxiety of the family and caregivers.

Another cited advantage of terminal weans is that they are perceived to diminish the moral burden of the family and caregivers, presumably because the terminal wean is perceived as being less "active" than terminal extubation. Whether this is an advantage or disadvantage remains controversial. There is a risk that terminal weans—particularly those in which the wean is prolonged over several days—may be perceived by families as bona fide attempts to have the patient successfully survive separation from the ventilator, even when this is not the expectation or intent of the clinicians. Terminal weans therefore should not be adopted as a means of avoiding difficult conversations with families about the patient's condition and prognosis.

In contrast to terminal weans, the principle advantages of terminal extubations are that they do not prolong the dying process and that they allow the patient to be free of an "unnatural" endotracheal tube. The process of terminal extubation also is morally transparent; the intentions of the clinicians are clear, and the process cannot be confused with a therapeutic wean.

Despite the tendency for clinicians to use only one of these approaches based upon their specialty training, the relative advantages and disadvantages of each suggest that both approaches have a role in end-of-life care, and that the technique used should be tailored to the needs of the patient, rather than just the preferences of the clinician.

PARALYTIC AGENTS. Neuromuscular blocking agents (NMBAs) are required occasionally for the management of critically ill patients, primarily to facilitate the use of nonphysiologic ventilatory modes such as high-frequency oscillation. When a decision is made to withdraw ventilator support from a patient who is paralyzed by these agents, there is a question as to whether the effects of the medication need to be reversed or allowed to wear off before the ventilator is withdrawn.

Neuromuscular blocking agents possess no sedative or analgesic activity and can provide no comfort to the patient when they are administered at the time of withdrawal of life support. Clinicians cannot plausibly maintain that their intention in administering these agents in these circumstances is to benefit the patient. Indeed, unless the patient is also treated with adequate sedation and analgesia, the NMBAs may mask the signs of acute air hunger associated with ventilator withdrawal, leaving the patient to endure the agony of suffocation in silence and isolation. While it is true that families may be distressed while observing a dying family member, the best way to relieve their suffering is by reassuring them of the patient's comfort through the use of adequate sedation and analgesia, rather than by simply paralyzing the patient (Truog et al., 2000).

PRACTICING PROCEDURES ON THE NEWLY DECEASED. Practicing procedures on newly deceased patients has been a source of controversy between physicians and society dating back at least to the Middle Ages. This is an especially relevant issue for pediatric critical-care medicine, where practitioners have an important obligation to practice and teach resuscitation procedures.

Some have argued that it is ethically justifiable to perform practice procedures on the newly dead without permission from the family because these procedures cannot harm the deceased, because there is a substantial societal benefit to be gained, and because families could not realistically be expected to discuss consent at such a difficult time (Orlowski, Kanoti, and Mehlman). Moreover, a study showed

that 39 percent of training programs in emergency and critical-care medicine use newly dead patients to teach various resuscitation procedures (for example, endotracheal intubation, central line placement, and pericardiocentesis). Few of these programs obtain either verbal or written consent from the families (Burns, Reardon, and Truog).

Despite the frequency of this practice without consent, some have argued that teaching procedures on newly deceased patients is ethical only when permission is first obtained from the family. Unquestionably, newly dead patients offer opportunities to practice resuscitation techniques that are difficult or impossible to learn in other ways without exposing living patients to additional risk. While seeking permission from family members to practice resuscitation procedures may generate additional stress at a time when the clinicians are most concerned with reducing it, they argue that this does not justify practicing without consent (Burns, Reardon, and Truog).

ROBERT D. TRUOG

SEE ALSO: *Adolescents; Autonomy; Beneficence; Children; Competence; Grief and Bereavement; Infants; Information Disclosure; Informed Consent; Life, Quality of; Life Sustaining Treatment and Euthanasia; Moral Status; Palliative Care and Hospice; Surrogate Decision Making*

BIBLIOGRAPHY

Burns, Jeffrey P.; Mitchell, Christine; Outwater, Kristen M.; et al. 2000. "End-of-Life Care in the Pediatric Intensive Care Unit after the Forgoing of Life-Sustaining Treatment." *Critical Care Medicine* 28: 3060–3066.

Burns, Jeffrey P.; Reardon, Frank E.; and Truog, Robert D. 1994. "Using Newly Deceased Patients to Teach Resuscitation Procedures." *New England Journal of Medicine* 331: 1652–1655.

Faber-Langendoen, Kathy. 1994. "The Clinical Management of Dying Patients Receiving Mechanical Ventilation: A Survey of Physician Practice." *Chest* 106: 880–888.

Glantz, Leonard H. 1998. "Research with Children." *American Journal of Law and Medicine* 24: 213–244.

Holder, Angela R. 1987. "Minors' Rights to Consent to Medical Care." *Journal of the American Medical Association* 257: 3400–3402.

Kohrman, Arthur; Clayton, Ellen Wright; Frader, Joel E.; et al. 1995. "Informed Consent, Parental Permission, and Assent in Pediatric Practice." *Pediatrics* 95: 314–317.

National Commission for the Protection of Human Subjects of Biomedical and Behavioral Research. 1977. *Research Involving Children: Report and Recommendations.* Washington, D.C.: U. S. Government Printing Office.

Orlowski, James P.; Kanoti, George A.; and Mehlman, Maxwell J. 1988. "The Ethics of Using Newly Dead Patients for Teaching and Practicing Intubation Techniques." *New England Journal of Medicine* 319: 439–441.

Prendergast, Thomas J., and Luce, John M. 1997. "Increasing Incidences of Withholding and Withdrawal of Life Support from the Critically Ill." *American Journal of Respiratory and Critical Care Medicine* 155: 15–20.

Truog, Robert D.; Cist, Alexandra F. M.; Brackett, Sharon E.; et al. 2001. "Recommendations for End-of-Life Care in the Intensive Care Unit: The Ethics Committee of the Society of Critical Care Medicine." *Critical Care Medicine* 29: 2332–2348.

Truog, Robert D.; Burns, Jeffrey P.; Mitchell, Christine; et al. 2000. "Pharmacologic Paralysis and Withdrawal of Mechanical Ventilation at the End of Life." *New England Journal of Medicine* 342: 508–511.

PEDIATRICS, OVERVIEW OF ETHICAL ISSUES IN

• • •

Pediatric ethics is a branch of bioethics that analyzes moral aspects of decisions made relating to the healthcare of children. Several matters distinguish pediatric from adult ethics, including issues of consent, confidentiality, genetic testing, end-of-life care, and justice.

Consent: Making Medical Decisions for Children

Decision making for children is a unique and challenging process. Adults generally make their own medical decisions through the process of informed consent, in which a competent adult capable of sufficient understanding is given adequate, clear information about the proposed intervention and granted the autonomy to make choices. Most children have not reached the developmental stage at which they can ethically or legally give informed consent. To further complicate matters, many parties may be involved in the decision-making process, including the patient, parents, family members, nurses, doctors, social workers, clergy, and the courts.

Beneficence is the foundation of decision making for children. This principle encourages identification of the child's best interest through a shared decision-making process involving the clinician, patient, and parents. Each member of this triad brings information that helps identify the child's best interest. The clinician provides a thorough understanding of the available medical evidence regarding the condition along with a repertoire of clinical knowledge and experience. The parents bring their intimate familiarity with the child and the family. As the child's primary caregivers, parents give informed consent by proxy (otherwise known as "informed permission") because they are usually best able to determine the child's best interest. Physicians have the responsibility to ensure that parental motivations are based on the child's needs rather than the parents' wishes. All of the tenets of informed consent apply to informed permission; however, the adult parents are the ones who ultimately make the decision instead of the child patient.

Children gradually develop the ability to understand a diagnosis and treatment plan as they approach adulthood. Hence, the older child's opinions deserve serious consideration and can be quite enlightening in the effort to identify the child's best interest. Although these older children may be legally unable to give informed consent, they may still express assent, which empowers them to the extent of their developmental abilities. Thus, the ideal decision-making scenario is a shared process: The physician provides information and recommendations, the parents give informed permission, and the patient gives assent to interventions in her best interest.

Confidentiality: Adolescent Issues

As part of the process of individuation, adolescents desire more privacy in their personal lives. At the same time, they are encountering increasingly complex and dangerous health issues. Not infrequently, issues of confidentiality arise within the physician/patient/parent triad, and management can be quite delicate in terms of the limits of confidentiality and the circumstances under which disclosure must occur. Although the specifics vary from state to state, the legal community gives adolescents who demonstrate some degree of maturity the discretion to make healthcare decisions for themselves and without the involvement of their parents regarding issues such as substance abuse, sexually transmitted diseases, pregnancy, contraception, and mental health. Variously known as emancipated minors, mature minors, or medically emancipated minors, some subgroups of adolescents are considered capable of providing informed consent for all forms of care by virtue of their life experiences, which may include financial independence, pregnancy, homelessness, or marriage. Because statutes governing adolescents vary, physicians should become familiar with the laws in their communities. In all cases, the primary duty of the physician is to optimize the adolescent's care by advocating for his best interest.

LIMITS OF CONFIDENTIALITY. All clinical interactions are by nature confidential. Because the adolescent is the patient, in most instances he or she must give permission to share information with parents or others. At the outset, the physician should establish an independent relationship with the adolescent, explaining to the patient and the parents both the breadth and the limits of confidentiality. In the event that the life of the patient or anyone else is in peril or the patient is being abused, the physician is mandated both ethically and legally to disclose this information to appropriate authorities. A critical role of the physician is to facilitate communication between the adolescent patient and the parents. Under most circumstances, the adolescent should be encouraged to involve the parents in her healthcare because they can ideally provide support on a continual basis. Conversely, the physician should also encourage the parents to embrace the adolescent's emerging sense of independence. Confidentiality in the physician–adolescent patient relationship must be a priority in the physician's effort to be a confidant and caregiver and to ultimately act in the patient's best interest.

Genetic Testing in Children

Genetic testing in children is generally more complex than other pediatric testing because the results have implications for other family members as well. Patients with certain genetic diagnoses, and their families, may suffer financial, psychological, or interpersonal prejudices that are not easily foreseeable. In spite of the awesome wealth of information the human genome can supply, both nature and nurture influence the health outcomes of any given person; and this form of testing runs the risk of assuming genetic determinism—exaggerating the genetic influences while devaluing the environmental ones. Deciding when to undertake a genetic evaluation in pediatrics can be a challenge. As with other medical decisions for children, physicians should use beneficence as their guide.

NEWBORN GENETIC SCREENING. Every state requires that newborns undergo screening to detect a number of metabolic and inherited conditions that can threaten the health of the child. The screening procedure reflects society's obligation to optimize health by detecting and treating particular infant or early childhood conditions. Theoretically, screening tests are carefully chosen to satisfy a number of criteria. Tests must be sensitive enough to identify cases among masses of screened newborns, specific enough to avoid the anxiety that comes from a multitude of falsely positive tests, and widely available. In addition, effective preventive or treatment interventions must be available that significantly alter the morbidity and mortality of the condition. Perhaps the most important criterion is that the test must provide a clear benefit for the child.

SCREENING CHILDREN FOR GENETIC DISEASES OF ADULTHOOD. Huntington's disease, breast cancer, and polycystic kidney disease are just a few of the exploding number of adult diseases for which genetic tests are available and can be performed in childhood or even in utero. Theoretically, identifying a predilection to such disease may lead to preemptive intervention to decrease the morbidity and mortality of the disease; but this supposition has not been confirmed in practice. Physicians faced with requests for this type of pediatric testing must proceed with great caution. The psychological and social impact of this information can be much greater than anticipated and may lead to discrimination by employers, insurers, and others. Performing these tests while remaining committed to the child's best interests can be troublesome. By definition, these tests detect diseases of adulthood; so if there is no intervention during childhood that can significantly alter the natural history of the disease, the testing may not be in the child's best interest. The testing may best be deferred until the child reaches adulthood and can make his own autonomous choice. Physicians faced with requests for genetic testing should keep all of these issues in mind when determining if testing is in the best interests of the child.

End-of-Life Issues

Caring for dying children is one of the most challenging responsibilities in pediatrics. The emotions engendered by anticipation of a child's death have a powerful impact on families and caregivers and may sometimes be an obstacle to the appropriate care of the child. Again, beneficence must guide any decisions at the end of life. Through a shared decision-making process, the clinician should obtain informed permission from the parents as well as patient assent, when possible, to optimize these interests. Careful, continual evaluation is critical so that when the burdens of treatment outweigh the benefits, the treatment plan can be appropriately modified.

WITHHOLDING AND WITHDRAWING SUPPORT. Clinicians and families often struggle at the point when they realize that neither the current interventions nor additional ones will alter the child's progression toward death. The inevitability of death then challenges the family and the healthcare team to change the goals from cure to palliation. Parents often fear that they would be taking an active role in hastening death by withholding or withdrawing support. Physicians must be prepared to help the family understand that palliation is not equivalent to giving up but instead part of the continuum of respect and consideration for the child. Parents and clinicians may feel that withholding support is somehow preferable to withdrawing support already in place. This distinction between not initiating an intervention and removal of an intervention is not ethically meaningful. Viewed in light of the changing goals of treatment and the child's best interest, either can be ethically sound.

Justice: The Example of Childhood Immunizations

The issue of immunizing infants and children highlights the role of justice in pediatric ethics. Parents frequently question the need for the immunizations recommended for their children. To address their concerns, the physician must know the risks and benefits of immunizations in order to identify the best interest of the child. Immunizations are generally intramuscular, painful injections; and the current immunization schedule recommends that the patient receive as many as four or five injections during one visit. Each vaccination has established side effects, and parents need to be aware of these. The list of available immunizations continues to change and grow and so do recent claims about vague associations between these vaccinations and diseases of unclear origin. Such claims have not been substantiated by careful medical research, yet the theories are still widely publicized and accessible.

Parents may be hesitant to immunize their children against diseases such as diphtheria and polio when the child's risk of contracting the disease is exceedingly low in the United States. Because of vaccine effectiveness, these diseases are currently uncommon. In past decades, however, these diseases affected thousands of American children and still overwhelm many in underprivileged societies. Countries such as Russia, whose established immunization programs have been compromised by political strife, are now experiencing epidemics of diseases that were previously under control. These events reinforce the idea that widespread vaccination confers immunity to the population as a whole and is likely the reason for the low prevalence of these devastating diseases in the United States. Nonetheless, humans live in a world community. Travel around the world is fairly easy, and transient and immigrant populations with different histories of disease exposure live throughout the United States.

Still, parents may argue that in a society with relatively low disease prevalence, their child should not be subjected to the pain, side effects, and inconvenience of immunization in order to protect the society at large; therefore, immunization is not in the child's best interest. Yet the American medical community continues to recommend routine vaccine administration. The ethical justification for this position requires a more comprehensive view of a child's best interest and includes consideration of the principle of justice. Just as there are limits to confidentiality, there are limits to pursuing the individual child's best interests. In the case of immunizations, justice imposes such a limitation. Broadly speaking, the principle of justice suggests that all members of a society must bear both the burdens and the benefits of coexistence. By not immunizing their children, parents may put their own children at only a small individual risk. But if the numbers of unimmunized American children grow, the entire population is at increased risk. Justice challenges the absolute sovereignty of the beneficence paradigm by suggesting that the child's best interest may be balanced by the needs of society, particularly when a particular action, or in this case inaction, puts the society in peril. In the case of immunizations, the child has the potential to benefit directly and also contributes to a safer society. These benefits outweigh the individual risk to the child. Optimal care for children goes beyond addressing the needs and interests of individual patients.

ERIC D. KODISH
ANNE LYREN

SEE ALSO: *Autonomy; Beneficence; Care; Children; Competence; Confidentiality; Family and Family Medicine; Infants; Informed Consent; Research Policy: Risk and Vulnerable Groups; Surrogate Decision Making*

BIBLIOGRAPHY

American Academy of Pediatrics Committee on Bioethics. 1996. "Ethics and the Care of Critically Ill Infants and Children." *Pediatrics* 98: 149–152.

Fleishman, et al. 1994. "Caring for Gravely Ill Children." *Pediatrics* 94(4): 433–439.

King, N.M. 1989. "Children as Decision Makers: Guidelines for Pediatricians." *Journal of Pediatrics*115: 10–16.

Nelson, L. J.; et al. 1992. "Ethics and the Provision of Futile, Harmful or Burdensome Treatment to Children." *Critical Care Medicine* 20: 427–433.

PEDIATRICS, PUBLIC HEALTH ISSUES IN

• • •

Public health and medicine represent separate and complementary approaches to the protection of health. While medicine focuses primarily on the health of individuals, public health concentrates on the health of populations. Government assumes primary responsibility for public health. Laws governing the water and food supply, controls on air pollution, legislative efforts to protect children from tobacco, mandatory immunization statutes, and the treatment of persons with sexually transmitted diseases, tuberculosis, or other communicable diseases are examples of how government may regulate environmental conditions and administer interventions that positively affect the health of a population.

Nearly every public health measure has the potential to impinge upon individual freedom. Balancing individual freedoms with the protection of a population's health represents perhaps the most important ethical issue related to public health and children. Compulsory immunization statutes illustrate these tradeoffs and the ethical issues surrounding public health interventions.

Compulsory Immunization and Children

Childhood immunization programs have been identified as one of the most effective health interventions of the twentieth century. The immunization of children effectively reduces the incidence of childhood disease. Alternatively, outbreaks of disease frequently occur when immunization rates fall (Rogers, Pilgrim, Gust, et al.). Disease prevention may be accomplished directly through the protection offered to vaccinated individuals and indirectly through a phenomenon known as *herd immunity*, in which unvaccinated individuals are protected from disease because they are surrounded by vaccinated individuals who neither contract nor spread the agent in question.

Immunization differs from most medical interventions in that it is administered to healthy individuals "to prevent diseases that often do not pose an immediate threat to the individual" (Wilson and Marcuse, p. 161). For childhood immunization programs to be successful, either parents must willingly agree to have their children vaccinated or immunization must be coerced. While some parents may object to immunization on religious or philosophical grounds, others may believe that immunization poses a risk to their children that is not justified by its benefits.

The government's authority in the public health arena arises primarily from its constitutionally sanctioned "police power" to protect the public's health, welfare, and safety (Dover). What is the ethical basis for the exercise of these police powers? In *On Liberty,* John Stuart Mill argued that "The only purpose for which power can rightfully be exercised over any member of a civilized community, against his will, is to prevent harm to others. His own good, either physical or moral, is not a sufficient warrant" (p. 13).

Mill's justification for interfering with the freedom of an individual has become known as the "harm principle." Philosopher Joel Feinberg has further refined the principle by arguing that to be justified, restriction of an individual's freedom must be effective at preventing the harm in question and no option that would be less intrusive to individual liberty would be equally effective at preventing the harm.

Public health authorities may therefore be justified in interfering with parental decisions regarding immunization in two situations. First, intervention may be justified under the *parens patriae* doctrine. Under this doctrine, states have the authority to protect and care for those who cannot care for themselves and may intervene when there is evidence that parental actions or decisions are likely to harm a child. Second, intervention may be justified as an exercise of government's police powers when immunization is necessary to protect the health of the population.

Parental Refusals and the Best Interests of Children

Parents who refuse immunization on behalf of their children may have valid and important reasons for doing so. While most mandatory vaccines are effective and safe, a small possibility of adverse reactions exists. A parent might reasonably conclude that refusing the pertussis vaccine is in the best interests of a child living in a community with a high immunization rate. In such a community, the prevalence of pertussis is sufficiently low that an unimmunized child would be unlikely to contract pertussis and, therefore, could be safely spared any possible risks associated with the vaccine. In fact, it has been argued that "any successful immunization program will inevitably create a situation, as the disease becomes rare, where the individual parent's choice is at odds with society's needs" (Anderson and May, p. 415).

The *parens patriae* doctrine recognizes that society has an obligation to ensure that the basic needs of its most vulnerable members are met. In general, parental decisions should be accepted unless they clearly fall outside the range of what would be a reasonable decision concerning the child's best interest. In those rare cases where the decision of a parent places the child at substantial risk of serious harm, state agencies may be obligated to intervene and provide the necessary immunization over the parents' objections. For example, where a child has sustained a deep and contaminated puncture wound, the state might justifiably override a parent's refusal of tetanus immunization.

In these cases, the state acts in loco parentis, in the place of the parents. While this role of the state has been recognized as constitutionally valid in the United States, courts have closely examined such actions, showing reluctance to require medical treatment over the objection of parents "except where immediate action is necessary or where the potential for harm is rather serious" (Wing, p. 32). With the exception of an epidemic, the *parens patriae* doctrine rarely provides sufficient justification for interference with parental decisions regarding immunization with most vaccines.

Community Interests and Public Health

The harm principle justifies an exercise of the state's police powers when an individual's action puts others at risk of harm. Parents who choose not to immunize their children increase the potential for harm to other persons in three important ways (Veatch). First, immunized individuals are harmed by the cost of medical care for those who choose not to immunize their children and whose children then contract preventable disease. Second, should an unimmunized child contract disease, they pose a potential threat to other unimmunized children. Finally, even in a fully immunized population, a small percentage of vaccinated individuals will remain susceptible to disease. These individuals derive important benefit from herd immunity and may be harmed by contracting disease from those who remain unvaccinated.

A parent's refusal to vaccinate a child also raises an important question of justice referred to as the problem of "free riders" (Veatch; Rogers et al.). When immunization rates are high and disease rates low, the risks of immunization may exceed or equal the risks of contracting disease. Some parents may rationally decide not to immunize their children, taking advantage of the benefit created by the participation of others in the immunization program. These individuals act unfairly to others in the community, reaping the benefits of an immunization program without sharing any of the risks.

Compulsory immunization laws in the United States have repeatedly been upheld as a reasonable exercise of the state's police power even in the absence of an epidemic, and even where these laws conflict with the religious beliefs of individuals (Dover).

When others are placed at substantial risk of serious harm, an individual's range of choices may be restricted. However, serious harm can be averted in most situations without compulsory immunization. Under the harm principle, compulsory immunization is clearly justifiable when widespread use of an effective vaccine could limit an epidemic. In all likelihood, however, compulsory immunization would be unnecessary under such conditions since it would clearly be in the self-interest of individuals to receive the vaccine both for themselves and their children. A noncompulsory immunization program would probably bring about a result similar to a compulsory program without infringing on liberties. Indeed, immunization rates in several countries without compulsory immunization laws suggest that self-interest in combination with effective education and public relations campaigns may be sufficient to achieve protection of most individuals within a population (Noah). On the other hand, in a highly immunized population, the risk posed by a small number of unimmunized children is not significant enough to justify state action (Ross and Aspinwall).

Justice and Public Health Interventions

Most vaccines carry a small but measurable risk. At a population level, the risk of currently accepted vaccines is almost always justified by the benefit of widespread immunization to the population. With the polio vaccine, for example, one person will suffer vaccine-induced paralytic disease per million people vaccinated, as opposed to some 5,000 people developing paralytic disease per million unvaccinated people. Yet there remains the problem that an occasional individual will bear significant burden for the benefit that is provided to the rest of the population by an immunization program.

Given the unequal sharing of the burdens associated with vaccine programs, it seems fair and reasonable that those who are protected by the immunization program be asked to bear some of the burden of those few who are injured by the program (Gelfand; Anderson and May; Rogers et al.). A tax-based system of compensation for vaccine-related injuries and expenses can easily be justified.

A similar argument can be made concerning the costs of the vaccine program itself. Since all individuals in the community, even those refusing to participate through immunization, benefit from the immunization program, the costs of the immunization program should be born by the public. The full series of childhood immunizations costs more than $500 and is not always covered by insurance. Charging individuals the cost of vaccines has a negative effect on immunization rates by offering a financial disincentive to vaccinate. At the same time, it allows "free riders" to avoid the financial costs of a program that benefits them. For those reasons, a strong argument can be made to fund immunization programs for all citizens through a tax-based system into which all citizens contribute (Diekema and Marcuse).

Public health interventions benefit all citizens. The harm principle justifies restrictions on individual liberty when individual decisions or actions put others at risk, when harm can be prevented by restricting individual liberty, and when no less restrictive alternative would be equally effective at preventing the harm. Justice requires that the burdens and benefits of public health intervention be shared equally across the population.

DOUGLAS S. DIEKEMA

SEE ALSO: *Abuse, Interpersonal; Autonomy; Beneficence; Blood Transfusion; Children; Healthcare Resources, Allocation of; Health Screening and Testing in the Public Health Context; Infants; Informed Consent*

BIBLIOGRAPHY

Anderson, Roy, and May, Robert. 1982. "The Logic of Vaccination." *New Scientist* 96(1332): 410–415.

Diekema, Douglas S., and Marcuse, Edgar K. 1998. "Ethical Issues in the Vaccination of Children." In *Primum non nocere Today,* 2nd edition, ed. G. Roberto Burgio and John D. Lantos. Amsterdam: Elsevier.

Dover, Thomas E. 1979. "An Evaluation of Immunization Regulations in Light of Religious Objections and the Developing Right of Privacy." *University of Dayton Law Review* 4(2): 401–424.

Feinberg, Joel. 1986. *Harm to Self: The Moral Limits of the Criminal Law.* New York: Oxford University Press.

Gelfand, Henry M. 1977. "Vaccination: An Acceptable Risk?" *Science* 195(4280): 728–29.

Mill, John Stuart. 1956. *On Liberty.* Indianapolis: Bobbs-Merrill.

Noah, Norman D. 1987. "Immunisation Before School Entry: Should There Be a Law?" *British Medical Journal* 294: 1270–1271.

Rogers, Anne; Pilgrim, David; Gust, Ian D.; et al. 1995. "The Pros and Cons of Immunisation." *Health Care Analysis* 3: 99–115.

Ross, Lainie Friedman, and Aspinwall, Timothy J. 1997. "Religious Exemptions to the Immunization Statutes: Balancing Public Health and Religious Freedom." *Journal of Law, Medicine & Ethics* 25: 202–209.

Veatch, Robert M. 1987. "The Ethics of Promoting Herd Immunity." *Family & Community Health* 10(1): 44–53.

Wilson, Christopher B., and Marcuse, Edgar K. 2001. "Vaccine Safety—Vaccine Benefits: Science and the Public's Perception." *Nature Reviews Immunology* 1: 160–165.

Wing, Kenneth R. 1990. *The Law and the Public's Health.* Ann Arbor, MI: Health Administration Press.

PHARMACEUTICAL INDUSTRY

• • •

In the public media and in discussions of healthcare ethics significant questions have been raised about some of the practices of the pharmaceutical industry in the early years of the twenty-first century. The increase in expenditures for medications in the United States appears to be one of the reasons for this attention. The expansion of direct-to-consumer advertising of prescription drugs, particularly on television, and the manner in which industry sales representatives relate to physicians are among the other factors that have focused attention on the industry.

Pharmaceutical companies are in the healthcare business. It therefore is not surprising that much of the interest in the ethics of the industry relates to the potential impact of company practices on the quality and cost of healthcare, access to healthcare, and the integrity of healthcare professionals. This entry discusses some of the major and recurring issues in studies of and commentaries on ethics and the pharmaceutical industry.

Relationships between Industry Representatives and Healthcare Professionals

Representatives of the pharmaceutical industry relate to healthcare professionals in a variety of ways, including personal visits with physicians, exhibits at professional meetings, industry-sponsored education on products, financial support for nonindustry educational programs, and employment of professionals as consultants. The general ethical concerns related to these relationships are whether the interactions are in the best interests of patients and the way the relationships should be managed or structured to prevent a negative impact on healthcare.

It has long been recognized in business ethics that when gifts are given by vendors or suppliers to purchasers, there is a serious risk of undermining the objectivity of the purchasers. Most corporate codes of ethics limit the kinds of gifts that may be offered and accepted to those of minimal or nominal value. Although physicians may not be purchasers as that term sometimes is understood, their decisions are directly related to the purchase of pharmaceutical products. As could be expected, therefore, the issue of gift giving has received particular attention in the context of efforts to prevent or limit inappropriate industry influence on healthcare professionals.

Studies consistently report that the acceptance of gifts or samples from pharmaceutical representatives is associated with the rapid prescription of a new drug, the prescription of fewer generic drugs, the use of more newer medications, and formulary requests for medications (Wazana). Although some healthcare professionals state that gifts and personal relationships do not influence their professional judgment about what is best for patients, research raises serious doubt about the validity of that assertion.

The responsibility to avoid practices that result in unnecessary conflicts of interest rests with both the industry and healthcare professionals. Professional healthcare providers have a responsibility to prevent other interests from compromising their ability to exercise independent objective judgment in their work, in other words, a responsibility to subordinate other interests to their commitment to provide good medical care. A pharmaceutical company, as a healthcare business, has a responsibility to interact with physicians and other healthcare professionals only in ways that do not lead to harm of patients or undermine the professionalism of medical practice.

By 2002 healthcare professionals, healthcare organizations, the pharmaceutical industry, and the federal government had begun major efforts to reform the interactions of company representatives with physicians in response to the concerns that have been identified here. Many hospitals developed policies clarifying and restricting the activities of industry representatives while on the hospital campus. The American Medical Association (AMA) undertook a major initiative to communicate its ethical guidelines on gifts to physicians, and the Ethics and Human Rights Committee of the American College of Physicians, and the American Society of Internal Medicine issued a position paper titled "Physician-Industry Relations" (Coyle). The industry trade

association, the Pharmaceutical Research and Manufacturers of America (PhRMA), published its voluntary "Code on Interactions with Healthcare Professionals" (Pharmaceutical Research and Manufacturers of America). The U.S. Department of Health and Human Services (2002) drafted standards for pharmaceutical companies, the first of this kind, for marketing products to healthcare professionals.

Although there were differences among these efforts, they all were designed to limit abuses without prohibiting all interaction between the industry and healthcare professionals. There is a widespread belief that continued interactions are valuable and benefit patients, especially through the information that is provided to healthcare professionals by the industry about new products and the risks and benefits of these products. It remains to be seen whether these reforms will prevent undue industry influence on doctors' prescribing behavior.

It also remains to be seen whether a system that permits drug companies to function as a significant source of physician education despite the fact that those companies have an organizational self-interest in selling their drugs (especially their most profitable drugs) will continue to be accepted as reasonable and ethically supportable. For many observers it is irresponsible to expect unbiased information about their own products from drug companies. Although pharmaceutical companies have an interest in promoting good healthcare, their marketing practices are designed to sell their products.

Industry Sponsorship of Research

Another issue that has received significant attention in healthcare ethics is sponsorship of medical research by the pharmaceutical industry. As in the issue of the relationship between doctors and the pharmaceutical industry, the concern is whether the nature of the relationship undermines professionalism and scientific objectivity, a concern expressed most frequently about clinical trials. The way a trial is designed and/or the relationship of the clinical researcher to the sponsor may result in research that is neither good science nor in the public interest.

Much attention has been paid to financial conflicts of interest that result from the relationship of investigators to the companies that manufacture the medication and/or sponsor their research. When investigators are paid consultants to or regularly receive speaker honoraria from a company, when they have significant personal funds invested in company stock, or when the research compensation arrangement is such that they personally benefit significantly, their scientific and professional objectivity and independence may be compromised. In these situations there is an incentive to avoid reporting findings that make it less likely that the company will do well selling the product or continue to hire the investigator.

Ethical reflection on conflicts of interest has indicated that in most instances actual conflicts of interest are unrecognized and/or unintentional. That is, professionals do not choose deliberately to go against their primary responsibility. Instead, the nature of the context inclines one to other interests, often without conscious awareness. Most efforts to prevent or mitigate the potential negative effects of conflicts of interest therefore go beyond appeals to individual ethical integrity. Policies, procedures, and other safeguards have to be put in place.

One response to the growing concern about the financial interest of investigators was a decision made by several major medical journals in 2001 to revise and strengthen their policies regarding financial disclosure by authors. Authors are required to disclose the sponsorship of their studies and any relevant financial associations. Editors can use that information in making decisions about publication and to inform readers of potential bias if an article is published.

Another response to concern about conflicts of interest was a task force report approved in 2001 by the Executive Council of the Association of American Medical Colleges (AAMC). The AAMC Taskforce on Financial Conflicts of Interest in Clinical Research developed guidelines for medical school policies on financial conflicts of interest. In addition to requirements for reporting and monitoring, the task force recommended that institutional policies assume that an individual who has a significant financial interest in a study involving human subjects should not do that research. This assumption may be overcome in individual cases, but the researcher should have to persuade an institutional committee that his or her involvement is in the best interests of the subjects.

Although most of the emphasis has been on the responsibility of investigators to avoid conflicts of interest, there is a concomitant responsibility on the part of companies that sponsor research to avoid such conflicts. Companies have a responsibility to ensure that trials assessing the safety and efficacy of their medications are scientifically sound. They can do this by adopting policies and practices designed to prevent obstacles to the independence and objectivity of investigators. In addition to avoiding conflicts of interest for the investigators, companies need to avoid the other reported threats to scientific independence, such as industry control over or delay of publication of study results. The ethical burden of doing good research falls on both the sponsors and the clinical investigators.

Direct-to-Consumer Advertising of Prescription Drugs

At the beginning of the twenty-first century the only countries that permitted direct-to-consumer (DTC) advertising of prescription drugs were the United States and New Zealand. In 1997 the U.S. Food and Drug Administration (FDA) adopted more permissive rules on mass media advertising of prescription drugs, and in the following years DTC advertising increased significantly in the United States. The 1997 regulations permitted advertisements for prescription drugs without detailed medical information on risks and side effects. The question of whether such advertising is ethically and socially responsible is widely debated.

The Institute of Medicine (1998) described problems with healthcare quality as including underuse (failure to provide proven effective medicine), overuse (unnecessary interventions or treatments not indicated by symptoms), and misuse (interventions causing preventable complications). The primary criticism of DTC advertising of prescription drugs is that it may contribute to overuse or misuse because patients demand and sometimes get prescriptions for medications that are not appropriate in their circumstances. This leads to poor-quality care. The unnecessary use of brand-name drugs also leads to unjustified increases in healthcare costs with all the implications for healthcare access that follow from rises in those costs. The primary ethical argument for DTC advertising is that it improves the quality of healthcare because patients, through their informed questions about specific medications, assist physicians in avoiding underuse or misuse. In addition, some argue that it gives patients a much more active role in their healthcare.

Other concerns have been raised about the impact of DTC advertising. One is whether such advertising more commonly contributes to valuable interaction or puts an undue strain on the patient–physician relationship. There is also serious concern about whether specific advertisements educate consumers or mislead them and oversimplify. There is also the question of whether in a culture in which such advertising is common the result will be a heightened expectation that physicians can and should prescribe pills to cure all ills.

One study found that prescription drugs that were advertised heavily accounted for a significant proportion of the increase in pharmaceutical spending in the year studied. The same study found that the number of prescriptions for the most heavily advertised drugs grew at a rate several times higher than that of prescriptions for other drugs (National Institute for Health Care Management). This study did not try to determine whether the public health benefited from or was harmed by the growth in prescriptions of the heavily advertised drugs. There appears to be evidence that DTC advertising leads to increased use of the drugs advertised in most cases, but it is not clear whether that use is medically appropriate and cost-effective and how the patient–doctor relationship is affected.

The controversy about whether DTC advertising is good for public health and healthcare is related to other questions about the nature of a good healthcare system. Those who advocate a more rigorous evidence-based foundation for decisions about medical treatment are not likely to welcome the influence of popular marketing tactics and techniques or that of patients who expect to get specific brand-name medications. The same thing is true of those who are seeking the most effective allocation of limited healthcare resources. In contrast, those who believe that patients are best served by a consumer-driven model of healthcare are likely to welcome the contribution of advertising to consumer initiative in interactions with professionals.

Many healthcare professionals have not accepted the claim that DTC advertising contributes to improved patient care. Patients who demand a particular brand-name drug are not necessarily better-informed patients. Some advertising does not even indicate the condition or symptoms a medication is designed to address; little if any of it describers the success rate of a drug or the necessary duration of use. Furthermore, there is often no independent evidence that a more expensive brand-name product (the type that typically is advertised) is sufficiently superior to generic medications to justify the use of limited healthcare resources.

The basic question may be whether medicines are enough like other commodities that it is appropriate to advertise them in a similar manner. One major difference is that unlike consumer products, they have to be prescribed by a licensed professional. If the objective of DTC prescription drug advertising is a better-informed public, the informational nature of the marketing will be of central importance. If the objective is to contribute to improvement in the quality of healthcare, the advertising will be designed to prevent misuse and overuse as well as underuse.

Other Issues

Whereas the three issues discussed above have received the most attention in the literature on healthcare ethics, several other questions have been raised about the practices and standards of the pharmaceutical industry. Three additional concerns are noted below as examples of those issues.

MISUSE OF THE PATENT SYSTEM. Pharmaceutical companies have been accused of "gaming the drug patent system."

(*New York Times*) The concern here is that drug companies are using questionable methods to extend the life of their most profitable patents. At least some of those methods are legal, taking advantage of existing interpretations of the law. One such method is to sue a generic company for infringing on patents for packaging or dosing schedules. Those suits automatically delay the introduction of the generic version into the marketplace for thirty months even if the suit is frivolous. Extending patent life may prove financially beneficial to the company but may be detrimental to public health by increasing healthcare costs and placing an unnecessary burden on available healthcare resources. The question is whether this is an ethically defensible practice for a health-related business even when it is legal.

PRICING. A related issue concerns pricing. The effort at the beginning of the twenty-first century to extend Medicare benefits to cover prescription drugs was driven in large part by the high cost of prescription drugs for many citizens over age sixty-five. The fact that the same drugs can be purchased in a neighboring country at a much lower price raises the question of whether the price in the United States is unnecessarily high. In addition, because the prices of pharmaceuticals are different for group purchasers from what they are in retail pharmacies, those who must purchase their prescription drugs at a local retail pharmacy pay the highest prices. This is a part of the bigger issue of equitable access to healthcare in the United States, but it also raises a serious question for the pharmaceutical industry: What constitutes fair pricing for prescription medicines?

RESEACH AND DEVELOPMENT. Pharmaceutical companies also have also been challenged in terms of their research and development agenda. There are two parts to this criticism: (1) that many of the drugs being developed are "me-too" medications, or prescription drugs that are slightly different formulations of existing drugs; and (2) that the new medications developed by the (multinational) industry are more likely to be lifestyle drugs for the wealthy world than drugs for serious diseases commonly found in poorer countries. Research programs in pharmaceutical companies on male impotence (Silverstein) and on baldness, for example, may have many more resources put into them than research programs on malaria. Because the industry both is a for-profit industry and accounts for a significant part of international efforts to meet the real healthcare needs of people, what is a responsible agenda for research and development?

Conclusion

A review of some of the ethical concerns about the pharmaceutical industry must focus on criticisms and questions related to industry practices. This focus does not deny that the industry has made significant contributions to public health through the development and marketing of important medications.

The concept of the stakeholder has come to occupy a central place in reflection on business ethics. Businesses have responsibilities to various stakeholders: all those who are affected significantly by company decisions and practices, including employees, investors, customers, suppliers, and the larger community. Although it is not always possible to satisfy the concerns and legitimate interests of all stakeholders all the time, it is not satisfactory to say that a company has only one key responsibility: to benefit the shareholders. Making the right decisions and keeping priorities straight when there have to be trade-offs in regard to different stakeholders is the hard work of business ethics.

Establishing the right priorities among stakeholder interests depends somewhat on the nature of the industry. Businesses in the healthcare industry, whether for-profit or not-for-profit, have a high-priority responsibility to protect public health and the integrity of the healthcare system. When specific practices of a health-related business appear to be placing the public health at unnecessary risk or to be undermining the public commitment to a good healthcare system, it is reasonable to question the ethical appropriateness of those practices. The variety and seriousness of the questions asked about practices of the pharmaceutical industry appear to indicate that for many people some industry practices mean unnecessarily risks for health and healthcare despite the industry's contributions to healthcare.

LEONARD J. WEBER

SEE ALSO: *Advertising; Commercialism in Scientific Research; Corporate Compliance; Pharmaceutics, Issues in Prescribing*

BIBLIOGRAPHY

Angell, Marcia. 2000a. "Is Academic Medicine for Sale?" *New England Journal of Medicine* 342: 1516–1518.

Angell, Marcia. 2000b. "The Pharmaceutical Industry—To Whom Is It Accountable?" *New England Journal of Medicine* 342: 1902–1904.

Blackett, Tom, and Robins, Rebecca, eds. 2001. *Brand Medicine: The Role of Branding in the Pharmaceutical Industry.* New York: Palgrave.

Bodenheimer, Thomas. 2000. "Uneasy Alliance—Clinical Investigators and the Pharmaceutical Industry." *New England Journal of Medicine* 342: 1539–1544.

Coyle, Susan L. (for the Ethics and Human Rights Committee, American College of Physicians, American Society of Internal Medicine). 2002. "Physician-Industry Relations." *Annals of Internal Medicine* 136: 396–406.

Holmer, Alan F. 2002. "Direct-to-Consumer Advertising—Strengthening Our Health Care System." *New England Journal of Medicine* 346: 526–528.

Institute of Medicine National Roundtable on Healthcare Quality. 1998. "The Urgent Need to Improve Health Care Quality." *Journal of the American Medical Association* 280: 1000–1005.

Kelch, Robert P. 2002. "Maintaining the Public Trust in Clinical Research." *New England Journal of Medicine* 346: 285–287.

New York Times. 2002. "Gaming the Drug Patent System." June 10, editorial, p. A24.

Silverstein, Ken. 1999. "Millions for Viagra, Pennies for Diseases of the Poor." *The Nation,* July 19, pp. 13–19.

U.S. Department of Health and Human Services, Office of Inspector General. 2002. "Draft OIG Compliance Program Guidance for Pharmaceutical Manufacturers." *Federal Register* 67: 62057–62067.

Wazana, Ashley. 2000. "Physicians and the Pharmaceutical Industry: Is a Gift Ever Just a Gift?" *Journal of the American Medical Association* 283: 373–380.

Wolfe, Sidney M. 2002. "Direct-to-Consumer Advertising—Education or Emotion Promotion?" *New England Journal of Medicine* 346: 524–526.

INTERNET RESOURCES

American Medical Association. 1990. "Gifts to Physicians from Industry." Updated 1998. Available from <http://www.ama-assn.org>.

National Institute for Health Care Management. 2001. "Prescription Drugs and Mass Media Advertising, 2001." Available from <http://www.nihcm.org>.

Pharmaceutical Research and Manufacturers of America. 2002. "PhRMA Code on Interactions with Healthcare Professionals." <http://www.phrma.org>.

PHARMACEUTICS, ISSUES IN PRESCRIBING

• • •

During much of the fourth quarter of the twentieth century, discussions of ethics in prescribing tended to focus on the physician–patient relationship, the quality of patient care, and on patient rights. By the turn of the century, another set of considerations began receiving consistent attention in the United States: issues raised for the prescribing clinician by some healthcare business practices. Most of the ethical issues related to prescribing decisions and behavior fit into one of these two, sometimes overlapping, categories.

Prescribing and the Clinician-Patient Relationship

In the traditional medical model of rational prescribing, the patient presents challenging symptoms that the physician investigates and then diagnoses a disease. Based on this diagnosis, the appropriate drug and/or non-drug treatment is prescribed. Emphasis is placed on accurate diagnosis and application of pharmacologic principles, which govern the use of safe and effective drugs to treat a disease (O'Hagan).

The prescribing of medication, which occurs in most physician–patient encounters, does not, however, always occur through the application of this rational model. Many prescriptions are written on the basis of careful diagnosis and assessment, but sometimes other factors are involved as well.

Patients often expect prescriptions. A friend or a family member may have experienced some benefit from a medication given for a similar symptom. Direct-to-consumer advertising has raised patient expectations, both that prescribed medications are needed and that they will be beneficial. The public is led to accept the principle that there is a pill for every ill (Morgan and Weintraub; O'Hagan). The physician is expected to "do something" for the patient. Patients may feel confident that something concrete has been offered when given a prescription. Regardless of how trivial the complaint may be, the patient's sick role is legitimated by a prescription. It validates the doctor visit and allows future visits for vague symptoms (Stimson; O'Hagan). It is quite possible, however, that physicians may be overestimating the extent to which patients actually desire medications (Frølund).

Physicians are regularly exposed to education and marketing that highlights the use of medications in patient care. Physicians frequently have little time to spend speaking with patients about non-drug regimens, which may contribute to the frequency of prescription writing. Many physicians, like many patients, expect that something will be done in a patient–doctor encounter. Prescribing is a common way for the physician to intervene. It also allays the physician concern that the patient may be unhappy if not given a prescription and go elsewhere for the medicine believed to be necessary (Schwartz, Soumerai, and Avorn).

Some have suggested that a prescription may even help the physician define the disease in situations where the diagnosis is uncertain (O'Hagan). "I prescribe an antibiotic, therefore the patient has a bacterial infection." Or "I prescribe a tranquilizer, so the symptoms must be due to anxiety." Reimbursement requirements of insurers may reinforce this attitude, since often a diagnosis is expected even if the physician is uncertain.

Clearly, it is more difficult not to prescribe than to prescribe. Medicines are generally viewed as good, and prescribing as a beneficent act. Nevertheless, there are some developments in American medicine in the beginning of the twenty-first century that place more emphasis on the risks associated with medications and on the importance of prescribing medications only when there is a good medical reason for do so. The Institute of Medicine in 1998 identified misuse (interventions causing preventable complications) and overuse (unnecessary interventions or treatment for clearly inappropriate indications) as healthcare quality problems, in addition to under-use (failure to provide proven effective interventions). The movement toward "evidence-based" healthcare, which stresses the importance of having a foundation in medical experience and research for interventions, discourages treatment that cannot be supported scientifically. The growing recognition of the risks of "polypharmacy" means that more emphasis is being placed on the harm done by multiple medications and their interactions (Colley and Lucas).

These and related developments have supported the efforts of some physicians (and others in healthcare) to highlight the ethical importance of avoiding unnecessary prescribing.

Placebos

The question of whether, or when, the prescribing of placebos is ethically acceptable has received considerable attention at least since the 1970s. Placebos can relieve symptoms and they are one way that physicians can please patients who expect a medication without prescribing unnecessary drugs. The use of placebos might appear, therefore, to benefit patients without much risk of harm (Schwartz et al.). The major objection to the use of placebos is based on the conviction that, however well they might work, prescribing placebos is a deception of patients and is a basic violation of their right to be informed about the diagnosis and the treatment (Bok). Long-term placebo treatment might divert attention from the cause of a patient's complaints, possibly resulting in a serious medical problem going unrecognized and untreated. In addition, the patient may lose trust in the physician upon recognizing the deception (Schwartz et al.).

The use of placebos received renewed attention near the end of the twentieth century in the United States with the movement to improve the management of patient pain. The use of placebos in response to patient request for pain relief became a focus of special concern. For many, prescribing placebos for pain relief is, in effect, a refusal to accept the patient's own perception of pain and was incompatible with a pain management program based on taking patient reports of pain seriously. Some hospitals developed policies prohibiting the use of placebos for symptoms of pain or for all treatment purposes, permitting placebos only as part of a clinical study approved by an institutional review board (IRB).

Healthcare Business Practices and the Writing of Prescriptions

As discussed above, some of the enduring concerns about ethics in prescribing focus on the quality of patient care and on the nature of the clinician–patient relationship. A commitment to professional competence and to professional integrity requires that these concerns continue to receive careful attention. In recent years, however, there has been a growing concern about another aspect of ethics in prescribing: the potential impact of different healthcare business practices on prescribing decisions and behavior. The practices of pharmaceutical companies and of health insurance plans are of particular interest in this regard.

Pharmaceutical companies invest heavily in marketing and most heavily of all in marketing to physicians (Johnson; Relman and Angell). Drug company representatives visit physician offices regularly and frequently, bringing information on their company's products, free samples, and gifts for the physician and staff. The sales representatives often have information on the physician's individual prescribing habits and are prepared to influence specific prescribing decisions (Kowalczyk).

As studies have demonstrated, physician prescribing is often affected by interactions with drug company representatives (Wazana). Drug companies market their products to provide patients with good and needed medicines, but they are also highly focused on profit and on market share. Physicians acquire some useful and important information from sales representatives, but they are at some risk of compromising their professional judgment by participating in these interactions. To protect the quality of healthcare, it is important to minimize the influence of (potentially) biased information and the influence of the personal interactions with sales representatives.

Influences can be present even when they are not recognized, when the individual is not aware of what is affecting a particular decision or action. Some physicians have decided that the best way of interacting with drug company representatives is not to see them at all (Griffith). While much of the concern about physician relationships with drug companies has been focused on the acceptance of gifts (American Medical Association; Coyle), the issue is more extensive than that. Marketing and objective education simply may be two quite different things.

The acceptance of free samples of medicines is also being questioned by some bioethicists. These medications are often used for patients with limited resources or to test whether a particular medication is effective for a specific patient. Once started, however, a medication is often difficult to change, even when it may not be the best for the patient or when the cost cannot be justified. Free samples are especially problematic when the sales representative rather then the physician decides which medications will be provided as samples.

Ethical challenges in prescribing are also raised by healthcare insurance industry practices. The use of formularies and a tiered schedule of pharmacy co-pays are two such practices. Healthcare plans publish lists of covered and of recommended medications for specific symptoms or diagnoses and provide physicians with clinical guidelines for recommended treatment. The insured are often charged different co-pays for different medications (for example, a lower out-of-pocket cost for generics, higher for recommended brand drugs, and highest for nonrecommended brand-name drugs).

Insurance plans are seeking to control costs through these practices. They are encouraging the use of the lowest cost medications or treatments appropriate. Physicians are free to prescribe whatever they think best, but they risk being identified as providers who are not following the plan's guidelines. In addition, their prescribing decisions have a direct impact on the patient's personal pharmacy expenses.

These practices raise the question of the clinicians' responsibility in regard to the cost of the medications they prescribe. Many physicians, at least until recently, have not routinely considered the cost when making medication decisions. In fact, based on the belief that the physician's responsibility is to do what is best for the individual patient under care, it has often been considered inappropriate to allow the cost of the treatment to play a significant role in the recommendation for medical treatment. This understanding of the meaning of patient advocacy was widely challenged at the beginning of the twenty-first century.

In a statement that has received considerable attention and support, James Sabin argued that physicians do have an ethical responsibility to act as stewards of society's healthcare resources. "As a clinician I believe it is ethically mandatory to recommend the least costly treatment unless I have substantial evidence that a more costly intervention is likely to yield a superior outcome" (Sabin, p. 859). If a physician's responsibility to patients includes taking cost into account, it makes good ethical sense to conform to an insurer's practice that promotes lower cost medications, whenever that "substantial evidence" of a more expensive medication being more effective does not exist.

Wise use of available medical resources is one rationale for physician attention to the cost of the medications prescribed. Another reason is respect for the patient role in making informed consent decisions. If patient out-of-pocket expenses are greater for one medication than another (because of lack of healthcare insurance coverage or because of a tiered co-pay system), the patient needs to know, in advance, the relative difference in price. The patient needs to know, as well, the prescriber's rationale for recommending a higher-cost drug, when that is the case. Without both pieces of information, the patient does not have all the information necessary to determine whether to consent to the recommended treatment.

Some cost-driven insurance company practices support (or are compatible with) high-quality prescribing decisions and some do not. The physician needs to distinguish between the two and act to protect the patients' best interests and their own professional integrity. Knowledge of the general costs of the medications that one prescribes is, it seems, an essential component of responsible practice.

The ethical considerations related to prescribing treatment, especially prescribing medications, can be expected to receive continuing attention—and perhaps significantly increased attention—in the early part of the twenty-first century.

DAVID T. LOWENTHAL
GEORGE J. CARANASOS (1995)
REVISED BY LEONARD J. WEBER

SEE ALSO: *Addiction and Dependence; Conflict of Interest; Informed Consent; Life, Quality of; Placebo; Pharmaceutical Industry; Psychopharmacology*

BIBLIOGRAPHY

Bok, Sissela. 1974. "The Ethics of Giving Placebos." *Scientific American* 231: 17–23.

Colley, C.A., and Lucas, L.M. 1993. "Polypharmacy: The Cure Becomes the Disease." *Journal of General Internal Medicine* 8: 278–283.

Coyle, Susan L., for the Ethics and Human Rights Committee, American College of Physicians—American Society of Internal Medicine. 2002. "Physician-Industry Relations." *Annals of Internal Medicine* 136: 396–406.

Frølund, Fleming. 1978. "Better Prescribing." *British Medical Journal* 2(6139): 741.

Griffith, David. 1999. "Reasons for Not Seeing Drug Representatives." *British Medical Journal* 319: 69–70.

Institute of Medicine National Roundtable on Healthcare Quality. 1998. "The Urgent Need to Improve Health Care Quality." *The Journal of the American Medical Association* 280: 1000–1005.

Johnson, Linda. 2003. "Drug Makers Continue to Bolster Sales Legions." *Associated Press* June 2, 2003.

Kowalczyk, Liz. 2003. "Drug Companies' Secret Reports Outrage Doctors." *The Boston Globe* May 25, 2003: A1.

Lowenthal, David T.; Levy, G.; Lavy, N. W.; McMahon, F. Gilbert; et al. 1990. "That None Should Be Denied." *Clinical Pharmacology and Therapeutics* 47(3): 422–423.

Morgan, John P., and Weintraub, Michael. 1974. "A Course on the Social Functions of Prescription Drugs: Seminar Syllabus and Bibliography." *Annals of Internal Medicine* 77(2): 217–222.

O'Hagan, J. J. 1984. "What Influences Our Prescribing?—Some Nonpharmacological Issues." *New Zealand Medical Journal* 97(756): 331–332.

Relman, Arnold S., and Angell, Marcia. 2002. "America's Other Drug Problem." *The New Republic* December 16, 2002: 27–41.

Ryde, David. 1976. "Does the Patient Really Need a Prescription?" *Practitioner* 216(1295): 557–559.

Sabin, James. 1994. "A Credo for Ethical Managed Care in Mental Health Practice." *Hospital and Community Psychiatry* 45(9): 859.

Schwartz, R. K.; Soumerai, S. B.; and Avorn, J. 1989. "Physician Motivations for Nonscientific Drug Prescribing." *Social Science and Medicine* 28(6): 577–582.

Stimson, G. V. 1976. "Doctor-Patient Interaction and Some Problems for Prescribing." *Journal of the Royal College of General Practitioners* 26(Suppl. 1): 88–96.

Wazana, Ashley. 2000. "Physicians and the Pharmaceutical Industry: Is a Gift Ever Just a Gift?" *The Journal of the American Medical Association* 283: 373–380.

INTERNET RESOURCE

American Medical Association. 2003. "Gifts to Physicians from Industry." Available from <http://www.ama-assn.org>.

PHYSICIAN-ASSISTED SUICIDE

SEE *Life Sustaining Treatment and Euthanasia: I. Ethical Aspects of*

PLACEBO

• • •

The terms *placebo* and *placebo effect* are quite difficult to define. Most commonsense definitions contain serious inconsistencies. For example, one commonly hears placebo defined as an "inert remedy"; but if a placebo were totally inert, there would be no point in giving it.

In Latin, *placebo* means "I shall please," but the effects of a placebo can be either positive or negative (the term *nocebo,* roughly meaning "I shall harm," is sometimes used to designate negative effects). Adolf Grünbaum emphasized that whether or not a remedy is a placebo is always relative to some biomedical theory. A sugar pill is a placebo for a migraine only because the biomedical theory agreed upon by all discussants denies any pharmacologic efficacy of small amounts of oral glucose in altering the pain of vascular headache.

Some find it useful to locate the species "placebo" under the genus "nonspecific therapy," by which they mean a therapy that strengthens the general resistance of the organism to disease of many sorts (as opposed to a therapy that removes the specific cause of a single disease or class of diseases). But the latter term may be as hard to define precisely as placebo is. Moreover, there may be an unspoken assumption that nonspecific therapies are synonymous with "therapies that operate through psychological rather than biological mechanisms." But this is clearly false; some psychological therapies may be very specific for certain diseases according to established psychiatric theories, and some biological therapies, notably diet and exercise, seem to be good candidates for "nonspecific" status.

For purposes of ethical analysis, placebo effect may be defined generally as the change in a patient's condition that results from the symbolic aspects of the encounter with a healer or with a healing setting, and not from the pharmacological or physiological properties of any remedy used. The term *symbolic* alludes not only to the psychological processes that occur within the patient but also to the social and cultural belief systems that form a background to the patient's thoughts and feelings and that give meaning to the healing process. A placebo, then, is a remedy administered either for purposes of eliciting the placebo effect or as a control in an experimental situation. Virtually any modality, including surgery and psychotherapy, can function as a placebo; the term is not confined to pills, capsules, or injections.

The practical goal of defining placebo effect as precisely as possible is to distinguish the changes it produces in the patient's condition from changes produced by other causes. In treatment, the two factors likely to be confused with placebo effects are the pharmacological or physiological effects of the therapy employed and the natural history of the illness. For example, if a patient with gastritis visits a physician, who recommends antacids, and the patient improves, the relief could have come from the pharmacological properties of the antacids, the natural tendency of gastritis to heal over time, the soothing symbolic effects of the physician consultation, or some combination of the three. The two-group design in a controlled experimental trial ("active" treatment versus placebo) allows the investigator to distinguish pharmacological or physiological effects from the placebo effects and the natural history of the illness. It does not allow a distinction to be made between natural history and placebo effects.

It is also helpful to distinguish a pure placebo, thought to have no pharmacological potency under any circumstances whatever, from an impure placebo, which has pharmacological potency under some circumstances. Common examples of impure placebos are vitamins administered to patients who have no documented deficiency and antibiotics administered to patients who have viral illnesses (which do not respond to antibiotics). In today's medical practice, impure placebos are probably used much more commonly than pure placebos.

Scientific Controversies

A number of works published in 2001 showed the controversy surrounding the science of the placebo effect. A careful meta-analysis of 114 randomized controlled trials concluded that the placebo effect does not exist in that context, and changes previously attributed to the placebo effect resulted from either natural history or random variation (Hróbjartsson and Gøtzsche). Other scientists reported further evidence that placebo effects in pain are mediated by endorphin release in the brain (Amanzio et al.) and that alteration in dopamine release in response to placebo therapy for Parkinson's disease can be detected by positron emission tomographic imaging of the brain (de la Fuente-Fernández et al.). The results of a conference on "The Science of the Placebo" sponsored by the U.S. National Institutes of Health (NIH) were published (Guess et al.), and the NIH announced that research programs would for the first time be devoted specifically to studying the mechanisms and extent of placebo effects. Readers were thus led to various conclusions: that the placebo effect is a myth; that scientists understand better how it works; and that further research into its mechanisms will be fruitful. The majority view appears to be that the "myth" dismissal is premature and that more study is needed.

At the biochemical and cellular level, placebo effects may induce organ changes via the release of catecholamines, endorphins, or immunoactive cells; all three have been shown to be very sensitive to a patient's psychological or emotional state. At the social and psychological level, one must identify aspects of the setting or of the human interaction that cause the patient to perceive the situation as a healing one, thereby releasing whatever biochemically active substances might be involved. It appears safe to claim that a positive change in the patient's health status is most likely to occur when at least three things happen: the patient receives a satisfying explanation of the illness and treatment, the patient feels cared for and supported, and the patient feels an enhanced sense of mastery and control over symptoms.

During the 1990s and early 2000s, the ethics of placebo-controlled trials has been both challenged (Rothman and Michels) and defended (Miller and Brody). Besides the ethical questions concerning whether it is permissible to deprive research subjects of an effective standard treatment, some researchers have questioned how much scientific benefit is added by the use of a placebo control as opposed to an active-treatment control (Freedman, Weijer, and Glass). Systematic reviews have claimed that at least for selected conditions, such as depression, studies conducted without placebo controls might be scientifically suboptimal (Walsh et al.).

Ethical Issues

In the traditional use of placebos, a pharmacologically inert pill might be administered to a patient under circumstances that encourage the belief that a powerful drug is being given. Many patients—the average of one-third is often cited, though this conceals a wide variation among different settings—will experience some degree of positive response (White, Tursky, and Schwartz). This traditional use is ethically questionable because the patient is deceived. Therefore, an ethical analysis of placebo use might proceed with two questions. First, is deception necessary to produce the patient benefit promised by the placebo effect? Second, are there nondeceptive uses of placebos?

If one wishes to use placebo effects for the benefit of patients, one can simply work to enhance those aspects of the patient encounter that have been scientifically correlated with symptom improvement. One can show care, offer explanations, and enhance perceived mastery and control in

many ways that require no deception whatever. Because, in the traditional use of placebos, the deception is justified by appeal to patients' benefit (Rawlinson), it is important to see that in almost all patient encounters, a nondeceptive alternative can produce the same result. Moreover, Sissela Bok argued, in her 1978 book, *Lying,* that the defender of the deception entailed in the traditional use of placebos makes two miscalculations: ignoring possible short-term harm (e.g., missing a diagnosis of serious disease because a placebo has temporarily relieved the patient's complaints) and failing to see how apparently trivial acts build up into collectively undesirable practices (e.g., overreliance on medication).

One may conclude that the traditional use of placebos in therapy can be justified only by very unusual circumstances (in which the use of a dummy pill is the only way to encourage the desired psychological state, for instance). By contrast, because reassuring patients and offering explanations and emotional support are part and parcel of good clinical care, one may argue that a physician has a positive ethical duty to try to enhance the placebo effect in every patient encounter (Connelly).

Counterarguments in defense of the traditional use focus on the claim that the deception is apparent rather than real (Spiro). It might be argued, for example, that if one gives the patient a placebo and says, "There, this will make you feel a lot better," one has not really lied. The increasing scientific interest in the placebo *effect* has triggered a resurgence of interest in administering *placebos* to patients, and some have claimed that placebo administration can be combined with respect for patients' rights and with appropriate informed consent (Brown). Perhaps the best reply to these counterarguments was put forth in a 1903 article by Richard C. Cabot: "A true impression, not certain words literally true," (Cabot, p. 345) is what the physician is obligated to promote in the patient. Most efforts at "informed consent" for placebo therapy still seem to rely on some element of equivocation, assuming that if the patient fully understood the pharmacologically inert nature of the remedy, no meaningful placebo effect would result.

Placebos may be employed in ways that do not entail deception and may therefore be fully licit. When placebos are used in controlled studies, it is generally possible to obtain a fully informed consent. It is also possible to use placebos in the therapy of individual patients in a way that avoids deception. One formal procedure for doing so has been termed the "N of 1 Trial," because it is basically a double-blind, controlled research trial performed on a single, informed subject (Guyatt et al.).

HOWARD BRODY (1995)
REVISED BY AUTHOR

SEE ALSO: *AIDS: Healthcare and Research Issues; Healing; Informed Consent; Pharmaceutics, Issues in Prescribing; Research Methodology; Research, Unethical*

BIBLIOGRAPHY

Amanzio, Martina; Pollo, Antonella; Maggi, Guiliano; and Benedetti, Fabrizio. 2001. "Response Variability to Analgesics: A Role for Non-specific Activation of Endogenous Opioids." *Pain* 90(3): 205–215.

Bok, Sissela. 1978. *Lying: Moral Choice in Public and Private Life.* New York: Pantheon.

Brody, Howard. 1982. "The Lie That Heals: The Ethics of Giving Placebos." *Annals of Internal Medicine* 97(1): 112–118.

Brody, Howard. 2000. "The Placebo Response: Recent Research and Implications for Family Medicine." *Journal of Family Practice* 49(7): 649–654.

Brown, Walter A. 1998. "Harnessing the Placebo Effect." *Hospital Practice* 33(7): 107–116.

Cabot, Richard C. 1903. "The Use of Truth and Falsehood in Medicine: An Experimental Study." *American Medicine* 5(9): 344–349. Reprinted in *Ethics in Medicine: Historical Perspectives and Contemporary Concerns,* ed. Stanley J. Reiser, Arthur J. Dyck, and William J. Curran. Cambridge, MA: MIT Press, 1977.

Connelly, Robert J. 1991. "Nursing Responsibility for the Placebo Effect." *Journal of Medicine and Philosophy* 16(3): 325–341.

de la Fuente-Fernández, Raúl; Ruth, Thomas J.; Sossi, Vesna; et al. 2001. "Expectation and Dopamine Release: Mechanism of the Placebo Effect in Parkinson's Disease." *Science* 293(5532): 1164–1165.

Freedman, Benjamin; Weijer, Charles; and Glass, Kathleen Cranley. 1996. "Placebo Orthodoxy in Clinical Research, I: Empirical and Methodological Myths." *Journal of Law, Medicine, and Ethics* 24(3): 243–251.

Grünbaum, Adolf. 1989. "The Placebo Concept in Medicine and Psychiatry." In *Non-specific Aspects of Treatment,* ed. Michael Shepherd and Normal Sartorius. Bern, Switzerland: Hans Huber.

Guess, Harry A.; Kleinman, Arthur; Kusek, John W.; and Engel, Linda L., eds. 2001. *The Science of the Placebo: Toward an Interdisciplinary Research Agenda.* London: BMJ Books.

Guyatt, Gordon; Sackett, David; Taylor, D. Wayne; et al. 1986. "Determining Optimal Therapy: Randomized Trials in Individual Patients." *New England Journal of Medicine* 314(14): 889–892.

Hróbjartsson, Asbjørn, and Gøtzsche, Peter C. 2001. "Is the Placebo Powerless? An Analysis of Clinical Trials Comparing Placebo with No Treatment." *New England Journal of Medicine* 344(21): 1594–1602.

Miller, Franklin G., and Brody, Howard. 2002. "What Makes Placebo-Controlled Trials Unethical?" *American Journal of Bioethics* 2(2): 3–9.

Rawlinson, Mary C. 1985. "Truth-Telling and Paternalism in the Clinic: Philosophical Reflections on the Use of Placebos in Medical Practice." In *Placebo: Theory, Research, and Mechanisms,* ed. Leonard White, Bernard Tursky, and Gary E. Schwartz. New York: Guilford Press.

Rothman, Kenneth J., and Michels, Karin B. 1994. "The Continued Unethical Use of Placebo Controls." *New England Journal of Medicine* 331(6): 394–398.

Spiro, Howard M. 1986. *Doctors, Patients, and Placebos.* New Haven, CT: Yale University Press.

Walsh, B. Timothy; Seidman, Stuart N.; Sysko, Robyn; and Gould, Madelyn. 2002. "Placebo Response in Studies of Major Depression: Variable, Substantial, and Growing." *Journal of the American Medical Association* 287(14): 1840–1847.

White, Leonard; Tursky, Bernard; and Schwartz, Gary E., eds. 1985. *Placebo: Theory, Research, and Mechanisms.* New York: Guilford Press.

POPULATION ETHICS

• • •

I. ELEMENTS OF POPULATION ETHICS: A. DEFINITION OF POPULATION ETHICS

Population studies deal with fertility, mortality, and migration. Fertility refers to human reproduction, mortality to death, and migration to the movement of people from one region to another. The articles on population ethics and population policies in this *Encyclopedia* take up only those aspects of fertility and migration with close links to healthcare and the life sciences, that is, to bioethics.

Population ethics has two main foundations: moral principles and factual information. Moral principles come from religious traditions, philosophy, declarations of human rights, and other sources. Factual information derives from careful analysis of what is happening or has happened in a given place or situation. Judgments about the ethics of population policies require the application of moral principles to cases based on solid, factual information. Vague principles or a poor understanding of how population programs really operate lead to questionable judgments about population ethics.

The articles on normative approaches and on religious traditions show similarities and differences in the moral principles applied to population policies. One major normative framework, accepted in principle by most countries, includes the universal statements on human rights developed by the United Nations. By endorsing and defining rights such as life, liberty, and welfare, the United Nations has established ethical standards applicable to all social programs, including those dealing with population. The major religious traditions of the world also have their own perspectives on fertility control and migration. Many of these are fully compatible with U.N. statements on human rights, but some are not. The main conflicts over population ethics arise when governments, most of which have officially accepted U.N. standards on human rights, violate those rights in their own population programs.

The articles on population policies apply moral principles to strategies used in fertility control, health standards required in that field, ethical issues in programs involving migration and refugees, and the work of donor agencies dealing with fertility control and migration and refugees. Strategies of fertility control can range from the application of force to information campaigns aimed at voluntary changes in attitudes and behavior. They include compulsion, which has been used to force China's one-child-per-couple policy; strong persuasion, such as the application of heavy government and community pressure on potential users of fertility control; financial incentives and disincentives given to users, field workers, and communities; and educational or information campaigns aimed at promoting greater acceptance of fertility control. The ethical issues are most serious with the use of compulsion and least serious, though still significant, with information campaigns.

Debates over whether rapid population growth poses problems for human societies also show the need for clear moral principles and solid factual understanding. Advocates enter those debates with different principles and factual information.

The moral principles guiding discussions about population problems include preventing environmental pollution (Ehrlich and Ehrlich); keeping population size within the carrying capacity of the world (Hardin); and promoting economic growth (World Bank). Each principle leads to a different focus on factual information. Those concerned with pollution analyze data about global warming, acid rain, and depletion of the ozone layer. Those proposing to keep population size within the carrying capacity of the world look, for example, at figures on population density. Students of economic growth consider the many links between birthrate and economic development, including relationships among fertility, education, and healthcare. Because each concern leads to a different meaning of a population problem and a different selection of information, it is difficult to compare one problem definition with another.

Two research practices have held back the development of an adequate factual base for population ethics. One practice begins with conclusions and then selects only those facts consistent with them. Analysts claiming that rapid population growth has had negative consequences for economic development often cite facts supporting that conclusion and leave out contrary evidence (World Bank). Those claiming benefits from rapid population growth do the same (Simon).

The second practice involves assigning more or less weight to population conditions than objective research would support. Some advocates of fertility control claim that rapid population growth has caused starvation and political instability in the developing countries. Such simple interpretations overlook the many other influences leading to those conditions, such as the lack of food in poor countries, corruption among political leaders, and ethnic conflicts.

The strategies countries use to control fertility have provoked the sharpest debates about population ethics. China and India have used outright coercion to promote sterilization or abortion. In China, women found to be pregnant with unauthorized children have been forced to undergo abortions (Aird). Between 1975 and 1977, police in some parts of India rounded up eligible men and required them to be sterilized (Gwatkin). Indonesia's use of strong community pressures to increase use of contraceptives has also been controversial. To gain new users the Indonesian government has relied on such methods as repeated visits to eligible women from village heads, family-planning workers, and members of Acceptors Clubs; pressure to accept intrauterine devices during "safaris" attended by prominent public officials; and promoting a positive image of small families.

Those defending coercion and heavy social pressures argue that countries such as China, India, and Indonesia require vigorous methods of fertility control to curb swelling populations. Voluntary methods, they say, will work too slowly to prevent damage to the economy and create impossible demands for a nation's schools and other public services. Critics respond that applying force and heavy pressure violates human rights and disregards international agreements on fertility control, such as the 1974 World Population Plan of Action (United Nations).

Policies on migration and refugees also raise questions of ethics. Under what conditions, if any, do residents of one country have the right to enter another? Are the moral claims of potential migrants stronger when they are facing starvation, persecution, or violence? Do countries have the right to bar or expel immigrants they see as harmful to their national interest, as the United States did with Haitian immigrants in the early 1990s? What obligations, if any, does a government have to undocumented aliens within its borders? Can it deny them healthcare services regularly available to its own citizens? What kinds of aid should donor agencies, such as the World Food Program or the International Committee for the Red Cross, provide to migrants, refugees, and displaced persons? And how should that aid be distributed?

Issues of medical risks and proper standards of healthcare arise in fertility control as well as migration and refugee programs. Family-planning programs sometimes put more emphasis on achieving numerical targets for clients than on safeguarding the freedom and health of users. Field workers may promote medically unsafe methods of fertility control, fail to disclose the risks of a given method, or be unavailable to deal with the side effects that do occur. Or they may insert the subdermal contraceptive Norplant and then refuse to remove it at the client's request (Ubinig). Fertility-control programs also differ in the health support they provide to users, such as local clinics to deal with minor problems or hospitals to handle serious complications.

Questions about standards for healthcare also arise in programs for refugees. Program managers often have to decide whether refugees should be sent back to countries from which they fled, where they may be tortured, imprisoned, or killed. If they are kept in camps, what should be done to prevent the high rates of illness sometimes seen in those settings? Possible preventive measures include providing adequate food, safe water, suitable shelter, sanitation, immunization of vulnerable groups, and a primary healthcare system.

International donor agencies, such as the World Bank, the United Nations Population Fund, and the U.S. Agency for International Development, also face moral choices in their assistance to fertility-control programs. Among those choices are whether donors should support programs known or thought to involve coercion, such as that in China; whether those organizations funding a variety of projects, such as the World Bank, should put pressure on countries to initiate fertility-control programs as a precondition for other aid; and how far and in what ways they should ensure that recipients of their funds provide honest explanations of methods to clients and adequate health support for complications or side effects.

In migration and refugee programs, ethical principles affect decisions about who receives assistance and who does not. Are those decisions based mainly on the health and welfare needs of those to be served or on other criteria, such as racial or ethnic politics? This question is particularly salient in countries where the government controls donor access to areas in which its political opponents want to be evacuated. Donors must likewise make moral choices in designing programs for migrants or refugees. In interventions for disaster relief, they must often choose between strategies providing rapid action by outsiders, such as building homes, or slower methods of educating residents in how to become more self-sufficient (Parker). Instead of constructing new homes after an earthquake, donors might show community members how to build their own homes using earthquake-resistant methods of construction. The result could be greater self-sufficiency and better protection against future disasters.

Population ethics thus involves the application of moral principles to what are often complex empirical situations. Its greatest challenges are to select principles that are broadly applicable to population issues, rather than those that advance some specific interest, and to explore their implications with an adequate factual understanding of the circumstances involved.

DONALD P. WARWICK (1995)
REVISED BY RONALD M. GREEN

SEE ALSO: *Abortion; Aging and the Aged; Autonomy; Behavior Control; Environmental Ethics; Ethics: Normative Ethical Theories; Fertility Control; Future Generations, Reproductive Technologies and Obligations to; Life, Quality of; Natural Law; Population Policies, Strategies for Fertility Control in; Race and Racism; Women, Historical and Cross-Cultural Perspectives;* and other *Population Ethics* subentries

BIBLIOGRAPHY

Aird, John Shields. 1990. *Slaughter of the Innocents: Coercive Birth Control in China.* Washington, D.C.: AEI Press.

Ehrlich, Paul R., and Ehrlich, Anne H. 1990. *The Population Explosion.* New York: Simon and Schuster.

Gwatkin, Davidson R. 1979. "Political Will and Family Planning: The Implications of India's Emergency Experience." *Population and Development Review* 5(1): 29–59.

Hardin, Garrett James. 1993. *Living within Limits: Ecology, Economics, and Population Taboos.* New York: Oxford University Press.

Parker, Ronald S. 1994. *The Achievement of Educational Objectives: A Study of the A2Z Relief and Development Agency's Projects and Procedures under Emergency Conditions.* Doctoral dissertation, Harvard Graduate School of Education, Harvard University.

Simon, Julian Lincoln. 1990. *Population Matters: People, Resources, Environment, and Immigration.* New Brunswick, NJ: Transaction Publishers.

Ubinig. 1991. "'The Price of Norplant Is TK. 2000! You Cannot Remove It.' Clients Are Refused Removal in Norplant Trial in Bangladesh." *Issues in Reproductive and Genetic Engineering: Journal of International Feminist Analysis* 4(1): 45–46.

United Nations. 1975. *Report of the United Nations World Population Conference, 1974.* E/CONF.60/19. New York: United Nations.

World Bank. 1984. *World Development Report 1984.* New York: Oxford University Press.

I. ELEMENTS OF POPULATION ETHICS: B. IS THERE A POPULATION PROBLEM?

Policy analysts, the popular press, and scholars often speak of "the population problem." This phrase usually means that the existence of too many people on the planet will cause difficulties or even catastrophes for individuals, couples, countries, or the world. It can also mean that a country or region has too few people for its economic, social, or political welfare.

The first definition argues that rapid population growth, large population size, or high population density can bring widespread poverty, famine, air pollution, poor public health, drought, more children than can be educated in national school systems, overcrowded cities, or other serious harms. Under the second definition, too few people can reduce a country's population below the number that the government wants, decrease the size of the labor force, change the size and mix of ethnic groups in ways that can cause conflict, or create a population with few young and many old people. In either case the location of the problem can be the world, geographic regions such as sub-Saharan Africa, single countries, cities, or other regions within a country.

Those stating that there is a population problem base their assertions on three elements: perceived threats to social, moral, or political values; factual evidence; and theories explaining how population creates the conditions that threaten values. Much of the confusion in discussion of population problems arises from ambiguity or disagreement about these three elements.

Every statement of a population problem explicitly or implicitly expresses concern about values such as preventing famine, having an adequate number of workers and jobs, and giving couples the opportunity to determine their family size. Whether the concern is with too many or too few people, those stating that there is a problem always mention or allude to some moral, social, or political value. They also directly cite factual evidence to support their case or imply that this evidence exists. The evidence may be quantitative, such as figures on the relationship between population size and the number of teachers and schools in a country, or qualitative, such as the judgments of political scientists on a country's strength in foreign affairs, or a combination of the two. And every claim that there is a population problem involves a theory or conceptual scheme showing the links between too many or too few people and indicators of the values at stake in the discussion. Economic theories, for example, may try to show how, specifically, rapid population growth has created or will create unemployment.

Confusion about whether there is a population problem arises when analysts are vague about the values advanced or threatened by population size; omit relevant factual evidence; or use theories that have little validity. Advocates are vague about values advanced or threatened when they state that there is a population problem without indicating the social, moral, or political goods affected by population size. Some writers simply take it for granted that the world is now too crowded and go on to say what should be done about it. Omitting relevant factual evidence leads to charges of bias in statements about population problems. So does the use of theories that aim more at making the case for a problem than at objectively weighing the influence of population conditions.

Whether or not there is a population problem is critical to the ethics of population control. If rapid or limited population growth, population size, and population density do indeed cause serious damage, societies and governments will have some ethical justification for trying to change those conditions. If, on the other hand, pronouncements about population problems fail to state the values affected, are selective in their choice of factual evidence, or rely on dubious theories, the ethical justification for policies to deal with those problems will be tenuous.

The following discussion illustrates the complexity of making statements about population problems by comparing four approaches: those of Paul and Anne Ehrlich, the World Bank, the U.S. National Academy of Sciences, and Julian Simon. It reviews the values at stake in each approach, the completeness of the factual evidence cited, and the theories invoked to link population conditions to outcomes reflecting the values of concern.

Approaches to the Population Problem

In *The Population Bomb* Paul Ehrlich made this statement about population growth:

> The battle to feed all of humanity is over. In the 1970s and 1980s millions of people will starve to death.... Although many lives could be saved through dramatic programs to "stretch" the carrying capacity of the earth by increasing food production and providing for more equitable distribution of whatever food is available ... these programs will only provide a stay of execution unless they are accompanied by determined and successful efforts at population control. (p. xi)

During the 1970s and 1980s, high birthrates did not produce the levels of starvation Ehrlich predicted, in part because of the Green Revolution, which led to much higher food production than in the 1960s. Nonetheless, in their 1990 book *The Population Explosion* Paul and Anne Ehrlich continued to argue that the human race would face starvation and widespread disease unless societies immediately controlled their birthrates.

> Human inaction has already condemned hundreds of millions more people to premature deaths from hunger and disease. The population connection must be made in the public mind. Action to end the population explosion *humanely* and start a gradual population *decline* must become a top item on the human agenda: the human birthrate must be lowered to slightly below the human deathrate as soon as possible. (pp. 22–23)

The authors blame overpopulation for starvation in Africa, homelessness and drug abuse in the United States, global warming, holes in the atmosphere's ozone layer, fires in tropical forests, sewage-blighted beaches, and drought-stricken farm fields.

The World Bank has taken a different approach to the population problem. The *World Development Report 1984* (World Bank) acknowledges that the evidence on this subject is complex but concludes that "population growth at

the rapid rates common in most of the developing world slows development" (p. 105). This statement echoes the remarks of the Bank's president in the foreword: "What governments and their peoples do today to influence our demographic future will set the terms for development strategy well into the next century" (p. iii). In the World Bank's view, high fertility and rapid population growth bring on a problem by creating conditions, such as lower-quality education, that block economic development.

In 1971 the National Academy of Sciences (NAS) claimed that rapid population growth causes serious harm to economic development in sixteen ways. It holds down growth in per capita income; leads to unemployment and underemployment; creates mass poverty; distorts international trade; aggravates political, religious, linguistic, and ethnic conflicts; retards the mental and physical development of children; and has other negative consequences.

Fifteen years later the NAS (National Research Council, 1986) issued a report that backs away from the earlier conclusions. According to that report, slower population growth may benefit developing countries, but there is little evidence for judging whether its impact will be large or small. Furthermore, the results of population growth will depend not only on numbers of people but also on the effectiveness of government administration, social institutions, and the resources of specific countries. Thus, over a decade and a half the NAS shifted from a negative to a more neutral assessment of the impact of demographic growth.

Julian Simon (1990) gives a much more optimistic view of population growth than do the Ehrlichs, the World Bank, and the NAS. He first questions what he calls myths about population and resources. For example, while some say that the food situation in developing countries is worsening, Simon holds that per capita food production has been increasing about 1 percent each year. Responding to arguments that higher population growth means lower per capita economic growth, Simon states: "Empirical studies find no statistical correlation between countries' population growth and their per capita economic growth, either over the long run or in recent decades" (p. 45). Simon also offers evidence challenging statements that the world is running out of natural resources and raw materials and that energy is becoming more scarce.

Simon argues that having additional children improves productivity in the more developed countries and raises the standard of living in less developed countries. Over a period of thirty to seventy years in the more developed countries, each additional person contributes to increased knowledge and technical progress by "inventing, adapting, and diffusing new productive knowledge" (p. 48). Over the same time period in the less developed countries, more children lead to more work done by parents, stimulate agricultural and industrial investment, and bring other benefits. Simon calls people "the ultimate resource" and holds that population growth increases that resource.

The four approaches have different notions of how population growth affects economies and societies. The Ehrlichs are consistently gloomy about the impact of population growth on human societies. The World Bank is seriously concerned about its effects, and generally negative in its conclusions, but willing to consider different points of view and some evidence challenging its position. Like the World Bank, the NAS focuses on population growth and economic development, but comes to very different conclusions in its 1971 and 1986 reports. Simon plays down the harms and underscores the advantages of population growth for economic development and social welfare.

Values, Evidence, and Theories

The statements just reviewed show the difficulty of having a coherent discussion about "the population problem." The main reason is that the authors are concerned about different values, do not use all available factual evidence, and base their conclusions on different conceptual schemes and theories.

For Paul and Anne Ehrlich, central values include avoiding starvation, protecting the environment, preserving the world's resources, and maintaining public health: "*The Population Explosion* is being written as ominous changes in the life support systems of civilization become more evident daily. It is being written in a world where hunger is rife and the prospects of famine and plague ever more imminent" (p. 10). The World Bank shows greater concern with promoting economic growth, providing the world with adequate food supplies, having public services such as health and education, and protecting the environment. Both reports of the NAS address similar values. The values guiding Julian Simon's work include showing the benefits of population growth for human welfare and economic development; removing or reducing popular fears about population growth and the availability of resources; and convincing the public that "life on earth is getting better, not worse" (p. 21).

What evidence do these writers use, and how representative is that evidence of all that was available? In *The Population Bomb,* Paul Ehrlich does not try to be objective. He opens his first chapter with these words:

> I have understood the population explosion intellectually for a long time. I came to understand it emotionally one stinking hot night in Delhi a few

years ago. My wife and daughter and I were returning to our hotel in an ancient taxi. The seats were hopping with fleas. The only functional gear was third. As we crawled through the city we entered a crowded slum area. The temperature was well over 100, and the air was a haze of dust and smoke. The streets seemed alive with people. People eating, people washing, people sleeping. People visiting, arguing, and screaming…. People defecating and urinating. People clinging to buses. People herding animals. People, people, people, people. (p. 5)

Ehrlich goes on to specify the nature of the problem, summarize what is being done to deal with it, state what needs to be done, and tell readers what they can do to help. The book makes its case more by an appeal to the moral and political concerns of its readers than by presenting factual evidence.

The Population Explosion has a more scholarly tone, but still limits the findings presented to those that would be widely interpreted as supporting the authors' claims about overpopulation. It has chapters on shortages of food in developing countries; the difficulties facing agriculture; greenhouse warming, acid rain, and other damages to Earth's ecosystems; and urban air pollution, crowding, and hazards to public health. The Ehrlichs adduce no evidence challenging or qualifying their conclusions. They conclude with a chapter showing what readers can do to stop the population explosion.

Like the Ehrlichs, Simon gives a one-sided presentation of his findings. He contrasts popular views of bad news about population with the "unpublicized, good-news truth" (p. 42) deriving from his own analysis. He summarizes commonly cited statements, such as that the food situation in developing countries is growing worse, and then offers his own view under the heading of *fact.* Instead of presenting a balanced summary of research findings, he tries to attack the popular belief with as many findings as he can assemble that will be widely interpreted as contrary.

The World Bank (1984) admits that judging the evidence about the consequences of population growth is not easy and summarizes some conflicting views on that subject. But it does not mention dozens of cross-national studies that contradict its main conclusion, including work by Simon Kuznets (1974) and Ester Boserup (1965, 1981). This research shows no relationship between the rates of growth of population size and the growth rates of per capita income. Nor does the Bank's report explore the possibility, put forth by Boserup and Simon, that population size, population growth rate, and population density contribute to technological progress. According to one reviewer, "the Report can be evaluated from two different perspectives: as a position paper making the best case for a point of view; or as a summary of current knowledge. It is clearly much more successful as the first than as the second" (Lee, p. 129).

The two reports by the NAS are also mainly concerned with economic growth, but they differ in their approach to the studies they cite. The 1971 report selects evidence that supports its conclusions about the negative consequences of population growth and neglects research whose findings challenge or contradict those conclusions. The 1986 study is much better balanced in its coverage of the evidence and more cautious in arriving at conclusions. The authors draw a clear distinction, for example, between conditions caused by population growth and those only associated with such growth.

The four approaches also differ in their use of theories and conceptual schemes. In *The Population Bomb*, Paul Ehrlich has no social-scientific theory; he argues almost entirely by assertion. He assumes that the connections between population growth and conditions such as starvation are evident and therefore need no conceptual or theoretical justification. As is the case with their choice of evidence, in *The Population Explosion* Paul and Anne Ehrlich select only those conceptual frameworks showing the negative consequences of population growth. The World Bank recognizes the diversity of theories about the impact of population growth, but chooses a model that eliminates the possibility of any positive effects, such as those mentioned by Julian Simon. The 1971 NAS report also relies heavily on conceptual models showing the harms done by population growth. The 1986 NAS report applies concepts and theories allowing for a fairer evaluation of the relationships between population growth and economic development.

Much of the debate about whether there is a population problem and what it means stems from the different values and concerns behind statements of problems; selective use of evidence; and choosing theories to support preestablished conclusions rather than to arrive at impartial conclusions. Until analysts remove the ideology and biases commonly found in discussions about population problems, the confusion will continue.

The Population Problem: Where and When?

Most discussions of the population problem focus on the world at large or regions such as developing countries. It is also possible to examine the impact of population growth, size, and density on single countries. This is the focus of the work done by the Population Division of the Department of International Economic and Social Affairs (DIESA) of the United Nations (Chamie). The Population Division assumes that, whatever the impact of population size, density,

and growth across the world, single countries will have different views on what those concepts mean to them. Since the mid-1970s DIESA has maintained the Population Policy Data Bank to assess the perceptions and policies of governments regarding fertility.

At the end of the 1980s, 44 percent of U.N. member countries reported that their fertility levels were too high and 12 percent that they were too low (Chamie). If one defines a population problem as a government's perception that its fertility is either too high or too low, then 56 percent of U.N. member countries had a problem. The response to that problem depended on whether the governments thought that their fertility was too high or too low.

The first group, usually in countries with low per capita incomes, often set up programs of birth control. Countries reporting that their fertility is too low, such as France, Greece, Hungary, and Switzerland, adopt financial incentives and other policies to encourage more births (McIntosh). Singapore has been unusual in shifting from the perception that it would have too many people to its current view that it requires higher fertility. These differing perspectives show the importance of asking where and why population is a problem. While many studies focus on the world or on developing countries, the research done by DIESA underscores the importance of opinions and policies in single nations.

The single countries mentioned show agreement on the definition of a population problem. The value of most concern is the government's perception of whether it has too many, too few, or the right number of people. This may be a limited way of defining a population problem, but it does have a consistent point of reference: the views of the government. The evidence used is also the same: the information collected for the Population Policy Data Bank. Conceptual frameworks and theories differ about the reasons for governments' perceptions of a population problem and about why they do or do not take action on population issues. But consistency in the value behind the data and in the evidence used makes it much easier to compare definitions of population problems than in the four approaches outlined earlier.

Another critical question about population growth, size, and density is how they will affect the future. Paul Ehrlich's *The Population Bomb* and William and Paul Paddock's *Famine 1975* (1967) show that confident predictions of disasters are often wrong. But that experience does not mean students of population problems should stop looking to the future. Instead, they should make their predictions but be modest enough to indicate that, because they do not know everything that will happen between the time of writing and the time of the predicted event, they may be mistaken about the predicted events.

A related question concerns the obligations of the present generation to future ones. Do people living now have a duty to preserve the world so that future societies and individuals will have the resources and health conditions currently available? There is no simple answer. Over time, serious problems, such as the pollution of London a century ago, have been resolved and new problems, such as the depletion of water supplies in some regions, have arisen.

Two principles can help reflection on this topic. First, U.N. organizations and governments should pay explicit attention to the long-term consequences of population policies. Rather than taking a passive stance in debates on this topic, they should encourage and, if necessary, subsidize research on how population growth, population size, and population density affect the future. Second, the present generation has no right to adopt or accept population policies likely to damage the health and welfare of future generations. These might include actions leading to widespread environmental pollution, deforestation, and poor conditions of public health.

Recommendations

How can students of population policy reduce the bias now seen in many discussions of population problems and provide a solid basis for comparing different statements of those problems?

First, commentators should explicitly state the geographic focus of their analysis. Is it the universe? All the countries in the world? Some region of the world, such as sub-Saharan Africa or South America? A single country? Regions within a single country, such as cities or rural areas? Or some combination of those options, such as a country as a whole and its urban and rural areas? Given the great differences in population, economic, social, and political conditions across nations, specifying the geographic focus would immediately help observers to see similarities and differences across the territory covered. Tables such as those in the World Bank's annual *World Development Report* would be helpful for that purpose.

Second, those discussing population problems should indicate the moral, social, or political values of concern in their analysis. This recommendation should apply whether the observer claims that the region being analyzed has too many, too few, or an adequate number of people. Values often found, explicitly or implicitly, in such analyses include

promoting economic growth; preserving the environment; preventing a decline in the region's population; increasing the size of the dominant ethnic group or changing the sizes of ethnic minorities; and maintaining the availability of schools and other social services for the region's inhabitants.

Third, scholarly analyses of population problems should use all relevant evidence rather than just studies that support the author's point of view. Discussions of population growth and economic development should make full use of the numerous cross-national comparisons on that subject. When, as often happens, the sources of evidence lead to different conclusions, that situation should be mentioned.

Fourth, those discussing population problems should specify the theories or conceptual frameworks guiding their analysis. It is particularly important to indicate how population conditions, such as growth rates and size, influence conditions such as economic growth or the availability of schools. Many publications have used conceptual models that attribute more influence to population than it deserves, partly because other relevant influences are not considered. Such is the case with the 1971 NAS study on the consequences of rapid population growth. By using a more thorough conceptual framework and considering a broader range of evidence, the 1986 NAS study in effect retracts many of the conclusions in the 1971 report.

Fifth, conclusions should be based on the results of careful conceptual or theoretical analysis and the weight of the evidence rather than on a priori judgments by the authors. Following this recommendation will often mean reporting contradictory or inconsistent evidence and arriving at qualified judgments. The greatest single source of confusion in present statements on population problems is a strong ideological bias in writing. This bias has led to vagueness about the values at stake, use of incomplete theories and conceptual schemes, citation only of those parts of the evidence consistent with the authors' preconceptions, and conclusions based more on ideology than on a fair assessment of the evidence.

Sixth, policy recommendations in statements about population problems should be based on the evidence presented rather than on the personal preferences of the authors or the donors who have supported them. For example, after a lengthy discussion of the links between population growth and economic development, the 1986 NAS report suggests that governments should establish family-planning programs. This recommendation has little to do with the main lines of the report, which says nothing about family planning. This practice is intellectually misleading, for it suggests that the policy suggestions flow directly from the scholarly analysis, which in this case they do not.

Conclusions

Is there a population problem? When the focus is on single countries, when the source of information is the Population Policy Data Bank maintained by the United Nations, and when the definition of the population problem is the government's opinion on whether it has too many, too few, or the right number of people, it is possible to answer that question. But when the focus is on the world as a whole, and authors are concerned with different values, use different theories and sources of evidence, and become advocates for a particular point of view, there is and can be no answer.

To have more comparable notions of population problems, authors must clearly identify the geographical region they are discussing; indicate the values of concern to them; use all available evidence; apply theories or conceptual schemes that consider all relevant influences; weigh the evidence objectively; and draw only those conclusions supported by their analysis. The ideological discourse seen in current discussions of population problems must give way to scholarly analysis. When these criteria are met, more accurate, less biased, and more comparable discussions of population problems will be available.

DONALD P. WARWICK (1995)

SEE ALSO: *Abortion; Aging and the Aged: Life Expectancy and Life Span; Children; Climate Change; Endangered Species and Biodiversity; Environmental Ethics; Epidemics; Fertility Control; Genetics and Environment in Human Health; Hazardous Wastes and Toxic Substances; International Health; Life, Quality of;* and other *Population Ethics* subentries

BIBLIOGRAPHY

Boserup, Ester. 1965. *The Conditions of Agricultural Growth: The Economics of Agrarian Change under Population Pressure.* Chicago: Aldine.

Boserup, Ester. 1981. *Population and Technological Change: A Study of Long-Term Trends.* Chicago: University of Chicago Press.

Chamie, Joseph. 1994. "Trends, Variations, and Contradictions in National Policies to Influence Fertility." *Population and Development Review* 20 (supp.): 37–50. Reprinted in *The New Politics of Population: Conflict and Consensus in Family Planning,* ed. Jason L. Finkle and C. Allison McIntosh. New York: Population Council.

Ehrlich, Paul R. 1971. (1968). *The Population Bomb,* rev. edition. New York: Ballantine.

Ehrlich, Paul R., and Ehrlich, Anne H. 1990. *The Population Explosion.* New York: Simon and Schuster.

Kuznets, Simon Smith. 1974. *Population, Capital and Growth: Selected Essays.* New York: Norton.

Lee, Ronald. 1985. "World Development Report 1984: Review Symposium." *Population and Development Review* 11(1): 127–130.

McIntosh, C. Allison. 1986. "Recent Pronatalist Policies in Western Europe." *Population and Development Review* 12 (supp.): 318–334.

National Academy of Sciences (U.S.). Office of the Foreign Secretary. 1971. *Rapid Population Growth: Consequences and Policy Implications.* Baltimore: Johns Hopkins University Press.

National Research Council (U.S.). Commission on Behavioral and Social Sciences Education. Committee on Population. Working Group on Population Growth and Economic Development. 1986. *Population Growth and Economic Development: Policy Questions.* Washington, D.C.: National Academy Press.

Paddock, William, and Paddock, Paul. 1967. *Famine 1975!* Boston: Little, Brown.

Simon, Julian L. 1990. *Population Matters: People, Resources, Environment, and Immigration.* Brunswick, NJ: Transaction.

World Bank. 1984. *World Development Report 1984.* New York: Oxford University Press.

I. ELEMENTS OF POPULATION ETHICS: C. HISTORY OF POPULATION THEORIES

Ancient and Medieval Theories

Like most general theories of Western civilization, those concerning population evolved first in ancient Greece. Both policies and their conceptual frameworks varied in their details, but there was much consistency from one city-state to another. The typical pronatalist policies were intended not to induce a growth in numbers but to prevent their decline (Stangeland, chap. 1; Hutchinson, chap. 2). In the ideal city-state that Plato pictured in *Laws,* the population was to be kept stable at 5,040 (the product of $1 \times 2 \times 3 \times 4 \times 5 \times 6 \times 7$) by encouraging or inhibiting fertility or by infanticide. If the population grew much beyond this optimum, the community was to establish colonies. To neglect measures that would keep the population more or less fixed, according to Aristotle, would "bring certain poverty on the citizens, and poverty is the cause of sedition and evil" (*Politics,* 2.9).

Greek thought on population, in sum, was characterized by an overriding concern with policy, and thus a relative indifference to empirical or conceptual analysis. Policy was to be applied, moreover, to aggregates ridiculously small by present-day standards. And whether the meaning of *population* was in accord with the modern sense is often not clear; in most instances the term may have referred only to citizens, thus omitting females, children, slaves, and aliens.

In its far larger arena, Rome's policy was more consistently pronatalist. As imperial hegemony spread from Italy throughout the Mediterranean basin and beyond, the center was troubled by moral decay, the dissolution of the family, and a slower growth of population. Successive pronatalist measures culminated in three enactments under Augustus (63 B.C.E.–14 C.E.), which punished celibacy and adultery and rewarded prolific couples (Stangeland, pp. 30–38). Since they had little apparent effect, the laws were repeatedly amended and finally repealed under Constantine (ca. 288–337).

As the empire gradually disintegrated, many came to believe that the end of the world was imminent, and various sects offered competing dogmas appropriate to the apocalypse. The early Christian church gradually developed its own doctrine with a compromise between libertine and ascetic, but emphasizing the latter (Noonan). Catholic thought reached its apogee in the *Summa Theologica* of Thomas Aquinas (ca. 1224–1274). For him, a marriage between Christians is not merely a means of obeying the injunction to replenish the earth but also a spiritual bond, a sacrament. The function of intercourse is procreation (Bourke).

Early Modern Theory

The dominant theme of the early modern period was the view that population growth is precarious and has to be fostered. Just as the mercantilist state hoarded gold, so it hoarded people, and for the same reason—to increase its economic, political, and military power. If rapid population growth resulted in what was termed "overcrowding," the mercantilist solution was to ship the surplus to colonies, where the settlers and their progeny could continue to aggrandize the state's power in another quarter of the globe.

Modern demography began with the efforts of mercantilist states to keep track of their populations (Glass). William Petty (1623–1687) was the first exponent of what he called "political arithmetic." John Graunt (1620–1674) constructed the first crude life table. Gregory King (1648–1712) calculated population estimates based on local enumerations, which he corrected for technical errors. On the Continent, Johann Peter Süssmilch (1707–1767) used Protestant parish records to estimate Prussia's fertility and mortality. Richard Cantillon (ca. 1680–1734) held that

internal migration, deaths, and especially marriages (and therefore births) varied according to the prevailing standard of living and the structure of the demand for labor. François Quesnay (1694–1774), who founded what was later called physiocratic thought, analyzed the implicit bounds to population growth.

The philosophes of eighteenth-century France varied greatly on many issues, but most also found reason to favor policies stimulating population growth. Charles-Louis de Secondat, Baron Montesquieu (1689–1755), believed that the entire world had undergone depopulation and recommended pronatalist decrees. According to Voltaire (1694–1778), a nation is fortunate if its population increases by as much as 5 percent per century. Louis de St.-Just (1767–1794) held that one can usually depend on nature "never to have more children than teats," but to keep the balance in the other direction requires the state's assistance. By this notion of an equitable family law, as inspired by Jean-Jacques Rousseau (1712–1778), marriages should be encouraged by state loans, and a couple that remained childless after several years ought to be forcibly separated.

The two utopians that Thomas Robert Malthus opposed in the first edition of his *Essay on the Principle of Population,* William Godwin (1756–1836) and Marie-Jean Caritat, Marquis de Condorcet (1743–1794), focused their attention on the wholly rational age they discerned just over the horizon. According to them, in a world from which diseases had been wholly eliminated, the span of life would have no assignable upper limit. People would devote themselves to more important tasks than, in Condorcet's words, "the puerile idea of filling the earth with useless and unhappy beings."

Malthus

Malthus summarized or contravened earlier ideas so effectively that, for more than a century and a half, subsequent theorists have generally taken him as a benchmark. Unfortunately, many references to "Malthusian" thought are based, at best, on the first edition of *Essay on the Principle of Population* rather than on the much enlarged and thoroughly revised later editions—or, at worst, on a total misunderstanding of what he stood for (Petersen, 1979, chap. 4).

Thomas Robert Malthus (1766–1834) was a professor at the newly founded East India College, occupying Britain's first chair in the new discipline of political economy. He spent much of his life collecting data on the relation between population and its social, economic, and natural environments, bringing his theory into accord with these facts and adjusting it to criticism. There were seven editions of the *Essay* in all.

According to the principle of population as expounded in the *Essay*, population, "when unchecked," doubles once every generation. Among "irrational animals" this potential is realized, and its "superabundant effects are repressed afterwards by want of room or nourishment." But rational human beings can consider the consequences of their reproductive potential and curb their natural drive. With humans, thus, there are two types of control of population growth: "preventive checks," the chaste postponement of marriage, and "positive checks," the deaths resulting from too large a population relative to its subsistence. Tension between numbers and food can have a beneficial effect: A man who postpones marrying until he is able to support a family is goaded by his sex drive to work hard, thus contributing to social progress. For this reason Malthus opposed contraceptives, for their use permits individual sexual gratification with no benefit to society.

Through the successive editions of the *Essay*, Malthus increasingly stressed the negative correlation between station in life and size of family. This, in his view, was the principal clue to solving what later became known as "the population problem." In order to bring the lower classes up to the self-control and social responsibility exercised by those with more money and education, Malthus asserted, the poor should be given more money and education. "The principal circumstances" that induce prospective parents to have fewer children are "liberty, security of property, the diffusion of knowledge, and a taste for the comforts of life." Those that tend to increase procreation are "despotism and ignorance." The thesis that upward mobility into the middle class effects a decline in fertility, though it is far less familiar than that relating population growth to food, is in retrospect Malthus's most important contribution.

For many decades Malthus's reputation was far below that of lesser social analysts. Recently it has become apparent that much of present-day demography was at least partly stimulated by Malthus and that those who denounced him as a false prophet had typically begun by misrepresenting his ideas.

Population Optima

Most of the populations that Malthus discussed tended to grow too rapidly relative to the available resources, and he recommended institutional checks to their fertility. But the extraordinarily rapid growth of the American colonies, whose population was doubling every twenty-five years, he held to be of great benefit. In other words, each country has an optimum size and rate of growth, depending on the social and economic conditions. Malthus neither used the term *optimum* nor developed the concept beyond an implicit statement, but he planted the seed of the theory. Malthus's principle that the population tends to increase by a geometrical ratio and food by an arithmetical ratio can be reformulated as a law of diminishing returns. If to a fixed acreage of land more and more labor is added, return per person may first rise but then will decline as the work force increases beyond its most efficient size. The first definition of "the optimum" was based on this schema: It is that population which under given conditions produces the highest per capita economic return.

Soon, however, the optimum came to mean simply "the best population," with each analyst furnishing a particular yardstick of what is "good." By this route the theory of population optimum could be regarded as a version of social choice theory, with a wide variety of open questions (Dasgupta). Should the population be related to the present institutional structure or to some supposed future ("socialism," for instance)? Should the criterion of "good" be economic welfare, military strength, the conservation of resources, or some combination of these? This conundrum is aggravated by the fact that optima vary greatly, according to the goal that society sets. And should the standard relate exclusively to the number of people or also to their age structure, rate of growth, level of skill, and other characteristics that affect how efficiently the society can operate?

Obviously, no judgment concerning "the optimum" can be very precise. Whether a country of western Europe, say, is underpopulated or overpopulated is less a demographic-economic measurement than a more or less arbitrary opinion. The norm can be applied meaningfully only at the extremes. The colonies that became the United States were definitely underpopulated, as Malthus pointed out. And in some of today's less developed countries, by the judgment of most demographers, the rapidly growing populations impede a rise in the people's well-being.

Migration

We are all born and we all die, but only some of us move from one place to another. Unlike fertility and mortality, migration is not a biological process. Indeed, many determinants of migration are political: Movements are subsidized, restricted, or forced, and the status of migrants in their new homeland depends on the state's laws on aliens. If we conceive of migration following the usual definition—as the relatively permanent movement of persons over a significant distance—the specifications "permanent" and "significant" must be set by more or less arbitrary criteria. Partly for this reason, migration statistics are generally imprecise and subject to capricious interpretation.

Migration changes the size of population and the rate of growth in the two areas involved, but usually not in the simple fashion that common sense suggests. Most migrants are young adults, and their movement changes the age structure, and thus the birth and death rates, in both areas. Given a sedentary population and a stimulus to emigrate, typically some leave and some do not. There is self-selection by age, sex, family status, and occupation, as well as possibly by intelligence, mental health, and independence of character. Since migration is not unitary, it cannot be analyzed in supracultural terms but must be differentiated even at the most abstract level with respect to the social conditions obtaining. Generalizations about migration, thus, developed mostly outside of standard population theories.

Demographic Transition

The number of people in the world is increasing at an unprecedented rate to unprecedented totals, and the basic reason is no mystery: Mortality has fallen sharply, and in many areas fertility has not. As originally formulated (e.g., Landry), this so-called demographic transition was conceived as taking place in three broad stages: (1) preindustrial societies, with high fertility more or less balanced by high mortality and a consequent low natural increase; (2) societies in transition, with continuing high fertility but declining mortality and a consequent rapid natural increase; and (3) modern societies, with both fertility and mortality stabilized at low levels and a consequent more or less static population. In its barest form this theory is one of the best-documented generalizations in the social sciences.

Collapsing the whole of human history into these three demographic types means, of course, that not only details but also important distinctions are passed over. When actual populations are reconstituted, so simplistic a theory often proves to be less a guide to research or policy than an invitation to misunderstanding. And this has been so concerning each of the three stages (Chesnais).

It is assumed that the mortality of primitive peoples was high relative to that in advanced societies, but estimates of the longevity in ancient times can hardly be very precise. Whether or not preindustrial peoples were warlike, lived in a favorable climate, developed cultural norms promoting cleanliness, and so on certainly influenced their death rates. And the usual formula—that since the mortality of primitive humans was high, their fertility must have been close to the physiological maximum if the group was to survive—is also questionable. From an early survey of contemporary primitive cultures, Alexander Carr-Saunders (1922) concluded that *all* of them included customs intended to restrict the increase of population. There is no reason a priori to postulate that all prehistoric peoples reproduced like unthinking animals, incurring the cost of a subsequent unnecessarily high mortality.

In stage two, the first steps toward a modern industrial society bring about a decline in mortality—but also often, contrary to the theory, a rise in fertility. Improved health can result in greater physiological ability to reproduce. Whatever means had been used to reduce population growth, such as infanticide in Tokugawa Japan, may not survive modernization. If the age at marriage had been set well past puberty, as in early modern western Europe, the institutions bolstering this norm often became less effective. Religious practices or taboos unintentionally inhibiting fertility, such as the one prohibiting the remarriage of widows in Hindu India, may dissipate. Most remarkably, family-planning programs can result in a rise in fertility, for if women are able to depend on controls later in their reproductive life, many begin childbearing at an earlier age. In short, the effect of modernization is partly to increase fertility and partly to decrease it (Heer).

Moreover, the early analysts of the demographic transition failed to forecast the decline of mortality in less-developed countries. Over the past two centuries or so, as the main advances were applied in medicine, surgery, public sanitation, agriculture, and nutrition, Western populations gradually improved in health and longevity. During the last several decades, however, some of the most recent techniques have been transferred to areas lacking most prior scientific controls; peoples cared for until recently by witch doctors acquired access to antibiotics. In Ceylon (now Sri Lanka), to take one striking example, the estimated expectation of life at birth increased from forty-three years in 1946 to fifty-two in 1947; the gain achieved in this one year had taken half a century in most Western countries.

Efforts to Reduce Fertility

Because of the continuing high fertility and the sharp decline of mortality in less-developed countries, their populations have grown at rates high enough to stimulate widespread control measures. Some of these programs have been successful, but many have achieved far less than their proponents hoped they would, in part because none has an appropriate theory underlying it.

Is a large and rapidly growing population indeed a problem? Leaders of the independence movements of pre-1940 European colonies held that their countries' poverty derived not from excessive procreation but from imperial misrule, and this view often persisted after independence. The very slow start of India's programs to check its population growth, for instance, was due in part to Jawaharlal Nehru's initial ambivalence. Among those who accept the thesis that too many people can impede modernization, proponents have often advocated *either* birth control *or* industrialization, as though one or the other were the sole relevant factor.

The theories underlying birth-control programs, often implicit rather than spelled out in papers, reports, or books, can be summed up in the following propositions:

1. *Elements of "traditional" society constitute the principal impediment to the spread of contraception.* But, as we have noted, most traditional cultures include antinatalist tendencies and, on the other hand, modern nationalism is often strongly pronatalist.

2. *The most important variable in any program is the contraceptive means to be used.* But the history of the West suggests that, given the will to reduce fertility, people will make effective use of whatever means are available to them—coitus interruptus and illegal abortion in France, postponed marriage or nonmarriage in Ireland, and so on.

3. *The agency through which contraception can be most effectively disseminated is the state.* But this contradicts, again, the history of the decline of Western fertility, where officialdom typically opposed the private neo-Malthusian leagues and their successors.

4. *Population policy can be equated essentially with family policy: That is, zero population growth can be realized by inducing each pair of parents to have an average of only two children.* But the rate of growth depends also on the proportion of the population that is of childbearing age, and in less-developed countries that is generally very high.

5. *It is so important that the population crisis be solved that policy-oriented action and knowledge-oriented research must be collapsed into a single operation.* This procedure violates the scientific canon that truth can be effectively sought only in a setting made as value-free as possible. As a consequence, field workers and analysts are encouraged to accept spurious results as valid, for it is very difficult to ascertain the actual sentiments and behavior patterns of respondents.

In sum, the many attempts to reduce fertility in less-developed countries have typically been made with little regard to what had been learned from the prior decline in family size in the industrial West. Perhaps the best link between the two is the wealth-flow theory, so designated by John Caldwell. The crucial factor is whether children are productively useful to their parents and care for them in their old age; if so, as in African cultures he studied, the incentive is to procreate to the maximum feasible. If, however, parents incur net costs for the long-term care and education of their children, who generally contribute little to household finances, the inevitable tendency is to reduce the number brought into the world. By concentrating on the family budget, Caldwell (1982) was able to elucidate both the historical decline of fertility in the West and the partial success of family-planning programs in less-developed countries.

Theories of Population in Totalitarian Countries

A focus on economic or cultural factors can mean that political influences on fertility are bypassed. More generally, theories developed in the democratic West are in many respects ill suited to analyze such past totalitarian societies as the Soviet Union and Nazi Germany. Though their cultures differed greatly, these two countries had certain features in common, many of which related to population theory and its application.

1. The Nazi party and the Communist party were defined as omnipotent, able to cope with any increase in population. According to the first Soviet delegate to the U.N. Population Commission, "I would consider it barbaric for the Commission to contemplate a limitation of marriages or of legitimate births, and this for any country whatsoever, at any period whatsoever. With an adequate social organization it is possible to face any increase in population" (quoted by Sauvy, vol. 1, p. 174; cf. Petersen, 1988).

2. Population theory had the same purpose as any other science—to bolster the power of the party in power (Besemeres). In particular, the need of the totalitarian state for labor was reflected in theories on how to maintain a high rate of population growth and in such applications as family subsidies.

3. Efforts to stimulate the birthrate, however, were hampered by the ruling party's hostility to the family, which by its legal and emotional links between generations helps to maintain a traditional opposition to radically new ideas and practices. Both Nazi Germany and the Soviet Union tried to establish institutions that could replace the family, such as brothels in which SS men could impregnate young women certified as racially pure, or the Soviet children's homes in which the state could convert orphans and the offspring of political dissidents into reliable instruments of the Communist party. But such substitutes never produced a large enough crop,

and policy toward the family therefore vacillated in both countries.

4. The need for a high fertility was enhanced by the recklessness with which sectors of the population designated as hostile or inferior were killed off. The terror most closely associated with the Nazis was the mass slaughter of Jews, based on the outpouring of writings on *Rassenkunde* (race science). More often Communists defined their victims as class enemies (though antagonism to ethnic minorities was also a constant element of Soviet life), but the difference was not fundamental: The slaughter began in different sectors of the population and was sometimes concentrated there, but in both cases it spread to the whole society (Hilberg; Conquest).

5. Totalitarian ideology was based on what in German is called *Stufenlehre,* a doctrine of stages. All analysis, all planning, began not in the empirical present but in the inevitable perfect future, homogenized into a "classless" (*Judenfrei,* "Jewless") sameness. The road to this paradise could be seen clearly only by the Nazi party and the Communist party, whose function was to move the rest of the population toward its destiny. The ruthless terror that was often needed was warranted, thus, by the glorious community that would ensue.

Conclusions

Intellectual history includes few population theories in the narrow sense; most theories were developed as usually minor adjuncts to systematic statements about the society or the economy. Even this thin conceptual framework, however, may have profound ethical implications, for long before anything scientific was known about the determinants and consequences of population growth, statesmen, theologians, and scholars proposed—and their societies sometimes adopted as policies—rules of behavior allegedly suitable to their environment.

Until the modern era, the usual policy orientation was pronatalist, for it was generally assumed both that more people were better than fewer and that realizing a faster growth required state aid. Though not the first to take a contrary position, Malthus was by far the most important. Paradoxically, the greatly increased concern with policy in recent decades has not been accompanied by a more precise definition of goals. The judgment of whether a population is too large or too small obviously depends on a reasonably precise designation of the optimum, which has remained perhaps the most controversial concept in demography.

In past times, tyrants and conquering armies slaughtered many aliens, variously defined, but the combination of ruthless nationalism with scientific means of disposing of "inferior" sectors of the population is an innovation of the twentieth century. Partly because of a reaction against totalitarian genocide, demographers have given less systematic attention than warranted to such population characteristics as health or skill, though in many contexts these may be more important than mere numbers.

In recent decades the most striking characteristic of demography has been the attempt to dispense with theory in the solution of population problems widely recognized as critical. The substitution of "concern" for competence has not led, however, to many successes. In spite of the proliferation of antinatalist programs in less-developed countries and of the numbers of potential parents who accept the contraceptives made available, the world's population continues to grow at a rapid rate.

WILLIAM PETERSEN (1995)

SEE ALSO: *Eugenics; Family and Family Medicine; Fertility Control; Infanticide; International Health; Public Health; Sustainable Development; Women, Historical and Cross-Cultural Perspectives;* and other *Population Ethics* subentries

BIBLIOGRAPHY

Besemeres, John F. 1980. *Socialist Population Politics: The Political Implications of Demographic Trends in the USSR and Eastern Europe.* White Plains, NY: M. E. Sharpe.

Bourke, Vernon J. 1967. "Thomas Aquinas, St." In *Encyclopedia of Philosophy,* vol. 8, pp. 105–116. New York: Macmillan.

Caldwell, John. 1982. *Theory of Fertility Decline.* New York: Academic Press.

Carr-Saunders, Alexander Morris. 1922. *The Population Problem: A Study in Human Evolution.* Oxford: Clarendon Press.

Chesnais, Jean-Claude. 1986. *La transition démographique: Étapes, formes, implications économiques: Étude de séries temporelles (1720–1984) relative à 67 pays.* Institut national d'études démographiques travaux et documents, cahier no. 113. Paris: Presses universitaires de France.

Conquest, Robert. 1990. *The Great Terror: A Reassessment.* New York: Oxford University Press.

Dasgupta, Partha. 1987. "The Ethical Foundations of Population Policy." In *Population Growth and Economic Development: Issues and Evidence,* pp. 631–659, ed. D. Gale Johnson and Ronald D. Lee. Madison: University of Wisconsin Press.

Glass, David V. 1973. *Numbering the People: The Eighteenth-Century Population Controversy and the Development of Census and Vital Statistics in Britain.* Farnborough, U.K.: Saxon House.

Heer, David M. 1966. "Economic Development and Fertility." *Demography* 3: 423–444.

Hilberg, Raul. 1973. *The Destruction of the European Jews.* New York: New Viewpoints.

Hutchinson, Edward Prince. 1967. *The Population Debate: The Development of Conflicting Theories up to 1900.* New York: Houghton Mifflin.

Landry, Adolphe. 1934. *La révolution démographique: Études et essais sur les problèmes de la population.* Paris: Librairie du Recueil Sirey.

Noonan, John Thomas, Jr. 1965. *Contraception: A History of Its Treatment by the Catholic Theologians and Canonists.* Cambridge, MA: Belknap Press.

Petersen, William. 1979. *Malthus.* Cambridge, MA: Harvard University Press.

Petersen, William. 1988. "Marxism and the Population Question: Theory and Practice." *Population and Development Review* 14 (supp.): 77–101, ed. Michael S. Teitelbaum and Jay M. Winter. Also published under the title *Population in Western Intellectual Traditions.* Cambridge, Eng.: Cambridge University Press, 1989.

Sauvy, Alfred. 1952. *Théorie générale de la population.* 2 vols. Paris: Presses universitaires de France.

Stangeland, Charles Emil. 1904. *Pre-Malthusian Doctrines of Population: A Study in the History of Economic Theory.* New York: Columbia University Press.

II. NORMATIVE APPROACHES

Population policies raise profound questions of ethics. Is China justified in using coercion to enforce its policy of one child per couple? Is it legitimate for government officials and community peers in Indonesia to apply strong pressure to promote birth control? Should U.S. judges be free to require the insertion of Norplant, a long-lasting, subdermal contraceptive, when sentencing women they consider unfit to be mothers (Feringa et al.)? Do the wealthiest nations of the world have a moral obligation to accept refugees from poor countries?

Answers to such questions require ethical principles applicable to population policies across all countries and cultures. Principles that reflect the standards of only one country or region, such as the United States or Europe, may not persuade leaders and peoples of other countries.

Three schools of thought have guided debates on these principles. The first argues that government programs of any kind must respect human rights as stated in the Universal Declaration of Human Rights adopted by the United Nations in 1948; the International Covenant on Economic, Social, and Cultural Rights (1976); the International Covenant on Civil and Political Rights (1976); and many related U.N. statements (Nickel; Claude and Weston). A second school holds that the morality of population interventions must be determined by the country that carries them out, for

it has the problem and best understands how to deal with it. This school accepts no universal standards of human rights. It considers attempts by others to impose such standards to be infringements on national sovereignty. The third school recognizes some or all of the human rights affirmed by the United Nations, but claims that when population growth or density create desperate economic or social problems for a country, its government has the right to limit individual reproductive freedom for the common good.

This article develops a framework of ethical principles based on the Universal Declaration of Human Rights, later U.N. statements on human rights, and regional declarations on the same subject, particularly the European Convention on Human Rights. It then applies those principles to population policies. It concludes by contrasting this approach with another ethical framework known as "stepladder ethics."

Five Key Principles

Ethical evaluation of population policies requires five principles to guide decisions as well as criteria for determining when one principle can be sacrificed for another.

Life heads the list, for without it people cannot benefit from the other four principles. Article 3 of the Universal Declaration of Human Rights states: "Everyone has the right to life, liberty and security of person." The International Covenant on Civil and Political Rights is more specific: "Every human being has the inherent right to life. This right shall be protected by law. No one shall be arbitrarily deprived of his life" (Part III, Article 6).

Life means not only being alive, but enjoying good health and having reasonable security against the actions of others that cause death, illness, severe pain, or disability. Policies on fertility control, migration, and refugees threaten this principle when they take no action to assist people facing starvation or slaughter and when they create incentives for female infanticide (Aird; Brown and Shue). Policies endanger health when they promote methods of fertility control, such as sterilizations, oral contraceptives, the intrauterine device (IUD), or injections, that can pose grave risks to physical well-being. Among such risks are cardiovascular diseases, tubal infertility, pelvic inflammatory disease, and septic abortion (National Research Council, 1989; Schearer). Fertility-control programs may also damage the health of users when they overlook sexually transmitted diseases, such as gonorrhea, or other reproductive-tract infections, including genital herpes, chancroid, genital warts, vaginal infections, and infections of the upper reproductive tract (Dixon-Mueller and Wasserheit).

Freedom is the capacity and opportunity to make reflective choices and to act on those choices. Freedom requires knowledge about the choices available, such as options for fertility control or migration; a chance to make choices without coercion or strong pressure from others; awareness that one is making choices and of the issues at stake in each; and the possibility of taking action to carry out the choices made (Warwick, 1982, 1990; Veatch). Restrictions on any of these conditions, such as ignorance of options, decisions made while an individual is being tortured, or barriers to acting on choices made, void or limit freedom.

U.N. statements strongly endorse freedom. According to the Universal Declaration, everyone has the right to freedom of thought, conscience, and religion (Article 18); freedom of opinion and expression (Article 19); freedom of peaceful assembly and association (Article 20); freedom from slavery and servitude (Article 4); and freedom from arbitrary interference with privacy, family, home, or correspondence (Article 12). Both the International Covenant on Economic, Social, and Cultural Rights and the International Covenant on Civil and Political Rights open with this statement: "All peoples have the right of self-determination. By virtue of that right they freely determine their political status and freely pursue their economic, social, and cultural development" (Part I, Article 1, in both covenants). In the World Population Plan of Action developed at the World Population Conference in 1974, delegates agreed to the following statement on reproductive freedom: "All couples and individuals have the basic right to decide freely and responsibly the number and spacing of their children and to have the information, education, and means to do so …" (World Population Conference, p. 7).

Welfare means a standard of living adequate to provide food, clothing, housing, healthcare, and education. Affirmed in Articles 25 and 26 of the Universal Declaration, this standard was both repeated and broadened in the International Covenant on Economic, Social, and Cultural Rights. That statement spoke specifically about the right to continuous improvement in living conditions; the steps needed to protect the right to be free from hunger; the right of everyone to the highest attainable standard of physical and mental health; the widest possible protection and assistance for the family; special protection for mothers before and after childbirth; and protection of children and young persons from social and economic exploitation, including work that threatens their lives or is harmful to their morals and health. The World Population Plan of Action of 1974 also explicitly tied population policies to human welfare: "The principal aim of social, economic, and cultural development, of which population goals and policies are integral parts, is to improve levels of living and the quality of life of the people" (World Population Conference, p. 7). Population programs, therefore, should not aim only to raise or lower fertility, reduce mortality, or control migration, but to be instruments for promoting human welfare.

Fairness refers to an equitable distribution of the benefits and harms from population policies. It does not require an equal distribution of benefits and harms, but it does demand that one individual or group should not receive disproportionate advantages or disadvantages from a given policy. The Universal Declaration strongly endorses fairness in Article 1: "All human beings are born free and equal in dignity and rights." Article 2 continues: "Everyone is entitled to all the rights and freedoms set forth in this Declaration, without distinction of any kind, such as race, colour, sex, language, religion, political or other opinion, national or social origin, property, birth, or other status." The 1967 U.N. Protocol Relating to the Status of Refugees established principles for determining fairness in refugee and immigration policies.

In 1972, Ugandan President Idi Amin Dada ordered the expulsion of between 40,000 and 50,000 Asians living in Uganda. His action is an extreme example of the unfairness seen when the costs of population policy are borne by a single ethnic group. India's use of coercion to promote sterilization among beggars and other poor people between 1975 and 1977 was another case of unfair policy implementation (Gwatkin). Other examples include the testing only in low-income areas of contraceptives designed for all women (Holmes et al.), and failing to tell uneducated candidates for sterilization how this operation is carried out, what it means for fertility, and what medical risks and side effects accompany it. In each of these cases the political, economic, social, and medical harms of population interventions fall more heavily on one group than another.

Truth telling requires accurate information about population policies and avoiding lies, misrepresentations, distortions, and evasions about their content, implementation, and consequences. Though truth telling is not explicitly stated in U.N. declarations of human rights, it is a prerequisite for the other four principles cited. Lies about policies of fertility control, migration, and refugees can jeopardize human life when they involve fatal risks, such as death from infections or from being shot in enemy territory. They limit freedom by depriving individuals of the knowledge necessary to make an informed choice, such as information about the side effects of sterilization. Lies harm welfare when they cause risk to one's income, education, or job prospects, and they violate fairness when they are more likely to be told to one group, such as the poor or an ethnic minority, than to others.

Life, freedom, welfare, fairness, and truth telling can conflict with each other. Faced with what they see as excessive population growth, government officials may claim that the common welfare demands restrictions on reproductive freedom and allows distortions of the truth, such as not disclosing the medical risks of contraceptives, in order to make birth control seem attractive. Also citing the national interest, political leaders may decide to exterminate members of a specific religion, such as Jews in German territory during World War II; expel an entire ethnic group from the country, as happened in Uganda; or put severe limits on the entry of immigrants they define as hostile to the national interest, as happened when the U.S. government used ships to block the entry of Haitian refugees in the early 1990s. All three policies subordinate fairness toward religious and ethnic groups to local definitions of the common welfare. Are such policies justified, or are there some principles that cannot be sacrificed to promote others?

The Universal Declaration puts no relative weights on the many rights it endorses. However, later agreements do set priorities among rights. In Article 15, the European Convention on Human Rights states that even in national emergencies, governments cannot use murder, torture, degrading punishments, slavery, or servitude. These rights thus hold the highest rank. Nothing, including government concerns about the damage due to population growth, can override them. The International Covenant on Civil and Political Rights, drafted after the European Convention, accepts all the rights that the Convention declares immune to being overridden and adds others, particularly freedom of thought, conscience, and religion. Henry Shue (1980) and James Nickel (1987) suggest comparable criteria for weighing human rights while Sissela Bok (1978) discusses the value of truth telling and the conditions under which it may be suspended.

Application to Population Interventions

The viability of any framework of population ethics depends on its ability to illuminate right and wrong in specific policies, strategies, and sets of actions. Policies set the directions for population interventions, strategies show the broad plans for following those directions, and actions indicate what happens in the field, whether intended or not. The ethics of the three are not necessarily the same. Policies may be stated in humane terms and yet be accompanied by strategies that are coercive. Strategies can be expressed in benign language but, through deliberate initiatives or neglect, lead to field actions that compromise truth, limit freedom, damage human welfare, and in extreme cases,

threaten life. Ethical analysis must pay close attention not only to official statements of policies and strategies, but also to how the programs they generate are carried out.

The five ethical principles will now be applied to three examples of interventions begun by population policies. In each case the aim will be to lay out the key principle or principles involved and to indicate how apparent tensions among principles might be resolved.

THE "POPULATION PROBLEM." Population policies usually begin with some notion of a problem. For strong advocates of fertility control, such as Paul Ehrlich and Anne Ehrlich (1990), the problem is captured in phrases such as "the population bomb" or "the population explosion." According to others, particularly Julian Simon (1981), population growth brings many benefits to society, including the stimulation of human creativity. And for some, fertility, migration, and refugees are complex phenomena that must be carefully studied and that may produce no catchwords that draw public attention.

Any definition of a population problem, or a statement that there is none, must be governed by the principle of truth telling. Those claiming a problem exists should indicate the good promoted or the evil created by fertility, migration, and refugees. What, precisely, has population done to make it qualify as a problem or a nonproblem?

Statements of a problem should also give a fair summary of the evidence bearing on the subject and its limitations. If the findings are drawn from simulations, or cover a small sample of the countries in the world, those points should be disclosed. Scholars violate truth telling when they say or imply that simulations done through a hypothetical model of reality are equivalent to data on what people or organizations actually do. Further, when scholars who write on population work for or are funded by organizations promoting or trying to prevent action on population, such as the World Bank or a right-to-life committee, can it be determined whether they have remained objective or have taken on the advocacy role of their sponsors? If scholars have merged research and advocacy, do they indicate where research stops and advocacy begins? Truth telling requires that all relevant information be presented, even when it may harm one's active endorsement of a policy.

Claims that a problem exists must next show the specific connection between research evidence and the good or evil that makes it a problem. That connection often proves elusive. Data showing that the poorest nations of the world have the highest fertility and the wealthiest nations the lowest fertility may seem to establish a link between population growth and economic development. Indeed, such data are commonly used to support claims of a "population bomb." Yet many studies have failed to show that rapid population growth holds back economic development in the industrialized or developing countries, and a few suggest that it may have advantages (Boserup; National Research Council, 1986). To meet the standard of truth telling, scholars should not, as often happens, cite only those studies that support the view of a population problem to which they subscribe and omit contrary evidence.

USING COERCION. China has used coercion to force some of its citizens to limit fertility. *Coercion* means using or threatening to use physical force or severe deprivation in order to make people do things they would not normally do. Governments apply physical force when they order armed police or military officers to take citizens against their will to clinics that perform abortion or sterilization, or when they credibly threaten with torture couples who have more than two children. They use severe deprivation when they require that poor citizens be sterilized before they can obtain a job or receive food supplies necessary for their own and their family's welfare; warn that parents with more than a certain number of children will be put in prison or have their houses demolished; or use other threats that carry serious risks to life, health, and welfare.

China has relied on coercion to carry out its one-child-per-couple policy (Aird). The Chinese government claims that its policies are voluntary, but its pressure on field workers to meet their targets, particularly in cities, has led to coercive implementation. According to Tyrene White: "Beijing's penetration to the household is awesome. In 1979 mobilization campaigns for 'voluntary' sterilizations, abortions, and adoption of contraceptive measures were widespread, and the fine line between persuasion and coercion was crossed frequently" (p. 315). Two other scholars comment: "During 1979 and in some subsequent years, in some urban areas and provinces, women pregnant with a second or higher order child were required to abort the pregnancies. Instances of mandatory sterilization were also reported" (Hardee-Cleaveland and Banister, p. 275).

China's use of coercion and heavy pressures to reduce fertility has, from indications, led to female infanticide and adoption (Johansson and Nygren). In traditional China, men had the basic duty of continuing the descent line of their fathers by having a son. This boy could carry on the family name, support his parents in their old age, and inherit their property. Failure to have a son showed ingratitude to one's ancestors and discredited men in their own communities. This tradition has continued to the present. If a man's only child is a daughter, he and his neighbors may feel that

he has not fulfilled one of his most basic duties in life. Yet a successful one-child policy would mean that many males could not have a son. Demographic analysis strongly suggests a clash between a couple's normal desire to keep and raise their daughters and the limits on having sons imposed by the country's policies on fertility control.

Terence Hull (1990) shows that in 1987 the sex ratios in China—the number of males per 100 females—were nearly 111, compared to an earlier reference norm of 106. Using comparable data, Sten Johansson and Ola Nygren (1991) estimate that from 1985 through 1987 the average number of missing girls (those normally expected to be in the population but, in fact, missing from it) was about 500,000 per year or 1,500,000 for those three years alone. These authors and others writing about the many millions of missing girls in China attribute this phenomenon to the one-child-per-couple policy. They offer four possible explanations: infanticide caused by deliberate actions of the parents or neglect leading to fatal illnesses; a higher proportion of abortions for female than male babies; births not properly registered with the authorities, usually because they were beyond the local quota for couples; and the practice of offering female children for adoption. The evidence offered by Johansson and Nygren suggests the presence of excess female infant deaths, whether from infanticide or other reasons; unregistered babies; and female adoption.

China's coercive policies show the severe tensions between limiting population for the common good and life, freedom, and fairness. If, in response to the one-child norm, Chinese couples have used female infanticide to raise their chances of having a son, compulsion clashes with the infant girl's right to life. Government officials may say that they never intended to encourage infanticide, but that statement does not absolve them of responsibility for the deaths that take place. A full ethical analysis of policies must take account not only of official declarations and intentions, but also of the actions to which they lead. If, as seems to be the case, the policy of one child per couple has led to infanticide, by U.N. standards of human rights this sacrifice of life cannot be justified by the argument that China's overpopulation demands stringent control of fertility. In social policies, life holds such a high value that it cannot be traded off for even the most compelling public claims.

Coercive policies also put unjustifiable limits on human freedom. Unlike life, freedom can be and often is restricted for the common good. Laws, tax regulations, and many other policies indicate what individuals and groups must and must not do. But forcing citizens to undergo sterilizations or abortions that they do not want, as has happened in China, violates the principles of liberty and human dignity endorsed in all U.N. declarations of human rights. The moral question is not whether individuals should be totally free to set their family size—which they are not in any country or culture—but whether some limits on reproductive choice violate human rights. Using force to promote small family sizes does violate those rights.

China's population interventions further raise the question of fairness. Policies leading directly or indirectly to female infanticide, the abortion of female children, or female adoption put a far heavier burden on girls than boys. Abortion and infanticide mean that, through the decisions of their parents, girls stand a lower chance than boys of being born or of surviving to be adults. With adoption, young girls survive but do not have the same opportunity as male children to be raised by their parents. All three outcomes violate fairness by providing more benefits to boys than to girls and more harms to girls than to boys.

INADEQUATE MEDICAL SUPPORT. Fertility control programs in low-income countries sometimes lead to a conflict between efficiency in delivering services and healthcare for those receiving the services. To raise efficiency, program managers may insist that field workers meet the targets set for them and threaten with severe punishments those who do not comply. During India's birth-control campaign between 1975 and 1977, which relied heavily on forced sterilization, the Chief Secretary of the state of Uttar Pradesh sent this telegraph to his subordinates: "… Failure to achieve monthly targets will not only result in the stoppage of salaries but also suspension and severest penalties. Galvanise entire administrative machinery forthwith and continue to report daily progress by … wireless to me and secretary to Chief Minister" (Gwatkin, p. 41).

Managers and staff working under such pressures often provide little or no health support for those receiving their services. In India during the period mentioned, hundreds of men died from infections that developed after hastily performed sterilizations with no medical follow-up (Gwatkin, p. 47). Other health hazards caused by fertility-control methods include severe, and sometimes fatal, upper reproductive-tract infections among women not properly screened for the intrauterine device; medical complications produced by using the Dalkon shield and high-dose oral contraceptives in developing countries when their risks were well-known in the United States and Europe; reproductive-tract infections among thousands of women in poor countries; and disruptions of the menstrual cycle, heavy bleeding or spotting, weight gain, depression, headaches, dizziness, fatigue, bloating, or loss of libido among women using the

injectable contraceptive Depo-Provera (National Research Council, 1989; Schearer).

Ethical Responsibilities of Fertility-Control Programs

Given these risks to life and health, officials responsible for fertility-control programs face three questions of ethics. The first question concerns the amount of information about the hazards of a particular method that should be disclosed by program staff to their clients. With heavy pressure from their superiors to meet their targets, field workers often emphasize the benefits of a method and conceal its risks. This practice violates the principle of freedom, which requires that clients have reasonable information about risks and benefits to make an informed choice about fertility control. Even when clients cannot grasp sophisticated explanations of medical hazards, they can be told what is at stake in language that they understand. When the risks not disclosed are serious, clients may also face threats to their life, their health, or their welfare.

The second ethical question concerns the adequacy of health services to deal with the hazards created by methods of fertility control. Some argue that, given the severity of the population problem, governments are morally justified in operating fertility-control services well ahead of health-support services. Others, particularly groups supporting the rights of women in family-planning programs, claim that this strategy not only violates human rights but produces a backlash against birth control. Clients who have not been told of any possible side effects or complications from the methods offered and who then suffer poor health can retaliate in many ways. They may discontinue the methods they have started, accept a method but not use it, start rumors about the physical dangers of birth control, stay away from family-planning clinics and field workers, enlist religious leaders or political parties to make fertility control a political issue, vote against the government in the next election, or, if they are truly angry, riot against the government in power. Many of these reactions followed India's use of coercion between 1975 and 1977.

The third ethical question is fairness in the distribution of medical harms and benefits among individuals and groups. This issue arises in the testing as well as the distribution of fertility-control methods. Beginning with the contraceptive pill, whose main evaluation was carried out in Puerto Rico, drug companies have often tested new methods of fertility control on poor individuals in developing countries. Government regulations on testing in those countries have been far less strict than in the United States. Moreover, the low-income individuals chosen for the testing asked few questions about what was being done and were unlikely to mount political protests or begin lawsuits to receive compensation for damage to their health. During the distribution of fertility-control methods, poor individuals in many countries likewise have received less adequate explanations and suffered more health hazards than those with higher incomes. As one example, for many years the U.S. government, citing health risks, banned the domestic use of the injectable contraceptive Depo-Provera. But it saw no problem including Depo-Provera as part of the contraceptive services in poor nations supported by U.S. foreign aid.

Four ethical guidelines help to resolve these conflicts. First, no program should knowingly threaten the life of its clients by using methods that can cause death or by failing to provide health services. If, as happened in India, sterilized males apply animal dung to areas of pain, and if that folk remedy proves fatal, fertility-control programs must take all possible steps to prevent its use.

Second, programs must offer healthcare for all users of methods with serious medical risks. In its villages, Indonesia has developed a simple system of healthcare often located in the home of the village head or another resident. Should clients show symptoms that cannot be treated there, they are referred to the nearest health clinic or hospital.

Third, clients must be told, in words they understand, about the risks as well as the benefits of fertility-control methods. To deny potential users information about risks unjustifiably limits their freedom of choice. Explanations need not be elaborate to be accurate, but they must be given.

Fourth, the distribution of risks and benefits from fertility-control programs should be fair, though not necessarily equal. Poor persons should not be the main candidates on whom fertility-control methods are tested, nor should some groups of citizens receive adequate health support while others receive little or none.

To promote user freedom and welfare, program designers and field workers can be trained to adopt the standards of quality suggested by Judith Bruce (1990). Quality care requires technical competence that gives accurate information to users in language they understand; informed consent that shows sensitivity to concerns about modesty among women and girls; pain management; and continuous rather than one-time service to clients. Instead of aiming only to avoid violations of human rights, which might attain that goal but result in mediocre care, staff can be taught to seek high client satisfaction with fertility-control services.

Stepladder Ethics: A Contrast

Ethical principles based on internationally accepted standards of human rights contrast sharply with the stepladder ethics proposed by Bernard Berelson and Jonathan Lieberson (1979). Berelson was president of the Population Council, a visible center of research, training, and advocacy on population policy, and Lieberson was a philosopher who served as adviser to the Population Council and taught at Columbia University. These two authors commanded attention and respect, and their article was the first and last systematic analysis of ethics to appear in *Population and Development Review*, the leading journal on population policy.

Berelson and Lieberson offered this pivotal statement about population ethics: "Employ less severe measures where possible and only ascend to harsher measures if the problem at hand, as a matter of (established) fact, is clearly grave enough to warrant it" (p. 596). They continued: "… The degree of coercive policy brought into play should be proportional to the degree of seriousness of the present problem and should be introduced only after less coercive means have been exhausted. Thus overt violence or other potentially injurious coercion is not to be used before noninjurious coercion has been exhausted" (p. 602). Their moral stepladder involves beginning with voluntary policies and, if they fail, moving up the scale of pressure on people to the point justified by the seriousness of the population problem. They do not mention fertility-control measures involving threats to life, but, by their logic, governments facing exceptionally severe problems from population growth would be allowed to use those methods as well.

The authors state that they are writing out of a Western, individualistic mode, and recognize that other countries draw ethical principles from different philosophical and political traditions. They do not mention U.N. declarations on human rights, or the widely varying views of the world's religions on methods of fertility control. They apply their Western code to the strategies adopted by countries whose local standards are very different from their own. Leaders in countries populated by Catholics, Buddhists, and Muslims, for instance, might vigorously challenge the principle of allowing governments to use any form of coercion in limiting fertility. Stepladder ethics provides no means of developing cross-national ethical principles whose morality derives mainly from religion or from assumptions that differ from those of the authors, including human rights.

Stepladder ethics thus differs greatly from principles based on universally accepted human rights. Norms such as life, freedom, fairness, and welfare provide a basis for developing ethical guidelines for population policies that apply to every society. Like all ethical principles, those norms need clear definition and are often violated in practice, but they open the way for discussion among persons from diverse political systems and religious traditions and beliefs.

Conclusions

To be applicable to the hundreds of countries and cultures across the world, population ethics must be based on widely shared norms. Principles drawing on the assumptions of a single society or culture will often be rejected by those from other backgrounds. Moreover, to be viable in helping decisions about population policies, the principles chosen should have priorities assigned to them. They must be able to answer one of the most challenging questions in ethics: Is it morally acceptable to sacrifice one principle, such as life, for another, such as the common welfare?

This entry proposes four principles based on international declarations of human rights: life, freedom, welfare, and fairness. It adds truth telling as a fifth principle valuable in itself and necessary in reaching the other four. When these principles clash, life receives first priority. In contrast to stepladder ethics, which grants no human rights, the ethical framework proposed here bans any method of population control with serious risks of death or those relying on torture, slavery, servitude, or other degrading punishments.

If adopted, this ethical framework would have the same advantages and limitations as all universal codes of human rights. The main advantage is that it can be used to educate policymakers and field workers on what is and is not morally acceptable in population programs. When a program violates its standards, U.N. organizations, including the Commission on Human Rights, or private groups, such as Amnesty International, could document the abuses of human rights and demand more humane policies or practices. As has already happened, universal codes can also stimulate geographic regions, such as Europe and Latin America, or major religions to examine human rights from other perspectives. S. M. Haider (1978) and his associates, for example, found many parallels and some differences between Islamic teaching and the Universal Declaration of Human Rights.

The key drawback to this framework is that, like other declarations of human rights, it might be viewed as noble in the abstract but unworkable in practice. Critics could say that it embodies foreign rather than national standards and takes no account of the difficulties with population control that face an overcrowded nation. Even so, it would give local and international advocates of human rights criteria that could be used to develop political and moral pressure to end abuses such as forced sterilization and abortion. And it would avoid the charge, leveled against stepladder ethics, that its ethical standards derive from one country or region, such as the West.

A normative framework based on internationally accepted standards of human rights offers no simple answers to the complex ethical difficulties found in population programs. It does, however, provide a foundation for discussing morality among those who hold widely different views about politics, religion, ethics, and culture. Without that foundation there will never be any serious analysis or lasting agreement about what should and should not be done in population policies and programs.

DONALD P. WARWICK

SEE ALSO: *Abortion; Adoption; Coercion; Embryo and Fetus: Religious Perspectives; Eugenics and Religious Law; Genetic Testing and Screening; Infanticide; Feminism; Fertility Control; Freedom and Free Will; Harm; Infanticide; Informed Consent; Justice; Life; Natural Law; Race and Racism; Rights, Human; Sexism;* and other *Population Ethics* subentries

BIBLIOGRAPHY

Aird, John S. 1990. *Slaughter of the Innocents: Coercive Birth Control in China.* Washington, D.C.: AEI Press.

Berelson, Bernard, and Lieberson, Jonathan. 1979. "Government Efforts to Influence Fertility: The Ethical Issues." *Population and Development Review* 5(4): 581–613.

Bok, Sissela. 1978. *Lying: Moral Choice in Public and Private Life.* New York: Pantheon Books.

Boserup, Ester. 1990. *Economic and Demographic Relationships in Development.* Baltimore: Johns Hopkins University Press.

Brown, Peter G., and Shue, Henry, eds. 1981. *Boundaries: National Autonomy and Its Limits.* Totowa, NJ: Rowman & Littlefield.

Bruce, Judith. 1990. "Fundamental Elements of the Quality of Care: A Simple Framework." *Studies in Family Planning* 21(2):61–91.

Claude, Richard Pierre, and Weston, Burns H., eds. 1989. *Human Rights in the World Community: Issues and Action.* Philadelphia: University of Pennsylvania Press.

Dixon-Mueller, Ruth, and Wasserheit, Judith N. 1991. *The Culture of Silence: Reproductive Tract Infections among Women in the Third World.* New York: International Women's Health Coalition.

Ehrlich, Paul R., and Ehrlich, Anne H. 1990. *The Population Explosion.* New York: Simon & Schuster.

Feringa, Barbara; Iden, Sara; and Rosenfield, Allan. 1992. "NORPLANT: Potential for Coercion." In *Norplant and Poor Women,* pp. 57–63, ed. Sarah-Ellen Samuels and Mark P. Smith. Menlo Park, CA: Henry J. Kaiser Family Foundation.

Gwatkin, Davidson R. 1979. "Political Will and Family Planning: The Implications of India's Emergency Experience." *Population and Development Review* 5(1): 29–59.

Haider, S. M. 1978. *Islamic Concept of Human Rights.* Lahore, Pakistan: Book House.

Hardee-Cleaveland, Karen, and Banister, Judith. 1988. "Fertility Policy and Implementation in China, 1986–1988." *Population and Development Review* 14(2): 245–286.

Holmes, Helen B.; Hoskins, Betty B.; and Gross, Michael, eds. 1980. *Birth Control and Controlling Birth: Women-Centered Perspectives.* Clifton, NJ: Humana Press.

Hull, Terence H. 1990. "Recent Trends in Sex Ratios at Birth in China." *Population and Development Review* 16(1): 63–83.

Johansson, Sten, and Nygren, Ola. 1991. "The Missing Girls of China: A New Demographic Account." *Population and Development Review* 17(1): 35–51.

National Research Council (U.S.). Working Group on the Health Consequences of Contraceptive Use and Controlled Fertility. 1989. *Contraception and Reproduction: Health Consequences for Women and Children in the Developing World.* Washington, D.C.: National Academy Press.

National Research Council (U.S.). Working Group on Population Growth and Economic Development. 1986. *Population Growth and Economic Development: Policy Questions.* Washington, D.C.: National Academy Press.

Nickel, James W. 1987. *Making Sense of Human Rights: Philosophical Reflections on the Universal Declaration of Human Rights.* Berkeley: University of California Press.

Schearer, S. Bruce. 1983. "Monetary and Health Costs of Contraception." In *Fertility Regulation and Institutional Influences,* pp. 103–122. Vol. 2 of *Determinants of Fertility in Developing Countries,* ed. Rodolfo A. Bulatao and Ronald D. Lee. New York: Academic Press.

Shue, Henry. 1980. *Basic Rights: Substance, Affluence, and U.S. Foreign Policy.* Princeton, NJ: Princeton University Press.

Simon, Julian L. 1981. *The Ultimate Resource.* Princeton, NJ: Princeton University Press.

Veatch, Robert M., ed. 1977. *Population Policy and Ethics: The American Experience.* New York: Irvington Publishers.

Warwick, Donald P. 1982. *Bitter Pills: Population Policies and Their Implementation in Eight Developing Countries.* New York: Cambridge University Press.

Warwick, Donald P. 1990. "The Ethics of Population Control." In *Population Policy: Contemporary Issues,* pp. 21–37, ed. Godfrey Roberts. New York: Praeger.

White, Tyrene. 1987. "Implementing the 'One-Child-per-Couple' Population Program in Rural China: National Goals and Local Politics." In *Policy Implementation in Post-Mao China,* pp. 284–317, ed. David M. Lampton. Berkeley: University of California Press.

World Population Conference. 1975. Report of the United Nations World Population Conference, 1974, Bucharest, 19–30 August, 1974. E/CONF.60/19. New York: United Nations.

III. RELIGIOUS TRADITIONS: A. INTRODUCTION

How and to what extent religion influences population policies and the practices of individuals, couples, and larger groups is a very complex question. Although specific religious teachings about marriage, ideal family size, and the permissibility of birth control or abortion would seem to bear on reproductive decision making, the actual effects of these religious beliefs and teachings are not easily assessed. Explicitly pronatalist doctrines that espouse the value of having many children and oppose birth limitation sometimes have little effect on reproductive behaviors or policies, while other aspects of religion, seemingly remote from reproductive decision making, may have powerful demographic effects.

Until recently, most major religions stressed marriage as a religiously sanctified state and were pronatalist in outlook; such teachings reflected the perilous demographic circumstances in which these religions were formed. Although Eastern Orthodox Christianity and most Protestant denominations have come to accept the use of contraception for family planning, other major traditions have concretized traditional religious pronatalism in specific beliefs that discourage the use of birth control. Roman Catholicism continues to prohibit contraception and sterilization; Orthodox Judaism forbids use of the condom or any male methods that prevent insemination. Classical Islam, Hinduism, and Confucianism, while more permissive regarding use of birth control, share the traditional religious bias in favor of marriage and large families. Although abortion has played an important role in societies that have undergone population stabilization, no historical religious tradition favors the use of abortion for purposes of limiting the size of the family.

Other features of religious practice and teaching would seem to have a strong pronatalist effect. Many traditions stress the importance of offspring, especially sons, in carrying out vital religious rituals and in maintaining family continuity. The *Rigveda* (VI.61.l), Hinduism's foundational sacred text, terms a son a *rnachyuta,* one who removes the moral debts of a father and spares him from hell. Recent studies suggest that preference for sons leads couples in India to continue building their family until they have a son

(Arnold, Choe, and Roy; Vlassoff). In Judaism, key rituals emphasize the importance of children, especially male offspring: a son's *bris,* or circumcision ceremony, is a major source of religious joy; children play an important part in the Passover service; and the *kaddish* rite for the dead is ideally performed by a surviving son.

In African tribal societies, veneration of the ancestors is a central religious activity. Whatever immortality awaits the individual after death depends on survivors' continued performance of family rites. Individuals without progeny are viewed as pitiful figures who may become marauding spirits after death (Molnos). Since ancestors profoundly affect the circumstances of the living, family prosperity and health require the existence of an ample number of descendants to maintain the family cult. In contrast to Western views, popular opinion in some African societies favors providing a scarce, lifesaving medical therapy to a bachelor over a family man (Kilner). This reflects the belief that an individual's religious and social significance is not established until he or she founds a family.

In addition to formal teachings, the whole tapestry of a religion's beliefs, its "bioethical sensibility" (Green), must be taken into account in understanding its bearing on demographic behaviors. Thus, although Judaism is historically pronatalist, it also tends to privilege women's interests in reproductive matters. This has led Jewish women to be among the most enthusiastic acceptors of female birth control measures. Popular religious beliefs, as opposed to formal teaching, must also be factored into thinking about reproductive behavior. Orthodox Islam, for example, does not actively prohibit the use of birth control, and most Muslims live under governments with official family planning programs (Omran). But popular attitudes about kismet, or fate, and the idea that Allah appoints each couple the children they have contribute to a widespread reluctance to adopt family-planning methods (Fagley; Knodel, Gray, Sriwatchacharin, et al.). In Africa and elsewhere, popular beliefs about reincarnation or the existence of "souls in heaven" awaiting birth contribute to a reluctance to employ birth control.

Teachings and practices regarding women are another significant aspect of religion that contributes to high birthrates. There is a growing body of evidence that women's autonomy is a key factor in promoting the practice of birth limitation (Dharmalingam and Morgan; Hindin). As a result, those aspects of religious belief and practice that reduce women's autonomy can contribute significantly to high fertility and population growth. Many features of traditional religions have this effect. For example, Hinduism regards women as of lower karmic status, able to effect spiritual ascent by having children and fulfilling family duties. In different ways, most other traditional religions echo these beliefs, removing women from the central sphere of political and religious life and locating whatever spiritual fulfillment that is available to them in the home (Ruether; Carmody).

Multiple demographic consequences follow from this history of marginalization of women and treatment of them as "second-class" religious citizens. Early marriage is associated with larger completed family size. Religious values that encourage child marriage, as in India, or that discourage women's education and career preparation before marriage are therefore major contributors to higher birthrates. The existence of highly differentiated social roles for men and women also may lead to larger completed family size, since sons and daughters are less "interchangeable" in terms of their ability to fulfill parental needs (Johnson and Burton). When religiously influenced values consign women to the home, their social, economic, and spiritual value comes to depend on their reproductive success. In polygynous African tribal societies, a woman's standing among her co-wives depends on the number of her children. Her material well-being also depends on the number of progeny she has to help her with home-based economic tasks and agriculture (Molnos). Although the consequences of religious teachings and institutional practices about gender have not been measured, they may be among the most important and persistent religious influences on fertility.

These beliefs and practices affect fertility through the behavior of individuals and couples. At the institutional and policy levels, religion can affect population through its impact on national and international family-planning programs. During the early 1970s, the Roman Catholic Church's opposition to contraception made it difficult for the governments of some Latin American nations to mount family-planning programs (McCoy). This opposition was vigorously expressed by the offical Vatican representative at the 1994 Cairo Conference on Population (Martino) and continues to influence Vatican responses to the population policies of the United Nations and other national and international bodies. Opposition to abortion by Roman Catholic and evangelical Christian groups has repeatedly led conservative U.S. administrations to deny support for international family-planning programs that offer abortion services or counseling. This was shown most recently at a December 2002 Bangkok Conference on Population when the administration of George W. Bush sought to strike from the conference's document endorsements of "reproductive health services" and "reproductive rights" because these can include abortion and abortion counseling in nations where this procedure is legal (Dao). In contrast to these oppositional positions, some religious pronouncements on behalf of responsible parenthood by religious leaders in Islamic countries may have contributed to the success of family-planning programs. On balance, it is not clear how much difference religious involvement in population policy or programs makes. For example, official Roman Catholic opposition to birth control and abortion has had little or no effect on altering the very low birthrates in Catholic countries such as Austria, Ireland, or Italy.

Whatever the influence of religion at the level of national policies, there is considerable evidence that explicit religious teachings about birth control or family size are only one of many factors that play a role in couples' reproductive decision making. Decades ago, sociologists noted that socioeconomic modernization is normally accompanied by a "demographic" transition—from the high birthrates of agricultural and traditional societies to the lower birthrates and family-planning practices of urbanized societies (United Nations). Once economic and social modernization begins, this demographic transition occurs regardless of the religious basis of the society, casting doubt on the importance of religion in reproductive behavior.

Demographers and social scientists have tried to determine the precise role played by religious, economic, or social factors in reproductive decision making, and the relative importance of these factors in influencing demographic behaviors. Three main hypotheses about the religion-fertility relationship have been advanced and variously tested by use of survey data or historical case studies (Johnson). The "characteristic" hypothesis stresses that socio-economic determinants are the primary causal factors in behavioral change, often eclipsing specific religious teachings about family size. For example, Joseph Chamie's 1981 study of fertility and religion in Lebanon shows that whatever their traditions teach, educated, urban, middle-class Catholic or Muslim couples make similar decisions about family size and reproduction; and lower-income, agricultural families have higher birthrates, regardless of their creed. In both cases, social and economic circumstances are determinative. The impact of purely religious doctrine on fertility appears significant only while a society is going through economic and social transition, when such doctrine may delay acceptance of birth control.

A second, "minority-group status" hypothesis holds that if a religious group is a minority and holds strong pronatalist views that are heightened by opportunities for group reinforcement, there may be some independent impact of religious teachings on fertility (Kennedy; Day; Williams and Zimmer). Studies of Mormons in the United States, for example, suggest that a pronatalism deeply rooted in Mormon theology and family values, and heightened by intragroup reinforcements, contributes to higher birthrates among Mormons than would be expected among groups of similar social and economic standing (Heaton and Calkins; Heaton).

Only the third, "particularistic theology" hypothesis sees religious belief as an independent causal variable affecting fertility. This hypothesis has drawn some support from studies of demographic patterns widely separated in time or geographical location (Brown and Guinnane; Knodel, et al.; Sanders).

Taken together there is good reason to believe that while religious teachings and doctrines have some direct influence on reproductive behavior and population growth rates, this influence is probably less than the amount of attention given inside and outside religious communities to specific teachings on marriage, birth control, or abortion would suggest. Furthermore, among religious teachings, those less directly related to reproductive decision making, especially the religiously sanctioned subordination of women, may have the most powerful impact on fertility.

RONALD M. GREEN (1995)
REVISED BY AUTHOR

SEE ALSO: *Authority in Religious Traditions; Eugenics; Family and Family Medicine; Feminism; Fertility Control; Infanticide; International Health; Public Health; Sustainable Development; Women, Historical and Cross-Cultural Perspectives;* and other *Population Ethics* subentries

BIBLIOGRAPHY

Arnold, Fred; Choe, Minja Kim; and Roy, T. K. 1998. "Son Preference, the Family Building Process and Child Mortality in India." *Population Studies* 52: 301–315.

Brown, John C., and Guinnane, Timothy W. 2002. "Fertility Transition in a Rural, Catholic Population: Bavaria, 1880–1910." *Population Studies* 56: 35–50.

Carmody, Denise L. 1989. *Women and World Religions.* Englewood Cliffs, NJ: Prentice-Hall.

Chamie, Joseph. 1981. *Religion and Fertility: Arab Christian-Muslim Differentials.* Cambridge, UK: Cambridge University Press.

Day, Lincoln H. 1984. "Minority-Group Status and Fertility: A More Detailed Test of the Hypothesis." *Sociological Quarterly* 25(4): 456–472.

Dharmalingam, A., and Morgan, Philip. 1996. "Women's Work, Autonomy, and Birth Control: Evidence from Two South Indian Villages." *Population Studies* 50: 187–201.

Fagley, Richard M. 1967. "Doctrines and Attitudes of Major Religions in Regard to Fertility." In *Proceedings of the World Population Conference: Belgrade, 30 August–10 September, 1965,* vol. 2, *Selected Papers and Summaries: Fertility; Family Planning; Mortality.* New York: United Nations, Department of Economic and Social Affairs.

Green, Ronald M. 1999. "Religion and Bioethics." In *Notes from a Narrow Ridge,* ed. Dena S. Davis and Laurie Zoloth-Dorfman. Frederick, MD: University Publishing Group.

Heaton, Tim B. 1986. "How Does Religion Influence Fertility? The Case of the Mormons." *Journal for the Scientific Study of Religion* 25(2): 248–258.

Heaton, Tim B., and Calkins, Sandra. 1983. "Family Size and Contraceptive Use among Mormons: 1965–76." *Review of Religious Research* 25(2): 102–113.

Hindin, Michelle J. 2000. "Women's Autonomy, Women's Status and Fertility-Related Behavior in Zimbabwe." *Population Research and Policy Review* 19: 255–282.

Johnson, Nan E. 1993. "Hindu and Christian Fertility in India: A Test of Three Hypotheses." *Social Biology* 40: 87–105.

Johnson, Nan E., and Burton, Linda M. 1989. "Religion and Reproduction in Philippine Society: A New Test of the Minority-Groups Status Hypothesis." In *Women in International Development,* Working Paper #178. East Lansing: Michigan State University.

Kennedy, Robert E., Jr. 1973. "Minority-Group Status and Fertility: The Irish." *American Sociological Review* 38(1): 85–96.

Kilner, John F. 1990. *Who Lives? Who Dies? Ethical Criteria in Patient Selection.* New Haven, CT: Yale University Press.

Knodel, John; Gray, Rossarin Soottipang; Sriwatchacharin, Porntip; and Peracca, Sara. 1999. "Religion and Reproduction: Muslims in Buddhist Thailand." *Population Studies* 53: 149–164.

McCoy, Terry L., ed. 1974. *The Dynamics of Population Policy in Latin America.* Cambridge, MA: Ballinger.

Molnos, Angela. 1968. *Attitudes toward Family Planning in East Africa.* Munich: Weltforum Verlag.

Omran, Abdel Rahim. 1992. *Family Planning in the Legacy of Islam.* London: Routledge.

Ruether, Rosemary Radford, ed. 1974. *Religion and Sexism: Images of Woman in the Jewish and Christian Traditions.* New York: Simon and Schuster.

Sanders, William. 1992. "Catholicism and the Economics of Fertility." *Population Studies* 46: 477–489.

United Nations /UNFPA Expert Group. 1979. *Demographic Transition and Socio-Economic Development.* New York: Author.

Vlassoff, Carol. 1991. "Progress and Stagnation: Changes in Fertility and Women's Position in an Indian Village." *Population Studies* 46: 195–212.

Williams, Linda B., and Zimmer, Basil G. 1990. "The Changing Influence of Religion on U.S. Fertility: The Evidence from Rhode Island." *Demography* 27(3): 475–481.

INTERNET RESOURCES

Dao, James. 2002. "At U.N. Family-Planning Talks, U.S. Raises Abortion Issue," *New York Times,* December 15, 2002. Online edition. Available from <http://www.nytimes.com/2002/12/15/international/15ABOR.html>.

Martino, Renato. "Statement by His Excellency, Archbishop Renato R. Martino, Permanent Observer of the Holy See Delegation at the International Conference on Population and Development, Cairo, 7 September 1994." Available from <http://www.columbia.edu/cu/augustine/arch/martino.txt>.

III. RELIGIOUS TRADITIONS:
B. ISLAMIC PERSPECTIVES

Population issues in Islam are the product of the interplay of faith and experience, Muslim belief and local social realities. Like Islam itself, in which unity of faith has been expressed by a diversity of practice, so the application of Islam to population issues has been conditioned by local circumstances and customs as well as personal piety. Understanding the issue of population control in Islam requires an appreciation both of the history of Islamic thought and practice and of its implementation in Muslim countries today.

The impact of Islam on population policies reflects the continuous interaction of religious teaching, local cultural traditions, and national politics. The diverse results of that interaction lead to great variation in the population policies of Muslim countries. Thus the government's approach to fertility control in Indonesia and Egypt differs greatly from that in Saudi Arabia and Iran. The first two have long had active fertility-control programs supported by senior Islamic officials. Saudi Arabia has no active family-planning program. Iran, for religious and political reasons, discontinued its family-planning program after the country's revolution in 1979 (Ross). However, in 1992, responding to severe economic and social conditions, including a rapid population growth, Iran reinstated its program with the approval of the religious leaders (*ulama*).

Muslim attitudes toward population control are influenced by beliefs and values concerning the nature and purpose of society, the family, marriage, procreation, and child rearing; they also reflect responses to several centuries of Western influence and dominance. The locus of Muslim norms and ethical standards is the Shari'a, Islamic law, which constitutes the blueprint for the ideal Islamic society. Shari'a consists of those rules and institutions that God has revealed in the Qur'an. In the early centuries of Islam, pious scholars in various Muslim capitals attempted to delineate God's law for the community. They produced a body of law that combined God's word with human interpretation and application of that word. The difference between the divine component of the law and human interpretations or applications of it has provided the rationale for legal change.

Islamic law is based upon four sources: the Qur'an, which Muslims believe is the literal and perfect word of God; the Sunnah, or example of the Prophet Muhammad; analogical reasoning; and the consensus of the community. Islamic law constitutes a comprehensive ideal that provides guidelines for personal and social life, a Muslim's duties to God (worship), and duties to society (social transactions). Jurists also recognized a number of subsidiary sources. Among the most relevant utilized for social and legal reform is public welfare. Sunni and Shi'ite Islam, the two major groups or traditions within the Islamic community, have a number of law schools, or schools of legal thought. Their laws, while in general agreement, nevertheless include a diversity of orientations, rules, and methods.

Muslim family law, covering marriage, divorce, and inheritance, has long been considered the heart of the Shari'a, an especially sacrosanct component of Islamic law. Historically, the family has been regarded as the basis of Muslim society. As the nucleus of the Islamic community, it is where the next generation receives its religious, social, and cultural training. In modern times, Muslim families, like those in much of the world, have undergone significant change. This is especially clear in the shift from extended to nuclear families as well as in greater educational and employment opportunities for women. These changes have been the subject of continued debate and legal reform.

Reforms in family or gender issues, from family law to population policies, have been widespread and the subject of controversy. During the latter part of the twentieth century, after Muslim nations had gained their independence from European colonial powers, many continued to look to the West for their models or paradigms of development. Political, economic, legal, and social changes were Western-inspired or -oriented, as were modern Muslim elites. As a result, social change, like political and legal reform, has often been judged both in terms of its relationship to the Islamic tradition and its law and within the context of reactions to Western influence, if not hegemony, in the Muslim world.

Marriage and the Family

Marriage in Islam is a sacred contract, though not a sacrament, between two individuals and also between their families (Esposito). Sexuality in Islam is centered on marriage and the family. The married state is the norm—indeed, the ideal—for all Muslims, prescribed by Islamic law and embodied in the life of Muhammad, the exemplar of Muslim life. Celibacy, while permitted if necessary, is not regarded as an ideal. Though procreation and the formation of the family are among the primary purposes of marriage,

Muslim jurists from early in Islamic history permitted contraception to limit the size of a family.

Islamic teachings on methods of fertility control depend on the method used. While open to the use of coitus interruptus and methods of contraception such as the pill, many Muslim scholars oppose any form of abortion; others accept it only to save the life of the mother during the first 120 days of pregnancy. Though some Islamic jurists accept sterilization to avoid having more children, most oppose this method unless it is a medical treatment.

Contraception

In contrast to the Christian and Jewish traditions, from earliest times the Islamic tradition showed acceptance of family planning and contraception. From the tenth to the twentieth centuries, the vast majority of legal scholars and all the major schools of law accepted coitus interruptus between a husband and wife. Early acceptance of birth control was built on a combination of sacred texts, biological knowledge, and reason (Musallam, 1978). The Qur'an contains no clear or explicit text regarding birth control. However, the traditions (*hadith*) of the Prophet do. Though some *hadith* forbid birth control, the majority permit it. Muslim jurists were able to construct an argument based on *hadith* and the biological knowledge of the times to declare birth control by means of coitus interruptus as licit. They argued that such means do not limit or counter God's power because they are not foolproof. Thus, if God wanted a woman to become pregnant, his will could and would prevail despite the practice of coitus interruptus.

The prominent religious scholar al-Ghazālī (d. 1111) is representative of the majority of Sunni Muslim jurists who accepted the use of contraception through coitus interruptus. For Ghazali, coitus interruptus was not only licit but also permissible, regardless of the need to practice it, because there was no explicit text in the Qur'an or Sunnah against it, nor was there clear judicial precedent based on an explicit text:

> We have ruled out its [coitus interruptus] … prohibition because, to establish prohibition, one has to have a text [from the Qur'an or Sunnah] or resort to analogous reasoning based on a precedence for which a text is available. In this case … there is neither a text nor a precedent for analogical reasoning. (Omran, p. 80)

The vast majority of Sunni and Shi'ite jurists believed that birth control through the use of coitus interruptus was permissible. However, because it deprived a woman of her right to children and to sexual satisfaction, her consent was required.

Despite the historical record of jurists regarding the permissibility of contraception, some scholars, such as Ibn Hazm (d. 1064), and local religious leaders viewed contraception as prohibited by Islam because they regarded increase in the number of Muslims as a Prophetic (Muhammad's) command. Though the Qur'an has no text that forbids contraception, critics of contraception interpret it to construct and legitimate their case. Among the major arguments offered are that it (1) constitutes infanticide, which is expressly forbidden by the Qur'an; (2) is contrary to belief in God's power and in divine providence, articulated in the Qur'an's teaching that God is the all-powerful creator and ruler or overseer of the world, and that he determines and controls the destiny of all (81: 29 and 11: 6); (3) ignores the Qur'anic mandate to trust or rely on God; and (4) ignores the necessary connection between marriage and procreation, the primary purpose of marriage.

In modern times, many Muslims, reacting to the impact of Western colonialism and imperialism, have argued that by diminishing the number of Muslims, contraception undermines the power of the Muslim community. More specifically, they charge that birth-control campaigns and programs are part of a Western conspiracy to limit development in the Muslim world and thus subdue Islam.

Modern Islamic Thought

The adoption of Western-inspired legal systems in many Muslim countries in the nineteenth and twentieth centuries limited the scope of Islamic law and the prestige and authority of religious scholars. However, because of the centrality of the family in Muslim society, in most countries family-law and family-planning issues continued to be strongly influenced by Islamic law and ethics. Consciousness of and concern over the implications of a population explosion in areas with limited and shrinking resources, the battle against poverty and illiteracy, urbanization, education and changing expectations, and the development of modern methods of contraception have made the issues of fertility control more prominent and contentious in Muslim societies. Government-sponsored family-planning programs and policies have become common in Muslim countries such as Indonesia, Egypt, Iran, and Bangladesh. Government intervention and implementation of such programs have met with mixed success. In many Muslim countries, when governments introduced fertility-control programs, they often looked to Islamic religious leaders to legitimate their programs and to mobilize popular support. Even when they did not support fertility control, Islamic scholars, viewing it as subject to Islamic law and as a critical area of social intervention, felt it was necessary for them to give moral guidance to Muslim believers.

Legal scholars have generally provided an Islamic rationale for various modern methods to control population growth. Modern Sunni and Shi'ite jurists, such as Lebanon's Sheikh Muhammad M. Shamsuddin, employing the legal principle of reasoning by analogy, have argued that since birth control in the form of coitus interruptus has been accepted for so long in Islam, then by analogy other, more modern forms of birth control that achieve the same effect are acceptable (Omran). Both individual jurists and assemblies of religious scholars have issued *fatwas* (formal legal opinions) that have endorsed contraception and in turn not only have informed the consciences of individual Muslims but also have been employed by governments from Egypt to Indonesia to support their birth-control policies and programs.

On the basis of the clear legal precedent of the acceptance of contraception in the form of coitus interruptus, modern jurists have argued for the permissibility of modern chemical and mechanical forms of birth control, such as the diaphragm, the contraceptive pill, and IUDs. Egypt's Sheikh M. S. Madkour, for example, citing the opinions of early jurists, wrote:

> We may say that the first mechanical method known as coitus interruptus, *al-azl* in Arabic, used by our ancestors to prevent pregnancy, corresponds to the device used these days by women and known as the diaphragm or ring to block the uterine aperture, or to another device used by men, the condom. Both are designed to prevent the semen from reaching the ovum and fertilizing it. The second method … for temporary contraception [is] … the contraceptive pill. Under this heading may also be included the injectables much advertised and supposed to be effective for several months … [and] every other beneficial drug which may be discovered by the medical profession for this purpose. The third … is the [IUD], … which … prevents the fertilized egg from attaching itself to the uterine wall, and the uterus expels it instead. (Omran, p. 81)

Sheikh Tantawi, the mufti of Egypt, senior official consultant on Islamic law, in his 1988 *fatwa* recognized several reasons for practicing contraception. Couples may wish to postpone or space the birth of children for financial reasons; others may wish to do so in order to provide a separate room for a son and daughter; even those who are well off but already have three children may wish to avoid another birth because they live in an overpopulated country (Omran).

Jurists have found many licit reasons for couples to practice contraception: to avoid pregnancy due to health risks to the wife or children resulting from repeated pregnancies, transmission of hereditary or infectious diseases, or genetic risks of inbreeding; economic hardship; to better provide for children's education; and even to preserve a wife's beauty (Omran).

Muslim jurists have addressed infertility within the context of family planning. They have tended to show the same openness and flexibility in their treatment of infertility. Thus, chemical and surgical treatment, as well as artificial insemination between a husband and wife, are permitted. Insemination of a wife with her husband's sperm or in vitro fertilization is allowed. However, procedures that involve someone other than a spouse, such as inseminating a woman with sperm from a man who is not her husband, are forbidden. Children who result from such procedures are regarded as illegitimate.

Sterilization and Abortion

As is the case with contraception, there is no clear text of the Qur'an or Sunnah that forbids sterilization. Although some diversity of opinion exists, the majority of jurists have maintained that sterilization for purposes of contraception, as opposed to its use for medical treatment, is forbidden. Whatever the debate among scholars, local Islamic leaders have tended to oppose sterilization. In recent years, a number of Sunni and Shi'ite jurists have called for a reconsideration of the legality of sterilization (Omran).

Abortion is a far more complex and contentious matter. There is a consensus among religious authorities that abortion after 120 days, when the fetus becomes "ensouled" and thus is a person, is absolutely prohibited except to save the mother's life. While many if not most jurists allow abortion as a means of contraception within 120 days of conception, this scholarly and theoretical position stands in sharp contrast with actual practice—abortion is condemned by most religious leaders and omitted from public-sector programs.

Religion, Government, and Population Issues

During the post–World War II period, governments in the Muslim world, faced with rapid population growth, cited religious, demographic, and nationalist reasons for instituting family-planning programs. Some utilized the prestige and authority of the religious establishment to legitimate family-planning policies. In Egypt, the government has often looked to the leadership and scholars of Cairo's al-Azhar University, a historic and authoritative international center of Islamic learning, for support. *Fatwas* obtained from experts (muftis) in Islamic law have played a prominent role in legitimating population policies throughout the Muslim world. However, differences often exist between official religious decrees and the more conservative responses of local religious leaders and popular beliefs. Since there is no organized church or hierarchy in Islam, and no clear text from revelation or consensus of scholars exists, local religious leaders and their followers are free to hold a variety of opinions.

Islam has legitimated and reinforced traditional pronatalist beliefs and practices in areas where social conditions have made large families desirable. Agricultural and pastoral societies have regarded large families as providing a source of labor, insurance against the loss of help due to high mortality or marriage, and social security in old age. Poverty, illiteracy, lack of educational and employment opportunities, and high mortality often foster and promote a belief in the necessity of a large family. Thus, many Muslims have been raised in a social context in which a primary emphasis on procreation in marriage and large families has been the traditional ideal and norm, a custom reinforced by the preaching and teaching of local religious leaders.

Local beliefs, attitudes, and values have reinforced high fertility rates. Values such as early marriage for women and emphasis on fertility and large families, in particular the importance of having a male child, pressure a young wife to gain the status of motherhood to "prove herself." Women also want to avoid the stigma of infertility and with it the possibility of divorce or of the husband taking a second wife. The importance of motherhood is reflected in the common practice in many Arab countries, once a woman has given birth to a male child, to call her by the name of that firstborn male child, that is, "mother of...."

Government-sponsored programs have varied considerably in their impact and effectiveness. Moderate-to-high contraceptive prevalence rates were indicated in 1994 for Turkey (63%), Tunisia (50%), Indonesia (50%), Algeria (36%), and Egypt (47%). Muslim countries with low rates reported in 1990 include Somalia (0%), Saudi Arabia (1%), Afghanistan (2%), and Yemen (2%) (Ross et al.). Bangladesh's poor performance has been attributed to a "population control battlefield" between contending religious and social forces (Hartmann); Indonesia, on the other hand, has been identified as a family-planning success story. Since the 1970s, Indonesia has used a carrot-and-stick approach of incentives and state pressure. This policy, combined with socioeconomic changes such as reduced infant mortality, increased educational levels, and rural-to-urban migration, has led to a significant decline in fertility (Hartmann).

Initially, many local religious leaders opposed family-planning programs on moral grounds and because they believed that growth in population was necessary in order to spread Islam. Efforts by the government, early in the program, to consult with religious leaders, and the government's decision to exclude sterilization and abortion from the program, helped counter the opposition.

The role and influence of religious leaders has varied and can often prove significant. The influence of Islam on people's acceptance or rejection of government-sponsored fertility-control programs depends not only on moral teachings of a religious tradition but also on how those teachings are interpreted to local people by religious leaders. If, as in Indonesia, many of those leaders support the program and use occasions such as marriage ceremonies to suggest the value of family planning, acceptance will typically be greater than if those leaders tell believers that using contraceptives to limit birth violates Islamic teaching. Postrevolution Shi'ite Iran provides a unique example of religious leaders, the *ulama,* functioning as both the executors and the formulators or legislators of new *fatwas* on family planning.

The Egyptian government has addressed the population question since the beginning of the rule of Gamal Abdel Nasser in 1952. Because of religious sensibilities, the government moved slowly, employing only the pill. Religious officials, from the government-appointed mufti of Egypt to the rector of the state-supported al-Azhar University, issued a series of *fatwas* endorsing the use of contraceptives. However, many think the religious establishment has been co-opted by the government. Thus, while Nasser and his successors could marshal the support of the religious establishment, local religious leaders continued to condemn contraception as immoral as well as contrary to Islam, and reinforced traditional emphasis on procreation and acceptance of the will of God, as did other opinion makers, such as midwives.

Like many other countries, Egypt has utilized a centralized, top-down approach, bypassing or ignoring local and regional realities. In 1953, Nasser was concerned that Egypt's population would leap to 44 million (Warwick, 1982). However, little was done about fertility control until the mid-1960s.

In Lebanon, religious sectarianism and communalism have both determined and limited the success of government policy. Lebanon was created as a confessional state whose delicate balance was based upon a system of proportional representation: Maronite Christians were dominant, followed by Sunni and Shi'ite Muslims and Druze. However, tensions between Christians and Muslims were exacerbated by the socioeconomic dominance and advancement of the Maronites, who had a lower fertility rate than the Muslims. By the mid-1970s, social realities proved explosive, and civil war broke out. The Shi'ite community, the poorest and most disenfranchised, had grown, and constituted one-third of Lebanon's population.

Given the precarious balance of power and social tensions, the Lebanese government for more than two decades shied away from any official promotion of family planning. However, while contraceptives remained illegal, the government indirectly supported private family-planning projects (Warwick, 1982).

Conclusion

Islam has a well-established body of teaching on fertility control that is closely linked to its views on marriage and the family. The interpretation of these teachings varies from country to country. The openness of individual Muslims to fertility control depends on many variables, including interpretations by local religious leaders of how it should be regarded by Muslims. Countries differ greatly in the extent to which Islamic religious leaders cooperate with government-sponsored fertility-control programs.

Much of the Muslim world faces rapid population growth in a situation of limited resources. Containment or reversal of this trend remains hampered by widespread poverty, illiteracy, and debates about the morality of birth control. In this struggle, the criticisms of local religious leaders combine with voices of many militant Muslims who attack government-sponsored family-planning programs and Western aid as a conspiracy to limit the size of the Muslim community in order to contain and dominate it more effectively.

JOHN L. ESPOSITO

SEE ALSO: *Abortion; Adoption; Coercion; Embryo and Fetus: Religious Perspectives; Eugenics and Religious Law; Feminism; Fertility Control; Freedom and Free Will; Genetic Testing and Screening; Harm; Infanticide; Informed Consent; Islam, Bioethics in; Justice; Life; Natural Law; Race and Racism; Rights, Human; Sexism; Women, Historical and Cross-Cultural Perspectives;* and other *Population Ethics* subentries

BIBLIOGRAPHY

Coulson, Noel James. 1964. *A History of Islamic Law.* Edinburgh: Edinburgh University Press.

Esposito, John L. 1980. *Women in Muslim Family Law.* Syracuse, NY: Syracuse University Press.

Hartmann, Betsy. 1987. *Reproductive Rights and Wrongs: The Global Politics of Population Control and Contraceptive Choice.* New York: Harper & Row.

Musallam, Basim F. 1978. "Population Ethics. Religious Traditions: Islamic Perspectives." In *Encyclopedia of Bioethics,* pp. 1264–1269, ed. Warren T. Reich. New York: Macmillan.

Musallam, Basim F. 1983. *Sex and Society in Islam: Birth Control Before the Nineteenth Century.* Cambridge, Eng.: Cambridge University Press.

Nazer, Isam R.; Karmī, Ḥasan S.; and Zayid, Mahmud Y., eds. 1974. *Islam and Family Planning.* 2 vols. Beirut: International Planned Parenthood Federation.

Omran, Abdel Rahim. 1992. *Family Planning in the Legacy of Islam.* London: Routledge.

Population Reference Bureau. 1994. *1994: World Population Data Sheet.* Washington, D.C.: Author.

Ross, John A.; Mauldin, W. Parker; Green, Steven R.; and Cooke, E. Romana. 1992. *Family Planning and Child Survival Programs as Assessed in 1991.* New York: Population Council.

Schieffelin, Olivia, ed. 1972. *Muslim Attitudes Towards Family Planning.* New York: Population Council.

Warwick, Donald P. 1982. *Bitter Pills: Population Policies and Their Implementation in Eight Developing Countries.* Cambridge, Eng.: Cambridge University Press.

Warwick, Donald P. 1986. "The Indonesian Family Planning Program: Government Influence and Client Choice." *Population and Development Review* 12(3): 453–490.

III. RELIGIOUS TRADITIONS: C. JEWISH PERSPECTIVES

Pronatalism is the contemporary word describing the classic Jewish tradition regarding fertility. To begin with the religious component of the Jewish culture, procreation is counted as a positive *mitzvah* (a commandment or virtue), given pride of place at the top of rabbinic formulations of Bible commandments. *P'ru ur'vu* ("Be fruitful and multiply," or better, "Be fruitful and increase"—more arithmetic than geometric) in the first chapter of Genesis is a general blessing to other creatures; for humans, it is a behavioral imperative to reproduce. Bible commentators explain this difference in terms of the human differential: The command mode is needed because humankind, created in the image of God, might seek to devote itself entirely to the spiritual and intellectual, and might neglect the material and physical. Accordingly, Scripture thus negates the antiprocreative or celibate views of some cultures. Alternatively, the commandment addresses the fact that only humans are aware of the consequences of sexual activity; they might seek to avoid the attendant responsibilities of procreation while indulging the sexual drive.

On another level, a rabbinic Bible commentary observes that, throughout the first chapter of Genesis, the seal of approval—the announcement that "the Lord saw that it was good"—is repeated for each element of creation. But after Adam was created, "the Lord said, 'It is not good that man [Adam] should be alone.'" Only that which can endure is good; if humankind does not procreate, it will not endure.

Nor will God himself endure, according to the Talmud, without us to acknowledge him: "Not to engage in procreation," we are told, "is to diminish the Divine image." That is why the verse "for in the image of God has He created man" (Gen. 9: 6) is followed immediately by the reaffirmation of Genesis 9: 7, "Be fruitful and increase" (*Yevamot* 63b). More to the point, when the later verse (Gen. 17: 7) introduces the Lord who will be "thy God and [that] of thy 'descendants after thee,'" the Talmud asks, "If there are no 'descendants after thee,' upon whom will the Divine Presence rest? Upon sticks and stones?" (*Yevamot* 64a). Without human progeny and continuity, there is no one to worship God. Without the physical body, there is no soul.

The biblical commandment is, as usual, spelled out in its details in *Mishnah* and *Gemara,* the two components of the Talmud, setting forth the *halakah,* the definitive legal ruling as formulated by the Codes. The *halakah* of "be fruitful" requires that a couple replace itself, that is, give birth to at least a son and a daughter. Having several sons or several daughters still does not fulfill the commandment. Yet, after the fact, the Talmud counts "grandchildren like children," so that parents with progeny of just one gender can be reassured that their children's children will help them measure up. Actually, even two children of different genders are only the bare minimum; in Maimonides' codification, the effort to procreate must continue. In *Tosafot,* authoritative critical commentaries from medieval France printed on the margin of the Talmud, the fear is expressed that letting the minimum number suffice could result in ethnic extinction (*Bava Batra* 60b). Infant mortality, as well as the possibility that the offspring may not live to adulthood or not reproduce, requires that more than one son and one daughter be conceived and born.

The duty to go far beyond the minimum has its rationale in the rabbinic dimension of the procreative *mitzvah,* where it is called, in brief, *la-shevet* or *la-erev.* (Deriving legal teaching from biblical books other than the Pentateuch is termed "rabbinic"; only the Five Books of Moses are the source of law called "biblical.") The biblical support for the first, *la-shevet,* is Isaiah (45: 18): "Not for void did He create the world, but for habitation [*la-shevet*] did He form it." The second, *la-erev*, comes from Ecclesiastes (11: 6): "In the morning sow thy seed, and in the evening [*la-erev*] do not withhold thy hand [from sowing], for you know not which will succeed, this or that, or whether they shall both alike be good." These verses strongly suggest a moral imperative to continue beyond the minimum.

The broader dimension of the *mitzvah* is very much an operative part thereof. To illustrate its legal implications, a Sefer Torah (scroll) belonging to an individual requires special care and may not ordinarily be sold for its proceeds. There are two exceptions: It may be sold (1) to finance tuition for the study of Torah, and (2) to dower a bride and thus enable her to marry and procreate. What if she already has a son and daughter? The power of the rabbinic extension of the *mitzvah* is now seen in the ruling that a Sefer Torah may be sold to finance the remarriage of that woman, so that she may fulfill *la-shevet* or *la-erev*.

The traditional pronatalist stance is vividly evident in modern-day rabbinic rulings with respect to reproductive technology. Just as illness or pathology are the targets of Judaism's mandate to heal, whereby Sabbath and dietary laws—and the rest of the Torah—are to be set aside to allow healing procedures to do their work, so barrenness and infertility are seen as pathological states to be overcome by aggressive therapies that may also supersede ritual laws. This equation of barrenness with illness means that fertility problems are to be overcome by such exigencies as in vitro or in utero fertilization, even artificial insemination or gestation by a host mother, for cases in which usual (or "natural") conception and birth are not possible. The principle of the primacy of fertility as a desideratum in a pronatalist tradition is given concrete form by the contemporary application of these legal provisions.

Another technical detail of Jewish law places the *mitzvah* (commandment) of procreation on the man rather than on the woman, though of course both are needed for procreation and both share in the *mitzvah* (virtue). This position may have its basis in the theoretical permissibility of polygamy or polygyny, whereby a man could marry more than one wife, but both paternity and maternity would still be known. The husband has to "worry about" the mitzvah's accomplishment. An actual sex-role difference derives from the "Be fruitful and increase" of Genesis, which goes on to say "Fill the earth and conquer it." The male is the conqueror, the aggressive one; the female, as the more passive, should not have to "go seeking in the marketplace" (*Yevamot* 65a). If that observation is rooted in anthropology, an explanation based more on ethics is offered by a Bible commentator of the twentieth century, Rabbi Meir Simcha

HaKohen (d. 1921): Both the pain and the risk of childbearing are borne by the woman, not the man. Since the Torah's "ways are ways of pleasantness, and all its paths are peace" (Prov. 3: 17), the Torah could not in fairness command a woman to undergo pain and assume risk; this must be her choice and it becomes her virtue. For the man, exposed to neither pain nor risk, there is both the command and the responsibility to heed the command (*Meshekh Hokhmah* to Gen. 1: 28).

The discussion of what is and what is not a commandment refers to the formulations of the Sinai Covenant, which did in most cases reaffirm the pre-Sinai imperatives of Genesis, and as such applies only to the covenanted Jewish community. What of the rest of the world? A system called "the Seven Commandments of the Children of Noah" was discerned by the Talmudic sages; it is derived from God's charge to Noah after the flood and applied to his descendants in the world at large. These commandments include basic moral imperatives against murder, incest, cruelty to animals, and a directive to establish general law and order. Hence, the Sinai legislation cannot be imposed on mankind in its specifics. Many Jewish teachers see the thrust of *la-shevet* as generally applicable, for that biblical verse holds forth the *telos,* or ultimate end, of the earth, that it be inhabited and populated.

Attitudes toward procreation among Jews were not, of course, shaped by the law alone. Pronatalism partakes of the personal and cultural: In the face of all God's promises, Abraham protests to God (Gen. 15: 2): "What canst Thou give me, seeing that I go childless?" The anguish of the barren woman is a recurrent theme in the Bible and beyond. On the other hand, fecundity is the most cherished blessing, exemplified idyllically in the Psalmist image (Ps. 128) of one "whose wife is a fruitful vine" and whose "children are as olive plants around the table" and whose ultimate satisfaction is the sight of "children [born] to thy children."

The natural impulse was buttressed by a national one. Historical circumstances of frequent massacres and forced conversions, with their resulting decimation of Jewish communities, added the impulse to compensate for losses to an existing instinct to procreate. The yearning for offspring was deepened, addressing positively the need to replenish depleted ranks. This contrasts to the response of despair reflected in an antiprocreative stance taken by some Christian sects in the face of evil. The Gnostics in the first century, the Manichees in the fifth century, and the Cathars in the twelfth century are among the groups that taught and lived by the belief that procreation is to be avoided in a world of evil unredeemed. Apprehensiveness about the eventual well-being of offspring, the Talmud teaches, should not be a reason for not bearing children. This was King Hezekiah's worry, to which the response of Isaiah (38: 1–10) is understood to mean: "The secrets of God are none of your business. You fulfill your duty [of procreation]" (*Berakhot* 10a).

In the post-Holocaust days, both the individual and the Jewish collectivity have been encouraged to make up for the physical losses of that tragic period. Nonetheless, realization of this impulse or teaching has not been evident across the board. In fact, the Jewish birthrate in the United States and other developed nations in recent decades was lower than, or as low as, that of the rest of the population. Upward socioeconomic mobility, and an increased pursuit of secular education and professional opportunity, has kept the birthrate down in assimilated families. Jews have, in fact, been visibly active in the movement for zero population growth, advancing a cause they consider ecologically necessary. Reform and, to a greater extent, Conservative Jews generally answer to the influence of Judaic tradition alongside social considerations, while Orthodox families register the highest rates of reproduction.

Contraception and Abortion

Sentiments toward procreation go hand in hand with views and practices of contraception and abortion. The *halakah* of contraception includes both the problem of method—whether or not a particular means completes the sexual union, or is not onanistic—and of motive—whether medical reasons or convenience are determinant. Contraception is clearly permitted where medically indicated, with even the less preferable methods. For nonmedical reasons, only methods such as rhythm or the pill may be used, providing the motive is acceptable. The preferable methods, such as the pill or Norplant, are not occlusive and not onanistic because sperm has an unimpeded trajectory. Coitus interruptus and the use of condoms are the least acceptable methods. But where AIDS, for example, is a threat, the condom's prophylactic properties take precedence, on the Talmudic principle that "[avoiding] danger is more serious than [avoiding] transgression" (*Chulin* 10a). This clear, medical permission means, incidentally, that in marital relations contraception is to be preferred over sexual abstinence.

Medical reasons are essentially what govern resort to abortion. The distinction is made between murder and killing of the fetus: If abortion were murder, it could only be considered if the life of the mother were at stake; as killing, or taking of only a potential human life, it can be considered to save her health or well-being, emotional as well as physical. As with contraception and pronatalism, Orthodoxy takes a less liberal position on abortion in theory and in practice than do the Conservative and Reform alignments.

The voluminous Responsa (formal replies to queries by rabbinic authorities) on these subjects are addressed to the individual couples and to their queries in deed. Global questions are also addressed, such as population control for ethical reasons as a concern for humanity and for available resources. The counsel of one rabbinic authority invoked the notion of "lifeboat ethics," whereby the lifeboat in which we all find ourselves, like Noah's Ark according to a Talmudic observation, must be kept from sinking as a result of overpopulation. The solicitude in halakic legislation for the welfare of existing children and their mother, before adding to one's family, was also invoked to argue for ecological responsibility.

Birthrate and the State of Israel

Advocacy of world population limitation is not contradicted by efforts to raise the Jewish birthrate. To the extent that growth globally threatens human well-being and Earth's ecology, it is an imperative concern for us all. But the Jewish people, constituting less than 1 percent of the world's population, would not adversely affect that picture even if their numbers doubled. Replacing Jewish losses would not upset the geophysical numerical balance; it would merely keep Judaism alive. Other minorities should similarly be allowed to maintain their existing numbers. Jewish aspirations, as reflected in synagogue liturgy, are not to become predominant in the world, but merely to "preserve the remnant of Israel."

That liturgical phrase refers, of course, to the People of Israel, but the State of Israel reflects similar concerns. At least one reason for the state's establishment in 1948 was demographic. When Palestine was ruled by British mandate, a "white paper" was issued that severely limited immigration by Jews, even hapless Holocaust survivors and internees of Europe's displaced-person camps. Whatever else sovereignty and independence provide, here they were necessary primarily to remove quotas and barriers to Jewish immigration.

After Israel was founded under the sponsorship of the United Nations and Jewish refugees were admitted, interior population growth was encouraged. The Hebrew word for immigration is *aliyah,* or ascendance to the Land of Israel. Now a new term was coined—*aliyah penimit,* or internal immigration—to refer to new births in Israel, encouraged as a patriotic act to build the nation and its defenses. Also, since the very raison d'etre of the establishment of the state was as a restored homeland and a haven of refuge, the Law of Return was promulgated. It called for the "ingathering of the exiles," inviting Jews to be rehabilitated in their ancestral home, and granting them automatic citizenship upon their arrival.

The politics of population power have been evident not only in control of the disputed territories of Judea and Samaria (West Bank) but also in Israel proper and in the peace efforts begun in 1993. Nationalists express the concern that a disproportionate increase in the Arab birthrate or Arab immigration could effectively dissipate the Jewish character of the world's only Jewish state. On the other hand, during the early 1990s, massive absorption of Jews from the former Soviet Union and from Ethiopia took place; this influx demonstrated the profound demographic and cultural, as well as political, consequences of population factors.

DAVID M. FELDMAN (1995)

SEE ALSO: *Abortion; Adoption; Coercion; Embryo and Fetus: Religious Perspectives; Eugenics and Religious Law; Feminism; Fertility Control; Freedom and Free Will; Genetic Testing and Screening; Harm; Infanticide; Informed Consent; Judaism, Bioethics in; Justice; Life; Natural Law; Race and Racism; Rights, Human; Sexism; Women, Historical and Cross-Cultural Perspectives;* and other *Population Ethics* subentries

BIBLIOGRAPHY

Feldman, David M. 1968. *Birth Control in Jewish Law: Marital Relations, Contraception, and Abortion as Set Forth in the Classic Texts of Jewish Law.* New York: New York University Press. Also in paperback as *Marital Relations, Birth Control, and Abortion in Jewish Law.* New York: Schocken Press, 1974.

Feldman, David M. 1986. *Health and Medicine in the Jewish Tradition: L'Hayyim—To Life.* New York: Crossroad.

Gold, Michael. 1988. *And Hannah Wept: Infertility, Adoption, and the Jewish Couple.* Philadelphia: Jewish Publication Society.

Goldstein, Sidney. 1992. "Contemporary Jewish Demography." In *Frontiers of Jewish Thought*, pp. 157–177, ed. Stephen T. Katz. Washington, D.C.: B'nai B'rith Books.

Rosenthal, Gilbert S. 1969. *Generations in Crisis: Judaism's Answers to the Dilemmas of Our Time.* New York: Bloch.

Tobin, Gary A., and Chenkin, Alvin. 1985. "Recent Jewish Community Population Studies: A Roundup." In *American Jewish Year Book, 1985,* pp. 154–178. Philadelphia: Jewish Publication Society.

III. RELIGIOUS TRADITIONS: D. ROMAN CATHOLIC PERSPECTIVES

Roman Catholic teaching on population is a complex blend of theological beliefs, ethical norms, and empirical judgments. The distinctive characteristic of Roman Catholic doctrine is the sustained and significant place its teaching on contraception has held in its population position. Indeed, the detailed discussion of contraception in Catholic moral theology at times conveys the impression that this one issue constitutes the whole Catholic position on population ethics.

It is necessary, therefore, to distinguish two related but not identical moral questions in Catholic theological ethics: the morality of contraception and the teaching on population policy. John Noonan's classic work on contraception identifies moments in the history of the tradition when demographic trends affected the official teaching of the church, but it points out that these instances do not stand out as major determinants in the development of Catholic doctrine on contraception (Noonan). Noonan's analysis illustrates the complexity of the Catholic response to falling birthrates in the late Roman Empire, in the medieval period, and again in the nineteenth century. During those periods the Catholic position criticized the idea of restraining population growth but did not assert that procreation of children should be fostered without regard to other values. The balancing factors in the Catholic position are the linking of procreation to education and the high status accorded virginity in Catholic life.

It is possible, therefore, to trace a relationship between contraception and population policy throughout Catholic teaching; yet until the twentieth century, the dominant idea is the prohibition of contraceptive and other birth-limiting practices, with the population issue treated as a minor theme. Even in Pius XI's encyclical *Casti Connubii* (1930), which Noonan describes as "a small summa on Christian marriage" (p. 426), the population issue receives only indirect reference. A systematic treatment of the morality of population policy as a distinct issue in its own right is not evident in Catholic thought until the time of Pius XII (Hollenbach). Beginning with Pius XII's address to the Italian Association of Catholic Midwives in 1951 and continuing through the teachings of Popes John XXIII and Paul VI, Vatican II, the Synod of Bishops (1971), and John Paul II, one can find an articulated ethical doctrine on population policy. The ethical teaching responds to two dimensions of the contemporary population debate: first, intensification of the debate about the relationship of population and resources; second, the move by governments and international institutions to design policies to affect demographic trends.

It is possible to distinguish in the Catholic teaching two species of moral analysis: One focuses on the context of population policy; the other, on the content of the procreative act. David Hollenbach distinguishes these two dimensions as the public and private aspects of Catholic teaching.

Population Policy

The public dimension is found generally in the social teaching of the church; the principal documents relating to population policy are *Gaudium et Spes* (1965) (Gremillion), *Populorum Progressio* (Paul VI, 1967), and the interventions of the Holy See on the occasions of international conferences about population, resources, and the environment. These documents manifest a social, structural analysis of the population issue, seeking to place demographic variables within a broadly defined socioeconomic context. The tenor and style of analysis is exemplified in Paul VI's message for the 1974 U.N. Population Year. The Pope's message argues for a broadly based approach to demographic problems with the category of social justice used as a principal theme (Paul VI, 1974a). This perspective is reaffirmed in the Holy See's intervention at the 1984 U.N. Population Conference (Schotte).

The main presupposition of all these statements is that the population problem is one strand of a larger fabric involving questions of political, economic, and social structure at the national and international levels. While acknowledging the existence of a population problem, this view asserts that it is morally wrong and practically ineffective to isolate population as a single factor, seeking to reduce population growth without simultaneously making those political and economic changes that will achieve a more equitable distribution of wealth and resources within nations and among nations (Rich; Paul VI, 1974a, 1974b).

The ethical categories used in analyzing the social aspect of the population problem are drawn from Catholic social teaching developed principally in the papal documents from 1891 to 1991 (Calvez and Perrin; Gremillion; Pavan; O'Brien and Shannon). The foundation of the argument is that the human person, endowed with the gifts of reason and free will, possesses a unique dignity or status in the world. The person, in Christian thought, is regarded as the pinnacle of God's creative action; the uniqueness of the person is argued in Catholic thought in both philosophical and theological terms. The dignity of the person is the source of a spectrum of rights and duties articulated as claims upon and responsibilities toward other persons and society as a whole. The distinguishing mark of the Catholic theory of rights, setting it apart from a classical, liberal argument, is the assertion of the social nature of the person. Society and state are necessary and natural institutions that are presupposed and required for full human development.

The strong social orientation of Catholic political philosophy holds that the way in which society, state, and subordinate social institutions are designed and structured is a moral question of the first order. Society and state are not self-justifying; they exist for the purpose of achieving the common good, defined as the protection and promotion of the rights and duties of each person in the society (Gremillion).

The central category used in evaluating the organization of social structures and institutions is social justice. This concept has roots in medieval Catholic teaching, but it has been developed and refined in the social encyclicals *Quadragesimo Anno* (1931) (O'Brien and Shannon) and *Mater et Magistra* (John XXIII, 1961), as well as in the third synodal document, "Justice in the World" (1971), and in the social teaching of John Paul II (O'Brien and Shannon). As social justice is used in these documents, it measures the role of key social institutions in procuring a fair distribution of wealth and resources nationally and internationally. In *Pacem in Terris,* the normative framework for assessing social institutions is expanded beyond justice to include truth, freedom, and charity (John XXIII, 1963).

The articulation of these categories in Catholic social teaching manifests two stages of development, both pertinent to a population ethic. The social teaching of the period from 1891 through the 1930s focuses on the nation as the unit of analysis; social justice principally means justice within the nation.

Beginning with Pius XII and continuing through John Paul II, the scope of analysis is broadened to focus on the international community. This move from assessing justice within the nation to justice among nations can be charted in the emergence of key concepts. John XXIII (1961) is the first to discuss the international common good as a standard for measuring national policies. The implication of this idea is that an adequate assessment of a state's policy must be calculated in terms of its impact on other states and peoples as well as upon its own citizens. For transnational questions like population and food policy, such a category of analysis opens a whole new set of questions. A similar expansion of a traditional category is found in "Justice in the World" in its discussion of international social justice (Gremillion). The concept explicitly addresses the structures through which states relate to each other in political and economic affairs. John Paul II develops the notion of solidarity as the ethical category that can direct the increasing interdependence of world politics and economics (O'Brien and Shannon).

At both the national and international levels, the categories of common good, social justice, and freedom of choice for individuals and families in society are used to define the population question. Among social institutions, the family, based on the covenant of marriage, holds a unique place in Catholic thought (Hollenbach). It is regarded as the basic cell or unit of society and the Catholic

Church. In the social hierarchy, reaching from the person through the state to the international community, no other association, save the Catholic Church itself, is accorded such status. The demands of the common good and the requirements of social justice are articulated in terms of providing the family and its members with those conditions of life that satisfy basic human needs, protect personal dignity, and allow human development through the exercise of rights and responsibilities in society.

High on the list of inviolable rights is that of marrying and having a family (Hollenbach). To protect this right and other such rights for each person, Catholic social teaching establishes two parameters: Positively, it calls upon the society to guarantee a basic minimum of material welfare, and negatively, it prohibits the state from any significant interference in the exercise of these rights. To summarize the public dimension of Catholic teaching, it accords primary attention to the context of the population question, focusing on the requirements of social justice that should be met as the first step in dealing with the relationship of resources and people. These requirements in specific form include questions of international trade, development assistance, agricultural reform, foreign-investment policies, consumption patterns, and the structure of social relationships within nations. In addition to these contextual issues in the population debate, Catholic teaching also includes a private dimension as regards the content of the procreative relationship.

The Teaching on Contraception

In contrast to the public teaching that focuses on societal structures, the tradition concerning private matters focuses upon the nature of the conjugal relationship and specifically upon the morality of the conjugal act. The principal issue involves analyzing permissible means of preventing contraception. The private aspect of the tradition is rooted in the extensive Catholic teaching on contraception, which has developed in very complex and detailed fashion since the second century (Noonan).

The modern expression of the private issues of the tradition is found in Pius XI's *Casti Connubii* (1930), Pius XII's *Address to the Italian Catholic Union of Midwives* (1954), Paul VI's *Humanae Vitae* (1968), and John Paul II's *Familiaris Consortio* (1982). The principal private issues in the tradition include the morality of abortion, contraception, and sterilization; in the official teaching, all are rejected as means of preventing conception of birth. The only sanctioned means of limiting conception is some form of natural family planning, that is, one that excludes contraceptives. In contrast to the discussion among theologians on the

public tradition, there is a very significant division between the official teaching on contraception and an analysis of contraception by theologians (Hoyt; Curran). While official teaching forbids all forms of contraception, many prominent theologians hold for the legitimacy of contraceptive techniques and the use of sterilization under specified conditions.

Population Policy and the Teaching on Contraception

The private dimension of the tradition on population policy has public implications; it seeks to prevent any public policy that would either constrain or induce individuals to procure an abortion or to use contraceptives or would prevent them from choosing to have children. There are themes of coherence and consistency between the public and private aspects of the Catholic tradition: Both are concerned with the procreative process as a sacred dimension of human relationships; both seek to preserve maximum freedom for the couple to determine when to exercise procreative rights; both stress that society and the state exist to serve their members, and the relationship of the state to citizens is articulated in terms of social justice and personal freedom.

Having acknowledged these elements of continuity, it is equally important to illustrate the tension that prevails between the public and private dimensions of Catholic teaching on population policy. The tension can be analyzed by examining two principal texts: *Populorum Progressio,* representing the public dimension, and *Humanae Vitae,* representing the private one (Paul VI, 1967, 1968). These texts, in turn, must be assessed in light of the teaching of John Paul II on population policy. Paragraph 37 of *Populorum Progressio* is a carefully articulated and expansive statement of Catholic teaching on population policy (Gremillion). The passage contains the following elements: (1) an acknowledgment that a population problem exists in the world; (2) an affirmation that governments have a right and competency to deal with the problem; (3) a prescription that governmental action must be in accord with the moral law. This specific treatment of population policy is couched in the context of Paul VI's most detailed statement of the need for international reform in the political and economic order. Hence, the paragraph presupposes that the social justice requirements are being addressed, and in that context the paragraph speaks to the question of measures to restrict population growth.

This passage is the clearest statement in Catholic teaching affirming the right of governments to intervene in the population question; left undefined, however, is the permissible scope of governmental intervention. The phrase that renders the policy ambiguous is that public intervention must be "in conformity with the moral law." In this area of public policy, what measures fall within the moral law? One way to clarify and specify the public tradition is to use *Humanae Vitae* as the guide for interpreting the moral law. The principal argument of the encyclical is that the moral law requires each and every act of intercourse to be open to procreation. A supporting reason offered for this position is that any compromise on this point opens the way to unregulated governmental intrusion into the sacred domain of family life (Gremillion). Presumably, then, the conjunction of *Humanae Vitae* and *Populorum Progressio* would limit the scope of governmental intervention to supporting and fostering only that means of population restraint approved in *Humanae Vitae*.

This is a restrictive reading of the texts; another view would stress the distinction between public and private dimensions of Catholic moral teaching as the key to interpreting Catholic teaching on population policy. This distinction is crucial in recognizing the different ethical norms used in Catholic thought for personal and social morality. A characteristic feature of Catholic social teaching is its sense of the multiple levels of society (Murray). The state is distinguished from society, and voluntary associations are distinguished from the state. Each principal part of the societal fabric is regarded as having a specific, limited role to play.

Two corollaries flow from this carefully delineated perspective on society. First, there is the recognition that personal conceptions of morality cannot be directly translated into requirements of social morality or public policy; to attempt to do so ignores the distinct nature of social and institutional relationships in society and thereby "makes wreckage not only of public policy but also of morality itself" (Murray, p. 286). Second, a recognition of two related but distinct levels of moral discourse—public and private—yields the jurisprudential distinction of moral law and civil law (Murray). While every human action and all human relationships fall under the moral law, only those that have a demonstrable effect on the public order and are open to state regulation without sacrificing other proportionately significant values are to be included under civil law or public policy. Since Catholic theology recognizes distinctions between public and private morality and between civil and moral law, it is possible for Catholic teaching to oppose an action or policy on moral grounds but not be inevitably committed to seek legal or political means to prevent its implementation.

The use of these distinctions between public and private morality and between civil and moral law could yield a more flexible reading of *Populorum Progressio*. First, such a reading would accent the state's right to intervene in the population question. Second, it would then treat the *Humanae Vitae* argument as being principally applicable in the area of personal morality and not an adequate framework for examining population policy. Third, it would acknowledge the disputed character of *Humanae Vitae* in the Catholic community, even as a norm of personal morality. The purpose of bringing to light the opposing Catholic views on papal teaching regarding contraception (as expressed in *Humanae Vitae*) would simply be to acknowledge that, when such dispute exists within the Catholic community, there is strong reason not to seek to make such a norm a standard of public policy in a pluralistic world. Finally, while not interjecting the specific prescriptions of *Humanae Vitae* into public debate, such a Catholic stance could still speak to the limits of permissible state intervention on population questions. The criteria for setting limits could be drawn from the human-rights standards of the public ethic in the tradition, including a stance against abortion (on human-rights grounds), protection of the person from coercion regarding procreative practice (particularly regarding sterilization), and a respect for religious and moral pluralism as a guide for governmental action.

This broadly designed "public" approach to population policy, one cast in terms of human rights and social justice, is defensible in terms of principles of Catholic moral theology. It is not, however, the direction Pope John Paul II has set for the church's approach to population questions since his election to the papacy in 1978. His approach has been to tie the public and private dimensions of policy more tightly together, thereby raising the visibility and role of the teaching on contraception in the overall direction of policy. The impact of John Paul's leadership can be found in his own teaching and in the positions the Holy See has taken in international conferences on population-related issues.

Teaching of John Paul II

John Paul's influence can be summarized in terms of four contributions. First, in his encyclical on Catholic moral theology *Veritatis Splendor* (1993), the pope reaffirmed the structure of moral argument that sustains traditional Catholic teaching, not only on abortion but also on sterilization and contraception. The encyclical did not break new ground on these issues, but the effect of it has been a call for greater restraint on theological dissent from the teaching on contraception and sterilization. The scope of *Veritatis Splendor* is much broader than specific issues of sexual morality; its influence on population policy lies in its resistance to an interpretation of Catholic teaching that would treat contraception as an internal issue of church discipline but not a position to be espoused in public policy. Prior to the encyclical, the pope's thinking was made clear in the Holy See's intervention at the 1984 U.N. Conference on Population at Mexico City. The Vatican's statement affirmed "that the Catholic Church has always rejected contraception as being morally illicit. That position has not changed but has been reaffirmed with new vigor" (Schotte, p. 207).

Second, the weight given to the private dimension of Catholic teaching does not, however, mean that John Paul II has forsaken the broader public dimensions of the teaching on population policy. Indeed, the second dimension of his contribution to population policy in the church has been to expand and develop the social justice theme espoused by Paul VI and the 1971 Synod of Bishops. John Paul's contribution is found in a series of encyclical letters, from *Redemptor Hominis* (1979) through *Centesimus Annus* (1991). In his social teaching, John Paul develops a moral vision rooted in human rights, including both political and economic rights, and shaped by principles of social justice and solidarity. The papal teaching takes the international community as the unit of analysis, and John Paul II argues that a broadly defined notion of human, economic, and social development should be the context for examining population questions. John Paul II substantially extends Paul VI's critique of international institutions and practices in the socioeconomic order. Like his predecessor, John Paul II primarily emphasizes deep and extensive changes in international economic policies as the response to demographic pressures. In *Sollicitudo Rei Socialis,* he argues that "one must denounce the existence of economic, financial and social mechanisms which … often function almost automatically, thus accentuating the situation of wealth for some and poverty for the rest" (O'Brien and Shannon, p. 404). In the same encyclical, John Paul II cites the need "for a solidarity which will take up interdependence and transfer it to the moral plane" (p. 411). In subsequent teaching, he explicates some of the policy demands of solidarity as they affect international distribution, problems of the Third World debt, and protection of human rights within nations and through the work of international institutions.

Third, a dimension of Catholic teaching which holds a prominent place in the pontificate of John Paul II is the relationship of migration and population. The teaching and the practice of the church both testify to a deep concern for the welfare of migrants and refugees. At the level of the Holy See, in the structure of national episcopal conferences, and in the work of dioceses and religious orders, the pastoral care of migrants and refugees holds a substantial place in the ministry of the church.

This ministry is supported by Catholic teaching on migration. The perspective on the right of the person to emigrate and immigrate is based on Catholic teaching on human rights and on the moral structure of the international order. The right of the person to emigrate places upon the international community, and states within it, the responsibility for developing fair policies regarding immigration. Catholic teaching does not assert an unlimited duty to receive migrants and refugees, but it does not specify particular limits either. The emphasis of the teaching falls on a duty of international solidarity that then must find expression in international and national policies regarding migrants and refugees. In John Paul II's teaching, "the state's task is to ensure that immigrant families do not lack what it ordinarily guarantees its own citizens as well as to protect them from any attempt at marginalization, intolerance or racism …" (John Paul II, 1994, p. 718).

This expansive conception of the duty of states to be open to the movement of populations when they are driven by war, famine, economic necessity, or human-rights violations provides another social instrumentality, along with the teaching on social justice, to complement the Vatican's restrictive policy regarding the limitation of population.

In summary, there is substantial continuity between Paul VI and John Paul II on the public dimensions of population policy. The public argument about human rights and social justice remains the context in which population policy is addressed. Within that context, however, there is a difference in the way John Paul II relates the public and private dimensions of Catholic teaching.

This is the fourth aspect of his teaching, and it does not point toward more active Catholic engagement concerning population issues. Paul VI had acknowledged the objective dimensions of demographic problems, and the duty of governments to address these; John Paul II places the emphasis in a different direction. He also acknowledges that population growth can create "difficulties for development," but his concern is principally about the abuses public agencies commit in pursuit of population policies (O'Brien and Shannon). There is undoubtedly a need for the multiple concerns expressed by the pope himself and by the Holy See in its 1984 intervention at Mexico City. The values and principles stressed in the Holy See's intervention at the Mexico City conference and reiterated in 1994 by Pope John Paul II in preparation for the U.N. Population Conference at Cairo—protection of the rights of the person and the family, resistance to conditioning economic assistance on the basis of population targets, restraints on the role of the state—are necessary for an ethically sound population policy. But there is less positive encouragement or guidance for the state or international agencies to take responsibility for population issues. The principal guidance for public authorities is to reject abortion, sterilization, and contraception in the implementation of population policy. These restrictions are matched with a statement of the duty states have to create conditions within which parents can make responsible choices about family size (e.g., John Paul II, 1994).

Clearly, any Catholic policy will oppose abortion because of the deeply held conviction that a human life is at stake, and it will be deeply suspicious of state intervention in any decisions and choices about procreation that are basic to the dignity and freedom of married couples. The question of whether all forms of contraception would have to be explicitly opposed, save that described in Catholic thought as "natural family planning," is what lay implicit in Paul VI's statement of 1967. John Paul's response is decisively in the direction of treating abortion, sterilization, and contraception in similar fashion; although different in nature, all three are to be opposed in population policy.

The basic lines of Catholic policy, in both its public and private dimensions, have been firmly set for centuries. The policy combines a powerful vision of economic justice and human rights with a comprehensive resistance to most specific measures of population limitation. At the level of implementation, does the policy framework allow for or manifest any differentiation? Two possibilities exist: at the level of pastoral care and the level of principles and rules of conduct.

The pastoral level involves the advice, counsel, and direction provided by the ministers of the church to Catholics as guidance for conscience. The pastoral level also involves the degree of activism that marks Catholic life on population issues at national and local levels of the church. The other possibility for differentiation would involve an attempt to change the basic principles of Catholic teaching in its public or private dimensions.

In his history of the teaching on contraception, John Noonan illustrates the fact that some difference has often marked the church's life between what has been prohibited at the level of principle and how distinctions were made to accommodate the specific conditions in the lives of individuals. In the years since *Humanae Vitae* (1968) was issued, substantial differences have existed between the principles of the encyclical and the choices individuals have made, often with advice from theologians or pastors. John Paul II has been vigorous in his attempt to close this gap. While pastoral practice undoubtedly affects the population issue, its primary impact is felt not at the level of church policy or involvement in the public debate on population issues but in the lives of individuals.

In terms of the principles of Catholic population policy, it is useful to compare the universal teaching and the role of the church within nations. It is clear that the church ministers in nations with very different approaches to population policy, some close to Catholic principles and others in direct opposition to either the public or private dimensions of Catholic teaching. It is also clear that in the period since the Second Vatican Council, there has been greater possibility in Catholic polity for national episcopal conferences to take initiatives in applying the church's teaching to specific local circumstances. Examples of this include Latin American hierarchies addressing human rights and economic justice, and the hierarchy of the United States engaging the issues of nuclear deterrence and economic policy.

Population policy, however, is not an area where much latitude exists for national or local voices. The Holy See, through its teaching office and its diplomatic engagement, is clearly the primary and predominant voice on population issues. National hierarchies may coexist with governmental programs that differ from Catholic teaching, but they seldom seek to challenge or change the principles of Catholic teaching to meet their local situations. Examples of national teaching that do seem to press for some change in the understanding or application of the teaching (particularly in its private dimensions) are recognized as rare exceptions. Such is the case of the Indonesian bishops who issued a statement in 1968 and then were required to provide clarification of their position in 1972 (Indonesian Bishops, 1972). The normal practice for episcopal conferences is to take the Holy See's principles as the premise of their position and then try to relate these principles to the broader policy debate in their own countries; this has been the policy followed by the U.S. bishops in their 1973 and 1994 statements on the population question (National Conference; U.S. Cardinals).

In the 1984 U.N. Conference on Population in Mexico City and in the preparatory debate leading to the 1994 Cairo conference, John Paul II has forcefully reasserted the papal role as the decisive voice on population issues. His position of tightly integrating the public and private dimensions of the teaching, and seeking to shape global policy in both areas, sets the standard for any other voice in the Catholic Church. No Catholic policy would forsake either the socioeconomic principles of justice or its opposition to abortion as a method of population limitation. The effect of John Paul II's leadership is to reaffirm these dimensions and to diminish the likelihood that any distinction will be made in the policy debate between the public and private dimensions of Catholic teaching (John Paul II, 1994).

J. BRYAN HEHIR (1995)

SEE ALSO: *Abortion; Adoption; Christianity, Bioethics in; Coercion; Embryo and Fetus: Religious Perspectives; Eugenics and Religious Law; Feminism; Fertility Control; Freedom and Free Will; Genetic Testing and Screening; Harm; Infanticide; Informed Consent; Justice; Life; Natural Law; Race and Racism; Rights, Human; Sexism; Women, Historical and Cross-Cultural Perspectives;* and other *Population Ethics* subentries

BIBLIOGRAPHY

Calvez, Jean-Yves, and Perrin, Jacques. 1961. *The Church and Social Justice: The Social Teaching of the Popes from Leo XIII to Pius XII (1878–1958),* tr. J. R. Kirwan. Chicago: Henry Regnery.

Curran, Charles E., ed. 1969. *Contraception: Authority and Dissent.* New York: Herder & Herder.

Ferree, William. 1948. *Introduction to Social Justice.* New York: Paulist Press.

Gremillion, Joseph, ed. 1976. *The Gospel of Peace and Justice: Catholic Social Teaching since Pope John.* Maryknoll, NY: Orbis Books. Cites many of the papal messages mentioned in this article.

Hollenbach, David. 1975. "The Right to Procreate and Its Social Limitations: A Systematic Study of Value Conflict in Roman Catholic Ethics." Ph.D. dissertation, Yale University.

Hoyt, Robert G., ed. 1968. *The Birth Control Debate.* Kansas City, MO: National Catholic Reporter.

Indonesian Bishops. 1973. (1972). "Population: Indonesian Bishops Statement." *Origins* 3(16): 250–251.

John XXIII. 1961. "Mater et Magistra: Christianity and Social Progress (May 15, 1961)." In *The Gospel of Peace and Justice: Catholic Social Teaching since Pope John,* pp. 143–200, ed. Joseph Gremillion. Maryknoll, NY: Orbis Books.

John XXIII. 1963. "Pacem in Terris: Peace on Earth (April 11, 1963)." In *The Gospel of Peace and Justice: Catholic Social Teaching since Pope John,* pp. 201–241, ed. Joseph Gremillion. Maryknoll, NY: Orbis Books.

John Paul II. 1979. *Redemptor Hominis: Redeemer of Man.* Washington, D.C.: U.S. Catholic Conference.

John Paul II. 1982. *Familiaris Consortio: The Role of the Christian Family in the Modern World.* Washington, D.C.: U.S. Catholic Conference.

John Paul II. 1993. "Veritatis Splendor: The Splendor of the Truth." *Origins* 23(18): 298–334.

John Paul II. 1994. "Population Conference Draft Document Criticized." *Origins* 23(41): 716–719.

Murray, John Courtney. 1960. *We Hold These Truths: Catholic Reflections on the American Proposition.* New York: Sheed & Ward.

National Conference of Catholic Bishops. 1973. "Statement on Population." In *Pastoral Letters of the United States Catholic Bishops,* pp. 380–383, ed. Hugh J. Nolan. Washington, D.C.: U.S. Catholic Conference.

Noonan, John Thomas, Jr. 1965. *Contraception: A History of Its Treatment by the Catholic Theologians and Canonists.* Cambridge, MA: Harvard University Press.

O'Brien, David J., and Shannon, Thomas A. 1992. *Catholic Social Thought: The Documentary Heritage.* Maryknoll, NY: Orbis Books.

Paul VI. 1967. "Populorum Progressio: On the Development of Peoples (March 26, 1967)." In *The Gospel of Peace and Justice: Catholic Social Teaching since Pope John,* pp. 387–415, ed. Joseph Gremillion. Maryknoll, NY: Orbis Books.

Paul VI. 1968. "Humanae Vitae: On the Regulation of Birth (July 25, 1968)." In *The Gospel of Peace and Justice: Catholic Social Teaching since Pope John,* pp. 427–444, ed. Joseph Gremillion. Maryknoll, NY: Orbis Books.

Paul VI. 1974a. "Paul VI/Population Year: The Common Future of the Human Race." *Origins* 3(43): 670–672. Message on the U.N. Population Year.

Paul VI. 1974b. "Address of His Holiness Pope Paul VI to the Participants of the World Food Conference, Rome (November 9, 1974)." In *The Gospel of Peace and Justice: Catholic Social Teaching since Pope John,* pp. 599–606, ed. Joseph Gremillion. Maryknoll, NY: Orbis Books.

Pavan, Pietro P. 1967. "Social Thought, Papal." In *New Catholic Encyclopedia,* 13: 352–361. New York: McGraw-Hill.

Pius XI. 1930. "Casti Connubii." *Acta Apostolicae Sedis* 22(13): 539–592.

Pius XII. 1954. "His Holiness Pope Pius XII's Discourse to Members of the Congress of the Italian Association of Catholic Midwives" (October 29, 1951). In *Catholic Documents: Containing Recent Pronouncements and Decisions of His Holiness Pope Pius XII.* London: Pontifical Court Club by the Salesian Press.

Rich, William. 1973. *Smaller Families Through Social and Economic Progress.* Washington: Overseas Development Council.

Schotte, Jan. 1984. "Perspectives on Population Policy." *Origins* 14(13): 205–208. Intervention of the Holy See at the U.N. International Conference on Population at Mexico City.

Synod of Bishops. Second General Assembly. 1971. "Justice in the World (November 30, 1971)." In *The Gospel of Peace and Justice: Catholic Social Teaching since Pope John,* pp. 513–529, ed. Joseph Gremillion. Maryknoll, NY: Orbis Books.

U.S. Cardinals and President of the National Conference of Catholic Bishops. 1994. "Letter to President Clinton." *Origins* 24: 58–59.

III. RELIGIOUS TRADITIONS: E. EASTERN ORTHODOX CHRISTIAN PERSPECTIVES

Population questions have not received a great deal of treatment in Orthodox theology or ethics. What little has been written comes out of other, related interests. Even in patristic times, population concerns usually appeared within the framework of discussion on Christian marriage and attendant issues, the most important of which was the place of procreation as a purpose, or even as *the* purpose, of marriage. The fourth-century writings of Saint John Chrysostom, for example, suggest that the purpose of marriage is in part determined by population considerations.

Recent Literature

The relevant Eastern Orthodox literature on the contemporary situation may be divided into two periods.

FIRST PERIOD: 1933–1969. During this time, Orthodox thinking discounted the threat of overpopulation, which was either ignored or seen as a dubious argument to support birth control. If it was taken seriously, it was perceived to be a false issue, unsupported by the evidence. This position aimed to undercut support for conception control, especially in regard to maintaining the strength of ethnic groups. Many traditionally Orthodox countries (e.g., Greece, Bulgaria, Romania, Serbia) were experiencing a reduced birthrate, which was often perceived as putting them at a political and military disadvantage in relation to neighboring countries. Hence, their interest was in increasing rather than decreasing their populations.

The first important work of this period appeared in 1933: Seraphim G. Papakostas's *To zetema tes teknogonias: To demographihon problema apo Christianikes apopseos* (The question of the procreation of children: The demographic problem from a Christian viewpoint), which places birth control and population concerns within family ethics. The population issue appears under the rubric "The Arguments of the Supporters [of birth control]," where the author holds that arguments drawn from the threat of overpopulation, financial considerations, the improvement of conditions of life for both individual and nation, and other such positions are inadequate to justify the practice of birth control. After discussing the relationship between population and cultivated land, Papakostas concludes that "the means of support are increasing faster than the population" (p. 53). Numerous factors contribute to overpopulation, he argues, and all must be functioning in order for it to occur. His conclusion is that "the danger of overpopulation is non-existent" (p. 57).

In 1937 the Holy Synod of the Church of Greece, its highest governing body, issued an encyclical against the practice of birth control that reflected Papakostas's views. (Papakostas was very likely the author of the encyclical.) Although the document treats birth control almost without reference to the population issue, the encyclical does characterize birth control as an agent of "permanent harm to the Greek Nation because of the reduction of the population."

A similar treatment of the subject, written by the *hegoumenos* (abbot) of one of the monasteries of Athos, Gabriel Dionysiatou, was published in 1957. In this work, *Malthousianismos: To englema tes genoktonias* (Malthusianism: The crime of genocide), concern with overpopulation is believed to be unwarranted. The author, however, does not foresee the progress of technology and the resulting increase of agricultural productivity and distribution. The study is based on the view that the primary purpose of marriage is the procreation of children.

SECOND PERIOD: 1970 TO THE PRESENT. The second period of the treatment of the population issue, beginning in 1970, continues to deal with its relationship to birth control. A significant number of writers now feel that birth control is not the unmitigated evil described in the previous period. Most have adopted their view not because of population issues but through a rejection of Augustinian understandings of sin and "concupiscence" and a more Eastern patristic understanding of the purposes of marriage. While the Western patristic approach drew moral teaching primarily from natural law, the Eastern view was based on a Trinitarian approach that emphasized the interpersonal dimensions of marriage.

Of great importance is Alexander Stavropoulos's *He ekklesia tes Hellados enanti tou problematos tes technogonias* (The Church of Greece and the question of the procreation of children), published in 1977. Using textual analysis, Stavropoulos shows that both Papkostas's work and the encyclical of 1937 were based not on patristic sources but on Western prototypes. As a result of Stavropoulos's work, the encyclical ceased to be considered an authoritative text for Orthodox theological and ethical reflection. Efforts were made to include the issue of conception control in the themes of a forthcoming Great and Holy Council of the Orthodox church, but eventually it was dropped.

Some Orthodox writers treat the issue on the basis of theological grounds without reference to population concerns (Meyendorff; Constantelos, 1975; Zapheiris, 1974, 1991; Harakas, 1982). During this period a revival of patristic thought and method in theology, emphasizing the importance of the interpersonal dimensions of Eastern Orthodox Christianity, has been instrumental in changing the attitude toward ethical issues as well. These theological developments focus on the human dimensions of Orthodox Trinitarian theological perspectives, since the doctrine of the Holy Trinity as "three persons in unity" is seen as paradigmatic for human beings, in that the goal of human life is growth toward Godlikeness.

Several new treatments of birth control in relation to population issues have appeared in this period. The debate now focuses on the actual (or the mistakenly perceived) danger of overpopulation. In *The Sacrament of Love,* Paul Evdokimov (1985) makes explicit reference to the danger of overpopulation as an argument for the use of birth control.

Similarly, Nicon Patrinacos (1975) deals with ethnic demographic implications, placing the population issue in historical perspective. Explaining the traditional emphasis on the procreative dimension of marriage, he notes: "As with all societies and nations of [the Byzantine] era, numbers were extremely important to the survival of the country and nation" (p. 3). He comments that many factors explain Orthodox emphasis on population increase: high infant mortality; population depletion resulting from frequent wars; and lack of adequate sanitary conditions, medical care, and food. Unlike the writers of the pre-1970 period, Patrinacos is convinced of the reality and dangers of the population explosion. Rather than discounting it, he takes it as one of the chief elements of his moral reasoning. He condemns as evasive and morally irresponsible those positions that ignore the issues created by overpopulation. He is convinced that "unlimited reproduction of our own kind has reached the point of impoverishing rather than enriching humanity" (p. 46).

Patrinacos holds that the command God gave to Adam and Eve to multiply and populate the Earth has been realized. The church must now provide new guidance: "Birth control is, in more than half of today's world, as important and as urgent as feeding the millions of starving. More births would mean more hunger, more pain, more deaths" (p. 48).

The revival of the patristic mind-set in Orthodox theology, with its emphasis on both divine and human relationality, makes untenable the older argument that the only or primary purpose of marriage is procreation. The theology of marriage has come to focus on the interpersonal unity and relationship of spouses. Studies by Megas Farantos (1983), Paul Evdokimov (1985), Haralambos Hatzopoulos (1990), Chrysostom Zapheiris (1991), W. Basil Zion (1992), and Stanley Harakas (1992), among others, reject the previous approach as not reflective of authentic Eastern Orthodox perspectives, and approve conception control within marriage. Some of these writers connect conception control to population issues.

Nicholas Bougatsos's 1994 work, *He rhythmise tes teknogonias: Orthodoxos kai Hellenike apopse* (The regulation of childbearing: Orthodox and Hellenic view), discounts the issue of overpopulation for Greece and Europe in general (it does not deal with population issues in the Third World). Nevertheless, Bougatsos argues that for theological reasons, different approaches to the issue of conception control are

ethically possible. These may include the practice of birth control by spouses for a number of reasons, among them the enhancement of interpersonal relations and growth in the unity of Christian marriage.

A Population Agenda for Orthodox Christian Ethics

The crucial differences between the earlier and later aspects of this discussion are traceable both to theological outlooks and to concern with issues of population. The foundations now exist for the development of an Orthodox population ethic, which might include a number of elements.

THEOLOGICAL APPROPRIATENESS OF POPULATION CONCERNS. It is true that "the Fathers of the Church were … uninterested in the economic implications of population growth … and early Christian writers can, indeed, hardly be considered to have had a population policy" (Callahan, p. 187). However, contemporary Orthodox ethics is concerned with population as both an imperative of present existential realities and a demand of the implications of the faith. Orthodox ethics cannot ignore the implications of the fact that there has been an enormous increase in the rate of world population growth, especially in the Third World. It cannot limit its teachings on conception control to the geographical areas where its members reside. Humanity must "maintain some balance between [its] numbers and the finite dimensions of this planet" (Freedman, p. 18).

THEOLOGY OF HUMAN DOMINION OVER THE EARTH. Theological anthropology has ecological and population implications. Traditionally, political implications have been discerned in humanity's creation in the image of God by finding parallels between the kingship of God and that of political leaders. The same doctrine requires human responsibility for creation, including ecological and population dimensions. Further, the dominion of humanity over the environment is an appropriate aspect of the Orthodox doctrine of divine providence in conjunction with the doctrine of "synergy," which calls for the cooperation of the human with the divine. Orthodox ethicists (e.g., Demetropoulos) have expressed some renewed interest in this approach.

ETHICAL DOCTRINE OF PHILANTHROPY. One of the chief theological and ethical categories of Eastern Christianity is *philanthropia*, a concept that transcends mere charity and includes the heartfelt identification of God, the church, and the individual Christian with all of humanity. *Philanthropia*, long a fruitful concept for Eastern Orthodox thought and life (Constantelos, 1968), has implications for population issues.

FERTILITY GUIDELINES. Orthodox personal ethics and the ethics of marriage and family have not adequately elucidated the implications of population realities. Both church leaders and scholars tend to leave such issues to "private conscience" or the "guidance of father confessors," although public teaching on the matter is now more widespread than it was earlier (Harakas, 1982; Meyendorff).

JUSTICE AND DISTRIBUTION POLICIES. The Orthodox churches tend to focus on national cultures and heritages. This is a result of their strong "incarnational" emphasis, based on the theological teaching in regard to the second person of the Holy Trinity, the Son, who took on full human nature and lived on Earth. The divine, as fully present in the created human reality of the one person Jesus Christ, becomes a model for all creation and relationships. Sacraments, icons, and church architecture are religious examples of this modeling in that in and through them the divine is made significant. Relationships, both formal and informal, are also imbued with the divine. Among these, marriage and marital relationships are thus understood incarnationally.

Global perspectives focusing on structural injustices, especially as they relate to population concerns, are equally incarnational concerns. The Orthodox Christian conscience has always had a universal dimension. Orthodox anthropology does not permit the view that equitable food distribution policies are utopian, nor that population concerns are limited to a single nation or region (Patrinacos).

AN ECUMENICAL APPROACH. Concern for population problems must be a shared endeavor. This may come closest to the original intent of Orthodox involvement in the ecumenical movement, the original justification of which was based on interchurch cooperation toward the solution of social problems. The ecumenical approach, however, must go beyond church cooperation and include collaboration with local and international agencies concerned with hunger and population problems.

POLICY AND PRACTICE. The recent direction in Orthodox thought has been to become more deeply involved in social issues. If this increased social involvement is to be put into practice seriously, Orthodox leaders will seek practical policy changes. For example, if birth control is to be considered by the Orthodox to be "one of the more effective means by which a balancing between eaters and food to be eaten, consumers and goods, and services and labor" can occur

(Patrinacos, p. 48), this implies a commitment to a positive emphasis on conception control, coupled with sex education founded on a deeply considered theology of marriage. In addition, the Orthodox church must develop acceptable practices to influence national and international policymaking, legislation, corporate decision making, and public opinion. Serious concern with population issues necessarily requires what has been called "eco-tactics" (De Bell)—what used to be called in Orthodox history "whispering in the ear of the Emperor in the name of Christ."

In conclusion, both the imperatives and the potentials for involvement by the Orthodox church in population concerns are found within its tradition.

STANLEY S. HARAKAS (1995)

SEE ALSO: *Abortion; Adoption; Christianity, Bioethics in; Coercion; Eastern Orthodox Christianity, Bioethics in; Embryo and Fetus: Religious Perspectives; Eugenics and Religious Law; Feminism; Fertility Control; Freedom and Free Will; Genetic Testing and Screening; Harm; Infanticide; Informed Consent; Justice; Life; Natural Law; Race and Racism; Rights, Human; Sexism; Women, Historical and Cross-Cultural Perspectives;* and other *Population Ethics* subentries

BIBLIOGRAPHY

Bougatsos, Nicholas. 1994. *He rhythmise tes teknogonias: Orthodoxos kai Hellenike apopse.* "Apostolike Diakonia" of the Church of Greece.

Callahan, Daniel, ed. 1970. *The American Population Debate.* Garden City, NY: Doubleday.

Constantelos, Demetrios J. 1968. *Byzantine Philanthropy and Social Welfare.* Rutgers Byzantine Series. New Brunswick, NJ: Rutgers University Press.

Constantelos, Demetrios J. 1975. *Marriage, Sexuality and Celibacy: A Greek Orthodox Perspective.* Minneapolis: Light and Life.

De Bell, Garrett, ed. 1970. *The Environmental Handbook.* New York: Ballantine Books.

Demetropoulos, Panagiotes C. 1970. *Orthodoxos Christianike ethike.* Athens: Author.

Evdokimov [Evdokimoff], Paul. 1985. *Sacrement de l'amour,* tr. Anthony P. Gythiel and Victoria Steadman under the title *The Sacrament of Love: The Nuptial Mystery in Light of the Orthodox Tradition.* Crestwood, NY: St. Vladimir's Seminary Press.

Farantos, Megas. 1983. "Ta antisylliptika kai ethike." In part 4 of *Dogmatika kai ethika,* pp. 337–344. Athens: Author.

Freedman, Ronald, ed. 1964. *Population: The Vital Revolution.* VOA Forum Series. Garden City, NY: DoubledayAnchor.

Gabriel, Dionysiatou. 1957. *Malthousianismos: To englema tes genoktonias.* Volos, Greece: Holy Mountain Library.

Harakas, Stanley. 1982. *Contemporary Moral Issues Facing the Orthodox Christian,* Newly rev. & exp. edition. Minneapolis, MN: Light and Life.

Harakas, Stanley. 1992. *Living the Faith: The Praxis of Eastern Orthodox Ethics.* Minneapolis, MN: Light and Life.

Hatzopoulos, Haralambos. 1990. *To hiero mysterion tou gamou: Oi miktoi gamoi.* Athens: Author.

Meyendorff, John. 1975. *Marriage: An Orthodox Perspective.* 2nd edition. Crestwood, NY: St. Vladimir's Seminary Press.

Papkostas, Seraphim. 1947 (1933). *To zetema tes teknogonias: To demographihon problema apo Christianikes apopseos.* Athens: Brotherhood of Theologians "Zoe."

Patrinacos, Nicon D. 1975. *The Orthodox Church on Birth Control.* Garwood, NJ: Graphic Arts Press.

Stavropoulos, Alexander. 1977. *He ekklesia tes Hellados enanti tou problematos tes tachnogonias.* Athens: Author.

Zapheiris, Chrysostom. 1974. "The Morality of Contraception: An Eastern Orthodox Opinion." *Journal of Ecumenical Studies* 11(4): 677–690.

Zapheiris, Chrysostom. 1991. *Ai ambloseis kai e Orthodoxos ekklesia: Theseis kai antitheseis.* Athens: Author.

Zion, William Basil. 1992. *Eros and Transformation: Sexuality and Marriage: An Eastern Orthodox Perspective.* Lanham, MD: University Press of America.

III. RELIGIOUS TRADITIONS: F. PROTESTANT PERSPECTIVES

Protestantism generally includes all Christian movements, denominations, and sects whose histories can be traced to or related to the sixteenth-century Reformers, especially Martin Luther and John Calvin. Hundreds of such Christian bodies exist worldwide. They represent very diverse theological orientations and forms of church discipline. It is possible to characterize a "mainstream" position on many theological and ethical issues held by major denominational families associated with the World Council of Churches (WCC), including Anglicanism (or Episcopalianism), Lutheranism, Presbyterianism, Methodism, Congregationalism, and various national united churches, such as the United Church of Canada and the Church of North India. Many other Protestant bodies, such as the Assemblies of God, Southern Baptists, and Jehovah's Witnesses are outside such a consensus. Even within the so-called mainline churches sharp differences exist. On many issues, some Protestants take positions completely at odds with others even within their own denominations while finding themselves in agreement with persons in other denominations or even with non-Christians. In recent years, there has been a sharp increase in numbers of Protestants in traditionally Roman Catholic Latin America, in Africa, and in parts of Asia. At the same time, there has been a marked falling off of active participation in the churches in such traditionally Protestant countries as Sweden and the United Kingdom.

It is therefore difficult to generalize about any one Protestant position on population ethics. This article focuses primarily on the mainstream churches and theologians for three reasons. First, these bodies represent the main currents of Protestant Christian history. Second, these bodies have taken the most explicit positions on population issues. Third, theologians representing these bodies present us with the clearest connections between distinctively Protestant theological emphases and ethical applications.

Early Protestant Thought on Population

The Reformers did not have theories about population as such, although their views on human sexual relations and procreation are relevant to discussions about methods of limiting population growth. Both Luther and Calvin understood sexual relations within marriage as a morally acceptable outlet for sexual drives quite apart from the purpose of procreation. Both, especially Calvin, also viewed sexual relations within marriage as an expression of loving companionship between a husband and wife (Fagley). Early Protestantism coincided in time with the decimation of Europe's population through the plague and the Hundred Years' War, so discussions of population during that period—which were mostly by secular writers—emphasized the need for population growth, not limitation. In contrast, Robert Malthus, whose demographic theories, published in 1798, first expressed alarm over excessive population growth rates, was a Protestant clergyman. His views derived more from economic thought than from Protestant theology, but the laissez-faire economic theories that exerted primary influence upon him may themselves have been encouraged by individualistic aspects of Protestant thought, especially the heightened importance of the "calling" each person has from God and the demand that each person respond, through faith, to God's grace (Weber).

Population issues were not intrinsically important to nineteenth-century Protestant thought except at three points. First, Malthus's pessimistic views of population growth were countered by various Protestant divines who considered them an impious reflection on the goodness of God's providence (Hutchinson). Second, in Anglo-Saxon countries, attitudes toward sexual relations during the Victorian era were often repressive. This gave rise to some rejection of contraceptive methods of birth control early in the twentieth century. Third, the nativist movement in North America, which sought to inhibit immigration from Roman Catholic countries, arose almost exclusively among Protestants. That movement exerted influence on subsequent anti-immigration legislation until the mid-twentieth century.

Theological Support for Family Planning

Protestant support for planned parenthood dates from early in the twentieth century. The early American movement in support of family planning and use of artificial methods of birth control, exemplified especially by Margaret Sanger (1883–1966, founder of Planned Parenthood), was more secular and humanist than Protestant, but it began to attract a serious following among Protestant thinkers and churches. The Lambeth Council of worldwide Anglicanism declared in 1930 that contraceptive methods could be justified when there is "a clearly felt moral obligation to limit or avoid parenthood and where there is a morally sound reason for avoiding complete abstinence" (Noonan, p. 125). During the thirty years thereafter, a strong consensus developed among mainline denominations and theologians in support of that position.

The preeminent Protestant theologian of that period, Karl Barth, wrote, "There is agreement to-day among all serious Christian moralists … that although the choice for or against generation and conception is not a matter for human caprice, it should not be left to chance and therefore lack the character of true decision, but must always be a matter of free obedience and therefore free consideration and decision" (Barth, p. 273). Artificial means of contraception must not, he wrote, be considered evil "just because they are so manifestly artificial" (Barth, p. 275). Dietrich Bonhoeffer, another European theologian of the midcentury, wrote, "It would not be right for blind impulse simply to run its course as it pleases and then to go on to claim to be particularly pleasing in the eyes of God; responsible reason must have a share in this decision" (p. 177). While Bonhoeffer strongly opposed abortion, on the grounds that in the pregnancy "God certainly intended to create a human being" (p. 176), he explicitly related support for planned parenthood to rapid population growth rates, which concerned him.

Barth's and Bonhoeffer's views are ultimately grounded in their respective views of creation. God's purposes for human life can be supported or obstructed by events in the natural order, including human interventions. When couples have children for which they are not prepared, this falls outside God's life-giving intentions. The same can be said of whole societies or of the world in general: Too rapid population growth can diminish the possibilities for humanity to find its God-intended fulfillment in the created order. Barth, therefore, did not limit his ethical perspective on family planning to decisions by individual couples about what is right for them. There was also the question of what

was best for society as a whole. Humankind, in his view, is no longer under the divine command of Genesis 1, "Be fruitful, and multiply."

A leading American liberal theologian, Albert C. Knudson, expressed typical American Protestant thought in insisting (1) that procreation is not the only purpose of sexual intercourse; (2) that "there is nothing in the use of contraceptives that is inconsistent with a sincere faith in Divine Providence," since there is no religious duty to let nature run its own course; and (3) that the general improvement in the standard of living requires lowering the rate of population growth (pp. 209–210).

The first two of these points have been so generally characteristic of mainline Protestant thought and official denominational statements that one is hard pressed to find exceptions. The third has been in some dispute.

The Evolution of Protestant Views in the Twentieth Century

We may broadly characterize three main periods in the middle to later twentieth-century Protestant church teaching on population matters.

The first period, roughly from the Lambeth statement of 1930 to the late 1960s, emphasized the companionate, love-enhancing possibilities of sexual intercourse within the bonds of marriage while deemphasizing the moral obligation of married couples to have children. Contraception was generally accepted as a morally legitimate means toward the end of expressing love within marriage for its own sake. Birth control, or "planned parenthood," was, however, considered mainly within the family unit. Couples should be able to have as many children as they wish: no more, no less. Since the real issue was whether people could decide to limit their family size by conscious decision and employing contraceptive means, the net effect of such teaching was to encourage a diminishing birth rate. But during this period comparatively little attention was given to the world population growth rate.

The second period, coinciding with the emergence of the environmental movement in the late 1960s and 1970s and the publication of neo-Malthusian literature on the "population explosion," found Protestant teaching focusing primarily on the dangers of population growth and a corresponding moral responsibility by societies to find ways to limit it. Many of the mainline church declarations date from this period, with revisions added in subsequent years.

The third period, beginning in the late 1970s and corresponding to the growth of the liberation theology movement (the movement that began in the 1960s and that emphasizes freedom from external oppression as a central theme of Christian faith), witnessed greater criticism of neo-Malthusianism as a way to avoid social justice issues in the distribution of the world's resources. There was less inclination to treat population growth rates themselves as the primary problem. During this period, the mainline denominations continued to affirm the importance of family planning and to recognize the morality of the use of contraceptive measures of birth control. But there was a growing tendency to consider population limitation as a by-product of increased social justice and economic prosperity rather than the reverse.

In the United States, this period also witnessed the rise of evangelical Christian movements critical of mainline denominations and of what was taken to be their laxness in sexual morality and family values. Evangelicals often deemphasized the population issue while reemphasizing the restriction of sexual intercourse to marriage and strongly opposing abortion. Evangelicals, as a force in U.S. politics, played a role in the decision by the administration of President Ronald Reagan to oppose the United Nations Fund for Population Activities at the Second World Conference on Population (Mexico City, 1984) and to withdraw funding from the International Planned Parenthood Federation.

Official Positions of Mainline Protestant Churches

Official statements by mainline denominations illustrate the continuing importance of views developed in each of these three periods.

Among the mainline denominations, the United Methodist Church developed what may be the most systematic position on population ethics. The principal outlines of its position were adopted in 1972 as part of a broader declaration of social principles. Subsequent revisions did not substantially modify this position, although various resolutions adopted by the denomination's General Conference show the influence of the third period of Protestant thinking. In its 1992 form the United Methodist statement cites the strains on food, mineral, and water supplies by growing populations and asserts, "People have the duty to consider the impact on the total world community of their decisions regarding childbearing, and should have access to information and appropriate means to limit their fertility, including voluntary sterilization" (p. 40). A 1980 resolution by that denomination adds a theological rationale: "Our goal in history is that everyone may have the conditions of existence necessary for the fulfillment of God's intentions for humanity. Our context in history is the preciousness of life and the love of God and all creation" (p. 345).

The United Methodists have also dealt at length with questions related to the migration of populations. While stopping short of supporting unlimited movement across national borders, the Methodist statement reminds its readers of biblical support for strangers and sojourners, and calls upon the leaders of all nations "to welcome generous numbers of persons and families dislocated by natural disasters, war, political turmoil, repression, persecution, discrimination, or economic hardship" (p. 510). This document also calls upon governments "to alleviate conditions and change internal politics that create a momentum for the migration of people over the world" while seeking "protection of the basic human rights of immigrants … for both documented and undocumented, permanent or transient refugees or immigrants" (pp. 509–510).

Another mainline denomination, the Presbyterian Church in the U.S.A. (and its predecessor denominations), advocated voluntary planned parenthood and population limitation as early as 1965. In that year, the General Assembly of the United Presbyterian Church in the United States of America (UPCUSA; one of the predecessor communions) called upon the United States to "assist countries who request help in the development of programs of voluntary planned parenthood as a practical and humane means of controlling fertility and population growth." In 1971, that body came to "recognize that reliance on individual desires and private decisions to effect voluntary [birth] control, however well supported by information and means, will not be sufficient to provide the necessary limitation of population growth unless there is a radical and rapid change in the attitudes and desires." This document challenged "the assumption that couples have the freedom to have as many children as they can support," asserting that "we can no longer justify bringing into existence as many children as we desire." In 1984, the Presbyterian General Assembly again voiced its awareness "of the increasing size of the world's population and conscious[ness] of the potential consequences of unlimited growth, of resource limitations, of insufficient public responses, and of unmet population needs." It called "upon the U.S. government to participate fully in the International Conference [on population] and to give generous and continuing financial and logistical support to United Nations programs designed to address specific population needs."

The American Baptist Churches adopted a policy statement in 1976 supporting "efforts to develop programs which encourage family planning in an environment of free individual choice." Subsequent declarations emphasized social and economic justice without much specific application to population questions. A 1988 resolution indicated the denomination's internal divisions on the abortion question while opposing abortion "as a means of avoiding responsibility for conception" or "as a primary means of birth control" (1988, p. 9).

The Friends Committee on National Legislation (FCNL) has long supported family planning, but that position receives comparatively little emphasis in statements adopted during what I have characterized as the third period in the evolution of Protestant views on population. A lengthy 1987 statement on a variety of social-political-economic issues, for instance, merely repeats the FCNL's "support for safe and non-coercive family planning as one element of an effective national population policy" (p. 5).

The same 1987 statement does, however, contain a much lengthier section dealing with immigration and refugees. That section expresses the belief that "the world should evolve toward a global community whose people can choose freely where they wish to live and work" (p. 6). The FCNL's "long-range ideal" is, therefore, "a world of open borders that ensures both asylum for refugees escaping oppression and freedom to migrate for those who hope to improve their living conditions" (p. 6). Such a world would require "a more equitable distribution of the world's wealth, more respect for human rights, and greater tolerance of differences than exist at present" (p. 6).

The Unitarian Universalist Association continues to support family planning as a response to "the crush of overpopulation" that "is frequently associated with increasing the pollution of the water, air, soil, and ozone shield, and further depleting the earth's finite resources" as well as being a factor in "aggressive and destructive behavior." This denomination, like the other mainline churches, supports full access to contraception while going further than most in its direct support for "the right to choose abortion" (p. 56).

This sampling of denominational statements on population-related issues in the latter third of the twentieth century suggests no diminution of commitment to planned parenthood and the full rights of access to contraceptive technologies. At the same time, churches devoted less attention to population issues during the 1980s and 1990s and seemed more reluctant to grant full moral legitimacy to abortion.

Protestant denominational statements do not generally enjoy the authoritative status of Roman Catholic papal encyclicals, though they do reflect deliberation by official bodies. When the official statements are seriously inconsistent with the deeper convictions of members, mechanisms are usually present to enact changes. That fact itself reflects a deep historic theme in most Protestant theology: God has immediate access to every believer. Consequently, the views of every church member, when expressed in good faith, must

be taken seriously. Not surprisingly, therefore, Protestant viewpoints on population policy and other issues can change without threat to the basic body of shared doctrine. It is more difficult to ascertain the extent to which denominational statements on such issues reflect nontheological sociocultural influences. But the deliberative process of decision making in Protestant churches generally affords ample opportunity, over time, for purely secular influences to be criticized on the basis of shared faith traditions.

Protestant Positions into the Twenty-first Century

Projecting the future of Protestant views on population, there seems little prospect that the basic commitments to planned parenthood will change during the period ahead. The amount of emphasis given to the issue may well vary, however, with perceptions of the effects of population growth rates and patterns of migration. Protestant churches worldwide will doubtless continue to reflect a wide variety of views on these and other subjects. Historically, however, Protestant views on such issues have tended to be framed in response to empirical problems and opportunities. Evidence mounts that the churches will increasingly have to respond to global environmental problems, and the continuing growth of world population will remain a significant factor in that (Nash). The churches' response to population migration may be even more interesting as the world moves into the twenty-first century. Toward the end of the twentieth century, ethnic nationalism was felt as a major political force in some parts of the world, such as the Middle East, the former Yugoslavia, and the former Soviet Union. Nevertheless, the growing integration of global economics, increased facilities for communication and transportation, and the conclusion of the Cold War between the United States and the Soviet Union all point toward greater pressure on the increasing irrelevance of national boundaries. While addressing problems related to population growth, religious bodies may find it equally necessary to respond to archaic restrictions of movement.

J. PHILIP WOGAMAN (1995)

SEE ALSO: *Abortion; Adoption; Christianity, Bioethics in; Coercion; Eastern Orthodox Christianity, Bioethics in; Embryo and Fetus: Religious Perspectives; Eugenics and Religious Law; Feminism; Fertility Control; Freedom and Free Will; Genetic Testing and Screening; Harm; Infanticide; Informed Consent; Justice; Life; Natural Law; Race and Racism; Rights, Human; Sexism; Women, Historical and Cross-Cultural Perspectives;* and other *Population Ethics* subentries

BIBLIOGRAPHY

American Baptist Churches in the U.S.A. 1976. Policy statement on hunger, Valley Forge, Pa.

American Baptist Churches in the U.S.A. 1988. Resolution concerning abortion and ministry in the local church, Valley Forge, Pa.

Bainton, Roland H. 1962. *Sex, Love and Marriage: A Christian Survey.* London: Collins.

Barth, Karl. 1968. *Church Dogmatics,* tr. Geoffrey W. Bromiley and Thomas F. Torrance. Edinburgh: T. & T. Clark.

Bonhoeffer, Dietrich. 1955. *Ethics,* tr. Neville Horton Smith. New York: Macmillan.

Fagley, Richard M. 1960. *The Population Explosion and Christian Responsibility.* New York: Oxford University Press.

Friends Committee on National Legislation (FCNL). 1988. *FCNL Washington Newsletter,* January.

Hutchinson, Edward P. 1967. *The Population Debate: The Development of Conflicting Theories up to 1900.* Boston: Houghton Mifflin.

Knudson, Albert C. 1943. *The Principles of Christian Ethics.* New York: Abingdon-Cokesbury Press.

Lucas, George R., Jr., and Ogletree, Thomas W., eds. 1976. *Lifeboat Ethics: The Moral Dilemmas of World Hunger.* San Francisco: Harper & Row.

Nash, James A. 1991. *Loving Nature: Ecological Integrity and Christian Responsibility.* Nashville, TN: Abingdon Press.

Noonan, John T., Jr. 1986. "Contraception." In *The Westminster Dictionary of Christian Ethics,* pp. 124–126, ed. James F. Childress and John Macquarrie. Philadelphia: Westminster Press.

Presbyterian Church in the U.S.A. 1991. *Social Policy Compilation.* Louisville, KY: Author.

Unitarian Universalist Association. 1990. *Resolutions of the Unitarian Universalist Association.* Boston: Author.

United Methodist Church. 1992. *The Book of Resolutions of the United Methodist Church,* ed. Neil M. Alexander. Nashville, TN: United Methodist Publishing House.

Weber, Max. 1950 (1904–1905). *The Protestant Ethic and the Spirit of Capitalism,* tr. Talcott Parsons. New York: Scribner.

Wogaman, J. Philip, ed. 1973. *The Population Crisis and Moral Responsibility.* Washington, D.C.: Public Affairs Press.

[*Note: Official declarations on population-related issues by Protestant and ecumenical church bodies are rarely available in libraries or in trade publication form. They generally can be obtained from denominational or ecumenical offices.*]

III. RELIGIOUS TRADITIONS: G. HINDU PERSPECTIVES

Hinduism includes a complex array of teachings related directly and indirectly to population dynamics (fertility, mortality, and migration) and to the ethics of population-related behavior. Its rich heritage spans millennia and embraces diverse populations. Hindus are found in many world regions, both within and beyond South Asia, its area of origin. Hinduism is the predominant religious tradition of India (for a general overview, see Hiltebeitel). It is practiced in one form or another by about 80 percent of the approximately 800 million people living there. Another 20 million Hindus live in nations other than India, including Fiji, Indonesia, Singapore, Guyana, Trinidad, Canada, the United States, and the United Kingdom. Diaspora Hindu communities increased in number and prominence in the United States beginning in the late 1960s, when the law was changed to allow immigration of educated professionals. The construction of major Hindu temples in such cities as Pittsburgh, Chicago, New York, and Washington, D.C., demonstrates the vitality of this international growth.

Basic Hindu teachings on population-related ethics and behavior will have different impacts depending on the context in which Hinduism is practiced. Within a particular locality, socioeconomic class, caste, and ethnicity are associated with differences in awareness of and adherence to Hindu religious teachings. Moreover, social resistance to certain aspects of orthodox Hindu religious teachings is being voiced around the world, particularly by ethnic minorities and women's groups.

This article first considers key aspects of Hindu religious teachings. It then focuses on Hindu values in India and how they contribute to demographic practices and outcomes. Last, it offers some observations on how members of Hindu communities in the United States are revising Hindu values related to population.

Hindu Teachings Related to Population

Several key teachings of Hinduism relate to population dynamics and have implications for how governments might formulate policy. A primary value is on *ahimsa* (this word combines the prefix *a,* "non," with *himsa,* "harm," thus meaning "nonviolence" or "nonkilling"). A well-known source of Hindu teachings on proper behavior, *The Laws of Manu* (Doniger and Smith), describes the model of four life stages (*ashramas*): student, householder, celibate, forest dweller. Manu's guidelines about marriage stipulate that the best form involves the father giving a virgin daughter, implying that the marriage is arranged by the parents of the bride and groom. Repeated statements in *The Laws of Manu* emphasize the importance for a woman of bearing offspring, especially sons. Other popular classical Hindu myths, such as in the epic *Mahabharata,* contain messages relevant to population. One is that the world is overpopulated, and that renunciation of the world is a valid means for release from personal, familial, and other worldly attachments. Celibacy is honored as reflecting a high level of self-control and spiritual attainment. Teachings about celibacy are linked with a strongly enunciated value on premarital chastity for females.

It is likely that these general teachings are known to Hindus throughout India and across most social divisions. It is also likely that links between people's knowledge of Hinduism and their population practices vary markedly across regions because India's demography differs dramatically by region and class (see Miller, 1981). Fertility is much higher in the northern plains than in the south and east. Mortality is more gender-differentiated in the northern plains, with excess female mortality, and is less severely skewed by gender in the south and east.

Thus we are confronted with a puzzle: Basic Hindu teachings are espoused by India's Hindu population more or less equally, but Hindu demography does not present a smooth pattern. We must therefore assume a loose linkage between Hindu teachings and demographic outcomes such as fertility rates and child survival by gender. In other words, as an explanatory variable affecting population dynamics, Hindu teachings are partial at most.

Population Issues in India

FERTILITY. Reproduction should, according to Hindu cultural norms, take place only within marriage. Stigma is attached to a premarital pregnancy, a situation that may bring serious consequences to the persons involved. A high premium is placed on marriage as a universal life stage through which, ideally, everyone should pass. As a householder, one marries, has children, and raises them. Reproduction is the primary goal of marriage. For Hindu women, the key to auspiciousness (a highly desired status for women that implies the opposite of stigma) involves being married, being devoted to one's husband, and bearing sons. All these values are clearly pronatal.

Hindu values support the bearing of children within marriage, and they emphasize the bearing of sons. Sons provide social security for their aged parents. The social security function of sons is especially marked in the northern Indian kinship system, which is followed strictly by Hindus and Jains. North Indian kinship rules stipulate that a daughter must marry a man from outside her natal village while a married son remains with his parents and brings a bride into his family. Another primary value of Hindus is to have a son light one's funeral pyre; a daughter cannot perform this task. The Sanskrit word for "hell" is *put*; the word for son, *putra,* means "the one who saves his ancestors from hell" (May and Heer, p. 200). Given mortality rates of the mid-1960s, demographers estimated that in order for a man to have a son who would be alive when he was sixty-five years old, his wife would have to bear seven children. Preference for male children operates to promote fertility and also plays a role in excess female mortality and indirect fertility reduction as discussed below. Desire for sons prompts families to keep trying until they have one, and then to have a second or third son as well.

The pervasiveness of the Hindu teachings on the value of having sons may be regionally variable in terms of intensity. Social surveys across the nation reveal that a stated preference for sons is stronger in the northern region than in the south and east (Dyson and Moore). This difference arises because socioeconomic factors such as the gender division of labor, marriage and kinship patterns, and the costs of marriage operate to affect the level of son preference (Miller, 1981; Dyson and Moore).

Other important fertility-reducing factors related to Hindu beliefs include ritually determined rules for sexual abstinence that limit the frequency of intercourse. One study found a total of 120 days mentioned for abstention (Nag). Such rules may be linked to a lower frequency of intercourse among Hindus than among Muslims, since the latter do not have such ritually proscribed days. Also important are the positive value placed on male self-control, including control of sexuality, and male anxiety about semen loss (Bottero). No one knows how much of an effect these conditions might have on the frequency of intercourse or actual reproductive rates, but one could posit at least some impact on both compared with non-Hindu populations.

Hindu views concerning widowhood may also lower fertility, since widows should not remarry and therefore should not reproduce (Mandelbaum). Restrictions on widow remarriage most significantly decreases fertility when women are widowed at a young age, as they often are in India.

Direct methods of fertility control, such as condoms, birth-control pills, or sterilization, are not antithetical to Hindu teaching since sexual intercourse is not seen solely as a means to achieve pregnancy. In contrast with this fairly liberal understanding, the famous leader of the independence movement and national hero, Mohandas Gandhi, supported abstinence as the only appropriate contraceptive.

Abortion for sociomedical reasons has long been legally allowed in India, except in the predominantly Muslim state of Kashmir (Chandrasekhar). In spite of legal provisions for abortion, safe services are lacking (Dixon-Mueller). This situation reflects the political priorities of the central and state governments more than religious doctrine.

Sex-selective abortion, a practice begun in the 1980s, is done almost exclusively to abort female fetuses. One study of a large number of hospital births in the Ludhiana area of the state of Punjab in northwestern India found that after 1983, when sex-selection became possible through amniocentesis, the sex ratio at birth rose from a normal of 105 boys per 100 girls to 117 boys per 100 girls in 1989 (Sachar et al.). Many feminist activists in India wish to maintain a woman's right to seek an abortion while striving to ban sex-selective abortion. The debate on prenatal sex selection in the public media in India has been largely secular.

MORTALITY. India is well known for its gender bias in survival of males and females. Hindu teachings that favor males provide the ideological justification for better treatment of males than females. But it is not possible to explain the scarcity of females relative to males in the Indian population solely on Hinduism. North India and neighboring Pakistan, which is predominantly Muslim, have similar gender patterns in mortality. Recent demographic data on China reveal substantial differences in mortality rates between males and females there as well. Economic, political, and social factors are important in explaining this phenomenon.

In the northern plains of India, son preference is linked with behavior termed "daughter neglect" (Miller, 1981, 1987). This neglect, which takes the form of biased allocations of food, medical care, and psychological attention, can be fatal. It skews the sex ratio among children as well as in the general population. In northern India, census data from the first part of the twentieth century indicated that unbalanced juvenile sex ratios favoring boys characterized all major religious groups in the area: Sikhs, Hindus, Muslims, and Jains. Son preference interacts with daughter neglect to create excess female child mortality. The indirect fertility-reducing effect of excess female child mortality is clear: If daughters experience higher mortality than sons, then the number of future childbearers is reduced in comparison with what would be the case without excess female child mortality. In such a demographic regime, the ratio of living sons to daughters is maintained over time, as brides are brought in from other villages and regions to marry sons; thus, no "shortage" of brides to produce future sons is perceived or experienced.

Hindu beliefs seem implicated in the high mortality rates of widows, which are caused by general neglect and nutritional deprivation (Chen and Drèze). More extremely, the low value placed on a woman once her husband has died relates to the uncommon practice of *sati,* the suicide of a Hindu widow on the funeral pyre of her husband. In general, the value of female self-sacrifice is long-standing in Hinduism, and it supports socialization patterns of girls that train them in self-denial of food and other resources.

MIGRATION. According to traditional Hindu teaching, migration beyond the boundaries of India was grounds for outcasting. Since the late nineteenth century, however, the rate of migration of Hindus outside of India has increased substantially (Madhavan), and anxiety about "outcasting" appears to be nonexistent among migrants. With international migration, Hindu traditions are being reshaped in local contexts.

The United States

In the United States, most Hindus are middle or upper class (Helweg and Helweg), although large populations, especially in New York City and New Jersey, are less well off. Among this employed and generally well-educated population, fertility rates are low, infant and child mortality rates are low, and longevity is high.

The value placed on having a son among the Hindu population of the United States is an important but unresearched question. Undocumented sources indicate numerous cases of demand for prenatal sex determination, in order to keep male fetuses, by South Asian immigrants in the United States and Canada. As of 1994, U.S. law prohibits abortion based on the sex of the fetus, but people circumvent this rule. They may have a test done ostensibly to reveal genetic abnormalities in the fetus and, in the process, find out its sex. If the fetus is female, they go to another doctor and present a story about genetic abnormalities in their family that cannot be proved or disproved because the relatives who are claimed to have the genetic problems are in South Asia. On this basis, the couple requests an abortion.

Within the teachings of Hinduism, nothing specifically argues against sex-selective abortion per se, since traditional teachings do not address the topic of abortion from a gender-specific perspective. This issue will pose a challenge for contemporary theologians and ethicists working within the Hindu tradition.

Another issue being quietly contested in the everyday lives of Hindus and Jains in the United States is premarital chastity. In opposition to the more liberal sexual mores among the general population, many Hindu and Jain parents apply pressures on their children, especially daughters, to maintain their virginity before marriage. Depending on how conservative the family is, more or less intergenerational conflict ensues.

Many Hindu and Jain communities have started Sunday schools (never a tradition in India) and summer camps where religious values are instilled in young children and teenagers. Such values include premarital chastity. At the same time, marked liberalizing changes are being made in some Hindu rituals in the United States, as a response to lowered fertility rates (many Hindu families have only one child) and an interest in treating daughters the same as sons. In the early 1990s, the Hindu-Jain temple of Pittsburgh held its first *upanayana* (sacred thread) ceremony for girls. Several liberal-minded leaders promoted this reform of Hindu tradition, which restricts the *upanayana* ceremony to boys of the upper castes.

The Challenge of Change

Neither Hinduism nor population dynamics is static. Contemporary movements in Hinduism range from conservative trends that could be termed fundamentalist to more liberal tendencies among some migrant communities. The greatest challenges to the study of the relationship between Hindu teachings and population lie in the following directions: the links that individuals make in their thinking between Hindu tenets and their own demographic practices; the reactions of Hindu theologians to new questions such as sex-selective abortion; and governments' policies in dealing with such problems as population growth and excess female mortality within a moral framework that would be acceptable to Hindu constituents.

BARBARA D. MILLER (1995)

SEE ALSO: *Abortion; Adoption; Coercion; Embryo and Fetus: Religious Perspectives; Eugenics and Religious Law; Feminism; Fertility Control; Freedom and Free Will; Genetic Testing and Screening; Harm; Hinduism, Bioethics in; Infanticide; Informed Consent; Justice; Life; Natural Law; Race and Racism; Rights, Human; Sexism; Women, Historical and Cross-Cultural Perspectives;* and other *Population Ethics* subentries

BIBLIOGRAPHY

Bottero, Alain. 1991. "Consumption by Semen Loss in India and Elsewhere." *Culture, Medicine, Psychiatry* 15(3): 303–320.

Chandrasekhar, Sripati. 1974. *Abortion in a Crowded World: The Problem of Abortion with Special Reference to India.* Seattle: University of Washington Press.

Chen, Marty, and Drèze, Jean. 1992. "Widows and Health in Rural North India." *Economic and Political Weekly of India* 27(43–44): W5–81–W5–92.

Dixon-Mueller, Ruth. 1990. "Abortion Policy and Women's Health in Developing Countries." *International Journal of Health Services* 20(2): 297–314.

Doniger, Wendy, and Smith, Brian K., tr. 1991. *The Laws of Manu.* New York: Penguin.

Dyson, Tim, and Moore, Mick. 1983. "On Kinship Structure, Female Autonomy, and Demographic Behavior in India." *Population and Development Review* 9(1): 35–60.

Helweg, Arthur W., and Helweg, Usha M. 1990. *An Immigrant Success Story: East Indians in America.* Philadelphia: University of Pennsylvania Press.

Hiltebeitel, Alf. 1987. "Hinduism." In vol. 6 of *The Encyclopedia of Religion,* pp. 336–360, ed. Mircea Eliade. New York: Macmillan.

Madhavan, M. C. 1985. "Indian Emigrants, Numbers, Characteristics, and Economic Impact." *Population and Development Review* 11(3): 457–481.

Mandelbaum, David G. 1974. *Human Fertility in India: Social Components and Policy Perspectives.* Berkeley: University of California Press.

May, David A., and Heer, David M. 1968. "Son Survivorship Motivation and Family Size in India: A Computer Simulation." *Population Studies* 22(2): 199–210.

Miller, Barbara D. 1981. *The Endangered Sex: Neglect of Female Children in Rural North India.* Ithaca, NY: Cornell University Press.

Miller, Barbara D. 1987. "Female Infanticide and Child Neglect in Rural North India." In *Child Survival: Anthropological Perspectives on the Treatment and Maltreatment of Children,* pp. 95–112, ed. Nancy Scheper-Hughes. Dordrecht, Netherlands: D. Reidel.

Nag, Moni. 1972. "Sex, Culture, and Human Fertility: India and the United States." *Current Anthropology* 13(2): 231–237.

Sachar, R. K.; Verma, J.; Prakash, V.; Chopra, A.; Adhlaka, R.; and Sofat, R. 1990. "The Unwelcome Sex: Female Feticide in India." *World Health Forum* 11(3): 309–310.

III. RELIGIOUS TRADITIONS: H. BUDDHIST PERSPECTIVES

Buddhism is a dominant cultural force in most parts of Asia. Theravada Buddhism, also known under the name of Hinayana or "Small Vehicle," prevails in such Southeast Asian countries as Sri Lanka, Thailand, Burma, Cambodia, and Laos; its sister sect, Mahayana Buddhism, or "Great Vehicle," is currently found in Tibet, Japan, Taiwan, and Korea. This article focuses on Theravada Buddhism, especially as practiced in Thailand.

Though Therevadins have their own sacred literature that distinguishes them from the rest of Buddhism, they do share certain central beliefs with other Buddhists. Among these beliefs are those concerned with *samasara, karma,* and *nirvana,* which are the key concepts of all forms of Buddhism. *Samasara* refers to the round of existence, or the cycle of rebirth, in which all beings revolve according to their *karma.* This perpetual cycle comprises three realms of rebirth, namely, the realm of desire (*kamaloka*), the realm of forms (*rupaloka*), and the formless realm (*arupaloka*). These realms have thirty-one subspheres containing different forms of life, such as humans (*manussa*); animals (*tirachan*); ghosts or unhappy departed beings with deformed bodies (*peta*); spirits or wandering ghostly beings (*bhuta*); hell-beings or tortured beings (*niraya*); titans (*asura*); and gods (*deva*). The realm of desire consists of the higher spheres of gods; the middle spheres, of sentient beings, humans, and animals; and the lower spheres, of ghosts, spirits, and hell-beings. The celestial realm of forms and the formless realm are the abodes of the most refined and subtle beings (*brahman*). Despite differences in life span, beings in all realms are subject to death and rebirth.

Karma means intentional, mental, verbal, or physical action and its result (*vipaka*). The sequence of actions, or deeds, and their effects, known as the law of *karma*, act both as the natural law of cause and effect (operating in the physical realm) and as the moral law (governing the moral sphere that regulates the movement of beings between rebirths). Rebirths of all beings are the natural results of their own deeds, good or bad, and not "rewards" or "punishment" imposed by a supernatural, omniscient ruling power. All beings reap what they sowed in the past, and all will be reborn according to the nature of their present deeds—they are "heirs" to their actions. When a being dies, the karmic result, acting as the individual life-force, passes to other lives, endlessly exalting or degrading successive rebirths. This life-force will become completely inactivated only with the cessation of craving (*tanha*), the inherent force of karmic action. Such cessation is referred to as nirvana and can be achieved through following the Middle Path (*Majima Patipada*) consisting of wisdom (*panna*), morality (*sila*), and concentration (*samadhi*).

Buddhist Concepts in Population Growth and Control

There is no fixed number for population in *samasara* existence. It is in a state of flux, with continual migration of beings from one realm to the others regulated by the law of *karma* and continuously readjusted to the nature and the quality of *samasara* dwellers. An increase of population in one realm means a decrease of population in others, and vice versa. Human rebirth is considered incomparably precious because the human realm is the only place where there is enough suffering to motivate humans to seek ways to transcend misery and enough freedom to act on their aspirations. In the higher and lower spheres, by contrast, beings are fully reaping the karmic results, good and bad: The gods are too absorbed in the blissful state to find ways

out of *samasara* existence while animals, ghosts, spirits, and hell-beings are in irremediable misery and have little freedom to do either good or evil. These suffering beings will gain the precious human rebirth only when the results of bad *karma* that led to their lower rebirths are exhausted. When this happens, the results of their previous good actions performed when they were human will lead them to better rebirths and, sooner or later, to the human level again.

From this view, an increase in the human population is desirable for it means more beings will have the rare human opportunity to transcend suffering. In theory, then, Buddhists should welcome population growth. But the fact that increasing numbers of Buddhists use contraceptives in countries such as Thailand, where 98 percent of the population is Buddhist, seems to indicate a different position. Family planning has been quite successful in both urban and rural areas of Thailand. Apart from the contributing factors of the economy, social change, and education, there are some Buddhist tenets that may account for the low fertility rate. The most important one is the emphasis on the quality of human life concomitant with the high value it gives to human rebirth.

In the Buddhist perspective, the rare human rebirth is meaningless if there is no quality in it. The value of life does not depend on its duration but on its quality. For life to be worth living, it should be lived with the ultimate purpose of attaining *nirvana*, the final emancipation. This goal, however, like all spiritual progress, cannot be achieved without a certain degree of material and economic security. Below the level of subsistence, human life lacks real meaning because it consists only of hunger, illness, and unrelieved misery. This emphasis on material necessities was made by the Buddha as a necessary condition for a truly enlightened, meaningful life. The Buddha himself once refused to preach to a starving man until his hunger had first been appeased. He also recommended that monks who lead the life of renunciation depend on the lay community for food, shelter, and clothing.

This emphasis on life's material necessities is an important part of the Buddhist perspectives on population control and thus needs to be considered together with the Buddhist endorsement of human rebirth. That is, human rebirth, though desirable, needs adequate supporting conditions (*upatthambhaka*) to enable it to be worthwhile. Since famine is one of the most powerful forces (*upapilaka*) working against spiritual development, Buddhism does not approve of population growth disproportionate to a society's available resources of food. Because of this, Buddhists in Thailand and other countries do not attribute large family size to good *karma*. Unlike the Hindu householder, who believes he must have sons to perform the prescribed rituals for him after his death, Buddhist parents are not anxious to have sons to be ordained as monks. Although ordination is considered a meritorious act that will ensure good rebirth after death, many other means of receiving merit are also available, including offering food to monks, listening to sermons, and building or repairing temples.

The lack of anxiety for sons or large families supports the practice of family planning among Thai Buddhists. Unlike abortion, which is still socially unacceptable in Thailand and not as widely practiced as it is in Japan, birth control is believed by Thai Buddhists to be in line with Buddhist teachings concerning marriage and family life. Though the Buddha considered celibate life superior to married life, he did not advise it for all his followers. Realizing that all humans were at different stages of spiritual evolution, he did not commend the same codes of conduct to all. To his lay followers who could not lead the austere life of monks and nuns, he recommended marriage but stressed spiritual progress, and not procreation, as its main goal. For those with children he devised a code of discipline, emphasizing responsible childbearing and child rearing.

For Thai Buddhists birth control, unlike abortion, does not transgress the Buddhist precept of nonkilling, nor does it interfere with the working of the law of *karma*. In Buddhist understanding, conception begins only when three factors merge: the coitus of the parents, the woman's generative capability, and the presence of the *gandhabba,* the karmic life force of one who has died. By preventing pregnancy, birth control makes human rebirth more difficult but it does not interfere with the operation of the law of *karma.*

From the Buddhist viewpoint, the fruition of good or bad *karma* requires the right supporting conditions; without them the karmic life-force cannot express itself. Only beings who are fully qualified for human rebirth can be reborn in the human realm. Under unfavorable physical conditions a being, though possessing the good *karma* to be reborn as a human being, must dwell in his or her sphere waiting until the opportune moment. Buddhism does not oblige parents to open the gate of human rebirth to all beings with good *karma* by having as many children as they can. The Buddhist concept of *karma* assigns to each person sole responsibility for his or her own life. According to the Buddhist analysis of human nature, one's sexual life is the outcome of the urge to satisfy one's sexual craving. Whether sexual activity produces children or not is a matter to be decided by the couples themselves. The autonomy of individuals to choose their own destiny and to be responsible for their own actions is a crucial element in Buddhist population ethics.

Self-restraint and the control of the senses and passions are recommended as important forms of population control and to prevent the sexual indulgence that widespread use of artificial means of birth control may lead to. Following this teaching, many Buddhists in Thailand, Sri Lanka, and Burma have contributed to population control by practicing sexual continence, leading celibate lives as monks or nuns, and using contraceptives.

PINIT RATANAKUL (1995)

SEE ALSO: *Abortion; Adoption; Buddhism, Bioethics in; Coercion; Embryo and Fetus, Religious Perspectives; Eugenics and Religious Law; Feminism; Fertility Control; Freedom and Free Will; Genetic Testing and Screening; Harm; Hinduism, Bioethics in; Infanticide; Informed Consent; Justice; Life; Natural Law; Race and Racism; Rights, Human; Sexism; Women, Historical and Cross-Cultural Perspectives;* and other *Population Ethics* subentries

BIBLIOGRAPHY

Chopra, Pran Nath. 1983. *Contribution of Buddhism to World Civilization and Culture.* New Delhi: S. Chand & Company.

Chulalongkorn University. Institute of Population Studies. 1991. *Population in Thailand in 25 Years (1965–1990).* Bangkok: Chulalongkorn University Press.

Gombrich, Richard, and Obeyesekere, Gananath. 1988. *Buddhism Transformed: Religious Change in Sri Lanka.* Princeton, NJ: Princeton University Press.

Harvey, Peter. 1990. *An Introduction to Buddhism: Teachings, History and Practices.* Cambridge, Eng.: Cambridge University Press.

LaFleur, William R. 1992. *Liquid Life: Abortion and Buddhism in Japan.* Princeton, NJ: Princeton University Press.

Smith, Bardwell. 1992. "Buddhism and Abortion in Contemporary Japan: Mizuko Kuyo and the Confrontation with Death." In *Buddhism, Sexuality, and Gender,* pp. 65–90, ed. José Ignacio Cabezon. Albany: State University of New York Press.

POPULATION POLICIES, DEMOGRAPHIC ASPECTS OF

• • •

Population projections made in the 1950s predicted the large expansion in human numbers that subsequently occurred in the second half of the twentieth century. When these projections were first published they led to widespread concern about the potential adverse consequences of rapid population growth for human welfare and the environment, especially in the poor countries of Asia, Latin America and Africa where growth was expected to be most rapid. As a result, in the 1960s and 1970s funding and technical assistance expanded enormously for developing country governments that were willing to take action. Efforts by these governments to curb rapid population growth focused on reducing high birth rates through the implementation of voluntary family planning programs. These programs aimed to provide information about and access to contraception to permit women and men to take control of their reproductive lives and avoid unwanted childbearing. Only rarely, most notably in China, has coercion been used. Newly available contraceptive methods, such as the pill and intrauterine device (IUD), greatly facilitated the delivery of family planning services. Successful implementation of such programs in a few countries in the early 1960s (for example, in Taiwan and Korea) encouraged other governments to follow this approach.

Rationale for Family Planning Programs

The choice of voluntary family planning programs as the principal policy instrument is based largely on the documentation of a substantial unsatisfied demand for contraception. In surveys, large proportions of married women in the developing world report that they do not want a pregnancy at the time of the interview. Some of these women want no more children because they have already achieved their desired family size, while others want to wait before having the next pregnancy. A substantial proportion of these women (more than one-half in some countries) risk pregnancy by not practicing effective contraception (including sterilization) and, as a result, unintended pregnancies are common. In the mid-1990s, 36 percent of all pregnancies in the developing world were unplanned and 20 percent ended in abortion (Alan Guttmacher Institute).

Why do apparently motivated individuals fail to practice contraception? The answer lies in a mixture of social and health service-related reasons. In the past, a lack of access to services or information was a dominant obstacle. But access in the geographic sense has improved with the widespread implementation of family planning programs and the expansion of the role of private-sector providers. These efforts have not eliminated all unmet need, however, because many service points still offer too few methods and little if any information, or they are otherwise deficient in quality. In addition, other factors—such as fear of side effects of contraceptive methods and overt or suspected disapproval of husbands/partners and other family members—are significant barriers to use in many societies.

The existence of this unmet need for contraception was first documented in the 1960s, and it convinced policymakers that family planning programs were needed and would be acceptable and effective. The health and human rights benefits of family planning and reproductive health programs have provided additional rationales for this policy approach, which was endorsed at the 1994 United Nations International Conference on Population and Development. The Programme of Action adopted by the participating governments encourages the expansion of reproductive health and family planning programs as a means to improve women's reproductive freedom and health. Coercion of any kind is strongly opposed.

Demographic Impact

Over the past three decades large changes in reproductive behavior have occurred in most of the developing world. Around 1960, only a tiny fraction of couples practiced contraception, and knowledge of methods was very limited. In contrast, contraceptive knowledge is now widespread and more than one-half of married women in the developing world are current users of contraception. The large majority of these current users rely on modern methods, including male and female sterilization, the IUD, and the pill.

As a consequence of this widespread adoption of contraception, birth rates have declined sharply. In the past, fertility was high and relatively stable at over 6 births per woman. Since a precipitous decline began in the 1960s, the fertility of the developing world has been reduced by almost one-half, reaching 3.1 births per woman in the years from 1995 to 2000 (United Nations). The largest fertility declines occurred in Asia (–52%) and Latin America (–55%) and the smallest in sub-Saharan Africa (–15%). On average, the pace of change in reproductive behavior in the developing world has been faster than was the case in Europe and North America in the late-nineteenth and early-twentieth centuries.

A key factor contributing to this rise in contraception has been the diffusion of information about and access to contraceptive methods, aided by a rapid expansion of family planning programs. Experiments have provided the most direct and convincing evidence of the value of well-designed family planning services. An example of a large and influential experiment is the one conducted in the Matlab district of rural Bangladesh (Cleland et al.). When this experiment began in the late 1970s, Bangladesh was one of the poorest and least developed countries, and there was considerable skepticism that reproductive behavior could be changed in such a setting. Comprehensive family planning and reproductive health services were provided in the treatment area of the experiment. A wide choice of methods was offered, the quality of referral and follow-up was improved, and a cadre of well-trained women replaced the traditional birth attendants as service providers. The results of these improvements in the quality of services were immediate and pronounced with contraceptive use rising sharply. No such change was observed in the comparison area. The differences between these two areas in contraceptive use and birth rates have been maintained over time. The success of the Matlab experiment demonstrated that appropriately designed services can reduce unmet need for contraception even in very traditional settings with low levels of development.

Despite the undoubtedly crucial role of family planning programs, they are not the only or even the principal cause of changes in reproductive behavior in the developing world. Instead, socioeconomic change is considered by most analysts to be the dominant driving force of the fertility transition. As traditional agricultural societies are transformed into modern industrial ones the cost of children (e.g., for education) and a decline in their value (e.g., for labor and old-age security) to parents leads to declines in desired family size. In addition, with fewer children dying at young ages, fewer births are needed to ensure the survival of the number of children that parents desire. A rise in human development and, in particular, improvements in health and education, appear to be the principal determinants of progress through the fertility transition (Jejeebhoy; Sen; Cleland). In fact, it is possible for poor populations to reach low fertility levels, provided literacy and life expectancy are high. Well-known examples of this occurred in Sri Lanka and the state of Kerala in India.

The primary role of family planning programs is and has been to reduce unintended births by assisting couples with the implementation of their preferences for smaller families through contraception and abortion. Family planning programs have accelerated fertility transitions, so that, on average, these transitions have occurred about a decade earlier than they would have without the programs. Because small changes in fertility have relatively large effects on long term population growth this acceleration of fertility decline attributable to programs probably has reduced the eventual population size of the developing world by a few billion (Bongaarts, 1997).

Demographic Causes of Future Population Growth

Despite recent fertility declines, population growth continues at a rapid pace throughout most of the developing world. According to United Nations projections, the expected increase in population of the developing world as a whole between 2000 and 2050 (from 4.87 to 8.14 billion) is about the same as the historically unprecedented increase that occurred between 1950 and 2000 (from 1.71 to 4.87). This future growth can be attributed to three demographic factors (Bongaarts, 1994).

First, the past decline still leaves average fertility about 50 percent above the two-child level per woman needed to bring about population stabilization. With more than two surviving children per woman, every generation is larger than the preceding one and as long as that is the case population growth will continue. High fertility can in turn be attributed to two distinct underlying causes: unwanted childbearing and a desired family size above two surviving children. Many couples continue to want large numbers of children, partly because of fears of child mortality and partly because of the need for a sufficient number of surviving children to assist them in family enterprises and support them in old age. In most developing countries, the completed family size desired by women still exceeds two children; in some areas, such as sub-Saharan Africa, desired family size is typically above four children.

Second, declines in death rates—historically the main cause of population growth—will almost certainly continue. Higher standards of living, better nutrition, greater investments in sanitation and clean water supplies, expanded access to health services, and wider application of public health measures such as immunization, will insure longer and healthier lives in most countries. The exceptions will be mostly in sub-Saharan African countries, where the AIDS epidemic is severest.

The third growth factor is what demographers call *population momentum.* This refers to the tendency for a population to keep growing even if fertility could immediately be brought to the replacement level of 2.1 births per woman with constant mortality and zero migration. Due to a young population age structure, the largest generation of adolescents in history will enter the childbearing years in the first decade of the twenty-first century. Even if each of these young women has only two children they will produce more than enough births to maintain population growth over the next few decades.

Population momentum is the most important of these three factors, contributing about one-half of projected future growth. Further large increases in the population of the developing world are therefore virtually certain.

Future Policy Options

To be effective, population policies should address all these sources of continuing growth, except declining mortality, by implementing several strategies.

REDUCE UNINTENDED PREGNANCIES BY EXPANDING HIGH QUALITY FAMILY PLANNING SERVICES. Unintended pregnancies occur when women and men who want to avoid pregnancy do not practice effective fertility regulation. Offering individuals and couples appropriate services is a priority of many governments in the developing world. Despite considerable progress over the last several decades, the coverage and quality of family planning services remain less than satisfactory in many countries. In addition, some countries have imposed demographic and provider targets on family planning programs, thus actively interfering with trust between clients and providers. To ensure that family planning programs appropriately assist individuals in reaching personal fertility goals, family planning should be a strictly voluntary service linked with other reproductive health services. The quality of most existing programs can be improved by extending services to under served areas, broadening the choice of methods available, (including safe pregnancy termination where it is legal), improving information exchanges between client and provider, promoting empathetic client/provider relationships, assuring the technical competence of providers, including men in programs, adding service elements to address related health problems, such as diagnosis and treatment of sexually transmitted diseases and treatment following unsafe abortion, and increasing public awareness of the value of and means available for fertility regulation, responsible/safe sex, and the location of services.

REDUCE HIGH DESIRED FERTILITY BY CREATING FAVORABLE CONDITIONS FOR SMALL FAMILIES. Even if unintended fertility could be reduced or eliminated, a desire for large families remains a key cause of population growth in many countries. Several social and economic measures have substantial effects on desired family size:

Increase Educational Attainment, Especially Among Girls. Mass education changes the value placed on large families and encourages parents to invest in fewer "higher quality" children. Higher levels of education are also associated with the spread of nontraditional roles and values, including less gender-restricted behaviors. Educated women want (and have) fewer children with higher survival rates.

Improve Child Health and Survival. No developing country has had a sustained fertility decline without a prior substantial decline in child mortality. A high child death rate discourages investments in children's health and education and encourages high fertility by requiring excess births to insure that at least the desired number of children will survive to adulthood.

Improve Women's Status and Provide Them with Economic Prospects and Social Identities Apart from Motherhood. Improvements in the economic, social, and legal status of girls and women is likely to increase their bargaining power over family reproductive and productive decisions. Increased women's autonomy reduces the dominance of husbands and other household members, the societal preference for males, and the value of children as insurance against adversity and as securers of women's social positions.

CURB THE MOMENTUM OF POPULATION GROWTH. While a young age structure—the key demographic cause of population momentum—is not amenable to modification, an option to reduce momentum is available that has received little attention in past policy debates. Further reductions in population growth can be achieved if the average age at which women begin childbearing rises (by delaying the first birth) and through wider spacing between births. Young women often have little choice about whether or not to have sexual relations, when or whom to marry, and whether to defer childbearing. Governments that wish to encourage later childbearing have several options at their disposal. Legislation to raise the age at marriage has been moderately effective in a few countries. However, legislation has the drawback that it forces rather than encourages changes in marriage customs. Indirect approaches are likely to be more effective. A greater investment in the education of girls, particularly at the secondary level, is the most obvious example. The longer girls stay in school, the later they marry and the greater the delay in childbearing. Delaying the onset of childbearing will therefore not only reduce population momentum, it also significantly improves individual welfare.

Well-designed population policies are broad in scope, socially desirable, and ethically sound. Mutually reinforcing investments in family planning, reproductive health, and a range of socioeconomic measures operate beneficially at both the macro and micro levels: The same measures that slow population growth increase productivity, and improve individual health and welfare.

JOHN BONGAARTS

SEE ALSO: *Fertility Control; International Health; Population Ethics; Population Policies, Strategies for Fertility Control*

BIBLIOGRAPHY

Alan Guttmacher Institute. 1999. *Sharing Responsibility: Women, Society and Abortion Worldwide.* New York: Author.

Bongaarts, John. 1994. "Population Policy Options in the Developing World." *Science* 263: 771–776.

Bongaarts, John 1997. "The Role of Family Planning Programmes in Contemporary Fertility Transitions." In *The Continuing Demographic Transition,* ed. Gavin W. Jones, John C. Caldwell, Robert M. Douglas, et al. Oxford: Oxford University Press.

Caldwell, John. C. 1980. "Mass Education as a Determinant of the Timing of Fertility Decline." *Population and Development Review* 6(2): 225–255.

Cleland, John. 2001. "The Effects of Improved Survival on Fertility: A Reassessment." In *Global Fertility Transition,* ed. Rodolfo A. Bulatao and John B. Casterline (supplement to *Population and Development Review* 27: 60–92.

Cleland, John; Phillips, James F.; Amin, Sajeda; et al. 1994. *The Determinants of Reproductive Change in Bangladesh: Success in a Challenging Environment.* Washington, D.C.: The World Bank.

Jejeebhoy, Shireen J. 1995. *Women's Education, Autonomy, and Reproductive Behaviour: Experience from Developing Countries.* Oxford: Clarendon Press.

Sen, Amartya. 1999. *Development as Freedom.* New York: Knopf.

United Nations. 2001. *World Population Prospects: The 2000 Revision.* New York: United Nations Population Division.

POPULATION POLICIES, MIGRATION AND REFUGEES IN

• • •

Global migration is as old as history, but its significance has waxed and waned over the centuries. In the late twentieth century, political, economic, and social factors have brought it once more to prominence; a 1993 United Nations Population Fund report asserted that migration "could become the human crisis of our age."

What accounts for the contemporary significance of global migration? For one thing, the world no longer contains politically unincorporated territories, so that every instance of migration is not only a move from some nation or other; it is a move to some nation or other. Nations are sovereign states whose recognized rights include the right to control their borders—the right, therefore, to decide who may enter their territory. Thus a decision to migrate to some place is a decision that, politically if not morally, is not for an individual alone to make; it requires the consent of the receiving country. In some cases, even the decision to migrate from a place has been taken out of the hands of the individual; some nations, that is, have claimed the authority to decide who may leave as well as who may enter.

There are further reasons for the increased significance and magnitude of international migration: explosive, uneven population growth in different nations; large disparities in economic wealth and economic development between countries; special interdependencies between particular countries; and advances in transportation and communications systems. Not surprisingly, people tend to move from crowded, poor countries to less crowded, richer ones where economic and other opportunities are better. The desire to migrate may be fostered by television and other mass media, which arouse awareness of opportunities in faraway places; the ability to migrate may be aided by transportation systems that make relocation easier. It has been said that the question is not why people migrate but why they do not migrate more often, given conditions in many "sending" countries and the basic economic principle that resources flow to optimal locations. Migration always involves both "push" factors that give people reason to want to leave a place and "pull" factors that attract them to someplace else.

International migration raises fundamental ethical questions about the moral significance of national boundaries and social communities, the nature and extent of human rights, and the circumstances in which people have moral obligations to aid others or to accept them into their communities. It also raises a host of empirical questions about the effects of migration on both sending and receiving countries and about the extent to which migration can be controlled. On the basis of our current knowledge, it cannot be said that the empirical questions are any more tractable than the ethical ones. Both the facts about migration, and the relevant moral principles, are highly controversial.

A Framework for Migration Issues

It seems a safe assumption that, other things being equal, most people would rather remain in their native countries than begin anew in a strange land. But other things are not always equal. The contemporary world is organized into nation-states possessing very different characteristics, a situation creating disequilibrium. Countries that are relatively rich, safe, or politically free tend to attract people—either as permanent residents or as temporary workers—from countries not possessing these features. Not only do individuals in such circumstances have reason to migrate, but the countries from which they come may view emigration as a way to relieve political or economic pressures. Moreover, receiving countries often have powerful economic interests in acquiring foreign labor. Disentangling the various interests at stake—between sending and receiving countries, and between different groups and classes within each—is a complex task.

The pressure point in contemporary discussions of migration centers primarily on its effects on receiving countries. It is perhaps a truism that if too many people come to those countries, they will eventually cease to be attractive either to their original inhabitants or to anyone else. But the question is how many are too many, and why? How should a receiving country decide which of those seeking entry ought to be admitted?

These questions are misleading if they suggest that an immigration policy is simply a way of implementing charity or beneficence. Immigrants, legal and illegal, serve important interests of receiving countries, or of significant groups within them. We can organize the issues at stake by elaborating four considerations appropriate to formulating an immigration policy—leaving aside, for the moment, the perspective of sending countries. First, what is at stake for those seeking entry? Second, is immigration the only way their needs can be met? Third, what costs and benefits—economic, social, cultural—are at stake for the receiving country as a whole and for particular groups within it? Should these costs and benefits be weighed differently depending on who bears them? Fourth, do receiving countries sometimes have moral obligations to accept potential immigrants—on the basis of past actions, a special relationship with the sending country, or general humanitarian grounds? We can begin to address this fourth question only after the first three have been explored.

Refugees, Immigrants, and Migrants

The first two considerations—what is at stake for those seeking entry, and the extent to which migration is the only way their needs can be met—are captured in the way different categories of people who migrate are usually described. The basic distinction is between refugees and immigrants.

According to the 1951 Convention Relating to the Status of Refugees and the 1967 Protocol Relating to the Status of Refugees, the definition accepted by the United Nations says a refugee is a person who, "owing to well-founded fear of being persecuted for reasons of race, religion, nationality, membership of a particular social group or political opinion, is outside the country of his nationality and is unable or, owing to such fear, is unwilling to avail himself of the protection of that country; or who, not having a nationality and being outside the country of his former habitual residence as a result of such events, is unable or, owing to such fear, is unwilling to return to it" (Article 1.A.2, in Goodwin-Gill, p. 253). Essentially this definition has been in force since shortly after World War II, in response to the upheavals surrounding that conflict.

The meaning of *immigrant* or *migrant* has traditionally been understood by contrast to refugees: Those who migrate are not fleeing political persecution. The difference between migrants and immigrants, furthermore, is not a formal one; but based on common usage, we may say that migrants relocate temporarily, or travel back and forth between their home country and another, while immigrants relocate permanently.

The suggestion is typically that immigrants move for economic betterment, with the implication that they are "pulled" rather than "pushed." But this implication, although often reasonable, is sometimes highly misleading. Even to speak of economic betterment misleadingly suggests an acceptable baseline from which one aims to improve; but many who migrate for economic reasons find themselves in desperate circumstances—as desperate, sometimes, as those of political refugees. The causes of migration may be natural disaster, external aggression, civil war, or internal oppression, all of which can severely affect even those who do not suffer direct political persecution. Furthermore, it may be that those who wish to migrate cannot be helped where they are. Recognizing these problems and the possible bias in the U.N. definition, the Organization of African Unity (OAU) in its 1969 Convention added the following to the definition of a refugee: "every person who, owing to external aggression, occupation, foreign domination or events seriously disturbing public order in either part or the whole of his country of origin or nationality, is compelled to leave his place of habitual residence in order to seek refuge in another place outside his country of origin or nationality" (Article I, Section 2). Thus, for example, "environmental refugees" may be forced to flee their homeland because of deforestation resulting from trading practices and the import strategies of rich countries or international institutions. The OAU definition accommodates the truth that in today's world—as Aristide Zolberg, Astri Suhrke, and Sergio Aguayo argue— "The causes of life-threatening conditions in the developing world stem from an interpenetration of national and transnational, or global, processes" (p. 33).

Why does it matter how we define *refugee*? The reason is that the term has special legal, moral, and emotional force; to be counted a refugee is to be treated as having a compelling claim to admission, whereas potential immigrants have a much weaker claim, in part because of the assumption that their needs can be met without relocation. Many countries are bound by international agreements forbidding *refoulement,* the forcible return of a refugee to his or her country. To exclude from the definition extremely pressing claims that do not result directly from persecution has a powerful influence on the lives and well-being of millions of people.

The definition of a refugee can be manipulated in other ways. Thus, although the United States helped draft the 1951 Convention Relating to the Status of Refugees, it did not ratify it, and adopted the U.N. definition only in the Refugee Act of 1980. Until that time, ideological considerations played a large part in U.S. policy; priority was given to those fleeing "Communist or Communist-dominated" societies. Even since 1980, ideological considerations have continued to influence U.S. refugee admissions. Of course, many of those seeking to migrate—for example, Mexicans to the United States, Turks to Germany—are not in desperate straits. They are poor compared to most people in the receiving countries, but they do not usually come from the poorest stratum of their own society; the poorest lack the physical, emotional, and economic resources to uproot themselves from their homes and begin again. What is at stake for these potential immigrants? A better life, a decent life—a life that most of those in the receiving countries would consider much superior to what is available in the sending countries, but one that it is in no way inappropriate to aim for. The life left behind, then, is not desperate, but it may not be acceptable either.

Costs and Benefits to Receiving Countries

No one would oppose immigration unless he or she believed it presented significant drawbacks or costs. Those who favor stricter limits on the number of immigrants, or stricter conditions of entry, typically argue that at certain levels (often current levels), immigration carries significant economic, social, or cultural costs. Sometimes the concern is primarily with those who enter illegally, either because it is believed that the flow of illegal immigrants inflates the number of outsiders to unacceptable limits, or because as illegal immigrants they pose special problems not posed by those admitted through legal channels.

A central debate concerns the effects of immigrant labor on jobs for natives. In the United States, the debate takes the following form: Some who wish to restrict immigration believe that immigrant labor displaces the worst-off native citizen groups and depresses wages (Briggs). Immigrants, it is said, will work for wages that citizens, possessing the elevated standards prevalent in more developed societies, find unacceptable. Illegal immigrants make things even worse, these critics argue, because they are fearful and thus willing to accept whatever they can get. Proponents of immigration argue, on the other hand, that immigrants do work that citizens consider too menial, such as domestic work and hard agricultural labor. In addition, they say, because the labor market is not a zero-sum game and because

immigrants are also consumers, they often stimulate the economy, thereby creating new jobs (Simon).

It is extremely difficult to sort out the various issues implicit in these claims and to derive conclusions with any degree of certainty. Immigration has multiple effects, and unequivocal conclusions about these effects lack plausibility. Most economists seem to agree that immigration increases aggregate national wealth, but that some displacement of low-skilled workers and depression of their wages do occur. For obvious reasons, the welfare of low-income citizens should be of special concern: Policies that make the worst-off even worse off are difficult to justify. But economists disagree about the magnitude of these problems, and many argue that in some occupations, immigrants and citizens do not compete.

In any case, it is easy to see how foreign labor serves business interests. This is especially true in industries dominated by undocumented migrant labor—those that are part of the "informal economy"—where workers' docility and fear are easy to exploit. In some industries, like the garment industry in the United States, women, who sometimes do "home work," are particularly at risk (Fernandez-Kelly and Garcia).

Another issue that is partly economic and partly social concerns the extent to which immigrants burden a society's social services and, particularly because of language deficiencies and cultural differences, its educational institutions. Even if new immigrants do utilize such services disproportionately—and this remains a point of controversy—they also contribute significantly to a nation's tax base. Some argue, furthermore, that countries with low population growth, like the United States and the nations of western Europe, will need immigrants to help pay for programs such as Medicare and Social Security for older citizens. In the United States, these costs and benefits cannot be easily weighed against each other, since for the most part social services are funded locally, and local jurisdictions are not reimbursed proportionately for the services they render. The countries of western Europe may face different and greater problems because of their more comprehensive social support systems.

Perhaps the most complex "costs" that immigration is said to impose are social and cultural. Several issues are relevant. For one thing, immigration sometimes produces conflict among ethnic groups. In part, this can arise because low-income native-born groups regard the newcomers—accurately or inaccurately—as competing for jobs and resources. But it may also occur when immigrants constitute "middleman minorities," a role played historically in many countries by Jews, Asian Indians, and Chinese (Portes and Rumbaut). Conflict of this kind exists today in the United States, for example, between African Americans and the Korean merchants who own shops in their communities.

Some critics argue that too many immigrants may threaten a society's distinctive way of life, diluting or destroying its identity and its institutions. This is a difficult criticism to assess, in part because the values said to be at stake are elusive and vague. Historically, immigrants have often been viewed with suspicion and fear (Higham), and sometimes the concern about culture amounts to no more than veiled xenophobia or racism. The immigration policies of many countries, such as the United States and Australia, have during extended periods excluded or severely limited the entry of non-northern European or nonwhite immigrants (Jones). When immigrant groups consist partly or largely of nonwhite peoples, as they often do today, it is difficult to avoid the suspicion that claims of cultural integrity contain a racial component.

Let us suppose that these attitudes do not exhaust the concern about cultural integrity. Then we are faced with difficult questions about what a culture is and how immigrant groups mix or assimilate into it, or do not (Gordon). It may be argued that the worry about cultural integrity rests on a misconception about culture. A culture is not an unchanging entity that is threatened by, and too inflexible to accommodate, influences from without or within. Especially in the contemporary world, cultures change. We can imagine radical, unacceptable changes that render the old culture unrecognizable; but the burden of proof is on the critic to show that immigrant groups cause such transformations.

In the United States, immigrant groups have shown a remarkable capacity to assimilate into the dominant culture. Historically, the nations of western Europe have had less experience with immigration than the United States; partly for that reason, the citizens of such a nation do not see themselves as part of a "melting pot," a "salad," or a "nation of immigrants," as Americans often do. Apart from this matter of self-conception, these societies are ethnically less heterogeneous than the United States. But one cannot conclude from this alone that they have more to fear from immigration.

Costs and Benefits to Sending Countries

Just as costs and benefits to receiving countries are controversial, so are those to sending countries. "Out-migration" serves to reduce economic and population pressures, but it can also cause "brain drain"—loss of some of the most productive members of a society—and it can reduce the

pressure for needed social, economic, and political reforms. On the other hand, some countries, such as the Philippines and El Salvador, now earn more from remittances sent home by migrants than from any export. Thus migration can produce important benefits to sending countries and to families within them.

But as important as these issues are, the central point of controversy today concerns the impact of migration on receiving countries. This is not unconnected with the fact that the moral and legal right to leave a place is generally accepted; debate centers on the right to enter. Thus, even if overall a decline in emigration benefited a sending country, few would endorse prohibitions against leaving. Thus the hard core of the argument—about what people or nations have the right to do or to prevent, about what strictures on mobility ought to be implemented—concerns the point of entry, not the point of exit. If immigration today is more imminently pressing than emigration, then the problems it poses—that is, problems in receiving countries—will be the engine that drives new approaches and policies. At the same time, as the world becomes increasingly interdependent economically, as well as in every other way, it is clear that there can be no "solution" to immigration that is not at the same time a solution to emigration. If people are to stop coming to the developed countries, conditions in their home countries will have to become more attractive. Policies are needed to weaken both the pulls and the pushes of migration.

Migration and Morality

Uncertainties about the effects of migration on sending and receiving countries and on particular groups within them; a sense that to a large extent these phenomena exemplify forces beyond our control; the legacy of political realism, according to which ethical considerations do not and should not operate in international relations—all of these may contribute to the view that moral questions have no place at all in discussions of migration.

But such questions cannot be avoided. In the case of refugees and others not officially designated as such but who are equally desperate, migration confronts us with clashes between the claims of some individuals both to survive and to attain basic levels of health and well-being, on the one hand, and the claims of nations, or individuals within them, to exclude these people from such basic goods by refusing them entry, on the other hand. Even when the needs of those seeking entry are not quite so stark, migration poses difficult questions about the relationship between rich and poor—both individuals and countries—and the nature of the moral ties between them. Do rich countries have an obligation to aid poor countries, either by accepting immigrants or by some other means? On what basis could such a moral obligation stand? And how far does it extend?

According to a commonly held view, nations have the right to prevent the entry of whomever they wish. But this claim needs further analysis. It may be uncontroversial that nations have the *legal* right to refuse entry to noncitizens and thus may use whatever criteria they like to decide admissions. Even this claim is somewhat misleading, however, because nations bound by agreements forbidding *refoulement* may not ordinarily expel refugees even if they have entered illegally. But refusing admission to those who have not yet entered does not constitute a violation of international law.

Yet a legal right is not a moral right, nor is it equivalent to what is morally right. Consider the well-known case of the *St. Louis.* In June 1939, the United States turned away a German vessel carrying more than 900 Jews fleeing Nazi Germany. They had been promised, then denied, visas by Cuba; proceeding up the U.S. coast, they requested refuge from the American government. These "boat people" were not inside U.S. territorial waters, and in any case, international agreements regarding refugees had not yet been established; thus there is no doubt that the United States was within its legal rights in refusing the refugees' appeal. But did it have a moral right to refuse their request? Or did it, on the contrary, have a moral obligation to provide at least a temporary haven?

Some people may shy away from speaking in terms of rights and obligations in this context. But few today would deny that the United States ought to have taken in the refugees, or that it was wrong and reprehensible for it to have refused. The moral principle underlying such a judgment might be expressed thus: If a person or a nation can prevent a great harm at little or no cost to itself, it is wrong not to do so.

This principle fits the case under discussion because taking in the St. Louis passengers, whose lives hung in the balance, would have had no adverse effects on the United States. The issues confronting us today, however, raise two kinds of questions not raised by this example. First, in most cases, those seeking entry are not as desperate as were the refugees from Nazi Germany. It might be argued that what is at issue in such cases is not preventing a great harm but providing a good, and that people are not obviously worthy of blame if they choose not to provide that good.

In any case, it is the second question raised by contemporary migration that more seriously challenges the relevance of the principle that one ought to act if one can do so with little or no cost to oneself. The great number of people who might be inclined to migrate—and who might be

encouraged to do so if they were aware that others have been admitted—calls into question the assumption that migration imposes no costs on countries that open their doors, or on particular groups or individuals within them. Debate continues about the economic, social, and cultural costs of migration. Some hold that the costs of migration at current levels are not significant, while others claim that it has adverse effects on the well-being of groups in the resident population. Thus, two critical empirical questions are at what point migration brings harm to groups in the receiving country, and which groups there are affected. The crucial moral question is whether and to what extent people in receiving countries should bear the costs of accommodating immigrants.

Haves and Have-Nots

Why, morally, should people in receiving countries bear any costs to promote immigration? Two kinds of reasons can be offered. First, it might be argued that it is wrong or indecent for some to have so much while others have so little, even if the haves are in no way responsible for the plight of the have-nots. Second, it can be argued that the haves owe something because they bear some responsibility for the situation of the have-nots, perhaps in virtue of some prior or current relationship between them. Let us consider these two kinds of reasons in turn.

From a moral point of view, the global distribution of wealth and poverty as it affects individuals is largely arbitrary. Whether one happens to be born in Sweden or Pakistan, Australia or Somalia, is a matter of chance, but it makes all the difference to a person's life prospects. What follows morally from this fact? There is little consensus. To some, it seems obvious that radical inequalities are unfair or otherwise unacceptable to the extent that they are undeserved. On this view, since people in rich countries are lucky to have been born there and those in poor countries are unlucky, and since these chance occurrences have much to do with how people fare in the world, something ought to be done to redistribute wealth from rich to poor. The same conclusion regarding the need for redistribution might be based not on the arbitrariness of birthplace but on a principle of humanitarianism or benevolence: Those who can help people in dire need ought to do so. Migration is one way to achieve redistribution. Whether and in what circumstances it is preferable to other approaches, such as humanitarian or development assistance to poor countries, will depend on a variety of factors.

But others draw no such conclusion from the moral arbitrariness of nationality. In part, their refusal may flow from the conviction that this line of thinking "proves too much": Not only does one not deserve to be born in a rich country, but one does not deserve to be born to rich parents, or to be endowed with superior genes. Taken to its logical conclusion, the critics say, this argument removes the grounds for all systems of rewards and punishments, and would mark the end of a free society. For this or other reasons, such critics insist that although it might be decent or nice or admirable for rich countries to share their wealth, the fact that birthplace is arbitrary implies no moral obligation to do so; and poor people or poor countries who do not receive such benefits have no cause for complaint.

Disagreement about what follows from the moral arbitrariness of nationality goes to the deepest questions about moral responsibility and social justice. Progress toward resolving these questions, if it can be achieved at all, is impossible without extensive and detailed argument. But there is another rationale for the conclusion that rich countries ought to make some sacrifices for the well-being of immigrants from poor countries—a rationale that does not depend on the moral arbitrariness of birthplace or on simple humanitarianism. This is the view that rich countries owe something to poor countries on the basis of past or present actions and relationships. For example, in 1974 the U.N. General Assembly's Declaration on the Establishment of a New International Economic Order argued that rich countries have "underdeveloped" poor countries: that it is because of colonialism and exploitation, at least in part, that there are now radical disparities in wealth and well-being among nations, and that poor countries are poorer than they would have been had there been no interaction. If this is true, then poor countries are owed something by way of reparations or compensation, not simply in virtue of benevolence.

There are several problems with such claims. Even if one agrees that rich countries did mistreat poor countries in various ways, it is difficult to know what the victims of such exploitation and harm would be like today in the absence of these actions. Without knowledge of this kind, it is almost impossible to decide what reparations or compensation are owed. Moreover, it is possible that in the absence of colonialism, some developing countries would not exist and would be even worse off than they are today. And some, such as Singapore, have fared well despite a colonial legacy.

An obligation may rest more specifically on a particular relationship between countries. For example, acceptance by the United States of large numbers of refugees and immigrants from Vietnam can be viewed as acknowledgment of the moral import of U.S. involvement in Vietnam and the U.S. debt to the Vietnamese people. American relations with

Mexico fit this principle as well, although in a less extreme form. Mexican labor was crucial to the growth of many American industries, and recruitment of Mexican labor by U.S. mining and railroad companies and by agricultural growers dates to the middle of the nineteenth century. European countries' use of "guest workers" can be understood similarly to generate obligations: Having brought workers to one's country when they were deemed necessary, one is not free to sever the relationship after the "guests" have set down roots.

Beyond "Us" and "Them"

Whether on grounds of the moral arbitrariness of nationality, general humanitarianism, or compensatory justice, it seems clear that developed countries, which tend to be the recipients of immigrants and refugees, have moral obligations to developing countries. To what extent such obligations are best fulfilled through migration requires further investigation: In some cases it will make more sense to move resources to people than to move people to resources.

More fundamental questions remain, however. How extensive are these moral obligations? How much ought people in rich countries to sacrifice, if that is necessary, to raise the welfare of poor and oppressed people to tolerable levels? It is clear that no general answers can be given to these questions. In part, the answers depend on how obligations to those outside one's country are to be weighed against obligations to those within. Does one not, it may be asked, owe more to the poor within one's own society than to those elsewhere? And is it not likely that serious commitment to fulfilling obligations to our fellow nationals will strain our resources and therefore our virtue as it is?

Perhaps we can find part of an answer to this question by addressing the concerns of those who view claims about the moral obligations of rich countries to poor countries as misplaced or pointless, because they believe that national policies are not based on such considerations, or even that they should not be. Obviously the foregoing discussion rejects this view. Nevertheless, it is important to see—both because it is true and because it may motivate those unmoved by considerations of morality—that "self-interest rightly understood," in Alexis de Tocqueville's phrase, may also serve to support policies that reduce global inequalities.

In what ways? With international economic interdependence ever increasing—and telecommunications and transportation systems rendering the world of the haves more accessible both psychologically and physically to the have-nots—in the long run, rich countries will be unable to keep their privileges to themselves without employing methods that are repellent, and perhaps ineffective. One might go further and say that the same factors that render the world more interdependent and the North more visible and immediate to the South also render the South more visible and immediate to the North. And so it will become more difficult for those in the North to maintain their humanity while denying their connections with distant strangers of whose suffering they are aware. The reasons that we have duties to those within our community, and that our well-being depends on the well-being of other members of our community, still stand. But the boundaries of our community now may have to be enlarged.

JUDITH LICHTENBERG (1995)
BIBLIOGRAPHY REVISED

SEE ALSO: *Immigration, Ethical and Health Issues of; Population Ethics; Race and Racism; Rights, Human; Warfare: Public Health and War*

BIBLIOGRAPHY

Biondi, Carrie Ann.1997. "Citizenship Old and New." *Contemporary Philosophy* 19(4–5): 20–25.

Black, Virginia. 1996. "Asylum: A Global Phenomenon." *Public Affairs Quarterly* 10(2): 85–101.

Briggs, Vernon M., Jr. 1992. *Mass Immigration and the National Interest.* Armonk, NY: M. E. Sharpe.

Brown, Peter G., and Shue, Henry, eds. 1981. *Boundaries: National Autonomy and Its Limits.* Totowa, NJ: Rowman and Littlefield.

Brown, Peter G., and Shue, Henry, eds. 1983. *The Border That Joins: Mexican Migrants and U.S. Responsibility.* Totowa, NJ: Rowman and Allanheld.

Convention Relating to the Status of Refugees. 1951. Reprinted in *The Refugee in International Law,* by Guy S. Goodwin-Gill. Oxford: Clarendon Press, 1983.

Dauvergne, Catherine. 1997. "Beyond Justice: The Consequences of Liberalism for Immigration Law." *Canadian Journal of Law and Jurisprudence* 10(2): 323–342.

Dummett, Michael. 2001. *On Immigration and Refugees.* New York: Routledge.

Fernandez-Kelly, M. Patricia, and Garcia, Anna M. 1989. "Informalization at the Core: Hispanic Women, Homework, and the Advanced Capitalist State." In *The Informal Economy: Studies in Advanced and Less Developed Countries,* pp. 247–264, ed. Alejandro Portes, Manuel Castells, and Lauren A. Benton. Baltimore: Johns Hopkins University Press.

Galbraith, John Kenneth. 1979. *The Nature of Mass Poverty.* Cambridge, MA: Harvard University Press.

Gans, Chaim. 1998. "Nationalism and Immigration." *Ethical Theory and Moral Practice* 1(2): 159–180.

Gibney, Matthew. 2003. *The Ethics and Politics of Asylum: Liberal Democracy and the Response to Refugees.* New York: Cambridge University Press.

Goodwin-Gill, Guy S. 1983. *The Refugee in International Law.* Oxford: Clarendon Press.

Gordon, Milton. 1964. *Assimilation in American Life: The Role of Race, Religion, and National Origins.* New York: Oxford University Press.

Higham, John. 1963. *Strangers in the Land: Patterns of American Nativism, 1860–1925.* New York: Atheneum.

Jones, Maldwyn Allen. 1992. *American Immigration.* 2nd edition. Chicago: University of Chicago Press.

Kershnar, Stephen. 2000. "There Is No Moral Right to Immigrate to the United States." *Public Affairs Quarterly* 14(2): 141–158.

Krulfeld, Ruth M., and MacDonald, Jeffery L., eds. 1998. *Power, Ethics, and Human Rights.* Totowa, NJ: Rowman & Littlefield.

Loescher, Gilburt D., and Scanlan, John. 1986. *Calculated Kindness: Refugees and America's Half-Open Door, 1945 to the Present.* New York: Free Press.

Mazur, Laurie Ann, ed. 1994. *Beyond the Numbers: A Reader on Population, Consumption, and the Environment.* Washington, D.C.: Island Press.

Muller, Thomas. 1993. *Immigrants and the American City.* New York: New York University Press.

Organization of African Unity. 1969. *Convention on Refugee Problems in Africa.* Reprinted in *The Refugee in International Law,* by Guy S. Goodwin-Gill. Oxford: Clarendon Press, 1983.

Portes, Alejandro, and Rumbaut, Ruben G. 1990. *Immigrant America: A Portrait.* Berkeley: University of California Press.

Protocol Relating to the Status of Refugees. 1967. Reprinted in *The Refugee in International Law,* by Guy S. Goodwin-Gill. Oxford: Clarendon Press.

Rothstein, Richard. 1993. "Immigration Dilemmas." *Dissent* 40: 455–462.

Schuck, Peter. 1993. "The New Immigration and the Old Civil Rights." *American Prospect* 15(3): 102–111.

Simon, Julian L. 1989. *The Economic Consequences of Immigration.* Oxford: Basil Blackwell.

Tomasi, Lydio, ed. Annual. *In Defense of the Alien: Proceedings of the Annual National Legal Conference on Immigration and Refugee Policy.* New York: Center for Migration Studies.

Wilbanks, Dana W. 1996. "Re-Creating America: The Ethics of U.S. Immigration and Refugee Policy in a Christian Perspective (Churches' Center for Theology and Public Policy)." Nashville, TN: Abington Press.

Yu, Henry. 2002. "Thinking Orientals: Migration, Contact, and Exoticism in Modern America." New York: Oxford University Press.

Zolberg, Aristide R.; Suhrke, Astri; and Aguayo, Sergio. 1989. *Escape from Violence: Conflict and the Refugee Crisis in the Developing World.* New York: Oxford University Press.

POPULATION POLICIES, STRATEGIES FOR FERTILITY CONTROL IN

• • •

Population wide fertility control has a history of both success and failure. That history has been fraught with ethical dilemmas rooted in issues of autonomy, responsibility, choice, community, the significance of reproduction, and the meaning of life, among many others, that have occurred in the context of a wide range of practical policies designed to limit or sometimes increase human reproduction.

Many early cultures, both Western and non-Western, have been aware of population pressures and have made attempts to prevent excessive population growth. However, the contemporary history of fertility control, responding to the economist Thomas Malthus's 1798 warnings, began in earnest in the mid-1960s, when some of the world's most populous nations, especially India and China, became aware of skyrocketing growth rates. From the mid-nineteenth century on, death rates had begun to decline. Developments in public sanitation, immunization, antibiotics, and medical technology began to reduce infant and child mortality and lengthen the average life span. Average family size in many cultures increased, and more offspring survived to reproductive age. In the latter half of the twentieth century, the world's population doubled in two generations, increasing from 3 billion in 1960 to 6 billion in 1999, and estimates of the population in 2050 ranged from 9 billion to 12 billion.

Despite these estimates of uncontrolled growth, in the early years of the twenty-first century global population growth rates began to decline, particularly in Europe, where by 2003 at least fourteen countries had below-replacement rates (that is, below 2.1 children per woman), in some cases well below that number. Average fertility rates in the less developed countries also fell, declining from 6.0 in the late 1960s, when fears of a "population explosion" were coming to the fore, to about 2.9 in 2003. Disputes over population policies and strategies for fertility control have continued to rage, although they have been tempered in the developed countries in recent years by the mistaken popular perception in which declining growth rates are conflated with declining growth. Despite declining fertility rates, absolute population growth remains high as a result of both above-replacement

birthrates in many populous parts of the world and enormous population momentum.

Ethical Issues in Population-Control Programs and Policies

The ethical issues raised by population-control programs are of two principal kinds: those concerned with specific means for controlling population growth and those which challenge the objective of limiting human fertility. The earlier population-control programs have been more vulnerable to criticism about the means used for limiting fertility; contemporary policies raise questions about the overall objectives of fertility control.

EARLY PROGRAMS: INDIA AND CHINA. In 1975, concerned by the prospect of uncontrolled population growth in an already very poor country, India launched a vigorous population-control program that encouraged vasectomy, a comparatively simple and inexpensive method for permanent fertility control. The program in India employed a broad system of incentives and penalties to secure cooperation. Its critics often focused on the violations of individual rights and procreative liberty it seemed to involve, especially when nonvoluntary or semivoluntary means were used to elicit consent, for example, "bribing" men with transistor radios, middle-of-the-night roundups coupled with fines, denial of benefits and wages, denial of educational opportunities, and other penalties. Hostility to the sterilization program was so substantial that it contributed to the downfall of Indira Gandhi's government in 1976, and the program essentially was dropped without an effective replacement.

In China concern with population growth also began in the mid-1960s, but it was not until 1979 that that country instituted an effective, if controversial, population-control program. Dubbed the "one-child" policy, that program introduced a system of birth limitations that were imposed in both urban areas and, less effectively, rural areas: With some exceptions couples were permitted to have only a single child. The few exceptions were made for couples whose first child died or was disabled and in some rural areas if the first child was a girl or the couple were members of a non-Han minority group. The one-child policy was imposed by means of a system of birth permits and local supervision of the menstrual cycles of village women, separate residences for young couples in different cities, delayed marriage ages, and the required use of indwelling contraceptives (especially the intrauterine device [IUD]) and required or forced abortion for supernumerary pregnancies.

Observers outside China typically identified two principal moral problems in the one-child policy: the sometimes draconian means by which regulations and penalties were imposed and the consequences for females in a culture with strong preferences for male offspring, including selective female abortion, female infanticide, and female abandonment and out-adoption. Although China has permitted considerable relaxation of the one-child policy—in particular, couples in which both the husband and the wife are only children are now allowed two children and couples who are able to pay a fine for a second child are often permitted to do so—but the one-child policy is still officially in force.

Although India's and China's population-control programs appear to have involved similar ethical abuses, including mandatory contraception and severe penalties for extranumerary children, there is a substantial ethical difference between them. India's system was a *targeted* system that worked by profiling categories of individuals on whom pressure for nonreproduction was to be put and was satisfied when a preset proportion of "acceptors" complied. China's policy, in contrast, has been imposed in a comparatively egalitarian way: The few exceptions aside, China's policy stipulated that at least in principle *all* couples were limited to having only one child. While China's policy was not easy to impose, especially at the outset, and the total fertility rate did not drop below 2 children per woman until 1990, the policy was egalitarian in intent. However, outside critics, in their haste to expose excesses such as forced abortion and female abandonment, typically have failed to notice the ethical conundrum at the center of China's policy: Although it is the most restrictive coercive population-limitation policy in any country, it is also the most fair.

Population policies in the developed world typically but not always have stressed voluntary fertility reduction. Zero population growth (ZPG) became a rallying cry as well as the name of an influential organization and an international family-planning movement dedicated to encouraging couples to have only two children; indeed, average family size in the United States and other developed nations declined dramatically to just above the replacement level. There has been some concern in the United States about manipulative and coercive fertility-control programs that have been suggested, recommended, or put into practice for various minority groups (for example, sterilization programs for Puerto Rican and Native American women that involved inadequate consent and proposals for bonuses or bribes to encourage black women on welfare to accept Norplant), but in general the developed nations have proceeded through the stages of the demographic transition, going from high birthrates and death rates, to high birthrates and low death rates, to low birthrates and low death rates at which population growth again stabilizes, largely as a result of voluntary fertility control.

DEVELOPMENT-BASED POLICIES. After denouncing abuses in policies such as those of India and China as well as other nations that attempted to limit population growth by nonvoluntary means, international attention turned to the pronounced association between more developed economies and lower fertility rates. With the once-a-decade United Nations Conference on Population and Development that was held in 1994 in Cairo, population policy began to shift toward encouraging development, which was understood as involving both macroeconomic changes such as moving from agrarian to industrial economies, improving infrastructure, and shifting the balance of trade to greater proportions of export commodities as well as changes in social agendas, especially more education for girls and improved economic status for women. With that shift would come the benefits of a modern consumer society, it was argued, with its advanced healthcare, social security policies, and other institutions, and people no longer would need to have many children to provide farm labor, foraging, or care and economic support in their old age.

The effort in the new development-based policies was understood as being aimed at stimulating mechanisms that would bring about the demographic transition in countries that had not undergone it, and so birthrates would drop, as death rates already had, and population growth would "level out" at a low, steady, globally supportable rate of about 2.1 children per woman. Because women in underdeveloped countries with high birthrates routinely reported having on average about two more children than they wanted, changes in the economic environment would make it possible for them to reduce fertility to accord with their desires.

Development-based fertility-lowering policies counted among their ethical advantages the fact that people in advanced industrial nations were willing to share a lifestyle— higher development with low fertility and small family size—that had brought them material advantages and were willing to foot much of the bill. Developed societies offered better nutrition, better healthcare, better infant and child survival rates, better education, better jobs, longer life spans, and better security in old age; those advantages were to be made possible for developing countries as well, and in the process fertility rates would decrease. Development-based population policies also seemed to have another moral advantage: They were aimed not at directly controlling population or restricting individuals' fertility but at changing people's background circumstances for the better, thus allowing them to choose to have fewer children. Thus, they seemed to have the moral advantage of favoring individual choice rather than manipulation (as in the Indian vasectomy-targeting scheme) or coercion (as in China's one-child policy).

However, development-based strategies for fertility reduction have raised at least three moral dilemmas. First, they function by disrupting existing cultures, changing traditional agrarian lifestyles into wage-labor ones, often leading rural villagers into the cities and the life of the urban poor and in the process changing gender roles, parent–child relationships, and community structures. Second, they move resources from developed countries into the economic restructuring of less-developed, high-fertility countries, not always in efficient ways, and in doing so often bring with them alien cultural and economic values.

Third, those models may have counterproductive results: Even if they reduce fertility, they may increase consumption, thus undercutting the Malthusian argument for population control. They exacerbate rather than reduce the so-called tragedy of the commons, in which individuals in economic competition exploit resources for their own self-interest and thus make communal restraint impossible. In terms of global resources and environmental impact, the original Malthusian rationale for population control, China's success with its one-child policy, for example, will be negated if all those single children want refrigerators and cars.

REPRODUCTIVE-HEALTH MODELS. Currently favored in programs in many countries, reproductive-health models of fertility control attempt to avoid many of the ethical problems associated with the early population-control programs and the development model. They avoid the targeting of "acceptors," instead attempting to provide access to contraception and reproductive healthcare to everyone; avoid birth ceilings and after-the-fact penalties for excess births; and do not attempt to change existing cultures' economic patterns, occupational roles, domestic relationships, and community structures.

Instead, the reproductive-health model attempts to provide women with full-range reproductive healthcare, including access not only to modern contraception but also to disease prevention; prenatal, perinatal, and postnatal healthcare; and other forms of healthcare and education that affect reproduction. They are designed to satisfy unmet needs for contraception rather than to force conception on unwilling users, keeping in mind that women in less developed, high-fertility societies routinely say that they would have wanted on average about two children fewer than they have. Many of these programs also seek to extend reproductive healthcare to men, including the provision of male contraception and the prevention of sexually transmitted diseases. Many programs that provide reproductive healthcare in less developed nations have been inventive in devising new, more effective forms of healthcare delivery: In Bangladesh, for example, healthcare workers are aware that village women may have difficulty reaching public clinics or may be prevented from visiting them and have developed systems of home delivery of contraceptives and other forms of reproductive healthcare.

Although reproductive-health models of fertility control have avoided many of the ethical problems of earlier programs, they have had other problems. Some nations with conservative administrations, including the United States, have refused to support programs that provide safe abortion services even when those services are recognized by local providers as essential to reproductive healthcare. Other points of dispute that have been raised primarily by the Catholic Church include the provision of condoms for disease prevention as well as contraception and the supplying of contraception and other reproductive-health services to unmarried adolescents and women. Those issues differ from the ethical dilemmas raised by the earlier programs in that they are politically freighted, occurring at the intersection of conservative political and religious thinking with progressive public-health-oriented concerns. Some view the fact that reproductive-health programs may involve contraception, abortion, and the provision of services to unmarried persons as an issue of troubling moral significance; for others there seems to be no moral problem.

Ethical Issues Concerning Fertility Encouragement

The most thoroughly explored issues in fertility theory involve global population growth and ways to control it without violating individual reproductive rights. In some parts of the world, however, including Europe and Japan, fertility rates have declined so dramatically that they are well below the replacement rate. Some of the apparent decline is an artifact of later-onset childbearing and longer child-spacing intervals, but some of it is real. Subreplacement societies are "graying," it often is said, and social security, health insurance, and other social systems are being stressed as very low birthrates coupled with much longer average life spans have produced comparatively few children but many elderly people.

The ethical issues that arise in this context involve fertility encouragement, usually in preference to more liberal immigration policies, and what measures a society may or should take to increase birthrates, if any, and for what reasons. It is becoming fashionable to speak of "population collapse," associating the prediction of population decline, particularly in Europe, with predicted economic collapse.

Some countries offer bonuses, generous maternity and paternity leave, and/or child support for having a baby.

Some engage in public advertising that promotes childbearing: "Sterben die Deutschen aus?" ("Are the Germans dying out?") asked one German subway poster. Although none of these programs repeat ethical abuses such as the requirement the former dictator Nicolae Ceausesçlu imposed on Romanian women that they bear at least five children, some attempt to influence individual reproductive behavior in many of the same ways in which advertising attempts to influence consumer choice.

The ethical issue here is whether individuals' reproductive lives should be influenced in the same ways and by the same means that manufacturers sell automobiles or laundry soap. There is also the question of whether public-service advertising to increase fertility is ethically analogous to public-service advertising to decrease fertility, as in "stop at one or two" billboards in Vietnam, soap operas favoring small family size in China, and similar measures in many other countries.

Averting "population collapse" is not the only motivation for a state, ethnic group, or religious group to encourage fertility increase. Many earlier societies and some contemporary ones, such as early Maoist China and contemporary Iraq, have encouraged high fertility as a source of military might and/or productive power: More children mean more soldiers and workers. Some religious groups have encouraged high fertility to, as detractors see it, increase denominational strength. It might be considered appropriate for some groups that have suffered genocide or other calamities to practice high fertility to recover their demographic strength. Examples include Armenians after their expulsion by the Turks, Jews after the Holocaust, African Americans after slavery, and New World Amerindians after European contact, when indigenous groups in North, Central, and South America were reduced not so much by warfare but by epidemics of European diseases such as measles, typhus, yellow fever, and smallpox that in many areas killed 80 to 90 percent of the population or resulted in complete extinction. In what sense a group may or should attempt to regain its earlier population size, when and how compensatory population gain should be measured, and what impact it may have on other groups inhabiting the same region are issues that invite further discussion.

Ethical Issues Concerning Technology in Fertility Control

New reproductive technologies play a major role in issues involving fertility control, especially new forms of contraception and pregnancy interruption. Three pose particularly complex ethical issues.

MALE CONTRACEPTION. With the exception of India's vasectomy program, virtually all programs for fertility control have focused on women. While a wide variety of modern contraceptive methods have been developed for women, until recently sexually active males had only three methods for controlling their contribution to reproduction: withdrawal, condoms, and vasectomy. A number of modern male contraceptive methods are under development, including vas-blocking methods, heat-based methods, and hormonal methods, and several can be expected to reach the market soon.

These methods raise a variety of ethical issues. Are different degrees of control over whether conception can occur appropriate to non-abstinent males and females? At least in areas where women have free access to it, female-controlled contraception has given women veto power over their own reproduction, something that is often held to be appropriate because reproduction occurs within women's bodies. Should males also have veto power over reproduction even though it does not affect them physically in the same way? Might the development of effective long-acting but reversible methods of male contraception herald an ethically problematic change in male/female reproductive roles, especially in roles that often are considered essential to female identity?

POSTCONCEPTION CONTRACEPTION. Among the various methods of female contraception, some function by preventing conception and others function by preventing implantation or interrupting an early pregnancy. Generating particularly vigorous ethical controversy have been "morning after" contraceptive modalities, not only "emergency contraception" that is effective for up to 120 hours but in particular abortifacient methods that interrupt pregnancy at up to seven weeks of gestation.

As with reproductive-health programs for fertility control, the problems here are the subject of political dispute, involving disagreements between those who oppose abortion altogether and those who do not or who find moral issues of abortion appropriately resolved privately or overridden by other moral concerns. Another issue posed by postconception technologies involves the timing of decisions about pregnancy: Should those decisions be made before conception, when one is not yet pregnant—that is, should they deal with a condition not yet established—or is there a moral and epistemological advantage to allowing conception and pregnancy to occur and then deciding whether to continue it? Opponents of abortion would insist on the former; the latter might be supported on the grounds that it gives the woman or couple a more realistic opportunity for full-fledged consent: Once pregnancy has begun, she can understand more fully the step she is taking, including the changes it brings about in her body, and then decide whether she wants to continue. Although this issue may seem bizarre to Western theorists of reproduction, it is pressing in countries, such as Soviet-era and post-Soviet Russia, in which abortion has been a principal method of fertility control. The total induced abortion rate for Moscow is about 6 (though for Russia as a whole it is 2.5) and decisions about pregnancy continuation often are made after rather than before the fact.

LONG-ACTING CONTRACEPTION. The ethical implications of the difference between short-acting, "time-of-need" contraceptive modalities such as the condom; the diaphragm; spermicidal foams, gels, and sponges; and other forms that require use at the time of sexual exposure as distinct from long-acting modalities that have a contraceptive effect over an extended period, such as the IUD, the subdermal implant, and the depot injection, also have been explored inadequately. The central theoretical difference involves the degree of user cooperation required to prevent conception. Short-acting, time-of-need modalities require user awareness and cooperation each time, every time, as do nontechnological methods of contraception such as withdrawal and the "rhythm method" of scheduled abstinence. In contrast, true long-acting contraception requires no user cooperation beyond the initial emplacement. This difference is obscured, however, by a variety of technologies that have a long-term chemical effect but require repeated dosing, such as oral contraceptives ("the pill"), as well as by permanent or difficult-to-reverse methods such as tubal ligation, quinacrine sterilization, and vasectomy.

The ethical issue that arises here concerns whether it is morally appropriate to "reverse the default" in human reproductive biology. Currently, sexual contact between a fertile male and a fertile female may permit conception *unless that is prevented;* if the default were reversed by having long-acting, indwelling but reversible contraception in place and if everybody used it, sexual contact would not permit conception *unless that were chosen.* The consequences of such a reversal for fertility control are potentially enormous: If everybody did it all the time—that is, used long-acting, reversible contraception except when he or she wanted to have a child—fertility rates would decline dramatically without a violation of reproductive rights.

Societal Interests in Fertility

The issue of societal interests in individual fertility has a greater scope than any of the issues discussed above. Society in general—that is, the global population as a whole—is composed of individual human beings, all of whom are the product of reproductive activity between earlier human beings: their parents, the providers of the male and female gametes involved. A very small proportion of this reproductive activity, at least in the developed world, involves artificial reproductive technologies such as in vitro fertilization, embryo storage and transfer, surrogacy, and cloning, and some involves arrangements between nonheterosexual couples, but most reproductive behavior takes place between a man and a woman, whose reproductive roles are influenced by the wide range of cultural settings in which their conjunction occurs.

The overarching ethical question is what weight the interests of their society or society in general should be given over people's personal choices about reproduction. Should concern about global population growth take precedence over individual reproductive behavior? Should the risks of population decline take priority over individual choice? Are pressures for increased fertility more or less defensible than pressures for fertility limitation? These larger issues invite extended exploration.

Population control measures are motivated principally by the Malthusian specter of global crowding, which traditionally is formulated as the threat that a population will outrun the carrying capacity of its site, that is, will consume more than can be replaced in its environment and thus eventually will exhaust its resources and die. The urgency of global fertility control often is underestimated by those who confuse declining growth rates with declining growth: Growth rates are falling in virtually all areas of the world, but as a result of immense population momentum in the latter decades of the twentieth century, total global population is still increasing rapidly. Nevertheless, the Malthusian specter does not answer the question of whether it is better to have fewer people with a higher standard of living or more people in far more modest circumstances. What should be the aim of population control?

As the philosopher Derek Parfit has discussed, different future scenarios may involve fewer people with a higher quality of life or more people with a lower quality of life, but as long as the quality of life is not so low that life is not worth living, it is not easy to say why a larger population of less fortunate people is not preferable to a smaller population of people with a higher quality of life. Parfit entertains what he calls the "repugnant conclusion" that for a large population with a high quality of life there always could be a much larger population with a much lower quality of life, a life barely worth living, but that such a future would be better.

Similarly, fewer people consuming more is not obviously better in terms of global environmental impact than more people consuming less and also is not obviously morally preferable to the opposite situation, assuming that the effect on environmental sustainability is equal. This philosophical puzzle raises deep cultural, political, and religious questions and perhaps will be the central challenge for theorists of fertility control in the future.

MARGARET PABST BATTIN

SEE ALSO: *Abortion; Autonomy; Eugenics; Eugenics and Religious Law; Family and Family Medicine; Feminism; Race and Racism; Sexism; Sustainable Development; Women, Historical and Cross-Cultural Perspectives*

BIBLIOGRAPHY

Battin, Margaret Pabst. 1997. "Color y Cultura: La anticoncepcion automatica y su impacto en la poblacion urbana negra Norteamericana y en la de paises en desarrollo," translated. *Perspectivas Bioeticas en las Americas* 2(1): 64–92.

Battin, Margaret Pabst. 1999. "Population Issues." In *Companion to Bioethics*, 2nd edition, ed. Peter Singer and Helga Kuhse. Oxford: Blackwell.

Bongaarts, John. 1994. "Population Policy Options in the Developing World." *Science* 263(5148): 771–776.

Bongaart, John. 1997. "The Role of Family Planning Programmes in Contemporary Fertility Transitions," In *The Continuing Demographic Transition*, ed. Gavin W. Jones, John C. Caldwell, Robert M. Douglas, and Rennie M. D'Souza. Oxford: Oxford University Press.

Bongaarts, John, and Bruce, Judith. 1995. "The Causes of Unmet Need for Conception and the Social Content of Services." *Studies in Family Planning* 26(2): 57–75.

Cohen, Joel E. 1995. *How Many People Can the Earth Support?* New York and London: W. W. Norton.

Cook, Noble David. 1998. *Born to Die: Disease and New World Conquest, 1492–1650.* Cambridge, Eng., and New York: Cambridge University Press.

Dixon-Mueller, Ruth. 1993. *Population Policy and Women's Rights: Transforming Reproductive Choice.* Westport, CT: Praeger.

Ehrlich, Paul R. 1968. *The Population Bomb.* New York: Ballantine.

Ehrlich, Paul R.; Ehrlich, Anne H.; and Daily, Gretchen C. 1995. *The Stork and the Plow: The Equity Answer to the Human Dilemma.* New York: G. P. Putnam's Sons.

Gardiner, Stephen M. 2001. "The Real Tragedy of the Commons." *Philosophy & Public Affairs* 30(4): 387–416.

Hardin, Garrett. 1993. *Living within Limits: Ecology, Economics, and Population Taboos.* New York and Oxford: Oxford University Press.

Harris, John, and Holm, Søren, eds. 1998. *The Future of Human Reproduction: Ethics, Choice and Regulation.* Oxford: Oxford University Press.

Hartman, Betsy. 1995. *Reproductive Rights and Wrongs: The Global Politics of Population Control.* Boston: South End Press.

MacDonald, Peter. 2000. "Gender Equity in Theories of Fertility Transition." *Population and Development Review* 26(3): 427–439.

Macklin, Ruth. 1981. "Ethics, Effectiveness, and Efficiency in Population Programs." In *Ethical Issues of Population and Culture, Economics, and International Assistance,* ed. Daniel Callahan and Philip G. Clark. New York: Irvington.

Maguire, Daniel C. 2003. *Sacred Rights: The Case for Contraception and Abortion in the World's Religions.* New York: Oxford University Press.

Malthus, Thomas Robert. 1872 (1798). *An Essay on the Principle of Population, as It Affects the Future Improvement of Society,* complete 1st edition and partial 7th edition. Reprinted in *On Population,* ed. Gertrude Himmelfarb. New York: Modern Library, 1960.

Nussbaum, Martha C. 1999. *Sex and Social Justice.* New York and Oxford: Oxford University Press.

Parfit, Derek. 1984. *Reasons and Persons.* Oxford: Clarendon Press.

Pope Paul VI. 1968. Encyclical Letter *Humanae Vitae,* July 25.

Sathar, Zeba Ayesha, and Phillips, James F., eds. 2001. *Fertility Transition in South Asia.* Oxford: Oxford University Press.

Sen, Amartya. 1999. *Development as Freedom.* New York: Knopf.

Sen, Gita; Germain, Adrienne; and Chen, Lincoln C., eds. 1994. *Population Policies Reconsidered: Health, Empowerment, and Rights.* Harvard Series on Population and International Health. Cambridge, MA: Harvard School of Public Health and International Women's Health Coalition, Harvard University Press.

Simon, Julian. 1981. *The Ultimate Resource.* Princeton, NJ: Princeton University Press.

United Nations. 1987. *World Population Policies.* New York: United Nations.

United Nations. 1995. "Program of Action of the 1994 International Conference on Population and Development." *Population and Development Review* 21(1): 187–213.

United Nations Population Fund. 2003. *State of the World Population 2002: People, Poverty and Possibility.* New York: United Nations Publications.

Veatch, Robert M. 1977. "Governmental Population Incentives: Ethical Issues at Stake." *Studies in Family Planning* 8(4): 100–108.

PRINCIPLISM

• • •

Since the mid-1970s, American bioethicists have tended to justify their proposed solutions to the moral problems arising in medical care and health policy by appealing to fairly abstract moral principles, such as respect for autonomy or beneficence, rather than to a particular moral tradition, such as a religion, or to a complex, philosophically articulated moral theory, such as consequentialism or deontology. This method has come to be called principlism, a label originally meant to be derogatory, but since embraced by its defenders.

Tom Beauchamp and James Childress present the canonical account of this method in their *Principles of Biomedical Ethics,* where they suggest that four principles—respect for autonomy, nonmaleficence, beneficence, and justice—provide the proper justificatory framework for bioethics. Because both Beauchamp and Childress were working at the Kennedy Institute of Ethics at Georgetown University in Washington, DC, while they were writing their book, principlism is sometimes called the "Georgetown approach" to bioethics.

A second, related source for principlism is the National Commission for the Protection of Human Subjects of Biomedical and Behavioral Research, with which both Beauchamp and Childress worked quite closely during the period they were drafting their book. The commissioners describe their method in what is known as the *Belmont Report* (after the location of a retreat held in 1976), where they present the set of principles that they relied upon to justify their policy recommendations. These principles more or less coincide with Beauchamp and Childress's, though the commissioners treat nonmaleficence as a subprinciple of beneficence.

Why Principles?

Moral thought can occur at several different levels of abstraction. Most concretely, there are the *judgments* people make in particular cases, when they say "this is the right thing to do here." Sometimes people justify these judgments by appealing to *rules* that offer general guidance about how to act in certain types of situations, such as "make only sincere promises" or "do not tell a lie." People can in turn justify a rule by showing how it falls under an even more general *principle* that links it with many other rules; not lying and making only sincere promises, for example, can both be seen as cases of respecting the autonomy of the persons one encounters. Finally, a *moral theory* is an attempt to systematize and justify a set of principles that applies comprehensively to all of the moral issues that people are confronted with.

Clinical bioethicists are in the business of making moral judgments when they help health professionals make decisions at the bedside, and many different kinds of bioethicists often help to formulate policies—a special kind of rule—to guide health professionals in their research and practice. It might seem that these judgments and policies are fully justified only to the extent that they are grounded in an ethical theory. The problem, however, is that philosophers have been unable to agree on what moral theory is best. Some, such as Beauchamp, favor consequentialist theories that take the promotion of the welfare of sentient beings as the fundamental aim of morality; others, such as Childress, favor versions of deontology, where certain types of actions are categorically proscribed no matter what the consequences; others favor yet other flavors of moral theory. This lack of consensus might seem to make the resolution of bioethical problems impossible, because it seems that bioethicists with different theoretical affinities will endorse different principles, different rules, and ultimately different concrete judgments.

But the commissioners discovered in their deliberations—a point that Beauchamp and Childress argue for more extensively—that despite differences at the level of theory, they could agree at the level of principles. The different theories converge on the same set of principles. The commissioners could thus appeal to members of this set to justify their policy recommendations, even while they differed on the principles' fundamental justification; though no one theory was satisfactory to all of them, each of them could turn to their preferred theory to defend the principles. Principlism is thus a practical response to the intractable debates found in moral philosophy: Because bioethicists deal with real-world problems, they should sidestep these academic debates by remaining one step down in the justificatory ladder.

The Four Principles

The first of Beauchamp and Childress's principles requires *respect for autonomy.* Autonomy is a controversial philosophical concept, but Beauchamp and Childress treat it largely in terms of autonomous choices or the intentional choices of agents who understand what they are undertaking and who are free from undue influences on their decisions. The principle of respect for autonomy requires others not to intervene when someone has made an autonomous choice, even if it is a choice that is thought to be imprudent or foolish. This principle, then, usually rules out health professionals' paternalistically interfering with the decision making of competent adults.

Beauchamp and Childress also argue that respecting autonomy requires that people take positive steps to promote and protect the capacity of agents to act autonomously. Health professionals are thus sometimes required to increase the options available to a patient or to work hard to make sure that patients are able to understand the decisions that confront them.

The most important bioethical rule to fall under the principle of respect for autonomy is the requirement for the informed consent of patients before health professionals intervene in their bodies. Health professionals must disclose to a patient the various possible courses of treatment for her condition and their likely outcomes; they must ensure that the patient understands this information; and they must let the patient make the decision for herself, so that she directs her medical care in light of her own values and preferences. By following the rules for informed consent, health professionals first enable a patient to make an autonomous choice, and then respect that choice by following the treatment directions she issues. Of course, the requirement for informed consent applies only to competent patients, because only they can make the autonomous choices that the principle requires others to respect.

Beauchamp and Childress's second principle is one of *nonmaleficence,* the requirement that health professionals not intentionally harm their patients. This principle encodes the ancient medical dictum, *primum non nocere* (above all do no harm). Because there are many different kinds of harm, the principle of nonmaleficence supports many different rules, such as: "Do not intentionally kill a patient," and "do not intentionally cause a patient unnecessary pain or suffering." This principle could, for example, require that treatment of a patient cease when it becomes a burden to her, even if that cessation hastens her death. This principle also plays an important role in research ethics, for it prohibits experimentation that is likely to harm subjects, even when they consent to it.

Whereas Beauchamp and Childress's second principle is largely negative, in that it prohibits a class of actions, their third principle, that of *beneficence,* is positive: It requires health professionals to act for the benefit of their patients, where "benefit" is construed with the same latitude that was used to interpret "harm" in the principle of nonmaleficence. The principle of beneficence requires health professionals to advocate on behalf of their patients in order to ensure that they receive appropriate care. It also mandates paternalistic intervention when, because of age, disability, or disease, a patient lacks the capacities for autonomous choice.

Beauchamp and Childress's fourth principle is the principle of *justice,* which they take to include distributive, criminal, and rectificatory forms of justice. The distributive version of this principle is especially relevant in bioethical issues having to do with the morality of institutions, where it requires that the benefits and burdens of the institution be shared fairly. This principle might require, for example, that the state provide a certain level of healthcare to all of its citizens. It also plays a significant role in evaluating the ethical dimension of a scheme for rationing scarce resources (such as organs for transplant or beds in an intensive care unit).

Beauchamp and Childress intend that each of these four principles be taken as only prima facie binding: The directives that flow from them are to be followed only when they do not clash with those arising from a different principle. Otherwise, a suitable resolution of the conflicting directives must be crafted.

Consider, for example, the question of what health professionals should do when they discover that a patient infected with the human immunodeficiency virus (HIV) is having unprotected sex with partners who are ignorant of his condition. First, respect for the patient's autonomy supports a policy of medical confidentiality, requiring health professionals not to reveal to others private information discovered in the course of caring for patients. According to this policy, health professionals should do nothing to warn the sexual partners of their HIV-positive patient, as doing so would violate his confidentiality. Second, if there is evidence that public disclosure of the patient's condition would harm him economically, socially, psychologically, or physically, the principle of nonmaleficence would also urge against interfering with his activities. Third, however, the principle of beneficence requires health professionals to benefit others by preventing harm to them, suggesting that they should warn the patient's sexual partners of their risk of infection. Finally, if the patient is intentionally trying to infect his partners with the disease, his behavior is criminal, and the principle of justice will require health professionals to notify the police; even if he is not intentionally trying to infect his patients, justice requires that everyone take responsibility for the public health, and so health professionals would have to alert public health authorities of his activity.

In this example, the four principles pull in two opposing directions. To resolve this conflict, note that the two principles discouraging health professionals from interfering with the patient's activities—respect for autonomy and nonmaleficence—also suggest that he should not be sexually active with partners who are ignorant of his infection: Respecting their autonomy requires that he give them the information they need to decide for themselves whether to be involved with him, and the principle of nonmaleficence requires that he not harm them by exposing them to possible infection. Accordingly, the moral requirement that health professionals protect third parties overrides their prima facie duties of noninterference. Principlism supports health professionals' duty to warn the unsuspecting sexual partners of the HIV-positive patient.

Criticisms

Critics have attacked the version of principlism Beauchamp and Childress developed in the first three editions of their book from opposite directions. On the one hand, K. Danner Clouser and Bernard Gert criticize Beauchamp and Childress for their failure to give a systematic organization to their principles. Because the principles are not justified by means of a single moral theory, Clouser and Gert worry that they offer no real guidance in cases where the principles clash. How can bioethicists justify choosing to favor the directions of one principle over those of another? In the situation explored above, for example, bioethicists might seem to be arbitrarily siding with the directive flowing from the principles of beneficence and justice, as opposed to that flowing from the principles of respect for autonomy and nonmaleficence.

On the other hand, Albert R. Jonsen and Stephen Toulmin argue that the move from specific cases to more general principles is of no help. Like Clouser and Gert, they think that the principles do not by themselves give sufficient guidance for bioethicists to resolve the problems that confront them. But unlike Clouser and Gert, Jonsen and Toulmin oppose developing a moral theory to integrate the principles, for Jonsen's experience on the National Commission helped him to realize that philosophical disagreement over moral theory is an inevitable consequence of any such attempt. Instead, Jonsen and Toulmin contend that bioethical problems are best resolved casuistically—not by appeal to principles but by reasoning analogically from settled cases to new situations. So, in the example above, bioethicists might argue that the case, *Tarasoff, Vitaly v. The Regents of the University of California,* which established the duty of psychiatrists to warn the potential victims of their violent patients, is sufficiently similar to the case of an HIV-positive patient whose sexual partners are ignorant of his condition to establish that health professionals have a similar duty to warn.

Beauchamp and Childress respond to both Clouser and Gert's and Jonsen and Toulmin's criticisms in the fourth and fifth editions of their book. Beauchamp and Childress agree that the four principles are, by themselves, too abstract to provide much guidance in particular cases. So they incorporate Jonsen and Toulmin's casuistical insight by suggesting that the use of the principles will first involve "specifying" them in light of the situation at hand and other

similar cases. Beauchamp and Childress respond to Clouser and Gert's criticism that they resolve conflicts between principles arbitrarily by saying that the specified versions of the principles can be "balanced" against one another to produce a final verdict in a manner akin to the "reflective equilibrium" that John Rawls described in his 1971 book, *A Theory of Justice.* That is, the proposed resolution of a bioethical problem is to be tested against other established moral principles, previously established cases, and empirical facts; if there is a lack of fit, then the principles are to be specified differently or rebalanced until there is mutual confirmation among all the relevant moral data.

In the case explored above, for example, before the conflicting principles were balanced, the principle of respect for autonomy was first specified to a rule requiring medical confidentiality; the principle of justice was specified in terms of the criminal justice protection against intentional bodily harm and the public health policy of preventing infectious disease; and so on. A full principlist justification of health professionals' duty to warn the sexual partners of their HIV-positive patients would show this requirement to be in reflective equilibrium with other limits to confidentiality, responses to other sexually transmitted diseases, and privacy rights in matters of sexuality.

Common Morality

In the fourth and fifth editions of their book, Beauchamp and Childress also introduce a new justification for their principlist methodology. Whereas in the earlier editions they justified their choice of principles in terms of the convergence of ethical theories on them, they now contended that the principles offer a "common morality" theory. This approach "takes its basic premises directly from the morality shared in common by the members of a society—that is, unphilosophical common sense and tradition" (Beauchamp and Childress, p. 100). The four principles are supposed to make explicit what is implicit in common morality as it applies to bioethics.

The earlier justification of the principles in terms of theory convergence has some affinity with this later common-morality justification because Beauchamp and Childress see the aim of ethical theory as systematizing and unifying the various facets of common morality. They take the incapacity of philosophers to agree on which ethical theory is best as a sign that each successfully captures some of common morality, but neglects other parts of it. Indeed, the common-morality justification of principlism improves on the convergence justification in at least one respect. Beauchamp and Childress devote most of their effort to establishing the convergence of only two theories—consequentialism and deontology—on their principles; but there are many other moral theories, some of which are given more attention in the later editions of their book, all of which should be shown to converge on the principles if this justification of principlism is to be successful.

The common-morality justification of principlism, however, leaves Beauchamp and Childress open to other objections. Why accept that these four principles fully characterize common morality as it applies to bioethics? Ronald Dworkin, for example, argues in a 1993 book that a commitment to a nonparochial version of the sanctity of life has as much of a place in common morality as any of the other four principles, but it is not accepted by Beauchamp and Childress as a guide for bioethical decision making.

H. Tristram Engelhardt Jr., in contrast, thinks that principlist approaches to bioethics are ideological, in that they allow bioethicists to force their own private moral outlook on others even while they pretend to be making judgments and formulating policies that are objective and fair to all. Engelhardt is skeptical about there being such a thing as *common* morality, holding instead that there are many different substantive moralities, no one of which should be used to solve bioethical problems that affect those in communities structured by different moral outlooks. He offers instead a libertarian approach to bioethics in which the rules governing the delivery of healthcare are justified only when patients and healthcare providers consent to them.

Perhaps Beauchamp and Childress's best reply to the criticism that they fail to take pluralism seriously would be for them to replace the common-morality justification of the principles with one modeled on the notion of an *overlapping consensus* that Rawls develops in his 1993 book, *Political Liberalism*. Rawls recognizes that people subscribe to conflicting moral outlooks, but he thinks that, at least at a basic level, policy problems can be solved by appealing to what people who disagree about the deep moral questions would nonetheless accept as the reasonable terms for their cooperation. Rawls thus appeals to *hypothetical* consent, instead of Engelhardt's appeal to *actual* consent. Similarly Beauchamp and Childress's four principles can be seen as what reasonable people would agree to as the fair terms for the provision of healthcare, despite their differing views on other moral questions. Many different moral doctrines would thus overlap by including a common commitment to the four principles as the appropriate norms for bioethics. Unlike Beauchamp and Childress's appeal to common morality or to the convergence of ethical theories on the principles, this alternative justification of them is based on the overlap of various moral outlooks, be they ethical theories, religions, or popular social movements.

Though the foundations of the principlist approach remain contested, it is likely to continue as the primary method used by American bioethicists. This is because principlism allows bioethicists to appeal to generally accepted norms to justify their resolutions of the problems they face, without requiring them to enter into abstruse philosophical debates about how best to understand morality.

DONALD C. AINSLIE

SEE ALSO: *Autonomy; Beneficence; Casuistry; Communitarianism and Bioethics; Confidentiality; Consensus, Role and Authority of; Contractiarianism in Bioethics; Ethics; Information Disclosure, Ethical Issues of; Justice*

BIBLIOGRAPHY

Ainslie, Donald C. 2002. "Bioethics and the Problem of Pluralism." *Social Philosophy and Policy* 19(2): 1–28.

Beauchamp, Tom, and Childress, James. 1979, 1983, 1989, 1994, 2001. *Principles of Biomedical Ethics,* 1st through 5th editions. New York: Oxford University Press.

Clouser, K. Danner, and Gert, Bernard. 1990. "A Critique of Principlism." *Journal of Medicine and Philosophy* 15(2): 219–236.

Daniels, Norman. 1996. *Justice and Justification: Reflective Equilibrium in Theory and Practice.* New York: Cambridge University Press.

Dworkin, Ronald. 1993. *Life's Dominion: An Argument about Abortion, Euthanasia, and Individual Freedom.* New York: Knopf.

Engelhardt, H. Tristram, Jr. 1996. *The Foundations of Bioethics,* 2nd edition. New York: Oxford University Press.

Gillon, Ranaan, ed. 1994. *Principles of Health Care Ethics.* New York: Wiley.

Jonsen, Albert R. 1998. *The Birth of Bioethics.* New York: Oxford University Press.

Jonsen, Albert R., and Toulmin, Stephen. 1988. *The Abuse of Casuistry.* Berkeley: University of California Press.

National Commission for the Protection of Human Subjects of Biomedical and Behavioral Research. 1979. *The Belmont Report: Ethical Principles and Guidelines for the Protection of Human Subjects of Research.* Washington, D.C.: U.S. Department of Health, Education, and Welfare.

Rawls, John. 1971. *A Theory of Justice.* Cambridge, MA: Harvard University Press.

Rawls, John. 1993. *Political Liberalism.* New York: Columbia University Press.

Richardson, Henry S. 1990. "Specifying Norms as a Way to Resolve Concrete Ethical Problems." *Philosophy and Public Affairs* 19(4): 279–310.

Tarasoff, Vitaly v. The Regents of the University of California, 529 P.2d 553, 118 Cal. Rptr. 129 (1974); 17 Cal.3d 425, 551 P.2d 334, 131 Cal.Rptr. 14 (1976).

PRISONERS AS RESEARCH SUBJECTS

• • •

Since the 1980s, virtually no prisoners in the United States have been used in biomedical experimentation that does not benefit prisoners as individuals or as a class. A principal reason is that ethical reflection on this topic in the 1970s not only decisively affected public policy but also shaped an enduring moral consensus in society.

A crucial year in that process was 1976. The Federal Bureau of Prisons announced an indefinite moratorium on nontherapeutic biomedical experimentation conducted in any federal prison. That same year, the board of directors of the American Correctional Association—the professional organization of U.S. prison officials at all levels of government—officially adopted a statement urging responsible bodies at federal, state, and local levels to eliminate the use of prisoners as subjects of medical pharmacological experimentation.

Most important, the U.S. National Commission for the Protection of Human Subjects of Biomedical and Behavioral Research (National Commission) recommended to the secretary of the Department of Health, Education and Welfare (now the Department of Health and Human Services, DHHS) that a moratorium on approving and funding prisoner experimentation be declared until certain specified minimum standards had been met by any prison allowing experimentation on inmates. The work of the National Commission deserves special attention because it was pivotal, at a critical moment in the 1970s, in articulating connections between moral principles and public policies concerning prisoner experimentation (U.S. National Commission, 1976a, 1976b).

Some debate continued over government regulations implementing the National Commission's recommendations, but by the 1980s, experimentation that was not therapeutic for the individual prisoner or prisoners as a class had virtually come to an end. With the crucial help of the National Commission, American society had reached a moral consensus already achieved by the rest of the world.

Practices

Such a consensus did not always exist. Rulers in ancient Persia permitted physicians to use prisoners as experimental subjects. Rome tested poisons on prisoners. European physicians in the eighteenth century used prisoners in experiments, exposing them—sometimes through injections—to venereal disease, cancers, typhoid, and scarlet fever.

In the United States, prisoners were used for experimentation from at least 1914, when white male convicts in Mississippi were used in pellagra experiments. During World War II, prisoner experimentation assumed a morally favorable aura when prisoners, to show their patriotism, signed up in large numbers for experimental studies. After reviewing this experimentation, several state commissions encouraged the use of prisoners (Beecher).

The American Medical Association (AMA) underscored the degree to which participation in medical experimentation was viewed as morally admirable. It adopted a resolution disapproving of the practice of permitting prisoners convicted of murder, rape, arson, kidnapping, treason, or other heinous crimes to participate in medical experimentation. They were not considered sufficiently virtuous to be part of such a noble enterprise (Katz).

After World War II, when it became known that Nazi physicians had used concentration camp prisoners in medical experiments that mutilated and killed their subjects—innocent Jewish citizens of all ages—Europe found the use of any incarcerated persons in experimentation morally repugnant. An early draft of the Declaration of Helsinki included the following provision: "Persons retained in prisons, penitentiaries, or reformatories—being 'captive groups'—should not be used as subjects of experiment; nor persons incapable of giving consent because of age, mental incapacity, or being in a position in which they are incapable of exercising the power of free choice" (U.S. National Commission, 1976a, essay 16, p. 4).

However, the provision was deleted from the final version of the 1964 Declaration, reportedly because of pressure from the United States. Not only did the United States have an extended history of approving prisoner experimentation, but during the post-World War II years there was a substantial increase in biomedical experiments, including those using prisoners.

The federal government funded a wide variety of biomedical and behavioral experiments using prisoners, including numerous studies on infectious diseases, and the Atomic Energy Commission (later absorbed by the Department of Energy) conducted experiments involving radiation of male prisoners' genitals. From 1970 to 1975, five of the six government agencies that supported experimentation—all within the Public Health Service of the Department of Health, Education and Welfare—used prisoners in 125 biomedical studies and 19 behavioral research projects (U.S. National Commission, 1976b).

The greatest use of prisoners was in initial tests of drugs, performed primarily by private drug companies. In 1962, following the thalidomide tragedy, the U.S. Congress passed legislation requiring that before drugs were released for therapeutic use, their safety and efficacy must be tested on humans. To ensure an increased and steady supply of experimental subjects, pharmaceutical companies built facilities within prisons.

Prisoners became the principal subjects in the United States for testing new drugs. By 1975, according to a survey conducted by the Pharmaceutical Manufacturers Association (whose members develop most of the prescription drugs in the United States), at least 3,600 U.S. prisoners were the first humans on whom the safety of new drugs was tested. Prisoners in the United States were even being used to test drugs for researchers in other countries.

Principles

When the National Commission conducted its deliberations on prisoners, the Department of Health, Education and Welfare was already on record as being enthusiastic about the advantage of using prisoners in research. The president of the Pharmaceutical Manufacturers Association testified before the National Commission that his organization believed there were few alternatives to using prisoners in drug tests. Given that factual assumption, the moral argument was made that the good of society required the use of prisoners.

In its *Report and Recommendations* the National Commission moved beyond the moral appeal to the good of society by challenging the factual assumption that prisoners were necessary for at least initial drug trials. The commission found several drug-testing programs in the United States that successfully used healthy, nonincarcerated volunteers (U.S. National Commission, 1976b). Thus prisoners were not essential for biomedical experimentation. Having established that empirical fact, the National Commission then devoted considerable attention to two of the three ethical principles it said should govern experimentation with human subjects.

RESPECT FOR PERSONS. According to the National Commission, the fundamental moral principle of respect for persons includes respect for their dignity and autonomy. Experimentation with autonomous persons demands obtaining their consent to participate. The basic principle of respect for persons thus justifies the bioethical guideline of informed consent. Debates arising from the moral principle of respect for persons revolve around whether prisoners can provide a sufficiently voluntary consent to participate in experimentation.

One line of reasoning argues that prisoners obviously are competent to volunteer for experiments. After all, conviction for a crime presupposes that the citizen has been found sufficiently competent to be held accountable for his or her acts. Also, the citizen who enters prison has had certain rights legally recognized, such as the right to sue for freedom of worship and even to obtain compensation for injuries sustained in prison jobs (McDonald).

According to this line of thinking, prison inmates participate in remunerated occupations that put them at some risk. No one challenges the capacity of prisoners to volunteer for these tasks—for example, stamping license plates in prison factories. Why should there be moral outrage at prisoners' choosing (they are permitted to refuse) to participate in medical experiments that admittedly provide financial inducements but also may do less physical harm?

Those who oppose prisoner experimentation argue that the relationship of persons to their bodies is very different from their relationship to their productive goods; the former comprises their relationship to themselves. There is a distinction between activities in which impinging on a person's body is accidental or unavoidable, as in a job, and those in which it is the very purpose of the activity, as in experimentation (Fried). The argument runs that since consent to a job is different from consent to experimentation, prisoners may be sufficiently free to consent to prison jobs but not sufficiently free to consent to experimentation.

Among those who cite the principle of free and informed consent as part of their opposition to the use of prisoners in experimentation, some argue that prisoners cannot in principle give a sufficiently free consent (American Civil Liberties Union). Others who oppose the use of prisoners in experimentation admit that in principle it might be possible for an inmate in some ideal correctional institution to give a sufficiently free and informed consent. However, they argue that in fact either the structure or the administration of the penal system in the United States makes it impossible for prisoners to give a sufficiently free consent to experimentation.

This argument relies on analyses of the basic structure of American prisons made by historians and sociologists. According to historians, the coercive structure of the American prison and its powerful impact on the attitudes of prisoners are not accidental. After the 1820s, foreign officials came to the United States to observe the unique lengths to which the country went in creating new institutions called *penitentiaries*. They were designed not only to incarcerate criminals but also to shape their behavior and their character (Rothman).

Those opposed to prisoner participation in experimentation argue that medical experiments cannot remain unaffected by the social environment of what sociologist Erving Goffman calls a "total institution," such as a penitentiary. In a total institution a single authority tightly controls the entire space and time of each person within it, including a series of abasements, degradations, and humiliations designed to convince inmates to accept the single authority's view of them. In such institutions the entire social environment is designed to elicit cooperation with the central authority. It is argued that in total institutions even the attractive and beneficial features of an activity such as experimentation can overcome the inmates' ability to give a sufficiently free consent (Goffman).

The National Commission's investigations revealed that in U.S. prisons there appeared to be limited alternatives to experimentation among available prison activities. Other activities were not conducted in comparably secure surroundings, and there appeared to be a paucity of meaningful, alternative ways for prisoners to express any altruism they might have. Most importantly, no other prison activity paid comparably. The National Commission learned of differences in payment between experimentation and other prison activities that ranged to well over ten to one. Not surprisingly, surveys showed that 70 percent of prisoner research subjects volunteered primarily for the money (Arnold et al.).

Ethicists who served on the National Commission, or as staff and consultants, have subsequently emphasized that the commission believed prisoners were able to consent to experimentation under some conceivable conditions. However, the actual and likely conditions of American prisons raised genuine questions concerning prisoners' being able to give sufficiently free and informed consent. A distinction between coercion and manipulation of a prisoner's consent may be useful, although even a manipulated consent to participation in experimentation may be impermissible (Beauchamp and Childress; Faden et al.).

JUSTICE. A significant contribution of the National Commission was making not only respect for persons but also justice central to ethical considerations of prisoner experimentation. A few voices defended the use of prisoners as a form of reparative justice. Prisoners, they said, have committed crimes against society, and it is inherently appropriate, as an act of reparation for those crimes, for prisoners to serve society by being used in research. Opponents of prisoner experimentation responded that society, through its legal system, had already pronounced sentence on prisoners for whatever crime they committed, and medical experimentation should not be considered a form of punishment.

The National Commission brushed past discussions of reparation to questions raised by comparative justice. The essence of comparative justice is that like cases or classes are to be treated alike, and different cases or classes are to be treated differently (Feinberg). Problems of remuneration immediately came to the fore. Considerations of justice would require paying prisoners participating in experiments the same as free volunteers. However, the amounts would be so much greater than remuneration otherwise available in prison that the payments could become so irresistible as to be coercive. Thus, in its final report, the National Commission included suggestions that researchers pay the same rate for prisoners to participate in experiments as they did for nonincarcerated volunteers; however, individual prisoners would receive the same amount they received for other prison jobs. The excess would go into a fund for the general benefit of prisoners, or into escrow accounts paid to each participant at the time of his or her release from prison (Branson).

Comparative justice leads in biomedical ethics to considerations of the selection of subjects for experimentation. With respect to nontherapeutic experimentation in particular, risks and benefits should be distributed equitably among classes and groups of experimental subjects. The implications of comparative justice specifically for the gender and race of prisoners selected for experimentation received some attention from the National Commission. It heard testimony from black prisoners that they did not have equal opportunity to participate in experiments. Better-educated whites were disproportionately enrolled in prisoner experimentation. In its report the National Commission also noted that less research was conducted in women's prisons than in men's.

More fundamental were concerns about the justice of selecting prisoners at all for research benefiting society generally. A principal moral concern was that prisoners bore a disproportionate share of the burdens of research benefiting society as a whole—for example, initial drug trials on humans.

Comparative justice refers not only to similarities but also to differences between groups. Unequal treatment—for example, permitting free subjects, but not prisoners, to participate in experimentation—can be justified when individuals or groups are different in relevant respects. Prison populations are significantly different from the free society.

Prisoners live in an institutional environment that is more coercive than that of free-living volunteers, and prisoners are less likely to receive equivalent healthcare. They also receive a minuscule percentage of the financial benefits given to free research subjects.

That prisoners are considered to be in so many relevant respects different from, and unequal to, the rest of society is a principal reason they are considered to be treated justly if they do not participate in research that does not benefit them directly.

Policies

In 1976, the National Commission recommended that research involving prisoners that posed more than minimal risk, that was not studying the process of incarceration, and that did not directly improve the health or well-being of individual prisoners should not be conducted unless the reasons for the research were compelling and "a high degree of voluntariness on the part of the prospective participants and openness on the part of the institution(s) to be involved would characterize the conduct of the research." The National Commission included a long list of acceptable prison conditions. Showing its concern for justice, the commission also said that research would have to satisfy "conditions of equity" (1976b, p. 16).

In 1978, the DHHS published final regulations on research involving prisoners that were more restrictive than the recommendations of the National Commission. The department threw up its hands at trying to find prisons that met the commission's conditions of openness, and prohibited research on prisoners that did not benefit them as individuals or as a class ("Additional DHHS Protections,").

DHHS limited research involving prisoners to: (1) studies, involving no more than minimal risk or inconvenience, of the possible causes, effects, and processes of incarceration and criminal behavior; (2) studies of prisons as institutional structures, or of prisoners as incarcerated persons; (3) research on particular conditions affecting prisoners as a class; and (4) research involving a therapy likely to benefit the prisoner subject. Minimal risk was defined as risk normally encountered by nonprisoners ("Additional DHHS Protections").

The Federal Bureau of Prisons has maintained a policy that is even more restrictive. It prohibits biomedical research and drug testing on its inmates unless an individual, sick federal prisoner could benefit directly from an experimental therapy. Even then, a federal prisoner can be enrolled in a relevant clinical trial only if the responsible physician recommends it, the experiment has been approved by the DHHS,

the prisoner consents, and the medical director of the Federal Bureau of Prisons approves the individual case.

The U.S. Food and Drug Administration (FDA), which has authority over private drug companies, announced regulations in 1980 that were essentially the same as those of DHHS. But in 1981 the FDA "stayed indefinitely" its proposed regulations concerning use of prisoners. As a result, as of 1993, no regulations were in place that would prevent private drug companies from arranging with somewhat less than half the state prisons of the United States to resume using prisoners as subjects of initial drug trials (Penslar).

However, drug companies have evidently taken to heart the view expressed in the FDA's proposed regulations that sponsors of research could never establish a compelling need to use prisoners ("Protection of Human Subjects"). Ethical discussion, most notably that of the National Commission, not only affected public policy. It also created a persistent moral consensus in society that prisoners should not be used in experimentation that does not specifically benefit them as individuals or as a class.

ROY BRANSON (1995)
BIBLIOGRAPHY REVISED

SEE ALSO: *Autonomy; Bioethics, African American Perspectives; Coercion; Eugenics: Historical Aspects; Freedom and Free Will; Holocaust; Informed Consent: Consent Issues in Human Research; Justice; Minorities as Research Subjects; Research, Human: Historical Aspects; Research, Unethical; Rights, Human; Utilitarianism and Bioethics*

BIBLIOGRAPHY

"Additional DHHS Protections Pertaining to Biomedical and Behavioral Research Involving Prisoners as Subjects." 1993. 45 Code of Federal Regulations 46, subpart C.

American Civil Liberties Union. National Prison Project. 1974. *Complaint before United States District Court of Maryland.* See also *Bailey v. Lally,* 481 F. Supp. 203 (D. Md. 1979).

Arnold, John D.; Martin, Daniel C.; and Boyer, Sarah E. 1970. "A Study of One Prison Population and Its Response to Medical Research." *Annals of the New York Academy of Sciences* 169(2): 463–470.

Beauchamp, Tom L., and Childress, James F. 1989. *Principles of Biomedical Ethics,* 3rd edition. New York: Oxford University Press.

Beecher, Henry K. 1970. "The Subject: Prisoners." In *Research and the Individual: Human Studies,* pp. 69–78. Boston: Little, Brown.

Branson, Roy. 1976. "Philosophical Perspectives on Experimentation with Prisoners." In *Research Involving Prisoners: Appendix to Report and Recommendations.* DHEW Publication no. (OS) 76–132. Bethesda, MD: U.S. National Commission for the Protection of Human Subjects of Biomedical and Behavioral Research.

Faden, Ruth R.; Beauchamp, Tom L.; and King, Nancy M. P. 1986. *A History and Theory of Informed Consent.* New York: Oxford University Press.

Federal Bureau of Prisons. 1990. *Health Services Manual,* Program statement 6000.3, pp. 6800–6818. Washington, D.C.: Federal Bureau of Prisons.

Feinberg, Joel. 1973. *Social Philosophy.* Englewood Cliffs, NJ: Prentice-Hall.

Fried, Charles. 1974. *Medical Experimentation: Personal Integrity and Social Policy.* Amsterdam: North-Holland.

Goffman, Erving. 1961. *Asylums: Essays on the Social Situation of Mental Patients and Other Inmates.* Chicago: Aldine.

Harkness, J. M. 1996. "Nuremberg and the Issue of Wartime Experiments on U.S. Prisoners: The Green Committee." *Journal of the American Medical Association* 276(20): 1672–1675.

Hornblum, Allen M. 1997. "They Were Cheap and Available: Prisoners as Research Subjects in Twentieth Century America." *British Medical Journal (Clinical Research Edition)* 315(7120): 1437–1441.

Hornblum, Allen M. 1998. *Acres of Skin: Human Experiments at Holmesburg Prison: A True Story of Abuse and Exploitation in the Name of Medical Science.* London: Routledge.

Katz, Jay, ed. 1972. *Experimentation with Human Beings: The Authority of the Investigator, Subject, Professions, and State in the Human Experimentation Process.* New York: Russell Sage.

Levine, Robert J. 1986. *Ethics and Regulation of Clinical Research.* 2nd edition. New Haven, CT: Yale University Press.

McCarthy, Colleen M. 1989. "Experimentation on Prisoners: The Inadequacy of Voluntary Consent." *New England Journal on Criminal and Civil Confinement* 15(1): 55–80.

McDonald, John C. 1967. "Why Prisoners Volunteer to Be Experimental Subjects." *Journal of the American Medical Association* 202(6): 511–512.

Penslar, Robin Levin. 1993. *Protecting Human Research Subjects: Institutional Review Board Guidebook,* 2nd edition. Bethesda, MD: National Institutes of Health, Office for Protection from Research Risks, Office of Extramural Research.

Pharmaceutical Manufacturers Association. 1976. "Survey: Use of Prisoners in Drug Testing." In *Research Involving Prisoners: Appendix to Report and Recommendations,* doc. no. 11, pp. 1–9. DHEW publication no. (OS) 76–132. Bethesda, MD: U.S. National Commission for the Protection of Human Subjects of Biomedical and Behavioral Research.

"Protection of Human Subjects: Prisoners Used as Research Subjects: Reproposal of Regulations." 1981. *Federal Register* 46, no. 245 (December 18): 61666–61671.

Reed, Joyce, 1999. "Regulatory Orphans: Juvenile Prisoners as Transvulnerable Research Subjects." *G IRB* 21(2): 9–14.

Rothman, David J. 1971. *The Discovery of the Asylum: Social Order and Disorder in the New Republic.* Boston: Little, Brown.

U.S. National Commission for the Protection of Human Subjects of Biomedical and Behavioral Research. 1976a. *Research Involving Prisoners: Appendix to Report and Recommendations.* DHEW publication no. (OS) 76–132. Bethesda, MD: Author.

U.S. National Commission for the Protection of Human Subjects of Biomedical and Behavioral Research. 1976b. *Research Involving Prisoners: Report and Recommendations.* DHEW publication no. (OS) 76–132. Bethesda, MD: Author.

PRISONERS, HEALTHCARE ISSUES OF

• • •

"It is but just that the public be required to care for the prisoner, who cannot, by reason of the deprivation of his liberty, care for himself" (*Spicer v. Williamson,* 1926).

Because of incarceration, the legal context of providing medical, dental, and mental health services is different in prisons and jails from that in the outside community. In no other setting are such services constitutionally guaranteed. Drawing upon the prohibition against "cruel and unusual punishment" in the Eighth Amendment to the Constitution (and the Due Process Clauses of the Fifth and Fourteenth Amendments for juveniles, pre-trial detainees, and federal prisoners), the courts require that institutions with custody of human beings provide for their basic necessities, including healthcare.

It was not always so. Historically, the correctional system in the United States has been largely protected from public scrutiny. Prisons were built far from population centers, and courts adopted a "hands off" doctrine regarding their administration (*Procunier v. Martinez,* 1974). Early cases in the 1970s, however, revealed horrendous medical conditions in which inmates were used without supervision to perform medical care on their fellows, including pulling teeth, suturing, and surgery. Dramatic instances were illustrated in which prisoners died neglected, covered in maggots, and lying in their own filth (*Newman v. Alabama,* 1974).

The present legal framework was established in the 1976 landmark decision of *Estelle v. Gamble,* in which the Supreme Court ruled that prisoners have a right to be free of "deliberate indifference to their serious health care needs." Although there has been some fine-tuning, the legal landscape has remained largely unchanged since that ruling.

In the hundreds of published cases following *Estelle v. Gamble,* three basic rights have emerged: the right to access to care, the right to care that is ordered, and the right to a professional medical judgment (Rold, 2001). The failure of correctional officials to honor these rights has resulted in protracted litigation, the awarding of damages and attorneys' fees, and the issuance of injunctions regarding the delivery of healthcare services.

To provide for constitutional care and to protect themselves from litigation, correctional administrators must adopt procedures to protect inmates' basic rights, including a functioning sick call system that uses properly trained healthcare staff, a means of addressing medical emergencies, a priority system so that those most in need of care receive it first, the development and maintenance of adequate medical records, liaison with outside resources for specialist and hospital care when needed, a system for staff development and training, and an ongoing effort at quality improvement. Jail wardens and prison superintendents and their chief medical officers must develop policies and procedures for meeting the special needs of disabled, elderly, and mentally ill inmates, as well as those with HIV infection and AIDS, and to preserve the confidentiality of medical information.

The Eighth Amendment

The Eighth Amendment, forbidding cruel and unusual punishment, presents a relatively narrow standard of liability. The Eighth Amendment does not render prison officials or staff liable in federal cases for malpractice or accidents, nor does it resolve professional disputes about the best choice of treatment. It does require, however, that sufficient resources be made available to protect the three basic rights.

While the constitutional standard does not require that an express intent to inflict pain be shown (*Wilson v. Seiter,* 1991), it does include an inquiry into the defendants' state of mind. A violation of the Eighth Amendment requires a "subjective" showing of "deliberate indifference." It is not enough that the defendant should have known or ought to have understood the danger to the inmate. The defendant must know of and disregard a substantial risk (*Farmer v. Brennan,* 1994). Such knowledge, however, can be inferred from the surrounding facts where the failure to respond to a clear risk is reckless.

In general, cost considerations are not valid defenses to a violation of the Eighth Amendment. Corrections officials must diagnose and treat illness and eradicate conditions of confinement that expose inmates to communicable disease and other identifiable health threats (*Jones v. Diamond,* 1981). Indeed, correctional facilities have been ordered to pay for the cost of medical procedures for indigent inmates,

such as an otherwise legal abortion, where the inmate was precluded by incarceration from any option other than carrying her fetus to term (*Monmouth County Correctional Institute Inmates v. Lanzano,* 1987). The Eighth Amendment does not afford inmates priority in the allocation of scarce medical resources, such as organ transplants; but it does require access to such resources for serious conditions on the basis of the same ethical and medical considerations for similarly situated patients who are not incarcerated (see Statement, United Network for Organ Sharing, 2001). Finally, the increasingly common practice of contracting with private healthcare corporations to provide healthcare services does not shield the correctional agency from fulfilling the constitutionally required dimensions of healthcare. The private contractor is likewise brought within the aegis of the Eighth Amendment (*West v. Atkins,* 1989).

THE RIGHT TO ACCESS TO CARE. The right to access to care is fundamental: When access is denied or delayed, the health staff does not know which patients need immediate attention and which patients need care that can wait. "A well-monitored and well-run access system is the best way to protect prisoners from unnecessary harm and suffering and, concomitantly, to protect prison officials from liability for denying access to needed medical care" (Winner).

The right to access to care includes access to both emergency and routine care. All institutions, of whatever size, must have the capacity to cope with emergencies and to provide for sick call. Access to specialists and to in-patient hospital treatment, where warranted by the patient's condition, are also guaranteed by the Eighth Amendment.

THE RIGHT TO CARE THAT IS ORDERED. Generally, courts assume that care would not have been ordered if it were not needed. Thus, once a healthcare professional orders treatment for a serious condition, the courts will protect, as a matter of constitutional law, the patient's right to receive that treatment without undue delay. The easiest way for an institution to lose a lawsuit is to fail to provide inmate patients with the care that its own staff has ordered.

THE RIGHT TO A PROFESSIONAL MEDICAL JUDGMENT. In general, the courts will not determine which of two equally efficacious treatment modalities should be chosen. The adjudication of constitutional claims is not the business of "second guessing" healthcare professionals. Rather, the courts seek to: "ensure that decisions concerning the nature and timing of medical care are made by medical personnel, using equipment designed for medical use, in locations conducive to medical functions, and for reasons that are purely medical" (Neisser).

By ensuring that professional judgment is actually exercised, however, the federal courts have not only protected the sphere of discretion surrounding medical practitioners' treatment and diagnostic decisions, but they have often enhanced it. At issue in a typical injunctive case are such matters as staffing, physical facilities, transportation, and sick call and follow-up procedures. When a court orders relief in these areas, it is assuring that the raw materials from which responsible professional judgment is formed and carried out are available to practitioners.

"Serious Medical Needs"

The Constitution requires that correctional officials provide medical care only for "serious medical needs." Generally, a medical need is "serious" if it "has been diagnosed by a physician as mandating treatment or … is so obvious that even a lay person would easily recognize the necessity for a doctor's attention" (*Duran v. Anaya,* 1986; *Ramos v. Lamm,* 1980). Conditions are also considered to be "serious" if they "cause pain, discomfort, or threat to good health" (*Dean v. Coughlin,* 1985). A condition need not be life-threatening to be deemed "serious," and many treatment plans that are labeled "elective" nevertheless are deemed "serious" within the meaning of *Estelle v. Gamble* (1976).

In general, courts consider three factors in determining whether correctional officials are being deliberately indifferent to "serious medical needs": (1) the amenability of the patient's condition to treatment; (2) the consequences to the patient if treatment does not occur; and (3) the likelihood of a favorable outcome. Within this mix, the court may also consider the length of the patient's anticipated incarceration. It is one thing to decline the provision of dentures or an artificial limb to an inmate with a three-day jail sentence. It is quite another to withhold such adjuncts to a patient serving twenty years to life (Rold, 1997).

The Role of Standards and Accreditation

Compliance with national standards and accreditation, while not dispositive on the outcome of litigation, are frequently regarded favorably by the courts. In the Arizona prison litigation (which ultimately reached the Supreme Court on the unrelated issue of inmates' claims of denial of access to the courts), experts for both sides relied on standards of the National Commission on Correctional Health Care in their testimony, the defendant prison officials' expert stating that "[t]here are no correctional health care standards that are more stringent or more difficult to fulfill than the National Commission on Correctional Health Care standards" (*Casey v. Lewis,* 1993) The standards of the National Commission

on Correctional Health are the only national standards devoted solely to healthcare delivery in corrections. They have been updated periodically as the standard of care evolves. The American Correctional Association (1990) and the Joint Commission on Accreditation of Health Care Organizations (2000) also have standards and accredit correctional facilities. The American Public Health Association (1986) also has detailed standards for prison and jail healthcare, although it does not accredit. While meeting standards is not a guarantee that a lawsuit against a correctional facility will fail, compliance with standards and facility accreditation have been noted by courts in the granting of summary judgment to defendants in individual prisoner damages cases (*Williams v. Ceorlock,* 1998; *Tumath v. County of Alameda,* 1996).

Confidentiality

Inmates have a constitutional right to privacy in their medical diagnoses and other healthcare records and information. That right is not violated by the reporting of medical findings in the ordinary course of prison medical care operations or probably even to prison and jail executives with a reason to know, but the "[c]asual, unjustified dissemination of confidential medical information to non-medical staff and other prisoners" is unconstitutional (*Woods v. White,* 1998; *Doe v. Coughlin,* 1988). "[T]he gratuitous disclosure of an inmate's confidential medical information as humor or gossip. . . is not reasonably related to a legitimate penological interest." (*Powell v. Schriver,* 1999).

In contrast, there are also occasions when a provider may have not only a prerogative, but a duty, to report or disclose confidential medical information to third parties. If a concrete risk to an identifiable person is revealed, and "disclosure is essential to avert danger," the revelation of a patient's private communication may be essential to protect peril to innocent persons. In such cases, however, disclosure must be done "discretely" and in a way that preserves the privacy of the patient "to the fullest extent compatible with the prevention of the threatened danger." (*Tarasoff v. Regents of the University of California,* 1976).

Informed Consent and the Right to Refuse Treatment

A mentally competent adult has the right to be informed of proposed medical treatment (and its likely benefits and risks) and the right to refuse medical treatment, including the direction that life-saving or other extraordinary measures be withdrawn in terminal cases (*Cruzan v. Missouri Department of Health,* 1990). As Judge Cardozo stated in the 1914

Schloendorff v. Society of New York Hospitals ruling: "Every human being of adult years and sound mind has a right to determine what shall be done with his own body." This right generally extends to prisoners as well (*White v. Napoleon,* 1990). On the other hand, in some cases life-sustaining care may be imposed. In *Commissioner of Corrections v. Myer* (1979), the court balanced the inmate patient's objections to treatment with the state's interest in orderly prison administration and ordered resumption of dialysis despite the patient's refusal. Temporary, forced administration of antipsychotic drugs over a prisoner's objection has also been allowed if preceded by administrative protections, including an impartial hearing that finds that the patient has a "mental disorder," is "gravely disabled," and "pose[s] a likelihood of serious harm to self or others" (*Washington v. Harper,* 1990).

Profound ethical issues can be presented, most acutely in the case of mentally ill inmates facing execution:

> [T]he determination of whether an inmate is "competent for execution" should be made by an independent expert and not by any health care professional regularly in the employ of ... the correctional institution .... This requirement does not diminish the responsibility of correctional health care personnel to treat any mental illness of death row inmates. (National Commission on Correctional Health Care, p. 75)

While the courts continue to explore this issue, the availability of an ethical advisory board for consultation with individual correctional systems is strongly recommended.

The right to refuse is, of course, the obverse of the right to informed consent, and each depends upon the genuine observance of the other (*White v. Napoleon,* 1990). Because of the environment, there are "reason[s] to be leery of refusals of care in prisons" (Anno), because the institutional environment often clouds issues of informed consent, making it difficult to distinguish between refusal of care by the staff. It is important in corrections to take steps to determine if a refusal of care is genuine. Some investigation of an inmate who does not appear for treatment should occur if the appointment were for a serious condition and a lapse in treatment might result in deterioration or a poor outcome.

Ethical Considerations

Correctional healthcare providers work in a "medically alien setting" (Wishart and Dubler). The mission of medical care is to diagnose, comfort, or cure; the goal of a prison or jail is to confine, to punish, and, ideally, to reform. There is an inevitable tension between these two purposes, because correctional facilities are "inherently coercive institutions that for security reasons must exercise nearly total control

over their residents lives and the activities within their confines" (*West v. Atkins,* 1988). This setting affects the way healthcare is practiced by professionals within institutions.

In addition to constitutional mandates and the range of medical/ethical problems complicated by the prison context, there is a series of ethical dilemmas peculiar to correctional settings, even though healthcare providers in correctional settings are bound by the same guidelines as their colleagues who work in more conventional medical spaces. They must promote the welfare of patients, advocate their medical needs, inform them about their diagnoses and prognoses, and protect their privacy. Providers in correctional settings, however, also face ethical challenges for which there are no parallels in the outside world because the prison setting exerts a continual pressure on professional judgment (Anno and Dubler).

Providers may be asked to act as impartial arbiters of potentially explosive or violent situations, to witness forced transfers, or to supervise punishment. It is assumed that their presence will prevent violence or that their skill and special status will render searches less painful and intrusive and the punishment less destructive. Acquiescing to these requests, however, may destroy the provider's ability to act independently as the patient's advocate. Such participation violates the particular provider–patient relationship, and by extension, relationships with other inmates (Anno and Dubler).

"No individual, however skilled and compassionate a doctor, can maintain a normal doctor-patient relationship with a man who the next day he may acquiesce in subjecting to solitary confinement" (Brazer). Other assignments that tend to undermine the provider–patient relationship include collecting forensic information for prosecutors, using restraints for nonmedical purposes, agreeing to endorse a "special diet" that is actually a nutritionally adequate yet inedible punishment, permitting a medical note about an inmate's noncompliance with a care plan or follow-up appointment to be used to trigger disciplinary action, agreeing to monitor a hunger strike, certifying that a prisoner has been successfully executed, or helping to determine whether an inmate is "competent" and sufficiently mentally intact and aware for execution.

Deciding how to respond to requests for such assistance is a difficult and complex task. The institutional pressures for provider participation may be enormous, yet many scholars and commentators have argued, consistent with comprehensive standards published by the National Commission on Correctional Health Care (2003) and by the American Public Health Association (1986), that if professional ethics would prohibit an action in a community setting, they prohibit it in a correctional setting as well.

Inmates are not passive in the process of receiving healthcare. The need for a medical note to obtain an assignment excuse and the lack of available common over-the-counter medications all encourage heavy use of the medical service. Prisoners, who are largely poor and did not have adequate access to medical, mental health, and dental care before incarceration, tend to have more significant health problems than a matched-age cohort. Prisoners may also view medical service personnel as more humane and caring than the rest of the prison staff and for this reason seek to spend inordinate amounts of time in their presence. Such use of the medical service to meet "nonmedical" needs, although perhaps a rational coping strategy in a dehumanizing environment, may elicit hostility from the medical staff (Wishart and Dubler). In short, correctional rules issued for administrative reasons (and not because of legal, medical, or ethical imperatives) continue to influence and challenge those who work in healthcare "inside the walls."

Conclusion

"No serious student of American correctional history can deny that litigation has provided the impetus for reform of medical practice in prisons and jails" (Nathan). Yet, as resources become increasingly scarce, government officials are constantly faced with doing more with less. Voluntary adoption of community and ethical standards and accreditation are a less tortuous road to reform, and, in the long run, are likely to be more successful and less divisive.

NANCY N. DUBLER (1995)
REVISED BY WILLIAM J. ROLD
NANCY N. DUBLER

SEE ALSO: *Coercion; Conflict of Interest; Death Penalty; Divided Loyalties in Mental Healthcare; Freedom and Free Will; Research Policy: Risk and Vulnerable Groups*

BIBLIOGRAPHY

American Correctional Association. 1990 (suppl. 1998). *Standards for Adult Correctional Institutions,* 3rd edition. Lanham, MD: Author.

American Pubic Health Association. 1986. *Standards for Health Services in Correctional Institutions,* 2nd edition. Washington, D.C.: Author

Anno, B. Jaye. 2001. *Correctional Health Care: Guidelines for the Management of an Adequate Delivery System.* Washington, D.C.: U. S. Department of Justice, National Institute of Corrections.

Anno, B. Jaye, and Dubler, Nancy Neveloff. 2001. "Ethical Considerations and the Interface with Custody." In *Correctional Health Care: Guidelines for the Management of an Adequate Delivery System,* ed. B. Jaye Anno. Washington, D.C.: U. S. Department of Justice, National Institute of Corrections.

Brazer, Margaret. 1982. "Prison Doctors and Their Involuntary Patients." *Public Law* 1982: 282–300.

Casey v. Lewis. 834 F. Supp. 1477, 1483–4. D. Ariz. (1993).

Commissioner of Corrections v. Myer. 399 N.E. 2d 452. Mass. (1979).

Cruzan v. Missouri Department of Health. 497 U.S. 261 (1990).

Dean v. Coughlin. 623 F. Supp. 392, 404. S.D.N.Y. (1985).

Doe v. Coughlin. 697 F. Supp. 1234. N.D.N.Y. (1988).

Duran v. Anaya. 624 F. Supp. 510, 524. D.N.M. (1986).

Estelle v. Gamble. 429 U.S. 97 (1976).

Farmer v. Brennan. 511 U.S. 825 (1994).

Joint Commission on Accreditation of Health Care Organizations. 2000. *Standards for Ambulatory Care.* Oakbrook, Terrace, IL: Author.

Jones v. Diamond. 636 F. 2d 1364. 5th Cir. (1981).

Monmouth County Correctional Institute Inmates v. Lanzano. 834 F. 2d 326. 3d Cir. (1987).

Nathan, Vincent. 1985. "Guest Editorial." *Journal of Prison Health* 5(1).

National Commission on Correctional Health Care. 1995b. "Position Statement on Competency for Execution." *Journal of Correctional Health Care* 1(2): 75.

Neisser, Eric. 1977. "Is There a Doctor in the Joint? The Search for Constitutional Standards for Prison Health Care." *Virginia Law Review* 63: 921, 956–957.

Newman v. Alabama. 503 F.2d 1320. 5th Cir. (1974).

Powell v. Schriver. 1999 WL 223434. 2d Cir. (1999).

Procunier v. Martinez. 416 U.S. 405, 416 (1974).

Ramos v. Lamm. 639 F. 2ed 559, 575. 10th Cir. (1980).

Rold, William J. 1997. "An Examination of Medical Necessity and the Law." *Correct Care* 11.

Rold, William J. 2001. "Legal Considerations in the Delivery of Health Care Services in Prisons and Jails." In *Correctional Health Care: Guidelines for the Management of an Adequate Delivery System,* ed. B. Jaye Anno. Washington, D.C.: U. S. Department of Justice, National Institute of Corrections.

Schloendorff v. Society of New York Hospitals. 211 N.Y. 125, 129 (1914).

Spicer v. Williamson. 132 S.E. 291, 293. N.C. (1926).

Tarasoff v. Regents of the University of California. 551 P. 2d 334, 337. Cal. (1976).

Tumath v. County of Alameda. 1996 WL 660611. N.D. Cal. (1996).

Washington v. Harper. 494 U.S. 210 (1990).

West v. Atkins. 487 U.S. 42, 57 n.15 (1988).

White v. Napoleon. 897 F. 2d 103, 113. 3d Dir. (1990).

Williams v. Ceorlock. 993 F. Supp. 1192. C.D. Ill. (1998).

Wilson v. Seiter. 501 U.S. 294 (1991).

Winner, Ellen. 1981. "An Introduction to the Constitutional Law of Prison Medical Care." *Journal of Prison Health* 67(1): 77.

Wishart, Margaret, and Dubler, Nancy Neveloff. 1983. *Health Care in Prisons, Jails, and Detention Centers: Some Legal and Ethical Dilemmas.* Washington, D.C.: National Science Foundation.

Woods v. White. 689 F. Supp 874. W.D. Wisc. (1988).

PRIVACY AND CONFIDENTIALITY IN RESEARCH

• • •

When people seek the help of healthcare providers, and thus become patients, they exchange some of their privacy for the chance to be healed, diagnosed, and protected from illness. Healthcare providers in turn promise to keep patients' private information confidential by sharing it only with those whose knowledge stands to benefit the patient, unless higher duties require that the promise be broken, or the patient has consented to other uses of the information. When private information is shared not for treatment purposes but in research, the exchange is necessarily different: Research subjects (even those who are also patients) are not the same as patients, and researchers are not the same as persons offering treatment (even if they are also clinicians). The research context may alter not only what information individuals consider private and the extent to which they are willing to share it, but also the potential harms and wrongs that may result from breaches of privacy and confidentiality.

Issues of privacy and confidentiality in human-subjects research can arise in three contexts. First, patient care can give rise to research questions, as when researchers wish to use data from patients' medical records or contact health providers for the names of patients with specific health problems to ask them to participate in research projects. Second, human subjects of biomedical, behavioral, or social science research, as well as persons and groups who may not be research subjects, can be affected in a variety of ways that implicate privacy and confidentiality by the gathering or the use of information for research purposes. Finally, clinical research involving subjects who are also patients has its own

particular risks to privacy and confidentiality, as when the media and the public claim a special interest in the first patient-subjects to receive a novel research intervention. In all of these circumstances we must examine the disclosure, sharing, and publication of information, and the interests of researcher, subject, and others, as well as the legal, policy, and practical protections that are available to preserve subjects' privacy and the confidentiality of their private information.

Privacy, as a right belonging to persons, and confidentiality, as an attribute of data that arises from a promise made by healthcare providers or researchers, can readily be seen as intimately related to the moral principles of autonomy, respect for persons, and beneficence, and to the requirement of informed consent. In the United States, federally funded research is governed by consolidated regulations for the protection of human subjects, known as the Common Rule, which require that all research collecting identifiable private information about living individuals be reviewed by an institutional review board. This review must minimize the risks that research poses to subjects, determine that the risks are reasonable in relation to anticipated benefits, ensure that informed consent is obtained, and, "when appropriate," require "adequate provisions to protect the privacy of subjects and to maintain the confidentiality of data." The required informed consent includes "a statement describing the extent, if any, to which confidentiality of records identifying the subject will be maintained" ("Federal Policy for the Protection of Human Subjects").

According to the Common Rule, if confidentiality is promised by researchers, they must be able to provide it; but confidentiality need not be promised, so long as subjects are informed that confidentiality is not offered and can freely choose to participate based on that knowledge. The *ethical baseline* thus provided by the Common Rule must then be supplemented by professional codes and other guidelines, as well as by existing federal, state, or local privacy laws (Annas, 2001; Symposium).

Privacy and Professional Codes

Many professional codes discuss the ethics of research and scholarly publication; the attention each gives to privacy and confidentiality necessarily varies, with each such code generally combining an aspirational morality with a particularized professional focus. For example, the Council for International Organizations of Medical Sciences' *International Guidelines for Ethical Review of Epidemiological Studies* (1991) contains an extensive discussion of confidentiality protection in large data sets, and its *International Ethical Guidelines for Biomedical Research Involving Human Subjects* (2002) includes a confidentiality provision addressing a broad range of data types, sources, uses, and risks of harm. In contrast, the World Medical Association's *Declaration of Helsinki* (2000) includes only a statement of the importance of respecting "the privacy of the subject [and] the confidentiality of the patient's information"; and the Nuremberg Code (Germany [Territory Under Allied Occupation …], 1949), devoted to the subject's right to consent, does not mention privacy or confidentiality at all.

PRIVACY AND HIPAA. In the United States, regulations implementing federal legislation designed to improve access to health insurance, the Health Insurance Portability and Accountability Act (HIPAA), may have considerable impact on privacy and confidentiality in research using health information. HIPAA's data privacy regulations apply to a specific set of users (*covered entities*) who generate and maintain personally identifiable health information. This group of users is not coextensive with federally funded researchers, and crosses professional boundaries; thus, HIPAA's privacy rule may have broader application in human subjects research than the federal regulations (Department of Health and Human Services [DHHS]).

In very general terms, the privacy rule's application to research means that personally identifiable health information may not be created or used for research by covered entities and their business associates unless the research subject has specifically authorized the use, the authorization requirement has been waived by a HIPAA privacy board or an institutional review board, or the use falls under a limited set of exceptions (Office of Civil Rights). In many respects, the privacy rule in research conceptually parallels the privacy and confidentiality concerns of institutional review boards and of federal research oversight agencies like the Office for Human Research Protections.

The HIPAA privacy rule may prove extremely helpful in addressing confidentiality problems in health research using large data sets (Barnes and Krauss; Durham). However, HIPAA's focused attention on personally identifiable health information in research may diminish attention to other types of risks to privacy and confidentiality that are posed by research but not considered by HIPAA, such as risks to groups, dignitary harms, or risks arising from interactions themselves, rather than from the resulting data. Because implementation of the HIPAA privacy rule is so new, whether and how it affects overall perspectives on research privacy remains to be seen (Annas, 2002; Kulynych and Korn).

Becoming a Research Subject

Usually, research subjects are enrolled in a study after giving their informed consent to participation. However, subjects in studies that examine information about which there is considered to be a lesser expectation of privacy (e.g., large-scale record abstraction that collects no identifying information, or studies observing public behavior) may never know that they have been the subjects of research. In fact, pursuant to the Common Rule, such studies may be exempted from review by an institutional review board. Violations of privacy may occur in such studies. For example, some subjects may not want researchers to read their records even though only aggregate data are recorded; and some subjects may feel wronged if they know their behavior is being observed for research purposes, even though many strangers who are not researchers observe the same behavior. However, the balance of benefits and harms is generally considered to warrant exempting such studies both from full consideration by an institutional review board and from the informed-consent requirements that would alert subjects to participation (Capron).

In addition, according to the Common Rule, some studies reviewed by institutional review boards may be considered appropriate for waiver or alteration of informed consent requirements. Factors used in determining whether waiving the informed consent requirement is acceptable include the magnitude and likelihood of the risks of harm to subjects in the study, and whether obtaining individual consent is considered impracticable. Large-scale database research that involves no direct contact with subjects, but in which researchers plan to retain information that identifies subjects in order to link, for example, information from a cancer registry to medical and other records and to stored tissue specimens presents an increasingly common scenario throughout the world. Investigators reason that they have no interest in the identities or characteristics of individual subjects, but need identifiers in order to gather, link, and analyze aggregate data. Seeking consent may be considered impracticable because of the cost and difficulty of reaching potential subjects, or because too many negative responses would result in a nonrepresentative sample, thus adversely affecting the validity of any findings. Confidentiality protections in such studies depend on ethically sensitive oversight and robust data security measures. (Berman; Bruppacher and Kaiser; Leufkens; Truter).

As in the case of research that is exempted from the informed consent requirement, research for which the consent requirement is waived may result in privacy violations if subjects would not wish investigators to see and use their personal information, even if only to link data sets. Breaches of confidentiality are of course also possible, but the risk may be lowered if adequate data security plans are in place, and identifying and potentially identifying information is destroyed as soon as it is no longer needed. Perhaps more basic, however, is the question whether sample validity overrides individuals' privacy interests in, at the very least, knowing that they are subjects. With the growth of large-scale research of this type, it is increasingly common to seek subjects' general consent to the prospective collection of data and specimens to be stored for future research (Annas, 2000; National Bioethics Advisory Commission, 1999).

All research requiring access to patients' medical records raises confidentiality concerns when the investigator is not also either a healthcare provider or other person with legitimate reason to inspect medical records. Perhaps the most significant concerns arise when patients are contacted to solicit their research participation by non-provider researchers using contact and diagnosis information they have obtained from medical records without patients' knowledge or permission. A variety of ways of balancing harms and benefits, and of reducing risks to confidentiality, are available to investigators and healthcare providers concerned about the interests of patients who are in the process of becoming research subjects (National Bioethics Advisory Commission, 2001; Office for Human Research Protections; Veatch).

The fact of study participation is generally treated as confidential information; this is especially important when the category of subjects or the purpose of the research carries potential social stigma (e.g., studies of HIV-positive patients, familial mental illness, genetic disease, or drug abuse). Inclusion in the subject pool may be enough to warrant confidentiality protection for potential subjects who decline to participate. Persons approached to participate in some studies may not want others to know that they fall into a category appropriate for inclusion. Others may be concerned that their participation may signal the existence of desirable information about them to employers, insurers, treating health professionals, or other authorities, placing the confidentiality of collected data at particular risk (Melton and Gray).

Privacy and the Researcher-Subject Relationship

Once enrolled, the subject is asked to disclose private information to a researcher. Such disclosure can take place in a variety of ways, from giving up tissue samples to answering extensive questions about personal history and psychology. The subject's judgment regarding the privacy of such information is highly dependent upon the circumstances. Someone enrolled in an addiction-control program may have little difficulty discussing alcohol consumption with health professionals in that program, but may have some hesitation about discussing it with a researcher collecting epidemiological information on the health of the person's county of residence, and even more when it is requested as part of a survey about the effects of television on perceptions about violence. Collection of genetic information may be of particular concern to subjects, because of heightened public awareness of how such information may be regarded and used (Sankar).

Sometimes revealing personal information (e.g., giving a blood sample, disclosing personal habits, recounting a past experience, or discussing physical limitations) can cause psychological or physical distress. According to the Common Rule, subjects must be informed when the research may be painful or address sensitive topics. Subjects must also be informed of their rights to refuse to answer individual questions and to terminate participation in the research at any time ("Federal Policy for the Protection of Human Subjects").

Interview studies raise an additional privacy concern when the information sought concerns persons other than the subject. For example, much survey research asks questions about the habits and activities of the subject's family, household, and associates. Some questions may concern sensitive topics or disfavored or illegal conduct. Although persons other than the subject are not named, they may be identifiable through naming of the relationship to the subject. In at least some such instances, these *secondary subjects* are research subjects in every respect, and their consent for participation should be sought unless criteria for waiver of consent are met (Botkin). Even if they are not identifiable, they may be wronged, simply because information about them is revealed without their consent or knowledge (Capron). It is likewise possible for some people or groups to become unexpected subjects if collection of information from them about study subjects incidentally reveals important information about the informants—as when studies of medical technologies or practices uncover information about healthcare providers who were not initially considered subjects (King, Henderson, and Stein; Veatch).

A similar concern can arise when others are asked to provide information about study subjects. In long-term studies, some subjects may become decisionally incapacitated, and investigators may turn to others, perhaps family members or institutional caregivers, to provide needed data.

This violation of subjects' privacy can be avoided by dropping these subjects from the study, or ameliorated by anticipating the problem and discussing with all subjects the designation of appropriate proxies should that become necessary (National Bioethics Advisory Commission, 1998).

The Promise of Confidentiality

The promise of confidentiality given by researchers to subjects extends not only to the information actually collected but also to whatever information the researcher encounters in the course of the data collection, regardless of whether that information is recorded. Thus, for example, when medical records are abstracted, information read by researchers as part of the abstraction process must be kept confidential, and information conveyed but not used in interviews similarly must not be divulged. Research projects that make use of record abstractors or interviewers generally require them to sign pledges of confidentiality promising that they will discuss no information outside the research project.

The information collected in human-subjects research needs protection not only from careless disclosure but also from intentional disclosure to those with a particular interest in the data. For example, study results may be offered as evidence in civil or criminal litigation, and both plaintiffs and defendants may seek to challenge the research by reexamining the data used or even by reinterviewing subjects. Criminal or social services authorities may seek access to study data that could inform them of ongoing violations. Health insurers may want to know whether those they insure have been tested for HIV or genetic disorders (Holder; Lansing; Symposium; Wing; Yolles et al.) In order to protect subjects from court-ordered disclosure of identifying information in civil, criminal, administrative, or other legal proceedings, federal certificates of confidentiality are available for human-subjects research that collects sensitive information which, if disclosed, could have adverse consequences for subjects or damage their financial standing, employability, insurability, or reputation. Certificates of confidentiality must be applied for by the investigator, and do not prevent voluntary disclosures by investigators; nonetheless, they can offer considerable protection for subjects (Office of Extramural Research).

Certificates of confidentiality have been expanded from their original focus on criminal justice questions, alcohol and drug use, and mental health, to encompass a broad range of research collecting sensitive information, including genetic information, information about sexual attitudes and preferences, information about sexually transmitted disease, behavioral research, and information about environmental or occupational exposures where litigation may be an issue. They preclude only the release of information that would identify specific individual research subjects and connect their identities with their data (Reatig). The concept of a researcher–subject privilege is not well established in the law, but courts that have considered requests for research data have generally required a strong showing of necessity and the deletion of all information that could lead to identification of subjects, even when the subjects' identities are a critical part of the request.

Confidential or Anonymous?

One way to ensure that confidentiality is not breached is to ensure that the information collected in research is anonymous—that is, that no information that could identify subjects is recorded or retained. Confidentiality can be preserved without anonymity by stripping collected data of identifying information but substituting a subject identification code and creating a secured *linkage file* that contains information connecting the subject's name and/or other identifying information to the code. The complexities of confidentiality protection can be considerable, especially in large projects, conducted at multiple sites that collect and manipulate data in hard copy or electronic formats, or both. Many different means of protecting confidentiality for different types of data have been devised (Berman; Schiedermayer).

Anonymous research virtually eliminates the risk of breaching confidentiality. However, anonymity may not be practicable or desirable. Researchers may wish to recontact subjects for a follow-up study, or may be conducting a long-term study that requires multiple contacts. Researchers may also wish to retain identifiers for subjects' benefit: Studies may collect health information, such as blood pressure or blood cholesterol levels, that subjects have been promised as an inducement to participation, or investigators may feel the need to inform subjects of potentially dangerous health situations that data collection may uncover. Finally, anonymity may too readily be considered a justification for not seeking participants' consent in studies that can be conducted without their knowledge (Bok).

Giving up anonymity in order to protect subjects' other interests can be highly problematic. HIV research provides an excellent example. Because of the stigma associated with the possibility of membership in an at-risk population and the difficulty in obtaining consents in sufficient numbers, some epidemiological researchers have conducted anonymous studies of the percentage of persons testing HIV-positive in large populations in order to obtain basic information about the spread of the disease. This makes it impossible to identify persons found to test positive, so that they can be counseled and treated. In effect, it precludes offering research subjects the opportunity to become patients.

Similar problems can arise in other research. For example, survey research that includes questions about family violence may uncover instances of recent or ongoing child abuse, but if survey answers have been rendered anonymous, even information gathered in *live* telephone or computer-assisted interviews may have insufficient detail to be reported to social services authorities, no matter how detailed the account of abuse given to investigators (King, Henderson, and Stein). How the tensions between public health goals in collecting data and protection and benefit for research subjects are addressed and resolved in such instances reflects continually shifting balances between the perceived need for epidemiological study, prospects for therapeutic intervention, and societal responses to particular health issues.

The Problem of Unexpected Information

Some researchers resist the idea of anonymous studies out of a felt obligation to offer information, counseling, and treatment to subjects found by the research to be in need of health services (Bayer et al.). But similar concerns can arise in confidential research as well. Studies using *gene-trolling* technologies like microarray techniques, which can quickly search a DNA sample for a wide range of disease-associated genes, can uncover potentially important health information that is unrelated to the stated goals of the research, thus surprising subjects who consented to research on one health problem with information about another (Berman; Collins). Additional challenges to privacy and confidentiality arise when the unexpected information has health implications for close relatives of the subject, who have not consented to participation and may know nothing about it. And if the research was conducted under a consent waiver, investigators may face the prospect of contacting people who have been involuntary subjects to give them bad news arising from their research participation.

Because the information derived from genetic research can have implications that go beyond those for subjects and their families, unexpected information may prove problematic for communities as well (Beskow; Rothstein). Even expected information may raise important concerns. The privacy interests of communities and groups may be directly and deliberately implicated by large-scale genetic research seeking information about the relationships between genetic characteristics and health outcomes, and both individual subjects and investigators may be ill-equipped to address and assess these risks of harm (Annas, 2000; Collins; Greely).

New Uses for Old Data

Data-sharing problems arise when researchers seek access to previously collected information. Researchers may seek to abstract information from the medical records of both currently and formerly hospitalized patients, or to perform additional tests on samples of blood or tissue obtained for diagnostic purposes. Study subjects may be approached by other researchers, or the data collected about them may be sought for new research uses. Stored research data may even yield information that is thought to be of therapeutic usefulness (Medical Research Council; Tribe).

Each of these examples raises one or more of several recurring problems: Is the new use one that was contemplated in the original consent? Is it one that the person would or would not be likely to find objectionable? Can the person be contacted for a new consent? If not, is proceeding without consent appropriate? If contact is necessary or desirable, does such a contact in itself constitute an unacceptable breach of confidentiality? The use of medical records and blood and tissue specimens for research has been addressed in a variety of ways, including: By asking patients at the time of hospital admission to give blanket consent to confidential or anonymous use of record data; by simply advising patients that such research may be undertaken with the approval of an institutional review board; by permitting researchers to contact patients for consent to specific uses, including long-term storage of identified or anonymized specimens for specified or unspecified research uses; and by using the treating physician to screen researchers' requests. Each of these solutions provides a different moral balance between the burden on researchers and the wrongs, harms, and benefits to subjects (Appelbaum et al.; National Bioethics Advisory Commission, 1999).

Where stored data have a potential therapeutic use, the situation is even more sensitive. A subject who participates in blood and tissue studies does not thereby consent to be contacted with a request to become a bone marrow donor for a specific patient. Such a contact could place considerable pressure on some subjects; others may want to have the opportunity to help, and may feel guilt at not having been afforded it. The temptation to compromise on privacy and confidentiality may be strong here. However, the argument that the needs of the patient should outweigh the privacy interests of a potential donor has not been embraced by the courts that have heard such cases (Davis, 1983; Lansing). As a result, this situation has been addressed, like the use of treatment information for research purposes, by asking research subjects whether they agree to be contacted later should a specific therapeutic need arise.

Publicity, Privacy, and Voice in Research

Publicity is most notably a problem for participants in innovative clinical trials, such as the first recipients of organ transplants, the first subjects to receive a novel intervention or vaccine for HIV infection, or the first subjects to experience an adverse event in a human gene transfer trial. The invasions of privacy threatened by the public interest in the lives of persons suffering from exotic diseases and undergoing unprecedented treatments may constitute civil wrongs if the media cannot claim First Amendment protection (Tribe).

The civil right to privacy is encompassed by several distinct courses of action, including the rights of private persons to be free from intrusion upon their solitude, to keep private information from being made public, and to prevent the publication of true information that places them in a *false light* (Warren and Brandeis). American society has changed greatly since this understanding of privacy was first outlined in law; yet finding a balance between protecting private information and sharing it remains a profound challenge (Goldman). Indeed, public interest in medical research is such that patient–subjects in clinical trials in high-profile emerging fields like gene transfer research are routinely informed that complete protection of their privacy may not be possible in the face of media interest.

A related threat to privacy and confidentiality is posed by the emphasis on narrative in research and teaching. Publication of research results is permitted, in professional and international codes and regulations, either when the subject has consented or when identifying information has been deleted or altered so as to preclude identification of the subject by readers and audiences, so long as the data are not misrepresented thereby (International Committee of Medical Journal Editors).

In many circumstances, such as in ethnographic research and increasingly in bioethics generally, it may not be possible to disguise case studies and other narratives adequately and still use them pedagogically (Davis, 1991). Well-known cases cannot be disguised at all. The scholarly community and the public have learned much from widespread discussion of Baby Fae, Barney Clark, Jesse Gelsinger, and many others, but not without costs to them and their families. And in less famous cases, even when a stripping of details is sufficient to disguise a patient–subject for a scholarly audience without misrepresenting the data, it may not be sufficient to disguise that person from family, associates, and treating health professionals who may chance to read a publication.

Finally, recognition of the subject by others may not constitute the only or the greatest wrong. Recognizing oneself in a public depiction can produce shame even when no one else knows. Although issues of consent and deception may be entangled with privacy and confidentiality in narrative research (Allen), subjects may be wronged and harmed regardless of whether the depiction is perceived to be accurate or distorted, and whether or not they have consented to the publication (King, Henderson, and Stein).

Some researchers address this complex problem by developing long-term collaborative relationships with subjects. Collaboration can reduce the exclusive control the researcher has over the story by including the subject's voice, but is not always possible, helpful, or desirable. Indeed, the ethics of telling stories has become a primary issue for bioethics itself (Chambers; Davis, 1991). As the problem of privacy and confidentiality in research shows, even in the face of the imperative to increase knowledge, it is important to consider whether some new knowledge is worth sacrificing privacy or confidentiality, and whether some knowledge comes at too great a cost to the rights and interests of those from whom we learn.

NANCY M. P. KING (1995)
REVISED BY AUTHOR

SEE ALSO: *AIDS: Healthcare and Research Issues; Confidentiality; Informed Consent: Consent Issues in Human Research; Law and Bioethics; Privacy in Healthcare; Research, Unethical; Research Ethics Committees; Research Methodology; Research Policy*

BIBLIOGRAPHY

Allen, Charlotte. 1997. "Spies Like Us: When Sociologists Deceive Their Subjects." *Lingua Franca* November: 31–39.

Annas, George J. 2000. "Rules for Research on Human Genetic Variation: Lessons from Iceland." *New England Journal of Medicine* 342(24): 1830–1833.

Annas, George J. 2001. "The Limits of State Laws to Protect Genetic Information." *New England Journal of Medicine* 345(5): 385–388.

Annas, George J. 2002. "Medical Privacy and Medical Research: Judging the New Federal Regulations." *New England Journal of Medicine* 346(3): 216–220.

Appelbaum, Paul S.; Roth, Loren H.; and Detre, Thomas. 1984. "Researchers' Access to Patient Records: An Analysis of the Ethical Problems." *Clinical Research* 32(4): 399–403.

Barnes, Mark, and Krauss, Sara. 2001. "The Effect of HIPAA on Human Subjects Research." *BNA's Health Law Reporter* 10(26): 1026–1034.

Bayer, Ronald; Lumey, L. H.; and Wan, Lourdes. 1990. "The American, British and Dutch Responses to Unlinked Anonymous HIV Seroprevalence Studies: An International Comparison." *AIDS* 4(4): 283–290.

Berman, Jules J. 2002. "Confidentiality Issues for Medical Data Miners." *Artificial Intelligence in Medicine* 26: 25–36.

Beskow, Laura M.; Burke, Wiley; Merz, Jon; et al. 2001. "Informed Consent for Population-Based Research Involving Genetics." *Journal of the American Medical Association* 286(18): 2315–2321.

Bok, Sissela. 1992. "Informed Consent in Tests of Patient Reliability." *Journal of the American Medical Association* 267(8): 1118–1119.

Botkin, Jeffrey R. 2001. "Protecting the Privacy of Family Members in Survey and Pedigree Research." *Journal of the American Medical Association* 285(2): 207–211.

Bruppacher, Rudolf, and Kaiser, Yolanda. 2001. "Ethical and Legal Considerations in a Swiss Study on the Quality of Pharmacotherapy in the City of Basel." *Pharmacoepidemiology and Drug Safety* 10: 685–688.

Capron, Alexander M. 1991. "Protection of Research Subjects: Do Special Rules Apply in Epidemiology?" *Journal of Clinical Epidemiology* 44(suppl. 1): 81S–89S.

Chambers, Tod S. 1999. *The Fiction of Bioethics : Cases as Literary Texts.* New York : Routledge.

Collins, Francis S. 1999. "Shattuck Lecture—Medical and Societal Consequences of the Human Genome Project." *New England Journal of Medicine* 341(1): 28–37.

Council for International Organizations of Medical Sciences. 1991. "International Guidelines for Ethical Review of Epidemiological Studies." *Law, Medicine and Health Care* 19(3,4): 247–258.

Davis, Dena S. 1983. "Case Study: 'Dear Mrs. X....'" *IRB* 5(6): 6–9.

Davis, Dena S. 1991. "Rich Cases: The Ethics of Thick Description." *Hastings Center Report* 21(4): 12–17.

Department of Health and Human Services. Aug. 14, 2002. Standards for Privacy of Individually Identifiable Health Information. 67 Fed. Reg. 53182–53273 (codified at 45 Code of Federal Regulations parts 160 and 164).

Durham, Mary L. 2003 "How Research Will Adapt to HIPAA: A View from Within the Healthcare Delivery System." *American Journal of Law and Medicine* 28(4): 491–502.

"Federal Policy for the Protection of Human Subjects: Notices and Rules." 1991. Federal Register 56: 117 (June 18); pp. 28001–28132. See pp. 28012–28018 for the text of the Common Rule adopted.

Germany (Territory under Allied Occupation, 1945–1955: U.S. Zone). Military Tribunals. 1949. "Permissible Medical Experiments." In vol. 2 of *Trials of War Criminals before the Nuremberg Military Tribunals under Control Council Law No. 10: Nuremberg, October 1946–1949,* pp. 181–184. Washington, D.C.: U.S. Government Printing Office.

Goldman, Janlori. 2001. "The New Federal Health Privacy Regulations; How Will States Take the Lead?" *Journal of Law, Medicine, and Ethics* 29(3, 4): 395–400.

Greely, Henry. 1998. "The Human Genome Diversity Project: Ethical, Legal, and Social Issues." In *Genetics: Issues of Social Justice,* ed. Ted Peters. Cleveland, OH: The Pilgrim Press.

Holder, Angela R. 1986. "The Biomedical Researcher and Subpoenas: Judicial Protection of Confidential Medical Data." *American Journal of Law and Medicine* 12: 405–421.

International Committee of Medical Journal Editors. 1991. "Statements from the International Committee of Medical Journal Editors." (Includes "Guidelines for the Protection of Patients' Right to Anonymity.") *Journal of the American Medical Association* 265(20): 2697–2698.

King, Nancy M. P.; Henderson, Gail E.; and Stein, Jane, eds. 1999. *Beyond Regulations: Ethics in Human Subjects Research.* Chapel Hill: University of North Carolina Press.

Kulynych, Jennifer, and Korn, David. 2002. "Use and Disclosure of Health Information in Genetic Research: Weighing the Impact of the New Federal Medical Privacy Rule." *American Journal of Law and Medicine* 28(2, 3): 309–324.

Lansing, Paul. 1984. "The Conflict of Patient Privacy and the Freedom of Information Act." *Journal of Health Politics, Policy and Law* 9(2): 315–324.

Leufkens, Hubert G. 2001. "Privacy Issues in Pharmacoepidemiology: The Importance of Weighing Costs and Benefits." *Pharmacoepidemiology and Drug Safety* 10: 659–662.

Medical Research Council. 1985. "Responsibility in the Use of Personal Medical Information for Research: Principles and Guide to Practice." *British Medical Journal* 290: 1120–1124.

Melton, Gary B., and Gray, Joni N. 1988. "Ethical Dilemmas in AIDS Research: Individual Privacy and Public Health." *American Psychologist* January: 60–64.

Reatig, Natalie. 1979. "Confidentiality Certificates: A Measure of Privacy Protection." *IRB* 1(3): 1–4.

Rothstein, Mark A. 2002. "The Role of IRBs in Research Involving Commercial Biobanks." *Journal of Law, Medicine and Ethics* 30(1): 105–108.

Sankar, Pamela. 2003. "Genetic Privacy." *Annual Review of Medicine* 54: 393–407.

Schiedermayer, David L. 1991. "Guarding Secrets and Keeping Counsel in the Computer Age." *Journal of Clinical Ethics* 2(1): 33–34.

Symposium. 2001. "Medical Confidentiality and Research." *Journal of Law, Medicine, and Ethics* 25(2, 3): 85–138.

Tribe, Laurence H. 1988. *American Constitutional Law,* 2nd edition. Mineola, NY: Foundation Press.

Truter, Ilse. 2001. "Ethical Issues Related to Retrospective Drug Utilization Studies in South Africa." *Pharmacoepidemiology and Drug Safety* 10: 679–683.

Veatch, Robert M. 1997. "Consent, Confidentiality, and Research." *New England Journal of Medicine* 336(12): 869–870.

Warren, Samuel D., and Brandeis, Louis D. 1890. "The Right to Privacy." *Harvard Law Review* 4: 193–220.

Wing, Steve. 2002. "Social Responsibility and Research Ethics in Community-Driven Studies of Industrialized Hog Production." *Environmental Health Perspectives* 110: 437–444.

Yolles, Bryan J.; Connors, Joseph C.; and Grufferman, Seymour. 1986. "Obtaining Access to Data from Government-Sponsored

Medical Research." *New England Journal of Medicine* 315(26): 1669–1672.

INTERNET RESOURCES

Council for International Organizations of Medical Sciences. 2002. "International Ethical Guidelines for Biomedical Research Involving Human Subjects." Available from <http://www.cioms.ch/frame_guidelines_nov_2002.htm>.

National Bioethics Advisory Commission. 1998. Research Involving Persons with Mental Disorders That May Affect Decisionmaking Capacity. Available from <www.bioethics.gov>.

National Bioethics Advisory Commission. 1999. Research Involving Human Biological Materials: Ethical Issues and Policy Guidance. Available from <www.bioethics.gov>.

National Bioethics Advisory Commission. 2001. Ethical and Policy Issues in Research Involving Human Participants. Available from <www.bioethics.gov>.

Office of Civil Rights, Department of Health and Human Services. 2002. "Guidance Explaining Significant Aspects of the Privacy Rule." Available from <www.hhs.gov/ocr/hipaa/privacy.html>.

Office of Extramural Research, National Institutes of Health. 2002. Certificates of Confidentiality Kiosk. Available from <http://grants1.nih.gov/grants/policy/coc/index.htm>.

Office for Human Research Protections. 1993. Protecting Human Research Subjects: Institutional Review Board Guidebook, chapter 3, section D. Available from <http://ohrp.osophs.dhhs.gov/irb/irb_guidebook.htm>.

World Medical Association. 2000. "Declaration of Helsinki: Recommendations Guiding Physicians in Biomedical Research Involving Human Subjects." Available from <http://www.wma.net/e/policy/17-c_e.html>.

PRIVACY IN HEALTHCARE

• • •

Privacy is a rich concept with a major role in the assessment of healthcare practices, policies, and law. It has become increasingly commonplace to ascribe important health-related privacy interests to individuals, families, and institutions and then to criticize public and private sector failures to protect those interests.

Privacy and Health Services

The word *privacy* has four major usages, corresponding to four distinct forms, dimensions, or conceptions of privacy: physical privacy, informational privacy, proprietary privacy,

and decisional privacy. Issues relating to all four pervade healthcare.

PHYSICAL PRIVACY. Under one popular usage of the term, *privacy* denotes freedom from contact with other people. The desire for limited physical accessibility—for seclusion and solitude conducive to peace of mind and intimacy—is a desire for privacy in this first sense. Members of the general public regard many social, business, and governmental contacts as privacy intrusions. These include door-to-door, street corner, telephone, and mail solicitation; some forms of sexual harassment; beeper and cellular telephone monitoring; and employers' performance, polygraph, drug, and alcohol testing. Common governmental practices are controversial for their threats to physical privacy, especially the use in foreign intelligence gathering and domestic surveillance of high-powered binoculars, concealed tape recorders, cameras, wiretaps, and thermal imaging. The loss of physical privacy is sometimes a concern when criminal-justice officials rely on body-cavity searches, prison-cell searches, and electronic monitoring of probationers; or when the police operate "checkpoints" to detect violations of curfew, seatbelt, drug, and drunk-driving laws.

Complete physical privacy is inconsistent with the demands of modern healthcare. The modern delivery of health services presupposes that patients and medical professionals mutually accept nudity, touching, and observation as unavoidable aspects of examination, treatment, surgery, and hospitalization. Typical patients willingly sacrifice the desire for bodily concealment and seclusion for a chance at better health. Yet patients often expect their physicians, nurses, and other caretakers to guard assiduously against unnecessary bodily exposure or contact. The examination gowns and pajamas worn by patients respond to the expectation of privacy, as well as the need for warmth.

Hospital patients—and their lawyers—have sometimes characterized unauthorized medical treatments as invasions of privacy, along with the bedside presence of inessential medical attendants, spectators, or cameras. The desire for physical privacy may lead patients who have a choice to select single over shared hospital rooms. Because for many Americans bodily exposure to persons of the opposite sex is a more significant loss of privacy than same-sex exposures, the desire for physical privacy has led some patients to prefer physicians or nurses of their own sex. Norms of quietude surrounding hospitals reflect the sentiment that patients have heightened physical and psychological needs for solitude and peace of mind.

INFORMATIONAL PRIVACY. Under a second popular usage, *privacy* is synonymous with secrecy, confidentiality, data protection, or anonymity. It requires limits on the accessibility of personal information. The expectations of privacy surrounding health information are especially high, but not unique. Significant expectations of privacy exist also for information related to employment, education, Social Security numbers, criminal arrest, library use, video rentals, motor vehicle registration, taxes, consumer credit, and banking.

Informational privacy concerns in the healthcare setting have traditionally focused on the confidentiality of the physician–patient relationship and on limiting access to medical and insurance records. The willingness of patients to speak openly about physical and mental health concerns depends, in part, on expectations of professional confidentiality. The administrative demands of managed care interject faceless decision makers into the context of physician care at a cost to privacy. Proposals for governmentally or institutionally mandated testing, reporting, and identification raise other informational privacy concerns. The public health community recognizes the potential threat to privacy and other important interests posed by nonanonymous AIDS testing or reporting and mandatory medical insurance identification cards.

Informational privacy in healthcare is not solely a matter of safeguarding information about individuals. By virtue of genetic ties, family members may share health conditions or predispositions. Progress by researchers toward the goal of mapping and sequencing the human genome has heightened ethical concerns about possible family, as opposed to individual, privacy interests in the information coded in a person's genetic materials (Powers).

Informational privacy requires appropriate forms of secrecy, sometimes defined as intentional concealment of fact (Bok); and confidentiality, defined as selective disclosure of fact to authorized persons (Allen, 1988). In institutional settings security requires mechanisms capable of limiting access to information, such as locked office doors and file cabinets. The security of health data shared on computers may require user identification passwords and encoding. In addition to security, concern about privacy of information overlaps with concern about what are sometimes called "fair information" practices. These include maintaining accurate information in confidence. The accuracy and security of information contained in health, insurance, adoption, and gene-research records potentially bears on the quality of healthcare and therefore holds special importance.

Managed care, the AIDS epidemic, and the Human Genome Project spawned numerous proposals for federal and state regulations governing health information. The federal government responded with the Health Insurance Portability and Accountability Act of 1996 (HIPAA). HIPAA included provisions encouraging uniform electronic transfer of medical information and required modern safeguards to protect both the security and confidentiality of medical data. HIPPA's initial privacy standards went into effect in April 2001 and did not preempt stronger state law privacy standards.

HIPAA covers government and private health plans, healthcare clearinghouses, and many healthcare-related service providers, such as firms that take care of patient billing. These firms must adopt privacy policies and inform patients of their privacy rights. They must also train staff to respect privacy and designate a privacy officer charged with privacy oversight responsibilities.

HIPAA requires special protections for individually identifiable health information disclosed orally, on paper, or electronically. Patients must be given notice of their privacy rights, access to their medical records, and a right to limit disclosures to third parties, subject to certain exceptions. For example, patients do not have the right under HIPAA to veto access to their medical records by public health officials, researchers, the courts, or emergency medical personnel or in certain other situations. Only psychotherapy notes used and created by psychotherapists are accorded a higher level of protection. Patients do have rights against the unauthorized disclosure of their medical information to third parties for employment personnel or marketing purposes. Although HIPAA does not authorize patients to sue for violations, it places enforcement powers in the hands of the Department of Health and Human Services, which may seek civil penalties and criminal punishments up to $250,000 and ten years in prison for the most egregious knowing violations of the statute.

PROPRIETARY PRIVACY. Concerns relating to the appropriation and ownership of human personality are increasingly framed as privacy concerns. Under a third usage, privacy can mean the appropriation of a repository of personal identity. These concerns have emerged in healthcare and health-research-related domains. According to American common law now recognized in a majority of states, to appropriate a person's name, likeness, or identity is a way of invading that person's privacy. Following this precedent, patients photographed without their consent may object to publication on privacy grounds. Moreover, because a person's genes are widely believed to be biologic keys to personal identity and sources of health information that should be properly controlled by the individual, a person whose DNA is appropriated without consent may likewise object on privacy grounds. In the 1990s, when the U.S. military first required active duty service members to undergo tissue sampling for possible future DNA testing in the

1990s, service members raised privacy objections that led the Department of Defense to strengthen safeguards against breaches of its DNA data banking system. After the Burlington Northern Santa Fe Railroad conducted secret DNA testing on employees to determine genetic predisposition to carpal tunnel syndrome, the company entered into a settlement with the Equal Employment Opportunity Commission in May 2002, agreeing to pay $2.2 million to affected workers.

DECISIONAL PRIVACY. Individuals, families, and domestic partners typically define some decisions as personal decisions and certain conduct as intimate conduct. Under its fourth usage, privacy denotes autonomous choices about the personal and intimate matters that constitute private lives. Decisional privacy signifies the ability to make one's own decisions and to act on those decisions, free from governmental or other unwanted interference. Decisional privacy concerns in the health context relate to responsibility for important decisions about treatment, the termination of treatment, and the allocation of scarce medical resources. Legal and ethical disagreements about who has the "right to decide" or the "right to choose" sometimes have turned collaborating patients, physicians, nurses, hospitals, families, researchers, and lawmakers into competitors and litigants.

In the United States, conceptions of decisional privacy have come to dominate discussions of government regulation of abortion and the treatment of patients who are severely disabled, terminally ill, or in a persistent vegetative state. In the context of so-called surrogate motherhood, privacy for infertile couples has meant the freedom to make legally enforceable agreements to procreate with the assistance of third parties. Gay men and lesbians invoke the ideal of privacy in their quest for the freedom to engage in consensual adult sexual relationships and marriage, free from the fear of criminal prosecution and legally sanctioned discrimination. Parents sometimes invoke "family privacy" to mean the freedom of heads of households to decide how those for whom they are responsible will be reared, educated, and medically assisted. Invocations to respect privacy accompany defenses of limited government and autonomous decision making respecting heterosexual sex, contraception, midwifery, women's prenatal conduct, use of experimental medical remedies, psychotropic drug therapy, organ sales and transplants, hunger striking, prostitution, and pornography.

Theories about Privacy

Theorists from disciplines that include philosophy, bioethics, and law have offered accounts of the meaning and value of privacy. Some of these accounts, though by no means all of them, have been prompted by a desire to clarify the assumptions and aims of health-related law and public policy.

DEFINITIONS OF PRIVACY. Contemporary theorists actively debate how precisely to define, value, and protect privacy (Cohen; Schoeman, 1992; Inness; Wacks; Allen, 1988). Although many acknowledge that privacy is used in distinguishable physical, informational, proprietary, and decisional senses, no single definition of privacy in any of its senses has gained universal acceptance. Nor has any theory of the value of privacy gained universal acceptance.

Scholars disagree about how to approach defining privacy (Allen, 1988). Some say privacy should be defined as a value or moral claim (Inness), others as a fact or a legal right (Gavison). Some say that definitions of privacy should prescribe ideal uses of the term (Gavison), others that definitions should describe actual usage (Allen, 1988). Debates over the definition of privacy may seem arcane. Yet the outcome of the debates bears importantly on the framing of ethical and legal issues raised by healthcare. For example, some theorists contend that the popular privacy arguments for abortion rights are unsound because they confuse privacy with liberty, autonomy, or freedom.

Proposed definitions of privacy range from the very expansive "being let alone," popularized by Louis Brandeis and Samuel Warren in an 1890 *Harvard Law Review* article, to Alan F. Westin's more specific "claim of individuals, groups or institutions to determine for themselves when, how, and to what extent information about them is communicated to others" (p. 7). Many definitions characterize privacy in its physical and informational senses as denoting conditions of restricted access to persons, their mental states, or information about them (Allen, 1988). According to Ruth Gavison, "[i]n perfect privacy no one has information about X, no one pays attention to X, and no one has physical access to X" (p. 428). So conceived, privacy functions as an umbrella concept, encompassing a family of concepts each of which denotes a form of limited access to others. There is disagreement about the composition of the privacy family's membership list. The list, however, arguably includes seclusion, solitude, anonymity, confidentiality, modesty, intimacy, reserve, and secrecy.

The debate over the relationship between the concepts of privacy and secrecy exemplifies the bewildering extent of disagreement about how to define privacy and related concepts. Although some scholars view secrecy as a form of privacy, others view privacy as a form of secrecy (Friedrich). Still others view them as distinct concepts. In a 1984 book titled *Secrets,* Sissela Bok argued that privacy and secrecy are wholly distinct concepts—the former referring to limited physical and information access, the latter to intentional concealment of information.

A number of definitions of privacy instead emphasize control, whether control over information or control over avenues of observation and physical contact (Fried; Westin). In the media-saturated and bureaucracy-dependent society of the United States, it is perhaps unsurprising that one scholar has suggested that privacy involves the possession of undocumented information (Parent, 1983a, 1983b). Other legal and moral theorists stress privacy as a social practice with normative functions (Inness). Jeffrey H. Reiman links privacy to the formation of individuality and personhood: "Privacy is a social ritual by means of which an individual's moral title to his own existence is conferred" (p. 39).

THE DECISIONAL PRIVACY CONTROVERSY. Perhaps the greatest source of definitional disagreement surrounding the concept of privacy has related to the decisional usage of privacy. Decisional privacy has been defined as control over intimate aspects of personal identity. In the United States, aspects of the human body, sex, reproduction, marriage, and family are generally considered as numbering among the intimacies of personal identity. The U.S. Supreme Court popularized the decisional usage of privacy in the 1960s, 1970s, and 1980s by characterizing laws restricting birth control, abortion, end-of-life medical decision making, marriage, and parental authority as burdening the right to privacy. Decisional privacy rights in the law presuppose a private sphere of conduct immune from state or federal regulation. Some scholars emphasize the ideal of privacy as the ideal of limited government (Rubenfeld).

Many theorists insist that privacy in the decisional sense is not properly understood as a sense of privacy at all (Gavison; Parent, 1983; McCloskey; Ely). They raise several arguments. First, they argue, as an aspect of liberty, freedom, or autonomy, decisional privacy stands apart from paradigmatic forms of privacy, such as seclusion, solitude, and anonymity. Second, if one speaks of "decisional" privacy, one loses the ability to treat privacy and liberty as distinct concepts. Confused, ambiguous uses of the concept of privacy in the U.S. Supreme Court's first contraception and abortion cases helped to raise this widespread objection.

Defenders of the decisional usage of the term *privacy* counter that decisional privacy is worthy of the name (DeCew, 1987). They emphasize that although decisional privacy denotes aspects of liberty, freedom, and autonomy, it denotes aspects of these that pertain to deeply felt conceptions of a private life beyond legitimate social involvement. Controversial or not, using "privacy" to denote a domain outside of legitimate social concern has become an entrenched practice in the United States.

THE PUBLIC AND THE PRIVATE IN POLITICAL THOUGHT. Linkage with the Greco-Roman heritage of Western law and political theory may provide a degree of historic and etymological validity to the controversial practice of referring to freedom from interference with personal life as "privacy." The decisional usage of privacy has origins in classical antiquity's distinction between private and public spheres.

The Greeks distinguished the "public" sphere of the polis, or city-state, from the "private" sphere of the *oikos,* or household. The Romans similarly distinguished *res publicae,* concerns of the community, from *res privatae,* concerns of individuals and families. The ancients celebrated the public sphere as the sphere of political freedom for citizens. The public realm was the sector in which select men—free men with property whose economic virtue had earned them citizenship and the right to participate in collective governance—could truly flourish. By contrast, the private realm was the sector of mundane economic and biologic necessity. Wives, children, and slaves populated the private economic sphere, living as subordinates and ancillaries to autonomous male caretakers.

The post-Enlightenment Western liberal tradition inherited the premise that social life ought to be organized into public and private spheres (Arendt; Habermas). It also inherited the premise that the private sphere is properly constituted by the home, the family, and intimate association. Nevertheless, whereas ancient thought tolerated the private and celebrated the public, modern liberal thought often reflects an opposing tendency: It tolerates the public as pervasive and necessary for collective welfare but celebrates the private as an essential expression of personal identity, freedom, and responsibility.

The political concept of a limited, tolerant government—elaborated by the English philosopher John Locke (1632–1704) and Thomas Jefferson as a requirement of natural rights, and by the nineteenth-century English philosopher and economist John Stuart Mill and the eighteenth-century Scottish economist Adam Smith as a requirement of utility—entails a nongovernmental, private sphere of autonomous individuals, families, and voluntary associations. Mill emphasized the importance of government tolerance, arguing that government is not well situated to assess the utility of "self-regarding" acts that potentially harm only the actors themselves. Self-regarding conduct "neither violates any specific duty to the public, nor occasions any perceptible hurt to any assignable individual except himself" (Mill, p. 80). It is, in other words, conduct that is restricted to an individual's own body and property and that may offend others but imposes no risk of significant harm on others. The contractarian political tradition of American democratic liberalism requires tolerance for religious minorities, political dissenters, and unpopular lifestyles. The ideal of tolerance is arguably the ultimate foundation of the case for sexual privacy for homosexuals and women seeking abortions (Richards).

The ideal of a private sphere free of government and other outside interference has currency, despite the reality that in the United States and other Western democracies, virtually every aspect of nominally private life is a focus of direct or indirect government regulation (Cohen). Marriage is considered a private relationship, yet governments require licenses and medical tests, impose age limits, and prohibit polygamous, incestuous, and same-sex marriages. Procreation and child rearing are considered private, but government child-abuse and neglect laws regulate, if at times inadequately, how parents, and possibly even pregnant women, must exercise their responsibilities. The ideal of a private sphere can be no more than an ideal of the ability of ordinary citizens to make choices that are relatively free of the most direct forms of governmental interference and constraint.

The worthiness of this ideal has been called into question in the United States, where problems of domestic and other private sector violence suggest a need for more rather than less involvement in the traditionally "private" spheres (Allen, 2003; Morris; MacKinnon). In addition, the ideal of a private sphere has been the ideal of a sphere of negative as opposed to positive freedom. The right to privacy in the context of contraception and abortion has meant a negative right against government decision making respecting procreation, not a positive right to governmental programs designed to make contraception and abortion services available to those who cannot afford to pay. Critics blame the emphasis on privacy and negative freedom for the failure of legal efforts to secure government funding of abortions for women who are poor.

ETHICAL VALUES. Physical and informational privacy practices serve to limit observation and disclosure deemed inimical to well-being. Psychologists have long emphasized the unhealthful effects of depriving individuals of opportunities for socially defined modes of privacy (Schneider). Many philosophers maintain that respecting physical, informational, and decisional privacy is paramount for respect for human dignity and personhood, moral autonomy, and workable community life (Schoeman, 1992; Allen, 1988; Kupfer; DeCew, 1986; Feinberg; Benn). Lawyers view the moral value of privacy as the basis of moral rights deserving legal protection (Greenawalt; Fried; Westin).

Scholarly disagreement about how best to characterize the ethical value of privacy is fundamental (Inness). One axis of disagreement concerns whether privacy denotes a value or a state of affairs. A second axis of disagreement concerns whether privacy, presumed to denote a state of affairs, refers to a state of affairs with necessary moral legitimacy or merely contingent moral legitimacy. A third axis of disagreement concerns whether the value of privacy, presumed to denote a state of affairs with only contingent moral legitimacy, should be measured against relevant consequentialist criteria, such as promoting aggregate happiness or efficiency; or deontological criteria, such as respect for personhood, personal identity, or humanity.

From the consequentialist perspective, privacy has value to the extent that it is useful in promoting, for example, aggregate happiness or the diverse interests of individuals, groups, or government. In this vein, scholars commonly argue that privacy has value because it functions to create or enhance human personhood in ways that promote liberal social and political institutions. Privacy practices promote individuality and the formation of self-concept presupposed by democratic self-government. Some accounts stress the utilitarian value to society of restraining government power in the spheres of what John Stuart Mill called "self-regarding" actions.

Scholars also argue that privacy has instrumental value relative to its role in creating and enhancing relationships. The traditional argument is that only in isolation from others can desirable forms of intimacy and friendship flourish; only if individuals and families can seclude themselves from others can the potentially stifling and emotionally explosive social demands of group life be abated. In reply, it is argued that privacy practices have facilitated both the mistreatment of women and children and the disregard for the ideal of aggregate as opposed to individual responsibility. The ethical challenge posed by these criticisms is to describe social arrangements that vigorously protect states of physical and informational privacy in the name of individuality, creativity, family, and free association, but that avoid the subordination and alienation often associated with modern Western liberal societies.

Scholars sometimes explain what they regard as the value of privacy by reference to the importance of personhood and personal dignity to individuals. These arguments draw connections between limited physical and informational access and/or the ability to make important decisions for oneself and the very idea of rational moral autonomy. In his contribution to the 1971 book, *Privacy,* Stanley I. Benn argued, for example, that the principle of respect for persons provides a moral reason for not interfering with personal privacy. David A. J. Richards, in his 1986 book, *Toleration and the Constitution,* argued, by appeal to the "social contract" metaphor, for legal privacy protections, stressing the fundamental value of government toleration of the choices individuals make for themselves pertaining to procreation, sexuality, and religion.

Privacy in the United States

The United States has a wealth of state and federal law protecting privacy. Recent federal law has increased legal safeguards for health information privacy at a time when Americans are increasingly open about formerly sensitive health matters.

CULTURAL AND HISTORICAL DIMENSIONS. Focusing on physical and informational privacy, anthropologist Barrington Moore observed in his 1984 book, *Privacy,* that both the desire for privacy and the ability to satisfy it are unequally distributed among and within human societies. Although some cultures do not emphasize privacy at all, privacy protection practices are found in virtually every human culture (Moore; Altman; Westin). Strikingly, what is treated as private can vary significantly from society to society (Pennock and Chapman). In one culture, defecation and sexual intercourse may be performed openly without embarrassment or shame; in another they are deeply private. One culture shields religious rites in secrecy, whereas another performs them on the commons. Female breasts and breastfeeding require concealment for modesty's sake in one place, but not another. Nuclear family problems are personal information in one society, but they are freely shared with leaders of one's tribe or village elsewhere.

The protection of personal privacy is among the most important public issues in the Western nations of the world (Flaherty; Schwartz and Reidenberg). These nations have in common large, well-developed bureaucracies and advanced information technologies (Bennett). Categories of data that western Europeans and North Americans deem personal include health information, criminal convictions, disciplinary measures, religious beliefs, political opinions, racial origin, trade union membership, sexual life, and intimate private life (Nugter).

U.S. culture is dominated by widely shared aspirations for lifestyles that afford frequent opportunities for privacy and intimacy. In families and friendships, though accountability for sensitive health information is the rule rather than the exception. Partners, kin, and friends rely on one another for health-related advice, comfort and care (Allen, 2003). Although the "taste" for privacy is strong in the United States, it competes with the principle of a "public right to know" reflected in the practices of government and the media. Commercial, professional, and personal relationships of many kinds presuppose a high degree of self-disclosure and physical contact. As a consequence, the

United States is not a country in which expectations of physical or informational privacy are easily satisfied.

American culture was not always dominated by articulated concern for privacy. Nor have deeply private lifestyles often been the norm. According to David H. Flaherty, Colonial lifestyle "left little room for privacy or nonconformity even among the free and the affluent" (Flaherty, p. 172). Concerns for physical and informational privacy achieved prominence as public issues for the first time in the nineteenth century, when a sharp increase in technology and industrialization had begun to transform the agrarian and mercantile culture to one of urban capitalism, and when the courts and legislatures began to expressly regulate marriage and family life (Garrow).

According to Alan Westin, nuclear family lifestyles, mobility in work and residence, and the decline of religious authority meant "greater situations of physical and psychological privacy" for mid- and late-nineteenth-century Americans (p. 21). Nevertheless, at about the same time that some middle-class and wealthy Americans were enjoying more privacy than ever before, a number of factors appear to have increased Americans' privacy-related anxieties. The simultaneous growth of crowded cities, the closing of the western frontier, the invention of commercial photography, and the rise of mass circulation newspapers may explain the emergence during the late nineteenth century of public concern about lost privacy (Allen and Mack; Copple).

The development in the early twentieth century of a social welfare bureaucracy and surveillance technologies may have further increased concerns about privacy. Indeed, the Supreme Court's first pronouncement about the right to privacy came in a dissenting opinion in *Olmstead v. United States* (1928), a case that validated telephonic eavesdropping by government. But the development of powerful computers capable of storing personal data appears to have spawned another, larger wave of concern about privacy in the 1960s and 1970s, the decades of origin for many of the major federal privacy laws that were in force in the early twenty-first century (Miller; Turkington and Allen). Finally, the rhetorical success of legal claims based on the "right to privacy" after 1965 in Supreme Court contraception and abortion cases spawned additional interest in fending off interference with choices people make respecting their bodies, healthcare, families, and lifestyles.

LEGAL DIMENSIONS. Near ubiquitous recognition of the importance of privacy is suggested by the language of key international human-rights documents. Privacy is mentioned, for example, in the Universal Declaration of Human

Rights, adopted by the United Nations General Assembly in 1948. Article 12 provides that "No one shall be subjected to arbitrary interference with his privacy, family, home, or correspondence, nor to attacks upon his honor and reputation" and that "Everyone has the right to the protection of the law against such interference or attacks" (Henkin et al., p. 144). In fact, the law of most modern legal systems prohibits, at least officially, physical privacy invasions and assaults on honor of the sort identified by Article 12. Western nations typically regulate several forms of physical, informational, and decisional privacy. Access to health-related information is limited by statute in most industrialized nations and the European Union (Nugter).

Great Britain and the United States share a common legal heritage and protect many of the same forms of privacy. Yet courts and legislatures in the United States have been more willing than their English counterparts to multiply the number of specific privacy protections. The reasons for this difference are unclear, although one explanation may be greater concerns in Britain about creating rights of uncertain application (Wacks). In the United States privacy interests are protected, often expressly, by tort law, the Constitution, and numerous federal and state statutes.

Tort law. The first privacy rights to be recognized expressly in United States law were rights of physical and informational privacy. The express right to privacy first came into existence through the common-law process of judicial recognition. Endorsed by Louis Brandeis and Samuel Warren in a famous 1890 *Harvard Law Review* article stressing the importance of freedom from unwanted publicity, the invasion of privacy tort was officially adopted by the Georgia Supreme Court in *Pavesich v. New England Life Insurance Company* (1905). Many other state courts eventually followed suit.

By 1960, William Prosser could identify, not one, but four common-law privacy rights recognized by courts in the United States. Today, most states have adopted one or more of Prosser's four privacy rights through their courts or legislatures. The influential *Restatement of the Law Second: Torts 2d* (American Law Institute), a summary and exposition of developments in personal injury law, embraced Prosser's analysis. In states that have adopted Prosser's analysis, a person may bring a privacy-invasion lawsuit claiming highly offensive conduct consisting of either:

1. interference with seclusion, solitude, and anonymity;
2. publication of embarrassing private facts;
3. publicity placing a person in a false light; or
4. appropriation of name, likeness, or identity.

In addition, most states permit privacy-invasion-related claims involving unauthorized publicity; breach of confidence or secrecy; and unfair business practices involving misappropriation, trade secret, trade name, and copyright violations. Plaintiffs have alleged invasion of privacy in cases related to health services. An Oregon physician was sued for disclosing the identity of an adult adoptee's birth mother. A New Yorker whose photograph appeared in a newspaper accompanying a story about an AIDS treatment facility sued the publisher.

Constitutional law. Although the U.S. Constitution makes no express mention of the term *privacy* itself, the constitutional law of the United States protects physical, informational, and decisional privacy interests. The First Amendment, the guarantor of freedom of speech and association, protects the physical and informational privacy concerns of exclusive clubs or political groups. In effect, the Supreme Court has held that the Fourth Amendment guarantees a right of physical privacy when it limits warrantless search and seizure, and that the Fifth Amendment guarantees a right of informational privacy when it limits compulsory disclosure and self-incrimination. Although the Supreme Court has never held as much, some judges and lawyers maintain that the Ninth Amendment, which provides that the "enumeration in the Constitution, of certain rights, shall not be construed to deny or disparage others retained by the people," implies decisional privacy rights. The Supreme Court has established First and Fourteenth Amendment limits on government record keeping and access to personal information. In *Whalen v. Roe* (1977), a major Supreme Court case involving a data bank of prescription drug users maintained by New York officials, the Court held that the First and Fourteenth Amendments require states seeking to deter drug abuse to implement confidentiality safeguards.

The U.S. Supreme Court and many lower courts have held that the Constitution protects decisional privacy respecting aspects of health, reproduction, sex, and family life, deriving this brand of privacy from what the court has termed the *penumbra* of the Bill of Rights and the Fourteenth Amendment. The Fourteenth Amendment, which provides that no state may deprive a person of liberty without due process, is the most frequently cited basis of the decisional privacy right protecting autonomous decision making respecting contraception, abortion, and the termination of medical treatment. *Griswold v. Connecticut* (1965) and *Roe v. Wade* (1973) established the right to contraception and abortion. The privacy doctrine that originated in the *Griswold* and *Roe* cases has come under repeated attack from critics who stress the absence of a textual basis for reproductive privacy rights. Some critics have urged that gender equality and equal protection of the laws, rather than privacy and liberty, are the core values served by reproductive rights.

In *Planned Parenthood of Southeast Pennsylvania v. Casey* (1992), the Supreme Court affirmed the essential holding of *Roe v. Wade,* reiterating the Fourteenth Amendment as protection for reproductive privacy. The Court backed away, however, from *Griswold*'s and *Roe*'s characterization of the right to privacy as a "fundamental" right that cannot be breached except where there is a truly "compelling" governmental interest. *Cruzan v. Director, Missouri Department of Health* (1990) recognized an adult patient's privacy right—not her parents'—to terminate life-sustaining medical treatment. Yet *Cruzan* and *Casey* applied weaker standards of review than *Roe v. Wade*. Abortion restrictions "rationally related" to a "legitimate state interest" that do not "unduly burden" the woman's constitutional right to privacy are valid. And restrictions on the right to refuse treatment that reasonably relate to a legitimate state interest are also valid.

Statutory law. The U.S. Congress enacted a number of federal statutes after 1970 to protect informational and physical privacy interests. The Privacy Act (1974), the Freedom of Information Act (1974), the Family and Educational Privacy Act (1974), the Right to Financial Privacy Act (1978), and Title V of the Financial Services Modernization Act (2001) protect information privacy by limiting access to personal information held in government, school, and bank records. The federal Employee Polygraph Protection Act protects workers from potentially incriminating self-disclosure in the workplace by limiting use of the lie-detector test. The Electronic Communications Privacy Act (1986) and other major federal statutes protect against intrusive searches using electronic surveillance, wiretapping, and other unauthorized access to telephones or computers. Proposed federal privacy statutes would limit access to genetic information about individuals. HIPAA requires the maintenance of the confidentiality and security of health-related information, including genetic health information.

State statutes in virtually every state address concerns about the privacy of information related to medical care, criminal histories, and adoption. Newer state statutory regulations include the decisional privacy protections of Virginia's Natural Death Act and Pennsylvania's Confidentiality of HIV-Related Information statute. Recently, state constitutions in Montana, California, and Florida have been amended or interpreted to require physical, informational, and decisional privacy protections. For example, in a pre-*Casey* decision, the Florida high court held that the state constitution protects decisional privacy to the same degree as *Roe v. Wade*.

Patients' privacy rights. One of the most important areas of health law is the broad field of patients' rights. Discussions of patients' rights include the physical, informational, and decisional privacy rights recognized under tort, constitutional, and statutory law. A Patients' Bill of Rights that would include privacy protections emerged as a policy initiative during the presidency of George W. Bush.

The oldest American legal case decided by reference to rights of privacy, *DeMay v. Roberts* (1881), vindicated interests in physical privacy and modesty. A Michigan husband and wife successfully sued a physician who permitted an "unprofessional young, unmarried man" to enter their home and help deliver their baby. A century later a married couple in Maine brought *Knight v. Penobscot Bay Medical Center* (1980), a similar, though unsuccessful, lawsuit claiming that a hospital violated the couple's privacy by permitting a layperson, the spouse of a nurse, to observe delivery of their child through a glass partition from a distance of 12 feet. The issue of whether women should be able to choose who is present at the birth of their children—including whether delivery is undertaken with the aid of a midwife, nurse practitioner, or physician—is clearly both a physical and a decisional privacy issue.

All patients generally may share the obstetrical patient's sense that adequate privacy is lacking in hospitals where well-intentioned medical, administrative, and support staff move freely in and out of (even nominally "private") in-patient wards. The feeling that one's privacy has been invaded may be especially acute in busy, crowded public hospitals serving low-income patients or in any hospital where groups of several physicians, interns, and medical students simultaneously conduct physical examinations and discussions at one's bedside. Some men and women report feeling their privacy invaded by having to share a room in an intensive-care unit with a person of the opposite sex. The law is unclear about the extent to which medical resources or the general written consent to treatment patients give upon admission to hospitals eliminates legitimate expectations of physical and informational privacy. Specific waivers of legal privacy claims may give patients clear notice of the privacy losses associated with treatment in teaching and research hospitals, but arguably they do not eliminate hospitals' ethical obligations to respect privacy to the extent possible.

Moral outrage over the discovery that healthcare providers have recorded, filmed, or photographed a patient for scholarly or research purposes occasionally results in litigation. Respect for privacy would appear to dictate obtaining prior consent to the publication of graphic images of a person, particularly if the person is identifiable in an image or is named in connection with its publication.

The legal importance of obtaining prior informed consent was underscored by the holding of the California court in a highly publicized case, *Moore v. Regents of University of California* (1990). John Moore brought a multimillion-dollar lawsuit when he discovered that University of California medical researchers who treated him for hairy cell leukemia had failed to disclose that "certain blood products and blood components were of great value in a number of commercial and scientific efforts." Moore's right to privacy claims were based on the notion that exploitation of his blood for commercial purposes was a highly offensive appropriation of a person's name, likeness, or identity compensable as an invasion of privacy under state tort law. According to the California court, a patient has a right to know the medical purpose of treatment and the treating physician's personal economic stake; otherwise treatment is battery, presumably no better than sterilizing a fertile woman or performing a cesarean section on a cancer patient without her consent.

As noted earlier, abortion, physician-assisted suicide, and the right to die are approached in the United States as patient privacy issues. Opponents of laws prohibiting abortions say that state and federal regulations should not prevent women from acting on their own decisions about whether to terminate pregnancy through medical abortion. On the other hand, it is also argued on privacy grounds that women should not be forced or counseled to abort for any reason, including where they are seropositive for the virus that causes AIDS. "Privacy" can signify freedom to choose the circumstances of death for oneself, a family member, or an intimate friend. It means the absence of criminal laws and bureaucratic procedures that constrain the choice to accelerate the death of a person who is terminally ill or to refuse artificial nutrition and hydration to preserve life in a person in a persistent vegetative state. The right to privacy may also prove to be the ethical refuge of supporters of physician-assisted suicide of nonterminally ill, fully competent adults. In *Vacco v. Quill* (1996) and *Washington v. Glucksberg* (1996), however, the U.S. Supreme Court ruled that states may outlaw physician-assisted suicide.

The privacy implications of nonvoluntary and routine AIDS testing of obstetrical patients, surgical patients, and newborns have been of great interest to public authorities and private healthcare providers for two reasons. First, nonconsensual testing is a prima facie denial of decisional privacy or autonomy. Some individuals prefer not to be tested and forced to confront the specter of terminal illness. And while this precise concern has never applied to newborns, newborn testing can reveal the HIV status of birth mothers. Second, where medical or insurance providers breach the confidentiality of an HIV- or AIDS-infected person, far-ranging implications for private lives and employment can follow because of prejudice and discrimination. In this context, policy analysts often assert that the individual interest in privacy is outweighed by societal interests, including the societal interest in controlling the spread of deadly disease through inappropriate handling of contaminated blood and other tissues. But societal interests do not always outweigh individual privacy rights.

The federal courts have upheld the mandatory AIDS-testing policies of the U.S. military and the nation's prisons. In *Glover v. Eastern Nebraska Community Office of Retardation* (1989), however, a federal court struck down a state requirement that all persons working closely with mentally retarded clients disclose their HIV and hepatitis B status and undergo periodic HIV and hepatitis B blood testing. Against the argument that persons working in highly regulated state agencies have lower expectations of privacy, the court stressed that constitutional values do not permit mandatory testing where the risk of disease transmission is extremely low. A similar weighing of the costs of testing against its benefits in view of the low risk of transmission may explain government reluctance to mandate AIDS testing for all dentists, physicians, and other healthcare providers who come in close contact with patients.

Conclusion

Privacy is likely to have an important role in bioethical discussions for some time. The English political philosopher James Fitzjames Stephen wrote in 1873 that "conduct which can be described as indecent is always in one way or another a violation of privacy" (p. 160). These words capture a truth about the broad usage the term *privacy* enjoys in the health field. Patients and those who care about them consider a diverse spectrum of "indecencies," ranging from maltreatment and breach of confidentiality to interference with decision making, as "invasions of privacy." Accordingly, the ethics, law, and politics of privacy have made what may be an indelible mark on the future of healthcare and health research.

ANITA L. ALLEN (1995)
REVISED BY AUTHOR

SEE ALSO: *Confidentiality; Privacy and Confidentiality in Research*

BIBLIOGRAPHY

Allen, Anita L. 1988. *Uneasy Access: Privacy for Women in a Free Society.* Totowa, NJ: Rowman and Littlefield.

Allen, Anita L. 2003. *Why Privacy Isn't Everything: Feminist Reflections on Personal Accountability.* Lanham, MD: Rowman and Littlefield.

Allen, Anita L., and Mack, Erin. 1990. "How Privacy Got Its Gender." *Northern Illinois University Law Review* 10(3): 441–478.

Altman, Irwin. 1977. "Privacy Regulation: Culturally Universal or Culturally Specific?" *Journal of Social Issues* 33(3): 66–74.

American Law Institute. 1986. *Restatement of the Law Second: Torts 2d.* St. Paul, MN: Author.

Arendt, Hannah. 1958. *The Human Condition.* Chicago: University of Chicago Press.

Benn, Stanley I. 1971. "Privacy, Freedom, and Respect for Persons." In *Privacy,* ed. J. Roland Pennock and John W. Chapman. New York: Atherton Press.

Bennett, Colin J. 1992. *Regulating Privacy: Data Protection and Public Policy in Europe and the United States.* Ithaca, NY: Cornell University Press.

Bennett, Rebecca, and Erin, Charles A. 1999. *HIV and AIDS: Testing Screening and Confidentiality.* Oxford: Oxford University Press.

Bloustein, Edward J. 1978. *Individual and Group Privacy.* New Brunswick, NJ: Transaction Books.

Bok, Sissela. 1984. *Secrets: On the Ethics of Concealment and Revelation.* Oxford: Oxford University Press.

Boone, C. Keith. 1983. "Privacy and Community." *Social Theory and Practice* 9(1): 1–30.

Brandeis, Louis, and Warren, Samuel. 1890. "The Right to Privacy." *Harvard Law Review* 4: 193–220.

Cohen, Jean L. 2002. *Regulating Intimacy: A New Legal Paradigm.* Princeton, NJ: Princeton University Press.

Copple, Robert F. 1989. "Privacy and the Frontier Thesis: An American Intersection of Self and Society." *American Journal of Jurisprudence* 34: 87–131.

Cruzan v. Director, Missouri Department of Health. 497 U.S. 261 (1990).

DeCew, Judith Wagner. 1986. "The Scope of Privacy in Law and Ethics." *Law and Philosophy* 5: 145–173.

DeCew, Judith Wagner. 1987. "Defending the 'Private' in Constitutional Privacy." *Journal of Value Inquiry* 21: 171–184.

DeMay v. Roberts. 46 Mich. 160, 9 N.W. 146 (1881).

Ely, John Hart. 1973. "The Wages of Crying Wolf: A Comment on *Roe v. Wade.*" *Yale Law Journal* 89: 920–949.

Etzoni, Amitai. 1999. *The Limits of Privacy.* New York: Basic.

Feinberg, Joel. 1983. "Autonomy, Sovereignty, and Privacy: Moral Ideals and the Constitution?" *Notre Dame Law Review* 58: 445–492.

Flaherty, David H. 1972. *Privacy in Colonial New England.* Charlottesville: University Press of Virginia.

Flaherty, David H. 1989. *Protecting Privacy in Surveillance Societies: The Federal Republic of Germany, Sweden, France, Canada, and the United States.* Chapel Hill: University of North Carolina Press.

Fried, Charles. 1968. "Privacy." *Yale Law Journal* 77: 475–493.

Friedrich, Carl. 1971. "Secrecy versus Privacy: The Democratic Dilemma." In *Privacy,* ed. J. Roland Pennock and John W. Chapman. New York: Atherton Press.

Garrow, David J. 1994. *Liberty and Sexuality: The Right to Privacy and the Making of Roe v. Wade.* New York: Macmillan.

Gavison, Ruth. 1980. "Privacy and the Limits of Law." *Yale Law Journal* 89(3): 421–471.

Gerstein, Robert S. 1978. "Intimacy and Privacy." *Ethics* 89: 76–81.

Glover v. Eastern Nebraska Community Office of Retardation. 867 F.2d 461 (1989).

Goldman, Janlori, and Hudson, Zoe. 2000. *Privacy: Report on the Privacy Policies and Practices of Health Web Sites.* Washington, D.C.: Georgetown University, Health Privacy Project.

Goston, Lawrence O., Hodge, James G., Jr., and Burghardt, Mira. 2002. "Balancing Communal Goods and Personal Privacy under a National Health Information Privacy Rule." *Saint Louis University Law Journal* 46: 5–35.

Greenawalt, Kent. 1974. "Privacy and Its Legal Protection." *Hastings Center Studies* 2(3): 45–68.

Griswold v. Connecticut. 381 U.S. 479; 85 Sup. Ct. 1678 (1965).

Habermas, Jurgen. 1989. *The Structural Transformation of the Public Sphere: An Inquiry into a Category of Bourgeois Society,* tr. Thomas Burger. Cambridge, MA: MIT Press.

Henkin, Louis; Pugh, Richard; Schachter, Oscar; et al. 1987. *Basic Documents Supplement to International Law: Cases and Materials.* St. Paul: MN: West Publishing.

Hodge, James G.; Gostin, Lawrence; and Jacobson, Peter D. 1999. "Legal Issues concerning Electronic Health Information Privacy." *Journal of the American Medical Association* 282: 1466–1471.

Humber, James M., and Almeder, Robert F. 2001. *Privacy in Health Care.* Totowa, NJ: Humana Press.

Inness, Julie C. 1992. *Privacy, Intimacy, and Isolation.* New York: Oxford University Press.

Institute of Medicine (U.S.). Committee on the Role of Institutional Review Boards in Health Services Research Data Privacy Protection. 2000. *Protecting Data Privacy in Health Services Research.* Washington, D.C.: National Academy Press.

Knight v. Penobscot Bay Medical Center. 420 A.2d 915 (1980).

Kupfer, Joseph. 1987. "Privacy, Autonomy, and Self-Concept." *American Philosophical Quarterly* 24(1): 81–89.

MacKinnon, Catherine A. 1991. "Reflections on Sex Equality under the Law." *Yale Law Journal* 100(5): 1281–1328.

McCloskey, H. J. 1980. "Privacy and the Right to Privacy." *Philosophy* 55: 17–38.

Mill, John Stuart. 1859 (reprint 1978). *On Liberty,* ed. Elizabeth Rapaport. Indianapolis, IN: Hackett.

Miller, Arthur R. 1971. *The Assault on Privacy: Computers, Data Banks, and Dossiers.* Ann Arbor: University of Michigan Press.

Moore, Barrington. 1984. *Privacy: Studies in Social and Cultural History.* Armonk, NY: M. E. Sharpe.

Moore v. Regents of University of California. 51 Cal.3d 120, 271 Cal. Rpt. 146, 793 P.2d 479 (1990).

Morris, Debra. 2000. "Privacy, Privation, Perversity: Toward New Representations of the Personal." *Signs: Journal of Women in Culture and Society* 25(2): 323–351.

Nugter, A. C. M. 1990. *Transborder Flow of Personal Data within the EC: A Comparative Analysis of the Privacy Statutes of the Federal Republic of Germany, France, the United Kingdom, and the Netherlands and Their Impact on the Private Sector.* Boston: Kluwer Law and Taxation Publishers.

Olmstead v. United States. 277 U.S. 438 (1928).

Parent, William A. 1983a. "A New Definition of Privacy for the Law." *Law and Philosophy* 2(3): 305–338.

Parent, William A. 1983b. "Recent Work on the Concept of Privacy." *American Philosophical Quarterly* 20(4): 341–355.

Pavesich v. New England Life Insurance Company. 122 Ga. 190; 50 S.E. 68 (1905).

Pennock, J. Roland, and Chapman, John W., eds. 1971. *Privacy.* New York: Atherton Press.

Planned Parenthood of Southeast Pennsylvania v. Casey. 112 Sup. Ct. 2791 (1992).

Powers, Madison. 1994. "Privacy and the Control of Genetic Information." In *The Genetic Frontier: Ethics, Law, and Policy,* ed. Mark S. Frankel and Albert Teich. Washington, D.C.: American Association for the Advancement of Science.

Prosser, William. 1960. "Privacy." *California Law Review* 48(3): 383–423.

Rachels, James. 1975. "Why Privacy Is Important." *Philosophy and Public Affairs* 4(4): 323–333.

Reiman, Jeffrey H. 1976. "Privacy, Intimacy, and Personhood." *Philosophy and Public Affairs* 6(1): 26–44.

Richards, David A. J. 1986. *Toleration and the Constitution.* Oxford: Oxford University Press.

Roe v. Wade. 410 U.S. 113; 35 L.Ed.2d 147; 93 Sup. Ct. 705 (1973).

Rubenfeld, Jed. 1989. "The Right to Privacy." *Harvard Law Review* 102: 737–806.

Scheppele, Kim L. 1988. *Legal Secrets: Equality and Efficiency in the Common Law.* Chicago: University of Chicago Press.

Schneider, Carl D. 1977. *Shame, Exposure, and Privacy.* Boston: Beacon.

Schoeman, Ferdinand David. 1992. *Privacy and Social Freedom.* Cambridge, UK: Cambridge University Press.

Schoeman, Ferdinand David, ed. 1984. *Philosophical Dimensions of Privacy: An Anthology.* Cambridge, UK: Cambridge University Press.

Schwartz, Paul, and Reidenberg, Joel. 1996. *Privacy and Data Protection.* Charlottesville, VA: Mitchie Law Publishers.

Stephen, James Fitzjames. 1873 (reprint 1967). *Liberty, Equality, Fraternity,* ed. R. J. White. Cambridge, UK: Cambridge University Press.

Storr, Anthony. 1988. *Solitude: A Return to the Self.* New York: Free Press.

Tefft, Stanton K., ed. 1980. *Secrecy: A Cross-Cultural Perspective.* New York: Human Sciences Press.

Turkington, Richard C., and Allen, Anita. 2002. *Privacy Law: Cases and Materials.* Minneapolis, MN: West Publishing Company.

United Nations. General Assembly. 1948. *Universal Declaration of Human Rights: Adopted the 10th December 1948 in Plenary Session by the General Assembly of the United Nations.* Available from the <www.unesco.org>.

Vacco v. Quill. 518 U.S. 1055 (1996).

Wacks, Raymond. 1989. *Personal Information: Privacy and the Law.* Oxford: Clarendon Press.

Washington v. Glucksberg. 518 U.S. 1057 (1996).

Westin, Alan F. 1967. *Privacy and Freedom.* New York: Atheneum.

Whalen v. Roe. 429 U.S. 589; 97 Sup. Ct. 869 (1977).

Young, John, ed. 1978. *Privacy.* Chichester, NY: Wiley.

PRIVATE OWNERSHIP OF INVENTIONS

• • •

As a historical matter, the Western tradition of protecting intellectual property has been justified by the argument for rights in tangible property put forth by the English philosopher John Locke (1632–1704): namely, that the individual who adds labor to a natural object should have rights in that object (Gordon). In the United States today, however, intellectual property rights are justified primarily on instrumental economic grounds, as a mechanism for inducing individuals to generate inventions that are expensive to create but easily copied once created. Because intellectual property protection prevents others from copying the invention, the inventor can capture as private value at least some portion of the social value represented by the invention. Although intellectual property encompasses patents, copyrights, and trade secrecy, patents represent the strongest form of intellectual property. Unlike a copyright, a patent protects the underlying idea behind the invention and not simply the particular expression the idea might take. Unlike trade secrecy, which protects only against misappropriation of the invention, patent protection also operates against those who may come up with the invention independently.

Public Funding and the Bayh-Dole Act

The most prominent alternative to intellectual property protection has been public funding. In the United States, public funding of science became particularly robust after World War II. By the turn of the twenty-first century, federal agencies such as the National Institutes of Health (NIH) were funding tens of billions of dollars of basic biomedical research each year. Although some of this research is performed intramurally, most of it is conducted extramurally, in university laboratories.

Until 1980, most federally funded research conducted in universities was put into the public domain. In 1979, for example, universities received only 264 patents (Mowery et al.). This figure has increased dramatically with the passage of the Bayh-Dole Act of 1980, which explicitly encourages university patenting. In 2000, universities received 3,764 patents. The rationale behind Bayh-Dole is not the conventional argument that patents are necessary to induce invention: In the case of federally funded invention, public funding has already provided the necessary invention incentive. Rather, the theory is that patent protection, coupled with exclusive licensing, is necessary to stimulate development of university research into commercially viable products.

As a consequence of Bayh-Dole, and the nearly simultaneous liberalization of patentability standards following the creation of a specialized patent appellate court in 1982, basic, or "upstream," biomedical research has increasingly become the subject of both university and private firm patents. Even when universities or private firms do not seek patents, they often impose proprietary restrictions on transfer of research tools, particularly research tools that are hard to replicate independently (NIH).

Impact of Proprietary Claims

For a number of reasons, these proprietary claims threaten to impede biomedical research. Most obviously, patents or other proprietary claims on upstream discoveries hinder subsequent research by permitting owners to charge a greater than competitive price. This feature of proprietary claims is particularly troubling for biomedical research given that researchers in nonprofit institutions, who are crucial to the progress of research, often cannot afford to pay large licensing fees. Upstream patents may also hinder biomedical research when a single broad patent gives a firm monopoly control over a significant new area of scientific territory. A monopolist is unlikely to see all of the different applications

of its broadly enabling patent. One response to this argument, that the profit-seeking owner of a pioneer patent will find it in its interest to license the discovery to as many follow-on improvers as possible, is belied by historical examples in many industries, including the electrical lighting, radio, automobile, and aircraft industries (Merges and Nelson). The transaction costs that arise when people are bargaining under conditions of imperfect information with current or potential scientific and commercial rivals are likely to be quite high (Rai). Transaction costs can also mount quickly when the basic research discoveries necessary for subsequent work are owned not just by one entity but by a number of different entities (Heller and Eisenberg). Notably, because under the patent law an initial broad patent on a pioneering discovery does not preclude a proliferation of upstream patents related to that discovery, the problems of broad patent scope and proliferating patent rights held by multiple owners can arise simultaneously.

Efforts and Arguments against Proprietary Claims

Various private and public sector efforts have attempted to mitigate the negative impact on research of broad and/or numerous proprietary rights. Developments in patent case law suggest, for example, that broad biotechnology patents will be struck down (*Regents of the University of California v. Eli Lilly & Co.*). In addition, federal funding agencies such as the NIH have urged universities to refrain from patenting, or at least licensing exclusively, research tools that are likely to be broadly enabling (NIH). In certain cases, actions by the private and public sector that have put genomic data into the public domain have also preempted the possible proliferation of proprietary rights on that data (SNP Consortium; NHGRI).

Another set of arguments concerns the impact of private ownership of inventions on stakeholders other than researchers. Some have argued that those who contribute the raw material for development of commercially successful inventions should, as a matter of equity, receive some portion of the commercial proceeds that proprietary rights on these inventions provide (Boyle). At a minimum, the sources of the raw material should be informed of the commercial intentions of those who use their material. These arguments have been made on behalf of patients with particular diseases who contribute genetic material for research (Palmer). Similar arguments have also been made on behalf of less-developed nations that are sources of commercially promising biological diversity or traditional knowledge. In the case of less-developed nations, the 1992 Convention on Biological Diversity specifically asserts that genetic resources belong to nation-states as an element of national sovereignty (Rosendal). Various contractual mechanisms are now being used to ensure the sharing of short- and long-term benefits between developed and developing countries (Reid et al.).

ARTI K. RAI

SEE ALSO: *Conflict of Interest; Patenting Organisms and Basic Research; Profit and Commercialism; Technology*

BIBLIOGRAPHY

Boyle, James. 1996. *Shamans, Software, and Spleens: Law and the Construction of the Information Society.* Cambridge, MA: Harvard University Press.

Gordon, Wendy. 1993. "A Property Right in Self-Expression: Equality and Individualism in the Natural Law of Intellectual Property." *Yale Law Journal* 102(7): 1533–1609.

Heller, Michael A., and Eisenberg, Rebecca S. 1998. "Can Patents Deter Innovation? The Anticommons in Biomedical Research." *Science* 280(5364): 698–701.

Merges, Robert P., and Nelson, Richard R. 1990. "On the Complex Economics of Patent Scope." *Columbia Law Review* 90(4): 839–916.

Mowery, David C.; Nelson, Richard R.; Sampat, Bhaven N.; and Ziedonis, Arvids A. 2001. "The Growth of Patents and Licensing by U.S. Universities: An Assessment of the Effects of the Bayh-Dole Act of 1980." *Research Policy* 30(1): 99–119.

National Institutes of Health (NIH). 1999. "Proposed Guidelines for Recipients of NIH Research Grants and Contracts on Obtaining and Disseminating Biomedical Research Resources." *Federal Register* 64(100): 28205–28209.

Palmer, Larry I. 2002. "Disease Management and Liability in the Human Genome Era." *Villanova Law Review* 47: 1–35.

Rai, Arti K. 1999. "Regulating Scientific Research: Intellectual Property Rights and the Norms of Science." *Northwestern University Law Review* 94(1): 77–152.

Regents of the University of California v. Eli Lilly & Co. 119 F.3d 1559 (Fed. Cir. 1997).

Reid, Walter V., et al. 1993. *Biodiversity Prospecting: Using Genetic Resources for Sustainable Development.* Washington, D.C.: World Resources Institute.

Rosendal, G. Kristin. 2000. *The Convention on Biological Diversity and Developing Countries.* Dordrecht, Netherlands: Kluwer Academic.

INTERNET RESOURCES

National Human Genome Research Institute (NHGRI). 1996. "Policy Regarding Intellectual Property of Human Genome Sequence." Available from <http://www.nhgri.nih.gov/Grant_info/Funding/Statements/>.

National Institutes of Health (NIH). 1998. Working Group on Research Tools. "Report of the National Institutes of Health (NIH) Working Group on Research Tools." Available from <http://www.nih.gov/news/researchtools/>.

SNP Consortium. 2003. Available from <http://snp.cshl.org>.

PROFESSIONAL-PATIENT RELATIONSHIP

• • •

I. Historical Perspectives

II. Sociological Perspectives

III. Ethical Issues

I. HISTORICAL PERSPECTIVES

The following article is a reprint of the first-edition article "Therapeutic Relationship: History of the Relationship" by the same author, with only minor changes.

We give the name "therapeutic relationship" to the link established between an individual (the patient) and another individual or group (the healers), with the aim of curing or relieving the disease suffered by the former. Our problem is to describe as exactly as possible the various forms this relationship has assumed throughout history.

The Empirico-Magical Stage

Ever since records have existed concerning the treatment of the sick, we may distinguish the following four chief forms: (1) the spontaneous or instinctive, (2) the empirical, (3) the magico-religious, and (4) the scientific. In all periods of history, all of these forms have had their practitioners. The mother who holds her feverish child on her lap, embracing it to protect it from the cold air, illustrates the first form, *spontaneous* or *instinctive* help. The second form, *empirical* help, consists in using a remedy because it has provided some relief in similar cases—that is, without asking why the remedy has those particular healing qualities. Medicine owes some very important discoveries to therapeutic empiricism. The treatment of wounds from firearms, discovered by chance by Ambrosio Paré (c. 1510–1590); the introduction of quinine into the Western world; and Edward Jenner's vaccination against smallpox are three superb examples.

Generically speaking, in *magico-religious* treatment both healer and patient believe that the cure is due to the action of "supernatural" or "divine" powers available for the purpose. In some cases the curative effectiveness of these powers depends on "who" uses them (medicine man, shaman, witch doctor, etc.); in others, on "how" they are applied (magic ritual); and in others, upon "where" the cure takes place (in localities "singled out" or "favored" for their healing powers—some shrine, island, or spring).

Since scientific treatment in the strict sense began in Greece in the fifth century B.C., we can definitely state that from the origin of the human race and for many thousand years thereafter, the therapeutic relationship was empirico-magical in character, with either the "empirical" or the "magical" element of the healing process dominant, according to circumstances. It is known that in the most highly developed pre-Hellenic cultures of ancient Egypt, China, and India, a form of medicine existed in which strictly "magical" or magico-religious elements were minor compared with the empirical and theoretical. However, a careful study of these three methods of understanding and practicing the care of the sick would reveal to some extent attitudes of the doctor that can only be called "magical" and that, above all, show a lack of principles capable of initiating a way toward purely "scientific" medicine.

The Ancient Scientific Stage

As Aristotle taught, treatment of the sick is scientific ("technical") in the strictest sense when it depends on the knowledge of why it is being done, what is being done, and by what means it takes effect (in other words, what is the disease, what remedy is being used, and by what therapeutic procedure is it administered). Thus the healer's ability to cure does not depend on the agent who applies the remedy, nor on the ceremony accompanying its application, nor on the privileged place where the cure takes place—that is, not on a magical "who," "how," or "where," but on a series of "whats" concerning the illness and its remedy.

Taking as their starting point the most important cosmological idea of the pre-Socratic philosophers—the idea of *physis,* or "nature"—the group of physicians, the Aesclepiades, known as Hippocratics, originated the technical concept of illness a century before Aristotle formulated the conceptual definitions just mentioned. Consequently, a doctor would try to cure a patient or to alleviate the patient's pain in the rational or scientifically definitive knowledge of the "nature" of humans, of illness in general, of the special disease he was treating, and of the remedy being used—while at the same time having the knowledge and skill to perform everything required by the treatment. This is not to say that Hippocratic medicine—apart from its inevitable deficiencies—was free from some serious errors and superstitious practice but to affirm that it already contained various principles: the notion of *physis* as the basis of all technical knowledge, the concept of medicine as *téchne iatriké,* the idea of a method of knowing whose first rule is the attentive sensory examination of the patient's body—as a result of which defects and errors would be gradually corrected.

From Hippocrates to Galen (A.D. 130?–200?)—while the ancient view of technical medicine remained in force—the therapeutic relationship can be described under four heads.

BASIS OF THE THERAPEUTIC RELATIONSHIP. Ideally considered, this basis is *philanthropia,* the "love of man," because, according to a famous saying, "Where there is love of man, *philanthropia,* there is love of the art [of healing], *philotechnia*" (Hippocrates, *Praeceptiones,* L.IX, 258). Of course, this saying belongs to a later, post-Stoic period; but the study of much earlier medical texts, such as the *Epidemias,* gives grounds for the belief that the Hippocratics, as they were called, practiced *philanthropia* before the word was invented. In any case, the "love of man" of ancient Greece was the same as "love of nature," of the divine *physis,* as is specifically and individually realized in the name given to the subject in question: *physiophilia.* It is not necessary to add that less noble interests, such as love of money and thirst for fame, in practice often obscured this ethical and technical ideal of "physiological philanthropy" as the basis of the therapeutic relationship.

DIAGNOSTIC ASPECT OF THE RELATIONSHIP. As scientific and effective "knowledge" was the first premise of the technical concept of medicine, the therapeutic relationship required—as it has of doctors since—that the Greek physician should reach a diagnosis by rational means. During the period in the history of medicine here called "ancient scientific," this diagnostic activity appears to have consisted of (1) a fourfold desire to discover whether the illness is determined by an insuperable and necessary cause (*kat'ananken*) or by some controllable contingency (*katà tychen*); to identify the typical form (*tropos, eidos*) of the suffering; to determine its causes, both remote and immediate (*aitia, prophasis*); and to establish a well-founded prognosis; (2) a series of exploratory maneuvers (*anamnesis,* study of the surroundings, examination of the patient's body by means of sight, touch, hearing, smell, and taste); and (3) adequate inductive reasoning (*logismos*).

CURATIVE ASPECT OF THE RELATIONSHIP. After some deliberation, the therapeutic activity of the Greek doctor was subjected to the following rules: (1) to help the patient, or at least to do no harm to the patient (Hippocrates, *Epidemias,* I, L.II, 634); (2) to refrain from interfering if the illness were incurable and inevitably mortal, because in that case the doctor, by intervening, would commit the sin of *hybris,* or rebellion against an edict of the divine and sovereign *physis;* and (3) insofar as possible, to attack the cause of the disease therapeutically. Diet, drugs, surgery, and to a lesser degree "psychotherapy" were the four great healing methods of ancient medicine.

ETHICAL AND SOCIAL ASPECTS OF THE THERAPEUTIC RELATIONSHIP. One must avoid the common error of seeing the oath contained in the *Corpus Hippocraticum* as the ethical code of Greek medicine; in all probability it was not in force outside the Pythagorean order (Edelstein). However, it is possible to trace the outline of the medical ethics and social medicine of the ancient Greeks:

1. The doctor's duties to the patient: to help or not to harm, to abstain from the impossible, to adjust the fees to the patient's income.

2. Duties toward other doctors: The ideal principle of regarding colleagues as brothers (Hippocrates, *Praeceptiones,* 4, IX, 258) was very infrequently infringed by the competitiveness of which doctors of antiquity are so often accused (Edelstein).

3. Duties toward self: A doctor should give attention to personal appearance and behave in a manner that would be called "beautiful and good" (Hippocrates, *Medicus,* L, IX, 204). To serve nature through the application of professional skill (Hippocrates, *Epidemias,* I, L.11, 636) should be the physician's paramount principle.

4. Duties to society: Though clearly stated by Plato (*Republic, Laws*), these are given much less importance in strictly medical writings; in any case (Plato, the Hippocratic treatise *On Diet*), it is certain that there was "medicine for the rich" and "medicine for the poor" in the ancient world.

Christianity and the Therapeutic Relationship

The propagation of Christianity was not motivated by the need to reform the conduct of doctor toward patient, insofar as this conduct could be held as technical, but because the medical technique prevailing at the time had been created by pagans. Because the Christian concept of love was relatively new, Christ's religious message influenced both the problem and the form taken by the therapeutic relationship in various ways.

Could the pagan medical technique have been accepted without more ado by Christians? Out of excessively vehement opposition to paganism, some of them—Tatian the Assyrian and Tertullian, for instance—gave a negative answer to this question. But the good sense of others prevailed in the end; and thus, from the fourth century to the increasingly strong anti-Galenism of the sixteenth and seventeenth centuries, the medicine of Christian peoples (e.g., in Byzantium and medieval Europe) showed a progressive intellectual effort to relate the art of healing, inherited from ancient Greece and culminating in the work of Galen, to the Christian worldview.

One can note the novelty of the Christian concept of love and its decisive effect on the form taken by the therapeutic relationship. When this was the direct, pure expression of the evangelical message—in other words, before Constantine's edict led to the primitive Christian communities' becoming involved with the civil power—there were two chief features of its structure.

IDEAL BASIS OF THE THERAPEUTIC RELATIONSHIP. We are no longer facing love of *physis* or universal "nature," as individualized in the sick person; rather, we are confronting his or her unique persona as a "neighbor" (parable of the good Samaritan). Moreover, in helping an ailing neighbor, one is helping Christ (Matt. 25: 39–40).

THE THERAPEUTIC RELATIONSHIP AS HELP. Herein lie the most significant new developments in primitive or pre-Constantinian Christianity.

1. In the assistance given to the sick person there should be no "natural limits," thus putting an end to the Hellenic imperative to refrain from therapy in cases of "necessarily" mortal or incurable disease. Here, although there is no place for therapeutic technique, the patient can always be helped by spiritual advice.

2. The egalitarian nature of treatment: No difference should be made between Greeks and barbarians, free people and slaves, friends and enemies.

3. The necessity of giving free help: Within a community governed by the principle that possessions are shared (see the texts of Acts of the Apostles), the basic motive of help for the sick was charity, not only on the part of the doctor but also on the part of other people (widows acting as nurses and, later, "deaconesses"). The Greek doctor would give free treatment in exchange for some favor received or to acquire prestige in the town (Hippocrates, *Praeceptiones,* L.IX, 258); the Christian doctor should give help free, on principle.

4. Such practices of the Christian religion as prayer and extreme unction were incorporated into the care of the sick.

The Medieval Scientific Stage

After Constantine's Edict of Milan (C.E. 312), the links between Christianity and the civil power became increasingly strong, and this gave rise to public awareness that the Christian life, such as was led outside the new conventual communities, was losing at least some of its original purity. This is shown by a brief examination of the two main politicosocial forms of Christianity, during the historical period that we call the Middle Ages, in the Byzantine Empire and medieval Europe. Exigencies of space allow no more than a mention of the third great cultural ambit of the Middle Ages: the world of Islam.

THERAPEUTIC RELATIONSHIP IN BYZANTIUM. The theocratic fusion between the Christian religion and civil power has never been stronger than in the Byzantine Empire; never has religious error or heresy been more methodically and sternly treated as "political crime." From this are derived the two main characteristics of the therapeutic relationship in Byzantine society: its doctrinal basis and its importance as help. The doctrinal basis of the therapeutic relationship in the Byzantine world was essentially the result of a juxtaposition that never turned out well. On the ethical plane, Byzantine medicine went on accepting and proclaiming the Christian concept of helping the sick; on the technical plane it accepted in principle everything described by the Greeks as "practical," and refused to acknowledge (as pagan and evil) the basic "theoretic" concepts of Hippocratic-Galenic medicine—for example, the notion of *physis* as "divine" and the denial or negation of a personal, spiritual God, creator of the world and transcending it. The doctors of Byzantium did not succeed in connecting the dogmas of their Christian faith with the scientific and philosophical basis of Hellenic *téchne iatriké*.

The most important contribution made by Byzantine Christianity to medical care was the creation of hospitals to treat poor invalids; among them was the famous "hospital city" of Caesarea, founded about the year 370. (Earlier institutions did not strictly deserve the name "hospitals.") In those institutions there were specialists, male and female nurses, surgeons, assistant doctors (*parabalani*), and servants. Charity was the ruling principle in their activity, but that did not prevent the distinction between "medicine for the rich" and "medicine for the poor" from being clearly observed in Byzantium. And finally, we must mention the

magical and pseudoreligious cures, which particularly attracted poorer patients.

THE THERAPEUTIC RELATIONSHIP IN MEDIEVAL EUROPE. The historical period we call the Middle Ages covers the millennium between the invasion of Rome by the Germanic races and the conquest of Constantinople by the Turks in 1453, and is far from uniform in character—suffice it to compare the life in a feudal castle in the ninth century with that of a Flemish or Italian town in the fifteenth. It is shown also by the gradual changes in the therapeutic relationship throughout this period.

Doctrinal basis of the therapeutic relationship. Two chief aspects must be distinguished—the technical and the ethical. Until the School of Salerno became famous (in the eleventh and twelfth centuries) and the Scholastic medicine of the thirteenth to fifteenth centuries was flourishing, medieval medicine hardly deserves the term *technical* or *scientific* in the strict sense. Mainly practiced by monks ("monastic medicine") either inside or outside monasteries, it was based solely on a certain amount of experience and the extremely scanty remains of ancient learning that had survived the destruction of the Roman Empire.

There was a marked change at the beginning of the twelfth century: Secular doctors with professional degrees became more common; from the time of Roger of Sicily in 1140, Greco-Arab learning began to spread from Salerno, or from Toledo, and became truly "technical" medicine, an authentic *ars medica*. By means of the intellectual resources provided by the theology and philosophy of the period, the Scholastic European doctors of the thirteenth and fourteenth centuries achieved something not attained by Byzantine medicine; they systematically adapted Hippocratic and Galenic thought to the needs of the Christian faith.

From the ethical point of view, medieval medicine continued to base itself ideally on the Christian concept of aid for the needy and sick—ideally because in practice the pressure of economic interest was not uncommon, nor, sometimes, free from corruption.

Diagnostic aspect of the therapeutic relationship. Though it had become impoverished and schematized in comparison with that of ancient Greece, the diagnostic relationship between doctor and patient—examination and establishment of "genus" and "species" of the affliction observed—remained much the same. Two techniques gained prominence and were gradually perfected: examination of the urine (*uroscopia*) and taking of the pulse. There were also two doctrinal guidelines to help the doctor pass from clinical experience to reasoning, treatises that systematically described the different species of disease (*de passionibus, de affectionibus*) and the didactic descriptions of individual cases of disease (*consilia*).

Curative aspect of the therapeutic relationship. From a technical standpoint the Middle Ages added little that was new to the treatment of the sick as taught by Greek and Arab doctors. Diet, the use of drugs, surgery, and "psychotherapy"—with a Christian orientation— remained the principal methods of treatment. As to theory, the chief concept of Galenic therapy, the "symptom" (*endeixis*), became latinized and scholasticized under the name of *insinuatio agendi*. On the other hand, the problem arose of how to harmonize "technical" requirements derived from the Galenic concept of symptoms with the "moral" rules imposed by the Christian idea of the person: the bond between *ars* and *caritas*. However, medieval physicians did not succeed in solving this delicate human problem coherently or systematically.

Ethical and social aspects of the therapeutic relationship. As to principles and ideals, medieval medical ethics are as faithfully Christian as the society to which they belong; but individual and social realization of this sincere Christianity was very different from that prevailing in pre-Constantine communities. Four reasons contribute to this:

1. The avarice of many clerical and secular doctors: "Doctor, do not be afraid of asking good fees from the rich," wrote Lanfranc in the eleventh century.

2. The growing interference of the civil power in regulating doctors' duties by means of ordinances— relating not only to the healer's technical behavior but also sometimes to his religious conduct— infringement of which was punished.

3. The frequent critico-burlesque attitude of society toward the doctor's greed for gain or lack of skill (John of Salisbury's *Metalogicus* and Petrarch's *Invectivae*).

4. The marked difference between "medicine for the rich" and "medicine for the poor"—in monasteries, the distance separating the *infirmarium* from the *hospitale pauperum*; in cities, the even greater gap between the treatment of those in power— politicians or churchmen, nearly all of whom had their own private doctors—and the almost purely religious treatment given to the unfortunates in hospital beds. Not everything in the Christian Middle Ages was in fact Christian.

Modern Scientific Stage: Christian Modernity

It is a platitude to say that the "modern world" began with the Renaissance or even in the fifteenth century. However, a thorough study of the various characteristics of this modernity—greater knowledge of classical antiquity, importance of worldly matters, new conceptions of science, rationalization of life, awareness of historical progress— clearly shows the roots of all these developments to be present in the transition from the thirteenth to the fourteenth century, when the voluntarism and nominalism of Franciscan thought (e.g., William of Occam, 1285?–1349?) began to influence European culture. When human freedom (and hence human creative ability) was seen as a person's chief similarity to God, the idea of "natural" and "necessary" limitations to human scientific and technical capacity with regard to the cosmos disappeared in principle, and the human mind began to entertain the idea of "indefinite progress." Science and modern techniques took their first steps, in the belief that knowledge of the sensible world consisted in creating abstract symbols—they would soon be called mathematical symbols—by means of which the external world could be understood and dominated. Many years had to pass, however, for these germinal concepts to be converted into strong, widespread social customs. Only in the secularized society of the eighteenth through the twentieth century would a great tree grow from the tiny seed of the fourteenth century.

Two periods must be distinguished in the history of the modern Euro-American world: In the first, from the fifteenth to the second half of the eighteenth century, by far the largest proportion of society was still nominally Christian, although the form of religion, whether Catholic or Protestant, was growing away from that of the Middle Ages; in the second, the nineteenth and twentieth centuries, society was becoming secularized.

BASIS OF THE THERAPEUTIC RELATIONSHIP. Whether Catholic or Protestant, modern Christian doctors still saw the injunction to give charitable help to those in need as the basic ideal of healing activity: They thought of Theophrastus Paracelsus, they remembered the ritual oath taken by newly graduated French doctors in front of the altar of Notre Dame. But the diversity of religions in Europe and America, and the growing esteem both for the reality of worldly values and for increasing civil power, led to two new features in this ideal: (1) greater respect for the personal religious life of the patient; and (2) an increasing and sharper separation between the spiritual and material worlds, the latter being known and governed by the beginnings of modern science and the technology founded upon it. Two examples of this spiritual–material separation will suffice: Hermann Boerhaave's teaching of the distinction between the mind and the body (*De distinctione mentis a corpore*) and Friedrich

Hoffmann's significant anthropological contrast between the physical (*cor corporale*) and the spiritual (*cor spirituale*).

DIAGNOSTIC ASPECT OF THE THERAPEUTIC RELATIONSHIP. The principle of understanding nature in order to master it (Francis Bacon, René Descartes) gained strength in modern society and led to the physician's concern to make diagnoses that were objectively correct. Very briefly, the following are the chief characteristics of the diagnostic aspect of the therapeutic relationship during this period:

1. Understanding of the disease being treated became more individualized, as was very clear in the form taken by case histories (Giovanni Battista Montanus, Boerhaave, etc.).

2. Numerical measurement gradually began to figure in examinations, leading to the first use of instruments such as watches and thermometers.

3. Diagnosis was increasingly used to guess at the existence of an anatomic lesion, which could be proved by an autopsy (Giovanni Maria Lancisi and Hippolyte Albertini, Hermann Boerhaave, Giovanni Battista Morgagni).

4. A more lively and objective interest was evinced in the influence of the social environment on the disease (Paracelsus, Bernardino Ramazzini, Johann Peter Frank).

CURATIVE ASPECT OF THE RELATIONSHIP. The spread and strength of the modern scientific mentality required a doctor who wished to keep up with the times to validate by experimentation the efficacy of the available remedies. On the other hand, awareness of human power over natural phenomena demanded a constant increase in the number and curative scope of those remedies. Paracelsus thought that every natural substance could be an efficacious medicament, if convenient means of using it could be discovered; God had disposed the world thus when it was created, and this the inquiring and inventive intelligence of the doctor should be able to make plain. Consequently, doctors no longer saw themselves as "servants of nature by means of their skill," as in ancient Greece but also during the Middle Ages in a Christian interpretation of the words as the true "collaborators of God." Whether Paracelsists or not, the most eminent doctors of the fifteenth to eighteenth centuries made use more or less consciously of this concept of therapeutic activity. But at the same time there was increasing distrust of the healing qualities assumed to belong to many of the remedies traditional practice had recommended.

The main therapeutic methods were still the four employed in Hippocratic medicine: diet (adapted to new ways of life), cure by drugs (enriched by various new medicines), surgery (whose technique had advanced considerably, from Ambrosio Paré to William Cheselden, Percival Pott, and Hunter), and, on a distinctly lower plane, psychotherapy, whose later triumph was unconsciously heralded by Franz Anton Mesmer at the end of the eighteenth century. The separation of healers into "doctors" (or "physicians") and "surgeons" was daily becoming more clear.

ETHICAL AND SOCIAL ASPECTS OF THE PROFESSIONAL-PATIENT RELATIONSHIP. Since both doctor and patient were Christians, it was natural for doctors to find their ethical principles in those of the Christian life; but at the same time, since the creation and rational order of the world had gained greater stature as explanations of the world, it was also natural for the form in which these principles were individually and socially realized to change to some extent. There should have been, and indeed there was, a relationship between religion and medicine that was both theoretical and practical. As religion was concerned with the life of the spirit and medicine with the life of the body (or what human knowledge tells us about the cosmos), the scientist and the physician did their best to discover and establish points of direct communication between those two worlds. In regard to theory, such communication was guaranteed by the "harmony" between Holy Writ and science, for example, in Francisco Valles's *Sacra philosophia* (sixteenth century) and Friedrich Hoffmann's *Dissertatio theologico-medica* (eighteenth century). Naturally, such communication and the bridge establishing it had to take a different form on the practical level. There the communication gave rise to "medical deontology," a collection of ethical precepts that were to be respected in the healer's technical activity. Examples of both early and mature forms of them are found in certain parts of the *Quaestiones medico-legales* of Paulo Zacchia (1621–1635) and the *Embriologia sacra* of Francesco Emmanuel Cangiamilla (1758).

Between the fifteenth and the seventeenth centuries, and therefore during the ancien régime, the bourgeois structure of society in Europe and America was being developed, and three distinct strata began to emerge: the "upper classes" (aristocrats, magnates of church and state, rich merchants), the "middle classes" (artisans, officials, and members of various professions), and the "lower classes" (laborers, the poor). Parallel strata could be observed in medical care. Ill persons of the upper classes were looked after in their luxurious homes and had a monopoly on more expensive treatments (one need only think of the distribution of quinine in the seventeenth century). The lower classes still went to hospitals for the poor, although during the eighteenth century those were altered or completely rebuilt on a larger scale. But the care of the sick inside those hospitals was far from acceptable (as to dirt, parasites, smell), as can be seen from denunciations by some socially and philanthropically sensitive doctors, like James René Tenon in 1788 and Howard in 1789. Nor was the medical care of the middle classes entirely satisfactory.

Modern Scientific Stage: Secularized Modernity

The process of secularizing society advanced at progressive speed during the nineteenth and twentieth centuries. Certainly there were still many Christians in the cities of Europe and America, but their individual and social style of living, their habits, were affected by this secularization; and it was in the eighteenth century that distinct groups came to be known as "intellectuals" and "aristocrats," and later (from the second half of the nineteenth century) a class came to be known as "proletarian."

Combined with this increasing secularization of behavior, we find that in the nineteenth century, life was becoming more technical, and in consequence of the industrial revolution an urban proletariat made its appearance. Submissive at first, the proletariat afterward organized itself as the "workers' movement" and asserted its rights more effectively, so that in one way or another it has decisively contributed to shaping the social scene of the twentieth century. How was the therapeutic relationship to be interpreted in this secularized world, part bourgeois, part proletarian?

DOCTRINAL BASIS OF THE RELATIONSHIP. As had been the case ever since Hippocratic medicine, the doctrinal basis of this relationship had two essential aspects, one ethical, the other scientific or technical. First, from an ethical standpoint, the ideal motive of medical care of the sick was "philanthropy," the feelings and the rules of conduct in which Christian charity was secularized. But modern philanthropy was radically different from the Hippocratic form (which had as its ultimate goal the divine *physis,* or universal nature), in that it was concerned with the "individual persona" of the patient—although the doctor's theory of humanity might not be formally "personalist." During the nineteenth and twentieth centuries many doctors have been "naturalist" in theory (in their scientific concept of human nature) and "personalist" in practice (in their therapeutic relation with the patient). Not until Marxist socialism did there appear a philanthropy based on the notions of "social or civil nature" and "state of nature." Second, from a

scientific point of view, the ideal basis of medical care was the concept of medicine as the application of pure natural science. "Medicine should be natural science—in other words, what the second half of the nineteenth century understood as natural science—or it will be nothing" was the oracular saying of Hermann Helmholtz. The sick person was *scientifically* considered as a fragment of the cosmos, acted on by biological evolution and governed by the laws of physics and chemistry. Scientifically, because in practice nearly all doctors obeyed the rule of Joseph Frédéric Bérard and Gluber: *Guérir parfois, soulager souvent, consoler toujours* (heal sometimes, relieve often, always console). This does not, of course, preclude the usual corruption of the medical profession—desire for gain, thirst for social prestige—often contaminating that philanthropic and scientific ideal.

DIAGNOSTIC ASPECT OF THE RELATIONSHIP. The diagnostic relationship with the patient now conformed to the following principles:

1. The patient was seen, above all, as an individual, capable of being rationally understood.

2. This understanding was increased by means of the instrumental aids to clinical examination (stethoscope, sphygmograph, ophthalmoscope, chemical analysis, X rays, etc.).

3. The disease was scientifically understood by applying rules that were anatomoclinical (diagnosis of anatomical lesions), physiopathological (diagnosis of disorders typical of the functional and material processes of life), or etiopathological (diagnosis of external causes, microbes, poison, etc., of the disease process); or the doctor could try to coordinate these three approaches.

4. Neurosis, whose frequency increased from the second half of the nineteenth century as a result of industrial civilization, was understood by natural scientific medicine by reference to anatomoclinical (Jean-Martin Charcot) or physiopathological rules (German practice since Friedrich Frerichs and Ludwig Traube).

5. To sum up, the diagnosis was, or tried to be, *at the same time* natural-scientific and individualist.

CURATIVE ASPECT OF THE RELATIONSHIP. When medicine was considered as applied natural science, the doctor's powers of healing (by experimental pharmacology, surgery enhanced by the development of anesthesia and antisepsis, synthesis of new drugs, serum therapy, vaccination, etc.) were progressively and wonderfully increased. Moreover, giving broad social expression to what was merely a slight and theoretical germ at the end of the thirteenth century and the beginning of the fourteenth, doctors freed themselves from the Hellenic concept of "natural force" (*ananke physeos*) and began to think of humans as not being, in principle, subject to diseases that were mortal or incurable "of necessity." What could not be cured today might well be curable tomorrow. In fact, the doctor ceased being "the servant of nature by means of skill" and became instead nature's "guardian, master, and sculptor."

Alongside dietetics, now scientifically regulated, increasingly rich therapy by drugs, and increasingly effective surgery, the psychotherapeutic element in treatment was acquiring more importance through several different methods and interpretations. In the history of this renewed importance of psychotherapy, the most distinguished names are those of the Englishmen Daniel Tuke, Alfred John Carpenter, and Hughes Bennet; the Frenchmen Jean-Martin Charcot and Bernheim; and, above all, Sigmund Freud, whose work had already reached maturity at the start of World War I in 1914.

ETHICAL AND SOCIAL ASPECTS OF THE RELATIONSHIP. Something has already been said about medical ethics in the society of the nineteenth and twentieth centuries. Like the society to which it belonged, this ethics became more secular, as is shown by the attempts to codify it, beginning with Percival's in 1803. From an ethical and social point of view, medical care was a service purchased at different prices or given free to the poor in hospitals supported by charity and inspired by the new philanthropy. The poor received medical care as a gift.

The sick were cared for in three different ambits.

1. *Hospitals* were supported by charity, the state, the municipality, or the church. Here the patient was one of two things in relation to the doctor: either an object that could be scientifically understood and modified, combined with a human being who was unknown and indifferent (if the doctor was a cold and matter-of-fact person), or an object that could be scientifically understood and modified, combined with a person suffering and in need of compassion (if the doctor was a person of feeling and carried out the rule of Bérard and Gluber).

2. *The patient's own home.* The patient visited at home was an object that could be scientifically understood and modified, combined with a well-known person—a friend.

3. *The doctor's private consulting room.* Here the patient was, according to circumstances, an object that could be scientifically understood and modified, combined with a person to whom the therapist was indifferent (purely "scientific" doctors); an object that could be understood and modified, combined with a person who paid the fee asked (doctors dominated by desire for gain); or an object that could be understood and modified, combined with a friend in need of compassion (generous, sympathetic doctors).

These three ambits, with certain exceptions, correspond to the three strata into which the bourgeois and proletarian society of the age are divided, and to the three socioeconomic methods of providing medical care: "medicine for the rich" (private consulting rooms for specialists), "medicine for the middle classes" (attendance in their homes), and "medicine for the poor and proletarians" (charitable hospitals). The injustice of this social organization of medicine becomes flagrant and untenable when the proletariat becomes conscious of its right to health and proper medical care, and when, one may add, medical treatment is both efficient and expensive.

Since the second half of the nineteenth century there has been a visible rebellion against this injustice with its politicosocial and clinical aspects. Since Turner Thackrah in 1831, Sir Edwin Chadwick in 1842, and Louis René Villermé in 1840, some doctors have denounced the terrible effects of industrial poverty on health; and workers' movements have included the right to put an end to this painful and unjustifiable situation in their programs for social reform. The great vogue of Friendly Societies in the United Kingdom between 1800 and 1875, the institution of the *zemstvo* system in tsarist Russia in 1867 after the liberation of the serfs, and the creation of *Krankenkassen* in Germany by Otto von Bismarck (1882–1884) are examples of the first medical results of the proletarian rebellion.

Among the clinical results of this rebellion may be counted the increase in neurotic forms of illness, which in some cases were direct consequences of social injustice and maladjustment. The "introduction of the subject in medicine" (von Weizsäcker's term), that is, the methodical study of the patient as an individual, both in diagnosis and treatment (penetration of hospitals by Freudian psychoanalysis and psychosomatic medicine) and in social pathology and medical sociology (Grotjahn and various English authors), constitutes the response of scientific medicine to the clinical rebellion of the sick against the medical care of the nineteenth century.

To the layperson as well as to the doctor of today, the present period begins with World War I. From that point on, the historian of yesterday must defer to the chronicler of the present day.

PEDRO LAÍN ENTRALGO (1995)
TRANSLATED BY FRANCES PARTRIDGE

SEE ALSO: *Beneficence; Care; Compassionate Love; Confidentiality; Healing; Hospital, Medieval and Renaissance History; Information Disclosure, Ethical Issues of; Informed Consent: History of Informed Consent; Medical Ethics, History of Europe; Medicine, Anthropology of; Medicine, Art of; Medicine, Philosophy of; Medicine, Profession of; Medicine, Sociology of; Nursing, Profession of; Trust; Virtue and Character;* and other *Professional-Patient Relationship* subentries

BIBLIOGRAPHY

Baas, Karl. 1915. "Uranfänge und Frühgeschichte der Krankenpflege." *Sudhoffs Archiv für Geschichte der Medizin* 8: 146–164.

Balint, Michael. 1964. *The Doctor, His Patient, and the Illness,* 2nd edition. New York: International Universities Press. First published 1957.

Blum, Richard H. 1960. *The Management of the Doctor-Patient Relationship.* Foreword by Joseph Sadusk and Rollen Waterson. New York: McGraw-Hill/Blakiston.

Christian, Paul. 1952. *Das Personverständnis im modernen medizinischen Denken: Schriften der Studiengemeinschaft der Evangelischen Akademien,* no. 1. Tübingen: J.C.B. Mohr.

Duffy, John. 1979. *Healers: A History of American Medicine.* Urbana: University of Illinois Press.

Edelstein, Ludwig. 1943. *The Hippocratic Oath: Text, Translation, and Interpretation.* Supplements to the *Bulletin of the History of Medicine* no. 1. Baltimore: Johns Hopkins University Press. Reprinted in *Ancient Medicine: Selected Papers of Ludwig Edelstein,* pp. 3–63, ed. Owsei Temkin and C. Lilian Temkin, tr. C. Lilian Temkin. Baltimore: Johns Hopkins University Press, 1967.

Field, Mark G. 1957. *Doctor and Patient in Soviet Russia.* Russian Research Center Studies, no. 29. Cambridge, MA: Harvard University Press.

Fleury, Mai L. 1984. *The Healing Bond: Human Relations Skills for Nurses and Other Health-Care Professionals.* Englewood Cliffs, NJ: Prentice-Hall.

Gracia, Diego. 1989a. "Los cambios en la relación médico-enfermo." *Medicina clínica* (Barcelona) 93: 100–102.

Gracia, Diego. 1989b. *Fundamentos de bioética.* Madrid: Eudema.

Gracia, Diego. 1991. *Procedimiento de decisión en ética clínica.* Madrid: Eudema.

Hippocrates. *Epidemias* I, L.II, 634 and 636. In Littré, *Oeuvres complètes d'Hippocrate,* vol. 2, pp. 634–637. Also in Jones, trans., *Hippocrates,* vol. 1, second constitution, par. 11, 11.10–12 and 13–14, pp. 164–165.

Hippocrates. *Medicus.* L. IX, 204. In Littré, *Oeuvres complètes d'Hippocrate,* vol. 9, pp. 204–207. Also in Jones, trans., *Hippocrates,* vol. 2, chap. 1, pp. 310–313.

Hippocrates. *Praeceptiones.* L. IX, 258. In Littré, *Oeuvres complètes d'Hippocrate,* vol. 9, pp. 258–263. Also in Jones, trans., *Hippocrates,* vol. 1, par. 6–7, pp. 318–323.

Hippocrates. *Regimen.* L. VI, 466. In Littré, *Oeuvres complètes d'Hippocrate,* vol. 6, pp. 466–663. Also in Jones, trans., *Hippocrates,* vol. 4, pp. 224–447.

Jones, William Henry Samuel, tr. 1923–1931. *Hippocrates.* 4 vols. Loeb Classical Library, ed. E. Capps, T. E. Page, and W. H. D. Rouse. London: William Heinemann; New York: G. P. Putnam's Sons. Greek and English.

Laín Entralgo, Pedro. 1958. *La curación por la palabra en la antigüedad clásica.* Madrid: Revista de Occidente, ed. and tr. L. J. Rather and John M. Sharp as *The Therapy of the Word in Classical Antiquity.* New Haven, CT: Yale University Press, 1970.

Laín Entralgo, Pedro. 1961. *Enfermedad y pecado: Medicina de hoy.* Barcelona: Ediciones Toray.

Laín Entralgo, Pedro. 1962. "La asistencia médica en la obra de Platón." In his *Marañón y el enfermo,* pp. 90–135. Madrid: Revista de Occidente.

Laín Entralgo, Pedro. 1964. *La relación médico-enfermo: Historia y teoría.* Madrid: Revista de Occidente.

Laín Entralgo, Pedro. 1969. *Doctor and Patient.* Translated by Frances Partridge. World University Library. London: Weidenfeld and Nicholson; New York: McGraw-Hill.

Laín Entralgo, Pedro. 1970. *La medicina hipocrática.* Madrid: Revista de Occidente.

Laín Entralgo, Pedro. 1972a. "El cristianismo primitivo y la medicina." In his *Historia universal de la medicina,* 3: 1–7. Barcelona: Salvat.

Laín Entralgo, Pedro. 1972b. *Sobre la amistad.* Colección Selecta, no. 41. Madrid: Revista de Occidente.

Littré, Emile, ed. and tr. 1839–1861. *Oeuvres complètes d'Hippocrate: Traduction nouvelle avec le texte grec en regard, collationné sur les manuscrits et toutes les éditions, accompagnée d'une introduction, de commentaires médicaux, de variantes et de notes philologiques; suivie d'une table générale des matières.* 10 vols. Paris: J. B. Baillière. Reprinted Amsterdam: Adolf M. Hakkert, 1961.

Majno, Guido. 1975. *Healing Hand: Man and Wound in the Ancient World.* Cambridge, MA: Harvard University Press.

Nutting, Mary Adelaide, and Dock, Lavinia L. 1907–1912. *A History of Nursing: The Evolution of Nursing Systems from the Earliest Times to the Foundation of the First English and American Training School for Nurses.* 4 vols. New York: G. P. Putnam, tr. Agnes Karll as *Geschichte der Krankenpflege: Die Entwicklung der Krankenpflege—Systeme von Urzeiten bis zur Gründung der ersten englischen und amerikanischen Pflegerinnenschulen.* 3 vols. Berlin: D. Reimer, 1910–1913.

Orr, Douglas W. 1954. "Transference and Countertransference: A Historical Survey." *Journal of the American Psychoanalytic Association* 2(4): 621–670.

Parsons, Talcott. 1951. "Illness and the Role of the Physician: A Sociological Perspective." *American Journal of Orthopsychiatry* 21: 452–460.

Pittenger, Robert E.; Hackett, Charles F.; and Danehy, John J. 1960. *The First Five Minutes: A Sample of Microscopic Interview Analysis.* Ithaca, NY: Paul Martineau.

Porter, Roy, ed. 1986. *Patients and Practitioners: Lay Perceptions of Medicine in Pre-Industrial Society.* New York: Cambridge University Press.

Reiser, Stanley J., and Anbar, Michael, eds. 1984. *The Machine at the Bedside: Strategies for Using Technology in Patient Care.* New York: Cambridge University Press.

Ritter-Röhr, Dorothea, ed. 1975. *Der Arzt, sein Patient, und die Gesellschaft.* Edition Suhrkamp, no. 746. Frankfurt am Main: Suhrkamp.

Rof Carballo, Juan. 1961. *Urdimbre afectiva y enfermedad: Introducción a una medicina dialógica.* Colección Hombre y Mundo. Barcelona: Editorial Labor.

Sigerist, Henry E. 1987. *History of Medicine.* 2 vols. New York: Oxford University Press.

Snyder, William U., and Snyder, B. June. 1961. *The Psychotherapy Relationship.* New York: Macmillan.

Szasz, Thomas S. 1958. "Scientific Method and Social Role in Medicine and Psychiatry." *Archives of Internal Medicine* 101: 228–238.

Valabrega, Jean-Paul. 1962. *La Relation thérapeutique: Malade et médecin.* Nouvelle Bibliothèque Scientifique. Paris: Flammarion.

Weiss, Georg. 1910. "Die ethischen Anschauungen im Corpus Hippocraticum." *Sudhoffs Archiv für Geschichte der Medizin* 4: 235–262.

Zborowski, Mark. 1952. "Cultural Components in Responses to Pain." *Journal of Social Issues* 8(4): 16–30.

II. SOCIOLOGICAL PERSPECTIVES

The purposes of this article are to provide a sociological perspective of the doctor–patient relationship by sketching the models of it as they have been developed by sociology, and to summarize contemporary sociological analysis. Both are essential for understanding the issues surrounding the therapeutic relationship today.

No other aspect of medicine has attracted more sociological analysis than the medical professional–patient relationship. From a classic view of the relation between doctor and patient "as a pure person-to-person relation" (Sigerist), the full range of psychosocial and sociocultural influences has been studied. Many of the most distinguished sociologists have used this particular problem to illustrate theories of the field. At the same time, the changing facts of technology, organization, and cost were charted as the necessary context for understanding the changes in professional–patient encounters.

There are also distinctive regional-cultural interpretations of the therapeutic relationship. European sociologists consistently have emphasized the significance of power (Foucault). This perspective makes the human body, and

hence the patient, the passive recipient of pathology, and sees the professional as an agent of the state (Rosen). David Armstrong, a British medical sociologist, has pointed out that in Britain, not until about 1970 was the importance of the "inherently problematic ... [aspects of the] ... doctor–patient relationship" recognized (Armstrong; Interdepartmental Committee on Medical Schools). Not until the Todd Report was history taking described as "a great deal more ... than simply asking a series of prescribed questions and checking the accuracy of the answers" (Great Britain). Essentially, Foucault viewed the clinical examination as a technique of surveillance. Beginning in the eighteenth century, such surveillance invoked a disciplinary power and required that the body (and hence the patient) be a discrete (passive) object. The change signaled by the Todd Report suggests "the beginnings of the fabrication of patient subjectivity" or, more simply, the activation of the patient (Armstrong).

Americans, on the other hand, have been preoccupied largely with the analysis of medicine as a profession, placing emphasis upon the role of the physician as a professional with resultant claims to autonomy and dominance (Freidson, 1970b). Initially, this perspective placed the patient in a primarily passive role. The American approach, however, has been to construct models that separate each role according to its structure—its reciprocal privileges and obligations—and its function for the society, defining the doctor as the legitimizer of illness and thereby the agent of social control, and the patient as an involuntary deviant who is allowed temporary exemptions from normal social expectations but is required to resume his or her place as soon as possible. Americans have assumed that within the framework of cultural expectations, behavior in these roles is voluntary. Europeans have directed their concern mainly to questions about how the rights and obligations of doctor and patient are inherent and controlled by the state.

These distinctive frames of reference for the analysis of medical relationships are reflected in very different systems for the delivery of health care. European nations, in both financing and service organization, have constructed systems that provide universal access to healthcare. Whether by a government-run national health service (the British model) or by national health insurance (the government guarantees the payment of fees for service by an essentially independent profession), the goal is to provide healthcare as a fundamental right for all citizens. The United States, virtually alone among modern industrialized nations—South Africa is its only companion state—has not guaranteed this right for the sick nor established the obligations of the caregiver, choosing instead to rely primarily on an implicit contract between the medical profession and the society. The latter arrangement, on the premises of individualism, claims that the doctor–patient relationship is sacred, based on the privileges of the professional to autonomy and the patient's right to choose his or her doctor. The alternative approach is based on the premise that in the therapeutic relationship, the behavior of the individuals—and their rights—depends upon social controls vested in the state. "Models," the Americans choose to call their explanations, signifying the fullness and reciprocity of the interaction between doctor and patient.

However, the intellectual distance between the continents has steadily grown smaller. When one traces the full history, the American and European interpretations can be seen gradually to converge. The starting point is in the 1930s, with all the major theories of sociological thought applied to the therapeutic relationship. Although the healing art is older than—and practiced by others than—the physician, the doctor's role has been the centerpiece. Other helping roles—the nurse, social worker, and various "allied health professionals"—have received attention (Aiken), but historically it is the therapist as a professional in modern society who has most interested the sociologist, and medicine is seen as the archetypal profession.

The result has been a changing portrait of both doctor and patient—from a dominantly psychological perspective to a sharp turn when Talcott Parsons introduced the social-system frame of reference (Parsons), shifting the analysis to the social roles of therapist and client, instilled in each individual by agents of socialization like the family and schools. The idea was that the qualities of patienthood were part of social development. We learn what to expect of physicians and how to behave as patients. Such roles were interpreted as "functional" components fashioned to maintain the society. Within this framework, the doctor's achieved high level of expertise is described as essential to modern scientific healthcare, and as a consequence, medical education is spotlighted. The medical school is seen as the principal source of attitudes and values as well as of training in skills and knowledge. That approach enhances the physician's image of awesome technological accomplishment and heroic personal attributes, while the patient is relegated to a subordinate, fragile state in which the only requirements are to be motivated to get well and to consult the physician toward that end.

The reaction to this approach, beginning in the 1960s, changed the role images dramatically: Complex bureaucratic forces were elevated to predominance over the voluntaristic choices of individuals (Starr). The "monopoly of dominance" replaced "technological achievement" as the more popular view of the doctor; the patient came to be viewed as "exploited" by the physician as much as or more than he or she was victimized by the primarily organic forces of illness. The doctor and patient became antagonists, each from a separate world, and their adversarial relationship was described as a "clash of perspectives" instead of a balanced, interdependent system.

In this changing approach, sociological thought has run parallel to the public's attitude toward the medical profession. The sociologists' picture of the physician, at first cautious and respectful, reflected the peak of public prestige and trust that allocated to doctors the privilege of virtually complete autonomy as "high priests in the temples of science" (Churchill). That pedestal was not an easy resting place, however. Physicians became the objects of public exhortation, government regulation, and legal attack.

The implications of the ethical standards by which physicians are judged are profound. After centuries of struggle to win the right to take risks, under conditions of uncertainty (Sigerist; Fox, 1957), in the "best interests of their patients," doctors now find themselves confronted by a fresh demand for accountability. The responsibility that was once assumed in trust is increasingly subject to the formal controls either of state-run systems or of various forms of peer review and medical audit. The added pressure of changing definitions of both the onset of life and its termination, stimulated by new technologies, has intensified the challenge to social values (Fox, 1979).

The therapeutic relationship is also responding to changes in the age profile, particularly of the populations of the United States and other modern industrial nations, and altered patterns of illness and disability. The challenge for physicians increasingly has become less a matter of cure and more of maintaining function (Mechanic, 1985).

At the same time, the sciences basic to medical practice—represented by modern molecular biology, genetics, and the neurosciences, together with computer-related technologies—have produced what has been called a "paradigmatic leap" that must profoundly affect the basic human relations of medical practice (Marston and Jones). As medical knowledge and technology have expanded, public expectations of physicians' expertise and caring have become higher than ever before, complicated by patient needs for a more active, sharing role in therapy.

The development of sociological interpretation of the therapeutic relationship must be viewed as an expansion rather than a linear growth. It is not possible to say that the models have emerged successively, each more valid than its predecessor. The theories represented are still hypothetical. We present them in historical order.

The System Model

FUNCTIONALISM. As applied to both biology and sociology, functional theory proposes that the relationships between the basic elements, whether chemical and physiological or social roles and institutions, are arranged in systems rather than as sums of their parts. Also basic in this conception is that the system is inherently driven toward equilibrium, a homeostatic balance that is reasserted whenever an intervention or change occurs. This dynamic toward balance and stability is the source of the term *functionalism.* It is assumed that living processes, including but not limited to the social, are dominated by relationships that function to maintain or reassert stability to the whole. Thus the terms *system, function,* and *equilibrium* are often used interchangeably: Functionalist theory is system theory.

Although not the first functionalist in social thought, Lawrence J. Henderson pioneered the application of an equilibrium model to the doctor–patient relationship (Henderson, 1935). This he did only in midcareer, after having established himself as an outstanding biological scientist by translating Willard Gibbs's model of physicochemical systems for use in the study of blood physiology. Known as the formulator of the acid-base equilibrium, he applied his functional model with simultaneous equations to explain the quantitative relationship of eight variables of the blood.

Functionalism in physics, chemistry, and biology replaced the linear, cause-and-effect positivism dominant in the nineteenth century. The introduction of this theoretical framework and its mathematical proofs had produced revolutionary effects in biology, and Henderson believed they would be duplicated in social science. The essence of his reasoning was expressed as follows:

Because every factor interacts in a social system, because everything, every property, every relation, is therefore in a state of mutual dependence with everything else, ordinary cause-and-effect analysis of events is rarely possible. In fact, it must be regarded as one of the two great sources of error in sociological work (Henderson, 1970, p. 29).

Henderson's application of the functionalist model to social systems produced a limited conception, and his model was mechanical and simplistic. As a result, his achievement in social science was mainly that of the seminal teacher: to inspire and challenge colleagues and students to take his model further.

Henderson's was soon followed by other interpretations of the social-system model. Illustrations and applications of the theory were drawn from all the major social institutions, especially the industrial and educational, but the doctor–patient relationship remained important. The major functional analysts of the therapeutic relationship, their illustrative examples, and their special contributions to knowledge are listed in Table 1.

Talcott Parsons, more than any other, carried forward the discussion of the doctor–patient relationship as a social system, giving it full expression as part of sociological theory. He argued that human social relationships can be described as patterns rooted in cultural expectation about the social roles of group members; that the fundamental process of behavior is communication; and that the integrity of the system is maintained by homeostasis, defined as a dynamic force that reacts to any change or intervention by reasserting a balance in the system that enables it to perform its intended function.

Parsons conceived of the doctor–patient relationship as a social-role interaction in which the sick role is voluntary; for instance, a person can be ill—say, with a cold—but choose not to be "sick," a status that invokes privileges and obligations determined by the cultural expectations of the society. The sick role is a form of social deviance that must be controlled to prevent the abuse of the dependency of illness. The professional role combines healing the patient and social control as the agent of the society. Accordingly, the sick role is temporary, undesirable, and socially disruptive. The professional is a technical expert who legitimizes the claim to illness and is responsible for returning the sick person to his or her normal role in society.

Criticisms of Parsons's views are of two distinct types. One is intellectual, challenging his theoretical premises and argument (Freidson, 1970a). The other is political, interpreting the work of both Henderson and Parsons as a conservative political response to the historical events of the early 1930s, particularly the Great Depression and the rise of communism (Gouldner).

The theoretical criticism of the model focuses on Parsons's emphasis on the asymmetry of the therapeutic situation—that is, the professional dominance versus the client's dependence—and in the distancing effect of that asymmetry. Parsons is interpreted as a defender of the technical elitism of the modern physician. His patients must be "controlled," lest they take advantage of the privileges of the sick role to prolong dependency; his physicians must be "protected" from emotional overinvolvement with their patients. The consequences, the criticism asserts, are not just to explain a role asymmetry based upon the achieved technical expertise of the professional, but also to categorize and label the roles so that the passive, dependent patient and the expert doctor become hardened stereotypes.

The continuous development of functionalist interpretations of the therapeutic relationship was broken abruptly

TABLE 1

Functional Models of the Doctor–Patient Relationship, Illustrative Cases, and Effects on the Field, 1930–1965

Models	Illustrative Examples	Effects on the Field
Lawrence J. Henderson 1935	Cancer patient: socioemotional determinants of system process	Established legitimacy of medical relationship as a subject of scientific inquiry
Talcott Parsons 1951	Institutional case: the profession a social system	Contributed to general theory of social behavior
Florence Kluckhohn, John Spiegel 1954	Psychiatric patients, studied according to cultural value orientation	Contributed to general theory of behavior, combining sociological with psychoanalytic concepts: transactional theory
William Caudill 1958	The hospitalized mental patient	Applied social-system theory to analysis of mental hospital; conceived hospital as a functional social system
Thomas Szasz, Marc Hollender 1956	Acute, ambulatory, and chronic diseases, to illustrate behavioral implication of biological symptoms	Operationalized role theory in medical terms; articulated system theory for education of physicians and to improve clinical practice
Michael Balint 1957	Ambulatory patient of general practitioner	Expanded biomedical model (in Great Britain) to include socioemotional; broke down mind-body dualism.
Samuel W. Bloom 1963	Diabetes, mental illness, and multiproblem patient to illustrate sociocultural determinants	Applied functional theory to health care in historical/ developmental terms
Kenneth Arrow 1963	The medical-care market	Adapted Pareto to general economic theory by conceptualizing optimum equilibrium as a theorem of competitive systems
Edward Suchman 1965	A population of "seriously ill" patients: a survey	Operationalized social-system explanation of health-services utilization

SOURCE: Adapted from Bloom and Speedling, 1989, p. 115.

in the 1960s with the appearance of studies that emphasized the structural, situational determinants and directly challenged the validity of the functional.

STRUCTURAL CONFLICT THEORY. Eliot Freidson is the major spokesman for the application of the structural conflict theory to the professional–patient relationship. The therapeutic interaction, he argued, is most effectively analyzed as a clash of perspectives. "The professional expects patients to accept what he recommends on his terms; patients seek services in their own terms. In that each seeks to gain his own terms, there is conflict" (Freidson, 1961, p. 171). The patient, in this formulation, is assumed to be governed by an interpersonal order equal in complexity to that of the professional. The asymmetry of Parsons's model underscoring the physician's technical expertise is discarded. The patient responds largely on the basis of current experience and sources of influence, not as a result of deeply embedded beliefs and expectation derived from long-term cultural socialization. Between doctor and patient, negotiation, not persuasion, occurs. The critical factor is structure, not function—the structural social positions based on the separate statuses and interests of the client and the professional. The deviance of the sick role, within this framework, becomes more central and more complex than in Parsons. A distinctive influence is assigned to stigma. For example, mental illness and sexually transmitted diseases, Freidson argues, are perceived by society on a variable scale of deviance and stigmatized accordingly; they are not lumped together as diseases that are beyond the control of the patient.

Freidson's critique of Parsons was very specific. First, the Parsons model sees the doctor–patient relationship from too limited a perspective, most essentially that of the physician; it does not pay attention to the varying expectations of all members of the "role-set," including the patients (or, more inclusively, their lay associates as well) and the nurses and other persons involved in the process of treatment. Second, expectations are presented by Parsons as though they are the primary influence on actual behavior; they are only an ideal standard against which actual behavior is judged. Third, influence does not inhere in the expectation but in the position of the person holding it; only from the structure of the situation and the limits imposed by it can one weigh the possibility of an expectation's being met. Fourth and most important, the functional model ignores the necessity of conflict in human relationships. Insofar as each person, the professional and the patient, seeks to gain his or her own terms from the other, there is conflict.

This approach spawned a succession of studies about the therapeutic situation. The major examples are listed in Table 2. Through these studies, the view of the patient was transformed. Fully equal to the physician, the patient might behave passively, influenced either by personality or by the structure of the situation. Nevertheless, the patient role was no longer inherently subordinate by virtue of the physician's technical expertise or of the patient's lack of adequate knowledge.

Neo-Marxism, Bureaucracy, and the Politics of Health

The high point of structural conflict theory occurred with the 1970 publication by Freidson of the second of his two books about the medical profession. Marxist critiques followed by Howard Waitzkin and Barbara Waterman in 1974 and by Vicente Navarro in 1975.

The new Marxism built its argument on the classic conception that social behavior is essentially organized according to principles of social stratification or social class, based on materialistic determinants, and inevitably dominated by one class, leading to monopolistic control of resources and markets by the dominant class and to the exploitation of subordinate groups for profit or gain of the more powerful class. Waitzkin illustrated what he called the "micropolitics" of the doctor–patient relationship, using the following types of cases: (1) a young worker with occupationally caused sterility; (2) neonatal death attributable to

neglect caused by poverty and racial discrimination; (3) an elderly man burdened by costs of technically oriented medicine. Waitzkin analyzed more than 300 taped doctor–patient interviews in an effort to demonstrate that medicine, like other social institutions, functions as part of the "ideologic state apparatus," with the doctor as the agent of ideology and social control. The micropolitics of the doctor–patient relationship, he argued, revealed contradictions that no current political system resolves (Waitzkin).

The boundaries between this view and that of the earlier structuralists were not as sharp as the demarcations with functionalism. Nevertheless, there are important differences. In Freidson, for example, there is no hint of patient exploitation. Nor does the drive among doctors for "professional autonomy and dominance," as described by the structuralists, mean anything similar to the Marxist description of the physician as a self-interested manager of health resources. What neo-Marxists like Waitzkin added to forecast subsequent trends was the analysis of how both doctor and patient have become captives of monopolistic trends in the healthcare industries.

The focus of the 1980s was on the same monopolistic big business, but with a different interpretation. Paul Starr (1982), for example, argued that rational behavior leads to large-scale privatization and the absorption of healthcare into the marketplace. He described the corporatization of the healthcare system of the United States in five dimensions:

1. Change in the type of ownership and control, shifting from nonprofit and governmental service organizations, especially hospitals, to for-profit healthcare companies.

2. Horizontal integration, the decline of freestanding institutions and the consequent shift in the locus of control from community boards to regional and national healthcare corporations.

3. Diversification and corporate restructuring, the shift from single-unit organizations operating in one market to conglomerates involved in a variety of healthcare markets.

4. Vertical integration, the shift from a single level of care organizations, like acute-care hospitals, to organizations that embrace the various phases and levels of care, such as health maintenance organizations (HMOs).

5. Industry concentration, the increasing concentration of control of health services in regional markets and the nation as a whole.

The implications of these trends, it was argued, are to depersonalize the therapeutic relationship and to change the nature of the social roles. The doctor, increasingly a salaried

TABLE 2

Models of the Doctor–Patient Relationship, Their Illustrative Cases, and Effects on the Field: Structuralism (Conflict Theory, Labeling), 1960–1975

Models	Illustrative Examples	Effects on the Field
Erwin Goffman 1961	Hospitalized mental patients	General theory of structured deviance; labeling; social stigma. Concepts: total institution, moral career of patients
Eliot Freidson 1961, 1970b	Health-care institutions; HMOs; the medical profession	General theory of conflict behavior determined by situational factors; clash of perspectives mediated by negotiation; professional autonomy and monopoly; patient networks
David Mechanic 1962	Illness behavior in various contexts	A multivariate theory: synthesized social psychological with situational variables; designed to operationalize for research; problem-oriented. Based on Volkart and W.I. Thomas. Health behavior as coping
Julius A. Roth 1963	Hospitalized tuberculosis patients	General theory: management of illness by normative timetables; institutional organization of illness response
Thomas Szasz 1964	Disabled patients, mental and physical	Critique of functionalism; contribution to deviance and labeling theory
Thomas Scheff 1966	Hospitalized mental patients	General theory of social deviance; labeling

SOURCE: Adapted from Bloom and Speedling, 1989, pp. 122–123

employee instead of an individual entrepreneur, is losing autonomy and, in effect, is becoming proletarianized. The patient, as a result of pressures to join large healthcare organizations, cannot freely choose a doctor or join with the doctor in certain decisions because cost control by the organization intervenes.

Such interpretations were buttressed by the increase in large-scale organizations for the delivery of healthcare, but the interest of scholars in psychosocial factors in therapeutic encounters continued to be strong. Compliance, the extent to which patients follow the recommendations of their therapists, for example, remained an important problem independent of the organizational framework for healthcare. Marshall Becker and Lois Maimon (1982) described a "health belief model" that made individual motivations and beliefs about the validity of treatment methods the central factors of health behavior. Attempts to quantify the sociobehavioral determinants of compliance preoccupied many researchers during the next two decades. The physician, at the same time, has been scrutinized in comparable empirical and quantitative detail as a "decision-maker" (Elstein et al.).

This quantitative trend is reflected in the training and assessment of medical students and residents. With the increasing orientation toward the use of measurements of clinical reasoning and behavior, didactic teaching and memorization are being replaced by problem-based learning and experiential learning situations such as simulations of clinical cases, called standardized patient (SP) methods (Woodward and Gerard). The goal of these efforts to change how physicians are trained is to create a more patient-oriented approach and, at the same time, influence doctors to become active, lifelong learners in order to maintain effectiveness under conditions of rapidly advancing basic medical sciences (Marston and Jones).

The Nonmedical Healing Professions

The history of the healing professions has been dominated by medicine. Although nurses, public-health workers, dentists, and social workers have been major contributors to the health of individuals and communities, their professional status and power have always been less than those of physicians. However, dramatic changes have expanded the need for the care of health and disease, challenging the monopoly of doctors. Constantly advancing technology applied to diagnosis and treatment, the increase in life expectancy and consequent growth of the elderly population, and changed patterns of illness and disability have forced physicians to depend on partnerships with members of other healing professions.

Nursing is the outstanding case in point. Nurses, although much more numerous than physicians (four nurses for every doctor), increasingly professionalized (over 100,000 have master's or doctorate degrees), and performing tasks in health settings previously restricted to physicians, continue to struggle for release from the view, argued by Freidson, that, following precedents established by Florence Nightingale more than a century ago, "All nursing work flowed from the doctor's orders … [so that] nursing became a formal part of the doctor's work, a technical trade.… Nursing thus was defined as a subordinate part of the technical division of labor surrounding medicine" (Freidson, 1970b, p. 61). There is some evidence that success in this struggle is at last being achieved.

Advanced-practice nurses, for example, are registered nurses with specialty training, usually at the master's degree level, in primary care (i.e., nurse practitioners and nurse-midwives) or acute care of in-patients (i.e., clinical nurse specialists). Mary Mundinger writes:

> The practice of nurse practitioners has been evaluated since 1965 when the role was developed by Henry Silver, M.D., and Loretta Ford, R.N. When measures of diagnostic certainty, management competence, or comprehensiveness, quality, and cost are used, virtually every study indicates that the primary care provided by nurse practitioners is equivalent or superior to that provided by physicians.… Over the past few years, state legislatures have broadened the authority of nurse practitioners to receive direct payment and write prescriptions, and the barriers to independence have fallen. As a result, nurse practitioners can establish independent practices that parallel those of primary care physicians (either solo or health maintenance organizations), or they can establish collaborative practices in which doctors and nurses care for patients together. (Mundinger, p. 211)

Initiatives from private foundations and the government have encouraged the professionalization of nursing and the other healing occupations, rewarding the creation of both educational and healthcare reforms that foster the creation of teams working together as equals. Nevertheless, these other professions remain in the shadow of medicine. As a consequence, nurses, probably the highest-status members

of the paramedicals, earn an average of less than a third of physicians' incomes; their training, except for the 5 percent who have earned higher degrees, is considerably shorter and less rigorous; and nursing is almost totally a women's profession, a fact that, regrettable though it is, remains a classic indicator of low occupational status.

However, as indicated by the testimony of Mary Mundinger above, the status of nursing as a profession has changed. Increasingly, nurses are both trained in and responsible for the complex knowledge and technical aspects of patient care. In 1960, 83 percent of new graduates were trained in hospitals, the rest in colleges and universities. By 1980, those figures had reversed.

We are witnessing, therefore, a historical development in nursing reminiscent of the changes that occurred in medicine in the 1910s. Like medicine in the post-Flexner era (1910 and following), nursing is seeking to increase its professionalism by extending its training in close association with the university. Included is new emphasis on biomedical science and research.

The value implications of these changes are of particular concern. Professionalism for nurses tends to emphasize intellectual and technical skills in an occupation whose major function has been as much the ministering of nurturant and humane care as technical prowess.

For the patient, the options seem to narrow as knowledge and technical skill increase. Whereas once it seemed reasonable to expect physicians to combine technical expertise with emotional sensitivity and skill, and nurses to complement them in both, now the patient gains equality and independence but with increasing emotional distance from caregivers.

Under the current conditions of healthcare, social workers would seem to have a strategic role. They are, after all, uniquely trained in the skills of interpersonal relations, and professionally are intended to function as the patient's advocate for well-being, both within the period of illness and in preparation for the recovery period. Yet, here, too, the pressures for professional status take an ironic toll. A trend toward private practice with fee-for-service financial rewards attracts social workers toward professional status on the medical model and away from the team model in which their function is to balance the technical with the social.

The same value dilemma confronts all the healing professions. A polarization has developed between two orientations, one centered on the *what* of healthcare and the other on the *how*. The former has been called a reductionistic approach, emphasizing biomedical knowledge and technology; the latter is the "social ecology" or "humanistic" approach.

The values of these two approaches are significantly different. The more traditional, reductionistic approach is dominated by faith that all problems of health and illness have rational solutions, and by a dedication to competence in practice and to a community of science that transcends personal interest. Patient, societal, and ethical issues are seen as matters of opinion not susceptible to rational discourse (Pellegrino; Fox, 1979).

The approach of social ecology, on the other hand, rests on a very different set of values. The social and behavioral sciences and even the humanities are here as pertinent as the biological sciences; students are selected on the basis of social concern and interest in people and their problems; emphasis is on caring as much as on curing. The community, not the university hospital, is the proper locus for the education of health professionals.

Although one can say that neither of these approaches has sought or gained exclusive dominance, their differences are important enough to generate partisan claims from each about the failures of the past, the needs of the future, and the implications for patients and society. Both the value of modern science and the critical need for enlightened social and ethical orientations can be found in the way national commissions are addressing the problems of today's healing professions (Marston and Jones).

Summary and Conclusions

The definition of the professions is the foundation of sociological analysis of the professional–patient relationship. Uniquely among modern occupations, a profession has been seen as an activity that requires extensive training based upon a continuously developing knowledge base coupled with the application of such knowledge for the general welfare of society. Therefore, although the rewards of professional life have been substantial, it is assumed that the professional is not free to exploit such skills and knowledge for personal gain alone, as other entrepreneurs may—the so-called principle of *caveat emptor* (let the buyer beware). On the contrary, the professional is granted unusual privileges involving access especially to the personal and biological privacy of patients, but only on an implicit contractual premise that such professional rights will conform to general rules of the welfare of society.

Medicine has been the primary subject of such analysis because it is seen as the archetype of professions. Virtually every person needs the help of healing occupations; the other classic professions, the law and the clergy, are not so ubiquitous. Therefore, a large sociological literature grew out of the study of medicine as a profession. However, the practice of medicine has changed radically in modern times and continues to change. Research in the biomedical sciences is usually considered the major driving force of this transformation, but changes in the social organization of the delivery of health services, the application side of the medical profession, have been no less dramatic.

In the wake of both the bioetchnological and application developments, new ethical issues have appeared and earlier ones have deepened. Bioethics as a separate discipline has grown significantly, very likely as a direct consequence of these changes. Sociology, meanwhile, has spawned its own forms of interest in medical ethics. In part, sociologists have followed the tradition of individualism, which interprets behavior as a social psychological process determined by the values individuals learn and carry with them into social encounters. A different perspective emphasizes the material technologies and organizational constraints that dominate the therapeutic relationship. For example, the bureaucratization of medicine has advanced, creating a situation in which both doctor and patient meet less as individuals than as members of groups. The resulting formalization has altered the emotional quality of the exchange and the nature of responsibility and accountability for those involved therein.

Conventional wisdom has suggested that the ethical problems of current therapeutic relationships are driven mainly by technical imperatives. Sociologists, in the main, however, have argued that bioethics is determined by the value context in which medical technology must be managed, not by the intrinsic qualities of the technology. The dilemmas—the extension of life at the sacrifice of quality of life, the increased efficiency of neonatology at the cost of disability—are seen as only part of the current medicoethical challenge. Equally important is the unequal access to the benefits of technological advancement for populations that are disadvantaged by poverty, by race, or by other sources of discrimination.

Pressures are increasing for comprehensive entitlement to medical care but, as in the past, the chances for such change remain in doubt. As analysts have noted, the proportion of national income that will be invested in healthcare is both a value judgment and a product of the political process. As a result, David Mechanic writes:

> When faced with competing claims on national resources, government finds it easier to restrain growth in programs affecting the poor and disabled, who constitute relatively weak constituencies, than to reduce subsidies shared by large, articulate, and sophisticated segments of the larger American public....The imminent risk we face is not a deterioration in medical care overall, but more a continuing erosion of access and appropriate care for our most unfortunate populations....

Between 1976 and 1984 the proportion of poor and near poor covered by the Medicaid program decreased from 65 to 52 percent. (Mechanic, 1985, p. 454)

In the pluralistic society that America epitomizes, attitudes have become polarized. At one extreme are those who view the system as basically sound and strongly support the conventional structure of medicine. At the other extreme are those "who view the delivery system as so flawed in its structure and priorities and so dominated by special interests that only major reorganization offers any promise of an equitable and effective delivery system in the future" (Mechanic, 1985, p. 190).

The struggle between these polar opposites will be strongly affected by the values that are basic to American thinking and that inevitably must be reconciled in the policy decisions that will be made. The trend at this time appears to be toward universal health insurance. The methods reinforce organizational development that fosters large corporate structures. Those who cling to the right to choose one's personal doctor, and believe that no healthcare system can function effectively otherwise, feel they have been put on the defensive against pressures for cost-effectiveness, even rationing, but nevertheless persevere in a time-honored American belief in individualism.

The contributions of sociologists, if they follow the patterns of the period since the 1940s, will continue to focus on the microrelations of medicine, especially the doctor–patient relationship (Stacey). They will also explore the ethics of human research, and issues of public policy such as equality of access to care and the role of the professions in determining the availability of medical and healthcare services (Sorenson and Swazey).

Renée Fox lists the primary values of American society as follows: individualism, contractual relations, veracity, the fair allocation of scarce resources, and the principle of benevolence. Individualism, for Fox, is "the primary value-complex on which the intellectual and moral edifice of bioethics rests" (Fox and Swazey, p. 352). It starts with a belief in the importance, uniqueness, dignity, and sovereignty of the individual. From this flows the assumption that every person has certain individual rights. Autonomy, self-determination, and privacy are fundamental. In addition, individuals are entitled to the opportunity to find, develop, and realize themselves and their self-interests. They are entitled to be and do as they see fit, so long as they do not violate the comparable rights of others.

Can these values be reconciled with the changes in modern American society, especially those that foster large organizational structures? Sociologists will certainly devote themselves to such questions, and include the fate of microrelations such as the professional–patient relationship.

SAMUEL W. BLOOM (1995)

SEE ALSO: *Autonomy; Beneficence; Care; Competence; Conscience, Rights of; Healing; Managed Care; Medical Codes and Oaths; Medicine, Anthropology of; Medicine, Profession of; Medicine, Sociology of; Nursing as a Profession; Patients' Rights; Profession and Professional Ethics;* and other *Professional-Patient Relationship* subentries

BIBLIOGRAPHY

Aiken, Linda H. 1983. "Nurses." In *The Handbook of Health, Health Care, and the Health Professions,* pp. 407–431, ed. David Mechanic. New York: Free Press.

Armstrong, David. 1982. "The Doctor-Patient Relationship: 1930–80." In *The Problem of Medical Knowledge: Examining the Social Construction of Medicine,* pp. 109–122, ed. Peter Wright and Andrew Treacher. Edinburgh: Edinburgh University Press.

Arrow, Kenneth J. 1963. "Uncertainty and the Welfare Economics of Medical Care." *American Economic Review* 53(5): 941–973.

Balint, Michael. 1964. *The Doctor, His Patient and the Illness,* 2nd edition., rev. and enl. London: Pitman Medical.

Becker, Marshall H., and Maimon, Lois A. 1983. "Models of Health-Related Behavior." In *The Handbook of Health, Health Care, and the Health Professions,* pp. 539–568, ed. David Mechanic. New York: Free Press.

Bloom, Samuel W. 1963. *The Doctor and His Patient: A Sociological Analysis.* New York: Russell Sage Foundation.

Bloom, Samuel W., and Speedling, Edward J. 1989. "The Education of Physicians: Training for What?" In *Medizin für die Medizin: Arzt und Ärztin zwischen Wissenschaft und Praxis. Festschrift für Hannes G. Pauli,* pp. 107–129, ed. Peter Saladin, Hans Jurg Schaufelberger, and Peter Schlappi. Basel: Halbing & Lichtenhahn.

Caudill, William A. 1958. *The Psychiatric Hospital as a Small Society.* Cambridge, MA: Harvard University Press.

Churchill, Edward D. 1949. "The Development of the Hospital." In *The Hospital in Contemporary Life,* ed. Nathaniel W. Faxon. Cambridge, MA: Harvard University Press.

Elstein, Arthur S.; Shulman, Lee S.; and Sprafka, Sarah A. 1978. *Medical Problem Solving: An Analysis of Clinical Reasoning.* Cambridge, MA: Harvard University Press.

Foucault, Michel. 1978. *The History of Sexuality,* tr. Robert Hurley. York: Pantheon.

Fox, Renée C. 1957. "Training for Uncertainty." In *The Student-Physician: Introductory Studies in the Sociology of Medical Education,* pp. 207–241, ed. Robert K. Merton, George G. Reader, and Patricia L. Kendall. Cambridge, MA: Harvard University Press.

Fox, Renée C. 1979. "Advanced Medical Technology—Social and Ethical Implications." In *Essays in Medical Sociology: Journeys into the Field,* pp. 413–461. New York: Wiley.

Fox, Reneé C., and Swazey, Judith P. 1984. "Medical Morality Is Not Bioethics—Medical Ethics in China and the United States." *Perspectives in Biology and Medicine* 27(3): 336–360.

Freidson, Eliot. 1961. *Patients' Views of Medical Practice: A Study of Subscribers to a Prepaid Medical Plan in the Bronx.* New York: Russell Sage Foundation.

Freidson, Eliot. 1970a. *Professional Dominance: The Social Structure of Medical Care.* New York: Aldine.

Freidson, Eliot. 1970b. *Profession of Medicine: A Study of the Sociology of Applied Knowledge.* New York: Dodd, Mead.

Goffman, Erving. 1961. *Asylums.* New York: Doubleday-Anchor.

Gouldner, Alvin W. 1970. *The Coming Crisis of Western Sociology: Essays on the Social Situation of Mental Patients and Other Inmates.* New York: Basic Books.

Great Britain. Royal Commission on Medical Education. 1968. *Royal Commission on Medical Education, 1965–1968: Report.* [Todd Report]. London: HMSO.

Henderson, Lawrence J. 1935. *Pareto's General Sociology: A Physiologist's Interpretation.* Cambridge, MA: Harvard University Press.

Henderson, Lawrence J. 1970. *On the Social System: Selected Writings,* ed. Bernard Barber. Chicago: University of Chicago Press.

Interdepartmental Committee on Medical Schools (Great Britain and Scotland). 1944. *Report of the Interdepartmental Committee on Medical Schools.* [Goodenough Report]. London: HMSO.

Kluckhohn, Florence R., and Spiegel, John P. 1954. *Integration and Conflict in Family Behavior.* Topeka, KS: Group for Advancement of Psychiatry.

Marston, Robert Q., and Jones, Roseann M., eds. 1992. *Medical Education in Transition.* Princeton, NJ: Robert Wood Johnson Foundation.

Mechanic, David. 1962. "The Concept of Illness Behavior." *Journal of Chronic Diseases* 15(2): 189–194.

Mechanic, David. 1968. *Medical Sociology: A Selective View.* New York: Free Press.

Mechanic, David. 1985. "Cost Containment and the Quality of Medical Care: Rationing Strategies in an Era of Constrained Resources." *Milbank Memorial Fund Quarterly/Health and Society* 63(3): 453–475.

Mundinger, Mary O. 1994. "Sounding Board: Advanced-Practice Nursing—Good Medicine for Physicians?" *New England Journal of Medicine* 330(3): 211–214.

Navarro, Vicente. 1975. "Social Policy Issues: An Explanation of the Composition, Nature, and Functions of the Present Health Sector of the United States." *Bulletin of the New York Academy of Medicine* 51(1): 199–234.

Parsons, Talcott. 1951. *The Social System.* New York: Free Press.

Pellegrino, Edmund D. 1978. "Medical Education." In vol. 2 of *Encyclopedia of Bioethics,* pp. 863–870. New York: Free Press.

Rosen, George, ed. 1974. *From Medical Police to Social Medicine: Essays on the History of Health Care.* New York: Science History Publications.

Roth, Julius A. 1963. *Timetables: Structuring the Passage of Time in Hospital Treatment and Other Careers.* Indianapolis, IN: Bobbs-Merrill.

Scheff, Thomas J. 1966. *Being Mentally Ill: A Sociological Theory.* Chicago: Aldine.

Sigerist, Henry Ernest. 1960. "The Physician's Profession Through the Ages." In *On the History of Medicine,* pp. 3–15, ed. Felix Marti-Ibanez. New York: MD Publications.

Sorenson, James R., and Swazey, Judith. 1989. "Sociological Perspectives on Ethical Issues in Medical and Health Care." In *Handbook of Medical Sociology,* 4th ed., pp. 492–507, ed. Howard E. Freeman and Sol Levine. Englewood Cliffs, NJ: Prentice-Hall.

Stacey, Margaret. 1985. "Medical Ethics and Medical Practice: A Social Science View." *Journal of Medical Ethics* 11(1): 14–18.

Starr, Paul. 1982. *The Social Transformation of American Medicine.* New York: Basic Books.

Suchman, Edward A. 1965. "Stages of Illness and Medical Care." *Journal of Health and Social Behavior* 6(3): 114–128.

Szasz, Thomas S. 1964. *The Myth of Mental Illness: Foundations of a Theory of Personal Conduct.* New York: Harper & Row.

Szasz, Thomas, and Hollender, Marc H. 1956. "A Contribution to the Philosophy of Medicine: The Basic Models of the Doctor-Patient Relationship." *AMA Archives of Internal Medicine* 97: 585–592.

Waitzkin, Howard. 1991. *The Politics of Medical Encounters: How Patients and Doctors Deal with Social Problems.* New Haven, CT: Yale University Press.

Waitzkin, Howard, and Waterman, Barbara. 1974. *The Exploitation of Illness in Capitalist Society.* Indianapolis, IN: Bobbs-Merrill.

Woodward, C., and Gerrard, B. 1985. "Evaluation of the Doctor-Patient Relationship." In *Assessing Clinical Competence,* ed. Vic Neufeld and Geoffrey R. Norman. New York: Springer.

III. ETHICAL ISSUES

Until recently in the history of healthcare, writing about and reflection on ethical issues in the health professional–patient relationship have focused primarily on the interactions and expectations of two individuals: a professional (traditionally, a physician) and a patient. The relationship usually is between a patient and a wide range of health professionals. Today, several basic ethical values, moral duties and rights, and virtues continue to be relevant to their interaction. The emphasis in this section of the entry is on concrete questions related to morality. Thus, enduring normative ethical foundations of the relationship as well as issues that have become relevant because of changes in the character of the relationship and the institutional settings in which it takes place will be discussed. In normative ethics, basic questions include, "What types of acts are morally right (or wrong)?" and "What are the morally praiseworthy (or blameworthy) virtues of the individuals or groups involved?"

Conduct, Virtue, and Context in the Professional-Patient Relationship

Normative ethical judgments about a relationship can be made on the basis of whether right conduct is exhibited by the parties toward each other, and whether praiseworthy character traits and dispositions (virtues) that ought to manifest themselves within the relationship are present. The context in which the relationship takes place also has moral relevance. Ethical issues can arise from any of the three.

CONDUCT-RELATED ISSUES. Issues related to morally right conduct in a relationship are understood through an examination of moral obligations and rights in the relationship. Today some of the most fundamental have been developed into general categories called *principles*. Several key principles that ought to be present in the professional–patient relationship are described later in this section.

VIRTUE-RELATED ISSUES. A second area of ethical issues is understood through an examination of the good or praiseworthy habits and dispositions of the parties in the relationship. Here the focus is less on the things people *do* and more on the types of people they *are*. Just as we can engage in reflection about ethical principles that help to elucidate right from wrong conduct, so can we make reasoned judgments about the character traits and attitudes that people ought to exhibit in a relationship. For example, we expect a person with virtue to be more disposed to honor another's values and to try to create a better community than would a person who lacks it. On this basis alone it is justifiable to place expectations of virtue on certain relationships. Some of the most basic virtues that have bearing on the professional–patient relationship also are discussed later in this section.

CONTEXTUAL CONSIDERATIONS. Issues involving judgments about the conduct and virtues that are morally appropriate may vary according to the larger social and institutional context in which the relationship takes place. One needs to assess, for example, the special peculiarities of the way in which the relationship was formed, the genesis of explicit or implicit expectations of the parties, the utility and function of the relationship, and the role of society's expectations.

A consideration of several dominant models that have been proposed to characterize this relationship will aid in the reader's understanding of the ethical issues discussed in this article.

Moral Models of the Relationship

Robert Veatch was one of the first contemporary bioethicists to seriously consider that various moral models exist. He offered four models of the physician–patient relationship: the *priestly model,* an explicitly paternalistic and value-laden approach in which the physician assumes competence not only for medical facts but also for naming and interpreting value dimensions of healthcare decisions on the patient's behalf; the *engineering model,* in which the physician acts as a scientist dealing with facts divorced from questions of value; the *collegial model,* in which physician and patient become *pals* assuming equality through mutual trust and loyalty; and the *contractual model,* which entails a mutual understanding of benefits and responsibilities incumbent on each person involved (Veatch, 1972).

In 1992, Ezekial Emanuel and Linda Emanuel, two physician bioethicists, also presented four models with some parallels, but set the context as one in which each model demonstrates the tension between patients's autonomy and their health as well as among various physician and patient values: In the *paternalistic model,* the physician independently acts on behalf of the patient's well-being; at the opposite pole, in the *informative model,* the patient receives all information and the physician serves as a technical expert only; in the *interpretive model,* the patient's life is viewed as a specific story or *narrative* from which a mutual understanding of appropriate goals and interventions are derived; and in the *deliberative model,* the physician, who provides the relevant information to the patient, also acts as a combined teacher-friend to empower the patient in ways that are consistent with the patient's health-related values.

Sheri Smith was among the first to distinguish models of the nurse–patient relationship, though others have followed. In the *surrogate mother* model, the nurse is morally obliged to assume ultimate responsibility for the well-being and care of an essentially passive patient; the *technician* model characterizes the nurse's responsibility as limited to competently applying technical knowledge and skills to meet the patient's needs; and the *contracted clinician* model defines the nurse's responsibility by the values and rights of the patient and assumes that the patient is capable of determining her or his own best interests (Smith).

In spite of important differences, the similarities among all three models are more important. They point to a progression over time from traditional paternalism to more mutuality and shared decision making. Several models support the idea of the professional as a patient (or client) advocate. The advocacy idea suggests that a patient's health-related rights must be protected and the health professional is in a unique—or at least opportune—position to protect these rights. Lively debate continues for and against adopting the advocacy idea as the central moral role of the health professional in relation to the patient (Bandman and Bandman).

U.S. law places the professional–patient relationship in the class of fiduciary relationships. In fiduciary relationships "each [person] must repose trust and confidence in the other and must exercise a corresponding degree of fairness and good faith," because the two persons cannot expect to have all of the usual facts that would allow them to contract as equals (Garner, p. 640). This law is used by the legal profession to help hold physicians (and, to varying degrees, other health professionals) accountable for the fact that they have the greater measure of power within the relationship and may not be able to equalize that power merely by disclosing relevant information to patients or their families. Trust is the bridge to the success of the relationship, and the burden is on the professional not only to engender the patient's trust but also to build a solid foundation of trustworthiness upon which the patient can depend.

The following discussion provides the reader with some basic components of ethical thought common to all of the models.

Ethical Principles in the Professional-Patient Relationship

Several ethical principles are relevant in an analysis of the professional–patient relationship and provide insight into its ethical foundations. Among the most important are respect for persons, nonmaleficence, beneficence, veracity, autonomy, and justice.

RESPECT FOR PERSONS. Respect for persons, highlighting the dignity of the patient as a person, is found in the preambles of most professional codes of ethics, mission statements of healthcare organizations, and patients's rights documents, as well as many other ethics writings. The principle assumes that persons have inherent or essential worth simply because they are human beings. Diverse philosophical, religious, and scientific understandings of the nature of persons provide a wide base upon which the health professions can ground this ideal (Lammers and Verhey). But the principle also presents challenges to health professionals: One is to discern categories of beings that are

persons; another is to discern practical direction from such a general ideal. For example, two health professionals may agree on a Judeo-Christian-Islamic interpretation that all persons have worth or dignity because they are equally children of God. They may follow the influential notion of the philosopher Immanuel Kant (1724–1804) that persons must be treated as ends and not as means to ends, yet the two may differ in their positions regarding the moral status of the fetus and come to different conclusions about whether a life-saving liver transplant should be given to a person who has an acute alcohol addiction. In spite of its difficulties, however, this principle makes a signal contribution to the understanding of the professional–patient relationship by counseling professionals against making hasty or arbitrary distinctions.

NONMALEFICENCE. The maxim to do no harm, *primum non nocere,* often is cited as the first ethical principle of medical practice. Its meaning and usefulness can be gleaned from the serious thought given to the concept in deontological (duty-oriented) approaches to moral philosophy. W. D. Ross argues that it is our stringent duty to inflict no harm intentionally, because to live in any other type of society would make each of us too vulnerable. This duty, he adds, is not covered by the duty to prevent or remove existing harm, or to do good (Ross).

The duty of nonmaleficence places the professional on alert that society reasonably expects him or her not to be an agent of harm. Debate about physician-assisted dying, euthanasia, and abortion often focuses on the interpretation of harm and the physician's, pharmacist's, nurse's or other health professional's role in participating in activities that cause harm. Discussion of maleficence must take into account that some types of harm are necessary in the name of a patient's greater good: For example, the patient undergoes the harm of the surgical knife in order to have the pathology removed.

BENEFICENCE. The principle of beneficence delineates conduct directed to the welfare of others and is pivotal in the understanding of the professional–patient relationship. Since its inception, the relationship has had its grounding in the idea that the professional's ethical priority is to further the welfare of a patient. Other worthy goals, such as furthering the knowledge about disease and its cure, or earning a just wage, or maintaining the efficiency or financial solvency of the institution, must take a lesser position on the scale of priorities.

Taken in combination with the principle of respect for persons, the principle of beneficence highlights that health professionals have a moral obligation to provide optimum care to all kinds of patients with whom they are in a professional relationship, assuming that the patient's problem lends itself to healthcare intervention and the professional is competent to treat the patient's type of condition. Therefore, the principle is put to the test when the professional is prejudiced against persons of a certain ethnicity, age, gender, religious conviction, sexual orientation, or any other characteristic, and therefore finds it difficult to give a full measure of attention to members of such groups. A health professional also may judge an individual patient *undesirable* on the basis of poor personal hygiene, irritating personality traits, or lifestyle choices. In each case, the health professional must regard the patient in the relationship as worthy of treatment however great a gulf exists between their respective values. If their differences create so great a barrier on the part of the professional that it prevents good care, he or she must attempt to assure that the patient receives it from someone else. In short, the health professional must focus on the person's needs whether the patient be model citizen or thief, old or young, man or woman, likable or not.

VERACITY. Philosophers may treat the principle of truth telling as a separate principle. More often today, however, it is conceived as derived from respect for persons (Veatch, 2003). However, treating it as a derived principle in this case only strengthens it since it is derived from such a fundamental moral premise of healthcare.

Given the moral stringency of truth telling, an interesting ethical quandary arises when it falls to the professional to convey bad news to patients and families. Health professionals long have believed that patients want professionals to help them maintain hope in the face of catastrophe. In 1932, Nicolai Hartman noted that for centuries this was interpreted as requiring the professional to protect patients from the truth at times, engaging, if necessary, in a *benevolent lie* and bearing responsibility for having breached the patient's moral expectation that veracity would be honored.

Today this belief has shifted, at least in some major subcultures of North America and Europe where the belief is that hope is enhanced by the patient's ability to take control of important life events. In other words, the fostering of hope is not dependent solely on whether the truth is shared directly with the patient. More determinative is the role of veracity in maintaining a patient's exercise of autonomy and capability to actively participate in decisions. This interpretation, however, does not necessarily lead to professional conduct consistent with it. For example, Nicholas Christakis observed that physicians tend to convey information about a poor prognosis in a way that avoids giving the worst aspects

and conforms to what the physician believes the patient's expectations are.

AUTONOMY AND SELF-DETERMINATION. In the tradition of medical ethics, discussion regarding autonomy did not focus on patient autonomy but on the professional's autonomy, the assumption being that freedom from impingement by others on his or her clinical judgment and practice was a key means to acting beneficently on behalf of the patient's best interests. However, there are numerous government regulations and other controls within healthcare today that restrict professional autonomy, causing thoughtful health professionals to worry whether they will be able to honor basic professional tenets of the professional–patient relationship.

By the beginning of the twentieth century the historical roots of libertarianism in the United States, first introduced as a political theory under the influence of such British thinkers as John Locke (1632–1704) and John Stuart Mill (1806–1873), had begun to seriously influence the character of the professional–patient relationship in the direction of honoring the patient's agency in healthcare decisions. Although related to the idea that the patient should have access to *the truth* in accordance with the principle of veracity, autonomy goes beyond that aspect.

The principle of autonomy provided a social groundwork for the introduction of the idea of patients' rights within the relationship. Applied to the patient's situation the principle evolved from being viewed as the patient's prerogative to refuse treatment to the negative right to refuse it, and finally to the positive right to play a central role in determining the course of treatment. For example, the increased emphasis on informed consent as the brokering chip in the relationship places a major focus on the patient's role as an active agent in treatment decisions. Today informed consent modes range from explicit or presumed consent in special situations to the more commonly discussed explicit consent. Moreover, in 1990 the U.S. Congress passed the Patient Self-Determination Act, which took the idea of patient autonomy as a right more deeply into the legal and life-span arenas. The law was a legislative mandate that patients have an opportunity to express their wishes about potential treatments in critical situations. This form of advance consent was buttressed through numerous cases and laws affirming use of living wills, durable power of attorney and other surrogate/proxy or substituted judgment mechanisms that are effective when the patient is unable to express his or her wishes on the spot.

In spite of the central role of patient autonomy in bioethics discourse and the medical-legal aspects of health professions' practice, lively discussion about its appropriate moral limits is growing (Schneierman).

For example, new attention is being devoted to tensions that develop when there is a serious disjuncture between the patient's expressed wishes and the professional's judgment of how best to carry out the professional obligations of beneficence and nonmaleficence. In other words, under what conditions is it morally permissible for the physician or other professional to go against the patient's informed preferences (hard paternalism) or not seek the patient's input (soft paternalism)?

The weight of moral opinion today supports at least four areas of paternalistic conduct. In the first instance the conduct is justified when the professional knows for a certainty that the intervention will harm the patient. (How *harm* is defined becomes extremely important. For instance, if death is judged an unacceptable harm the professional may engage in a kind of vitalism that imposes additional suffering on a dying patient). A second situation exists when the intervention being sought goes beyond or against the public moral mandate of medicine and the other health professions. Third, professionals need not be held hostage to patient wishes that will be of no benefit whatsoever to the patient even if it does no harm. The idea of futility, though imperfectly developed to date, is an attempt to provide criteria for setting boundaries that will prevent these potential misuses of healthcare. And fourth, a request by a patient that the professional engage in a clinically indicated and legally sanctioned option that is morally repugnant to the professional may cause moral distress for the professional and can be denied. In this case, although he or she is not morally obligated to personally participate in the intervention, the patient must be placed in the hands of another competent professional who can more sympathetically assess the patient's informed wishes.

Two critical concerns are being raised regarding the centrality of patient autonomy in the professional–patient relationship. The first addresses an increased awareness of the importance of diversity by professionals In order to meet the moral mandates of cultural sensitivity and cultural competence, the professional must have a deep understanding of how various cultures conceptualize individual, family and clan roles in regards to decision making (Hyun). In some groups the professional's insistence on the patient's individual informed consent is morally and socially antithetical to healing or other appropriate reasons for seeking out professional attention. A second concern arises in instances of high medical/clinical uncertainty. The professional's disposition to shared decision making often falters, likely due to a fear that an admission of uncertainty will undermine the patient's or family's confidence or create additional stress for them (Parascandola, Hawkins, and Danis). Both of these concerns warrant careful attention and research.

JUSTICE. The principle of justice, stated simply, is that each should get his or her due. What is *due* must be derived from the high moral standards of healthcare and the information available about what will create the most benefit. At the level of the professional–patient relationship, this has several implications. First, its relationship to beneficence is apparent: The patient can expect to be treated fairly. Persons seeking treatment should not be given advantage on the basis of arbitrary favoritism or be left out on the basis of arbitrary dislike. The rules will be applied consistently, taking into account legitimate departures from the norm. For instance, a procedural rule of first come, first served will be applied except in cases where greater need morally requires that the rule be flexible enough to allow for valid exceptions.

The principle of justice raises important ethical issues related to the allocation of scarce resources. Health professionals abide by a duty of beneficence, but that duty does not entail the prerogative of automatically providing a disproportionate amount of a scarce resource to any one person, even if that person's need could warrant receiving all of it. The resulting allocation may have a relatively deleterious effect on one or more other patients because their optimum benefits are compromised. For example, a nursing shortage on a unit may require the nurses to make difficult (though not arbitrary) decisions about patient-care priorities.

Compensation for harm also derives from our understanding of what justice requires. A patient who is harmed in the relationship through, say, professional error, has a right to know that the harm has occurred and may wish to seek compensation for the harm.

Serious barriers to justice often arise outside of the relationship. Societal discrimination against patients on the basis of race, ethnicity, religion, sex, and age are well documented, and continue to contribute to serious disparities in the distribution of U.S. healthcare benefits and burdens in spite of legislation designed to prevent them (Garner). Other barriers are imposed by today's bureaucratic context of healthcare: institutional mechanisms and societal arrangements designed to foster efficiency, profit, or other goals, but not the patient's well-being (Stein). The relationship does not stand in isolation from these influences, all of which have profound effects on it.

The health professional who is committed to upholding the profession's moral ideals must work not only to preserve justice within the relationship directly but also to remove barriers to it on a broader scale so that the appropriate ends of healthcare can be realized.

Conflicts among Principles

As illustrated by the issue of paternalism in truth-telling situations and the compromise of beneficence in situations of scarce resources, conflicts among this set of general principles inevitably arise in everyday professional–patient relationship situations. In actual situations, professionals usually can use the basic moral ideas imbedded in the principles as guides to set priorities consistent with the values of healthcare, the professions's moral codes and standards, and patients's informed preferences. At the same time, not all conflicts can be resolved and sometimes principles seem to remove us a step further from the immediacy of the situation.

Virtue in the Professional-Patient relationship

Cognizant of the limitations in an ethics based entirely on conduct, Aristotle in *Nichomachean Ethics* suggested the alternative of a focus on *virtues* by those who are decision-makers so that they approach moral conflict in the right frame of mind and heart. A life of moral virtue is characterized by dispositions and attitudes that can be cultivated into habits of preparedness that enable a person to act in ways that further the good of a relationship or community. Aristotle also underscored the importance of the person's desire to become a good person, which in turn requires knowledge of ultimate goods and ends. Aristotle did not divorce virtue from the realm of feelings and emotions, suggesting instead that acts arising out of various dispositions will give pleasure and that, at the same time, ethical action resulting from a virtuous disposition requires the exercise of reason.

Since the late twentieth century, several leading ethicists have led a lively re-examination of the virtues that should be expressed by health professionals. Notable among them are Edmund Pellegrino and David Thomasma who propose that the contemporary reappraisal is not an attempt to demean the emphasis on rights-and-duty-based ethics, "but a recognition that rights and duties notwithstanding, their moral effectiveness still turns on dispositions and character traits of our fellow men and women" (Pellegrino and Thomasma, p. 113).

A challenge throughout the ages has been to identify dispositions that the professional should cultivate so as to further the good and proper ends of healthcare. Many virtues have been proposed, among them benevolence and kindliness, compassion, integrity, honesty, fairness, conscientiousness, fidelity beyond duty, and humility.

These virtues are as appropriate in today's professional–patient relationship as they have always been. However, some things about the relationship are understood differently today than in the past, and our understanding of human relationships in general continues to undergo new evaluation. It is not surprising that our understanding of the virtues also continues to evolve. The following two illustrations of this evolution by no means exhaust the important work that is being conducted in this area.

BENEVOLENCE AND CONSIDERATIONS OF TRUST. The traditional professional virtue of benevolence or kindness has enjoyed a long history in the writings on the professional–patient relationship. This character trait evokes pictures of a physician, midwife, or nurse sitting quietly at the bedside, reassuring a patient, an image consistent with a period in which the professional was viewed as a kindly person who used the limited technologies available to minister to the clinical and emotional needs of a trusting, mostly passive patient. Today the notion of benevolence must be refined to adapt to a relationship in which patients are active participants in the interaction, suggesting that kindness met by blind trust taken alone are not adequate ingredients for the tasks of this relationship to be accomplished. At the very least an adequate notion of professional benevolence today must include an examination of how the professional's trustworthiness figures in the professional–patient relationship.

For example, traditionally confidentiality focused on the physician's duty. To the extent that the physician had cultivated a benevolent disposition toward the patient, the duty would come more naturally. Today the moral focus has shifted to the patient, particularly to his or her right to expect confidentiality. Only trustworthiness based on the professional's authentic commitment to respecting the patient's rights and dignity assures the patient that he or she is in the hands of a benevolent professional.

Benevolence as traditionally understood is challenged further by a revitalized emphasis on professionalism in the medical profession. In this broader conceptualization benevolence commitments explicitly include competence, honesty, confidentiality, maintenance of appropriate boundaries, improvement of the quality of and access to care, and management of conflicts of interest, to name some. Moreover, a rise in the literature on such dimensions of the physician's moral role as that of dealing positively with professionals' errors (Kohn et al.) and fatigue (Gaba and Howard) are expanding the scope of what benevolence entails today.

COMPASSION AND CONSIDERATIONS OF CARING. Compassion also has long been viewed as a virtue that should characterize the professional–patient relationship. Compassion often has been interpreted according to its etymological root, "to suffer with." Theories vary about what, exactly, this means in the healthcare context, but one central theme is that healing is enhanced when professionals exhibit a disposition and ability to sympathize deeply with the patient's plight. The cultivation of this disposition leads the professional to recognize that the key issue is not only "Have I done my duty?" (e.g., truth telling) but also "Have I been sensitive to the effect my approach will have?" (e.g., how, when, by whom, and where this information should be disclosed). The central notion of *caring* in the professional–patient relationship sheds light on important ways in which the virtue of compassion might manifest itself in the everyday work of professionals. Among contemporary bioethicists Warren Reich makes an important contribution to the understanding of compassion by relating different modes of compassion to different phases of a patient's suffering. Care in the relationship between health professional and patient also has been seen as an activity that reflects an attitude of sensitivity to the patient's deepest values and concerns.

Anne Bishop and John Scudder propose that "Being compassionate is not something that human beings can achieve by an act of will. It is possible, however, to be open to compassion, to be situated so that compassion is likely to be evoked…" (p. 81). They conclude that professionals who do not feel compassion but have a deep desire to show caring (i.e., *feel called to care*) can actually express care by a focus on fostering the patient's well-being as well as a commitment to full participation in being an excellent practitioner. In some current approaches to professional care, compassion or other virtues are not invoked at all; rather the emphasis turns exclusively to conduct and behaviors that various professions describe as *caring behaviors* with the goal of incorporating them into an assessment of measurable outcomes in patient management (Galt). This latter approach diverges dramatically from the traditional and most contemporary research on the role of care and its relationship to compassion in the larger ethical context of the professional–patient relationship. There have also been serious caveats raised about a professional ethic based primarily on the concept of care.

Aware of problems created by sexism, and that caring and the care-giving role are associated with women, social devaluation of professions that promote care as a centerpiece of their identity could follow to the patient's detriment (Nelson). Therefore, when a health professional expresses care to a patient he or she may also appear to condone injustices that derive from being in a society that devalues women in a care-giving role (Condon). At the same time,

recipients of care may be forced into stereotyped roles of *dependency*. Eva Feder Kittay calls for a reassessment of the dichotomy often viewed as existing between caregiver and care receiver. Clearly, the role of care and its relationship to compassion warrants continued attention.

Existential Dimensions of the Patient's Experience: Implications for the Professional-Patient Relationship

The existential dimensions of the patient's experience also deserve consideration in the relationship. *Existential,* as used here, refers to the human quest for meaning in the face of our limitations, among them illness and death. Especially significant are new insights regarding the health professional's role in exploring the existential meaning of illness for a patient.

One aspect of the exploration has focused on the professional's desire and ability to individualize the patient's situation and story: Respect in the relationship rests on a premise that health professionals are called into a particular relationship with patients because of the importance of the illness experience to the patient, and the medium of that relationship is the patient's story (Purtilo and Haddad). The notion of patients's *patterns* is the term used by Margaret Newman to describe what has value—is meaningful—in a patient's life. The professional's skill in helping the patient recognize aspects of him- or herself that the person may not even be conscious of is the professional's act of *pattern recognition.* The professional, acting as facilitator, can show how the pieces fit. Once identified, professional and patient can work together toward mutually agreed upon health goals. Bishop and Scudder capture the essence of the professional's position in this task as being a *caring presence,* a "personal presence that assures others of another's concern for their well-being" (Bishop and Scudder, p. 41).

Narratives, the patient's and the professional's, are the professional's means of gaining insight into the existential complexities of the professional–patient relationship (Greenhalgh and Horwitz). Sociologist Arthur W. Frank, drawing partially on his own illness experiences (from *patienthood* to *survivorship* roles), powerfully illustrates how the moral responsibility of survivorship is to reconstruct, *put back together,* a life that had been altered by interventions and professional interactions. Through that process the wounded also becomes healer, but the process requires the mutual effort of professional and patient. When the professional, through narrative, shows to the patient a personality with emotions, likes and dislikes, fears and dreams, hopes and faults, the patient has a greater opportunity to understand that there is a *person* in the professional role, not just a bundle of competencies and technical skills. The patient becomes more trusting that his or her own personality has a chance of being taken seriously (Purtilo).

Howard Brody, a physician bioethicist, notes that the challenge does not lie only in the professional's desire and willingness to hear and respect the patient's story. Even those who are so disposed may meet barriers because both professional and patient believe that the professional holds the key to knowing the *real problem* (i.e., the medical problem). The power differential built into the structure of the relationship means that the professional is believed to be empowered to impute the *real* meaning of the patient's story. A concentrated effort must be made to overcome such a barrier (Brody). Merging from such thinking and reflection on the existential aspects of the relationship and its key members are new materials for refining their encounter, new ethical dimensions to build on the traditional foundations of moral obligations, rights, and virtues. The healing quest will be for the discovery of the patient's lost or changed self, not just for removal of a disease that resides in that person, and the recognition that in the deepest sense each party is affected by the relationship.

Mechanisms for Resolving Ethical Conflict in the Professional-Patient Relationship

Ethical issues in the professional–patient relationship are receiving more attention in the everyday environments of healthcare. Inevitably, differences in judgment, even deeply held differences, arise between professional and patient (or the patient's family). *Conflict* does not always denote a feeling of animosity. Often it signals a frustration shared by all involved in not knowing the best way to proceed.

There are several mechanisms designed to assist patients in such situations. First, the patient representative or patient ombudsperson is an employee of the provider institution who is charged with being available to patients and their families when dissatisfaction or questions arise. This advocate may learn that a patient or family believes that the patient is being harmed by receiving substandard treatment. While not all such situations involve ethical issues, many do. The advocate may act as a direct liaison between the parties or may refer the issue to one of the other mechanisms designed to provide assistance.

Second, ethics consultants are being hired by many major hospitals. Their charge is to deal with ethical issues regarding patient-care decisions. Depending on the institution, the ethics consultation service may be accessed by the physician, nurse or other professional, patient, or patient's family. Usually the consultant meets with all the relevant parties to help them identify the ethical issues involved,

reason about the issues, and make recommendations for how to weigh conflicting priorities. The consultant does not make the final decision, which is correctly left to be decided within the professional–patient relationship.

Third, clinical ethics committees are present in many healthcare environments. Usually multidisciplinary, they function in a manner similar to the ethics consultant. Sometimes an ethics consultant will be called first, and if he or she thinks that the issue merits further deliberation by several different disciplines and personalities, may call the ethics committee together.

Everyone would agree that whenever possible, prevention is the best approach to moral conflict in a professional or institutional setting. The professional's diligence in communication, technical competence, and caring are keys to conflict prevention, as well as powerful instruments for resolution of conflict when it does occur in the professional–patient relationship.

RUTH B. PURTILO (1995)
REVISED BY AUTHOR

SEE ALSO: *Authority; Autonomy; Beneficence; Care; Compassionate Love; Confidentiality; Conflict of Interest; Informed Consent; Justice; Medical Codes and Oaths; Medicine, Art of; Narrative; Paternalism; Profession and Professional Ethics; Rights, Human; Trust; Virtue and Character;* and other *Professional-Patient Relationship* subentries

BIBLIOGRAPHY

ABIM Foundation. 2002. "Medical Professionalism in the New Millenium: A Physicians Charter. ABIM Foundation. American Board of Internal Medicine. ACP-ASIM Foundation. American College of Physicians-American Society of Internal Medicine. European Federation of Internal Medicine." *Annals of Internal Medicine* 136: 243–246.

Bandman, Elsie, and Bandman, Betran. 2002. "Models of Professional Relationships." In *Nursing Ethics through the Lifespan,* 4th edition. Upper Saddle River, NJ: Pearson Education, Inc.

Bishop, Ann, and Scudder, John. 2001. "Caring Presence." In *Nursing Ethics: Holistic Caring Practice,* 2nd edition. Sudbury, Canada: Jones and Bartlett.

Brody, Howard. 2002. *Stories of Sickness,* 2nd edition. New York: Oxford University Press

Christakis, Nicholas A. 1999. *Death Foretold: Prophecy and Prognosis in Medical Care.* Chicago: University of Chicago Press.

Condon, Esther H. 1991. "Nursing and the Caring Metaphor: Gender and Political Influences on and Ethics of Care." *Nursing Outlook* 40(1): 14–19.

Emanuel, Ezekiel J., and Emanuel, Linda L. 1992. "Four Models of the Physician-Patient Relationship." *Journal of the American Medical Association.* 267(16): 221–225.

Frank, Arthur W. 1995. *The Wounded Story Teller: Body, Illness and Ethics.* Chicago: University of Chicago Press.

Gaba, David M., and Howard, Steven K. 2002. "Fatigue among Clinicians and the Safety of Patients." *New England Journal of Medicine* 347(16): 1249–1255.

Galt, Kimberly A. 2000. "The Need to Define *Care* in Pharmaceutical Care: An Examination across Research, Practice and Education." *American Journal of Pharmaceutical Education* 64: 223–233.

Garner, Bryan A., ed. 1999. *Blacks Law Dictionary.* 7th edition. St. Paul, Minnesota: West Group.

Greenhalgh, T., and Hurwitz, B. 1998. "Why Study Narrative?" In *Narrative Based Medicine: Dialogue and Discourse in Clinical Practice,* ed. T. Greenhalgh and B. Hurwitz. London: BMJ Books.

Hartman, Nicolai. 1932. "Truthfulness and Uprightness." In *Ethics,* vol.2, tr. Stanton Coit. New York: Humanities Press.

Hyun, Insoo. 2002. "Waiver of Informed Consent, Cultural Sensitivity, and the Problem of Unjust Families and Traditions." *Hasting Center Report* 32(5): 14–22.

Kittay, Eva Feder. 2000. *Loves Labor: Essays on Women, Equality and Dependency.* New York: Routledge Press.

Kohn, L. T.; Corrigan, J. M.; and Donaldson, M. S., eds. 2000. *To Err is Human: Building a Safer Health System.* Washington, D.C.: National Academy Press.

Lammers, Stephen E., and Verhay, Allen, eds. 1998. *On Moral Medicine: Theological Perspectives in Medical Ethics,* 2nd edition. Grand Rapids, MI: William B. Eerdmans.

May, William F. 2000. *The Physician's Covenant: Images of the Healer in Medical Ethics.* Lexington, KY: Westminster/John Know Press.

Nelson, Hilde Lindemann. 1992. "Against Caring." *Journal of Clinical Ethics* 3(1): 8–15.

Newman, Margaret A. 2002. "The Pattern That Connects." *Advances in Nursing Science* 24(3): 1–7.

Parascandola, Mark; Hawkins, Jennifer; and Danis, Marion. 2002. "Patient Autonomy and the Challenge of Clinical Uncertainty." *Kennedy Institute of Ethics Journal.* 12(3): 245–264.

Pellegrino Edmund, and Thomasma, David. 1993. *The Virtues in Medical Practice.* New York: Oxford University Press.

Purtilo, Ruth B. 1999. *Ethical Dimensions in the Health Professions,* 3rd edition. Philadelphia: W. B. Saunders.

Purtilo, Ruth B., and Haddad, Amy M. 2002. *Health Professional and Patient Interaction,* 6th edition. Philadelphia: W.B. Saunders.

Reich, Warren T. 1989. "Spreading of Suffering: A Moral Account of Compassion." *Soundings* 72: 83–108.

Ross, William D. 1930. *The Right and the Good.* Oxford: Clarendon Press.

Schneider, Carl 1998. *The Practice of Autonomy: Patients, Doctors, and Medical Decisions.* New York: Oxford University Press.

Smedley, Brian D.; Stith, Adrienne Y.; and Nelson, Alan R., eds. 2002. *Unequal Treatment: Confronting Racial and Ethnic Disparities in Health Care.* Washington, D.C.: National Academy Press.

Smith, Sheri. 1980. "Three Models of the Nurse-Patient Relationship." In *Nursing: Images and Ideals: Opening Dialogue with the Humanities,* ed. Stuart Spicker and Sally Gadow. New York: Springer.

Stein, Janice G. 2001. *The Gulf of Efficiency.* Toronto: Anansi.

Veatch, Robert M. 1972. "Models for Ethical Medicine in a Revolutionary Age." *Hastings Center Report* 2(3): 5–7.

Veatch, Robert M. 2003. *The Basics of Bioethics,* 2nd edition. Upper Saddle River, NJ: Prentice Hall.

PROFESSION AND PROFESSIONAL ETHICS

• • •

Among any society's most important institutions are the social structures by which the society controls the use of specialized knowledge and skills. This is particularly true when highly valued aspects of human life depend on such expertise, and all the more so if acquiring such expertise requires lengthy theoretical education and intensive training in its practical application under the supervision of those already expert, thus rendering the knowledge and skill in its application unavoidably exclusive.

Social control over the use of such knowledge and skills is important because the members of the expert group could use their exclusive expertise solely for their own benefit or even hold society hostage to their expertise. But those who might exert such control, if they are outside the expert group, cannot depend on their understanding of this expertise precisely because they lack the relevant knowledge and practical training. How, then, can a society control the use of important, specialized expertise and render those outside the expert group secure so that they will be able to enjoy the values that depend on it? One of the most important social structures developed to this end is the institution of profession.

In many people's minds, it is by publicly taking an oath that a person becomes a professional and acquires specifically professional obligations; and indeed the term *profession* does come to us from the Latin *professio* that comes in turn from the Greek verb *prophaino,* "to declare publicly." But it is not the oath that classically concludes professional training that creates professionals or produces their special obligations. It is in their presenting themselves to others as possessors and practitioners of a profession's expertise that they *declare publicly* that they are members of a profession and accept its ethical commitments as their own. The oath that many new professionals take is rather a reminder to those beginning professional practice that important ethical commitments go with it and a public assurance to the larger community by the new practitioners that they understand and accept this reality.

In the minds of many mature professionals, it was not the formal oath nor any other public activity that made them professionals, but rather their personal sense of vocation, of a calling or of being called, to this way of life. There is something truly admirable in this view of profession because professional practice is ethically challenging enough that only those with a deep sense of personal ethical commitment will manage its challenges well. But it would be a serious mistake to put all the focus on the person of the committed professional and none on the important social systems in which such a person functions. First, the content of the ethic of each profession—that is, the ethic that the committed professional is called to practice—is the content of an ongoing dialogue between the profession as a whole and the larger community within which it practices. Second, every professional's practice is necessarily practice in conjunction with someone served, frequently a capable, independent decision maker and always someone whose well-being is not fully defined by the values of the profession. The vocation or calling of the committed professional is precisely a social vocation, a calling to ethical relationships with those served in the context of the whole profession's proper relationship to the larger community.

The practice of specialized expertise and the special moral commitments associated with professional practice are what most differentiate a profession from other occupations. All the ways in which people spend their time earning a living involve skills and knowledge of value to others and involve relationships with others that have ethical significance, at a minimum the prohibition of coercion and the requirement that people honor their contracts that characterizes marketplace relationships. But the analysis just offered indicates that specifically professional practice involves a particular combination of institutionalized expertise and special ethical obligations over and above the obligations of the marketplace. It is these characteristics taken together that differentiate professions from other occupations.

The Key Features of a Profession

A few social philosophers and a large number of sociologists, following Émile Durkheim (1858–1917), a Frenchman, and Talcott Parsons (1902–1979), an American, have studied the institution of profession in depth and have attempted to identify its essential elements. This is not easy because so many groups have been eager to appropriate the title of profession in order to enjoy the social rewards that go with it. In addition, the terms *profession* and *professional* have both normative and descriptive uses in ordinary discourse. Nevertheless, by looking for common features among the most obvious examples of this institution, such as medicine, law, and dentistry, a useful listing of characteristic features is possible.

IMPORTANT AND EXCLUSIVE EXPERTISE. For an occupational group to be a profession, it must provide its clients with something the larger community judges extremely valuable, either because of its intrinsic value or because it is a necessary precondition of any person's achievement of valued goals, or both. Health and the preservation of life, to take two commonly identified goals of the health professions, are held by almost everyone to be values of the highest order, either as intrinsic values or as necessary preconditions of people's achievement of whatever else they value. In a similar way, security of one's property and person against the errors of others and against the adverse workings of government and the legal system, as one defensible description of the goal of the legal profession, is also widely valued as a precondition of achieving whatever other goals one has.

The expertise of a profession has both cognitive (theoretical and factual) and practical (the fruits of experiential learning) components that are of sufficient subtlety and complexity that only persons who have been specifically and extensively educated in them, by persons already expert, can be depended upon to bring about the relevant benefits for those whom the occupation serves. In the practical division of a society's labors, this makes possession of such expertise exclusive to a relatively small group.

Moreover, for the same reason, only persons fully educated in both knowledge and practice of a profession's expertise can be relied on to judge correctly the need for expert intervention in a given situation or to judge the quality of such an intervention as it is being carried out. Such judgments by those not so trained are not dependable. Because of the importance of what is at stake, it is not sufficient to judge the performance solely on the basis of its long-term outcomes, even when the nonexpert can accomplish such a judgment unaided. Long-term outcomes will not be known for some time, and the risk of negative consequences in the meantime, in a matter of great importance, is too great.

The expertise of a profession involves not only specialized and complex knowledge, both theoretical and practical, but also the application of this knowledge. This is the reason that mastery of a profession's expertise requires experiential as well as cognitive education. This is also why the members of a profession are said to "practice" its expertise. A profession is not made up simply of experts; it is made up of practitioners of a body of expertise.

INTERNAL AND EXTERNAL RECOGNITION. A profession, as an occupational group made exclusive by reason of its particular body of expertise, is also characterized by a set of internal relationships of which the most important is a mutual recognition of expertise on the part of its members. These internal relationships may remain informal or may become quite formal, as when a community of experts who mutually recognize each other's expertise establishes a formal organization. The expression "the profession of medicine" thus refers most properly to all those expert in the practice of medicine, mutually recognized as such by one another, within whatever geographic limits are relevant. This same expression is also used, however, to refer either to the chief national organization of such persons, the American Medical Association (AMA), or to some larger set of associations, including the AMA, to which physicians would likely belong. Nevertheless, it is not the formal character of association among experts, but the fact of their mutual recognition of expertise, that is most important here. Other expressions—for example, "organized medicine"—are available to refer to formally constituted groups.

The expertise of a profession is also recognized by the members of the larger community. This recognition may remain quite informal, or the external recognition of a profession's expertise may be expressed in formal actions of the larger community, such as certification, licensure, and so on, that confer formal authority in matters of the profession's expertise to an organized group of professionals. A group may be given, for example, exclusive authority to determine the degree of expertise needed by those who intend to practice it and to test the expertise of those who wish to do so. Such authorization often includes a grant of exclusive authority to train and certify new members of the profession as well. But, as with internal recognition, it is the reality of the community's recognition of the group's expertise that is essential to the character of a profession, not the degree to which it has been formalized.

AUTONOMY IN MATTERS OF EXPERT PRACTICE. Because the activity of a profession is so valued by those it serves, and because proper performance and dependable judgments about performance depend upon expertise that is unavoidably exclusive and therefore not available to the ordinary person, those served by a profession routinely grant its members extensive autonomy in the performance of the profession's practice. The term *autonomy* has a number of important uses in moral discourse and often appears when issues in bioethics are under discussion. Here, however, this term refers specifically to the acceptance by others of professionals' judgments as determinative on any matter that is within the range of the relevant profession's expertise. Such autonomy can characterize three kinds of judgments by professionals.

First, such according of autonomy depends on the assumption that each member of the expert community possesses the relevant professional expertise and is therefore a dependable provider of its benefits. Professional autonomy here extends to three arenas of professional practice: (1) determining the specific needs of the person seeking services in matters within the range of the profession's expertise; (2) determining the likely outcomes of various courses of action that might be undertaken in response to these needs; and (3) judging which of the possible courses of action is most likely to best meet these needs.

Consider, for example, the encounter between a physician or a dentist and a patient. The patient often accepts without question the doctor's judgments regarding these three things: (1) the nature of the patient's present condition and of the patient's need for care, if any (diagnosis); (2) the possible courses of action that might be undertaken in response and their likely outcomes (prognosis); and (3) the likelihood that one of these courses of action will meet the patient's needs better than the others (treatment recommendation).

In addition to these items, professionals also make judgments about the intermediate, instrumental steps involved in carrying out the chosen course of action. But these judgments can be and frequently are relegated to another party, such as a technician. Such a person, while capable of making judgments about properly applying instrumental actions already identified as needed, is not necessarily capable of dependably judging the need for these actions or which of the possible actions will best meet the need.

Although those who seek professional services ordinarily grant autonomy of this sort to the professional, they do not ordinarily do so simply on the basis of their individual judgments of the expertise of the individual professional. Instead they make their judgments on the basis of a more complex set of factors including the community's (external) recognition of the professional group's expertise and the professional group's (internal) recognition of the expertise of the particular professional. Thus, even though this grant of professional autonomy ordinarily takes place principally in the interaction of an individual in need and a particular professional, its full meaning can be understood only against the social background of the institution of profession.

A second kind of judgment sometimes accorded autonomy by the larger community concerns the various features of the situation in which the encounter between professional and the person seeking professional services takes place. Professionals often seek and the larger community and individuals seeking professional service often grant professionals considerable additional autonomy in determining the immediate circumstances of their practice.

The extent of this aspect of professional autonomy depends on answers to two questions: What aspects of the immediate circumstances of practice significantly affect the quality of professional performance? And what additional factors do members of the profession also prefer to control, either for their convenience or out of a conviction, possibly unexamined or even mistaken, that they affect the quality of professional performance?

For example, physicians, not their patients, typically control much of the daily routine of medical practice. In the marketplace, this control could easily be explained as the producers' control of the product they offer. But physicians ordinarily justify such preferred patterns on the grounds that they maximize their service to their patients. Patients in turn typically change their daily schedules accordingly even if they are doubtful that the inconveniences they accept are in fact the only way that physicians can best serve all of their patients.

Third, professionals' ability to make dependable judgments for their clients is also conditioned by other, still more remote situational factors over which professionals may seek, and the larger community may grant, some measure of control. To an even greater degree than autonomy in making practice judgments and in controlling the immediate circumstances of practice, autonomy of this third kind is ordinarily granted not to individual members of a profession but to organized groups of professionals.

For example, physicians' opposition to health insurance programs in the middle of the twentieth century and their later opposition to federally funded healthcare programs for the needy were efforts to preserve the medical community's then-preferred economic structure for healthcare distribution, namely, the fee-for-service marketplace. At one time, physicians also exercised almost total control over hospitals in the United States. They believed that their preferred economic and institutional arrangements for hospitals were the best way to produce healthcare for their patients. For a

number of years, the larger community accepted this rationale and granted physicians a great deal of control of healthcare economics and healthcare institutions, with dramatic changes in this regard coming only in the last decade of the twentieth century. Regarding these changes, however, note that the lessening of physicians' control of these aspects of healthcare has not entailed any lessening of the professional autonomy of physicians in matters central to their expertise, the first category of professional autonomy discussed above.

THE OBLIGATIONS OF PROFESSIONS AND PROFESSIONALS. The final and, for present purposes, the most important feature of the institution of profession is that membership in a profession implies the acceptance by its members of a set of ethical standards of professional practice. Contrasting what may be termed a "normative" picture of a profession with what may be termed a "commercial" picture may make this point clear.

According to the commercial picture, practicing a profession is no different in principle from selling one's wares in the marketplace. The professional has a product to sell and makes the appropriate and needed agreements with interested purchasers. Beyond some fundamental obligation not to coerce, cheat, or defraud others, the professional would have no other obligations to anyone except those voluntarily undertaken with specific individuals or groups. According to the commercial picture, in other words, there are no specifically professional values or obligations in any profession. There is nothing to which a person is obligated precisely because she is a professional.

Some commentators consider the commercial picture to be an accurate description of what professions are like, whereas others maintain that professionals or the community at large would be better off if professions conformed to this view more thoroughly (Sade; Kuskey). But recall that all professional groups have a corner on some valuable form of knowledge within a society. Wherever this is the case, there is power—power to control the knowledge itself and, especially, power over the aspects of human life that depend upon this knowledge. Now compare how various powerful groups are dealt with in U.S. society. Contrast professionals with politicians, for example.

Experience has taught that politicians will be tempted to misuse their power. Consequently, Americans want to keep a close eye on them. This is arguably one reason why Americans accept without too much complaint the terribly inefficient system of periodic reelection, to take one example—the system enables the populace to keep close watch over those with political power. This may also be why Americans tolerate the excesses of a free press, because a free press means that it will be that much harder for politicians to misuse their power.

But the professions, though they do face some measure of regulation through licensing boards and the like, are subjected to remarkably little oversight in U.S. society. In fact, even when there is regulation, professions are generally regulated by their own members, not the larger community. How does the community assure itself that the power of the professions will not be misused? The answer is: by means of the institutions of professional obligation.

When a person enters a profession, he undertakes obligations, obligations whose content has been worked out and is continually being affirmed or adjusted through an ongoing dialogue between the expert group and the larger community. In other words, there are conventional obligations, over and above obligations incurred in other human relationships, that both individuals and groups have simply because they are members of a profession. Professions and professionals have obligations, and the content of these obligations for each profession comprise the "professional ethics" of that profession. In this way, the way in which a profession functions within the larger community is inherently normative. That is, the institution of profession is such that for each profession there are ethical standards that apply both to the actions of the whole professional group and to the actions of each member of the profession.

The Chief Categories of Professional Norms

Although most professions have articulated a code of ethics or other statement of the norms of their professional practice, such statements are never complete or fully authoritative. They are, at best, good partial representations of the content of the profession's norms and obligations. The full content of these norms is the fruit of an ongoing dialogue between the expert group and the larger community, on whose recognition of expertise and grant of professional autonomy the expert group depends for its status as a profession. Therefore, the effort to answer such questions as "What professional norms apply to this situation?" and "What is a member of this profession obligated to do in this situation?" must include asking what the larger community understands those norms and obligations to be, rather than looking only at the views of the professional group or some organization(s) within it.

Determining a profession's norms is therefore a much subtler enterprise than it might seem. Even the well-known moral categories of autonomy, beneficence, maleficence, and justice are only a useful starting point. Another way to examine a profession's norms is in terms of nine categories of

professional obligation that have been identified from studies of numerous professional groups (Ozar and Sokol). Each of these categories provides a set of questions about a profession's norms for use in personal reflection on one's obligations, in scholarly study, and in professional ethics education.

Briefly stated, the nine categories of questions about professional obligation are:

1. Who is (are) this profession's chief client(s)?
2. What are the central values of this profession?
3. What is the ideal relationship between a member of this profession and a client?
4. What sacrifices are required of members of this profession and in what respects do the obligations of this profession take priority over other morally relevant considerations affecting its members?
5. What are the norms of competence for this profession?
6. What is the ideal relationship between the members of this profession and co-professionals?
7. What is the ideal relationship between the members of this profession and the larger community?
8. What ought the members of this profession do to make access to the profession's services available to everyone who needs them?
9. What are the members of this profession obligated to do to preserve the integrity of their commitment to its values and to educate others about them?

THE CHIEF CLIENT. Every profession has a chief client or clients, which is a category or categories of persons whose well-being the profession and its members are chiefly committed to serving. (The English language does not have a satisfactory generic noun to refer to the person or class of persons whom a profession serves. *Beneficiary* is etymologically correct but is clumsy and typically associated with trusts or insurance. *Client* is too commercial in its connotations, but it seems better than any other term for present purposes.)

For some professions, the identification of the chief client seems quite easy. Surely, one might say, the chief client of a physician and a nurse, for example, is the patient. But who is the chief client of a lawyer? Is it simply the party whose case the lawyer represents or to whom the lawyer gives advice? Lawyers are told and they announce in their self-descriptions and codes of conduct that they have obligations to the whole justice system; therefore, there are things that they as professionals may not ethically do, even if doing them would advance the situation of the party they represent or advise. So it appears that the answer to the question about the chief client of the legal profession is complex, involving not only the persons lawyers represent or advise but also the whole justice system and/or perhaps the whole larger community served by that system.

Once this sort of complexity about the chief client is noticed, even those cases that initially appear simple prove more complex. The physician and the nurse must attend not only to the patient before them, for example, but also to those in the waiting room or to the other patients on the hospital unit, and so on. In fact, they have some obligations to all the patients in the institution where they work, or to all their patients of record if they are in private practice. They also have significant obligations to the public as a whole; for example, they are obligated to practice with caution so as not to spread infection from patients they are caring for either to themselves or to other patients.

In all cases, this question about the chief client is one of the first questions that must be asked if a particular profession's obligations are to become clear: Whom does the profession principally serve?

THE CENTRAL VALUES OF THE PROFESSION. Every profession is focused only on certain aspects of the well-being of its clients. The professions' rhetoric to the contrary, no professional group is expected by the larger community to be expert in their clients' whole well-being or to secure for its clients everything that is of value to them. There is, rather, a certain set of values that are the focus of each profession's expertise, and it is the job and obligation of that profession to work to secure these values for its clients. These values can be called the profession's central values.

Most professions are committed to pursuing more than one central value for clients. For example, whatever other values are central for a given profession, the value of client autonomy is ordinarily a central value as well. Efficiency in the use of resources may have a similar standing. In any case, if there is more than one central value for a given profession, the question can then be asked whether these values are all equal in rank, or whether the members of the profession are committed to choosing them in some ranked order when they cannot all be realized at once.

For example, the values proposed as the central values that the dental profession is committed to pursuing for its patients, in order of decreasing importance, are: life and general health; oral health (understood as appropriate and pain-free oral functioning); patient autonomy (i.e., patient control), whenever practicable, over what happens to her body; preferred patterns of dental practice; aesthetic considerations; and efficiency in the use of resources (Ozar and Sokol).

Every profession needs to ask and answer the question: What are its central values? What specific aspects of human well-being is it the task of each member of this profession to secure for clients? And if there are more than one, which takes precedence?

THE IDEAL RELATIONSHIP BETWEEN PROFESSIONAL AND CLIENT. The point of the relationship between a professional and a client is to bring about certain values for the client that cannot be achieved without the expertise of the professional. To achieve this, the professional and the client must both make a number of judgments and choices about the professional's interventions. This third category of professional norms addresses the proper roles of the professional and the client as they make these judgments and choices.

At least four general models of such relationships can be distinguished:

1. In a "commercial model," only the minimal morality of the marketplace governs. In other words, neither party has any obligations beyond a general prohibition on coercion and fraud, unless and until individuals freely contract together to be obligated toward each other in specific additional ways.

2. In a "guild model," the emphasis is on the professional's expertise and the client's lack of it, so that the professional alone is the active member in all judgments and choices about professional services for the client.

3. In an "agent model," the expertise of the professional is simply placed at the service of the values and goals of the client without interference by any competing goals or values, including values to which the profession is committed from the start.

4. In an "interactive model," both parties have irreplaceable contributions to make in the decision-making process. The professional offers expertise to help meet the client's needs and has a commitment to the profession's central values, and the client brings his own values and priorities as well as the value of his self-determination. Ideally, the two parties judge together what professional interventions will most benefit the client and choose together to carry them out.

In addition, because the ideal relationship is described in regard to fully functioning adults, a profession's norms must also include how its members are to interact with clients who are not capable of full participation in decision making about professional interventions. Such clients might include children, the developmentally disabled, and persons whose capacity to participate is diminished by fear, illness, or other conditions.

SACRIFICE AND THE RELATIVE PRIORITY OF THE CLIENT'S WELL-BEING. Most sociologists who study professions mention "commitment to service" or "commitment to the public" as one of the characteristic features of a profession. Similarly, most professional organizations' codes of ethics and other self-descriptions give clients' best interests or service to the public a prominent place. But these expressions are subject to many different interpretations with significantly different implications for actual practice.

Consider, for example, what could be called a "minimalist" interpretation of this general norm. According to this interpretation, a professional would have an obligation to consider the well-being of the client as only one of the professional's most important concerns. This is called a minimalist interpretation because if any less consideration than this were given, the client's well-being could not be said to have any priority at all for the professional.

On the other hand, according to a "maximalist" interpretation, the professional has an obligation to place the well-being of clients ahead of every other consideration, both the professional's own interests and all other obligations or concerns that the professional might have.

It is doubtful that either of these interpretations accurately represents what the larger community wants or understands in this matter. Professional obligation almost certainly requires that members of a profession accept certain sacrifices of other interests in the interest of their clients. On the other hand, even if it were only for the sake of assuring a continued supply of professionals to meet its needs in the future, the larger community certainly would not actually require the commitment of a member of any profession to be absolute or to impose the utmost of sacrifices for the sake of the client's well-being in all circumstances. The actual content of professional obligation in this respect lies somewhere in the middle.

Each professional group therefore has, as an element of its obligations worked out over time in dialogue with the larger community, an obligation to accept certain kinds of sacrifices, certain degrees of risk in certain matters, and so on. For health professionals there is a degree of risk of infection, accepted in order to serve their clients. In other professions it may be primarily a risk of financial loss, social loss, or criticism. In any case, it should be a part of reflection on every profession's ethics and a part of all professional ethics education to raise this issue and to try to identify the kinds and degrees of risk that are part of that profession's obligations.

COMPETENCE. Every professional is obligated both to acquire and to maintain the expertise needed to undertake her professional tasks, and every professional is obligated to undertake only those tasks that are within her competence.

Competence is probably the most obvious category of professional obligation. It is also the easiest to describe in a general way. For if a professional fails to apply his expertise, or fails to obtain the expertise for undertaking some task, these failures directly contradict both the point of being an expert and the very foundation of the larger community's award of decision-making power to the professional in the first place.

But determining what counts as competence on the part of a member of a given profession, both in general and in relation to specific tasks, is a complex matter. In practice, and almost of necessity, detailed judgments about requisite expertise are left to those who are expert—to the profession itself. But the larger community usually requires that explanations be given regarding the general reasoning involved. In particular, the community should understand the risk–benefit judgments involved in every determination of minimal competence. For as the level of competence identified as the minimum acceptable in some matter is raised, the relative availability of that level of expertise to the profession's clients will fall, and these trade-offs should be made in dialogue with the larger community, not unilaterally by members of the profession alone.

IDEAL RELATIONSHIPS BETWEEN CO-PROFESSIONALS. Each profession also has norms, mostly implicit and unexamined, concerning the proper relationship among members of the same profession in various matters and also among members of different professions when they are dealing with the same client. Some elements of the proper relationship between a family practitioner and a renal specialist, for example, are not matters of etiquette, but they bear directly on the medical profession's ability to achieve its proper ends. The same is true of relationships between physicians and nurses, dentists and dental hygienists, dentists and physicians, and so on, when they are caring for the same patient, and between architects and engineers when serving the same client.

Some aspects of these relationships are dictated by each professional's obligation not to practice beyond her competence and so to seek assistance from other professionals when a particular matter requires expertise that the first professional does not possess. But other aspects of co-professional relationships are also governed by professional norms, though they are rarely explicit. For example, how should co-professionals communicate with a client about their differing recommendations for the client when these differences derive not from differing interpretations of the facts, but from differing philosophies of practice within their different professions or from their professions' different or differently ranked central values?

THE RELATIONSHIP BETWEEN THE PROFESSION AND THE LARGER COMMUNITY. The activities of every profession also involve diverse relationships between the profession as a group, or its individual members, and persons who are neither co-professionals nor clients. These relationships may involve the larger community as a whole, various significant subgroups, or specific individuals. Every profession, precisely because it is permitted to be self-regulating, for example, owes the larger community the effort needed to carry out this task conscientiously. This includes providing and monitoring educational programs and institutions in which new members of the profession receive their formation as professionals; monitoring the collective activities of members of the profession in their various professional organizations to make sure that these organizations act in ways consistent with the other professional obligations of the members; and having measures in place to monitor and correct incompetent or other professionally inappropriate practice on the part of individual members of the group.

Each profession has an educational obligation to the larger community. The reason is that both through actions of its individual members and through collective actions, every profession functions as the principal educator of the community regarding those elements of the profession's expertise that the lay community needs to understand in order to function effectively in ordinary life. Thus, for example, the health professions have obligations regarding public education in matters of ordinary health self-care and hygiene; and the engineering and scientific professions have obligations to educate regarding safety practices that the lay community needs to know in daily life.

A more subtle kind of obligation in relation to the larger community has to do with the content of key value concepts that become part of the public culture and play crucial roles in people's private lives and especially in public policy, but whose content is significantly influenced by the members of a profession or of a group of professions. For example, the engineering professions have a powerful formative influence on the culturally dominant notions of safety and physical risk; the health professions are more responsible than any other group for educating the public about what it means to be healthy; and so on. This is an area of professional obligation to the larger community that has received little attention but is of continuing ethical significance.

ACCESS TO PROFESSIONAL SERVICES. Professional services are distributed within a society by a complex system of economic, legal, and social structures. These structures principally determine who in the society will have access to the services of the professions when they need them. But because every professional is committed to the values that are central to his profession, no professional can consistently be indifferent when a significant number of people in the society need professional assistance to achieve these values and their need remains unmet.

There is, however, no single best answer to the question, "What ought I do when the society's distribution system leaves people in need of my profession's services without access to them?" Individual professionals will respond to this aspect of their professional obligation in different ways. For some it will involve pro bono or charity service of one sort or another. For others it will involve advocacy for changes in the distribution system or for publicly funded programs to provide services for the underserved. Others may focus on the value judgments being made by public decision makers who are arguably giving too low a priority to the kinds of well-being the profession provides. But in any case, access to the profession's services on the part of those in the society who need them is a matter that deserves special notice and explicit attention in the articulation of every profession's ethic.

INTEGRITY AND EDUCATION. Finally, there is that very subtle component of conduct by which a person communicates to others what she stands for, not only in the person's acts themselves but also in how these acts are chosen and in how the person presents herself to others in carrying them out. The two words that seem to communicate the core of this concern are *integrity* and *education,* especially when the two words are paired.

Each profession stands for, or "professes," certain values that it is committed to bringing about both for its clients individually and for the community at large. But a professional's personal priorities may communicate a different set of values, even though the professional's choices of interventions for clients and his efforts to secure appropriate relationships with clients all conform to accepted standards. Concern with this kind of communication to their patients and to the general public, for example, motivates some health professionals to establish in their personal lives patterns of healthy living consonant with what they say to their patients. Failure to attend to this element of professional commitment also makes illegal personal activities on the part of lawyers somehow doubly wrong.

Professionals may be obligated, then, to do some things and to refrain from doing others in order to remain true to the values that their profession stands for and thereby to educate others in these values by their own example.

There are undoubtedly other useful ways of dividing the general topic of professional obligation besides these nine categories. The point is that conceptual tools such as the key features of the institution of profession and the principal categories of professional obligation can assist professionals in determining their own obligations in general and in particular cases, and can assist scholars and educators of professional ethics to gain a clearer understanding of professional practice and of the ethical standards that apply to it.

Alternative Views of Profession

The account just given explains the institution of profession in terms of its function in society, as a means by which a society secures the benefits of specialized expertise for its members and prevents or at least limits its misuse by those who possess it. Like every account of a thing's function, this account is both descriptive and normative. It describes how professions and their members act, at least for the most part, and it identifies sets of standards by which their successes and failures to act in those ways are to be judged.

The principal alternative ways of explaining the institution of profession can be described under four headings: historical, critical functionalist, radical democratic, and personalist. Each of these approaches separates the descriptive and normative elements that are interwoven in a functionalist account, with the first and second stressing the descriptive elements and the third and fourth the normative elements.

Historical explanations of the institution of profession identify, through historical study, a developmental pattern that brings an occupational group to the point of being considered a profession. This pattern is then used normatively to determine whether particular occupational groups qualify as professions and what patterns of conduct by these groups conform or do not conform to the pattern. Some historical studies of professions do not purport to explain the institution of profession, of course, but simply tell part of its story without attempting to draw normative conclusions. Historical explanations may depend, at least initially, on some functionalist account of profession or on the selection of certain occupations, in their contemporary form or otherwise, as endpoints or at least markers of the developmental process being studied. But once a developmental explanation has been formulated, it can then be offered to replace functionalist accounts on the grounds that these are excessively idealized and are not adequately descriptive of the current or historical conduct of relevant groups. For example, the medical profession in the mid-twentieth century has

been described as the product of a process of monopolization, or gradual acquisition of control by an exclusive group over a segment of market activity over the years (Berlant). The institution of profession generally has been described as a specialized mechanism for maintaining economic power and class-based status and dominance (Larson).

Some critics of the professions formulate a functionalist account of the institution for themselves, or accept someone else's, and then use its normative content to critique current patterns of conduct of individuals and organizations within a particular profession or across the professions generally (Freidson). Other functionalist critics argue that currently accepted functionalist accounts are so idealized—that is, pay so little attention to the gap between what is described as the profession's function and the profession's actual conduct— that they leave unchallenged actual or potential harm to the community by the professions or at least do not call upon the professions strongly enough to correct their inadequacies for the community's sake. Therefore, an alternative account of the function of professions and professionals is proposed, and its implications for professional conduct are identified (Kultgen).

Radical democratic critics of the institution of profession believe that any society that accepts this institution makes a profound mistake. It is central to the institution of profession that the possession of expertise is a basis of power and that one element of that power is a grant of autonomy to those possessed of it. By institutionalizing deep inequalities of power and autonomy in this way, these critics argue, a society makes the achievement of genuine democracy almost impossible. According to the radical democrat, the failures in conduct pointed out by functionalist critics and the developmental patterns leading to monopoly and to other forms of economic and class-based inequality that the historical critics point out are not historically contingent events but the inevitable outcomes of the inherently undemocratic constitution of the institution of profession. For these thinkers the solution, on which the well-being of the human community depends, is to do away with the institution of profession and all other institutions grounded on undemocratic premises (Illich, 1973, 1976).

The personalist explanation of profession identifies the individual professional's act of personal commitment upon entering a profession as the basis of everything morally significant about the institution of profession. As centuries ago a solemn vow initiated a person's membership into a profession—a vestige of which remains, for example, in the ceremony in which new physicians speak the Hippocratic Oath—so today the act of personal commitment by each member of a profession is what brings the profession continually into being and gives it its character. The contents of a profession's norms are determined by the contents of these personal acts of commitment; and the professional who falls short in conduct fails above all to honor her own commitment to serve others, rather than failing to follow a norm created and sustained principally, according to the account proposed here, by the mutual effort of the profession and the community at large (Pellegrino; Pellegrino and Thomasma).

Each of these approaches stresses a feature of the institution of profession that standard functionalist accounts are held to overlook or underestimate: the developmental patterns by which professions and professionals are formed; the extent to which professions' and professionals' actual conduct falls short of the functionalist's proposed norms; the undemocratic character of exclusive expertise; and the centrality of the act of commitment by which a person becomes a professional. More complex functionalist accounts could incorporate much that is stressed in these other approaches, as more complex versions of each of them could incorporate emphases and concerns from the others. From the point of view of understanding professions as they exist, in other words, each of these approaches teaches something of importance and all deserve careful study.

Changing Times, Changing Standards, Changing Concepts

It is not only the conduct of individuals and groups, as measured by professional norms, that can fall short of what ought to be. Professional norms themselves can fall short of what they ought to be, particularly when important characteristics of a society undergo change. There was a time, for example, when the general level of education in the United States may well have justified an ethics in which the ideal patient–practitioner relationship for physicians and dentists conformed to the guild model rather than the interactive model, whereas the latter has become normative for these professions in the years since the 1970s.

A profession's norms and the institution of profession itself are human constructs and, like all things of human making, they can fall short of their intended goals, and the goals themselves can change with changing times. When norms and institutions are no longer able to do the tasks that a society needs them to do, then the society is justified in trying to change them. But social structures such as professions are inherently conservative, in the root sense of that word; they exist to preserve a mode of acting or of organizing conduct that has proven fruitful, and they preserve it by forming in their participants strong habits of perceiving, judging, and acting in ways that support it.

So when times and expectations change, or people's values or abilities change, or the surrounding social institutions change, then it is important to reexamine the relevant norms and institutions to see if they are still appropriate and to change them if they are not, even if this involves a major transformation of a particular profession's norms across many of the nine categories. One of the weaknesses of functionalist accounts of the institution of profession in the minds of critics is that such accounts seem to say that whatever is the case is what ought to be the case. But, like the other four approaches, the functionalist account is simply a conceptual tool whose purpose is to help a society understand what it has when it has a particular profession with a particular set of norms so that the society can then make a judgment on whether that is the profession that ought to exist.

In an analogous way, the new professional enters a profession whose norms are already in place. This does not mean that these norms cannot be changed, but they achieve their content by means of an ongoing dialogue between the profession and the larger community, and they change their content in the same way. So the new professional cannot create the contents of his professional obligations out of whole cloth. Yet, even in the individual case, the norms of the profession are not the ultimate determiners of right and wrong. If these norms are in conflict with one another or with other important moral considerations, or if they are severely defective in some way, then the professional must form his own conscience to decide how to act. Situations arise in which conscientious disobedience of a professional norm is what a person's moral judgment requires when all things about a situation are considered.

By what standards should a society judge a profession's norms when their adequacy to the society's needs is in question? By what standard should the institution of profession itself be judged? By what standard should the individual professional form her own conscience when conflict or severe doubt about the adequacy of a professional norm in a particular case suggests that conscientious disobedience may be the correct path? Surely not by the norms of the profession, because these are precisely what are being challenged when such questions arise. It is to the deeper values and standards of human conduct and social life that individuals must turn at such times, for it is upon them that the norms of professions rest for their moral force in the first place.

As is true for many other human institutions, if the institution of profession did not exist, it or something like it would need to be invented in order for people to live together effectively. For no one person can master all the knowledge and skills on which the achievement of so many important values in human life depend. But, like other human institutions, the institution of profession as a whole, and each individual profession, and each normative feature of each profession, requires regular ethical scrutiny to make sure it continues to fulfill the purposes for which it was made. One of the principal roles of the field of bioethics and its practitioners is to provide the members of the health professions and the larger community with effective conceptual tools to employ in this scrutiny.

DAVID T. OZAR (1995)
REVISED BY AUTHOR

SEE ALSO: *Care; Compassionate Love; Competency; Confidentiality; Conflict of Interest; Divided Loyalties in Mental Healthcare; Impaired Professionals; Information Disclosure, Ethical Issues of; Informed Consent; Medicine, Profession of; Professional-Patient Relationship; Nursing, Profession of; Teams, Healthcare; Psychiatry, Abuses of; Sexual Ethics and Professional Standards*

BIBLIOGRAPHY

Abbott, Andrew. 1988. *The System of Professions: An Essay on the Division of Expert Labor.* Chicago: University of Chicago Press.

Applbaum, Arthur Isak. 1999. *Ethics for Adversaries: The Morality of Roles in Public and Professional Life.* Princeton, NJ: Princeton University Press.

Bayles, Michael D. 1989. *Professional Ethics,* 2nd edition. Belmont, CA: Wadsworth.

Berlant, Jeffrey Lionel. 1975. *Profession and Monopoly: A Study of Medicine in the United States and Great Britain.* Berkeley: University of California Press.

Brincat, Cynthia A., and Wike, Victoria S. 2000. *Morality and the Professional Life: Values at Work.* Upper Saddle River, NJ: Prentice-Hall.

Burrage, Michael, and Torstendahl, Rolf, eds. 1990. *Professions in Theory and History: Rethinking the Study of the Professions.* London: Sage.

Camenisch, Paul F. 1983. *Grounding Professional Ethics in a Pluralistic Society.* New York: Haven Publications.

Davis, Michael, and Stark, Andrew. 2001. *Conflict of Interest in the Professions.* New York: Oxford University Press.

Derber, Charles; Schwartz, William A.; and Magress, Yale. 1990. *Power in the Highest Degree: Professionals and the Rise of a New Mandarin Order.* New York: Oxford University Press.

Durkheim, Émile. 1960. *The Division of Labor in Society,* tr. George Simpson. New York: Free Press.

Etzioni, Amitai, ed. 1969. *The Semi-professions and Their Organization: Teachers, Nurses, Social Workers.* New York: Free Press.

Freidson, Eliot. 1970. *Profession of Medicine: A Study of the Sociology of Applied Knowledge.* New York: Dodd, Mead.

Freidson, Eliot. 1986. *Professional Powers: A Study of the Institutionalization of Formal Knowledge.* Chicago: University of Chicago Press.

Freidson, Eliot. 1994. *Professionalism Reborn: Theory, Prophecy, and Policy.* Chicago: University of Chicago Press.

Freidson, Eliot. 2001. *Professionalism, the Third Logic: On the Practice of Knowledge.* Chicago: University of Chicago Press.

Gardner, Howard; Csikszentmihalyi, Mihaly; and Damon, William. 2001. *Good Work: When Excellence and Ethics Meet.* New York: Basic.

Goldman, Alan H. 1980. *The Moral Foundations of Professional Ethics.* Totowa, NJ: Rowman and Littlefield.

Greenwood, Ernest. 1957. "Attributes of a Profession." *Social Work* 2(3): 45–55.

Hughes, Everett C. 1965. "Professions." In *The Professions in America,* ed. Kenneth S. Lynn. Boston: Houghton Mifflin.

Illich, Ivan. 1973. *Tools for Conviviality.* New York: Harper and Row.

Illich, Ivan. 1976. *Medical Nemesis: The Expropriation of Health.* New York: Pantheon.

Koehn, Daryl. 1994. *The Ground of Professional Ethics.* London: Routledge.

Kultgen, John. 1988. *Ethics and Professionalism.* Philadelphia: University of Pennsylvania Press.

Kuskey, Garvan F. 1973. "Health Care, Human Rights, and Government Intervention." *California Dental Association Journal* 1(1): 10–13.

Larson, Magali Sarfatti. 1977. *The Rise of Professionalism: A Sociological Analysis.* Berkeley: University of California Press.

Luban, David. 1988. *Lawyers and Justice: An Ethical Study.* Princeton, NJ: Princeton University Press.

Martin, Mike. 2000. *Meaningful Work: Rethinking Professional Ethics.* New York: Oxford University Press.

May, William F. 2001. *Beleaguered Rulers: The Public Obligation of the Professional.* Louisville, KY: Westminster John Knox Press.

Millerson, Geoffrey. 1974. *The Qualifying Associations: A Study in Professionalization.* New York: Humanities Press.

Ozar, David T. 1993. "Building Awareness of Ethical Standards and Conduct." In *Educating Professionals: Responding to New Expectations for Competence and Accountability,* ed. Lynn Curry and Jon F. Wergin. San Francisco: Jossey-Bass.

Ozar, David T., and Sokol, David J. 2002. *Dental Ethics at Chairside: Professional Principles and Practical Applications,* 2nd edition. Washington, D.C.: Georgetown University Press.

Parsons, Talcott. 1951. *The Social System.* New York: Free Press.

Parsons, Talcott. 1954. *Essays in Sociological Theory,* rev. edition. Glencoe, IL: Free Press.

Pellegrino, Edmund D. 1979. "Toward a Reconstruction of Medical Morality: The Primacy of the Act of Profession and the Fact of Illness." *Journal of Medicine and Philosophy* 4(1): 32–56.

Pellegrino, Edmund D., and Thomasma, David C. 1988. *For the Patient's Good: The Restoration of Beneficence in Health Care.* New York: Oxford University Press.

Rest, James R., and Narváez, Darcia. 1994. *Moral Development in the Professions: Psychology and Applied Ethics.* Hillsdale, NJ: Erlbaum.

Rest, James R.; Narváez, Darcia; Bebeau, Muriel J.; and Thoma, Stephen J. 1999. *Postconventional Moral Thinking: A Neo-Kohlbergian Approach.* Hillsdale, NJ: Erlbaum.

Sade, Robert M. 1971. "Medical Care as a Right: A Refutation." *New England Journal of Medicine* 285(23): 1288–1292.

Starr, Paul. 1982. *The Social Transformation of American Medicine.* New York: Basic.

Wilensky, Harold L. 1964. "The Professionalization of Everyone?" *American Journal of Sociology* 70(2): 137–158.

Wolgast, Elizabeth. 1992. *Ethics of an Artificial Person: Lost Responsibility in Professions and Organizations.* Stanford, CA: Stanford University Press.

Wueste, Daniel E. 1994. *Professional Ethics and Social Responsibility.* Lanham, MD: Rowman and Littlefield.

Znaniecki, Florian. 1968. *The Social Role of the Man of Knowledge.* New York: Harper and Row.

PROFIT AND COMMERCIALISM

• • •

The practice of medicine is clearly a profession, as usually defined. In some senses it is also a business. However, the extent to which the professional behavior of physicians ought to be influenced by business considerations is a matter of debate (Veatch). A more general but closely related question is the degree to which business values should control the healthcare system (Gray).

Physicians in private practice must generate income to pay their costs and earn a livelihood. In this sense, profit (the excess of gross revenues over costs) is as economically important in the fee-for-service practice of medicine as it is in the conduct of a business. But some have carried the analogy further and have maintained that the payment of a fee is an essential part of the professional relation between physicians and patients, because this relation is in effect a commercial contract between the supplier of a service (the physician) and the purchaser of a service (the patient). Although the service is professional, and therefore involves more constraints and responsibilities for the supplier than does an ordinary market transaction, this interpretation of medical practice effectively blurs most of the distinctions

between medicine and business (Sade). This argument further asserts that physicians may choose to offer their services to indigent patients gratis or at reduced rates, but their professional status does not require them to do so. Nor are physicians required to ignore or minimize their own economic interests when making professional decisions, provided their treatment is medically appropriate (Engelhardt and Rie).

Opposed to this point of view is the perhaps more traditional interpretation that regards medical practice primarily as a ministering function—a commitment to serve the needs of patients without concern for self-interest (Relman, 1992). According to this interpretation, profit may be an economic necessity in fee-for-service practice, in the aggregate if not in each individual case, but a de facto contract binding all physicians establishes an overriding obligation to serve those in need of medical care regardless of their ability to pay. Furthermore, fee for service is not considered to be a critical, or even an important, feature of professional practice. In this view, the contract between doctor and patient is basically ethical, not commercial, and is seen as part of a broader commitment that physicians make to society in exchange for licensure, authority, and the many other benefits bestowed on them by the state.

Although there has always been an uneasy tension between these two perspectives, until recently the traditional view of the ethical obligations of the medical profession generally prevailed. Most people considered medical care to be a social good, not an economic commodity, and most physicians and medical professional organizations acted as if they agreed. For example, the version of the American Medical Association's (AMA) ethical code prevailing from 1957 to 1980 said: "The practice of medicine should not be commercialized nor treated as a commodity in trade" (AMA Judicial Council, 1969, p. 28). Advertising was discouraged, and physicians were advised to limit the source of their professional incomes to services to patients rendered by them or under their supervision (AMA Judicial Council, 1969).

A similar view of the role of hospitals as essentially not-for-profit social institutions was widely accepted. Although many small proprietary hospitals existed in the early part of the twentieth century, until fairly recently virtually all hospitals larger than seventy-five beds were public or private, not-for-profit institutions that considered their primary mission to be public service. Most of the private, not-for-profit (voluntary) hospitals admitted patients—particularly those who were acutely or seriously ill—without regard to income, and many accepted less than full payment from patients with limited means. They sometimes operated at a deficit and depended on philanthropy, public contributions, or other non-patient-derived income to continue operation. The public hospitals, of course, were tax supported and were not expected to meet their expenses from patient revenues.

Beginning in the late 1960s, however, a new commercial spirit began to permeate the healthcare system (Relman, 1980; Gray). It started with the hospitals but soon spread rapidly to virtually every other part of the system. In response to the growing opportunities for profit resulting from the expansion of government-supported health insurance through Medicare and Medicaid in the 1960s and employment-based private health insurance, large chains of investor-owned hospitals sprang up in many communities. Other types of for-profit medical facilities and services soon followed, attracted by the seemingly unlimited opportunities for financial gain. Today about 15 percent of all private general hospitals and the majority of private nursing homes, psychiatric hospitals, and free-standing ambulatory care and diagnostic facilities are owned by for-profit corporations. When the Clinton administration's proposals for health insurance reform failed in 1994, for-profit companies selling managed care insurance quickly filled the breach. By the beginning of the twenty-first century, the great majority of private health insurance plans were owned by investor-owned companies. So were most private indemnity health insurance companies, and most healthcare management and consulting services. Together with the new and rapidly-growing biotechnology companies and the traditional pharmaceutical and medical supplies and equipment industries, these for-profit businesses constitute a vast commercial network with a pervasive and powerful influence on the U.S. healthcare system. In no other country is so much of the healthcare delivery and insurance system operated by investor-owned corporations, and in no other country does private business have so large a stake in healthcare policy.

Even the not-for-profit voluntary hospitals have become infused with the entrepreneurial spirit. Overexpansion of hospital capacity and competition from investor-owned healthcare facilities, both in-patient and ambulatory, forced voluntary hospitals to become more competitive. Private managed care insurance and federal insurance programs have pressured the not-for-profit hospitals to accept lower payments. As a result, their marketing and advertising efforts, and their preoccupation with the generation of revenue, are almost indistinguishable from those of their investor-owned competitors. Care of the indigent, once considered a prime responsibility of voluntary as well as public hospitals, has been increasingly shifted to public institutions. Pressures to control costs have led to reductions in hospital staff and shortened lengths of stay, which may adversely affect quality of care.

Practitioners first began to feel economic pressures in the decade of the 1980s, and these pressures have increased since then, forcing them, like the hospitals, into more entrepreneurial behavior. The numbers of competing specialists have grown rapidly, while available fee-for-service patients have become more scarce and insurance companies have shifted from unquestioning payment of the doctor's bill to increasingly stringent efforts to control expenses through capitated and discounted payment, and through managed care. Medicare fees are also being reduced. To protect their income, many physicians began to act like competing businesspeople seeking more customers and more ways to deliver profitable services (Relman, 1988). Physicians have also become interested in opportunities to increase their revenues through partnership in, or ownership of, healthcare facilities and through financial arrangements with companies supplying the drugs, devices, or diagnostic services they prescribe for their patients. In many parts of the United States, practicing physicians refer their patients to free-standing diagnostic or ambulatory surgery facilities in which the physicians hold financial interest—a practice called *self-referral.*

In 1975 the U.S. Supreme Court declared that the reach of antitrust law extended to the professions (*Goldfarb v. Virginia State Bar,* 1975), and shortly thereafter the AMA was legally enjoined from interfering with the advertising and marketing practices in which increasing numbers of physicians were engaged. In response to the growing view that healthcare was a competitive marketplace and physicians were essentially small independent entrepreneurs, the AMA retreated in the 1980s from its earlier proscriptions against commercialization. Its 1982 revised ethical code says nothing about the distinction between medical practice and trade; instead, there is a statement that competition is "not only ethical but is encouraged" (AMA Judicial Council, 1982, p. 22). Advertising was sanctioned provided it was not misleading, and the earlier restriction on sources of professional income was removed. Self-referral and other kinds of economic interests by physicians in the medical products they prescribe were said to be ethical, provided the financial interest was disclosed to patients and did not influence medical judgment. The most recent AMA position (AMA, 1998, p. 121) puts additional restraints on self-referral, but does not prohibit it altogether.

Ethical issues aside, does the commercialization of the healthcare system bestow any special benefit on patients or on society in general? In most sectors of the economy, free market competition among suppliers of goods and services helps to control prices and encourages quality. Although suppliers promote consumption through marketing and advertising, the cost-conscious choices of consumers largely determine the number of units purchased and the total expenditures allotted to each product. Goods and services are distributed primarily according to consumers' desires, their judgments about price and quality, and their ability to pay—all of which is believed to serve useful social purposes.

But the healthcare sector is quite different from most other parts of the economy, and the consequences of market competition are not the same. Consumers (patients) can make relatively few independent and informed purchasing decisions because they must rely so heavily on advice from their physicians. And because of third-party payment, neither the consumer nor the provider of services (the physician) is much constrained by cost. Physicians largely determine the distribution and use of services. Professional judgment of the patient's medical needs is the primary consideration, but the economic benefits to the physician and the healthcare institution also play a role, particularly when the medical needs are optional or uncertain. Therefore, when healthcare that is paid on a fee-for-service basis becomes commercialized, competition serves not to limit but to increase expenditures, because providers have greater economic incentives to offer their services to patients who are, for the most part, dependent and unresisting consumers. Profit motives thus intensify inflation in a healthcare system unless it has effective cost-control mechanisms.

On the other hand, when payment for medical services is made in advance, as in HMOs and other kinds of prepaid managed care, economic incentives tend to force physicians and hospitals to reduce, rather than increase, their allocation of elective services to patients. In such a system insurers and providers profit most when medical expenditures are kept to a minimum. Commercialization of managed care thus raises concerns about cutting corners and underserving patients' needs, just as the commercialization of fee-for-service care raises concerns about excessive and unnecessary services. In both cases, there is the risk that the profit motive may influence professional judgment and make it more difficult for physicians to act in the best interests of their patients.

Furthermore, a commercialized healthcare system has little concern for the needs of the uninsured and the underinsured. Unless government intervenes, those without means to pay are denied access to all but emergency care. The steadily rising number of uninsured and underinsured patients testifies to the social indifference of a profit-oriented medical marketplace and to the inability of tax-supported institutions to accept the growing burden of the medically indigent. It is currently estimated that about 15 percent of the U.S. population has no medical insurance and that at least as many are seriously underinsured. Efforts by providers of medical care to remain economically viable may require them not only to restrict charity but also to promote profitable services, which may not be those most needed by the community.

Proponents of commercialization in healthcare argue that it rewards innovation and technological development. They say that one of the benefits of an expanding medical marketplace is stimulation of applied research and development, leading to the more rapid introduction and dissemination of useful new products. However, there is no reason to believe that the pace of worthwhile innovation would be significantly slowed in a system that encouraged research and development but allowed industry to market only properly tested new products, and restrained entrepreneurialism in the delivery of medical care. The current dominance of the United States in the development of new medical technology is probably the result more of substantial public support of medical research than of the commercialization of the healthcare system.

Avocates of for-profit healthcare also claim that market competition and commercial incentives improve the quality and efficiency of medical services. What little data there are on comparative quality seem to suggest the opposite. For example, studies of the quality of care in investor-owned hospitals (Devereaux et al.), kidney dialysis centers (Garg et al.) and nursing homes (Harrington et al.) show serious deficiencies in comparison with similar but not-for-profit facilities. The efficiency of medical care, on the one hand, is hard to define and measure. Some suggest that efficiency means the delivery of medically acceptable care at lower cost to the payer, but there simply aren't any good studies that would allow comparison of for-profit and not-for-profit services by that kind of measure. However, administrative and total costs in for-profit hospitals have been reported to be higher than in their not-for-profit counterparts (Woolhandler and Himmelstein).

In short, defenders of commercialism in healthcare have no firm empirical support for their arguments. Instead, their position is largely based on the assumption that market incentives will improve services in healthcare, just as they are supposed to do in ordinary commerce. However, as already noted, there is reason to question that assumption. This issue has been hotly debated ever since the introduction of managed care. Those who believe that the era of the "corporate practice of medicine" has arrived assert that old-fashioned medical professionalism is becoming obsolete (Robinson), but there are still influential voices defending the traditional ethical values (Freidson).

It remains to be seen whether commercialism in medicine will continue to grow and ultimately dominate the U.S. healthcare system. Those who believe medical care is a business like any other regard such an outcome as desirable and necessary for the achievement of optimal efficiency. On the other hand, those who believe medical care is primarily a social rather than an economic good hope that the present trend toward commercialism will be resisted and in the long run reversed. They believe the ultimate solution of the healthcare problems in the United States will be found through social action and community responsibility.

ARNOLD S. RELMAN (1995)
REVISED BY AUTHOR

SEE ALSO: *Advertising; Commercialism in Scientific Research; Economic Concepts in Healthcare; Health Insurance; Healthcare Institutions; Managed Care; Pharmaceutical Industry*

BIBLIOGRAPHY

American Medical Association Council on Ethical and Judicial Affairs. 1992. *Code of Medical Ethics: Annotated Current Opinions Including the Principles of Medical Ethics, Fundamental Elements of the Patient–Physician Relationship, and Rules of the Council on Ethical and Judicial Affairs.* Chicago: Author.

American Medical Association Council on Ethical and Judicial Affairs. 1998. *Code of Medical Ethics 1998–1999.* Chicago: Author.

American Medical Association Judicial Council. 1969. *Opinions and Reports of the Judicial Council.* Chicago: Author.

American Medical Association Judicial Council. 1982. *Current Opinions of the Judicial Council of the American Medical Association: Including the Principles of Medical Ethics and Rules of the Judicial Council.* Chicago: Author.

Devereaux, P. J.; Choi, P. T. L.; Lacchetti, C.; et al. 2002. "A Systematic Review and Meta-Analysis of Studies Comparing Mortality Rates of Private For-Profit and Private Not-for-Profit Hospitals." *Canadian Medical Assocation Journal* 166(11): 1399–1406.

Engelhardt, H. Tristram, Jr., and Michael A. Rie. 1988. "Morality for the Medical–Industrial Complex: A Code of Ethics for the Mass Marketing of Health Care." *New England Journal of Medicine* 319(16): 1086–1089.

Freidson, E. 2001. *Professionalism: The Third Logic.* Chicago, IL: University of Chicago Press.

Garg, Pushkal P.; Frick, Kevin D.; Diener-West, Marie; et al. 1999. "Effect of the Ownership of Dialysis Facilities on Patients' Survival and Referral for Transplantation." *New England Journal of Medicine* 341(22): 1653–1660.

Goldfarb v. Virginia State Bar. 421 U.S. 773 (1975).

Gray, Bradford H. 1991. *The Profit Motive and Patient Care: The Changing Accountability of Doctors and Hospitals.* Cambridge, MA: Harvard University Press.

Harrington, Charlene; Woolhandler, Steffie; Mullan, Joseph; et al. 2001. "Does Investor Ownership of Nursing Homes Compromise the Quality of Care?" *American Journal of Public Health* 91(9): 1452–1455.

Relman, Arnold S. 1980. "The New Medical–Industrial Complex." *New England Journal of Medicine* 303(17): 963–970.

Relman, Arnold S. 1988. "Medicine as a Profession and a Business." In *The Tanner Lectures on Human Values,* Vol. 8, ed. Sterling S. McMurrin. Salt Lake City: University of Utah Press.

Relman, Arnold S. 1992. "What Market Values Are Doing to Medicine." *Atlantic Monthly* 269(3): 98–106.

Robinson, J. C. 1999. *The Corporate Practice of Medicine.* Berkeley, CA: University of California Press.

Sade, Robert M. 1971. "Medical Care as a Right: A Refutation." *New England Journal of Medicine* 285(23): 1288–1292.

Veatch, Robert M. 1983. "Ethical Dilemmas of For-Profit Enterprise in Health Care." In *The New Health Care for Profit: Doctors and Hospitals in a Competitive Environment,* ed. Bradford H. Gray. Washington, D.C.: National Academy Press.

Woolhandler, Steffie, and Himmelstein, David U. 1997. "Costs of Care and Administration at For-Profit and Other Hospitals in the United States." *New England Journal of Medicine* 336(11): 769–774.

PSYCHIATRY, ABUSES OF

• • •

Abuse of psychiatry conjures up a situation in which a psychiatrist acts improperly, causing a patient to experience some sort of harm. The concept is more complex than it appears to be at first sight. This article examines psychiatric abuse in an effort to determine its accurate meaning so that steps can be taken to eliminate or prevent it.

Historical Background

Evidence has emerged of such practices as the abuse of psychiatry for political purposes in the former Soviet Union (Bloch and Reddaway, 1977, 1984), a similar pattern in Cuba designed to suppress political dissent (Brown and Lago), the deployment of psychiatric knowledge in torture and interrogation in Northern Ireland in 1971 (Bloch, 1990), and pursuit of financial profit as a priority in Japanese private psychiatric hospitals (Harding). The tragic perversion of psychiatry during the Nazi era, in which tens of thousands of chronic psychiatric and mentally retarded patients were gassed to death, and similar numbers were sterilized, is the most gross instance of abuse (Burleigh; Müller-Hill).

Commentary on psychiatric abuse has also referred to its prevalence elsewhere particularly in the United States and South Africa. But, as will become evident in the section on definition, care must be taken to distinguish between intentional misapplication of psychiatric knowledge, skills, and technology and inadequate or negligent practice. In the South African case, the policy of apartheid involved massive inequity in the provision of mental health services, with blacks allocated substantially lesser resources compared with whites despite equivalent need. On the other hand, the allegation of the misuse of psychiatry to squelch black political activism never had any basis (Bloch, 1984).

In the United States, discriminatory practices have also occurred but due to economic rather than explicitly political forces. With millions of Americans unable to afford health insurance and inadequate budgets for public psychiatric services, the result has been substandard care in state mental hospitals, particularly for minority groups and the poor (frequently the same population) (Green and Bloch; Torrey).

The abuse of psychiatry for political or other purposes in the United States has been sporadic, the examples of the poet Ezra Pound (1885–1972) and General Edwin Walker (1909–1993) being especially well known. In the case of Pound, psychiatry was recruited to deal with a politically sensitive situation. A celebrated poet, indicted for treason following his pro-Axis broadcasts in Italy during World War II, Pound faced possible execution. Although the evidence was equivocal, Pound was judged incompetent to stand trial on grounds of insanity and transferred to St. Elizabeth's Psychiatric Hospital where he spent the next thirteen years. The indictment was later dismissed and Pound released. Whether psychiatry was misused to extricate the U.S. government from a quandary or Pound was deluded and this accounted for his wartime behavior remains a baffling issue. Suffice to say, the case demonstrates the vulnerability of psychiatry to political exploitation.

Similar factors prevailed in the case of Edwin Walker, a decorated major general in the American army who adopted an extreme right-wing position during the civil rights campaigns of the 1950s and the 1960s. His competence became a matter of dispute after he had been charged with offenses related to his activism. Although declared competent to stand trial (the case was later dismissed for technical reasons), the possibility of the government's recourse to psychiatry to deal more conveniently with a *troublemaker* cannot be ruled out (Stone).

A final comment in this brief historical context concerns criticism of psychiatry for its patronizing attitude toward women. The dramatic case of Mrs. E. P. W. Packard in 1860 illustrates how prejudice may undermine clinical judgment. Upon the insistence of her husband, a fundamentalist clergyman, that she harbored dangerous religious beliefs, Mrs. Packard was committed to a mental hospital, where she remained confined for three years. Upon her release, she launched a campaign against the expression of opinions as a basis for psychiatric detention (Musto).

Over a century later in 1972, Phyllis Chesler was among the first to argue that psychiatry's view of women was so distorted as to impair its objectivity. Other feminist perspectives followed (e.g., Showalter; Luepnitz). According to this view, a male-dominated profession too readily regards women not conforming to stereotypic roles as psychologically suspect, even disturbed. Freud's contribution to gender psychology has no doubt been influential in the maintenance of such attitudes.

Definitions

Psychiatric abuse can be defined according to specified criteria and differentiated from other undesirable activities, which are best termed *malpractice. Abuse* refers to the intentional, improper application of the knowledge, skills, and technology of psychiatry for a purpose other than serving the patient's interests or to harm, in diverse ways, people who do not warrant psychiatric status in the first instance. Abuse is invariably perpetrated by psychiatrists (and other mental health professionals) in collaboration with other persons or agencies, such as a state security service or political authority and, then, usually as part of a totalitarian system.

Such institutional abuse is always unethical in that the protagonist intentionally carries out an act in the knowledge that the act is intrinsically wrong (whether or not it turns out to harm), explicitly violating professional ethics. A psychiatrist who acts in this way, claiming that he is obliged to follow the orders of superiors and in that sense is heteronymous, is inexcusably rejecting a responsibility to ensure that regulations serve good, not bad, professional goals. In these circumstances, even if psychiatrists covertly seek to ameliorate the welfare of the patient, claiming that this is the sole means to maintain an ethical stance, their behavior, by virtue of colluding in an abusive practice, becomes an inherent part of the abuse.

Reference to institutional abuse, on which this article focuses, does not negate the possibility of individual psychiatrists abusing one or more of their own patients. A similar ethical violation takes place in both cases, psychiatrists in the latter exploiting patients to meet their personal needs on the pretext that the practice applied is clinically indicated. A clear-cut example is sexual involvement, but other forms of abuse of power intrinsic to the psychiatrist–patient relationship, such as financial and religious, are relevant here. This sort of abuse may mar any doctor–patient relationship, but the not uncommon situation in psychiatric treatment of an excessively vulnerable patient seeking comfort from an ostensibly all-caring professional is arguably more conducive to its occurrence than in other medical spheres.

Abuse can also be perpetrated by a psychiatrist in conjunction with, or acceding to, attempts by lay people to exploit the discipline for nonmedical purposes. Consider this example: A husband who knows that his wife is not mentally ill, but is determined to gain custody over their children in an impending legal tussle, persuades a psychiatrist to commit her to a mental hospital. His interests are other than the welfare of his wife; he desires to wield power over her for his own purposes and recruits the psychiatrist as an accessory (Robitscher).

Malpractice is distinguishable from abuse with respect to intent. Although the term is used in diverse ways, an alternative remains elusive; *inadequate practice* comes closest in meaning. A psychiatrist who does not set out to use knowledge, skills, or technology improperly but who deploys these in an unskilled fashion is engaging in malpractice. An example is prescribing psychotropic drugs for patients upon the request of nursing staff, who claim they are otherwise unable to manage "difficult behavior," in cases where patients do not need such medication. Psychiatrists do not pervert their science in these circumstances but fail to adhere to a standard of practice that requires the application of drugs only when clinically indicated. Malpractice should be differentiated from "errors in clinical judgment" when that judgment has been made in good faith. Psychiatrists, like any other professionals, are prone to err on occasion. Although the consequences may simulate the effects of malpractice, malpractice is not actually carried out.

The Vulnerability of Psychiatry to Abuse

Abuse is more common in psychiatry than elsewhere in medicine, probably because it is inherently more vulnerable to it in at least three respects: (1) its boundaries remain ill-defined; (2) diagnosis is often made in the absence of objective criteria; and (3) the psychiatrist is granted immense power by society to determine the fate of other people, even to the extent of detaining them in hospital or imposing treatment on them.

The lack of a well-demarcated conceptual boundary in psychiatry leads to a correspondingly ill-defined role for its practitioners. Debate has long continued among psychiatrists themselves, and in the wider community, as to what

constitutes their legitimate role (Dyer). Attitudes vary considerably, even to the point of contradiction. The following views, expressed by former presidents of the American Psychiatric Association, reflect this diversity. In 1969 Ewald Busse argued for a limited role whereby psychiatrists restrict their focus to the suffering patient, and services are accordingly confined to reducing pain and discomfort. In 1970 his colleague Raymond Waggoner had a much wider perspective, calling upon the profession to pursue "fundamental social goals," and for psychiatrists to be visionaries.

Definitions of health and ill health are pertinent to the above positions. Thus, a *visionary* outlook brings psychiatrists into the domain of social policy. Their potential participation in a context beyond hospital and clinic is boundless, leading to professional judgements, ostensibly derived from expertise, on social issues like unemployment, racism, poverty, torture, religious cults, child-rearing practices, sexual expression, and indigenous rights. Psychiatrists may assume roles, including those of social commentator, political activist and lobbyist, that extend well beyond the traditional role of clinician.

Whatever the role adopted, psychiatrists are buffeted by the demands of multiple loyalties. They are caught ineluctably between responsibilities to patients and to society, the latter potentially including, among others, a patient's family, an employer, the courts, prison officials, and military authorities. In these circumstances they have to weigh the interests of patients against those of social agencies. In so doing, they may be subject to such intense pressure as to subordinate themselves to social forces, and so neglect their obligation to patients.

Psychiatry's role is more clear-cut when limited to an exclusively medical function. But this depends on the psychiatrist's ability to conduct diagnostic assessments that are relatively objective and value-free—for example, in the case of a person with a brain disorder like Alzheimer's Disease. This brings us to the second feature of psychiatry that contributes to its vulnerability to abuse, lack of objective criteria in clinical evaluation.

Although psychiatry has evolved as a scientific discipline for over a century and a half, including progress in classification, the discipline still faces the key question of what constitutes mental illness (Fulford, 1989). No satisfactory criteria exist to define precisely many of the conditions with which psychiatry deals. Compared with those in other medical fields, many currently used psychiatric diagnoses derive from clinical observation alone, and lack identifiable pathophysiological correlates. Objective tests to confirm the presence of a psychiatric condition are rare.

Moreover, in the diagnostic task psychiatrists rely in uncomfortably large measure on social criteria and value judgments. As the British sociologist Kathleen Jones reminds us, society would not be able to determine what was normal if it failed to designate certain acts and certain people as abnormal or antisocial. William Fulford and Walter Reich have contributed handsomely to the question of what constitutes a mental disorder by dissecting the complex process psychiatrists use to determine whether a diagnosis should be applied to a specific constellation of mental or behavioral features. Fulford (1999) stresses the place of values in clinical practice overall, positing that diagnoses in both physical and psychological medicine are an admixture of the factual and the evaluative. For him the concept of mental illness is on the same logical platform as the concept of physical illness.

Reich makes explicit the vulnerability of the diagnostic process in psychiatry to error given its reliance on subjective criteria, the intrusion of bias and prejudice and shifting criteria leading to inconsistency and frequent change. Consider the illustrative diagnostic controversies which buttress Reich's contentions: the deletion of homosexuality as a condition following a poll of members of the American Psychiatric Association in 1973; intense debates over whether a concept like attention-deficit hyperactivity in children or in adults is valid; and the question of whether antisocial personality disorder is a valid disorder of personality functioning or mere social deviance (and therefore belongs within the sphere of crime and delinquency). Many more examples could be added to this list.

In the context of an ill-defined professional framework and the vague criteria for diagnosis, the psychiatrist is sanctioned by law to manage the situation in which a person suffers or is suspected of suffering from mental illness that may require enforced hospitalization and/or treatment to protect a person's welfare or that of others (Peele and Chodoff). This is an awesome responsibility in that a person may be deprived of his liberty, lose basic civil rights, and be subject to a range of legal regulations.

Although commitment statutes in many jurisdictions, particularly those pertaining to determining the risk of dangerousness to self and/or others, have been rigorously scrutinized, a disconcerting uncertainty persists as to what constitute relevant criteria. Psychiatrists are caught in a dilemma of having to arrive at a judgment about a person's clinical needs and protecting her civil rights at the same time. The civil libertarian would insist that an inalienable right to liberty should be guaranteed above all other considerations whereas those with a paternalistic outlook would aver that society, through its legally sanctioned agents, has an obligation periodically to take measures, undesirable as they may be, to protect patient, society, or both from harm.

Soviet Psychiatric Abuse

In summary, ill-defined boundaries, the subjective basis of assessment, and the authority to treat a person involuntarily combine to make psychiatry especially vulnerable to abuse. The most clear-cut illustration of this was the use of psychiatry in the former Soviet Union to suppress political, religious, and other forms of dissent. These practices have been analyzed at length by several observers (Bloch and Reddaway 1977, 1984; see also Bukovsky; Plyushch).

Soviet psychiatry's boundaries were drawn in such a way that made the entire discipline subordinate to the pervasive influence, overt and covert, of the Soviet state and, more particularly, of the Communist Party. The monolithic form of the administrative structure, with power wielded by a small, compliant group of psychiatrists, allowed a political authority to mould the functions of all Soviet psychiatrists. Even if professional boundaries had been clearer, the totalitarian nature of the Soviet state prevented psychiatrists from functioning autonomously. The fact that boundaries were blurred made it all the easier for the state to exert control and influence the profession in terms of its ideology. The Soviet government's avowal that the interests of society were as pertinent as those of the individual paved the way for the principle of respect for autonomy to be undermined.

The Soviet abuse is a blatant reminder that psychiatrists may function in a state whose interests do not serve those of the society. The corollary is obvious—psychiatrists must act independently with regard to ethical standards.

The lack of objective criteria for diagnostic evaluation permitted the evolution of an idiosyncratic taxonomic scheme in Soviet psychiatry for virtually four decades. Andrei Snezhnevsky rapidly ascended to the pinnacle of the psychiatric establishment during the 1950s, and from that impregnable position launched a unique classificatory system of mental illness. A crucial result was the profound shift in the way schizophrenia was conceptualized. Snezhnevsky advanced several claims, among them the notion that since the illness could be present in a person showing minimal features, schizophrenia was much more common than previously thought. A form of the illness, *sluggish schizophrenia,* named thus because of its slow progression, accounted for the wider limits placed on the use of the diagnosis. When suppression of dissent by psychiatric means escalated in the 1960s, the label *sluggish schizophrenia,* was commonly applied to political, religious, and other dissidents whom the state wished to disempower and punish (Reich; Bloch and Reddaway, 1977).

Although this framework was not originally devised to curb dissent, the vagueness of its concepts enabled application of a disease label to people whom psychiatrists elsewhere would have regarded as normal, mildly eccentric or, at worst, *neurotic.*

The inadequacy of criteria to appraise the risk of harm of a person to himself and/or to others makes psychiatry open to the improper use of its sanction to detain. As an element of the Soviet pattern, the notion of "social danger" was promulgated. In a letter to the Western press in 1973 (Guardian), the psychiatric establishment, fending off allegations that psychiatry was being misused, asserted that in a proportion of patients, their disease process could result in antisocial activity, including "disturbances of public order, dissemination of slander, and manifestations of aggressive intentions." They commented further on the "seeming normality" of these patients when they committed dangerous acts. Aggression in the mentally ill leading to self-harm or harm to others was conflated with disturbance of public order and slander. Well-documented cases of dissenters in Soviet hospitals pointed to an obvious conclusion: Psychiatrists there had broadened the concept of dangerousness in an ethically dubious way.

Chinese Abuse

The allegation of the systematic, political abuse of psychiatry in China, comparable to what occurred in the former Soviet Union, has been widely debated since Robin Munro, a Research Fellow in the University of London and formerly an observer of the human rights situation in China employed by Human Rights Watch, produced a report detailing most methodically its prevalence and procedures (Munro, 2001; Dangerous Minds).

According to Munro, a small number of political dissenters were arrested as *enemies of the state,* diagnosed with a major psychiatric disorder and then compulsorily hospitalized as far back as the 1950s. Having stumbled across evidence of this practice in 1989 in a Chinese textbook on legal aspects of psychiatry, Munro scrutinized the *official* psychiatric literature—books and journals in the main—only to find repeated references to *political* patients. In one series of forensic psychiatric assessments, no less than one in five related to *counterrevolutionary behavior.*

The Cultural Revolution from 1966 to 1976 saw further ethical disarray in psychiatry. On the one hand, genuine patients forced by the Red Guards into confessing that they were truly counterrevolutionary, were thereupon promptly imprisoned or even executed. Conversely, genuine political dissidents were dispatched to institutions for the criminally insane. As one prominent forensic psychiatrist, Zheng Zhanpei, put it in 1988, the turmoil within Chinese psychiatry "… had to do with the particular historical circumstances of the time" (Munro, 2002, p.102). Munro

provides extracts from Chinese psychiatric publications during this turbulent period which reveal just how politicized the profession became. For instance, mental illness was seen as being bound up with the class struggle and, given the tussle between the proletariat and capitalist positions, most patients had a bourgeois outlook.

Following the Cultural Revolution, the Soviet pattern of abuse returned but became more prominent in the late 1990s in association with the state-led campaign to stamp out the religious Falun Gong movement. As the pressure began to mount against the movement's members, so a proportion of them were falsely detained in general psychiatric hospitals under the rubric of a newly devised psychiatric condition with the bizarre title of "evil cult-induced mental disorder."

The response of Western psychiatrists to Munro's findings and conclusions have differed substantially, ranging from total incredulity that any country would be silly enough to repeat the Soviet saga and thus earn universal disapproval and condemnation to a solid conviction that the allegations are well-founded.

The Royal College of Psychiatrists for instance resolved at its 2001 Annual General Meeting to call on the World Psychiatric Association to organize a fact-finding visit to China.

How prominent Western figures in psychiatry have arrived at their conclusions, one way or the other, is difficult to fathom. Alan Stone, Professor of Law and Psychiatry at Harvard University, sharply criticizes Munro's research and regards Chinese psychiatrists as more victims than victimizers. It is relevant here that Stone remains adamant that Soviet psychiatrists also did not misuse their knowledge and skills to curb dissent. Sing Lee, and Arthur Kleinman, a distinguished anthropologist and psychiatrist, also at Harvard, similarly argue that "… there is simply no evidence of systematic abuse of mental hospitals for reasons of political oppression by the profession as a whole" (p.124) although they do concede that some psychiatrists are more open to "abusive practices" (p.124) when under police or Communist Party pressure.

Among psychiatrists who contend that abuse almost certainly has taken place and continues are Jim Birley, past President of the Royal College of Psychiatrists, who opines thus: "There is certainly a strong case, more than a suspicion, that psychiatry is once again being used for political purposes" (p. 147); and Sunny Lu and Viviana Galli, two American psychiatrists, who have provided a detailed account of the role of Chinese psychiatrists in dealing with the Falun Gong specifically. The latter conclude that the psychiatric gambit is part of a "… comprehensive and brutal campaign to *eradicate* Falun Gong" (p. 129).

Western psychiatrists and human rights organizations had to toil long and hard before the abuse of psychiatry ceased in the former Soviet Union. The toll of suffering was tragically high as thousands of dissenters were victimized through psychiatry. In the case of the Chinese allegations, a similar delay should not ensue.

Preventing Abuse

Legislation, professional self-regulation, establishment of watchdog committees, and adherence to appropriate codes of ethics are complementary means to deal with and prevent psychiatric abuse. Legislation has the potential to safeguard patients's civil rights, hold psychiatrists accountable, and specifically define their functions. Such mental health laws promote patients's rights and protect them from abusive psychiatry, and set requirements of practice whose transgression is tantamount to illegal conduct (e.g., Mental Health Act, 1986).

Peer review and quality assurance may help identify ethically suspect judgments or actions. Many national associations of psychiatrists have procedures to discipline members who violate principles of clinical care: informal warning, reprimand, suspension, or expulsion (see for example, Royal Australian and New Zealand College of Psychiatrists). The Royal College of Psychiatrists in Britain and the American Psychiatric Association have developed procedures to investigate abuse.

As a professional collective, psychiatrists, both nationally and internationally, need to maintain vigilance when governmental or nongovernmental entities try to exploit them to apply their knowledge and skills for purposes other than serving the interests of patients and the community at large. Psychiatrists operating in totalitarian states may not be in an equivalent position without jeopardizing their professional or personal interests. For instance, Semyon Gluzman and Anatoly Koryagin experienced years of incarceration for condemning the misuse of psychiatry in the former Soviet Union.

As part of their ethics, psychiatrists have an obligation to protest against the misuse of their profession wherever and whenever it occurs. Such action points to a political role psychiatrists may be required to play.

Finally, psychiatrists need to familiarize themselves with, and adhere to, relevant ethical codes, from the Oath of Hippocrates which stipulates that the doctor will "keep [the sick] from harm and injustice," to their own national and international codes, many of which affirm that they should never use their professional authority to maltreat people.

The 1998 ethical code of the Royal Australian and New Zealand College of Psychiatrists explicitly covers abuse by incorporating the principle that "Psychiatrists shall not allow the misuse of their professional knowledge and skills." A series of annotations follows which deal with such issues as never diagnosing a person as mentally ill solely on the basis of political, religious, ideological, moral, or philosophical belief; the impermissibility of using nonconformity with a society's prevailing values as the determining factor in diagnosis; and the unacceptability of participation in torture and executions.

Conclusion

The history of psychiatry has been dreadfully tarnished by the occurrence of gross abuses, the Soviet and Nazi cases being especially prominent. Attention to such cases has led to greater ethical sensitivity among psychiatrists and beyond. Although this may serve as a safeguard against abuse now and in the future, both the profession and society need to maintain a vigorous defense against any malignant force that is tempted to exploit psychiatry and thus jeopardize its integrity.

SIDNEY BLOCH (1995)
REVISED BY AUTHOR

SEE ALSO: *Autonomy; Coercion; Deep Brain Stimulation; Electroconvulsive Therapy; Holocaust; Informed Consent: Issues of Consent in Mental Healthcare; Insanity and Insanity Defense; Institutionalization and Deinstitutionalization; Mental Illness: Conception of Mental Illness; Mental Illness: Cultural Perspectives; Mental Institutions, Commitment to; Mistakes, Medical; Paternalism; Patients' Rights; Psychosurgery, Medical and Historical Aspects of; Race and Racism; Technology; Women, Historical and Cross-Cultural Perspectives*

BIBLIOGRAPHY

Birley, Jim. 2002. "Political Abuse of Psychiatry in the Soviet Union and China: A Rough Guide for Bystanders." *Journal of the American Academy of Psychiatry and the Law* 30: 145–147.

Bloch, Sidney. 1984. "Apartheid and Psychiatry." *Lancet* ii: 1252–1253.

Bloch, Sidney. 1990. "Interrogation and Torture." In *Principles and Practice of Forensic Psychiatry,* ed. Robert Bluglass and Paul Bowden. Edinburgh: Churchill Livingstone.

Bloch, Sidney, and Reddaway, Peter. 1977. *Russia's Political Hospitals: The Abuse of Psychiatry in the Soviet Union.* London: Gollancz.

Bloch, Sidney, and Reddaway, Peter. 1984. *Soviet Psychiatric Abuse: The Shadow over World Psychiatry.* London: Gollancz.

Brown, Charles, and Lago, Armando M. 1991. *The Politics of Psychiatry in Revolutionary Cuba.* New Brunswick, NJ: Transaction.

Bukovsky, Vladimir. 1978. *To Build a Castle: My Life as a Dissenter.* New York: Viking.

Burleigh Michael. 1988. *Death and Deliverance.* Cambridge, Eng.: Cambridge University Press.

Busse, Ewald W. 1969. "APA's Role in Influencing the Evolution of a Health Care Delivery System." *American Journal of Psychiatry* 126: 739–744.

Chesler, Phyllis. 1972. *Women and Madness.* Garden City, NY: Doubleday.

Dangerous Minds. *Political Psychiatry in China Today and its Origins in the Mao Era.* New York: Human Rights Watch and Geneva Initiative on Psychiatry.

Dyer, Allen R. 1988. *Ethics and Psychiatry: Toward Professional Definition.* Washington, D.C.: American Psychiatric Press.

Fulford, William. 1989. *Moral Theory and Medical Practice.* Cambridge, Eng.: Cambridge University Press.

Fulford, William. 1999. "The Concept of Disease." In *Psychiatric Ethics,* 3rd edition, ed. Sidney Bloch, Paul Chodoff, and Stephen Green. Oxford: Oxford University Press.

Green, Stephen, and Bloch, Sidney. 2001. "Working in a Flawed Mental Health Care System: An Ethical Challenge." *American Journal of Psychiatry* 158: 1378–1383.

Harding, Timothy. 1991. "Ethical Issues in the Delivery of Mental Health Services: Abuses in Japan." In *Psychiatric Ethics,* 2nd edition, ed. Sidney Bloch and Paul Chodoff. Oxford: Oxford University Press.

Jones, Kathleen. 1978. "Society Looks at the Psychiatrist." *British Journal of Psychiatry* 132: 321–332.

Lee, Sing, and Kleinman, Arthur. 2002. "Psychiatry in its Political and Professional Contexts: A Response to Robin Munro." *Journal of the American Academy of Psychiatry and the Law* 30: 120–125.

Lu, Sunny, and Galli, Viviana. 2002. "Psychiatric Abuse of Falun Gong Practitioners in China." *Journal of the American Academy of Psychiatry and the Law* 30: 126–130.

Luepnitz, Deborah 2002. *The Family Interpreted: Psychoanalysis, Family Therapy and Feminism.* New York: Basic Books.

Mental Health Act 1986. Act No. 59/1986. Reprinted incorporating amendments as at 19 June 1997. Melbourne: State of Victoria, Australia.

Müller-Hill, B. 1988. *Murderous Science.* Oxford: Oxford University Press.

Munro, Robin. 2001. "Judicial Psychiatry in China and Its Political Abuses." *Columbia Journal of Asian Law* 14: 1–128.

Munro, Robin. 2002. "Political Psychiatry in Post-Mao China and its Origins in the Cultural Resolution." *Journal of the American Academy of Psychiatry and the Law* 30: 97–106.

Musto, David. 1999. "A Historical Perspective." *In Psychiatric Ethics,* 3rd edition, ed. Sidney Bloch, Paul Chodoff, and Stephen Green. Oxford: Oxford University Press.

Peele, Roger, and Chodoff, Paul. 1999. "The Ethics of Involuntary Treatment and Deinstitutionalization." In *Psychiatric Ethics,* 3rd edition, ed. Sidney Bloch, Paul Chodoff, and Stephen Green. Oxford: Oxford University Press.

Plyushch, L. 1979. *History's Carnival.* New York: Harcourt Brace Jovanovich.

Reich, Walter. 1999. "Psychiatric Diagnosis as an Ethical Problem." In *Psychiatric Ethics,* 3rd edition, ed. Sidney Bloch, Paul Chodoff, and Stephen Green. Oxford: Oxford University Press.

Robitscher, Jonas B. 1980. *The Powers of Psychiatry.* Boston: Houghton Mifflin.

Royal Australian and New Zealand College of Psychiatrists. *Code of Ethics,* 2nd edition. Melbourne: Author.

Showalter, Elaine. 1987. *The Female Malady: Women, Madness and English Culture, 1830–1980.* London: Virago.

Guardian "Soviet Psychiatry: The Doctors Reply." September 29, 1973. Letters.

Stone, Alan. 1984. *Law, Psychiatry, and Morality: Essays and Analysis.* Washington, D.C.: American Psychiatric Press.

Stone, Alan. 2002. "Psychiatrists on the Side of the Angels: The Falun Gong and Soviet Jewry." *Journal of the American Academy of Psychiatry and the Law* 30: 107–111.

Torrey, F. 1997. *Out of the Shadows: Confronting America's Mental Illness Crisis.* New York: Wiley.

Waggoner, Raymond W. 1970. "The Presidential Address: Cultural Dissonance and Psychiatry." *American Journal of Psychiatry* 127: 1–8.

World Psychiatric Association. 1991. "Declaration of Hawaii." In *Psychiatric Ethics,* 3rd edition, ed. Sidney Bloch, Paul Chodoff, and Stephen Green. Oxford: Oxford University Press.

PSYCHOANALYSIS AND DYNAMIC THERAPIES

• • •

The term *psychoanalysis,* in its narrow sense refers to a method of psychological therapy originally developed by Sigmund Freud around the turn of the twentieth century and now practiced by analysts trained in the intellectual and clinical tradition that has followed Freud. The earliest psychoanalytic investigations led to revolutionary discoveries about the working of the mind, and therefore the term *psychoanalysis* refers also, in a broader sense, to the accumulated body of findings and theories about human mental functioning that have resulted from clinical psychoanalysis, and that are available to guide psychoanalysts in continuing their work.

The issue of the ethical implications of psychoanalysis was not one that greatly preoccupied Freud. He considered ethics to be the reflection of the cultural super-ego at a given moment in history, a "therapeutic attempt" to come to terms with human aggression (1930), and would no doubt have regarded the present concern with bioethics in this light. An examination of its principles and practices may help to show how current ethical reflection is relevant to psychoanalysis.

Clinical psychoanalysis is used as a treatment for a variety of psychological conditions, including both specific symptoms and more general personality problems. The treatment involves individual meetings with an analyst, several times per week, over a period of several years. The patient usually lies on a couch and is instructed to say whatever comes to mind (a technique called free association), including symptoms, life events, memories, fantasies, dreams, physical sensations, and feelings about the analyst. The analyst listens to this material, and eventually interprets it as revealing conflicts between emotional forces ("dynamic" conflicts) of which the patient had previously been unconscious. Feelings about the analyst, called transference feelings, are particularly important for this purpose, since these feelings are unconsciously transferred onto the analyst from significant persons in the patient's past, and can be used to interpret and rework current conflicts derived from these past relationships.

Psychoanalytic theory has been continually revised and expanded since its inception. Its earliest form was codified in Freud's major work, *The Interpretation of Dreams* (1900). In this volume he presented the topographic theory, which emphasized the division of the mind into conscious and unconscious realms, and explained not only neurotic symptoms but also normal phenomena, such as dreams and slips of the tongue, as the results of unconscious wishes breaking through, in disguised and distorted form, into consciousness. Psychoanalytic techniques, such as free association and the use of the couch, were intended to maximize the possibility of such breakthroughs. In this way, unconscious wishes could be interpreted and made conscious, and the symptoms resulting from those wishes could be relieved.

Dreams, errors, and symptoms remain useful sources of interpretable material for the modern analyst, but topographic theory has been subsumed by later theoretical developments. Freud's 1923 work "The Ego and the Id" presented a structural theory, in which the mind includes three agencies: the id, ego, and superego. Each agency has wishes and directions of its own, and they often come into conflict with each other. Neurotic symptoms, as well as character traits, are interpreted as the results of conflicts among these structures, and the goal of analysis is to strengthen the ego, the structure responsible for resolving conflicts within the mind and negotiating compromises between internal wishes and external reality.

Structural theory forms the core of a theoretical tradition known as "ego psychology," one of the dominant schools of thought in modern psychoanalysis, along with object-relations theory and self psychology. Object-relations theory places greater emphasis on the effects of early relationships, most importantly with the mother. It holds that pathological early relationships are internalized and unconsciously repeated, causing problems in later relationships. Self psychology emphasizes the role of early trauma and parental failure in preventing the establishment of a stable and coherent self. Proponents of these theories hold that they are more serviceable than structural theory for the treatment of seriously disturbed patients, those whose pathological early lives prevented the formation of stable mental structures.

The applicability of clinical psychoanalysis is limited by a number of practical and psychological factors. There are many patients for whom psychoanalytic ideas and insights might be useful, but who cannot be treated with clinical psychoanalysis because they cannot afford the time or money required, because they are interested only in more limited treatment for well-circumscribed problems, or because they do not have the necessary psychological resources, such as curiosity about the mind, access to dreams and fantasies, and an ability to tolerate frustration. The term *dynamic therapies* refers to a variety of psychotherapeutic techniques that have evolved for use in these situations.

The dynamic therapies, which are now considered the treatment of choice in some situations, are similar to psychoanalysis in that they involve regular meetings between patient and therapist in which talking is the primary therapeutic activity, an effort is made to understand the unconscious origins of the patient's problems, the patient's relationship to the therapist is used as an important source of information and a vehicle for change, and the practitioner is guided by psychoanalytic ideas about the working of the mind, including the idea that psychological problems are caused by "dynamic" conflict between unconscious forces. The dynamic therapies differ from psychoanalysis in that they are usually less intensive and involve less frequent meetings, the patient usually sits in a chair facing the therapist, the overall duration of the treatment may be shorter, the treatment may be focused on more specific goals, and the therapist is more likely to use techniques that offer emotional support to the patient as well as exploration of the unconscious. To the extent that the dynamic therapies are derivatives of psychoanalysis, similar considerations of ethics and values apply to both. This article will focus on ethical and value-related issues in psychoanalysis, with the understanding that similar considerations apply to the other dynamic therapies.

Training and Practice

Freud was trained as a neurologist, but most medical psychoanalysts have been psychiatrists. Freud believed that a medical background was not necessary for analysts (1926), and in Europe it has been common for nonphysicians to become analysts. In the United States analysis was for many years seen primarily as a subspecialty of psychiatry, but recently some nonphysicians have been admitted to analytic training.

Training in psychoanalysis begins after the completion of professional school and specialty training, and includes classroom education, a personal analysis of the trainee, and the treatment of several analytic cases under the supervision of senior analysts. Becoming a psychoanalyst involves not only mastering theory and technique but also becoming a member of a nonmedical profession, and accepting that profession's ethical judgments. The psychoanalytic profession's formal organization, the International Psychoanalytical Association, and its component associations, articulate and enforce ethical standards for the profession, as well as standards for training and procedures for certifying the skills of psychoanalysts. However, these bodies have no legal authority and cannot prevent nonmembers from calling themselves psychoanalysts.

The field of psychotherapy is much less organized and regulated. Individuals from many different professional backgrounds are free to call themselves therapists. Those individuals may be answerable to the standards of their own professions, but there is no overarching set of standards for training or ethical practice in psychotherapy.

Clinical Theory Versus Theory of the Mind

Over the decades, psychoanalysis has evolved two related but quite different bodies of theory. The first, "clinical theory," is a set of ideas about how the process of psychoanalysis works and a set of principles about how the analyst should behave. The second, comprising ideas about the working of the human mind that have resulted from psychoanalytic investigations in the past, might be broadly termed a psychoanalytic "theory of the mind"; this body of theory includes ideas about normal development, about the nature and origins of psychopathology, and about the structure and functioning of the mind (a branch of theory termed *metapsychology*). For the purpose of ethical analysis, these two bodies of theory present quite different challenges. Psychoanalytic clinical theory strives to remain value-neutral, while the psychoanalytic theory of the mind embodies a host of value-laden assumptions about normality and deviance, health and sickness, and the relationship of the individual to society, many of which have been challenged by critics of psychoanalysis.

Freud argued that psychoanalysis was a scientific method of investigation, and therefore neutral with respect to values (1927). The assertion that clinical analysis is value-neutral is related to the tenet in clinical theory that the analyst is guided by the principles of abstinence (Freud, 1915a) and neutrality (Freud, 1919; LaPlanche and Pontalis). The principle of abstinence enjoins the analyst from indulging in any kind of gratification (for patient or analyst) other than the satisfactions of analysis itself; sexual contact between analyst and patient, extra-analytic friendship, and nonanalytic emotional support are all proscribed.

The principle of neutrality dictates, in terms of structural theory, that the analyst should occupy a position equidistant from the competing forces in the mind (Freud, 1946), analyzing the conflict between them but not trying to influence the outcome of that conflict. In lay terms, the principle of neutrality means that the analyst should not try to influence the patient to adopt any particular set of values, or to conduct his or her life in any particular way; the analyst's job is only to analyze conflicts and remove inhibitions. Neurotic inhibitions limit the patient's freedom, and their successful removal liberates the patient to live however he or she chooses.

The Limits of Neutrality

The attitude of neutrality is not easy to adopt or to maintain. It requires that the analyst first become aware of his or her own values and preferences, unconscious as well as conscious, and then exert a constant and vigilant self-discipline, in order not to let these personal values influence the conduct of analysis. Much of the analyst's lengthy training, especially the personal analysis that he or she must undergo, is directed toward this end. However, it can be argued that absolute neutrality is not possible, even with a thorough personal analysis and a consistent adherence to the principle. The process of psychoanalysis necessarily embodies certain values, both in its selection of patients and in the ideals that inhere in the process itself.

The analyst can adopt the attitude of neutrality only if certain preconditions are met in the patient. Patient and analyst must have a common view of reality, at least in a broad way, for the analyst will probably find it impossible to remain neutral with respect to frankly psychotic ideas. Similarly, if the patient's illness is of the type that produces serious danger to the patient or others, the analyst may be unable to remain neutral with respect to that danger, and may instead intervene to protect the values of life and health, concluding that these medical and therapeutic values take precedence over analytic goals in this situation. In order to adopt an attitude of neutrality, the analyst must also believe that the patient possesses an adequately sound moral character; if the analyst believes the patient to be an evil person, neutrality will be impossible. It is part of the individual analyst's clinical and ethical responsibility to become aware of the kinds of patients with whom he or she has particular difficulty. Thus, some of the preconditions in the selection of patients for analysis embody value-laden assumptions that limit the scope of the principle of neutrality.

Moreover, the process of analysis itself can be seen to embody certain values that are not universally held and deviate from absolute neutrality (Michels and Oldham). Psychoanalysis assumes that insight is a goal worth pursuing; that it is always better to know things, especially about oneself, than not to know them; and that greater knowledge will ultimately lead to decreased suffering. This is a common belief, but by no means an unquestionable one; indeed, the Greek drama on which Freud based much of his theory of the mind, Sophocles's *Oedipus Rex,* primarily concerns the question whether knowledge or insight is an unmitigated good.

Clinical analysis also embodies the value of individuality; it is a process in which an individual patient spends a great deal of time, energy, and money exploring his or her individual mind and personal history in order, ultimately, to achieve greater individual happiness. This is not to say that relationships with others are neglected, or that the individual is encouraged to promote his or her welfare at the expense of others. However, to members of other cultures, especially non-Western ones, the idea of devoting so much attention to the individual alone, rather than as a member of the group, would seem strange and inappropriate. Thus the principle of neutrality, while central in clinical theory, is limited in its scope; the process requires that patient and analyst share certain value-laden assumptions about the perception of reality, about morally acceptable behavior, and about the importance of individuality and insight.

Limitations on the Analyst's Role

The principles of abstinence and neutrality dictate that the analyst may not assume other roles in the patient's life. As noted above, nonprofessional contacts, such as sexual, social, or business relationships, or exchanging gifts with patients, are inconsistent with analytic abstinence. Certain other professional functions, which might well be beneficial, are still proscribed because they are inconsistent with neutrality, and therefore are not analytic. For example, advising the patient on life decisions or on how to manage relationships with important others, as one might do in a supportive psychotherapy, would constitute a deviation from analytic neutrality. Similarly, certain assessment or advocacy functions, such as testifying on a patient's behalf in a legal proceeding, would violate the analytic role. In certain circumstances, such violations are inescapable or necessary; if an analytic patient becomes suicidally depressed, the analyst may have to intervene in a nonabstinent and nonneutral fashion. However, such a situation is best understood not as an exception to the principles of analysis but as a point at which other values, such as preserving life, override the importance of analysis, and the analyst chooses temporarily to suspend analysis in order to serve other goals.

The Analyst's Obligations

In the broadest sense, the analyst's primary obligation is to give good treatment. In practice, this means ensuring that he or she is well-trained; that his or her skills remain current and consistent with professional standards, by keeping up with the analytic literature and being involved with professional associations; selecting patients for analysis carefully, to be sure that they have the psychological resources necessary for analysis, and that there is no more appropriate treatment for each patient's condition; and conducting the analysis under the guidance of the principles of neutrality and abstinence. By adhering to these guidelines, the analyst will fulfill most of his or her ethical obligations. However, certain obligations deserve particular notice.

COUNTERTRANSFERENCE. Just as the patient in a successful analysis predictably develops intense transference feelings about the analyst, the analyst predictably develops intense feelings about the patient, which are called countertransference. These feelings may be positive or negative, and their specific content will be determined both by the nature of the patient's transference and by the analyst's own history and unconscious dynamics. In any case, countertransference feelings, especially unconscious ones, constitute the most serious challenge to analytic neutrality.

The ability to recognize and manage countertransference feelings is both an essential goal of analytic training and supervision, and an ongoing ethical obligation for the practicing analyst.

SEXUAL MISCONDUCT. A very common variety of transference and countertransference involves erotic attraction between patient and analyst. The analyst is under a strict ethical obligation to strive to recognize the transferential origin of this attraction and, in any event, to refrain from acting on it (Freud, 1915a). Sexual contact between doctor and patient is prohibited in general medicine, as stated in the Hippocratic Oath, and in psychiatry, but there are additional reasons for this rule in psychoanalysis. In general medicine and psychiatry, the patient is in a dependent position, and the chance that the patient's needs could be exploited for the doctor's sexual satisfaction is so great that the American Medical Association (AMA) has seen fit to ban sex between physicians and their current patients (Council on Ethical and Judicial Affairs). In 1993 the American Psychiatric Association (APA) went further and stated in their *Principles of Medical Ethics: With Annotations Especially Applicable to Psychiatry* that "Sexual activity with a current or former patient is unethical" (p. 4).

In psychoanalysis, the same argument about dependency and exploitation applies, but another and more encompassing argument exists as well. The conduct of psychoanalysis rests on the proposition that the treatment is conducted in words only, not in action; the patient is free to say or imagine anything, because no action will ensue. If this principle is violated and the patient and analyst act on their erotic attraction to each other, either during or long after the analysis, the credibility of the treatment itself is seriously damaged, and the interests of those who might benefit from analysis in the future are thus harmed. Accordingly, the American Psychoanalytic Association, recognizing that the unconscious is timeless (Freud, 1915b), absolutely prohibits sexual contact between analyst and patient, with no special exemption for a postanalytic relationship (1983).

CONFIDENTIALITY. The analyst's obligation to respect the patient's confidentiality derives not specifically from the principles of clinical psychoanalysis but from the general principle of confidentiality recognized in both physician–patient and therapist–client relationships. However, the principle assumes special importance in psychoanalysis, since the analyst specifically instructs the patient to hold no information back, and thereby acquires the obligation to treat the patient's communications with full respect for privacy.

Psychoanalysis and Social Values: Common Criticisms

CRITICISMS OF THE THEORY OF THE MIND. Many of the value-laden assumptions embodied in the psychoanalytic theory of the mind have been attacked as promoting negative stereotypes and producing destructive social consequences. For example, feminist critics have argued that the psychoanalytic theory of female development and psychology offers a negative view of women as psychologically inferior to men. The argument is based on Freud's early position that women do not experience castration anxiety in the same way men do, and are therefore less likely to develop a rigorous superego. This criticism is generally accurate with respect to Freud's original theory, which was very much a product of the culture in which he lived and his personal predilections. However, psychoanalytic ideas about female psychology and social roles have been extensively revised since that time, with the result that current psychoanalytic theorizing on the subject offers a much fuller, more positive, and more nuanced view of both male and female development and psychology.

Similarly, spokespersons for the gay community have argued that psychoanalysis treats gays unfairly and advances a biased view that homosexuality is invariably a pathological outcome of disturbed development. This criticism could only be directed at organized psychoanalysis after Freud, since Freud himself argued strongly that homosexuality need not be considered a form of pathology (1905). Debate on the subject has been intense over the last decades, involving such questions as whether homosexuality has significant concurrence with certain forms of psychopathology, especially narcissistic disorders; whether the psychopathology seen in homosexuals can be understood as a result of familial and social condemnation of biologically determined orientation; whether heterosexuality can or should be a goal of analytic treatment; and whether homosexuals are acceptable candidates for training as analysts. As far as the American Psychoanalytic Association is involved, the issue has been formally settled by a position statement affirming that "same-gender sexual orientation cannot be assumed to represent a deficit in personality development or the expression of psychopathology," and disavowing "efforts to 'convert' or 'repair' an individual's sexual orientation" (American Psychoanalytic Association, 2000; for the history of this debate, see also Bayer).

Another important criticism of psychoanalysis, deriving largely from the circumstances of Freud's personality and culture, is that it is hostile to religion. Freud himself made clear his belief that religion was nothing more than a cultural neurosis (1927). For many years, psychoanalysis and religion saw each other as enemies, but in recent decades this situation has changed. Analysts have come to recognize religion as an important domain of human mental activity, not to be lightly dismissed, and theologians have become increasingly interested in the use of psychoanalytic insights in their thinking and pastoral practice.

The concept of "psychic reality" is both a central tenet of psychoanalytic theory and a source of some important criticisms of that theory. The concept appeared when Freud revised his theory about the role of childhood seduction in causing neurosis; at first, he believed his patients' frequent stories of being sexually abused as children were historically accurate, but later he came to appreciate the psychological importance of fantasies and wishes as capable of producing neurosis even in the absence of actual seduction. Critics have argued that psychoanalytic theory went too far in this direction, presenting a view in which all memories of childhood sexual abuse were dismissed as fantasies, and that this development was responsible for long-standing and widespread denial, until recently, of the extent of actual sexual abuse of children.

Finally, psychoanalysis has been criticized by the antipsychiatry movement as a form of mind control. Spokespeople for this movement are opposed to all psychiatric practice as a tool of social control that imposes on patients a view of reality acceptable to the politically powerful. As a particularly influential form of psychiatric treatment, these critics argue, psychoanalysis is very effective in imposing the analyst's view of reality on the unsuspecting patient. Whether this general criticism is valid or not, the behavior it describes is clearly inconsistent with analytic neutrality and good analytic practice.

CRITICISMS OF CLINICAL THEORY AND PRACTICE. Various ethical objections have been raised against clinical psychoanalysis, concerning both its status as a form of treatment and the effects it has on individuals and on society.

Critics have argued that it is impossible for a patient to give informed consent to analysis, since the patient cannot possibly appreciate beforehand what an exploration of the unconscious will involve. This situation is analogous to other investigative procedures in medicine, in which neither patient nor doctor can know beforehand what will be found, and the patient can be informed only as to the risks and potential benefits of the procedure itself, with the understanding that the findings cannot be predicted. In clinical analysis, the patient's act of giving consent is ongoing

throughout the treatment. Opponents of psychoanalysis, including many prominent psychiatrists, have argued extensively that it is unethical to offer a treatment, like psychoanalytic therapy, the value of which has not been demonstrated in controlled statistical studies, when other treatments are available that have been shown by such studies to be effective (Klerman). However, the vast majority of treatments and practices in clinical medicine have not yet been proven effective in this rigorous fashion. The fact that psychoanalysis still awaits such proof requires only that the prospective patient be informed of what is known about the treatment's effectiveness, and of other treatments that might be available.

A related issue arises from a concerted attack on psychoanalysis as science (see, for example, the work of Adolf Grunbaum) that has worked against the support of psychoanalytic treatment in a climate of managed care and health maintenance organizations (HMOs) (Gunderson and Gabbard). One aspect of this problem is the difficulty of research for the purpose of empirical validation in a situation that "allows the presence of no third person" (Freud, 1926). Indeed, some early studies may have crossed the line later to be laid down by committees on experimentation with human subjects (Wallerstein). But the negative effects of outside observers on therapy may have been overestimated (Busch et al.), and comparative studies of dynamic and other therapies for specific disorders seem to promise new support for their effectiveness (Barber and Crits-Christoph).

With respect to the effects of analysis, critics have argued that it discourages spontaneity, encourages dependence and self-centeredness, excuses evil or criminal behavior, and medicalizes human relationships. For the most part, these criticisms describe expectable complications and distortions of the analytic process, or inappropriate applications of analytic principles outside of analytic treatment, rather than the process of analysis as it should be conducted.

The idea that analysis discourages spontaneity by requiring that the patient substitute thought for action presents a common and analyzable distortion of the process. While it is true that analysis requires substituting thought for action during the analytic hour, it does not follow that the patient is expected to behave this way outside the hour. In fact, an inhibition of spontaneity outside of analysis would usually be seen as a manifestation of obsessional pathology, in which thought is substituted for action, or as an enactment of the transference, and in any case as an indication for further analytic work. Similarly, the idea that the focus on oneself required in the analytic hour should extend to the rest of life is a miscarriage of analysis, requiring interpretation and correction.

The argument that analysis encourages dependency results from the fact that a dependent transference toward the analyst commonly develops, since the patient's relationship to important others in the past will often have been a dependent one, or that the experience of a dependent time of life is remembered when regression occurs in the analysis. However, analysis itself neither encourages nor discourages dependency; it encourages only the emergence and resolution of the transference, whatever its content may be. If the patient is reluctant to relinquish this dependent posture, that development is an interpretable distortion. Some varieties of dynamic therapy, in contrast, may encourage dependency as the cost of attaining important therapeutic goals.

Debates about the insanity defense in criminal proceedings have often involved a misapplication of the psychoanalytic principle of neutrality. Critics argue that by trying to make all behavior understandable in terms of the interplay of unconscious forces, psychoanalysis has removed the sense of personal responsibility for behavior. However, as described above, the principle of neutrality is employed only in a very specific setting, the psychoanalytic hour, and only with a well-selected population and for a specific limited purpose. Analysts do not encourage the adoption of an attitude of neutrality outside of clinical psychoanalysis (Gaylin).

The argument that psychoanalysis tends inappropriately to medicalize problems in human life and relationships is based partly on a peculiar historical association between analysis and medicine. Freud was a physician, as were his earliest disciples, but the psychoanalytic movement in Europe rapidly expanded to include nonmedical practitioners. In the United States, analysis has been dominated by the medical profession, though the 1991 decision of the American Psychoanalytic Association to approve full training for nonmedical candidates presages a significant increase in the proportion and influence of nonmedical analysts in the United States. The distinction between prescribing analysis and conducting analysis may be useful in elucidating the proper relationship between medicine and analysis. The act of prescribing psychoanalysis as the treatment of choice for a particular patient is a medical act, since it requires diagnosing the patient's problem and knowing the possible alternative treatments; but the act of conducting the analysis, while it requires good clinical judgment, does not require medical knowledge or training.

Finally, psychotherapeutic practices have come under scrutiny because of a widespread feeling that medicine in general and psychiatry in particular have paid insufficient attention to the real needs and sensitivities of patients as individual human beings. This feeling has been articulated in part by advocacy groups like the National Alliance for the Mentally Ill (NAMI), but has also been evidenced in independent critiques of the profession by writers who have claimed that it is out of its depth and "omits the moral dimension of living" (Lomas) or that it is in disorder and desperately needs a "culture of responsibility" (Luhrmann). Such manifestations of the moral and social preoccupations of the current cultural epoch can only be welcomed; they represent challenges that it is in everyone's interest to meet openly and honestly.

PUBLIC-HEALTH ISSUES. Some criticisms of psychoanalysis contend that it is a luxury for the rich, is suitable only for a tiny minority of the most prosperous and least disturbed members of society, and consumes a vast amount of medical resources that could be put to better use meeting the needs of the poor and the seriously mentally ill. Psychoanalysts offer several rebuttals. First, it is not true that the problems of psychoanalytic patients are trivial; while analysis does require certain particular psychological strengths, patients in analysis can be seriously impaired and genuinely suffering in many ways, and analysis can provide significant relief to them. Second, the benefits of psychoanalysis extend well beyond the patients who are treated with full analysis. Many other forms of treatment, including the dynamic therapies and even pharmacotherapy and general medical treatment, can be rendered more effective if the practitioner understands and makes use of psychoanalytic insights about human motivation. Finally, analysts recognize that few individuals can afford to pay a standard psychiatric fee several times per week over many years, and many analysts are willing to reduce their fees to enable a wider range of people to benefit from psychoanalytic treatment. These financial problems could be mitigated if systems of reimbursement paid fairly for cognitive and interpersonal services in comparison with surgical and invasive procedures. But such decisions are usually governed by political and economic concerns rather than by ethical imperatives.

Conclusion

Until the 1960s, psychoanalysis was the dominant theory and psychoanalytically derived therapies were the most common treatment in the mental health professions. Since then the dominance has waned, partly as a result of economic forces leading to the development of briefer treatments, and partly as the result of the rise of biological psychiatry and the development of effective pharmacologic treatments. In recent decades only a small fraction of psychiatrists have chosen to become psychoanalysts, and only a small fraction of patients are treated with full psychoanalysis. However, the influence of analytic theories and findings continues to be felt throughout the fields of psychiatry, psychotherapy, and medicine. It is likely that there will remain a population of patients who have problems of sufficient breadth and depth, and who can support its financial costs, who will choose psychoanalysis and its related therapies as their treatments of choice.

KEVIN V. KELLY (1995)
REVISED BY PETER CAWS

SEE ALSO: *Behavior Control; Behaviorism; Behavior Modification Therapies; Freedom and Free Will; Mental Health; Mental Illness; Psychiatry, Abuses of*

BIBLIOGRAPHY

American Psychiatric Association (APA). 1993. *Principles of Medical Ethics: With Annotations Especially Applicable to Psychiatry.* Washington, D.C.: Author.

American Psychoanalytic Association. 1983. *Principles of Ethics for Psychoanalysts and Provisions for Implementation of the Principles of Ethics for Psychoanalysts.* New York: Author.

American Psychoanalytic Association. 2000. "Committee on Gay and Lesbian Issues: Position Statement on Reparative Therapy." New York: Author.

Appelbaum, Paul S., and Jorgenson, Linda. 1991. "Psychotherapist-Patient Sexual Contact after Termination of Treatment: An Analysis and a Proposal." *American Journal of Psychiatry* 148(11): 1466–1473.

Barber, Jacques P., and Crits-Christoph, Paul, eds. 1995. *Dynamic Therapies for Psychiatric Disorders (Axis I).* New York: Basic Books.

Bayer, Ronald. 1987. *Homosexuality and American Psychiatry: The Politics of Diagnosis.* Princeton, NJ: Princeton University Press.

Busch, Fredric N.; Milrod, Barbara L.; Shapiro, Theodore; et al. 2001. "How Treating Psychoanalysts Respond to Psychotherapy Research Constraints." *Journal of the American Psychoanalytic Association* 49(3): 961–984.

Council on Ethical and Judicial Affairs, American Medical Association. 1991. "Sexual Misconduct in the Practice of Medicine." *Journal of the American Medical Association* 266(19): 2741–2745.

Freud, Anna. 1946. *The Ego and the Mechanisms of Defense.* New York: International Universities Press.

Freud, Sigmund. 1886–1940 (reprint, 1953–1974). *The Standard Edition of the Complete Psychological Works of Sigmund Freud,* 24 vols., tr. and ed. James Strachey, Anna Freud, Alix Strachey, and Alan Tyson. London: Hogarth.

Freud, Sigmund. 1900. *The Interpretation of Dreams.* In *The Standard Edition of the Complete Psychological Works of Sigmund Freud,* vols. 4 and 5. London: Hogarth.

Freud, Sigmund. 1905. "Three Essays on the Theory of Sexuality." In *The Standard Edition of the Complete Psychological Works of Sigmund Freud,* vol. 7. London: Hogarth.

Freud, Sigmund. 1915a. "Observations on Transference-Love." In *The Standard Edition of the Complete Psychological Works of Sigmund Freud,* vol. 12. London: Hogarth.

Freud, Sigmund. 1915b. "The Unconscious." In *The Standard Edition of the Complete Psychological Works of Sigmund Freud,* vol. 14. London: Hogarth.

Freud, Sigmund. 1919. "Lines of Advance in Psychoanalytic Therapy." In *The Standard Edition of the Complete Psychological Works of Sigmund Freud,* vol. 17. London: Hogarth.

Freud, Sigmund. 1923. "The Ego and the Id." In *The Standard Edition of the Complete Psychological Works of Sigmund Freud,* vol. 19. London: Hogarth.

Freud, Sigmund. 1925. "An Autobiographical Study." In *The Standard Edition of the Complete Psychological Works of Sigmund Freud,* vol. 20. London: Hogarth.

Freud, Sigmund. 1926. "The Question of Lay Analysis." In *The Standard Edition of the Complete Psychological Works of Sigmund Freud,* vol. 20. London: Hogarth.

Freud, Sigmund. 1927. "The Future of an Illusion." In *The Standard Edition of the Complete Psychological Works of Sigmund Freud,* vol. 21. London: Hogarth.

Freud, Sigmund. 1930. "Civilization and Its Discontents." In *The Standard Edition of the Complete Psychological Works of Sigmund Freud,* vol. 21. London: Hogarth.

Gaylin, Willard. 1982. *The Killing of Bonnie Garland: A Question of Justice.* New York: Simon and Schuster.

Grunbaum, Adolf. 1984. *The Foundations of Psychoanalysis: A Philosophical Critique.* Berkeley: University of California Press.

Gunderson, John G., and Gabbard, Glen O. 1999. "Making the Case for Psychoanalytic Therapies in the Current Psychiatric Environment." *Journal of the American Psychoanalytic Association* 47(3): 679–740.

Klerman, Gerald L. 1990. "The Psychiatric Patient's Right to Effective Treatment: Implications of *Osheroff v. Chestnut Lodge.*" *American Journal of Psychiatry* 147(4): 409–418.

LaPlanche, Jean, and Pontalis, J. B. 1973. *The Language of Psychoanalysis,* tr. D. Nicholson-Smith. New York: W. W. Norton.

Lomas, Peter. 1999. *Doing Good? Psychotherapy Out of Its Depth.* Oxford, UK: Oxford University Press.

Luhrmann, T. M. 2000. *Of Two Minds: The Growing Disorder in American Psychiatry.* New York: Alfred A. Knopf.

Michels, Robert, and Oldham, John M. 1983. "Value Judgments in Psychoanalytic Theory and Practice." *Psychoanalytic Inquiry* 3(4): 599–608.

Wallerstein, Robert S. 1986. *Forty-two Lives in Treatment: A Study of Psychoanalysis and Psychotherapy (The Report of the Psychotherapy Research Project of the Menninger Foundation, 1965–1962).* New York: The Guilford Press.

PSYCHOPHARMACOLOGY

• • •

Psychopharmacology is the study of drugs used to treat disturbances in mood, behavior, and mental functioning across a broad range of illnesses and conditions. While many drugs used in general medicine (e.g., antihypertensives, hormonal therapies) can cause behavioral changes or psychological symptoms, psychopharmacologic agents are used specifically for their behavioral or mental effects. The classes of psychopharmacologic medications include the following: antipsychotics, antidepressants, antianxiety agents, and mood stabilizers. There are numerous ethical issues in psychopharmacology. This entry focuses on issues related to consent to treatment, the inclusion of severely mentally ill persons in psychopharmacologic research, involuntary outpatient treatment, and the cost of newer psychotropic medications.

The main classes of psychopharmacologic agents, which are antipsychotics, antidepressants, antianxiety agents, and mood stabilizers, are discussed below. Under each category, the U.S. Food and Drug Administration (FDA) approved drugs as well as their therapeutic and adverse effects are described. Cognitive enhancers (e.g., donepezil or Aricept), used to treat Alzheimer disease, are not included in this entry.

Antipsychotics

As the first effective medications to be introduced into treatment of psychosis, antipsychotic drugs revolutionized the treatment of schizophrenia and other severe psychiatric disorders. Prior to the introduction of the first antipsychotic (i.e., chlorpromazine [Thorazine]) in 1952, the principal treatment for a person with schizophrenia was long-term hospitalization. Often this hospitalization was aimed primarily at protecting society from patients with mental illness. The arrival of antipsychotic medications that could actually reduce psychiatric symptoms heralded a new era in the history of mental healthcare. Over the ensuing years, care for schizophrenia and other psychotic disorders changed from a largely custodial, institution-based system to a more community-based model emphasizing treatment and rehabilitation of individuals with psychiatric disorders (Grob).

Although they have been used to treat a variety of psychiatric conditions, antipsychotic drugs are primarily intended for psychotic disorders, the best example being schizophrenia. Schizophrenia affects approximately 1 percent of the population worldwide, and the vast majority of patients receive antipsychotic medication. Antipsychotics are especially useful in treating the hallucinations (perceptual disturbances such as hearing voices or seeing things), delusions (fixed false beliefs), and disorganized behavior. In addition antipsychotics can reduce the associated agitation, hostility, and unsafe behaviors that frequently impact the quality of life of patients, family members, and caregivers of persons with schizophrenia. Antipsychotic medications can reduce the symptoms of schizophrenia but do not cure the underlying illness, so a person who stops taking his medications is likely to have a relapse. In addition symptoms such as social withdrawal, loss of motivation, reduced emotional expression, and slowed thinking often persist, despite the use of antipsychotics.

There are different types of antipsychotics, each with a distinct chemical structure. With the advent of a newer generation of antipsychotics beginning in the late 1980s, drugs are now categorized as either *conventional* or *atypical*. The conventional agents were the only drugs available for treating schizophrenia for the first thirty-five years of the pharmacologic treatment era.

Conventional antipsychotics block receptors for a chemical messenger called dopamine in certain areas of the brain that are believed to mediate psychotic behavior. Hence increased dopamine activity is believed to be associated with psychosis, whereas blocking dopamine is believed to reduce psychosis. At the same time, blocking dopamine in other areas of the brain can produce uncomfortable muscular symptoms (stiffness, rigidity, tremor, restlessness) as well as abnormal breast milk production and sexual dysfunction.

The newer atypical antipsychotics may be of greater clinical benefit compared to the conventional antipsychotics. These atypical antipsychotics have fewer side effects and are better tolerated by patients. Patients may be more likely to take the newer medications regularly (Dolder et al.) and these medications may facilitate improved emotional expression, motivation, and social interaction in patients with schizophrenia.

ADVERSE EFFECTS. In the short term, dopamine receptors in brain regions responsible for involuntary movement system often produces rigidity, tremor, slowing of movement, and an unpleasant feeling of muscular restlessness. Over the long term, a substantial proportion of patients treated with conventional antipsychotics develop tardive dyskinesia, a potentially irreversible neurological disorder of involuntary movements of the mouth, face, neck, and body. The condition can be quite incapacitating, and there is currently no effective treatment. Each additional year of antipsychotic exposure increases a person's chance of developing tardive dyskinesia. Elderly patients are particularly at risk for this condition, especially if there is a pre-existing movement disorder such as drug induced parkinsonism (Jeste et al., 1999b; 1999a).

The newer antipsychotics have been found to be much less likely to induce abnormal movements including tardive dyskinesia. To that end, clozapine (Clozaril), the first atypical agent to become available in the United States, is recommended for patients who either have not responded to other antipsychotic medications or have developed severe abnormal movements or tardive dyskinesia while taking other agents. The use of Clozaril has been limited by other unpleasant adverse effects such as excessive sedation, weight gain, low blood pressure, cognitive clouding, blurred vision, hypersalivation, and increased risk of seizures. In addition Clozaril has a rare tendency to cause a drop in the white blood cell count, which can be potentially life-threatening. For that reason, any patient who begins treatment with Clozaril is required to have a blood test every week to monitor his or her white blood cell count.

In the late 1990s and early 2000s, five other atypical antipsychotics were approved by the FDA: risperidone (Risperdal), olanzapine (Zyprexa), quetiapine (Seroquel), ziprasidone (Geodon), and aripiprazole (Abilify). Each agent has a somewhat unique side effect profile. Some of the newer agents have been found to be associated with metabolic changes such as weight gain, development of diabetes and lipid abnormalities, and risk for serious cardiac arrhythmia. Additional experience with the newer agents over the coming years will provide a better knowledge base regarding their more serious side effects.

Antidepressants

The arrival of antidepressant drugs closely followed that of antipsychotics, and eventually paved the way for a new approach to the treatment of depression. Like the antipsychotics, antidepressants have contributed to reduced hospitalization and a move to a more rehabilitative model of treatment. The tricyclic antidepressants (TCAs), named for their three-ring chemical structure, were found to block the reuptake of the chemical messengers (i.e., neurotransmitters) norepinephrine and serotonin at the junction between nerve cells. Ordinarily unused neurotransmitter substance is taken back into the cell to be reused, a process known as reuptake (Stahl). By blocking reuptake, tricyclic antidepressant agents were found to make more neurotransmitters available to the nerve cell. A second class of antidepressants blocks monoamine oxidase, the enzyme that degrades both norepinephrine and

serotonin; drugs belonging to this class became known as monoamine oxidase inhibitors (MAOIs).

Despite the therapeutic effects of these drugs, their use is complicated by adverse effects. Like the conventional antipsychotics, these agents frequently produce sedation, hypotension, and anticholinergic effects. These side effects can be particularly problematic for older individuals who may be cognitively impaired and at risk for falls. In addition these agents can be lethal in overdose, as they cause serious cardiac arrhythmias. Nevertheless clinical experience with these medications ultimately led to the current prevailing theory of depression as a deficiency in certain neurotransmitters in predisposed individuals.

The introduction of fluoxetine (Prozac) in 1985 was arguably the single most influential development in contemporary treatment of depression. As the first in a family of new antidepressants, Prozac revolutionized the treatment of psychiatric illness. Because of its significantly improved side effect profile, Prozac provided a more convenient treatment alternative for patients. With the improved safety and tolerability of antidepressants beginning with Prozac, depression has come to be understood even by the lay public as a treatable medical condition frequently compared to diabetes or hypertension. This has been a critical step in destigmatizing depression as a mental illness. Moreover it has made possible improved recognition and treatment of depression as well as other psychiatric disorders in the United States and worldwide.

The newer family of antidepressants ushered in by Prozac became known as selective serotonin reuptake inhibitors (SSRIs). In contrast to the TCAs and MAOIs that act on both serotonin and norepinephrine, SSRIs primarily increase the availability of serotonin. The SSRIs have fewer side effects than the older antidepressants, are easier for physicians to dose, and do not have the risk of heart conduction problems that TCAs have, nor do the SSRIs require special dietary restrictions like the MAOIs. Although they were developed for the treatment of depression, SSRIs have become widely used for the treatment of various conditions including certain anxiety disorders, eating disorders, and disorders of impulse control.

There are five other SSRIs currently available in the United States: sertraline (Zoloft), paroxetine (Paxil), citalopram (Celexa), and fluvoxamine (Luvox), and escitalopram (Lexapro). All are FDA approved for depression with the exception of Luvox, which is indicated for obsessive-compulsive disorder. All SSRIs are equally effective for the treatment of depression and the choice of an agent is largely dependent on other effects (see below). The availability of different agents allows clinicians to customize treatment to some extent. For example a patient with prominent apathy and fatigue may benefit from an antidepressant that is activating, such as Prozac. Conversely a patient with severe insomnia and anxiety may be better served by an agent that is more sedating, such as Paxil.

Since the arrival of SSRIs, several newer antidepressants have been developed with unique mechanisms of action. Venlafaxine (Effexor), nefazodone (Serzone), bupropion (Wellbutrin), and mirtazapine (Remeron) are antidepressants that were designed with the benefit of even more recent pharmacological knowledge. Effexor is an agent that exerts its effect on different neurotransmitters according to the dosage selected by the clinician. At lower doses, its effect is mediated primarily via increasing serotonin, whereas at higher doses of the drug, norepinephrine and dopamine effects predominate. Lower doses tend to be appropriate for milder depressive states and higher doses for more severe disorders.

ADVERSE EFFECTS. Adverse effects of antidepressants can be problematic. The TCAs tend to produce dry mouth, constipation, and sedation, but the sedative effect can be used to treat the insomnia that frequently accompanies depression. In cases of overdose, MAOIs and TCAs can produce dangerous cardiac arrhythmias. MAOIs can also produce serious blood pressure elevations if they are combined with certain other drugs or tyramine-rich foods such as aged cheese or meats. Patients on MAOIs must adhere to strict dietary guidelines in order to prevent problems.

The SSRI antidepressants produce a characteristic spectrum of adverse effects including nausea, diarrhea, weight loss, headache, insomnia, agitation, and fatigue. Many of these effects resolve within 2 to 3 weeks of treatment, and patients are generally advised to continue taking their medication to see if the unwanted effects dissipate over time. These compounds can also cause sexual side effects such as reduced sexual interest as well as difficulty in achieving orgasm. Other less common effects include tremor, rash, and easy bruising. Although they tend to be relatively safe in overdose, SSRIs can produce serious adverse effects if combined with other serotonin-containing drugs (i.e., serotonin syndrome). Serotonin syndrome is characterized by symptoms such as confusion, tremors, sweating, fever, and incoordination. It may become potentially life threatening if not recognized and appropriately treated.

Other non-SSRI antidepressants have somewhat unique side effects. The side effects of Effexor are similar to those of an SSRI at lower doses, and it causes an increase in blood pressure in a small percentage of patients. Serzone tends to be sedating and many patients prefer to take it at bedtime, especially if they have insomnia. It can interact with many commonly used medications including certain antihistamines, antibiotics, and anti-fungal agents, causing potentially dangerous cardiac arrhythmias. Wellbutrin is a stimulant-like agent that can produce agitation and insomnia in susceptible individuals. It has the potential to increase the risk for seizures in a small percentage of patients. It is the antidepressant least likely to cause weight gain and sexual dysfunction and has been successfully used to improve sexual function in some patients. Remeron is sedating and can also produce significant weight gain. It tends to be prescribed at bedtime for patients with insomnia.

Antianxiety agents

Antianxiety drugs are used to treat primary anxiety disorders such as panic attacks, phobias, obsessive-compulsive disorder (OCD), and post-traumatic stress disorder (PTSD), as well as anxiety that accompanies depression. In addition these medications are used to treat anxiety associated with various emergency medical conditions (e.g., myocardial infarction). Alcohol is the oldest antianxiety agent. Medical use of anxiolytics began with barbiturates and propanediols, drugs with sedative and anxiety-reducing effects, but these agents also slowed thinking and decreased alertness.

In the late 1960s, benzodiazepines were introduced as drugs that reduced anxiety but preserved cognitive function and physical activity. These drugs include diazepam (Valium), lorazepam (Ativan), and alprazolam (Xanax). Benzodiazepines are believed to stimulate another neurotransmitter, gamma aminobutyric acid (GABA), which plays an inhibitory role in brain function, lessening arousal and anxiety. Benzodiazepines are safer compared to the earlier antianxiety drugs. Nevertheless they do have significant cognitive and sedating effects that limit their use. Moreover benzodiazepines produce tolerance and withdrawal symptoms, which defines them as potential drugs of abuse. Their effects tend to dissipate over time, leading to the need for increases in dosage and increased potential for toxicity.

Scientists have searched for antianxiety drugs that do not produce tolerance or addiction. Currently the SSRI antidepressants are the preferred agents for treating anxiety disorders including panic attacks, phobias, and OCD. They have been found to reduce effectively symptoms of anxiety and do not lead to dependence syndromes. However these agents often require several weeks before beginning to exert therapeutic effects. They are not useful for emergency situations, but rather, for ongoing management and prevention of recurrent distressing symptoms. Buspirone (Buspar) is another agent that affects serotonin and was developed for the treatment of anxiety disorders. Like the SSRIs, it has a role in maintenance treatment rather than for acute intervention in anxiety disorders. Benzodiazepines continue to be the most frequently used agents for acute anxiety because of their immediate effects.

ADVERSE EFFECTS. The adverse effects of SSRIs have been described in the previous section. Regarding benzodiazepines, several side effects are generally extensions of their therapeutic effects: sedation, impaired cognitive or motor performance, tolerance, and physical dependency (addiction); the sedative effects impair driving and attention to mechanical tasks. However untreated anxiety or insomnia can produce serious problems in these same areas. Thus clinicians must carefully weigh the risks and benefits of prescribing benzodiazepines. Their safety profile is better compared to that of barbiturates. Nevertheless physical addiction can occur, and if abruptly discontinued, a withdrawal state can result.

Benzodiazepine withdrawal is rather similar to withdrawal from alcohol. It is characterized by anxiety, restlessness, agitation, and insomnia, as well as increased heart rate, sweating, tremors, and blood pressure elevation. An example of a withdrawal reaction is the so-called "rebound insomnia" associated with the discontinuation of short-acting benzodiazepines (e.g., triazolam) as a sleep-aid. In more severe cases, withdrawal from benzodiazepines can lead to a seizure. This syndrome typically develops two or three days after abrupt cessation of benzodiazepines, especially shorter-acting agents such as Xanax. It is characterized by an acute confusional state with fluctuating level of consciousness, disorientation, hallucinations, paranoia, agitation, and often seizures. Without appropriate medical management, this syndrome can be life threatening. During short-term, low-dose therapy, the risk is low; however patients with prior drug abuse or alcoholism are at an increased risk for these problems as are patients who take higher doses over longer periods of time.

Mood Stabilizers

Mood stabilizing agents are primarily indicated for the treatment of bipolar disorder, previously known as manic-depressive illness. Bipolar disorder is typically characterized by alternating episodes of depression and mania. Whereas depression is a state of low mood, hopelessness, low motivation and energy, and slowed activity, mania is a state of elevated or euphoric mood, increased energy, inflated self-esteem, racing thoughts, and a tendency to become involved in excessive, often unrealistic, and even unnecessarily risky activities. Like other psychiatric disorders, there are various

forms of bipolar disorder. Some patients experience primarily depressive episodes with only occasional manias, while other patients may experience almost continuous mania, with very little depression. Whatever form the disorder takes, mood stabilizing agents are intended to reduce the frequency and severity of the mood episodes, and thereby reduce functional impairment.

The first mood stabilizer was lithium carbonate, a naturally occurring salt introduced into clinical use in the 1960s. For many years it was the preferred treatment for bipolar disorder, although its mechanism of action has never been well understood. It is effective for both depression and mania and has been shown to reduce the risk of suicide in patients with bipolar disorder. It has a variety of toxic side effects that limit its tolerability (see below). In addition, lithium has a very narrow therapeutic range, in terms of blood levels, below which it may be ineffective and above which it causes toxic side effects. A number of commonly prescribed medications can interact with lithium and increase its serum level. Therefore any patient taking lithium requires regular monitoring of serum levels in order to maintain safety and efficacy with this drug.

Because of its side effects and safety issues, today fewer patients are being treated with lithium as other options have become available. Most of the other mood stabilizers are anticonvulsants initially developed for seizure control. Carbamazepine (Tegretol) and valproate (Depakote) were the earliest drugs of this class. Depakote has become the first-line medication for bipolar disorder, particularly for patients who have rapid cycling of moods or episodes with combined symptoms of depression and mania (i.e., mixed episodes). Although they have been well studied and demonstrated to be effective, similar to lithium, both of these agents have side effects and potential for toxicity (although not as narrow a margin for toxicity as that of lithium). Several newer anticonvulsants have therefore been studied and introduced for mood stabilization. These include gabapentin (Neurontin), lamotrigine (Lamictal), topiramate (Topamax), and oxcarbazepine (Trileptal). Although they appear to be better tolerated overall, the efficacy of these newer agents is not yet as well established as that of the older mood stabilizers.

ADVERSE EFFECTS. Lithium is associated with numerous side effects including cognitive slowing, gastrointestinal upset, weight gain, tremor, excessive thirst and urination, acne, and rash. Long-term use of lithium is known to be particularly toxic to the thyroid and kidneys. When the level of lithium in the serum becomes high, patients develop signs of neurological toxicity, such as slurred speech, impairment in gait and coordination, worsening tremor, and sedation.

Lithium toxicity is considered a medical emergency requiring hospitalization, intravenous hydration, and often hemodialysis to prevent irreversible kidney failure.

The most common early side effects of Depakote are sedation and gastrointestinal upset, both of which tend to subside or decrease within a few weeks. Other reported side effects include weight gain, dizziness, tremor, and hair loss. Depakote frequently induces an elevation in the liver enzymes, which is usually benign, but requires monitoring because of the rare possibility of liver toxicity. Depakote may also lower serum platelets. Tegretol too can be toxic to the liver and bone marrow and therefore requires serum monitoring. It also produces sedation and dizziness, as well as cognitive slowing. In rare instances, it is associated with the development of a severe allergic reaction involving the skin. Elevation of Tegretol levels beyond a certain level can produce neurotoxicity with coordination and gait impairment, and abnormal eye movements. Tegretol has a tendency to reduce the levels of other medications, such as oral contraceptives.

Side effects of the newer anticonvulsants include sedation and dizziness. Lamictal is associated with the development of a life-threatening rash in rare cases. Topimax is associated with weight loss and cognitive slowing.

Ethical Dilemmas in Psychopharmacology

CONSENT TO TREATMENT. A principal ethical dilemma of treating people with mental illnesses is that many patients are impaired by their condition, but need to make an informed choice as to their treatment and its risks and benefits. For example, antipsychotic drugs may be prescribed to a psychotic patient who is paranoid, especially about drugs he is asked to take. The prescriber faces the dilemma of determining how reasonable the patient's ability is to accept or refuse treatment for an illness that impairs his ability to process reality, leading him to suspect all those who try to help him, and even to constitute a risk to self or others.

A basic tenant of medical care is that a competent patient has the right to refuse treatment of any kind. Unfortunately, determining competency can be difficult, and state laws have not clearly defined competency in regard to psychotic disorders. One study demonstrated that the most severely psychotic patients refused treatment more frequently than did patients who are less symptomatic (Marder et al.). For patients who are a danger to themselves (e.g., refusing to eat) or to others (e.g., attacking feared persecutors), both common sense and state statutes permit temporary involuntary medication treatment. However when a patient who is very ill and hospitalized for a mental illness refuses medications, but is not a danger to herself or others, it can be very difficult to provide optimal care. Many physicians involve the family in this decision, but this approach poses risks too. From the perspective of the paranoid patient, an alliance between a doctor and the family may make the patient even more suspicious of the physician. Often the psychiatrist is forced to involve the court system in determining whether a patient is competent to refuse treatment. Although a judge may allow involuntary treatment, these competency hearings may delay decision making for weeks, and are expensive for both the patient and the treating physician or facility.

CONSENT TO PARTICIPATE IN PSYCHOPHARMACOLOGIC RESEARCH. Conducting research on new psychopharmacologic treatments poses ethical dilemmas. For serious mental illnesses such as schizophrenia, current treatment is beneficial in reducing the symptoms, but many patients continue to have significant impairments. Improved treatments are needed, especially for the patients with the most severe psychopathology. In addition to knowing whether the new treatments will help those patients with the most severe symptoms, research into the new treatments needs to include the full range of patients. A critical component of conducting ethical research is obtaining informed consent from potential research subjects. Often those patients with the most severe psychopathology also have the greatest impairment in their ability to provide informed consent to be a research subject (Kim et al.).

Informed consent includes four key components: understanding, appreciating, reasoning, and expressing a choice. Patients with schizophrenia are more likely to have impairments with one or more of these four areas of decision making. At the same time, it is important to emphasize that having a psychiatric illness is by no means synonymous with having impaired decision-making capacity to consent for research. In studies of the decisional abilities of patients with schizophrenia, for example, the majority of non-hospitalized patients have not been found to be impaired on measures of their capacity to consent (Jeste et al., 2003).

Including patients with severe mental illness in studies of new medications, when the patient's ability to give informed consent to be a research volunteer is impaired due to the illness, is a major ethical challenge. In 1998, the National Bioethics Advisory Commission (NBAC) issued a report entitled "research involving persons with mental disorders that may affect decision making capacity." This report recommended additional special protections for research that involved persons with mental disorders. Critics of the NBAC report have expressed concern that the report's recommended additional special protections, specifically a proposed moratorium on research studies that posed greater than minimal risk until a new "special standing panel" or "national IRB" could review each study, which could impede important biomedical research, including neuroimaging and genetic linkage studies (Shore and Hyman). Another criticism of the NBAC report was that many medical illnesses, not just mental illnesses, can impair a person's decision-making capacity. By focusing on persons with psychiatric disorders, the NBAC report's recommendations risk increasing the stigma associated with mental illnesses (Appelbaum). One area of current research focuses on ways to enhance the process of informed consent so patients with more severe psychopathology can participate in research. As new potential treatments for schizophrenia become available, a key question will be finding ethical ways of determining whether these medications help the most severely ill patients.

SPECIAL POPULATIONS: ELDERLY PATIENTS. Certain segments of mentally ill populations are at a particularly high risk of problems with decisional capacity. These include children, elderly persons, and non-English speaking ethnic minority groups. Below one such group—that is, elderly patients with serious mental illnesses in need of pharmacotherapy—is considered.

It is anticipated that the numbers of older persons with psychiatric disorders will increase substantially within the next three decades (Jeste et al., 1999a). Yet most investigations of the efficacy and safety of pharmacologic treatments for these illnesses have focused on younger adults. Hence there will be a need for a marked growth of geriatric psychopharmacologic research in the immediate future. As mentioned above, an important issue in intervention research is ensuring that the patient has adequate decision-making capacity for participation in such research. Older psychiatric patients are at a risk of lacking decisional capacity by virtue of their aging-associated cognitive deficits and physical comorbidity, which are compounded by complex medication regimens. At the same time it is critical to stress that considerable heterogeneity exists among older persons with mental illnesses. Moreover the capacity to consent may vary from one protocol to another. It is clear that empirical research into assessing and possibly improving decisional capacity is needed in older people with severe mental illness.

One model of a multidisciplinary collaboration that is necessary for facilitating such research is the Bioethics Unit of an Intervention Research Center (Jeste et al., 2003). This Unit was developed in the last half of the 1990s. It includes geriatric psychiatrists, psychologists, bioethicists, lawyers,

and most importantly, a Community Advisory Board comprised of patient participants in research, their family members, patient advocates, and mental health workers in the community not affiliated with the research team. The members of the Bioethics Unit have conducted several studies of decisional capacity and of ways to improve the process of giving information to the research participants by educational means (e.g., repeating the information) or by use of techniques such as PowerPoint slide presentation of the consent material (Dunn et al.; Palmer et al.). As of mid-2003, those investigations suggest that older individuals with psychotic disorders vary considerably in their decisional capacity, and many (but not all) subjects are fully capable of consenting to research projects. Additionally the patients's comprehension of the consent material can be improved significantly through repetition and user-friendly presentation of the information. It thus appears that, even in older seriously mentally ill individuals, decisional capacity for a given research protocol is not necessarily an unmodifiable trait, but can be enhanced with improvements in consenting procedures. Research at the Bioethics Unit has also demonstrated that the Community Advisory Board is very helpful in ensuring community equipoise—for example, the community's perspective of the relative risk: benefit ratio of a research protocol.

INVOLUNTARY TREATMENT. One of the most controversial areas in psychiatry is involuntary outpatient treatment. The field of psychiatry has long held that benevolent coercion is necessary to treat some people with serious mental illnesses such as schizophrenia and bipolar disorder, and most experts would agree that involuntary treatment for a person who is imminently suicidal or homicidal is justified. However it is much less clear whether a person with a serious mental illness who stops his medications and decompensates, becoming homeless or requiring rehospitalization, may be treated against his or her will to prevent this decompensation. In the early-twenty-first century, there are many people with serious mental illnesses who are unable or unwilling to receive outpatient mental health treatment, and some of these patients end up being homeless, incarcerated, or hospitalized multiple times. Involuntary outpatient treatment has been advocated as a means to improve the mental healthcare of these patients (Swartz et al.; Torrey and Zdanowicz).

Most states have provisions for involuntary outpatient treatment, which is usually court-ordered. This involuntary outpatient treatment is often used for patients who are being released from a psychiatric hospital and have a past record of stopping their medications, decompensating, and being rehospitalized. Depending on the particular state, this involuntary treatment may or may not include forced administration of medications. Proponents of involuntary outpatient treatment argue that it can help a patient to remain compliant with treatment (or face re-hospitalization), and at the same time, force the mental health systems to provide a patient with needed treatment. Opponents of involuntary outpatient treatment argue that it unnecessarily restricts the rights of people with mental illnesses, and that improved access to comprehensive outpatient services can accomplish the same goals as involuntary outpatient treatment (Allen and Smith).

DRUG THERAPY AND RESOURCE ALLOCATION. Since the mid-1990s the cost of pharmaceuticals has received increasing attention. Pharmaceutical costs are currently the fastest rising component of healthcare costs; between 1987 and 1996 per capita spending on psychotropic medications increased by 254 percent, while spending on all mental health and substance abuse treatments only increased by 30 percent (Zuvekas). This increase has many causes, including an increasing awareness and acceptance of treatment for mental illnesses, and a large number of newer psychiatric medications that have fewer side effects and may be more effective, but are significantly more expensive. For example there are five new *atypical* antipsychotic medications that have been introduced in the past decade. These medications have fewer short-term and long-term side effects, but cost much more than the older antipsychotic medications. The newer medications cost approximately $300 to $400 per month. This compares with about $15 to $50 per month for the older antipsychotic medications. There is some evidence that over one to two years the atypical antipsychotic medications are *cost neutral* due to lower rates of relapse and fewer psychiatric hospitalizations (Csernansky and Schuchart). Similarly the newer antidepressants are also more expensive (at $80 to $90 per month) than the older antidepressants ($10 to $15 per month). It should be kept in mind that the recent increase in cost of medications is not restricted to psychiatric medications; lipid lowering agents cost $70 to $90 per month, Viagra runs $8 to $9 per pill and common triple-drug treatments for HIV can cost $1000 to $1250 per month (drugstore.com).

Optimistically a balancing of the needs of the patient, the government's ability to pay, and market forces may provide the optimal solution. From a clinical and ethical perspective, it is necessary to ensure that patients who would benefit from a new psychotropic drug should not be denied that medication. However people without prescription drug benefits as part of their healthcare insurance are often unable to afford to pay for their medications and many state Medicaid plans and private insurance companies have created medication formularies that restrict the medications which a patient can receive. Many psychiatrists, patients, and patient advocates believe that these restrictions on which medications can be used to treat a serious mental illness could cause an exacerbation of symptoms and may require more intensive, institutional-based care in the future, ultimately resulting in greater cost. Among the important issues that arise in the debate over the cost of newer psychiatric medications include: Who decides whether a new medication, which is safer but more expensive, should be used: the patient, the physician, the insurance company, or the government?

Conclusion

Psychopharmacologic medications have undergone a major transformation since the mid-1990s. In 2003, medications have fewer side effects, are easier to take, and may be more effective. On the other hand, these medications are significantly more expensive. The development of these newer medications has highlighted the challenge of ethically studying new treatments for people with serious mental illness. In addition these new medications have not solved the longstanding dilemma of consent for psychotropic medication treatment or administering psychiatric treatment involuntarily. Finally weighing the cost versus benefit of these newer (more expensive) medications has been receiving growing attention.

DAVID P. FOLSOM
JEREMY SABLE
DILIP V. JESTE

SEE ALSO: *Behavior Control; Health Insurance; Life, Quality of; Mental Health; Mental Illness; Patients' Responsibilities; Pharmaceutics, Issues in Prescribing; Profit and Commercialism; Psychiatry, Abuses of*

BIBLIOGRAPHY

Allen, M., and Smith, V. F. 2001. "Opening Pandora's Box: The Practical and Legal Dangers of Involuntary Outpatient Commitment." *Psychiatric Services* 52: 342–346.

Appelbaum, Paul S. 1999. "Competence to Consent to Research: A Critique of the Recommendation of the National Bioethics Advisory Commission." *Accounts Res.* 7(2–4): 265–276.

Csernansky, J. G., and Schuchart, E. K. 2002. "Relapse and Rehospitalisation Rates in Patients with Schizophrenia: Effects of Second Generation Antipsychotics." *CNS Drugs* 16: 473–484.

Dolder, C. R.; Lacro, J. P.; Dunn, L. B.; et al. 2002. "Medication Adherence: Is There a Difference Between Typical and Atypical Agents?" *American Journal of Psychiatry* 159: 103–108.

Dunn, L. B.; Lindamer, L. A.; Palmer B. W.; et al. 2002. "Improving Understanding of Research Consent in Middle-Aged and Elderly Patients with Psychotic Disorders." *American Journal of Geriatric Psychiatry* 10: 142–150.

Grob, G. 1994. *The Mad among Us: A History of the Care of America's Mentally Ill.* New York: Free Press.

Jeste, Dilip V.; Alexopoulos, G. S.; Bartels, S. J.; et al. 1999. "Consensus Statement: The Upcoming Crisis in Geriatric Mental Health: Challenges and Opportunities." *Archives of General Psychiatry* 56: 848–853.

Jeste, Dilip V.; Dunn, L. B.; Palmer, B. W.; et al. 2003. "A Collaborative Model for Research on Decision Capacity and Informed Consent in Older Patients with Schizophrenia: Bioethics Unit of a Geriatric Psychiatry Intervention Research Center." *Psychopharmacology*

Jeste, Dilip V.; Gilbert, P. L.; McAdams, L. A.; et al. 1995. "Considering Neuroleptic Maintenance and Taper on a Continuum: Need for Individual Rather than Dogmatic Approach." *Archives of General Psychiatry* 52: 209–212.

Jeste, Dilip V.; Rockwell, E.; Harris, M. J.; et al. 1999. "Conventional vs. Newer Antipsychotics in Elderly Patients." *American Journal of Geriatric Psychiatry* 7: 70–76.

Kim, S. Y. H.; Karlawish, J. H. T.; and Caine, E. D. 2002. "Current State of Research on Decision-Making Competence of Cognitively Impaired Elderly Persons." *American Journal of Geriatric Psychiatry* 10: 151–165.

Marder, S. R.; Mebane, A.; Chien, C. P.; et al. 1983. "A Comparison of Patients Who Refuse and Consent to Neuroleptic Treatment." *American Journal of Psychiatry* 140: 470–472.

Palmer, B. W.; Nayak, G. V.; Dunn, L. B.; et al. 2002. "Treatment-Related Decision-Making Capacity in Middle-Aged and Older Patients with Psychosis: A Preliminary Study Using the MacCAT-T and HCAT." *American Journal of Geriatric Psychiatry* 10: 207–211.

Shore, David, and Hyman Steven E. 1999. "An NIMH Commentary on the NBAC Report." *Biological Psychiatry* 46(8): 1013–1016.

Stahl, S. M. 1997. *Psychopharmacology of Antidepressants.* London: Martin Dunitz Ltd.

Swartz, M. S.; Swanson, J. W.; Wagner, H. R.; et al. 2001. "Effects of Involuntary Outpatient Commitment and Depot Antipsychotics on Treatment Adherence in Persons with Severe Mental Illness." *Journal of Nervous and Mental Disease* 189: 583–592.

Torrey, E. F., and Zdanowicz, M. 2001, "Outpatient Commitment: What, Why, and for Whom." *Psychiatric Services* 52: 337–341.

Zuvekas, S. H. 2001. "Trends in Mental Health Services Use and Spending, 1987–1996." *Health Affairs* 20: 214–221.

INTERNET RESOURCES

drugstore.com. 2003. Available from <www.drugstore.com>.

National Bioethics Advisory Commission. 1998. "Research Involving Persons with Mental Disorders That May Affect Decisionmaking Capacity." Available from <http://www.george-town.edu/research/nrcbl/nbac/capacity/TOC.htm>.

PSYCHOSURGERY, ETHICAL ASPECTS OF

• • •

As long as patients with problems of feeling, thinking, and behavior are assumed to be capable of making a free and informed decision on the question of a brain operation intended to improve some aspect of their mental state, there is no logical reason to object to such treatment. Ethical and legal problems regarding psychosurgery should arise primarily because of issues relating to consent to treatment, about which there certainly can be argument.

The Peculiar Case of Psychosurgery

The peculiar problem of psychosurgery arises in part because the brain, which is the instrument of consent, is also understood to be the source of the disability that requires cure. In itself, this is scarcely an objection. Perhaps no one gives a second thought to the specific justification for obtaining consent to the removal of a brain tumor, even if the patient is confused and a proxy consent is necessary. In contrast, it is plausible that much of the hesitation and obstruction that attend discussions of consent to psychosurgery are based upon an unwillingness to view mental illness in the same way as physical illness. Frequently, equality of treatment is denied for all sorts of psychological illness compared with physical illness, as can be seen in numerous health insurance policies. With respect to psychosurgery, there is concern that informed consent must depend upon the adequate function of a large part or wide area of the brain, and there is a valid fear that such function is liable to be absent in those to whom the operation is offered.

Even more aptly, it may be supposed that the effect to be abolished is a prime source of virtue, so that if leukotomy (the cutting of the white matter in the brain; also known as lobotomy) abates guilt it may also impair admirable features of the personality. While there can be sympathy with some of these concerns, they are judgmental questions for which practical answers can be demanded. They ought not to operate as presumptive justifications for refusing practical treatment to anyone. Sometimes there are practical problems in ensuring that the consent of a particular patient to a particular procedure is genuinely free. Nevertheless, psychosurgery attracted enough hostile comment from various quarters to lead to the creation in the United States of the National Commission for the Protection of Human Subjects of Biomedical and Behavioral Research to look into this topic and related issues after "Widespread expression of public and congressional concern ... including allegations that these procedures were ... being used for 'Social Control' of dissidents and violence-prone individuals and ... were performed disproportionately on members of minority populations" (HEW, p. 53242). Thus, the ethical issues of psychosurgery must be considered against a historical background of success.

The commission demonstrated that there was no substance to the claims being made. For example, only 100 procedures meeting the definition of psychosurgery were being performed annually in the United States in the years leading up to 1977 (when the commission issued its report on psychosurgery). It also determined that no significant psychological deficits were attributable to the psychosurgery undertaken; that the treatment was efficacious in more than half of the case studies; that there was no evidence that the procedure had been used for psychosocial control; and that only a few operations were conducted on minority or disadvantaged populations. Correspondence with the most active psychosurgeons in the United States revealed that out of 600 patients, only one was black, two were Asian, and six were Hispanic Americans. Between 1970 and 1980 only seven operations were reported to have been performed on children, and only three prisoners underwent psychosurgery. In fact, psychosurgery was largely limited to middle-class individuals. In a 1988 study, English investigators E. S. Hussain, H. Freeman, and R. A. C. Jones showed that psychosurgery provided valuable benefits for a selected small group within a cohort of patients from a defined population, particularly those with depression, agoraphobia, obsessional neurosis, and certain aspects of schizophrenia. Such findings show that the ethical aspects of psychosurgery have to do with the conditions under which it is offered, not with the inherent nature of the procedure.

Axioms and Rules

In psychiatric practice, there are some common axioms and some derivative rules. The following may apply to psychosurgery (Merskey, 1991):

1. Ordinarily, medical advice is just advice, and the patient is not obliged to follow it. Even the imposition of treatment to save life (e.g., a surgical operation for kidney disease or cancer) is ethically and legally permissible only if the patient consents.

2. Children and others in a condition that precludes them from deciding rationally may have decisions made for them by people, usually their next of kin, who have appropriate concern for their interests and welfare.

3. Special care is needed when decisions are made for children and other incompetent persons. Careful scrutiny of the status and motives of the person who makes the decision for the patient is necessary. Given that care, treatment can be ethically undertaken.

4. Ethical actions may or may not be sanctioned by law. The legality of a physician's conduct is a separate issue from its ethical basis.

5. Coercive treatments for the benefit of a third party are unethical, and healthcare professionals should not use behavior modification, drugs, or lobotomy against an individual's wishes to prevent that person from hurting someone else.

6. Likewise, coercive treatment for the benefit of society rather than the patient is repugnant to ethical physicians.

7. Patients may consent to treatment that benefits either themselves or others, but there are peculiar difficulties in confirming the presence of free consent in some circumstances, particularly with prisoners.

Overall, the critical issue for the physician is to recognize whether the problem receiving attention is one that is seen by the patient as needing treatment or whether it is seen by others as requiring treatment in the patient's interest. The relationship of physicians to patients is principally based on an implicit contract that the physician will care for the patient provided that the physician is not expected to violate the legal and ethical interests of other people in order to provide that care (Merskey, 1986). Given these presuppositions, the issues surrounding brain surgery can be considered with and without consent in mind.

Brain Surgery with Consent

The easiest case in which to accept the validity of leukotomy is the relief of severe depression. While leukotomy and related operations such as cingulotomy (destruction of a part of the medial portion of the cerebral hemispheres) are now rarely required for this purpose, a patient with this protracted and life-threatening condition may wish to undergo a surgical operation with relatively small risk in order to relieve the condition. Prior to the introduction of physical methods of treatment, there was a high death rate in patients with severe depression (Huston and Locher).

When leukotomy was more common in the 1950s and 1960s, a written agreement might not have been obtained—schizophrenic patients are notoriously unwilling to sign documents—but the patient was not actively opposed. Relatives would support the procedure, and, at least in Britain, the relatives' consent was accepted as legally sufficient. A large number of chronic schizophrenic patients in some countries were submitted to bilateral standard leukotomy operations under the above conditions. If operations failed to relieve fully the schizophrenic illness, at least they reduced agitation or aggressive outbursts and produced a more manageable state in some extremely disturbed patients. Was this process used for "social control?" The available options included locked or padded rooms and physical restraint. Though most psychiatrists did not regard these options favorably, leukotomy operations were not necessarily undertaken to provide otherwise unattainable control but rather to provide the patient with a quieter and easier life. If the patient did not object, and if he or she was substantially disturbed and likely to benefit from the operation, there could be no reasonable objection to such treatment, given the consent of those most likely to have the patient's best interests at heart. It remains the case that such treatment is still appropriate in the same circumstances.

Although the numbers of brain operations for depression, anxiety, and obsessive-compulsive disorder decreased in the 1970s and remained low in the 1980s and the 1990s, their accuracy was much enhanced by the use of stereotactic surgery for movement disorders (especially Parkinson's disease), intractable pain (usually cancer), and the modern developments from leukotomy. Such surgery, undertaken with the help of a fixed framework attached to the cranium, radiological control through magnetic resonance imaging, and radiofrequency ablation of the chosen area, has provided very acceptable results for a number of patients with depression, anxiety, and obsessive-compulsive disorders.

Four related operations stand out as having been the most successful and as having been usefully employed since the 1970s in the treatment of depression, anxiety, and obsessive-compulsive disorder: subcaudate trachtotomy, the implantation of pellets of radioactive yttrium below the head of the caudate nucleus to destroy the neighboring tissue over some six to eight weeks; cingulotomy, the bilateral destruction of the cingulate gyrus; anterior capsulotomy, ablation of the anterior limb of the internal capsule; and limbic leukotomy, in which lesions are placed in the orbito-fronto thalmic and limbic circuits. In 2001 Robert P. Feldman, Ronald L. Alterman, and James T. Gooderich detailed success rates and complications with these methods and described their neuroanatomical bases and physiological implications. In 1997 P. Sachdev and J. Sachdev concisely reviewed psychiatric considerations and the social setting.

With the improvements in technique and results, the discussion of ethical issues appears to have been reduced to a minimum. Only a few centers are known to perform these operations in Australia and New Zealand, Canada, Sweden, the United Kingdom, and the United States. In their 1988 book, *Physical Treatments in Psychiatry,* Leslie G. Kiloh, J. Sydney Smith, and Gordon F. Johnson observed that in 854 stereotactic operations the operative mortality rate was 0.1 percent, the rate for epilepsy was 0.4 percent, marked personality change affected 0.4 percent of patients, and mild personality change affected 3 percent. With a complication rate of this order, and results generally in which 50 percent of patients get considerable benefit and the majority get some benefit, the operations present a rate of risk that is highly acceptable for most individuals who have suffered from disabling chronic depression, anxiety, or obsessive-compulsive disorder for many years. Of the four operations, anterior capsulotomy appears to have the best results overall.

In addition to the treatment of depression and schizophrenia, stereotactic neurosurgical operations—especially amygdalotomy (the amygdala being the gray matter of the brain's frontal lobe)—have been used for the control of aggression, which may be directed against the patient's own self or at others (Kiloh et al.). Also, such an operation was sometimes considered for a number of chronic self-mutilators. The availability and relatively specific effect of serotonin reuptake inhibitor drugs have eased the symptoms of many patients who were prone to self-damage. That medication might produce such a radical change in self-harm means that a surgical operation when medication fails can be seen as a logical and reasonable effort to modify an aberrant portion of the brain. Many patients with such tendencies are not intellectually retarded and have no organic brain damage. Nevertheless, although most of them can respond to antidepressant medication, others need more radical treatment, suggesting that psychosurgery still has a role to play for a few patients.

Psychosurgery for individuals who are dangerous only to others but who might be willing to consent is the most difficult issue in this field. If the patient can consent, one might ask why the person should not be allowed the treatment? This problem is exemplified by the 1973 case of *Kaimowitz v. Department of Mental Health.* A patient who had behaved aggressively, but was a prisoner, consented to treatment but was refused it on the grounds that his consent in prison could not be truly free. The patient, who had spent eighteen years in prison for murder, had satisfied an "informed consent" review committee comprising a law professor, a priest, and an accountant that he wanted the operation. A suit was brought by an attorney, Kaimowitz, and others belonging to a medical committee for human rights who had never consulted the prisoner. The lawyer appointed by the courts to represent the prisoner thought that the prisoner desperately wanted the operation. Coincidentally, the prisoner's appointed lawyer satisfied the court that his client was held unconstitutionally as a prisoner. He went free, but the discussion continued on the question of whether as a prisoner he had given free informed consent to psychiatric surgery. The court held that he could not have. Once the prisoner was released, he changed his mind about wanting the operation. According to Robert A. Burt (1975), imprisonment and medical surveillance at least contributed to the prisoner's consent without any attempt having been made by physicians to press the prisoner to agree. Some commentators have argued that no prisoner's consent should be accepted for psychosurgery if its purpose is to alter the type of behavior that caused imprisonment. To guard against the possibility that a prisoner might be deprived of the right to medical care, some framework should be contemplated that would provide for exceptions. Exceptions would include independent professional examination of the individual's motives as well as separation of the question of release from the outcome of the operation.

Incompetent Patients

Certain incompetent patients might undergo surgery provided that it can be demonstrated that the action is not against their wishes. This would apply particularly to schizophrenic patients, who might accept a surgical operation but would never be able to comprehend or fill out a form requiring them to indicate informed consent. Patients should not undergo surgery if they give the merest hint of refusal.

Children with significant brain damage may benefit from psychosurgery, not so much to treat epilepsy caused by the brain damage as for the reduction of aggressive behavior against either themselves or others (Balasubramaniam and Kanaka). If the interests of the child are paramount, then the child should not be deprived of the possibility of beneficial surgery, even though the child is either unable to consent or appears hostile to almost any physical intervention by nursing staff or attendants. This would apply both to patients who gravely damage themselves—and sometimes have been kept for weeks or months in canvas clothing to protect themselves from such injury—and to patients who, while retarded and clearly incompetent, attack others if allowed the minimum opportunity for human contact. Such a

patient also may benefit if a paternalistic approach to treatment is recognized, acknowledged, and followed.

Nevertheless, there is no justification for the forcible use of psychosurgery with individuals who are thought to be political prisoners by the family, the patient's proxies, the treating doctor, or indeed any rational contemporary.

In summary, psychosurgery should never be forced, but it might be performed on noncompetent individuals or prisoners without their formal consent, subject to stringent safeguards that require extensive consideration.

HAROLD MERSKEY (1995)
REVISED BY AUTHOR

SEE ALSO: *Autonomy; Coercion; Deep Brain Stimulation; Electroconvulsive Therapy; Holocaust; Informed Consent: Issues of Consent in Mental Healthcare; Insanity and Insanity Defense; Institutionalization and Deinstitutionalization; Mental Illness: Conception of Mental Illness; Mental Illness: Cultural Perspectives; Mental Institutions, Commitment to; Mistakes, Medical; Narrative; Paternalism; Patients' Rights; Psychiatry, Abuses of; Psychosurgery, Medical and Historical Aspects of; Race and Racism; Technology; Women, Historical and Cross-Cultural Perspectives*

BIBLIOGRAPHY

Balasubramaniam, V., and Kanaka, T. S. 1975. "Amygdalotomy and Hypothalamotomy—A Comparative Study." *Confinia Neurologica* 37(1–3): 195–201.

Burt, Robert A. 1975. "Why We Should Keep Prisoners from the Doctors." *Hastings Center Report* 5(1): 25–34.

Fabrega, Horacio, Jr. 1974. *Disease and Social Behavior: An Interdisciplinary Perspective.* Cambridge, MA: MIT Press.

Feldman, Robert P.; Alterman, Ronald L.; and Gooderich, James T. 2001. "Contemporary Psychosurgery and a Look to the Future." *Journal of Neurosurgery* 95(6): 944–956.

Greenblatt, Steven Jay. 1977. "The Ethics and Legality of Psychosurgery." *New York Law School Law Review* 22(4): 961–980.

Hussain, E. S.; Freeman, H.; and Jones, R. A. C. 1988. "A Cohort Study of Psychosurgery Cases from a Defined Population." *Journal of Neurology, Neurosurgery, and Psychiatry* 51: 345–352.

Huston, P. E., and Locher, L. M. 1948. "Involutional Psychosis: Course When Untreated and When Treated with ECT." *Archives of Neurology and Psychiatry* 59(3): 385–394.

Kaimowitz v. Department of Mental Health. Civil Action No. 73–19434-AW (Wayne County, Mich., Cir. Ct. 1973). Reprinted in *Operating on the Mind: The Psychosurgery Conflict*, ed. Willard M. Gaylin, Joel S. Meister, and Robert C. Neville. New York: Basic, 1975.

Kiloh, Leslie G.; Gye, R. S.; Rushworth, R. G.; et al. 1974. "Stereotactic Amygdaloidotomy for Aggressive Behaviour." *Journal of Neurology, Neurosurgery, and Psychiatry* 37: 437–444.

Kiloh, Leslie G.; Smith, J. Sydney; and Johnson, Gordon F. 1988. *Physical Treatments in Psychiatry.* Melbourne: Blackwell Scientific.

Merskey, Harold. 1986. "Variable Meanings for the Definition of Disease." *Journal of Medicine and Philosophy* 11(3): 215–232.

Merskey, Harold. 1991. "Ethical Aspects of the Physical Manipulation of the Brain." In *Psychiatric Ethics,* 2nd edition, ed. Sidney Bloch and Paul Chodoff. New York: Oxford University Press.

Sachdev, P., and Sachdev, J. 1997. "Sixty Years of Psychosurgery: Its Present Status and Its Future." *Australian and New Zealand Journal of Psychiatry* 31: 457–464.

U.S. Department of Health, Education, and Welfare (HEW). Public Health Service. 1978. "Determination of the Secretary Regarding the Recommendation on Psychosurgery of the National Commission for the Protection of Human Subjects of Biomedical and Behavioral Research." *Federal Register* 43(21): 53242–53244.

U.S. National Commission for the Protection of Human Subjects of Biomedical and Behavioral Research. 1977. *Appendix, Psychosurgery.* Washington, D.C.: U.S. Government Printing Office.

U.S. National Commission for the Protection of Human Subjects of Biomedical and Behavioral Research. 1977. *Psychosurgery: Report and Recommendations.* Washington, D.C.: U.S. Government Printing Office.

PSYCHOSURGERY, MEDICAL AND HISTORICAL ASPECTS OF

• • •

Psychosurgery is the surgical removal or destruction of brain tissue with the intent of normalizing behavior in otherwise disabling psychiatric disorders. The patients selected for treatment generally have certain types of symptoms rather than being a part of entire nosological groups or diagnostic categories. Examples of such symptoms include phobias, anxieties, depressions, obsessive compulsions, and affective components of schizophrenia—behaviors that include, but are not limited to, incapacitating alterations in mood with loss of interest in usually pleasurable activities; persistent and irrational fear of an object, activity, or situation; or feelings of apprehension or dread about the future. Routine neurosurgical procedures are employed, including cutting, burning, or irradiation of brain tissue. Neurosurgical procedures for psychosurgical purposes are performed in the absence of definable, structural brain changes such as tumors, vascular malformations, or post-traumatic scarring. Surgical intervention in the brain for the purpose of treating a structural lesion, or other definable pathology such as an epileptic focus or tumor, would not be considered psychosurgery even if the procedure resulted in some behavioral alteration. Regarding pain relieving procedures employing some of these techniques, there is no clear consensus. Such procedures clearly are designed to alter the perception of pain, thereby altering the behavioral response to that pain. Pain relieving procedures have not been included in most discussions of psychosurgery unless they are specifically oriented toward altering an emotional or affective disorder associated with the pain.

Mechanisms

The best results of treating psychiatric disease by neurosurgical interventions follow destruction of some part of the frontal lobes or their connections to other brain structures. The limbic system—that portion of the brain including the white-matter fiber tracts (consisting of nerve fibers covered with myelin and hence white in appearance) of the corpus callosum (connecting the two hemispheres of the brain), the cingulate, the fornicate, and the angulate gyri, and the amygdala and hippocampus of the temporal lobes, as well as the deeper nuclei (consisting of cell bodies or gray matter), the thalamus, and the hypothalamus—is now generally accepted to control behavior and the emotions. While the relationship of these structures to behavior and emotions is accepted, the specific functions of the various segments have not been identified with any certainty. The present state of knowledge about the physiological mechanisms for the control of normal emotions, to say nothing of the mechanisms involved in affective disorders, can only be characterized as rudimentary and empirical. Hence, there is no pathophysiological rationale for selecting targets for psychosurgical procedures. There is no good answer at present to the question of how these treatments work. It is, therefore, of critical importance to prospectively evaluate outcomes of treatment in relation to the initial patient symptoms.

The Development of Psychosurgery

Psychosurgery began in the 1930s in the Yale University laboratory of neurophysiologist John Fulton. Based on a growing background of knowledge from animal experiments using selective destruction of frontal lobe areas, combined with behavioral training from a number of laboratories, and on a specific observation from Ivan Pavlov (1928) concerning the production of neurotic behavior in dogs presented with confusing reinforcement symbols, he and his colleague Carlyle Jacobsen conducted behavioral experiments on two chimpanzees trained to solve complex problems in order to obtain food rewards. When frustrated with attempts to obtain food, they became agitated and aggressive. Fulton and Jacobsen then performed frontal lobectomies, literally cutting out the anterior frontal lobes of the brain, and noted that the animals became immune to frustration, although they performed assigned tests slightly less well.

Fulton and Jacobsen reported their observations at a 1935 London neuroscience meeting (Fulton and Jacobsen; see also Fulton, 1942, 1951). In attendance was a noted Portuguese neuroscientist, Egas Moniz, who, with his neurosurgical colleague Almeida Lima, performed the first procedures in humans a few months thereafter. The initial operation involved placing two holes through the skull three centimeters from the midline over the frontal area, with injection of alcohol to destroy the brain substance. In subsequent operations a wire loop was used to cut the frontal lobe connections. Thus they modified the Fulton procedure, performing only a frontal lobotomy or, as Moniz termed it, a *leukotomy* (cutting of the white matter). Moniz was awarded the 1949 Nobel Prize for his discovery of the therapeutic value of prefrontal leukotomy in certain psychoses.

Neuropsychiatrist Walter Freeman of the United States also attended the London conference. He and his neurosurgical colleague James Watts introduced psychosurgery to the United States. They pioneered the *lobotomy*, in which frontal lobe connections to the surrounding brain were severed initially by an open neurosurgical approach called *craniotomy*, using suction to sever the fibers. The demographics of the over 600 patients reported on by Freeman and Watts are not easily summarized. Many were institutionalized but many others were cared for at home and referred by their psychiatrists. The majority were women. All of these patients were considered disabled by their illness. However, Freeman felt the procedure was too costly, being primarily governmentally funded through the state-run mental institutions, and required too much skill to use on a broad scale to empty the wards of the large mental institutions. Freeman was very much a community psychiatrist and saw it as his mission to empty the back wards of state mental hospitals.

Around 1945, Freeman introduced a procedure described by the Italian neurosurgeon Amarro Fiamberti, in which the surgeon introduced a sharp probe (originally an ice pick) through the roof of the eye socket (orbit) into the frontal lobe white matter and oscillated it back and forth, thus severing the nerve fibers; this was called a *transorbital lobotomy* (Freeman and Watts). Watts, who performed the traditional procedure, felt Fiamberti's procedure violated any sense of neurosurgical dignity. The so-called "ice pick

lobotomy" could easily be performed, and it is estimated that by 1955 over 40,000 had been done in the United States. Freeman, a nonsurgeon, alone performed or supervised over 3,500 operations in 19 states and 10 foreign countries (National Commission for the Protection of Human Subjects of Biomedical and Behavioral Research). The indications were broad, including almost any patient confined to an institution, predominantly schizophrenics. While as effective as open craniotomy, the procedure was undertaken at a much greater risk of immediate complications resulting in neurologic sequelae, such as paralysis or epilepsy. Long-term psychological results were often associated with intellectual and emotional changes, such as a withdrawn and flattened affect. However, more patients were able to be discharged from the institutions because of the procedure than previously had been possible (Mettler; Tow; Petrie).

With the introduction of the drug chlorpromazine in 1952, use of psychopharmacologic agents (drugs designed to treat the symptoms of psychiatric illness) ended the era of lobotomies. Chlorpromazine resulted in the sedation of agitated patients and alleviation of psychotic behaviors, such that patients could be managed better both in and out of institutions. In the 1960s, with the advent of antidepressant medication, the number of psychosurgical procedures declined even further. Although they were performed far less frequently, they continued to be used from time to time because of their demonstrated beneficial effects in many intractable patients who were not helped by traditional therapy.

In 1947, Ernest Spiegel and Henry Wycis introduced a technique for precisely locating points or targets within the human brain, thereby allowing destruction of specific tissue with minimal disruption of the surrounding brain (Spiegel and Wycis). This technique, still the technique of choice, is called *stereotaxic surgery*. Stereotaxis employs precise calculation of locations within the brain using internal, radiographically determined reference points, thus allowing placement of a probe or beam of radiation with great accuracy. At about the same time, John Fulton reasoned that an optimum site of a lesion to treat psychiatric illness should be located in one quadrant of the frontal lobe and could be quite small. Stereotaxic surgery ushered in the modern era of psychosurgery by making possible treatment of psychiatric disease through very small, precisely located lesions.

As knowledge of the limbic structures became more precise, neurosurgeons began directing their efforts to cutting selected fiber tracts that connected the frontal lobes with specific limbic structures by using stereotaxis. Although surgeons could not specify how destruction of small brain areas worked to alleviate the symptoms of psychiatric disease, it did work. Complications from surgery declined significantly. The safety and efficacy of psychosurgery improved greatly. Stereotaxic psychosurgical technique gained in popularity by the late 1960s, when mental-health professionals recognized that the medications used to treat psychic disease did not help everyone and often had significant side effects.

Psychosurgery suffered a dramatic decline in the United States, similar to that coinciding with the advent of psychotropic medication, beginning in the 1970s. Those who viewed psychosurgery as mutilation of the brain leveled much criticism at those who were performing the procedures. The most vocal opponent was Peter Breggin (Breggin, 1972). Trained in a tradition that denied the authenticity of mental illness as a disease, he argued vehemently that all surgical treatments mutilated the brain and destroyed function. No scientific data were presented to substantiate his claims, but they did serve to raise public awareness about psychosurgery. The case against psychosurgery was aided by the speculation of Vernon Mark and Frank Ervin that the techniques might be helpful in controlling criminal or violent behavior, thereby raising the specter of political control (Mark and Ervin).

The debate generated a politically stressful environment, with the most vocal groups being against the treatment. There developed a desire on the part of American psychiatrists and neurosurgeons to avoid controversy over this form of treatment. The result was a dramatic decline in the use of psychosurgery techniques. Between 1949 and 1952, approximately 5,000 lobotomies were performed each year in the United States, largely by itinerant physicians lacking neurosurgical training. The commission established by Congress to investigate psychosurgery estimated that in 1971 and 1972, 140 neurosurgeons had performed a total of approximately 400 to 500 operations a year (National Commission for the Protection of Human Subjects of Biomedical and Behavioral Research). In 1987, Harvard University neurosurgeon Thomas Ballantine reported on a group of 474 psychosurgical patients treated over the previous twenty-five years (about 18 per year); most procedures had occurred in the late 1960s and early 1970s (Ballantine and Giriunas). More specific reports from which the current incidence of psychosurgical procedures in the United States might be calculated are lacking.

Current Safety and Effectiveness

Psychosurgery, in spite of declining frequency due to nonmedical reasons, benefited from the more precise definition and understanding of the types of patients who were likely to be helped by this surgery. This process occurred simultaneously with the development of psychosurgery, as psychiatry made advances in the understanding of mental illness. One important consideration is consent to treatment. Informed consent for mentally ill patients may be possible if the impairment does not extend to rendering the patient "incompetent" in the legal sense. But whether a mentally ill or incarcerated person can ever give a voluntary informed consent is doubtful, as mental competence and autonomy are such arbitrary notions. The integrity of the physician is the most effective guarantee of a patient's rights.

Currently, in selecting who should be treated, an appropriate psychiatric diagnosis revealing symptoms amenable to relief by psychosurgery is required. Appropriate candidates include chronically and severely depressed individuals with a preexisting history of obsessive-compulsive personality traits; chronically anxious patients whose psychic pain is incapacitating; and increasingly incapacitating obsessive-compulsive neuroses associated with depression. All other treatments deemed appropriate for the diagnosis, including the use of appropriate doses of psychopharmacologic medication, should be tried before psychosurgery is contemplated. Incapacity produced by the illness should be disabling and persistent. There should be no contraindications, either physical or mental, to the performance of the procedure.

Technique

Modern stereotaxic psychosurgery consists of producing lesions by heating electrodes in the target areas to coagulate the tissue or, more recently, by the destruction of a target area by focused radiation utilizing either a linear accelerator radiation source or a focusable cobalt radiation source known as the gamma knife. Either technique requires fixing a head frame to the patient's skull with pins, inserted under local anesthesia. Some type of imaging—magnetic resonance scanning, computed tomographic scanning, or the introduction of air into the fluid space of the brain for contrast and using radiographs (ventriculography)—defines the target within the brain. When heat is used, the surgeon places a burr hole through the skull over the target area and introduces a probe into the target. A radio frequency current is applied to the probe and the lesion is produced. The production of the lesion is painless. The radiation lesion technique requires no opening of the skull. The patient is transported to the instrument used and is exposed to a focused beam of radiation. This also is painless. Following the production of the lesion, the patient is returned to the hospital room and usually discharged the following day. The onset of the effects of the heat lesion is virtually immediate, while the radiation may take as long as six months to produce the final result. Both lesions are irreversible.

Targets

Primarily four areas of the limbic system are currently utilized as targets. The procedures, named for the target areas, are cingulotomy, subcaudate tractotomy, limbic leukotomy, and amygdalotomy. Cingulotomy places the lesion in the cingulate gyrus of the brain, located on the inside of the frontal lobes. One or both of these structures may be lesioned, primarily for relief of depression and/or obsession; the procedure has a reported 75 percent recovered or markedly improved result in depression and 56 percent in obsession. Subcaudate tractotomy is performed just below the nucleus of the brain, called the caudate nucleus, in the white-matter fiber tracts connecting with frontal lobe structures. The primary indications for this procedure are depression, anxiety, and obsession; it has a recovered or improved rate of 68 percent for depression, 63 percent for anxiety, and 53 percent for obsession. Limbic leukotomy is a lesion placed in the white-matter tracts of the frontal lobe connecting to the nucleus called the thalamus. This lesion has been used for depression, anxiety, and obsession, with recovery or improvement in 61 percent for depression, 63 percent for anxiety, and 84 percent for obsession. Amygdalotomy places a lesion in the amygdaloid nucleus of cell bodies located in the temporal lobe and integrally connected to the limbic system structures. Unlike the other targets, amygdalotomy is used primarily for aggression, with a 76 percent markedly improved or recovered outcome (Maxwell).

Complications

The incidence of complications for each procedure is extremely low when compared with the morbidity and mortality of the old frontal leukotomy of Freeman and Watts (Mettler; Tow; Petrie). Significant neurologic complications, such as paralysis or epilepsy, and psychological complications, such as persistent behavioral or personality changes, occur in much less than 1 percent of cases (Ballantine and Giriunas).

The one aspect of the old frontal lobotomy that has remained in the minds of those caring for these patients is the generally placid affect, loss of initiative, and decline in intellectual function that was frequently seen. Reports of neuropsychological studies of patients undergoing modern psychosurgical procedures have indicated no significant damage to higher brain functions such as recognizable personality. Relief of disabling and intractable behavioral symptoms is followed by impressively improved overall function with preservation of personality (Mindus and Jenike; Bridges). However, neuropsychological instruments designed to measure cognition may not be sensitive enough to detect subtle emotional impairments. Currently available methods of testing support the conclusion that limited procedures such as cingulotomy, subcaudate tractotomy, limbic leukotomy, and amygdalotomy result in minimal intellectual and cognitive changes for the patient while reducing disabling symptoms such as depression.

Issues of Patient Selection

In the 1970s, amid concern about violence in the ghettos, some political activists, black and white, made accusations that psychosurgery was being used as a tool of the establishment to exercise political and social control, specifically of minorities and women (Mason; Carver). These accusations arose from publicity regarding proposed but never undertaken research projects, to be supported by federal funds, that focused on the psychosurgical treatment of irrational and spontaneously violent behavior arising from epilepsy in the limbic system. In addition, the issue of social control and racism in the application of psychosurgery became public when, with the establishment in Los Angeles of a Center for the Prevention of Violence, one of the researchers who had proposed a study of psychosurgery and violence joined the staff. At about this time, reports of psychosurgery performed on black patients in Mississippi were published (Andy and Jurko). These were institutionalized, severely disturbed, mentally retarded children; the neurosurgeon defended the practice on the basis that the psychosurgery was indicated medically as a treatment of last resort, and that the preponderance of black patients reflected the composition of the total patient group and not prejudice. There were those in the psychiatric community who felt that the levels of psychiatric care, the availability of qualified staff, and the availability of alternative treatment in this facility were below even minimal standards, thus calling into question the use of psychosurgery. The possibility of de facto racism existed.

No reliable evidence to support charges of intentional racism in the use of psychosurgery has been presented. There is no case of a responsible individual or group claiming that psychosurgery has actually been used for purposes of political action, social control, or acting out of personal prejudices against minority groups or women. However, there are no reliable data with respect to the incidence of psychosurgery performed on whites or blacks, males or females; such reports as are available give no support to the charge that minority groups of any category have been subjected to operations specifically on the basis of membership in such a group.

With respect to legally committed or otherwise involuntarily institutionalized patients, the issue of valid or proxy consent is a difficult one. However, it is generally acknowledged that there are some patients in this category who may benefit from psychosurgical procedures. As issues of autonomy versus community are studied and elaborated, new ethical grounds for consent in this population should arise (Beauchamp et al.).

Recent Developments

Since the mid-1990s, the use of functional neurosurgery to access the cingulate gyrus, subcaudate tractotomy, limbic leukotomy, and anterior capsulotomy targets has seen a renaissance of interest (Christie; Lichterman; Snaith). Although efficacy continues to be estimated at 30 to 70 percent of persons treated, depending on diagnosis, the difficulty of evaluating the efficacy of such procedures cannot be overemphasized and researchers have placed an emphasis on developing methods to better assess efficacy (Binder and Iskandar). Several factors have made these determinations difficult. Most reports have been long-term retrospective analyses using methods that did not remain constant over the period studied. Most evaluations since the mid-1990s describe shorter follow-up periods but are prospective in design, and feature more well-defined diagnostic populations, but suffer from the problem that the persons selecting the patients and performing the outcomes analysis also selected the persons to be treated. Estimates of outcomes have been difficult to compare between studies. The most difficult problem has been determining appropriate control groups. A randomized, double blind, prospective study of surgical versus non-surgical treatments is definitely needed. The ability to perform such a procedure is constrained by the ethics of withholding treatment in the population of persons selected for treatment, the practical difficulty of identifying controls with severe disease who are not surgical candidates, and the ethics of sham open neurosurgical procedures, which carry significant risk. In the absence of such studies, the best current evidence of efficacy remains in the pre- and post-operative evaluation of individuals.

With the increased interest in psychosurgical procedures, now more favorably referred to as functional neurosurgery for psychiatric disorders, clinical practice guidelines have been developed to assist physicians who are contemplating surgical intervention for their patients (March et al.). Such guidelines identify the availability of surgical therapy for psychiatric disorders and the make explicit the order of treatment. The guidelines help referring psychiatrists with selection criteria and indications. Obsessive-compulsive disorders, treatment resistant affective disorders, and anxiety were the accepted indications for surgical treatment in the early 2000s. Personality disorders and psychotic disorders are relative contraindications.

Several technical advances have contributed to the increasing interest in these procedures. More precise delineation of the anatomical substrate of psychiatric disorders has been progressing, for example the relationship of the amygdala to human fear (Adolphs et al.). Researchers have compared the activation of certain structures during obsessive-compulsive states to resting states using imaging techniques, and similar studies have been done for psychosis and bipolar disorder. Such information begins to confirm that the targets selected for functional neurosurgery are indeed related to the diseases being treated. Such information is also teaching that surgical destruction of brain target areas may not be the only way to affect these anatomical locations. Surgical interventions that might augment nervous system function such as electrical stimulation, implantation of mini-pumps or drug-secreting capsules, transplantation cells, and implantation of genetically modified vectors for gene delivery are all being explored. Researchers have also performed deep brain electrical stimulation for obsessive-compulsive disorder and Tourette's syndrome.

Conclusion

There is substantial evidence that twenty-first century stereotaxic techniques, involving smaller, more discrete lesions in the brain, avoid the unwanted outcomes seen in many patients treated by earlier psychosurgical procedures. In addition, there is sufficient evidence that certain procedures do offer potential benefit to the patient who has failed to respond to other known therapies. These procedures do not appear to produce adverse psychological changes.

JOHN C. OAKLEY (1995)
REVISED BY AUTHOR

SEE ALSO: *Autonomy; Coercion; Deep Brain Stimulation; Electroconvulsive Therapy; Holocaust; Informed Consent: Issues of Consent in Mental Healthcare; Insanity and Insanity Defense; Institutionalization and Deinstitutionalization; Mental Illness: Conception of Mental Illness; Mental Illness: Cultural Perspectives; Mental Institutions, Commitment to; Mistakes, Medical; Narrative; Paternalism; Patients' Rights; Psychiatry, Abuses of; Psychosurgery, Ethical Aspects of; Race and Racism; Technology; Women, Historical and Cross-Cultural Perspectives*

BIBLIOGRAPHY

Adolphs, R.; Tranel, D.; Damasio, H.; and Damasio, A. R. 1995. "Fear and the Human Amygdala." *Journal of Neuroscience* 15: 5879–5891.

Andy, Orlando J., and Jurko, Marion F. 1972. "Thalamotomy for Hyperresponsive Syndrome: Lesions in the Centermedian and Intralaminar Nuclei." In *Psychosurgery: Proceedings of the Second International Conference on Psychosurgery,* ed. Edward Robert Hitchcock, Lauri Laitinen, and Kjeld Vaernet. Springfield, IL: Charles C. Thomas.

Ballantine, H. Thomas, and Giriunas, Ida E. 1988. "Treatment of Intractable Psychiatric Illness and Chronic Pain by Stereotactic Cingulotomy." In *Operative Neurosurgical Techniques: Indications, Methods, and Results,* 2nd edition, vol. 2, ed. Henry H. Schmidek and William Herbert Sweet. Philadelphia: Saunders.

Beauchamp, Tom L.; Bok, Sissela; Veatch, Robert M.; and Dresser, Rebecca. 1994. "Public and Private: Redrawing Boundaries." *Hastings Center Report* (May/June): 18–22.

Binder, Devin K., and Iskandar, Bermans J. 2000. "Modern Neurosurgery for Psychiatric Disorders." *Neurosurgery* 47: 9–23.

Breggin, Peter K. 1972a. "Psychosurgery for the Control of Violence." *Congressional Record,* 92nd Cong., 2nd sess., 118, pt. 9: 11396–11402.

Breggin, Peter K. 1972b. "The Return of Lobotomy and Psychosurgery." *Congressional Record,* 118, pt. 5: 5567–5577.

Bridges, Paul. 1990. "Psychosurgery Revisited." *Journal of Neuropsychiatry and Clinical Neuroscience* 2(3): 326–331.

Carver, James. 1973. "Psychosurgery: A Matter of Class and Racial Oppression." *Daily World* (New York), October 10.

Christie, B. 1996. "Neurosurgery for Mentally Ill Given Go Ahead in Scotland." *British Medical Journal* 13: 644.

Freeman, Walter, and Watts, James W. 1950. *Psychosurgery in the Treatment of Mental Disorders and Intractable Pain,* 2nd edition. Springfield, IL: Charles C. Thomas.

Fulton, John. 1942. *Physiology of the Nervous System.* New York: Oxford University Press.

Fulton, John. 1951. *Frontal Lobotomy and Affective Behavior: A Neurophysical Analysis.* New York: Norton.

Fulton, John, and Jacobsen, Carlyle. 1935. "The Functions of the Frontal Lobes: A Comparative Study in Monkeys, Chimpanzees and Man." *Advances in Modern Biology* 4: 113–123.

Lichterman, B. L. 1993. "On the History of Psychosurgery in Russia." *Acta Neurochir* (Wien) 125: 1–4.

March, J. S.; Frances, A.; Carpenter, D.; Kahn, D. A. 1997. "Treatment of Obsessive-Compulsive Disorder." *Journal of Clinical Psychiatry* 58(suppl. 4): 1–72.

Mark, Vernon H., and Ervin, Frank R. 1970. *Violence and the Brain.* New York: Harper & Row.

Mason, B. J. 1973. "Brain Surgery to Control Behavior." *Ebony* (February): 62–64, 76.

Maxwell, Robert E. 1993. "Behavioral Modification." In *Brain Surgery: Complication Avoidance and Management,* vol. 2, ed. Michael L. J. Apuzzo. New York: Churchill Livingstone.

Mettler, Fred A., ed. 1952. *Psychosurgical Problem.* Philadelphia: Blakiston.

Mindus, Per, and Jenike, Michael A. 1992. "Neurosurgical Treatment of Malignant Obsessive Compulsive Disorder." *Psychiatric Clinics of North America* 15(4): 921–938.

Moniz, Egas. 1936. *Tentatives opératoires dans le traitement de certaines psychoses.* Paris: Masson.

National Commission for the Protection of Human Subjects of Biomedical and Behavioral Research. 1977. "Use of Psychosurgery in Practice and Research: Report and Recommendations of the National Commission for the Protection of Human Subjects of Biomedical and Behavioral Research." *Federal Register* 42(99): 26318–26332.

Pavlov, Ivan. 1928. *Lectures on Conditional Reflexes.* New York: International Publishing.

Petrie, Asenath. 1952. *Personality and the Frontal Lobes: An Investigation of the Psychological Effects of Different Types of Leucotomy.* London: Routledge & Kegan Paul.

Spiegel, Ernest A., and Wycis, Henry T. 1952. *Stereoencephalotomy: Thalamotomy and Related Procedures.* New York: Grune and Stratton.

Snaith, R. P. 1997. "Surgery for Mental Illness Has Been Proved Effective." *British Medical Journal* 314: 75.

Tow, Peter Macdonald. 1955. *Personality Changes Following Frontal Leucotomy: A Clinical and Experimental Study of the Functions of the Frontal Lobe in Man.* London: Oxford University Press.

Valenstein, Elliot S. 1986. *Great and Desperate Cure: The Rise and Decline of Psychosurgery and Other Radical Treatments for Mental Illness.* New York: Basic Books.

PUBLIC HEALTH

• • •

I. DETERMINANTS

The current preoccupation with medical science and its application as the primary determinant of health derives largely from the enormously successful experience with applying microbiology in the battle against ill health. Identification of specific microorganisms as agents of epidemic communicable diseases, and means of controlling them, aroused expectations of finding "magic bullets" for most of humanity's ills. Further discoveries, such as insulin for diabetes and chemicals effective against certain forms of cancer, have encouraged the notion. Using the term *health provider* to mean a physician epitomizes this view.

However, dependence on medicine as the source of health tends to obscure far more fundamental influences on health. For millennia it has been evident that living conditions and the response to them largely determine people's health. Therefore, people have sought to extend life and improve health not only as individuals but also through communal efforts in the societies of which they are a part. These social efforts to enhance the health of whole populations have come to be called public health, "what we, as a society, do collectively to assure the conditions in which people can be healthy" (Institute of Medicine, p. 1). In modern times, government plays the leading role in this endeavor, supplemented by other endeavors organized to advance the health of the public. Making medical services available to people is only one way in which modern industrialized societies address health challenges; other measures include assuring a healthful environment and encouraging healthful behavior by individuals. To carry out its mission, public health must establish effective linkage with other efforts for social advancement, particularly in welfare and education.

Public health measures its progress by the health status of the population it serves. Thus, knowing the determinants of the public's health (which is also known as public health) is essential to the field.

Advances in Health, 1800–2000

The period since 1800 has brought the most spectacular health improvement in human history. From the time of the hunter-gatherers thousands of years ago until the industrial revolution around 1800, Mark Cohen estimates that life expectancy at birth ranged consistently between twenty and fifty years, most commonly about twenty-five to thirty years (Cohen). At the end of the twentieth century, life expectancy exceeds sixty-five years in most parts of the world and seventy-five years in western Europe, North America, and Japan.

In the United States, for example, life expectancy was only forty-seven years when the twentieth century began. By the late 1980s it had reached seventy-five years, according to the National Center for Health Statistics (1990). To a considerable extent that advance was due to declining infant mortality, from more than 100 per 1,000 in 1900 to less than 10 per 1,000 in the late 1980s, and to the control of communicable diseases, which take their major toll during the early years of life. Since 1960, however, relatively greater extension of life has occurred in the later years. From 1900 to 1960 life expectancy at birth increased twenty-two years, but only one-tenth of that expansion came after age sixty-five. Since 1960, on the other hand, more than half of the five years gained in life expectancy at birth have come beyond age sixty-five.

Table 1 lists specific diseases, and their trends, that have affected residents of the United States since 1900. Medical students in the early 1900s learned about pneumonia as "the old man's friend" and tuberculosis as "the captain of the men of death." Heart disease at the start of the century largely came from rheumatic fever, whereas now atherosclerosis accounts overwhelmingly for heart disease. Population aging considerably influences death rates from cancer and heart disease. Even when adjusted for age, however, cancer mortality has been increasing, mainly because of the twentieth-century epidemic of lung cancer. A rare form of the disease in 1900, respiratory cancer increased to constitute about one-tenth of all cancer deaths in 1950 and almost one-third as the century closed. Other measures of health status, such as survival to age sixty-five, reveal the role of violence and injury in certain human populations, such as young males in the United States.

Historical Determinants of Health

Health may be viewed as the human side of a dynamic equilibrium between the organism and its environment; that interface is the place where health is mainly determined.

The genetic structure with which humans enter the world will generally allow survival for about eighty-five years, according to James Fries (1980). In some people, of course, hereditary abnormalities interfere with and/or shorten life, while others live more than eighty-five years in reasonably good health. Beyond these biological influences, since food and oxygen are the most critical elements for human life and since oxygen is only rarely inadequate, nutrition constitutes a paramount factor in health. From earliest times to the present, inadequate food has been a major threat to health. In fact, society has evolved largely to supply enough food for people—for example, through migration and the development of agriculture.

Not infrequently, however, huge numbers of people have been trapped in starvation through ecological and social catastrophes—both in ancient times and more recently, as in the Irish potato blight of the late 1840s and in slavery in the United States, and now in certain African nations and among the homeless in America. Moreover, beyond gross lack of calories, deficiencies of vitamins and

TABLE 1

Crude Death Rates per 100,000, Selected Causes, U.S. Registration Area, 1900–1988						
Cause of Death	*1900*	*1920*	*1940*	*1970*	*1980*	*1988*
Pneumonia	153	82	25	31	24	32
Tuberculosis	94	113	46	3	1	1
Diphtheria	40	15	1			
Organic heart disease	123	151	296	362	336	312
Cancer	64	83	125	163	184	199
Diabetes	11	16	27	19	15	16

SOURCE: Linder, Forrest E., and Grove, Robert D., 1943; Stieglitz, Edward J., 1945; U.S. Bureau of the Census, 1990.

other micronutrients cause incalculable damage to health—incalculable because scurvy, rickets, and pellagra may be only the most striking clinical manifestations of severe damage to health.

Industrialization, even though it has improved the standard of living in many respects, has also precipitated some devastating health events. In the early 1800s, when people flocked from the countryside to factory towns and cities in search of a better life, they found crowded housing, gross lack of sanitation, and exhausting work (even for children), as well as food deficiencies. These living conditions produced the "crowd" diseases, epidemics spread by intestinal and respiratory discharges that debilitated many people and caused high mortality. Though all segments of society were affected, the poor suffered then, as throughout history, most severely from the adverse conditions.

While medical science has helped in overcoming the communicable disease epidemics since 1800, other factors have been even more important. John and Sonja McKinley have estimated that at most 3.5 percent of the total decline in mortality (from influenza, pneumonia, diphtheria, whooping cough, and poliomyelitis) since 1900 could be ascribed to medical measures (McKinley and McKinley). Thomas McKeown has demonstrated that medical science barely affected the decline of tuberculosis (McKeown).

During the twentieth century a constellation of noncommunicable diseases, led by cardiovascular disease and cancer, has supplanted the epidemic communicable diseases as the foremost health problem in industrialized countries (despite the current public attention to AIDS); and increasingly such noncommunicable diseases are affecting the rest of the world. Again, the circumstances of life and the way people behave in them are the major determinants. For example, the first to indulge in excessive calories, fats, cigarettes, and physical inactivity were affluent men, and accordingly they suffered consequent ischemic heart disease

first. Poor men—for example, blacks in the United States—only later had considerable access to those relevant factors; their epidemic of ischemic heart disease came later and is persisting longer.

Major Current Influences on Health

Epidemiological studies have delineated key factors in the rise and the start of the decline of twentieth-century noncommunicable diseases. Most noteworthy, in 1964 an advisory committee to the U.S. surgeon general summarized the growing evidence that "Cigarette smoking is causally related to lung cancer in men … the most important of the causes of chronic bronchitis in the United States … [and is associated with] … a higher death rate from coronary artery disease …" (U.S. Surgeon General's Advisory Committee, pp. 31–32).

Studying a sample of the Alameda County, California, population, Nedra Belloc and Lester Breslow demonstrated the strong relationship of seven health practices to health status and subsequent total mortality: eating moderately, sleeping seven to eight hours, using alcohol moderately if at all, not smoking, eating breakfast, not snacking, and having at least moderate physical activity (Belloc and Breslow). Men who followed all seven health practices enjoyed physical health equal to that of men thirty years younger who reported two or fewer. Forty-five-year-old men who followed none to three of the health practices had a longevity of sixty-seven years; four to five, seventy-three years; and six to seven, seventy-eight years, thus yielding an advantage of eleven years, depending upon health behavior. Lisa Berkman and Lester Breslow reported further that the extent of one's social network likewise substantially predicted physical health status and mortality (Berkman and Breslow). A 1974 official Canadian document, the LaLonde Report, proposed a health field concept. According to the latter, four broad elements comprise the health field: human biology, environment, and lifestyle, and healthcare organization. Further, the LaLonde Report asserted that "Improvements in the [social as well as physical] environment and an abatement in the level of risks imposed upon themselves by individuals, taken together, constitute the most promising ways by which further advances can be made."

The growing emphasis on the way people live as an important health factor in the industrial (and postindustrial) world must be considered carefully in relation to social responsibility for lifestyle. Otherwise, that emphasis can properly be termed "victim blaming." A 1952 report to the president of the United States, *Building America's Health,* noted that "Recognition of the significance of individual responsibility for health does not discharge the obligation of a society which is interested in the health of its citizenry. Such recognition, in fact, increases social responsibility for health" (President's Commission on Health Needs of the Nation, vol. 1, p. 2). As the Ottawa Charter for Health Promotion stated, "Health promotion is the process of enabling people to increase control over and to improve their health. … [It] … demands coordinated action by all concerned: by governments, by health and other social and economic sectors, by non-governmental and voluntary organizations, by local authorities, by industry, and by the media" (International World Health Organization Conference, p. 1).

As it becomes clear that we are able to raise life expectancy to some sort of biological limit, it may well be that public health rather than gross national product (GNP) will constitute the criterion for national success. Using public health as a standard for this success would help illuminate how GNP masks the staggering toll of ill health found among low-income or very poor Americans, many of whom, like American Indians or African Americans, have been disproportionately disadvantaged for generations. Achieving that reorientation of values will require a new approach to the food, alcohol, tobacco, medical, and other industries whose products and services are pertinent to health. Health ethics now entails concern for issues beyond matters in which the physician–patient relationship predominates. How to deal effectively with the "right" to addict young people throughout the world to tobacco and to expose others to one's intoxicated behavior, and similar public-health issues, are coming to the fore. Social action reflecting experience and thought concerning such questions will determine health in the future, just as assuring safe water and milk determined health in the past.

LESTER BRESLOW (1995)
BIBLIOGRAPHY REVISED

SEE ALSO: *Hazardous Wastes and Toxic Substances; Health and Disease: History of Concepts; Health Screening and Testing in the Public Health Context; Injury and Injury Control; Lifestyles and Public Health; Public Health Law; Sexual Behavior, Social Control of; Warfare: Public Health and War;* and other *Public Health* subentries

BIBLIOGRAPHY

Belloc, Nedra B., and Breslow, Lester. 1972. "Relationship of Physical Health Status and Health Practices." *Preventive Medicine* 1(3): 409–421.

Berkman, Lisa L., and Breslow, Lester. 1983. *Health and Ways of Living: The Alameda County Study.* New York: Oxford University Press.

Cohen, Mark N. 1989. *Health and the Rise of Civilization.* New Haven, CT: Yale University Press.

Fries, James. 1980. "Aging, Natural Death, and the Compression of Morbidity." *New England Journal of Medicine* 303(3): 130–135.

Institute of Medicine (U.S.). Committee for the Study of the Future of Public Health. 1988. *The Future of Public Health.* Washington, D.C.: National Academy of Sciences.

International World Health Organization Conference on Health Promotion. 1986. *Ottawa Charter for Health Promotion.* Ottawa: Author. Sponsored by WHO, Health and Welfare Canada, and Canadian Public Health Association.

LaLonde, Marc. 1974. *A New Perspective on the Health of Canadians: A Working Document.* Ottawa: Government of Canada.

Linder, Forest E., and Grove, Robert D. 1943. *Vital Statistics Rates in the United States, 1900–1940.* Washington, D.C.: U.S. Government Printing Office.

McKeown, Thomas. 1988. *The Origins of Human Disease.* Oxford: Basil Blackwell.

McKinley, John B., and McKinley, Sonja M. 1977. "The Questionable Contribution of Medical Measures to the Decline of Mortality in the United States in the Twentieth Century." *Milbank Memorial Fund Quarterly* 55(3): 405–428.

Stieglitz, Edward J. 1945. *A Future for Preventive Medicine.* New York: Commonwealth Fund.

U.S. Bureau of the Census. 1990. *Statistical Abstract of the United States, 1990,* 11th edition. Wshington, D.C.: U.S. Dept. of Commerce, Bureau of the Census.

U.S. Department of Health and Human Services. Public Health Service. Centers for Disease Control and National Center for Health Statistics. 1991. *Health, United States, 1990.* Hyattsville, MD: Author.

U.S. President's Commission on Health Needs of the Nation. 1952. *Building America's Health.* 5 vols. Washington, D.C.: U.S. Government Printing Office.

U.S. Surgeon General's Advisory Committee on Smoking and Health. 1964. *Smoking and Health: Report.* Public Health Service Pub. no. 1103. Washington, D.C.: U.S. Government Printing Office.

II. HISTORY

Public health may be defined as the collective action by a community or society to protect and promote the health and welfare of its members. In a world where sickness and accidents were attributed to spirits, the welfare of the tribe and its individual members depended upon paying proper homage to the spiritual realm. Since public-health measures are based upon the level of existing medical knowledge or prevailing assumptions, the observance of taboos and rituals by early tribal societies represents a form of public health. The origins of modern public health lie in efforts to prevent pestilential diseases, but in the past centuries public health has broadened its aims and now applies the findings of social and scientific fields to promoting physical and mental well-being.

Public health in its modern sense arose as a phenomenon of urbanization. As towns and cities emerged, communal living created special problems relating to food, water, sanitation, and disease. In an urban environment, the responsibility for providing safe food and water and disposing of garbage and human wastes could no longer be left to individual initiative, and what were essentially public-health regulations appeared. Both health and aesthetics supplied the motive for these early sanitary regulations, since foul odors were associated with the miasmic theory of disease, a belief that some obnoxious gaseous substance was the cause of epidemic disease.

The classical civilizations evolved relatively sophisticated public health measures. In the second millennium B.C.E. the Minoans developed elaborate plumbing systems that included flush toilets. The great Roman aqueducts that were built between 312 B.C.E. and about 100 C.E., sections of which still survive, are familiar to all; but what is not so well known is that the Roman water systems, at least the one for Rome, differentiated between water for common use and that for drinking. The decline of the Western Roman Empire meant a return to a rural society, and it was not until the rise of towns and cities in the medieval period that public-health measures were reinstituted. The need to live within the town walls for safety intensified crowding and its concomitant sanitary and health problems. In the medieval period fear of two horrible diseases, leprosy and bubonic plague (the Black Death), was responsible for the practice of isolating the sick and instituting quarantines to keep the sickness at bay. Victims of leprosy were literally read out of society, and the first quarantine laws appeared in 1348 in response to the spread of the Black Death.

The late Renaissance and early modern period witnessed two developments that helped pave the way for the institutionalization of public health. The first of these was the concept of mercantilism, which, among other factors, counted population as a source of a nation's wealth. The second was the development of what was termed political arithmetic. Morbidity and mortality statistics are basic to understanding the health of a population and to determining health policy. Two Englishmen, William Petty (1623–1687) and John Graunt (1620–1674), were among the first to recognize this need. They urged the collection of statistics pertaining to health and social matters in order to promote a more healthy and productive population. The astronomer Edmund Halley in 1693 published a life expectancy table that made possible the first life insurance company. Later, life and industrial insurance companies in the United States were to play a role in promoting public health.

John Locke (1632–1704) in 1690 published his classic treatise, *Essay on Human Understanding,* in which he asserted that human beings were the product of their environment. By applying intelligence to social problems and creating a better society, it would be possible to improve humankind. The French philosophers Denis Diderot, Jean Le Rond d'Alembert, Voltaire, and Jean-Jacques Rousseau carried the idea even further by assuming the perfectibility of humanity. Joining this assumption to the mercantilist principle that a growing and healthy population strengthened the power of the state, the "benevolent despots" of the eighteenth century sought to impose public-health measures by fiat. This form of public health, in which administrators issued decrees relating to health and sanitation, was called "medical police" or medical policy; and its leading exponent was Johann Peter Frank, whose six-volume *Complete System of Medical Policy* (1779–1817) dealt with virtually all aspects of public health, from sanitation to the health of workers.

In Britain, the Civil War and the Glorious Revolution of 1688 had made the British people suspicious of the central government; consequently, much administration was kept at the local level. As in the United States, the major impulse for public-health reform came in the nineteenth century and was led by middle-class reformers motivated by a mixture of Christian benevolence, humanitarianism, and rationalism. The dislocations resulting from economic changes in the eighteenth and early nineteenth centuries created a large impoverished class and led to efforts by humanitarians to reduce the enormous mortality among infants, to alleviate the suffering of prisoners and the insane, and to fight against widespread alcoholism among the working class.

By the early nineteenth century, the industrial revolution was drawing thousands of workers from rural areas into crowded city slums, compounding the growing urban sanitary problems. In Britain, the harsh conditions of the poorly paid men, women, and children working long hours in the newly spawned factories and mills came to the attention of several humane individuals, and, under the leadership of Lord Ashley, a series of factory acts was enacted. The first of these, passed in 1833, restricted the working hours of children below the age of eighteen to twelve per day and sixty-nine per week. In the legislative battle for this law, parliamentary hearings drew attention to the atrocious living conditions of the workers and their high rates of sickness and death. The hearings also showed that the excessive use of alcohol and opium was a means of escape for workers condemned to lifelong toil in a brutalizing environment.

Meanwhile, the physicians C. Turner Thackrah, James Philips Kay, Thomas Southwood Smith, and Neil Arnott were drawing attention to the need for health reform. They were fortunate in enlisting Edwin Chadwick (1801–1890) in their cause. Chadwick was a single-minded reformer who dedicated himself to promoting the welfare of the working class. His investigations and reports on behalf of government commissions, culminating in his report for the Health of Towns Commission, were largely responsible for the passage of the Public Health Act of 1848. This measure marks the first step in the institutionalization of public health in the West.

In France the work of Louis René Villerme (1782–1863) roughly paralleled that of Chadwick. Like the latter, his morbidity and mortality statistics demonstrated the close correlation between health and living standards, and led the French government to establish a national public-health advisory committee in 1848. The committee, which included professionals such as physicians, chemists, pharmacists, and veterinarians, was purely an advisory body. Although it dealt with a wide range of public-health issues, from epidemics to industrial health, it was devoid of all powers, and the successive French governments did little to strengthen it during the rest of the century.

The industrial revolution and its concomitant problems arrived late in the United States, but by 1800 cities were beginning to establish temporary boards of health. The chief impetus for these early health agencies came from a series of yellow fever epidemics that struck port cities from South Carolina to New England in the years from 1793 to 1806. These boards were appointed whenever yellow fever threatened or was present. With medical opinion divided as to whether the disease was an imported contagion or the result of a miasma arising from foul, putrefying substances or some other source, the health officials played safe by promptly quarantining incoming vessels and instituting large-scale sanitary programs. Privies were cleaned, dead animals removed from the streets, stagnant pools drained, and slaughterers, tanners, and other members of the "noxious" trades required to cleanse their premises. After 1806 the danger from yellow fever in the region north of Norfolk,

Virginia, receded, and health boards virtually disappeared. The appearance in 1832 of the first of three great epidemic waves of Asiatic cholera that swept through the United States revived these temporary boards, but generally they functioned only in times of emergencies.

By the 1830s and 1840s, American cities were beginning to experience the worst aspects of the industrial revolution. Rural Americans and immigrants flooded into urban areas that were ill prepared to handle the influx. Housing and sanitary conditions deteriorated, and morbidity and mortality rose. The movement to remedy these conditions was initiated largely by physicians, most notably by Benjamin W. McCready, whose 1837 essay drew attention to the deplorable health conditions in the workplace and the slums housing the workers, and by John H. Griscom, whose 1845 report, *The Sanitary Condition of the Laboring Population of New York,* laid the basis for establishing the first effective municipal health department in the United States. In other cities, too, physicians led the reform movement: Wilson Jewell in Philadelphia, Edwin Miller Snow in Providence, Edward Jarvis in Boston, and Edward H. Barton and J. C. Simmonds in New Orleans.

The outstanding layman in the early health movement was Lemuel Shattuck of Boston, who pioneered in the collection of vital statistics and promoted sanitary reform. The success of the early reformers in drawing public attention to the need for action led in the 1850s and 1860s to the appearance of civic sanitary organizations and agencies such as the New York Association for Improving the Condition of the Poor. As in England, the public health movement was both a humanitarian and a moral crusade. A few reformers emphasized improving the morals of the poor, but most recognized that immorality and intemperance were closely associated with the crowded and brutally degraded living conditions of the poor.

In 1857, an abortive attempt was made to unite the health reformers at the national level when Wilson Jewell of Philadelphia summoned a national quarantine convention. The original purpose was to respond to the danger from yellow fever, a disease still ravaging southern ports and threatening the Mississippi Valley. In the first meeting the delegates generally agreed on the necessity to standardize state quarantine laws, but many of them felt that the real need was complete sanitary reform. In the following three annual meetings, sentiment among the delegates swung in favor of a program affecting all areas of community health. At the 1860 meeting a resolution was passed suggesting that the delegates form a national health association. The outbreak of the Civil War ended these hopes, and a national organization awaited the postwar years.

Although the Civil War temporarily set back a nationwide organization of public health leaders, it stimulated the health movement. Wartime experiences in army camps and hospitals demonstrated the value of cleanliness and proper food and housing. In addition, the U.S. Sanitary Commission, a civilian body given official status at the outset of the war, introduced thousands of Union soldiers to the principles of personal and public hygiene. Leading members of this commission also played a key role in establishing the New York Metropolitan Board of Health in 1866, an agency that set the pattern for municipal health departments throughout the United States. Four years later, the Massachusetts State Board of Health, the first effective state health agency, came into existence. The founding of the American Public Health Association in 1872 indicated that the institutionalization of public health in the United States was under way.

Until the 1870s, the only action by the federal government relating to health had been the creation of the U.S. Marine Hospital Service in 1798. Although designed to provide medical care for sick sailors, for much of the nineteenth century it served primarily as a form of political patronage. Two yellow fever epidemics, one in 1873 and a major one in 1878 that spread far up the Mississippi River Valley, resulted in the federal government's briefly moving into the area of public health. Responding to widespread alarm, in 1879 Congress established the National Board of Health. The board was given little authority and limited funds, and was expected to act primarily in an advisory capacity. It immediately encountered strong opposition from the U.S. Marine Hospital Service, which was seeking to expand into the health area, and from state and municipal health officials reluctant to surrender any of their authority. The board performed quite well, promoting scientific health studies, assisting local health boards, and encouraging standardization of local quarantine laws. Nonetheless, political pressure led to its demise in 1883. During the nineteenth century Congress voted substantial funds to promote the health of domestic animals and fowls but virtually nothing for human health.

The Progressive movement at the turn of the century promoted political reform, economic efficiency, and social justice and, in the process, gave an impetus to U.S. public health. By the early twentieth century, public health in all developed countries was both professionalized and institutionalized. The bacteriological revolution had provided a new basis for action by health authorities, shifting the emphasis away from sanitation and environmental considerations and toward utilizing the newly developed antitoxins and vaccines to cure and prevent the great epidemic disorders of earlier years. Advances in technology and improvements in civic administration enabled health departments to spin off to separate agencies many former responsibilities, such as street cleaning and garbage removal, inspecting housing, and supervising water supplies and sewage removal. Their place was taken by new concerns: maternal and child care, the health of schoolchildren, the development of laboratory techniques for diagnostic purposes, and the health of people in rural areas. The major gains during the first forty years of the twentieth century were the elimination or drastic reduction of smallpox, measles, diphtheria, scarlet fever, tuberculosis, and other killer diseases.

Until the bacteriological revolution and the advances in basic sciences in the last decades of the nineteenth century, the medical profession, particularly in the United States, was viewed with considerable skepticism. In an effort to improve their status, physicians took an active role in the early publichealth movement, and in England and on the Continent they gained control of it. The institutionalization of public health in the United States, however, assumed a different form, in part because the American Public Health Association from its founding in 1872 included sanitary engineers, bacteriologists, and other nonphysician members. In the early twentieth century, as public health moved into the area of school, maternal, and child health, health officials recognized the inadequacy of the medical care available to the lower-income groups and began establishing clinics. The medical profession by this time had gained control of hospitals and medical education, and dominated medical care. Recognizing that clinics represented a threat to the lucrative fee system, the American Medical Association used its political power to force public-health agencies out of direct healthcare. Health departments in general were restricted to supplying free vaccines to physicians, referring patients screened by public-health doctors or nurses, gathering statistics, and dealing with community health problems.

As the great killer diseases of former times were brought under control in the first forty years of the twentieth century, health authorities began turning their attention to chronic and constitutional disorders and to the long-neglected area of occupational hazards. Although the danger from miasmas had been dismissed, the post–World War II period saw a rising concern over the environment. The thousands of new chemicals polluting the air and water presented subtle but potentially serious dangers to health, and radiation introduced still another possible threat. In addition, stimulated in part by the psychiatric problems uncovered during the war years, public health was broadened to include community mental health.

The development of sulfa drugs and antibiotics in the World War II period seemed to have ended contagious diseases as major public-health problems. Even venereal disorders appeared to be in full retreat by the 1950s. Within another decade the situation began to change. The success of the new "miracle drugs"—such as penicillin—in curing venereal disorders led physicians to prescribe antibiotics for almost every form of infection, whether the cause was bacterial or viral. The result was the rapid creation of resistant strains of pathogenic organisms. The emergence of resistant forms of syphilis and gonorrhea coincided with the sexual revolution of the 1960s and contributed notably to a sharp rise in the incidence of venereal diseases. Since the 1970s new or newly diagnosed disorders such as genital herpes, Legionnaire's disease, Lyme disease, and acquired immunodeficiency syndrome (AIDS) have appeared, further confirming that infectious diseases remain a serious public-health threat.

Of the above disorders, AIDS best epitomizes the interrelationship between the social and biological factors in defining and dealing with disease. In the U.S., public fears aroused by the rising incidence of AIDS have led to the ostracizing of its victims, demands that physicians and health workers be tested, and pressure upon Congress to divert funds from other medical research to investigate AIDS. The public reaction to this new and fatal disorder has antecedents going far back in history. Bubonic plague, smallpox, yellow fever, and Asiatic cholera all evoked a similar response. In the nineteenth century, Asiatic cholera victims were not infrequently dumped from river boats and left to die on the banks. AIDS bears an additional burden because it is equated with sexual immorality, a venereal disorder compounded by its association with homosexuality. Since the eighteenth century any disease associated with sexual activity has been equated with immorality. As late as 1897 Howard Kelly of Johns Hopkins objected in the American Medical Association's annual meeting to a discussion of "the hygiene of the sexual act," on the grounds that the subject "was attended with filth."

AIDS also illustrates the perennial question of the rights of the individual versus those of society. When, as was true for most of history, epidemic diseases were strange, inexplicable occurrences, isolating or casting out the sick or effectively quarantining an infected area was taken for granted. Pesthouses in the colonial period were designed more to protect the town than to provide care for the sick. When inoculation for smallpox was introduced into the United States in 1721, the early laws forbade its use on the justifiable grounds that it would spread the disease. In the nineteenth century, laws requiring vaccination were bitterly opposed by many citizens, with antivaccination societies flourishing in a number of areas.

Public-health regulations by their nature are designed to restrict certain activities on the part of individuals. The 1867 annual report of the New York City Health Board declared: "The Health Department of a great commercial district which encounters no obstacles and meets no opposition, may safely be declared unworthy of public confidence." The vast majority of health regulations affect private property or place an extra cost on individuals or businesses; hence they have invariably led to protests. In New York and New Orleans, when health officials designated certain buildings as hospitals during yellow fever epidemics, mobs rioted and burned them to the ground. During an 1894 smallpox epidemic in Milwaukee, the Health Department sought to isolate cases and vaccinate all individuals in the infected areas. The result was rioting and the dismissal of the health officer. Health officers are government officials subject to political pressures; they must always seek a balance between what needs to be done and what can be done.

Limiting the right of individuals to practice medicine, requiring vaccinations, setting standards for food processing, and requiring physical examinations for food handlers, or establishing sanitary regulations with respect to housing or other property is an assertion that the community's health transcends individual or property rights. Laws requiring physicians to report contagious diseases have always raised strong objections from the medical profession, whether they involved reporting yellow fever in the eighteenth and nineteenth centuries or venereal disease in the twentieth century. When the New York City Health Department issued an order requiring the reporting of tuberculosis cases, the city's medical societies were outraged and appealed to the state legislature to restrict the powers of the Board of Health. In contrast, when on several occasions the New York City Board of Health ordered the evacuation of many blocks during the early yellow fever outbreaks, no one objected, nor were any protests made in 1907 when the New York City Health Department decided that in the interest of public welfare Mary Mallon (Typhoid Mary) should be kept on North Brother Island in the East River, where she remained until her death in 1938. Since medical experiments on the poor had long been taken for granted, neither physicians nor laymen, black or white, objected to the 1932 Tuskegee syphilis experiment, funded by the U.S. Public Health Service and designed to study the course of untreated syphilis in blacks.

The latter decades of the twentieth century have seen an increasing sensitivity to individual rights. The most obvious example is the deinstitutionalization of the mentally sick, who now constitute a large portion of the homeless. The question arises of whether individuals, the homeless in particular, have the right to refuse treatment for mental illness or contagious disorders. The presence in the community of cases of tuberculosis and other communicable diseases represents a threat both to the individual concerned and to the citizens at large. The main issue—as alcoholism, drug addiction, and smoking illustrate—is not whether the government should regulate individual conduct but the degree to which it does so.

As the United States moves toward revising its healthcare system, decisions must be made as to the role of public-health agencies. Maternal and child care for the lowest income groups and preventive medicine have traditionally been in the domain of public health. At present the vaccination of children is left to private medicine or state and local authorities, with the result that thousands of children remain unprotected. These responsibilities should, and probably will, be of major concern in a comprehensive healthcare system. In devising a new health system, will public-health departments expand their work in these areas or surrender them? Or should public health be incorporated into a comprehensive healthcare system? Whatever the case, serious thought must be given to formulating any major changes in the nation's healthcare system.

JOHN DUFFY (1995)

SEE ALSO: *Coercion; Environmental Health; Hazardous Wastes and Toxic Substances; Health and Disease: History of Concepts; Health Screening and Testing in the Public Health Context; Injury and Injury Control; Lifestyles and Public Health; Public Health Law; Sexual Behavior, Social Control of; Warfare: Public Health and War;* and other *Public Health* subentries

BIBLIOGRAPHY

Duffy, John. 1953. *Epidemics in Colonial America.* Baton Rouge: Louisiana State University Press.

Duffy, John. 1968–1974. *A History of Public Health in New York City.* 2 vols. New York: Russell Sage Foundation.

Duffy, John. 1971. "Social Impact of Disease in the Late Nineteenth Century." *Bulletin of the New York Academy of Medicine,* 2nd ser., 47(7): 797–810.

Duffy, John. 1979. "The American Medical Profession and Public Health: From Support to Ambivalence." *Bulletin of the History of Medicine* 53(1): 1–22.

Duffy, John. 1982. "The Physician as a Moral Force in American History." In *New Knowledge in the Biomedical Sciences: Some Moral Implications of Its Acquisition, Possession, and Use,* pp. 3–21, ed. William B. Bondeson, H. Tristram Engelhardt, Jr., Stuart F. Spicker, and Joseph M. White, Jr. Dordrecht, Netherlands: D. Reidel.

Duffy, John. 1990. *The Sanitarians: A History of American Public Health.* Urbana: University of Illinois Press.

Griscom, John H. 1845. *The Sanitary Condition of the Laboring Population of New York: With Suggestions for Its Improvement....* New York: Harper & Brothers.

Lubove, Roy, ed. 1966. *Social Welfare in Transition: Selected English Documents, 1834–1909.* Pittsburgh: University of Pittsburgh Press.

McCulloch, Samuel C., ed. 1950. *British Humanitarianism: Essays Honoring Frank J. Klingberg.* Philadelphia: Church Historical Society.

Meckel, Richard A. 1990. *"Save the Babies": American Public Health Reform and the Prevention of Infant Mortality, 1850–1929.* Baltimore: Johns Hopkins University Press.

Melosi, Martin V., ed. 1980. *Pollution and Reform in American Cities, 1870–1930.* Austin: University of Texas Press.

Rosen, George. 1974. *From Medical Police to Social Medicine: Essays on the History of Health Care,* pp. 120–158. New York: Science History Publications.

Rosen, George. 1975. *Preventive Medicine in the United States, 1900–1975: Trends and Interpretations.* New York: Science History Publications.

Rosenberg, Charles E. 1962. *The Cholera Years: The United States in 1832, 1849, and 1866.* Chicago: University of Chicago Press.

Shattuck, Lemuel; Banks, Nathaniel P., Jr.; and Abbott, Jehiel. 1948. *Report of the Sanitary Commission of Massachusetts, 1850.* Foreword by Charles-Edward Amory Winslow. Cambridge, MA: Harvard University Press.

Starr, Paul. 1982. *The Social Transformation of American Medicine: The Rise of a Sovereign Profession and the Making of a Vast Industry.* New York: Basic Books.

Williams, Ralph Chester. 1951. *The United States Public Health Service, 1798–1950.* Washington, D.C.: Commissioned Officers Association, U.S. Public Health Service.

Wing, Kenneth R. 1985. *The Law and the Public's Health,* 2nd edition. Ann Arbor, MI: Health Administration Press.

III. PHILOSOPHY

Public health is the prevention of disease and premature death through organized community effort. While this community effort is often led by government, many nongovernment and quasi-public institutions play key roles in promoting the public's health. Public health as an idea is one of the most influential of our time, and has been an important force in changing the shape of the modern world and enlarging government's scope, if not its size, since the middle of the nineteenth century. The general idea that government and communities can systematically discover, anticipate, and relieve disease and social distress through collective choice and organization is relatively new in human history. It involves the complex and related developments of collections and analysis of statistics, the understanding of variations in disease patterns in human societies (usually called epidemiology), and government of sufficient scale and capacity to exploit these findings.

Public health's focus on populations and communities is its most distinctive feature and the primary source of its philosophical interest. The community perspective produces a way of thinking about disease and early death and their prevention, that often runs counter to the categories and assumptions of much of modern bioethics and other disciplines as well. Public health as an organized practice views disease and premature death from the standpoint of the community and its capacity for self-examination, reorganization, and modification. The community perspective, far from neglecting the welfare of individuals, strengthens society's ability to discover the causes of disease in individuals, and society's capacity to devise flexible and rapid means for controlling disease and preventable death. Bioethics has been interested mainly in the intersection of the worlds of public health and the individual and his or her autonomy, and far less in public health as a method, seeing this as falling outside its sphere into the world of practice, and into the realm of contingency, experience, and practical action (Dewey).

Considerations for a Philosophy of Public Health

Public health as a method bears a strong resemblance to pragmatism, with its emphasis on probabilistic and fallibilistic ways of knowing, on exploiting experience and action, and on the centrality of knowing and acting in the context of communities, institutions, and practices (Bernstein; Rorty). While it is true that public health has many roots in utilitarianism (the English reformer E. H. Chadwick was once a literary secretary to Jeremy Bentham), public health came of age in the United States and Europe during the late nineteenth century and the early decades of the twentieth century, when the causes and methods for preventing many deadly diseases were discovered.

At the same time, philosophy and the social sciences began to revolt against the formalism of previous centuries (Dewey), and in both the United States and Europe, in philosophy and the social sciences, the search for fundamental truths gave way to empiricism and pragmatism, to a greater stress on the parallels between social science and philosophy, and to courses of action guided by both results and experience (Feffer; Anderson). After World War II there was in the United States a marked retreat to the earlier formalism with the rise of analytic philosophy and the return to social contract ideas, factors in the tendency of bioethics and philosophy to ignore the more pragmatic way of public health. This is not to say that public health as an organized practice needs no further philosophical elaboration or justification, or that it can ignore questions about the limits of

health policy in restricting liberty or the coherence of public health's use of the idea of the common good. It is simply to say that public health does not need first to be translated into utilitarianism or contract theory to become a social philosophy.

A philosophy of public health must accomplish four things. First, it must give a central place to the unique approach and method of public health, with its distinctive emphasis on community, and on the central role of the scientific method in formulating courses of action for social improvement. Second, a philosophy of public health must give priority to prevention, and must challenge and revise explanations for health problems with the community perspective, which is essential to effective prevention. Third, a philosophy of public health must set out and defend an adequate definition of the common good, taking into account public health's pursuit of the common well-being— measured in terms of rates of disease and early death—as the object of group or common action. Fourth, while the philosophy of public health must acknowledge the claims of individual autonomy and justify actions that limit liberty and autonomy, it must do so in a way that leaves the community perspective and the common good intact.

Health by Design: The Idea of Prevention

Prevention is the major focus in public health, and it involves as a minimum the imaginative redesign of social environments and communities to better promote health and safety, as well as the replacement of older models of the problems that need to be solved. A major part of the battle in public health, especially in applying public-health methods to modern problems of chronic disease, injury, and alcohol and other drug problems, is to redescribe these problems in terms of the community perspective, countering the individualism, so widely prevalent in much of philosophy and social science, that serves as a powerful obstacle to effective prevention.

Two recent examples make this point. In the case of alcohol, since the 1970s there has been a shift away from purely individual or agent-focused explanations for alcohol problems, based on the capacities, dispositions, and motivations of individuals who drink, and subsequently experience problems, factors like "loss of control" over drinking. With the public-health perspective, the focus is on the exposure of whole societies to alcohol, on the varying levels of total consumption among groups, and on such factors as price, hours of sale, and age limits in causing rates of problems. This approach does not seek so much to explain alcoholism (why some people drink addictively) but why rates of alcoholism rise or fall among communities, or over time (Moore and Gerstein).

In a similar way, highway safety since the early 1960s has witnessed a shift from individual capacities ("driver error," "driver negligence," "failure to yield the right-of-way," and factors beyond the control of agents, such as "acts of God") toward such factors as the exposure of drivers to highway hazards, miles driven annually, types of roads driven on, and the safe or unsafe character of the automobile. Exposure is a key variable in this redescription and often results in counterintuitive insights. For example, researchers have noted that "driver education programs" in the United States probably raise the level of death and injury because they expose more young people to the hazards of driving at an early age.

Public health has many similarities to modern applied systems theory and the policy sciences, with their stress on nonreductionism, on policy or systems knowledge rather than disciplinary knowledge, on systems-level (community-level) analysis, and on promoting change through novel interventions with high leverage potential, often deployed at places located far from the primary cause of the problems.

It is common to find public-health specialists, in their attempt to fashion new means of reducing disease, speaking of "agents," "hosts," and "environments," translating individual descriptions of problems into community descriptions. According to the interpretation of William Haddon, Jr., this framework's "agents" are "exchanges" of hazardous chemicals, ionizing sources, drugs, or kinetic energy, suffered by individual "hosts." The environment is the larger social and physical terrain of hazardous agents and hosts. The purpose of this strange language is to provoke new ways of thinking about old problems, and to give public-health designers free play in their imaginative search for new and innovative ways of reducing dangers, ways that are both effective and ultimately politically feasible. All three elements—hosts, agents, and environment—are potential targets for change and modification, with no priority given any one (Haddon).

This search for new societal arrangements is often expressed as the search for "conditions" that promote health or prevent disease, a point found in the Institute of Medicine's report *The Future of Public Health,* and its definition of the mission of public health: "the fulfillment of society's interest in assuring the conditions in which people can be healthy" (Institute of Medicine).

In one way or another, public health concerns collective choice. Public health is about how much alcohol is permitted in society (per capita consumption levels), about the frequency of highway crashes, about the number of drownings in a state or nation, and about the changes in environment, legislation, and public attitudes that will directly affect those statistics. This emphasis on social organization and social arrangements in public health does not reduce public health to a species of social causation. For example, to use the link between general consumption levels and occurrence rates of cirrhosis is not to say that society causes specific individuals to drink heavily or alcoholically. It is to say that because we have learned through scientific studies that society, through alcohol policy, can influence the levels and kinds of problems in society, it is accurate to say that society influences these problems, and can and should seek, within the context of democratic discussion and debate, to sharply reduce them.

Public Health and the Common Good

In the public-health view, the common good in public health means the good of individuals taken together as a group, as communities, or in terms of aggregate health and safety; this aggregate health, expressed as so many thousands of lives saved, is the object of organized government or community effort. The common good does not mean that each individual has the same or identical good in health and safety, or even the same interests. An individual with a genetic predisposition for colon cancer does not have the same interest in health and safety as another who lacks such genetic makeup. Yet both can be said to have a common interest in measures to promote health and safety and to reduce general risks to health and safety that all face, including risks from cancer. This is another way of saying that individuals can face threats to health and safety alone and in groups, using group efforts to reduce those threats.

The common good expressed in aggregate terms does not refer to a good that is separate from, and set over against, the good of the individuals who constitute a group at risk. It is rather that the good of the group is jointly consumed, producing a common benefit of thousands of lives saved and many thousands more who will avoid injury or disease. This common benefit of lives saved (and avoidance of disease) is taken as the expression of the common good and is the object or purpose of collective or common action.

For most public-health problems, the aggregate savings in lives is far smaller than the number of individuals at risk and whose liberty is to be limited. Put another way, and for most public-health problems, the group that benefits from protections is a much smaller subset of the group that is at risk. Thus, all who are at risk and whose liberty is limited by public-health legislation do not benefit; the benefit accrues for an unknown and unaccountable minority of the larger at-risk group. Because this good is expressed in the form of statistical lives, it is viewed as a savings for the community. Thus, it is not wrong to think of public-health measures as undertaken by a community for the sake of a common good, that is, the thousands whose lives will actually be saved. The slogan for public health should not be "The life you save may be your own," but rather, "The lives we save together may include your own."

Geoffrey Rose refers to the fact that communities benefit more from public health than individuals as the "prevention paradox" (Rose). The prevention paradox states that most modern public-health risks are sufficiently low and widely distributed—indeed, they often stem from mass behavior like driving automobiles, drinking, smoking—and that despite the fact that millions engage in the activity, savings in lives will measure only in the tens of thousands in any period.

Public Health and Autonomy

Some have used John Stuart Mill's famous point in *On Liberty* that only individuals can know their own good (Mill, 1975) to criticize many public-health measures—such as laws that require people to wear seat belts in automobiles and helmets when riding motorcycles, and requiring fluoride in the water supply—as paternalistic. These laws threaten the autonomy of individuals, and also threaten to usher in an era of vast, paternal, preventive government. Ronald Dworkin argues that "laws that promote the common interest insult no man ... while laws that constrain one man, on the grounds that he is incompetent to judge are profoundly insulting" (Dworkin, 1977, p. 263). Dworkin is here arguing that seat-belt laws or higher taxes on alcohol are not in the common interest, and are therefore insulting. Unlike Mill, he believes that the class of these kinds of laws and restrictions is actually quite small.

Those who support public-health restrictions on individual liberty, but who wish to avoid a strong paternalist position, can do so in basically two ways. They can argue that public-health measures are only mildly paternalistic. This is the "weak paternalism" thesis (Dworkin, 1972; Feinberg). In this view, public-health measures are not strongly intrusive, and they save thousands of lives. Most philosophers today seem to embrace this view. The second and more controversial view is that public-health interventions are not at all paternalistic (Beauchamp, 1988) because the good produced is not a private or individual good, but rather a common good produced by common action. In this view, the citizen sees himself or herself as living in a world in which common action, after public and democratic discussion, often promotes public health, and while individuals may potentially benefit from these actions, the community or the common good will assuredly benefit.

The differences between these two basically supportive perspectives on most public-health legislation cannot easily be reconciled, but their differences should not be exaggerated. Both sides agree that any restriction on liberty and autonomy needs justification. The only disagreement is over who is benefiting from this restriction and whether the good is private or common.

In the public-health perspective, the conception of autonomy is one of a basic autonomy, not an absolute autonomy. A basic autonomy can be overridden on evidence that restrictions are minimal, acceptable, and will produce a substantial savings in lives. The guardians of basic autonomy are the democratic process and elected officials, such as legislators or chief executives. This makes many nervous, yet the long history of the struggle for public-health legislation is, on balance, reassuring. Because most public-health legislation necessitates the burdens placed on large numbers of individuals, including powerful interests, to benefit small numbers of individuals, the political path to successful public-health legislation is strewn with political roadblocks that are likely powerful deterrents to overzealous public-health activists. This emphasis on relying on the processes of democratic communities reflects the pragmatism of public health as philosophy, and its interest in political theory. Also, Richard Flathman, a political theorist, notes that governments rarely promote the good of a single individual (Flathman).

Public Health and Social Justice

An enduring theme in public health is the attempt to persuade democratic bodies to legislate rules for economic production and distribution that are safer and more benign. Community public-health interests frequently oppose powerful, well-organized entities such as corporations and interest groups. Public health as an interest of the community often causes deep conflict among elected officials, who are also strongly enjoined to promote economic prosperity.

The struggle for the common health and safety is further complicated by the fact that the redistribution of the burdens of health and safety protection is on behalf of "statistical lives." Thus the struggle of public health has many resemblances to the struggle for social justice in society (Beauchamp, 1976) in that they both work on behalf of the less numerous and less powerful against the power of the market and its masters. The idea of social justice influences public health, for instance, as it battles the human immunodeficiency virus (HIV) epidemic, to modify its traditional methods of fighting epidemics (Bayer), using new weapons like confidentiality and privacy to fight societal discrimination and prejudice toward the victims of the widespread epidemic.

Democracy, Public Discussion, and Public Health

Much of public health is concerned with providing and/or regulating information and education. These activities typically encounter far fewer ethical conflicts than does legislation that limits individual liberty or property in order to promote health and safety. Yet even here the distinctive footprint of public health as a social practice can be detected. Progress against cigarette smoking has been made in the United States during the decades after World War II not so much through regulating or banning smoking as through communicating the discovery by public-health researchers of the links between smoking and disease. The subsequent public discussion and controversies surrounding a series of reports by U.S. surgeons general (and also by health officials in other nations) widely publicized the links between smoking and lung cancer and heart disease. The further publicity surrounding the role of tobacco in public policy and other related controversies produced a growing awareness of smoking as a social problem. This publicity, coupled with the ban on television advertising of cigarettes, produced sharp declines in smoking rates (Warner), in advance of more recent and controversial moves to ban smoking in public areas.

Here again, the unique emphasis in public health is to use the discovery of threats to the common health as part of the "hubbub" of democracy. Such controversy can be used to affect public opinion and discussion (including a growing social disapproval of smoking) as principal forces for promoting change in individual and mass behavior (Beauchamp, 1988). Public dialogue, in turn, moves public health into the new territories of promoting more information and speech and of countering advertising's role in limiting information.

Conclusion

The idea of public health as philosophy involves the elaboration of its core ideas of promoting fallibilistic and probabilistic ways of knowing, of learning from experience and action, of imaginatively proposing new designs to social environments to promote health and safety, and, above all, of focusing on prevention and community approaches everywhere possible. While public health proponents have been successful in ensuring that their methods are central to the study of health problems, working closely with scientists studying disease from an epidemiological perspective (and in the future from a more molecular and genetic perspective), they have been less successful in having public health's group approach accepted as philosophy. While it is true that public health is one of those "second languages" of community (Bellah et al.), it has yet to be widely appreciated among philosophers and social scientists as a distinctive method

with a distinctive philosophical perspective on common health problems, one that bears a strong resemblance to pragmatist perspectives on action and experience.

Finally, as health reform has increasingly dominated the public agenda in the United States, it is likely that public-health lessons will be more widely appreciated for two reasons: to prevent disease and reduce the burden and costs of illness, and, equally important, to remind the larger society that medicine and public health alike promote a common good, a lesson that is central to public health's distinguished history.

DAN E. BEAUCHAMP (1995)

SEE ALSO: *Autonomy; Coercion; Eugenics; Genetic Testing and Screening; Hazardous Wastes and Toxic Substances; Health and Disease: History of Concepts; Health Screening and Testing in the Public Health Context; Injury and Injury Control; Lifestyles and Public Health; Public Health Law; Sexual Behavior, Social Control of; Warfare: Public Health and War;* and other *Public Health* subentries

BIBLIOGRAPHY

Anderson, Charles W. 1990. *Pragmatic Liberalism.* Chicago: University of Chicago Press.

Bayer, Ronald. 1988. *Private Acts, Social Consequences: AIDS and the Politics of Public Health.* New Brunswick, NJ: Rutgers University Press.

Beauchamp, Dan E. 1976. "Public Health as Social Justice." *Inquiry* 13(1): 3–14.

Beauchamp, Dan E. 1988. *The Health of the Republic: Epidemics, Medicine, and Moralism as Challenges to Democracy.* Philadelphia: Temple University Press.

Bellah, Robert N.; Madsen, Richard; Sullivan, William M.; Swidler, Ann; and Tipton, Steven. 1985. *Habits of the Heart: Individualism and Commitment in American Life.* Berkeley: University of California Press.

Bernstein, Richard J. 1992. *The New Constellation: The Ethical-Political Horizons of Modernity/Postmodernity.* Cambridge, MA: MIT Press.

Dewey, John. 1929. *The Quest for Certainty: A Study of the Relation of Knowledge and Action.* New York: Minton, Balch.

Dworkin, Gerald. 1972. "Paternalism." *Monist* 56(1): 64–84.

Dworkin, Ronald M. 1977. *Taking Rights Seriously.* Cambridge, MA: Harvard University Press.

Feffer, Andrew. 1993. *The Chicago Pragmatists and American Progressivism.* Ithaca, NY: Cornell University Press.

Feinberg, Joel. 1973. *Social Philosophy.* Englewood Cliffs, NJ: Prentice-Hall.

Flathman, Richard E. 1966. *The Public Interest: An Essay Concerning the Normative Discourse of Politics.* New York: Wiley.

Gusfield, Joseph R. 1981. *The Culture of Public Problems: Drinking-Driving and the Symbolic Order.* Chicago: University of Chicago Press.

Haddon, William, Jr. 1973. "Energy Damage and the Ten Countermeasure Strategies." *Journal of Trauma* 13(4): 321–331.

Institute of Medicine. 1988. *The Future of Public Health.* Washington, D.C.: National Academy Press.

Mill, John Stuart. 1975 (1850). *On Liberty,* ed. David Spitz. New York: W. W. Norton.

Moore, Mark H., and Gerstein, Dean R. 1981. *Alcohol and Public Policy: Beyond the Shadow of Prohibition.* Washington, D.C.: National Academy Press.

Rorty, Richard. 1982. *Consequences of Pragmatism: Essays, 1972–1980.* Minneapolis: University of Minnesota Press.

Rose, Geoffrey. 1985. "Sick Individuals and Sick Populations." *International Journal of Epidemiology* 14(1): 32–38.

Selznick, Philip. 1992. *The Moral Commonwealth: Social Theory and the Promise of Community.* Berkeley: University of California Press.

Warner, Kenneth E. 1986. *Selling Smoke: Cigarette Advertising and Public Health.* Washington, D.C.: American Public Health Association.

IV. METHODS

Epidemiology is basic to modern public health. It provides, for example, the rational basis for health planning, the justification for allocating funding, and the basis for deciding whether or not to introduce or change preventive health policies. Finally, it plays a fundamental role in making decisions concerning optimal treatment regimens through its involvement in the clinical evaluation process.

Epidemiology is distinct from medical science in that epidemiology's focus is on population health, opposed to medicine's focus on the individual patient. While medicine seeks to heal the individual who, by virtue of being susceptible, becomes ill, epidemiology seeks to identify the underlying cause that results in illness among those who are susceptible. With an underlying cause identified, it becomes possible to intervene at the source of the chain of events that leads to illness among people who are susceptible. Removal of the cause can directly result in preventing those who are susceptible from being exposed to it in the first place and thereby from becoming ill.

Epidemiology focuses on large numbers of people comprising populations or communities. It is a quantitative (as opposed to a qualitative) science whose methods are heavily dependent on the application of biostatistical principles and on advances in biostatistical methods. As with other quantitative sciences, epidemiology requires the counting, classification, and analysis of sizable amounts of data. In order to derive meaning from large amounts of data, statistical techniques are used to produce various kinds of summaries. These techniques are known as biostatistics in the health and/or biological sciences.

Through the early 1940s, prior to the advent of antibiotics at the time of World War II, epidemiologists were occupied almost exclusively with controlling infectious diseases. Success resulted in better control of infectious diseases; improved living standards, especially in developed countries; and increased life expectancy of the population. Consequently, epidemiology expanded from its preoccupation with infectious diseases to include noninfectious diseases.

The notion that noninfectious and, by extension, chronic diseases can be prevented by eliminating their causes, analogous to the prevention of infectious diseases, is a relatively new concept. Hence, the modern role of epidemiology, from the public health perspective, is to identify appropriate interventions for consideration by policymakers for controlling disease at the source and thereby promoting health in the community.

The linking of epidemiology and biostatistics has become a hallmark of modern epidemiology in both its research and its practice areas of activity. Research in epidemiology tends to embrace activities of an experimental nature, while the practice domain tends to focus on disease surveillance and monitoring activities. Regardless of the domain, biostatistics provides the analytic tools used in epidemiology.

Scientific discovery in the laboratory should ultimately have practical application at the bedside. Results of epidemiologic investigations made on a population or on clearly defined subgroups of the population ought to benefit individuals. Because the results of population-based research are couched in terms of probabilities, the application of epidemiologic studies to the individual is not direct. Nevertheless, the identification of risk factor information in the absence of a biologically identified cause of a disease has been instrumental for prevention programs. Furthermore, physicians can apply probabilities in deciding therapeutic options.

The Scope of Epidemiologic Activity

Epidemiologic studies are necessary to provide both valid and reliable data not only concerning the distribution of diseases in populations, but also on the impact of social, economic, environmental, and other factors on the health of populations. In addition, epidemiologic data are often fundamental in making future projections of disease burden, crucial for planning purposes.

Concerning professional ethics, in the physician–patient "medical" relationship, the physician assumes a patient advocacy role; epidemiologists, on the other hand, assume a population/community advocacy role. Ethical guidelines that have been developed for medicine therefore have little relevance to epidemiology. Obligations assumed under these two different models must be explicit for trust to exist between professionals and the public.

Since the 1960s, epidemiology has undergone dramatic growth, paralleling to some extent the growth and development of computers. In North America, for example, the sex distribution and training of epidemiologists has changed over this period. Previously, epidemiologists were predominantly male, but today about half, especially those engaged in research, are women. Also, about half of today's epidemiologists were never trained as physicians.

The absolute numbers of epidemiologists have grown exponentially and the development of advanced computer technology has enabled epidemiologists to work with and share increasingly larger databases and to apply sophisticated multivariate statistical adjustment techniques via the use of computer software. But while technology has led to important advances in epidemiology, the complex issues of ensuring both integrity in science and ethical conduct among scientists have yet to be adequately addressed. There is increasing recognition of the need for guidelines to ensure professional accountability to the public in whose service epidemiologists work.

Classical epidemiology—as distinct from clinical evaluation—is primarily an observational science; it studies the events of daily life among the members of the various subgroups that comprise a community. Unlike controlled experiments, epidemiologic research measures events associated with populations whose lifestyles, work habits, and other characteristics have evolved outside the epidemiologist's control. Because uncontrollable and unknown risk factors can impact study outcomes radically, they must be accounted for if demonstrated contrasts, comparisons, and differences are attributed to these. Epidemiologic methods include various approaches for ensuring appropriate analysis of observational events. Professional epidemiologists are cognizant of the strengths, weaknesses, and limitations of the various methodologic options in light of the complexities associated with the conduct of uncontrolled experiments.

The closest epidemiology comes to the conduct of a controlled experiment is in the randomized controlled trial (RCT). However, RCTs can be justified only on the basis of substantial preexisting information concerning the intervention of interest (e.g., a particular therapy). Preexisting information usually is derived from the conduct of studies utilizing designs that are nonexperimental in nature (i.e., from the realm of natural experiments). Only where justification exists can human beings be subjected to random allocation in a clinical trial. Natural experiments in observational research include descriptive, ecological, retrospective case-control, and prospective cohort designs.

Diseases associated with aging, including cancer, diabetes, and cardiovascular diseases, have required greater attention. Because epidemiology provides the methodology for rational approaches to interventions, epidemiology is fundamental to disease prevention. Interventions based on epidemiological studies have taken the form of health promotion programs, such as campaigns for smoking cessation, no drinking and driving, and condom use in sexual intercourse. The onset in 1981 of the acquired immunodeficiency syndrome (AIDS) pandemic, however, reminded epidemiologists that infectious diseases are not necessarily a thing of the past.

With escalating healthcare costs in Canada, the United States, and elsewhere, epidemiology is playing a major role through providing the evaluative methodology for assessing cost-effective interventions for rational healthcare planning. Epidemiologists establish health goals by assessing health status indicators for a population; they identify target levels for reduced morbidity, disability, and mortality. These activities have implications for resource allocation which bear directly on the ethical principle of distributive justice. Indeed, numerous jurisdictions are attempting to identify those illnesses for which free health coverage should be provided by the "state" based on prevailing population values. Epidemiology assists in these determinations through expertise in survey methodology, health-status indicators, and disease classification.

From the foregoing, it is clear that epidemiology plays a major role in health-policy decisions, which involve, among others, substantial financial resources. "Health" is big business. Concerns arose during the 1980s about the possible influence of individuals and/or groups whose vested interests could bias outcome(s), motivated by financial profit and/or professional prestige. Conflicting-interest issues have been of concern not only in the interpretation of epidemiologic studies in favor of any one interest group's position but even in limiting or blocking the potential to conduct the best possible epidemiologic study for addressing a health concern.

The legal aspects—in terms of civil, administrative, and criminal law—are profound. With utilitarian goals in mind (i.e., doing the greatest good for the largest number of people), the courts usually have invoked the collective good over individual freedoms (e.g., in legislation concerning vaccination, quarantine, seat belts, and smoke-free public indoor environments in both Canada and the United States).

In general, governments prefer that professions regulate themselves. Professional organizations are expected to do what is necessary to minimize scientific misconduct and ensure professional etiquette among employers, sponsors, colleagues, and clients.

A Historic and Ongoing Concern: Privacy

Any epidemiologic investigation conducted under the auspices of an institution (e.g., a university, hospital, or government office) is likely to be subjected to ethical review by a committee. The committee usually comprises members of various disciplines as well as a lay representative.

Not only can ethics review committees examine the nature of the question to be addressed by the investigation, but they also may determine the appropriateness of the methods being proposed. Generally, however, the main focus tends to be on the possible harms versus benefits to those who will participate in the study; that is, with issues of privacy, informed consent, and confidentiality, and most important, that none of the procedures expected of the subjects/participants will cause them harm.

Scientific peer review concentrates on the aptness of the proposed scientific research methods, including the scientific relevance of the proposed research question, assessment of potential bias and confounding, adequacy of the proposed size of the study and associated statistical power, and recognized limitations impacting on the interpretation of the study. These two distinct but related areas of concern are seldom brought to the attention of a single expert other than the principal investigator, and perhaps also his or her research team. Without the support of both groups, the proposal usually cannot proceed into action.

Because the data epidemiologists rely on can be personally sensitive, governments have enacted privacy legislation to protect its citizens. Only with special permission from the custodians of these data bases can epidemiologists gain access—usually controlled—to the data banks essential to the conduct of health research. Some agencies also impose an oath of secrecy on the researcher.

One protection that researchers are expected to exercise (in their publication of results from access to health records in the public domain) is the anonymity of all persons studied. In addition, the identification of small areas or groups of people must be avoided also to ensure anonymity and thereby the protection of individual privacy. Individual or group stigmatization is to be avoided. Any infringement

of the public trust could have repercussions, including legal penalties to the researcher involved. Furthermore, the epidemiologic research enterprise could be placed in jeopardy by engendering a loss of trust in research by the very communities whose support (both financial and possibly also participatory) is needed for investigation purposes.

Professional training, in conjunction with well-publicized guidelines, is likely to minimize any risk of infringement. In addition, the epidemiologist has an obligation not only to respect the right to privacy of personal data, but to ensure that co-workers are equally vigilant. "Whistleblowing" also must be encouraged and those doing so must be protected from any form of reprisal. Most professional ethics guidelines/codes require that attention be drawn to the person who elects to perform contrary to normative standards of professional practice.

In 1991, European Community government officials developed a set of proposals concerning rights to privacy. Unfortunately, if enacted, these proposals could serve to make it virtually impossible to conduct epidemiologic research that depends on access to these data banks. The proposals ensure that personal information provided for one purpose cannot be used for another purpose without prior consent. Similar legislative proposals were mounted in the United States in the mid-1970s, but were defeated. Hence, epidemiologists and biostatisticians worldwide have a duty to remain vigilant of legislative proposals that might, directly or indirectly, adversely impact research for the public's health. They must be organized enough to provide input to such legislative proposals. Ultimately, it is the public-health interest that must prevail.

Current Issues

ETHICS GUIDELINES. The first stated need for guidelines on the ethical conduct of epidemiologists was printed in 1985. Despite considerable debate within the profession in North America, through 1987, little movement was made. It was at the International Epidemiological Association's (IEA) 1987 XIth Scientific Meeting in Helsinki, Finland, that the proposal to develop guidelines was adopted. By 1990, further discussion had advanced the thinking on this subject and a first draft of IEA guidelines was published.

A milestone conference on the subject of ethics in epidemiology had stimulated the discussion in 1989. The conference had been organized by the United States' Industrial Epidemiology Forum. The organizers had compiled a set of ethics guidelines and a commentary; these subsequently were published in the conference proceedings in

1991. Since then, the Council for International Organizations of Medical Sciences (CIOMS) has published *International Guidelines for Ethical Review of Epidemiological Studies* together with a compendium conference proceedings which contributed to the development of these guidelines. In addition, CIOMS published *International Ethical Guidelines for Biomedical Research Involving Human Subjects*. (CIOMS, 1991, 1993).

In November 1991, the American College of Epidemiology was accorded the leadership role among the North American epidemiology bodies to further ethics initiatives in this region of the world. Other groups of epidemiologists with specialty interests are contributing to this process (e.g., environmental epidemiologists).

The Industrial Epidemiology Forum's Guidelines, modeled on those developed some years earlier by the International Statistical Institute, are organized as follows:

I. *Obligations to the subjects of research*

to protect their welfare, ensuring no physical or mental harm through their participation;

to obtain their informed consent, ensuring the fullest possible understanding of any risks and benefits associated with participation;

to protect their privacy, ensuring no stigmatization resulting from information provided through their participation;

to maintain confidential information, ensuring the privacy of the participant.

II. *Obligations to society*

to avoid conflicting interests, recognizing that vested interests could bias research in ways that fail to serve the goal of seeking truth;

to avoid partiality by openly recognizing one's biases;

to widen the scope of epidemiology by teaching its methods to interested candidates;

to pursue responsibilities with due diligence;

to maintain public confidence in the profession by ensuring that both the strengths as well as the limitations of the profession are disclosed.

III. *Obligations to funders and employers*

to specify obligations, ensuring that the values and principles to which epidemiologists are expected to abide are clearly understood;

to protect privileged information, respecting the need of employers and providers of information to have reasonable time to assess the implications of research utilizing their data to their interests prior to disseminating the results from such a study.

IV. *Obligations to colleagues*

to report methods and results for wider peer review;

to confront unacceptable behavior and conditions, ensuring ethical conduct in support of the public interest;

to communicate ethical requirements, thereby ensuring accountability of the profession to the public.

Loreen Herwaldt (1993) has extended the guidelines set forth by the Industrial Epidemiology Forum by identifying principles having special relevance to hospital infection control officers and clinical practice.

While guidelines, commentaries, and case studies are recognized as essential to ethical conduct, they are insufficient. They must be taught, learned, discussed, challenged, and revised in light of case studies, if they are to affect behavior. Finally, mechanisms for dealing with allegations of breaches of conduct need to be established with remedies that serve to mitigate any wrongs.

CONFLICTING INTERESTS. Objectivity is required both on the part of the epidemiologist who is proposing a research project or submitting a manuscript for publication and on the part of the scientific peer review committee members. A conflict of interest arises when a reviewer has a vested interest in the subject under review that can either positively or negatively impact on the review decision. When a reviewer has a conflict of interest—whether at the scientific approval stage, the ethics review stage, or the publication stage—this must be declared and such reviewer's comments should be considered in this light in any final decision.

Reviewers have an obligation never to use, or to discuss with others, the ideas conveyed in a proposalmanuscript without full attribution to the person who proposed them. To do otherwise would misappropriate the intellectual property of another. In addition, if the reviewer is in a position to execute another's proposal, whether funded or not, such work should not proceed without the prior written permission of the person whose idea it was.

SCREENING FOR DISEASE AND HIV ANTIBODY. As a means of secondary prevention, early detection of disease through screening programs is well recognized. The AIDS pandemic, however, has presented new challenges well documented by Ronald Bayer and his colleagues, whose concern has been more with the stigmatization of individuals or groups. Access to test results by, for example, employers, landlords, or insurance companies has been of concern to infected people who fear job or housing loss and noninsurability. In research involving sexual practices, for example, the investigator requires special legal protection not only to render data inaccessible under subpoena but also to disclose such issues as the sexual abuse of children to child welfare authorities. Since valid responses must be obtained from persons volunteering for research if epidemiologic studies are to be useful, the right to privacy by the person being studied has to be secured in order for the person to participate honestly in the study.

In its initial years, testing for the human immunodeficiency virus (HIV) antibody was intended (together with self-exclusion) to secure the safety of the donated blood supply. Shortly thereafter, however, there were mandates for the testing of population subgroups believed to be at high risk of infection. It was postulated that the HIV antibody test could separate those truly positive from those truly negative, after which one could identify or physically separate the positives from the negatives. (The Cuban model, applied since early in the epidemic, has required that all persons found to be HIV-antibody positive be confined to a common residence and thus be barred from associating with persons who are not HIV-antibody positive.) Unfortunately, no test provides 100 percent sensitivity and specificity for HIV antibody or any other test. Furthermore, a "window period" exists between time of exposure and infection with HIV and the actual development of antibody. This window period can range from about three weeks to several months during which time the individual would test negative when in fact he or she could transmit the virus. This example demonstrates how epidemiology can assist in the rational presentation of facts, thus preventing misinterpretation by the media and/or lobby groups not fully informed of the scientific facts and how to interpret them.

NOTIFICATION. When special subgroups are identified for a study, the results of that study should be provided to the participants. Specifically, in occupational cohort studies, it is recommended in the United States that study participants be informed of any exposure to health risks uncovered through the study. The question that remains relates to the welfare of other workers who may be exposed to similar risk factors and who therefore could be at the same level of risk as those workers who were actually studied. If the cohort study that initially identified the risk was well-designed, it might be possible to extrapolate the research findings to other subgroups at risk in similar occupations, as well as to former employees. These latter two potentially at-risk groups are not currently included in the United States' National Institute for Occupational Safety and Health (NIOSH) guidelines.

Technologies continue to grow for determining individual susceptibility to illness that arises from workplace exposure to hazardous substances. If employers were privy to such information, they could exclude a job applicant on the grounds of wishing to protect the individual and at the same time to protect themselves from potential litigation. The tension arises between the obligation for full disclosure by the job applicant/worker on the one hand, and the obligation of the employer to provide a safe workplace. Some employers have argued that to render a workplace safe could be economically impractical. The controversy continues. Women, for example, face restrictions on employment in certain industries for fear by employers of liability—based on the existing body of knowledge about exposure to certain substances during pregnancy—if pregnancy should result in any abnormality at birth.

One mechanism for disseminating information involves community participation at all stages of a study, from hypothesis formulation through proposal development, review, conduct, analysis, write-up, and interpretation. In this way, community values are integrated into the research. Some occupational health studies have succeeded simply by establishing steering committees. These include not only scientists but also labor and management. Government involvement on a steering committee may also be appropriate.

WOMEN AND MINORITIES. The U.S. National Institutes of Health has stated that research has focused disproportionately on white male subjects (Dresser). Results from studies on males are generalized to other population subgroups (i.e., to women and racial minorities) when the results, in fact, may not be generalizable. Such inferences may not only be misleading for the health of women and minorities but also could create harm through the potentially inappropriate application of findings from studies on white males to other groups in the United States. Therefore, it has now been mandated in the United States that women and minorities be included in all research programs whenever possible (NIH/ADAMHA).

It is difficult to quarrel with the concerns and remedies noted above. However, epidemiology is undertaken in populations not only where the problem to be investigated arises but also in populations that are large enough to satisfy statistical considerations. That is, access to exposed populations is what motivates and justifies epidemiologists to design and conduct a study. Statistical power is a function of the prevalence of exposure in a population. If a large enough number of women or minorities is not exposed to a given agent (e.g., chemical or pathogen) of interest, then their inclusion in studies could be unproductive, consequently wasting resources. Clearly, the researcher must be cognizant of the limits to which inferences can be drawn from any study; it is up to those formulating policy, however, to provide the incentives needed to encourage and enable the address of researchable questions of relevance to groups other than white males.

Assessment to Date and Future Directions

Only recently have ethics guidelines been drafted for epidemiologists, whereas statisticians had broached the subject and developed guidelines in the 1980s. Physicians have been concerned with professional standards of practice in North America since the late nineteenth century. Although epidemiologists indeed may be entering the ethics discussion later than their counterparts, the relative recency of the profession must, of course, be considered. In their favor, epidemiologists are making efforts not only to develop ethics guidelines but also to integrate ethics into their teaching programs and into continuing professional education more generally. Ultimately, the expectation is that grass-roots involvement will maximize the likelihood of adherence to guidelines; the greater accountability of the profession to the public in whose interest epidemiology functions will be more assured.

Of growing concern are issues of self-interest and conflicting interests that sometimes take precedence over the public interest. Greater attention is being given to the consequences of research for destructive purposes through possible harm to the ecosystem and the advancement of militarism. Unless the professions are conversant with the principles of ethics, technological advances will continue to outstrip the ability of professions to respond; the professions' role will continue to be one manifesting a reactive as opposed to a proactive position.

COLIN L. SOSKOLNE (1995)
BIBLIOGRAPHY REVISED

SEE ALSO: *AIDS: Public Health Issues; Coercion; Conflict of Interest; Economic Concepts in Healthcare; Epidemics; Information Disclosure, Ethical Aspects of; Informed Consent; Minorities as Research Subjects; Occupational Safety and Health; Privacy and Confidentiality in Research; Profession and Professional Ethics; Public Policy and Bioethics; Research, Unethical; Technology; Whistleblowing;* and other *Public Health* subentries

BIBLIOGRAPHY

Bankowski, Z.; Bryant, John H.; and Last, John M. 1991. *Ethics and Epidemiology: International Guidelines. Proceedings of the XXVth CIOMS Conference, Geneva, Switzerland, 7–9 November, 1990.* Geneva: Council for International Organizations of Medical Sciences.

Bayer, Ronald. 1993. "The Ethics of Blinded HIV Surveillance Testing." *American Journal of Public Health* 83(4): 496–497.

Bayer, Ronald; Dubler, Nancy N.; and Landesman, Sheldon. 1993. "The Dual Epidemics of Tuberculosis and AIDS: Ethical and Policy Issues in Screening and Treatment." *American Journal of Public Health* 83(5): 649–654.

Bayer, Ronald, and Fairchild-Carrino, Amy. 1993. "AIDS and the Limits of Control: Public Health Orders, Quarantine, and Recalcitrant Behavior." *American Journal of Public Health* 83(10): 1471–1476.

Bayer, Ronald, and Toomey, Kathleen E. 1992. "HIV Prevention and the Two Faces of Partner Notification." *American Journal of Public Health* 82(8): 1158–1164.

Beauchamp, Tom L.; Cook, Ralph R.; Fayerweather, William E.; Raabe, Gerhard K.; Thar, William E.; Cowles, Sally R.; and Spivey, Gary H. 1991. "Ethical Guidelines for Epidemiologists." *Journal of Clinical Epidemiology* 44 (suppl. 1): 151S–169S.

Coughlin, Steven S., and Beauchamp, Tom L., eds. 1998. *Ethics and Epidemiology.* New York: Oxford University Press.

Council for International Organizations of Medical Sciences (CIOMS). 1991. *International Guidelines for Ethical Review of Epidemiological Studies.* Geneva: Author.

Council for International Organizations of Medical Sciences (CIOMS). 1993. *International Ethical Guidelines for Biomedical Research Involving Human Subjects.* Geneva: Author.

Darragh, Martina, and McCarrick, Pat Milmoe. 1998. "Public Health Ethics: Health by the Numbers." *Kennedy Institute of Ethics Journal* 8(3): 339–358.

Dresser, Rebecca. 1992. "Wanted: Single, White Male for Medical Research." *Hastings Center Report* 22(1): 24–29.

Elston, Robert C.; Olson, Jane M.; and Palmer, Lyle, eds. 2002. *Biostatistical Genetics and Genetic Epidemiology.* Hoboken, NJ: John Wiley & Sons.

Fawcett, Eric. 1993. "Working Group on Ethical Considerations in Science and Scholarship." *Accountability in Research* 3: 69–72.

Fayerweather, William E.; Higginson, John; and Beauchamp, Tom L., eds. 1991. "Industrial Epidemiology Forum's Conference on Ethics in Epidemiology." *Journal of Clinical Epidemiology* 44 (suppl.). Special issue.

Gordis, Leon, and Gold, Ellen. 1980. "Privacy, Confidentiality, and the Use of Medical Records in Research." *Science* 207(4427): 153–156.

Gordis, Leon; Gold, Ellen; and Seltser, Raymond. 1977. "Privacy Protection in Epidemiologic and Medical Research: A Challenge and a Responsibility." *American Journal of Epidemiology* 105(3): 163–168.

Herwaldt, Loreen A. 1993. "National Issues and Future Concerns." In *Prevention and Control of Nosocomial Infections,* 2nd edition, ed. Richard P. Wenzel. Baltimore: Williams & Wilkins.

Hoffman, Richard E. 1984. "The Use of Epidemiologic Data in the Courts." *American Journal of Epidemiology* 120(2): 190–202.

Jekel, James F.; Katz, David L.; and Elmore, Joann G. 2001. *Epidemiology, Biostatistics, and Preventive Medicine.* Philadelphia, PA: W B Saunders.

Jowell, Roger. 1986. "The Codification of Statistical Ethics." *Journal of Official Statistics* 2(3): 217–253.

Lachmann, Peter J. 1998. "Public Health and Bioethics." *Journal of Medicine and Philosophy* 23(3): 297–302.

Lappe, Marc. 1986. "Ethics and Public Health." In *Maxcy-Rosenau Public Health and Preventive Medicine,* 12th edition, pp. 1867–1877, ed. John M. Last. Norwalk, CT: Appleton-Century-Crofts.

Last, John M. 1987. "Ethical Issues in Public Health." In *Public Health and Human Ecology,* pp. 351–370. East Norwalk, CT: Appleton & Lange.

Last, John M. 1991. "Guidelines on Ethics for Epidemiologists." *International Journal of Epidemiology* 19(1): 226–229.

Lilienfeld, Abraham, and Lilienfeld, David E. 1982. "Epidemiology and the Public Health Movement: A Historical Perspective." *Journal of Public Health Policy* 3(2): 140–149.

Mann, Jonathan M. 1997. "Medicine and Public Health, Ethics and Human Rights." *Hastings Center Report* 27(3): 6–13.

National Institutes of Health. 1991. "NIH/ADAMHA Policy Concerning Inclusion of Women in Study Populations." *NIH Guide* 20(32): 1–3.

Oleske, Denise M., ed. 2001. *Epidemiology and the Delivery of Health Care Services: Methods and Applications.* New York: Kluwer Academic Publishers.

Rose, Geoffrey. 1985. "Sick Individuals and Sick Populations." *International Journal of Epidemiology* 14(1): 32–38.

Rose, Geoffrey. 1989. "High-Risk and Population Strategies of Prevention: Ethical Considerations." *Annals of Medicine* 21(6): 409–413.

Rosen, George. 1958. *A History of Public Health.* New York: MD Publications.

Rothman, Kenneth J. 1981. "The Rise and Fall of Epidemiology, 1950–2000 A.D." *New England Journal of Medicine* 304(10): 600–602.

Russel, Elizabeth, and Westrin, Claes-Goran. 1992. "Ethical Issues in Epidemiological Research." In *Medicine and Health: Workshop on Issues on the Harmonization of Protocols for Epidemiological Research in Europe, Florence, June 30 to July 2, 1991.* ed. Manuel Hallen and K. Vuylsteek. Commission of the European Communities, COMAC Epidemiology EUR 14596 EN.

Schulte, Paul A. 1991. "Ethical Issues in the Communication of Results." *Journal of Clinical Epidemiology* 44 (suppl. 1): 57S–61S.

Severson, Richard K.; Heuser, Linda; and Davis, Scott. 1988. "Recontacting Study Participants in Epidemiologic Research." *American Journal of Epidemiology* 127(6): 1318–1320.

Soskolne, Colin L. 1985. "Epidemiological Research, Interest Groups, and the Review Process." *Journal of Public Health Policy* 6(2): 173–184.

Soskolne, Colin L. 1986. "Scientific and Ethical Conflicts in Cancer Studies Involving Human Subjects." *Women and Health* 11(3–4): 197–215.

Soskolne, Colin L. 1989. "Epidemiology: Questions of Science, Ethics, Morality, and Law." *American Journal of Epidemiology* 129(1): 1–18.

Soskolne, Colin L. 1991. "Ethical Decision-Making in Epidemiology: The Case Study Approach." *Journal of Clinical Epidemiology* 44 (suppl. 1): 125S–130S.

Soskolne, Colin L. 1991–1992. "Rationalizing Professional Conduct: Ethics in Disease Control." *Public Health Reviews* 19(1–4): 311–321.

Soskolne, Colin L. 1992. "Reader Questions Extensive Funding for Women's Health." *New Epidemiology Monitor* 13(10): 7.

Soskolne, Colin L. 1993a. "Ethics and Policy Lost in Headline." *New Epidemiology Monitor* 14(1): 7.

Soskolne, Colin L. 1993b. "Introduction to Misconduct in Science and Scientific Duties." *Journal of Exposure Analysis and Environmental Epidemiology* 3 (suppl. 1): 245–252.

Soskolne, Colin L., ed. 1993c. *Journal of Exposure Analysis and Environmental Epidemiology* 3 (suppl. 1): 297–320. Special issue, "Questions from the Delegates and Answers by the Panelists Concerning 'Ethics and Law in Environmental Epidemiology.'"

Soskolne, Colin L., and Last, John M. 1993. "CMA Epidemiology Guidelines." *Journal of Occupational Medicine* 35(2): 97–98.

Stolley, Paul D. 1985. "Faith, Evidence, and the Epidemiologist." *Journal of Public Health Policy* 6(1): 37–42.

Susser, Mervyn. 1977. "Judgment and Causal Inference: Criteria in Epidemiologic Studies." *American Journal of Epidemiology* 105(1): 1–15.

Susser, Mervyn. 1985. "Epidemiology in the United States after World War II: The Evolution of Technique." *Epidemiologic Reviews* 7: 147–177.

Susser, Mervyn; Stein, Zena; and Kline, Jennie. 1978. "Ethics in Epidemiology." *Annals of the American Academy of Political and Social Science* 437: 128–141.

Teich, Albert H., and Frankel, Mark S. 1992. *Good Science and Responsible Scientists: Meeting the Challenge of Fraud and Misconduct in Science.* Washington, D.C.: American Association for the Advancement of Science.

Terris, Milton. 1979. "The Epidemiologic Tradition: The Wade Hampton Frost Lecture." *Public Health Reports* 94(3): 203–209.

Terris, Milton. 1987. "Epidemiology and the Public Health Movement." *Journal of Public Health Policy* 8(3): 315–329.

Vineis, Paolo, and Soskolne, Colin L. 1993. "Cancer Risk Assessment and Management: An Ethical Perspective." *Journal of Occupational Medicine* 35(9): 902–908.

Weed, Douglas L. 1997. "Underdetermination and Incommensurability in Contemporary Epidemiology." *Kennedy Institute of Ethics Journal* 7(2): 107–127.

Weed, Douglas L., and Trock, Bruce. 1988. "Interactions and Public Health Decisions." *Journal of Clinical Epidemiology* 41(2): 207–209.

Westrin, Claes-Goran. 1993. "Ethical, Legal, and Political Problems Affecting Epidemiology in European Countries." *IRB* 15(3): 6–8.

Westrin, Claes-Goran; Nilstun, Tore; Smedby, Bjorn; and Haglund, Bengt. 1992. "Epidemiology and Moral Philosophy." *Journal of Medical Ethics* 18(4): 193–196.

PUBLIC HEALTH LAW

• • •

I. The Law of Public Health

II. Legal Moralism and Public Health

I. THE LAW OF PUBLIC HEALTH

Public health law is used to regulate activities and facilities to protect human health and establish institutions and programs that advance health and well-being. Its development has long been informed by the shared political and philosophical beliefs that provide a reason for government generally: to advance the common good and protect people's health, safety, and welfare. Public health law has changed over the years to reflect technological, scientific, and medical advances and respond to new threats and hazards. Societal and legal developments continue to create new ethical problems and challenges.

Historical Background

In the eighteenth and nineteenth centuries public health was largely a matter of protecting the public against communicable diseases and preventing epidemics. Concerns about food and waste sanitation, health and safety in the workplace, and other issues arose late in the nineteenth century and the early twentieth century. As a result of recurring epidemics of cholera, yellow fever, smallpox, typhus, typhoid, dysentery, diphtheria, and scarlet fever, states and municipalities created boards of health to protect people against disease (Rosen).

Because little was known about the causes of disease, quarantine—the separation of persons who could infect others—became, in the absence of immunization and other preventive measures, the primary mode of control. As the understanding of the bacterial cause and spread of disease grew, other preventive measures followed, including the control of food handlers to prevent typhoid carriers from working in food establishments, the prevention of persons with tuberculosis from working as teachers or nursemaids, and the prohibition of industrial work in the home to prevent the dissemination of tuberculosis through home-made clothing. Other regulations forbade spitting in public places and carrying soiled laundry on public conveyances such as the subway system in New York (Rosen).

The basis for early state and local legislation was the state's police power to protect people's safety, health, and welfare. The police power constitutes the reason for the establishment of state governments: to advance the public good and protect people from one another. This is a broad and inherent power because it is part of the social contract (Bentham, 1969a, 1969b).

The police power was relied on long before public health became a concern. For example, in 1837 the courts relied on police power to support a state law authorizing the construction of a second bridge across the Charles River that interfered with an alleged earlier franchise held by the owners of an old bridge (*Proprietors of Charles River Bridge v. Proprietors of Warren Bridge*). In 1851 the courts relied on police power to uphold state legislation limiting an owner's use of his property in Boston Harbor because that use would interfere with navigation (*Commonwealth v. Alger*). In 1876 the police power provided the basis for a state law to regulate grain elevator charges (*Munn v. Illinois*).

The broad thrust of police power to advance and protect community interests was developed further in early public health cases that upheld state regulation of retail liquor sales over the objection that that regulation interfered with the use of private property (*Crowley v. Christiansen*). In those early cases the claims of public interest under the police power overcame the assertion of private property interests protected under constitutional due process. Later cases involving the discriminatory regulation of laundries in wood-frame buildings (*Yick Wo v. Hopkins*) and the establishment of a quarantine district in a way that included and burdened a larger number of Chinese immigrants (*Jew Ho v. Williamson*) firmly applied the police power to protect public health, safety, and morals while upholding individual interests protected by the Fourteenth Amendment of the U.S. Constitution.

In the twentieth century public health law in the United States increasingly dealt with the resolution of tensions between the exercise of state police power and the protection of personal liberties through the due process clause of the Fourteenth Amendment and other parts of the Bill of Rights. In the landmark case *Jacobson v. Massachusetts* in 1905 the U.S. Supreme Court upheld the city of Cambridge and the state of Massachusetts in exercising the police power to compel Jacobson to undergo a smallpox vaccination not for his own protection but to prevent him from infecting others if he became infected in a smallpox epidemic. Jacobson argued that the law denied him due process and the equal protection of the law. The Court upheld the state's exercise of the police power by applying a standard of reasonableness that followed the utilitarian principle of the greatest protection for society at the least cost to the individual. Thus, the state's chosen method of control (vaccination) was adopted to achieve the end sought (an end to the epidemic) and was seen by the Court as a reasonable price to be paid by the individual in those circumstances (Bentham, 1969b).

In cases in which the exercise of police power allegedly violated property rights other analytic approaches were applied. In some of those cases reliance on constitutional principles was not articulated because the common law had long dealt with inappropriate uses of private property. For example, it is a well-established legal principle that citizens have a right to enjoin or abate a nuisance: A condition that is unwholesome or filthy and adversely affects neighboring property owners. The ancient principle of *sic utere tuo ut alienum non laedas* ("use your property so as not to hurt another") often was applied in private disputes and cited in constitutional decisions. States and municipalities began to designate such conditions as abatable nuisances, and public authorities could prohibit or abate them. Some conditions that were considered nuisances were referred to in *Commonwealth v. Alger* (1851), including warehouses for the storage of gunpowder near habitations or highways, wooden buildings of excessive height in populous neighborhoods and similar structures not covered with incombustible materials, buildings used as hospitals for contagious diseases, the use of buildings to carry on noxious or offensive trades, and the raising of a dam that caused stagnant waters emitting dangerous fumes to spread over meadows near inhabited villages.

A contemporary listing would include garbage dumps, sites for the disposal of hazardous wastes, paint spray plants, and fat-rendering plants. In *Mugler v. Kansas* (1887) the defendant was enjoined from using his property to operate a brewery, a proscribed use. The equitable rule of *sic utere* also calls for a balancing of equities, that is, a balancing of the benefit denied to the defendant against the benefit derived by the community in stopping undesirable uses of the property.

Public Health Law and the Eugenics Movement

The father of eugenics was Sir Francis Galton (1822–1911), a cousin of Charles Darwin who self-identified as a philosopher of natural science. One of his works was titled "Genius, an Inquiry into Its Laws and Consequences" (Pickens). Galton's work reflected the worst aspects of nineteenth-century Enlightenment thought, including the fundamental

error that acquired characteristics can be transmitted by heredity. Eugenicists believed that the human race could be improved and social ills eliminated through selective procreation to eliminate defective germplasm from the national genetic germ pool.

Between 1900 and 1970 some 100 statutes based on eugenic theory were adopted by state legislatures to improve the nation through selective mating and to eradicate disease, crime, poverty, and other social ills by preventing the reproduction of socially deviant individuals. In the late nineteenth century and early twentieth century people worried about the future health of a growing and diverse population and held Malthusian fears about the adverse impact of overpopulation. That message was carried in the *American Journal of Eugenics,* which was published in July 1907 until 1910, and by two other journals, both publications of the American Eugenics Society, namely *Eugenics: A Journal of Race Betterment* from October 1929 to February 1931 and *Eugenical News* published from January 1916, continuing publication until December 1953 (Lombardo). The eugenics movement coincided with the development of the twentieth-century interest in broader public health protection, but it contributed to racial divisions and undermined the scientifically sound genetic research of the twentieth century.

The American eugenics movement was championed by the Eugenics Record Office of Cold Spring Harbor, Long Island, which collaborated with other groups that objected to the large numbers of immigrants from central and eastern Europe between 1880 and 1924. It supported the Immigrant Restriction (Johnson-Reed) Act of 1924 (Chase), which restricted immigration by Russian and Polish Jews, Italians, and other central Europeans, who were said to have a greater number of inborn undesirable qualities, including insanity, feeblemindedness, dependency, criminal behavior, deformities, and tuberculosis, than did the older Nordic and Anglo-Saxon stock. The act imposed severe immigration quotas to maintain the national racial and ethnic balance. A misguided effort of the Progressive Era, it applied so-called scientific approaches to manage the ills of society. Endorsing a form of social Darwinism, it extolled the Anglo-Saxon heritage and encouraged prejudice against inferior races and persons of color because the unlimited immigration of those groups would dilute the native stock with defective germplasm. Its "quarantine mentality" sought to separate the healthy from the ill or abnormal (Markel, Kühl).

The work of Charles B. Davenport and the Eugenics Record Office was supported by prominent citizens and some members of Congress who relied on pseudo-scientific charts, tables, and graphs illustrating the genetic inferiority of those immigrants. The organization favored the sterilization of hereditary paupers, criminals, the feebleminded, tuberculars, the shiftless, and ne'er-do-wells (Chase). At the turn of the century states began enacting involuntary sterilization laws to deal with idiots and imbecile children, hereditary criminals, and other genetically defective persons as well as sexual perverts, drug fiends, drunkards, epileptics, and others considered ill or degenerate. By 1931 about thirty states had enacted compulsory sterilization laws that covered mostly the "insane" and "feebleminded" and frequently "epileptics." Those laws were applied in the sentencing process and in institutional treatment and covered recent immigrants and others who were functionally illiterate or did poorly on intelligence tests. Although most of those laws were not enforced in all the states, by January 1935 some 20,000 people in the United States had been sterilized involuntarily, mostly in California. The California law was not repealed until 1979 (Hubbard and Wald). Nineteen states had laws that permitted the sterilization of mentally retarded persons without a clear definition of that category (Reilly).

In 1927 Justice Oliver Wendel Holmes wrote the opinion in *Buck v. Bell*, a case that has influenced law and genetics for many years. The opinion concluded with the assertion, "Three generations of imbeciles are enough." The case involved a law in Massachusetts that authorized the involuntary sterilization of feebleminded persons in state institutions. Carrie Buck was ordered sterilized because she was the feebleminded daughter of a feebleminded mother and had given birth in the institution to a feebleminded daughter. The sentence was carried out shortly after the decision in 1927. Subsequent investigation seemed to show that none of the three generations of women involved in the case were feebleminded (Gaylord). Never overruled, the decision was discredited by *Skinner v. Oklahoma*, which invalidated a law that provided for the sterilization of repeat offenders convicted of crimes of "moral turpitude."

The history of the eugenics movement was recalled by opponents of the U.S. Human Genome Project who compared it with the outrages of the Nazi holocaust, which used racist theories to justify compulsory sterilization and the murder of six million persons who were viewed as subhuman (Caplan). Citing *Buck v. Bell*, American opponents of the Human Genome Project also relied on other instances of involuntary sterilization, such as the cases that arose out of abuses in the U.S. sickle cell anemia program in the 1970s. Another instance of misguided medicine cited in the context of racist eugenics is the so-called Tuskegee Institute Study, which involved the intentional failure for many years to treat African Americans in Macon County, Alabama, who were suffering from syphilis (Duster; King; Hubbard and Wald).

Scholarly writings opposing the Human Genome Project and other genetic research do not assert that those projects attempt to advance eugenic principles but insist that in a racist society genetic investigation will exacerbate existing racial divisions and that even if such projects yield medically useful results, they will be used to benefit the dominant group rather than groups that have been discriminated against. In the course of mapping and sequencing the human genome, correlations will emerge between genetic characteristics and race or ethnicity that will be misused. Those writers also believe that genetic studies overemphasize genetic factors in human development and downplay the importance of environmental influences.

The only beneficial aspect of eugenics was personified by Margaret Sanger. Born in 1879, Sanger became a feminist activist as well as a socialist. After 1911 she pursued her interest in sex education and women's health. Sanger believed that frequent and unwanted pregnancies, sometimes including miscarriages and self-induced abortion, burdened women's lives, personal development, and freedom. Some of her books on female sexuality, social hygiene, and venereal disease were seized by postal authorities as obscene, and her career frequently was interrupted by arrests and imprisonment on obscenity charges. Later, focusing on the development of family-planning and birth control clinics, she argued that prenatal care and the limitation of pregnancies would result in healthier babies as well as healthier and more fulfilled women.

The idea that sex need not lead to conception and that women freed of the burdens of unwanted pregnancies could enjoy sex ran afoul of the 1873 federal Comstock law and state obscenity laws. In 1914 her books on birth control and contraception led to her indictment for violating postal obscenity laws. Sanger later continued her efforts at birth control advocacy by founding the American Birth Control League and connected those efforts with a part of the nativist U.S. eugenics movement that sought birth control for persons with mental or physical genetically transmitted defects, seeking the forced sterilization of mentally incompetent persons. Although Sanger did not advocate positive eugenics or limitations on population growth based on race, ethnicity, or class, her reputation was damaged by the growing development of race-based eugenics.

In 1936 the ruling by the U.S. Court of Appeals in *U.S. v. One Package of Japanese Pessaries* that physicians were exempted from the ban on the importation of birth control materials supported Sanger's efforts. Though ahead of her time, she never gained public funding for birth control as a public health measure. In 1939 the American Birth Control League and Sanger's Birth Control Clinical Research Bureau became the Birth Control Federation of America, which in 1942 became the Planned Parenthood Federation of America. The words *birth control* were considered too radical to be included in the name of the organization.

In 1952 Sanger and others founded the International Planned Parenthood Federation (IPPF) to address global overpopulation. She believed that reducing the number of unwanted children would make it easier to allocate economic and social resources. Sanger worked with the American and British medical establishments to develop an effective and inexpensive female contraceptive. That was accomplished in the 1950s when Gregory Pincus developed an effective anovulant, the birth control pill; Sanger had helped secure funding for this effort. Sanger died in 1966, soon after the Supreme Court's 1965 decision in *Griswold v. Connecticut,* which allowed the use of birth control information by unmarried and married couples.

Although the legislation it spawned remained on the books, by the 1930s and 1940s the eugenics movement no longer fit the economic and political changes in society and in scientific attitudes. The simplistic view that heredity would produce copies of earlier generations and their acquired characteristics unaffected by nurture and environment was abandoned. Moreover, the search for the perfect contraceptive was successful at a time when the pressures that created the eugenics movement had abated. At the beginning of the 1940s birth control research and eugenics in both Britain and in America gave way to the pressing concerns of World War II and the needs of the Third World (Soloway).

Expansion of Public Health Law

With the entry of the federal government into public health in the twentieth century, public health law expanded and there were significant changes in the exercise of governmental powers and the tasks assigned to public health law. The federal government has no plenary police powers (it lacks the power to provide for health, safety, and welfare), yet it plays a major role in the creation and execution of public health policies through the exercise of the powers delegated to it by the states under Article I of the U.S. Constitution. Those powers include the power to regulate interstate and foreign commerce and to tax and spend for the general welfare. The Food, Drug, and Cosmetic Act enacted in 1938 demonstrates the use of the federal commerce power in the regulation of public health. Congress not only regulates trade in and the interstate transport of food, drugs, and cosmetics but also authorizes the U.S. Food and Drug Administration (FDA) to set standards for and monitor the quality of that merchandise. Through the FDA the federal government also regulates the safety and efficacy of drugs and pharmaceuticals with a detailed mechanism of administrative controls, including the power to adopt standards to inspect pharmacies and supervise food and drug regulation. Interstate commerce regulation also includes the control of harmful emissions from automobile engines, showing that interstate commerce controls affecting public health may be designated environmental controls even though their primary purpose is the advancement of public health. To exercise the commerce power the federal government usually acts directly through a federal agency such as the FDA or the U.S. Environmental Protection Agency (EPA).

Taxing and spending power represents a less direct exercise of federal powers. An early example of the use of that power in public health was the 1944 Hill Burton Hospital Construction Program, under which the federal government grants funds to a state or municipality for hospital construction programs and nonprofit community hospitals (Grad, 1990). As a condition of the grant the state or local government must comply with federal regulations, including facility and personnel requirements, and provide free services for indigent persons. Another ongoing grant-in-aid program is the program under Subchapter II of the Federal Water Pollution Control Act Amendments of 1972 for the construction of public waste-treatment works by states and municipalities. This program has helped clean up waterways and develop improved sewers in cities. Grant-in-aid programs have been used widely to support infrastructure developments to advance public health. Under those programs the federal government requires states to pass regulations and carry out construction, enforcement, and compliance activities to meet the conditions of a grant.

Federal public health activities under the commerce power are analogous to state exercise of the police power in that they command and control certain activities. Like exercises of state police power, they must meet the constitutional requirements of due process and equal protection. Their philosophical basis is largely utilitarian, seeking a balance between the public interest and the protection of private entrepreneurial interests in development and property. Federal public health activities under the taxing and spending power may advance similar concerns, but to the extent that they involve the distribution of federal funds, other concerns, such as those relating to fairness in distribution, also play a role. John Rawls argues that if the principle of equal liberty is met, as well as that of equality of opportunity, the difference principle permits inequalities in the distribution of social and economic goods if those inequalities will benefit everyone, especially the least advantaged (Rawls). Distribution formulas for the sharing of federal funds by responding to areas with greater needs satisfy that formulation.

Relationship between State and Federal Public Health Law

The relationship between state and federal public health law is not a simple hierarchical one. Although under Article VI, Section 2, of the U.S. Constitution federal law is the supreme law of the land, in cases of conflict between federal and state law, federal law trumps state law only if Congress has the jurisdiction to pass such a law. In the case of public health law, federal jurisdiction generally is defined by the interstate commerce power. In the past the federal commerce power generally was viewed as broad enough to cover virtually any law Congress decided to pass. However, a series of close decisions by the Supreme Court has limited congressional power to subjects that are clearly related to interstate commerce. The Court has invalidated laws involving gun control and violence against women. Other decisions have addressed the issue of whether the federal exercise of regulatory power was sufficiently related to the area of interstate commerce. This stringent limitation on federal power and correlative limitations on state judicial power were enhanced by decisions interpreting the reach of states' Eleventh Amendment immunity from lawsuits. In another effort to increase state powers the Court has held that although an activity may be federally regulated, Congress lacks the power to subject nonconsenting states to private suits for damages and other relief in state courts. Thus, under the Americans with Disabilities Act the Court held that the Eleventh Amendment limits private actions by state employees for damages under the federal law. The Court also has held that the Constitution does not permit private lawsuits to recover damages from nonconsenting states for the violation of federal rights even when the suits are brought in state courts (*Alden v. Maine*). Those cases indicate that the subject matter of public health does not change the Court's rules concerning the protection of states' rights.

Major Public Health Approaches

There are two major approaches to the protection of public health. The first and older one uses regulatory enforcement programs that range from epidemiological controls and protection against unwholesome living conditions to the identification and removal of poisons in the environment. Included are protection of the food and water supplies and protection against hazards and poisons in the workplace. Programs to protect the public against hazards from the generation of nuclear energy and efforts to prevent the destruction of the stratospheric ozone layer by the dissemination of hydrofluorocarbons and other destructive gases are included in this area.

Although public health regulation and enforcement have grown enormously, that expansion has been exceeded by the second area of public health protection: public health services. The government provides services to advance the health of the public, including the provision of well-baby clinics, family-planning clinics, community mental health programs, and government-sponsored research institutions that provide special services.

Both regulatory enforcement programs and service programs must meet constitutional requirements. In general, equal protection under the Fourteenth Amendment specifies that the same degree of fairness apply in the provisions of benefits and services as applies in the imposition of obligations and duties. As a result government agencies carefully consider allocation factors in the distribution of services to determine how priorities should be set between public health and other needs and determine the priority of certain health-related needs. Finally, institutions often must determine specific allocations among individuals with different health and other needs (Rawls). Political considerations such as pressure from physicians and other service providers or from consumers also have an effect on the process.

In addition to direct service programs, Medicare and Medicaid, both of which were established in 1965, pay or reimburse medical costs. Medicare is an offshoot of Social Security. Focused on the reimbursement of fees for service, it subsidizes the healthcare costs of Social Security recipients, primarily the disabled and persons age sixty-five and older. Initially paid for by employer and employee contributions, Medicare became an entitlement program because employees had secured contractual rights to social insurance through their contributions. Medicaid is a federal grant-in-aid program financed by federal and state contributions to provide medical care for "medically indigent" persons whose family income level is so low that they cannot pay for their own medical care. Both Medicare and Medicaid are managed federally by the Health Care Financing Administration.

Government involvement is dominant in these programs; because the government reimburses medical providers for services rendered, it is directly involved in regulating the quality of those services. Medicaid may be viewed as a welfare program that takes the place of earlier provision of care for the poor through charitable or public institutions. Medicare, based on contractual entitlements, was created with the expectation that employees would die soon after reaching the retirement age of sixty-five. However, the increasing longevity of the covered population and the substantial increase in the cost of health services have led to persistent political criticism. Such programs are not novel. State financing of healthcare costs began in Germany in the late nineteenth century, and many European nations, including Great Britain, the Netherlands, the Scandinavian countries, and Austria, have continued to provide healthcare even though their gross national products and industrial bases are considerably smaller than those of the United States.

In the United States there is no right to healthcare or to treatment under federal or state law except insofar as specific reimbursement provisions have been provided by law. There is no constitutional entitlement to healthcare. However, a number of writers have suggested an egalitarian right to healthcare, claiming that everyone who has an equal need for healthcare services or resources must have equal access to them. This sometimes has been asserted as a corollary of a general egalitarian welfare right that requires the distribution of resources to assure that everyone's lifetime net welfare is equal (Buchanan; Veatch). This expansion of welfare rights, including the right to healthcare, last failed to become part of American law during the second term of the Clinton adminstration when the universal health insurance proposal by the committee headed by First Lady Hillary Clinton was not adopted. However, in June of 2003, new efforts were underway to include "universal" health insurance as part of the law had not as of 1994 become part of American law. Any such proposal would be rejected by those who hold the so-called libertarian point of view, which regards as inappropriate all social ordering that does not rely on the allocation of goods and services through market processes (Buchanan; Nozick).

It is difficult to formulate a single philosophical basis for federal involvement in the multiplicity of public health programs. Twentieth-century federal public health programs were based on detailed programmatic legislation that not only established new rules of law but also created new governmental structures to manage the new areas of governmental control (Grad, 1985). Those new structures are exemplified by the FDA, the EPA, and agencies that manage social insurance programs such as Medicare and Medicaid. In every instance the agency is given broad rule-making powers that must be exercised in accordance with the general purposes of the statute. In statutes intended to protect society against toxic substances and hazardous waste the general purpose may be "to protect health and the environment."

In regard to such legislative instructions one might refer to the principle *sic utere* or to the broader principle of preventing harm to others, but that would not be historically or analytically correct because those principles were intended to govern persons in their private relationships or their relationships within a relatively small community. Modern public health programs, in contrast, address broader national or even global problems. Moreover, the emphasis of earlier approaches was generally on preventing harm, whereas modern programmatic legislation often seeks to advance public benefits. The utilitarian rationale of protecting the health interests of the public at the lowest possible cost to the individual seems the most appropriate. The purposes of public health programs are legislatively defined. Legislation is political and therefore majoritarian in its nature, unlike the judicially established bases for protection under common law articulated by judges and intended primarily to resolve individual disputes.

Public Health and AIDS

The emergence of AIDS in the 1980s demonstrated the tension between the protection of individual rights and the enforcement of broadly applicable police-power measures to protect public health. Another significant challenge was the threat of a multidrug-resistant form of tuberculosis in the late 1980s and 1990s. Communicable diseases generally are reportable under health codes, and those reports to a health department are normally protective of the patient's privacy. Special confidentiality protections are particularly applicable to reports of sexually transmitted diseases and, in earlier times, tuberculosis. Special privacy protections originated in the protection of patients against stigma because a report of certain diseases was regarded as a social disgrace. The knowledge that the report of a communicable disease might result in stigmatization and discrimination was undesirable from the point of view of public health because patients were less likely to seek treatment if their confidentiality was breached.

When AIDS emerged in 1981, most other communicable diseases no longer represented major public health problems, and the history of reports to health departments and the possibility of contact investigations to trace potentially exposed persons, particularly in the area of sexually transmitted diseases, had been forgotten. Constitutional protection of privacy as a part of due process had developed earlier in the context of the right of a pregnant woman to choose to terminate her pregnancy. Privacy protections and related protections of personal autonomy are asserted to protect against the disclosure of human immunodeficiency virus (HIV) status even though AIDS is now a reportable disease in all the states.

Because transmission of HIV was associated first with homosexual intercourse and later with intravenous drug use, there were compelling reasons to protect the identity of persons who were HIV-positive. Privacy protections also interfered with giving notice of exposure and risk to persons who had been exposed because that information, unless disclosed voluntarily, inevitably would breach the patient's confidentiality. Patient privacy continued to have broad legal protection, and the tension between the protection of individual privacy and the need for public information in order to protect the public health is a continuing one, even though there is today in 2003 both greater tolerance of what had earlier been considered deviant sexual behavior. Many more persons freely acknowledge their sexual preferences and "come out of the closet." At the same time, the medical and public view of HIV/AIDS has changed in view of the decline in HIV morbidity and mortality during the late 1990s, attributable to combination antiretroviral therapy. This decline appears to have ended, and in 2003 new outbreaks of primary and secondary syphilis among men who have sex with men and increases in newly diagnosed human immunodeficiency virus (HIV) infections among such men and among heterosexuals have been increasing. As a result there are new concerns that HIV incidence may be increasing. Earlier programs focused on prevention efforts targeted at persons at risk for becoming infected with HIV and on programs to reduce sexual and drug using risk behavior. More recent efforts are focused in 2003 on prevention efforts for persons living with HIV. During 1981 to 2001, an estimated 1.3 to 1.4 million persons in the United States were infected with HIV, and 816,149 cases of AIDS and 467,910 deaths were reported to CDC. During the late 1990s, after the introduction of combination antiretroviral therapy, the number of new AIDS cases and deaths among adults and adolescents declined substantially. The annual number of incident AIDS cases and deaths have remained stable since 1998, at approximately 40,000 and 16,000, respectively. The number of children in whom AIDS attributed to perinatal HIV transmission was diagnosed peaked in 1992 at 954 and declined 89 percent to 101 in 2001. (Morbidity and Mortality Weekly Report, 2003).

The *Morbidity and Mortality Weekly Report* (2003) notes that since early 1990 an estimated 40,000 new HIV infections have occurred annually in the United States and the number of persons living with HIV continues to increase. Of an estimated 850,000 to 950,000 persons living with HIV an estimated 180,000 to 280,000 (25%) are unaware of their serostatus. The report points to new and faster tests for HIV which create a new prospect for expanding testing, identification, and treatment of HIV infections. Thus, testing and more information will be used to reduce

the number of HIV infections by working with persons diagnosed with HIV and their partners. There will consequently be increased emphasis on partner notification (Morbidity and Mortality Weekly Report; CDC; HIV/AIDS Surveilance Report, 2001).

It is notable that the new program returns to the earlier methods applied to deal with sexually transmitted diseases (STDs) such as routine screening, identification of new cases, partner notification, and prevention services for those who are infected. The change in approach is a reversal of earlier emphasis on privacy where for sometime a New York physician who diagnosed a patient as HIV positive could, but was not under any legal compulsion, to inform the patient's spouse or other sexual partners.

Because persons who are HIV-positive and have a defective immune system are more likely to contract tuberculosis than are others, the recurrence of tuberculosis in a multidrug-resistant form creates a situation in which the disclosure of a patient's affliction with tuberculosis may be regarded, often erroneously, as an indication of positive HIV status, aggravating the problem of maintaining confidentiality. Privacy is now an aspect of personhood, and protection against the invasion of privacy—in this case the invasion of informational privacy—is constitutionally granted by the Fifth Amendment (Tribe). Ethical protection of privacy is based on privacy as an aspect of personhood that is protectable to the same extent that a person's physical integrity is. Violations of privacy are ethically justifiable only if disclosure serves a greater good. Thus, whether a patient's HIV status should be disclosed to others depends on the need of those persons to know and the uses and benefits that may result from the disclosure (Bayer).

Public Health and Bioterrorism

The use of passenger aircraft as guided missiles to destroy the World Trade Center on September 11, 2001, did not change the task of public health but created an urgent need to plan for disasters. Terrorists target civilian populations, and the means and the impact are likely to be unexpected, deeply hurtful, and unrestrained by humane concerns. Civilian populations in dense urban centers are vulnerable because in those areas disease and terror spread readily.

Bioterrorism involves the use of pathogens—disease-causing organisms such as bacteria and viral agents—as weapons to attack civilian populations and armies to weaken their health and resistance. Pathogens may be spread by using advanced technology, but simple devices such as giving smallpox-contaminated blankets to Native Americans during the French and Indian Wars of 1763 can serve the same purpose. During World War II and the Cold War period virtually all the major powers worked to develop biological weapons (Evans et al.).

Before September 11, 2001, public health commentators thought that a significant bioterrorist attack was not likely. Because it was impossible to predict the nature and extent of an attack, preparations could be both costly and inadequate. After a simulation by the U.S. Department of Justice at the request of Congress in Denver in May 2000 in which a hypothetical terrorist sprayed airborne plague bacteria at a concert, a survey of hospital emergency departments showed that as few as 50 casualties could not be well served. The simulation called attention to the infrastructure weaknesses of many public health systems, noting inadequacies of capacity, underfunding, and inability to recognize a new epidemic.

Although bioterrorism events such as the anthrax cases in 2001 may be small-scale, a bioterrorism attack could leave hundreds of thousands dead or incapacitated. In the anthrax event, which involved contaminated letters and resulted in five deaths, it took several days for the first case to be diagnosed. Only later was it recognized that one form of respiratory anthrax could be released from sealed envelopes. The old notion that physicians are the first line of defense for public health was proved again because only physicians know to diagnose diseases, determine who has been exposed and to what agent, and determine who will have to be quarantined.

The period immediately after a bioterrorist attack is crucial for saving lives and managing public panic. An adequate response at the local level is essential, and local agencies must be equipped for an effective response. Although the federal government plans to spend billions of dollars to increase the stockpile of antibiotics and vaccines and develop protection and treatments against bioterrorism agents, funds are needed for infrastructure improvements of state and especially local public health departments to put those materials to use. In addition to stockpiling vaccines and medications, more needs to be done to enable local health agencies to function and respond in the first twelve hours after an attack. Aside from bioterrorism readiness, the capacity for full local responses also will upgrade the public healthcare system because if a local public healthcare system were more fully integrated, it could respond more effectively to bioterrorism, or to such unexpected developments as the emergence of new highly communicable and potentially deadly disease, SARS (severe acute respiratory syndrome).

The threat of bioterrorism by itself may cause major disruptions. Past experiences with bioterrorism show the need for infrastructure changes to facilitate immediate responses. Those responses require the ability to provide the public with accurate and consistent information. Public health must use its long experience in addressing and responding to naturally occurring infectious diseases in large populations to deal with the challenges of bioterrorism, but this may be difficult to undertake in view of other demands on the system. Agencies must be capable of responding both to actual illnesses of exposed persons and to psychogenic casualties and also must be aware of the likelihood of injury to healthcare workers. Because bioterrorism is a crime, law enforcement agencies may be involved. Teamwork is needed with a cross section of public health professions, and public health physicians must learn to recognize diseases that may be related to bioterrorism. The Centers for Disease Control and Prevention's (CDC) National Electronic Disease Surveillance System project provides funds to help states develop electronic modalities to speed reporting.

An immediate response is essential to address events that cause large numbers of casualties, but states also must have an independent ability to cope with smaller-scale events during the first twelve to forty-eight hours after a bioterrorism attack. State and local agencies must develop plans to prevent the spread of infection from bioterrorism agents. Guidance is provided by the CDC in the "Model State Emergency Powers Act" and "Smallpox Plan and Guidelines" to deal with the complex challenges of controlling communicable disease initiated by bioterrorism.

Planning is necessary for the stockpiling of antibiotics as well as to deal with the economic impact of bioterrorism, which is likely to be very high. The economic impact of the release of a Category 1 agent might range from $500 million to $26.2 billion per 100,000 persons exposed, depending on the agent. Public health agencies must ensure that future means and projections are adequate to respond to the risks involved and that adequate information and a capacity for a quick response are available.

Smallpox is a very effective agent for bioterrorism because in nonimmune persons the mortality rate can approach 30 percent and because person-to-person airborne transmission may occur rapidly. There is no effective antiviral therapy against smallpox because the disease effectively was eradicated by 1977 through a World Health Organization program. Serious viral diseases occur in specific locations, and physicians outside their normal locales are likely to mistake them for other local ailments. Other diagnostic difficulties arise because those cultures may be hard to culture from humans and may pose risks to laboratory personnel. Few practitioners have ever seen a case of smallpox, and cases are likely to be mistaken for more common diseases. There is also substantial resistance to smallpox immunization because of possible adverse reactions that have received broad publicity even though they occur very infrequently. Immunization is possible for smallpox, but there are few immunization strategies for other viral diseases. Viral agents as weapons of mass destruction pose major risks because they are highly contagious in susceptible populations and have a high rate of fatality (Bronze et al.).

Because pathogens used for bioterrorism may be spread without being observed immediately, infectious agents may not be discovered until it is too late to respond. Detectors that consist of electronic chips that can detect pathogens through the use of antibodies or DNA are being developed, and an important question will be to determine where to place those devices, which apply a new and expensive technology (Casgrande).

Bioterrorism is analogous to what has been referred to as ecoterrorism, which uses existing industrial and ecological hazards against populations near atomic power plants or other plants that use or store dangerous substances. Attacks on such plants that result in the release of hazardous substances may equal or exceed the consequences of bioterrorism (Prenders and Thomas). The consequences of accidental releases of hazardous substances in Bhopal, India, have made people aware of the potential of intentional releases through acts of terrorism.

Conclusion

Public health law is a developing field that is based on established principles and legal tradition yet is contemporary and responsive to current needs. Based on the police power of the state and federal powers delegated under the U.S. Constitution, public health law has experienced a significant expansion through its inclusion of fields such as the law of mental health, the law of occupational health and safety, major aspects of environmental law, and the growing area of legal developments related to genetic disease. Although the domain of public health law has expanded, it has retained its essential purpose of advancing the public good at the least cost to individual freedom.

FRANK P. GRAD (1995)
REVISED BY AUTHOR

SEE ALSO: *AIDS: Public Health Issues; Bioterrorism; Coercion; Conscience, Rights of; Environmental Policy and Law; Epidemics; Eugenics; Health Screening and Testing in the Public Health Context; Paternalism; Public Health*

BIBLIOGRAPHY

Alden v. Maine. U.S. 706 (1999).

Arras, John, and Hunt, Robert. 1983. *Ethical Issues in Modern Medicine,* 2nd edition. Palo Alto, CA: Mayfield.

Bayer, Ronald. 1989. *Private Acts, Social Consequences: AIDS and the Politics of Public Health.* New York: Free Press.

Beauchamp, Tom L., and Childress, James F. 1983. *Principles of Biomedical Ethics,* 2nd edition. New York: Oxford University Press.

Bentham, Jeremy. 1969a. "A Fragment on Government." In *A Bentham Reader,* ed. Mary Peter Mack. New York: Pegasus.

Bentham, Jeremy 1969b. "An Introduction to the Principles of Morals and Legislation." In *A Bentham Reader,* ed. Mary Peter Mack. New York: Pegasus.

Bronze, Michael S.; Huycke, Mark M.; Machado, Linda L.; Voskuhl, Gene W; and Greenfield, Ronald A. 2002. "Viral Agents as Biological Weapons and Agents of Bioterrorism." *American Journal of Medical Sciences* 323(6): 316–325.

Buchanan, Allen. 1989. "Health-Care Delivery and Resource Allocation." In *Medical Ethics,* ed. Robert M. Veatch. Boston: Jones and Bartlett.

Buck v. Bell. U.S. 200 (1927).

Caplan, Arthur L., ed. 1992. *When Medicine Went Bad: Bioethics and the Holocaust.* Totowa, NJ: Humana Press.

Casagrande, Rocco. 2002. "Technology against Terror." *Scientific American* 287(4): 82.

Chase, Alan. 1977. *The Legacy of Malthus: The Social Cost of the New Scientific Racism.* New York: Knopf.

Commonwealth v. Alger. 61 Mass. 53 (1851).

Crowley v. Christiansen. 137 U.S. 86 (1890).

Duster, Troy. 1990. *Back Door to Eugenics.* New York: Routledge.

Evans, R. Gregory; Crutcher, James M.; Shadel, Brooke; Clements, Bruce; and Bronze, Michael S. 2002. "Terrorism from a Public Health Perspective." *American Journal of Medical Sciences* 323(6): 291–297.

Gaylord, C. Lester 1978. "The Sterilization of Carrie Buck." *Case & Com* 83(5): 18–20, 21–26.

Grad, Frank P. 1985. "The Ascendancy of Legislation: Legal Problem Solving in Our Time." *Dalhousie Law Journal* 9(2): 228–260.

Grad, Frank P. 1986. "Public Health Law." In *Public Health and Preventive Medicine,* 12th edition, ed. John M. Last. Norwalk, CT: Appleton-Century-Crofts.

Grad, Frank P. 1990. *The Public Health Law Manual,* 2nd edition. Washington, D.C.: American Public Health Association.

Griswold v. Connecticut. 381 U.S. 479 (1965).

Henkin, Louis. 1974. "Privacy and Autonomy." *Columbia Law Review* 74(7): 1410–1433.

Hubbard, Ruth, and Wald, Elijah. 1993. *Exploding the Gene Myth: How Genetic Information Is Produced and Manipulated by Scientists, Physicians, Employers, Insurance Companies, Educators, and Law Enforcers.* Boston: Beacon Press.

Jacobson v. Massachusetts. 197 U.S. 11 (1905).

Jew Ho v. Williamson. 103 F.10 Circuit Court, N.D. Cal. (1900).

King, Patricia. "The Past as Prologue: Race, Class, and Gene Discrimination." In *Gene Mapping: Using Law and Ethics as Guides,* ed. George Annas and Sherman Ellis. New York: Oxford University Press.

Kühl, Stefan. 1994. *The Nazi Connection: Eugenics, American Racism, and German National Socialism.* New York: Oxford University Press.

Lombardo, Paul A. "Medicine, Eugenics, and the Supreme Court: From Coercive Sterilization to Reproductive Freedom." *Journal of Contemporary Law and Policy* 13(1): 1–25.

Markel, Howard. 1992. "The Stigma of Disease: Implications of Genetic Screening." *American Journal of Medicine* 93: 209–211.

Mugler v. Kansas. 123 U.S. 623 (1887).

Munn v. Illinois. 94 U.S. 113 (1876).

Nozick, Robert. 1974. *Anarchy, State, and Utopia.* New York: Basic Books.

Pickens, Donald K. 1968. *Eugenics and the Progressives.* Nashville, TN: Vanderbilt University Press.

Prenders, Michael J., and Thomas, William L. "Ecoterror: Rethinking Environmental Security after September 11." *Natural Resources and Environment* 17(2).

Proprietors of the Charles River Bridge v. Proprietors of the Warren Bridge. 36 U.S. 420 (1837).

Rawls, John. 1971. *A Theory of Justice.* Cambridge, MA: Harvard University Press.

Reilly, Philip. 1991. *The Surgical Solution: A History of Involuntary Sterilization in the United States.* Baltimore: Johns Hopkins University Press.

Rosen, George. 1958. *The History of Public Health.* New York: MD Publications.

Skinner v. Oklahoma. U.S. 535 (1942).

Soloway, Richard A. "The 'Perfect Contraceptive': Eugenics and Birth Control Research in Britain and America in the Interwar Years." *Journal of Contemporary History* 30(4): 637–664.

Tribe, Laurence H. 1978. "Rights of Privacy and Personhood." In *American Constitutional Law.* Mineola, NY: Foundation Press.

U.S. v. One Package of Japanese Pessaries. 86 F.2d 737 (2d Cir. 1936).

VanDeVeer, Donald, and Regan, Tom, eds. 1987. *Health Care Ethics: An Introduction.* Philadelphia: Temple University Press.

Veatch, Robert M. 1981. *A Theory of Medical Ethics.* New York: Basic Books.

Yick Wo v. Hopkins. 118 U.S. 356 (1886).

II. LEGAL MORALISM AND PUBLIC HEALTH

Modern public health, which uses organized community effort, law, and regulation to save lives and prevent disease, has long been entangled with legal moralism, which uses the same measures to protect society against behavior that is viewed in some quarters as "offensive, degrading, vicious, sinful, corrupt, or otherwise immoral" (Schur and Bedau, p. 1). "Morals offenses" have "included mainly sex offenses, such as adultery, fornication, sodomy, incest and prostitution, but also a miscellany of nonsexual offenses" (Feinberg). Legal moralism has cultural and religious origins, but its deepest roots are in purity rituals codified in religious and secular codes (Douglas). Purity rituals are avoidance rituals designed to make the environment and the community safe from the threat of uncleanness and contamination and to promote social order. These codes governed diet, sexual conduct, bodily cleanliness, and avoidance of contamination.

In its most expansive expression legal moralism is the belief that these behavioral codes, regulations, and legal proscriptions are foundational to a social order. To the moralist, drug taking, vice, crime, and sexual promiscuity not only harm the self and others but also threaten, through contagion and example, to loosen the bonds that hold society together. It is the connection between the proscribed conduct or practice and the theories about how the spread of this conduct threatens social order that so often results in the confusion of public health and moralism. Because moralism is often expressed in terms of public-health theories of contagion, it has proved difficult to separate the two modes of thought.

The belief that immorality is contagious also often includes the belief that immorality causes disease. Barbara Gutmann Rosenkrantz's authoritative history of public health in Massachusetts cites a review of Lemuel Shattuck's 1850 report on the health of the state, noting that the "sanitary movement does not merely relate to the lives and health of the community; it is also a means of moral reform.... The ultimate connection between filth and vice has been noted by all writers upon this subject" (Rosenkrantz, p. 2).

Moralism in public health arises when society or groups in society respond to a health crisis more by voicing objections to a social practice or to a group engaged in that practice than by rationally assessing the dangers of disease and the best ways to prevent its spread. The parallels between theories of disease causation found in public health and legal moralism are often challenged and overturned by scientific theories of disease causation. While public-health campaigns and officials have often addressed problems moralistically in the past, the long-term trend indicates a separation of the two ways of thinking. Moralism has also suffered attacks from religious groups that emphasize social justice or inwardness more than adherence to religious rules. Finally, moralism is challenged by the modern and postmodern tolerance of a wider range of sexual expression and by the spreading support for political liberties and rights of privacy for all citizens, even those accused of immoral practices.

Moralism's most potent threat to public health comes from the ways in which epidemics and moral dissolution are believed to be inextricably tied together. This entanglement makes the victims of new outbreaks of certain diseases seem a threat to society itself. It also leads to powerful drives to stigmatize and shame the epidemic's victims, in the use of legislation and regulation to invoke shame and public denunciation for a category of persons or in what have been called "status degradation ceremonies" (Garfinkel). The current struggle in the fight against acquired immunodeficiency syndrome (AIDS) is the best-known contemporary example of the confusion between moralism and public health. Thus, the purpose of the policies of the United States in incarcerating prostitutes during World War I was not just to prevent the spread of syphilis and venereal disease but also to shame and punish a class of individuals and to close and solidify the ranks of a nation going to war (Brandt). This moral campaign of imprisonment took priority over the use of new medical treatments for syphilis and gonorrhea, which, while still primitive, were surely more effective.

Modern public-health problems, especially those of a contagious or epidemic nature, provide a constant temptation for legislators, health officials, and the public to confuse the ends of preventing harm to individuals and communities and of proscribing immorality. Yet it would be wrong to conclude that all proscriptions of a practice or behavior are tantamount to moralism. Moralism and social disapproval are not the same thing, even though the latter may be an echo of the former. Social disapproval or even indignation about a practice remains a potent ally of many public-health campaigns.

Public Health and Alcohol Policy

Legal moralism has played a prominent role in alcohol policy, particularly in movements to prohibit all drinking in the United States, in England, and in the Nordic countries. The history of alcohol policy, more than that of most public-health problems, reveals the difficulty in separating health issues from moralizing claims. It also reveals how some of the ways we seek to avoid moralism can be counter to science and to the health and safety of the public.

In the United States, Prohibition, or the outlaw of the manufacture and sale of alcoholic beverages, was enforced from 1917 until 1933. The Prohibition movement is a fascinating intermingling of progressive and scientific thinking, moralism, and religious fundamentalism. For example, the Progressive period in U.S. history (roughly 1890 to 1920) was not just a period when the states began to expand their powers over child labor, over the working conditions of adults, or of assuring safe food and water by strengthening

the regulatory power of the states over private property; it was also a period that witnessed the rise of movements to protect the decency and purity of the public through antipornography legislation, crackdowns on prostitution (especially during World War I), and American Prohibition (Brandt). There is little doubt that the various reform movements that culminated in the passage of the Prohibition amendment brought to the nation's attention a social problem (drunkenness, the saloon, and an overly powerful liquor interest) that demanded state and federal legislation. Also, the record shows clearly that the results of Prohibition, measured solely in public-health terms, were sharply reduced overall consumption of alcohol and related steep declines in serious public-health problems like cirrhosis, admittance to public hospitals for alcohol-related disorders, and the like (Moore and Gerstein; Beauchamp).

The strong secular and progressive side to the movement for Prohibition saw the saloon as a great social problem, one that undermined the public health and safety and promoted domestic violence and crimes against women. Both the movements for women's suffrage and the movement against slavery frequently were headed by leaders who also advocated Prohibition. Yet this began to change in the last decade of the nineteenth century. The women's movement had focused its energies on winning suffrage, and the movement against slavery had long since been replaced by Reconstruction. During the concluding decades of the agitation for Prohibition, the first two decades of the twentieth century, support for Prohibition came primarily from Protestant churches; national Prohibition's justification shifted more and more toward the moralistic claim that drink was the root of most of society's evil. (Moralism is often characterized by inflated claims of the evils or dangers from a substance or a practice, even in very small quantities or isolated and scattered acts.) The intertwining of moralism and public policy, especially for alcohol and drug taking, seems more common in nations where fundamentalist forms of Protestantism that stress adherence to religiously sanctioned behaviors are widespread, or in Muslim nations, where similar fundamentalism obtains; Catholic societies have never had successful Prohibition movements (although temperance movements are found in Ireland).

The backlash to Prohibition produced theories of alcoholism that sought both to deny its moralistic forebears and to establish a new and scientific theory of causation, called the disease concept of alcoholism. This was the belief that alcoholism was caused by an inability to control drinking. In parallel fashion, and also to separate itself from a discredited past, the new alcoholism movement denied the public-health benefits of Prohibition, and as late as the 1960s leading national experts claimed that Prohibition caused people to drink more. The links between what a society drinks generally and the level of alcohol problems were viewed as part of a neoprohibitionist agenda.

The attempt to purge society of moralistic remnants of Prohibition has often been met with surprises. For example, there were strong drives to prohibit alcohol in Norway, Sweden, and Finland during the 1920s and 1930s. Only Sweden avoided Prohibition, in a narrow national referendum vote. In Finland, during the late 1960s and 1970s, the drive to eliminate the rural remnants of their national prohibition legislation of the 1930s led to a sharp relaxation of drinking laws throughout society and the elimination of prohibition in rural areas. The experts believed that restrictions actually encouraged drinking of distilled beverages in unsocialized ways and that by eliminating prohibition, drinking would actually decrease. Yet the measures to liberalize drinking were followed by steep increases in drinking rates and associated problems such as public drunkenness (Beauchamp). Subsequently, state authorities and their advisers retreated from a too-uncritical relaxation of drinking legislation, shifting the justification for alcohol policy more toward a public-health model that accepted limits on all drinking as a necessary part of a sound policy and as not necessarily moralistic.

Western democracies during the 1970s and 1980s witnessed declines in drinking rates, attributed by experts to a growing cultural conservatism and a widening awareness of the public-health consequences of heavy drinking and high levels of per capita consumption. This new period was likely also solidified by the fact that heavy drinking became socially and even morally undesirable, just as smoking became morally undesirable. While drunkenness and addiction were still viewed less punitively, the public began to register its strong disapproval of heavy drinking, especially when it posed risks to others, such as in drinking and driving, or any drinking at all by teenagers. More broadly, the era when drinking itself was not seen as the problem was replaced with a period in which all drinking remains somewhat under a public-health cloud. The evidence that some forms of drinking might promote a healthier heart has caused that cloud to lift only a little.

Smoking and Public Health

At the turn of the twentieth century, smoking was treated as morally offensive. Churches proscribed cigarette smoking and urged public action. But the long-term popularity of smoking spread too quickly, and the campaign was eventually abandoned. Soon smoking was regarded as cosmopolitan and modern. Cigarette smoking rates grew and became widely and culturally approved (Warner). In the 1950s epidemiological studies appeared in the United States and England noting the link between smoking and lung cancer and the possible links with heart disease. The U.S. Surgeon General issued a widely discussed report compiling very strong and extensive research suggesting that smoking was one of the most lethal hazards of our times.

The social climate against smoking began to turn in the late 1960s and 1970s. Antismoking sentiment rose, and cigarette advertising on television was banned. The risks of smoking for third parties was noted. Communities and entire states began to legislate against smoking in public places. Higher taxes on cigarette smoking were advocated. Smoking rates in most industrial societies fell, but most impressively in the United States. This sharp decline is not only due to the extensive public discussion devoted to the hazards of smoking but also to the growing sense of social and even moral disapproval of smoking by the larger society. This social disapproval was sometimes seen as a resurgence of moralism. But there is scant evidence that the strong current of disapproval against smoking adds up to moralism.

Moralism and the AIDS Epidemic

As Allan Brandt notes, the battle against venereal diseases in the first decades of the twentieth century and the rise of AIDS more recently give evidence that moralism remains a powerful element in the social construction of society's definition of these diseases. Early in the twentieth century, syphilis was a symbol of a "society characterized by a corrupt sexuality. Venereal disease has typically been used as a symbol of pollution and contamination, [and of] … a decaying social order. Venereal disease makes clear the persistent association of disease with dirt and uncleanness as well" (Brandt, p. 5).

The most serious challenge to modern public health by legal moralism entered with the AIDS epidemic and HIV-related diseases. Because anal sex and frequent sex with multiple partners heightens the risk of transmission of the HIV virus and because intravenous drug use also seriously elevates the risk of infection from contaminated needles, legislation that seeks to regulate these behaviors—which are widely proscribed in many states—is always open to the charge of moralism.

Early in the epidemic in the United States, bathhouses frequented by homosexual patrons became targets of public-health regulations. Many in the gay community charged that the measures were aimed less at fighting the epidemic than at proscribing homosexuality. These advocates argued, quite plausibly, that the regulations would have little impact on the course of the epidemic in San Francisco or New York, the two cities where conflicts primarily arose. This was because the bathhouses were the site of only a fraction of the proscribed behaviors. Advocates also argued that city officials and state public-health authorities had caved in to political pressures (Bayer, 1991b).

The same charge of moralism and discrimination was also brought when public-health officials attempted to introduce methods of identifying the sexual partners of those who were AIDS victims, or when state medical societies sought legislation to make AIDS and HIV diseases reportable to state health authorities (Bayer, 1991b). (All states require private physicians to report certain communicable diseases to state health officials.) Ronald Bayer, in his book *Private Acts, Social Consequences* (1991b), has provided the best chronicle of the clash between public-health legislation and the civil libertarians defending AIDS victims. As Bayer says, "These two abstractions, liberty and communal welfare, are always in a state of tension in public health policy" (1991b, p. 16).

It is likely, however, that the AIDS epidemic has permanently altered the landscape of public-health policy, and not just in the United States. No longer will it be possible to easily equate public health only with the use of powers to restrict power and liberty to promote the public health or to see the realms of public health and individual liberty as radically distinct. The growing awareness is that a sound public-health policy requires more than restrictions on liberty and property to promote the communal welfare. It also may require the expansion of private liberties and rights for groups suffering social discrimination based on moralism.

DAN E. BEAUCHAMP (1995)

SEE ALSO: *Abortion; AIDS; Body; Cloning; Conflict of Interest; Death, Definition and Determination of; Embryo and Fetus; Fertility Control; Informed Consent: Legal and Ethical Issues of Consent in Healthcare; Law and Morality; Life Sustaining Treatment and Euthanasia; Maternal-Fetal Relationship; Public Health; Sexual Behavior, Social Control of;* and other *Public Health Law* subentry

BIBLIOGRAPHY

Bayer, Ronald. 1991a. "AIDS: The Politics of Prevention and Neglect." *Health Affairs* 10(1): 87–97.

Bayer, Ronald. 1991b. *Private Acts, Social Consequences: AIDS and the Politics of Public Health.* New Brunswick, N.J.: Rutgers University Press.

Beauchamp, Dan E. 1980. *Beyond Alcoholism: Alcohol and Public Health Policy.* Philadelphia: Temple University Press.

Beauchamp, Dan E. 1988. *The Health of the Republic: Epidemics, Medicine, and Moralism as Challenges to Democracy.* Philadelphia: Temple University Press.

Brandt, Allan M. 1987. *No Magic Bullet: A Social History of Venereal Disease in the United States since 1880.* New York: Oxford University Press.

Devlin, Patrick. 1959. *The Enforcement of Morals.* London: Oxford University Press.

Douglas, Mary. 1966. *Purity and Danger: An Analysis of the Concepts of Pollution and Taboo.* London: Routledge.

Feinberg, Joel. 1973. *Social Philosophy.* Englewood Cliffs, NJ: Prentice-Hall.

Garfinkel, Harold. 1956. "Conditions of Successful Status Degradation Ceremonies." *American Journal of Sociology* 61(5): 420–424.

Gusfield, Joseph R. 1963. *Symbolic Crusade: Status Politics and the American Temperance Crusade.* Urbana: University of Illinois Press.

Hart, H. L. A. 1963. *Law, Liberty, and Morality.* New York: Vintage.

Moore, Mark H., and Gerstein, Dean, eds. 1981. *Alcohol and Public Policy: Beyond the Shadow of Prohibition.* Washington, D.C.: National Academy Press.

Rosenkrantz, Barbara Gutmann. 1972. *Public Health and the State: Changing Views in Massachusetts, 1842–1936.* Cambridge, MA: Harvard University Press.

Schur, Edwin M., and Bedau, Hugo Adam. 1974. *Victimless Crimes: Two Sides of a Controversy.* Englewood Cliffs, NJ: Prentice-Hall.

Shattuck, Lemuel. 1948. *Report of the Sanitary Commission of Massachusetts, 1850.* Cambridge, MA: Harvard University Press.

Warner, Kenneth E. 1986. *Selling Smoke: Cigarette Advertising and Public Health.* Washington, D.C.: American Public Health Association.

PUBLIC POLICY AND BIOETHICS

• • •

There are at least two ways of understanding the relation of public policy to bioethics. The first, focusing on public policy *in* bioethics, involves the public laws (both statutory and case law), policies, regulations, and guidelines that bear on ethical aspects of medical practice and healthcare. These are public in the sense that they emanate from some publicly accountable governmental process, as opposed to private or professional policy; in addition, nonpublic institutions such as hospitals can adopt their own policies to conform to public policy. In this sense, legal requirements to obtain informed consent for treatment, federal regulations requiring approval of a research protocol by an institution's human subjects committee, and the lack in the United States of any governmental means of ensuring universal access to healthcare for all citizens represent public policy bearing on ethical aspects of medical and research practice.

When the relation of public policy to bioethics is understood in this way, the question arises as to the extent to which bioethics issues have been and should be matters of explicit public policy. Physician–patient relations, for example, may be taken to be a largely private matter to be worked out by physicians and patients outside of the public sphere, as they were to a great extent in the early part of the twentieth century, or to be a matter of professional concern by physicians in professional settings, but not the subject of and regulated by public policy. Alternatively, such issues might be seen, as they increasingly were in the United States in the 1970s and 1980s, as an appropriate concern of public policy. Thus, public policy in bioethics includes what governments choose not to do, as well as what they do, in bioethics.

The second understanding of the relation of public policy to bioethics focuses on public-policy bodies that have been influential in shaping bioethics, public policy on bioethics issues, and healthcare practice. Understood in this way, the subject is the manner and extent to which bodies in the United States, such as the President's Commission for the Study of Ethical Problems in Medicine and Biomedical and Behavioral Research (hereafter President's Commission) or the National Bioethics Advisory Commission (NBAC), or international bodies, such as the United Nations Educational, Scientific and Cultural Organization (UNESCO) or the World Health Organization (WHO), have shaped bioethics and medicine. Why have the United States and many other countries frequently turned to such bodies in the development of public policy in bioethics? How have such bodies functioned? What has been their impact?

This entry addresses both of these understandings of the relation between public policy and bioethics. A general thesis of this entry is that bioethics and public policy have influenced one another. The field of bioethics has helped shape and has been shaped by both public policy in bioethics and a variety of public policymaking institutions in bioethics.

The Relation between Substantive Public Policy and Bioethics

As bioethics in the United States and elsewhere during the 1970s and 1980s became an area of great public and professional concern, many standard bioethical issues began to be addressed, not just in classrooms or between doctors

and patients, but also in explicit public debates and policies. One of the most prominent examples, cardiopulmonary resuscitation (CPR), illustrates a relatively common pattern of this development of public policy on important bioethics issues. First, a new technology was developed; in this case and not atypically, it was a form of life-sustaining treatment. Originally the technology was developed for and applied in a relatively narrow range of cases in which there was clear expected benefit: saving otherwise healthy people who had suffered unexpected cardiac or respiratory arrest. CPR later came to be used in a wider range of cases, including many patients for whom its expected success and benefit were questionable. The reason for the wider use was that the conditions under which CPR was applied precluded taking time to make thoughtful decisions about whether to employ it once a patient was in need of it.

Reports of widely varied practices, including some that were ethically problematic at best and certainly did not represent sound general practice, led many hospitals to develop formal policies concerning resuscitation. In particular, the general interest in "do not resuscitate" (DNR) orders led to scholarly studies of the use of CPR and of DNR orders. Public bodies such as the President's Commission addressed the issue and developed recommendations about institutional policies, and the Joint Commission on Accreditation of Healthcare Institutions required institutions to have a policy regarding DNR orders. In this case, a public-policy response to an identified and significant ethical problem in medical practice led to both a public and a professional policy response.

In other cases, public-policy initiatives have sought to increase the use of a practice generally deemed desirable. For example, the U.S. Patient Self-Determination Act of 1991 was intended to increase the use and effectiveness of advance directives by requiring institutions receiving federal funds both to inform patients at admission of their rights under state law to use advance directives, and to have policies in place for implementing them.

Public policy regarding life-sustaining treatment and the care of the dying reflects as well as any issue the mutual interaction and development of bioethics scholarship and public policy. The Karen Ann Quinlan case first focused public attention in the United States on issues of life-sustaining treatment. In the landmark *Quinlan* ruling in 1976, the New Jersey Supreme Court held that an incompetent patient retained a right to refuse life-sustaining medical care, a right that could be exercised by a surrogate, in this case a parent, acting for the patient. The next fifteen years were filled with intense activity on these issues in both the public-policy and scholarly arenas of bioethics. In addition to books on the topic, many articles appeared in bioethics journals such as the *Hastings Center Report* and in medical journals such as the *New England Journal of Medicine;* at the same time, state courts around the country were addressing many legal cases concerned with life-sustaining treatment and the care of the dying. Other public-policy bodies issued extensive studies, such as the President's Commission's report *Deciding to Forego Life-Sustaining Treatment* (1983a), and briefer policy statements on the subject came from professional bodies such as the American Medical Association (AMA). The President's Commission's report drew explicitly on a wide range of bioethics scholarly work on life-sustaining treatment decisions, as well as on closely related legal scholarship and healthcare research. Court decisions frequently appealed not only to legal scholarship but also to the growing bioethics literature.

The bioethics literature on life-sustaining treatment issues was influenced by these court cases in two important ways. First, the attention many of these legal cases received served as a relatively direct stimulus for much bioethics commentary and analysis of the arguments made in the opinions. Because there was generally little specific statutory law constraining the judicial rulings, they often appealed in part to explicitly ethical arguments. Second, and at a deeper level, the President's Commission's report and many legal decisions greatly influenced debates on life-sustaining treatment and played a major role in the degree and nature of the consensus that emerged during the 1980s. This was true especially for specific issues such as the moral importance of differences between stopping and not starting life-sustaining treatment and between ordinary and extraordinary treatment, as well as on broader issues such as the nature and importance of the moral values of individual autonomy and well-being in guiding life-sustaining treatment decisions. The issue of forgoing life-sustaining nutrition and hydration is a particularly good illustration. Here, the debate in the bioethics literature began, not coincidentally, at about the same time that nutrition and hydration cases were being brought to a number of courts. Because the bioethics literature and the court decisions are best understood as profoundly interdependent parts of a single debate on which significant consensus was emerging, the bioethics literature and the court decisions were unlikely to veer in sharply conflicting directions on the permissibility of forgoing nutrition and hydration.

From its inception, bioethics has had a micro focus, especially on individual doctor–patient issues, and a macro focus on ethical issues in health policy, especially justice in healthcare. The micro issues were predominant in bioethics during the 1970s and much of the 1980s, and will, no doubt, continue to be important. But as health-policy debates in the United States focus on access to healthcare,

containment of healthcare costs, and rationing of healthcare, the macro focus of bioethics is likely to become increasingly prominent. On these macroethical issues in health policy, the profound interaction of bioethics and public policy is even more evident. Unlike many doctor–patient issues, which could to a significant extent be worked out between individual doctors and patients, questions of justice in healthcare can be adequately addressed only at an institutional and policy level. Bioethics scholarship on these questions of justice that hopes to influence public policy and practice must address questions about the design of social, political, and professional institutions and practices. These are public-policy issues at their very core, which means that more profound mutual influences between bioethics and public policy can be expected in the future.

The Role of Public Policymaking Bodies in Bioethics: U.S. Commissions and Efforts

In the United States and throughout much of the rest of the world, public policy bodies have been established in bioethics to study and issue reports on bioethics issues. These public commissions have varied considerably in their nature, roles, and effectiveness.

THE NATIONAL COMMISSION. In 1974 the U.S. Congress established the U.S. National Commission for the Protection of Human Subjects of Biomedical and Behavioral Research (hereafter National Commission). Two important factors led to the creation of this first public, national body to shape bioethics thinking and practice in the United States.

First, the character of biomedical research had changed significantly in the preceding three decades. Before World War II, such research was carried out largely in small-scale therapeutic settings in which researchers tended to be well known to and trusted by their patients/subjects and the surrounding community. During and following the war, however, the scale of this research expanded greatly as public expectations about the potential benefits of medical research grew. Biomedical researchers increasingly were distinct from clinicians caring for patients, and the unknown investigator replaced the well-known and trusted clinician.

Second, public concern with research abuses had increased. The shocking abuses of human subjects by Nazi doctors during World War II had earlier drawn public attention to these issues. In 1966 a member of the faculty of Harvard Medical School, Henry K. Beecher, published an article in the *New England Journal of Medicine,* detailing twenty-three instances of published research in which the treatment of human subjects was at best ethically problematic. Around the same time some especially egregious cases of research abuse received wide public attention, such as the Tuskegee Syphilis Study, in which African-American men infected with syphilis were left untreated in order to study the natural course of the disease.

The National Commission's work has shaped law, federal regulatory oversight, and institutional oversight of research practice. The National Commission consisted of eleven commissioners and a professional staff. The commission held public hearings, sponsored a wide range of studies and scholarly papers, and eventually issued reports on the use of different groups of human subjects—children, prisoners, the mentally infirm, and fetuses—in research. The legislation establishing the National Commission required the secretary of the U.S. Department of Health, Education, and Welfare (forerunner of the Department of Health and Human Services) to implement the National Commission's recommendations or offer a public justification for not doing so. In some cases, the commission's reports led to the virtual elimination of research with particular classes of subjects, such as prisoners, whereas in other cases, they led to the development of special rules for the involvement of particular classes of subjects, such as children. The final report of the National Commission—the *Belmont Report* (1978a)—had a great impact on bioethics because it addressed the moral principles that underlay the various reports on particular aspects of research. Here, the principles of respect for persons, beneficence, and justice were enunciated; these same principles later figured prominently in Tom L. Beauchamp and James F. Childress's *Principles of Biomedical Ethics* (first published in 1979), probably the most widely read and influential scholarly work in bioethics.

The National Commission stressed the moral principle of respect for persons and the implications of this principle: that subjects should be enrolled in research only with their free and informed consent and with their confidentiality properly protected. The work of the National Commission continues to form the ethical basis for the federal government's regulatory oversight of research involving the use of human subjects, carried out by the Office for Human Research Protections within the Department of Health and Human Services (HHS).

THE PRESIDENT'S COMMISSION. When the National Commission concluded its work in 1979, the Congress established the President's Commission with a substantially broader mandate. During the four years of its existence, this commission issued ten book-length reports on a wide variety of topics in bioethics, including the definition of death, the compensation of injured research subjects, genetic screening and counseling, genetic engineering, informed consent in

medical treatment, decisions about life-sustaining treatment, access to healthcare, whistle-blowing in research, and protection of research subjects. Like the National Commission, the President's Commission had public commissioners and a full-time professional staff representing a wide variety of academic disciplines.

Because of the diverse nature of the topics addressed by the President's Commission, its reports had different kinds of impacts on bioethics. For example, *Defining Death* (1981) contributed to the adoption of a uniform brain-death standard for death by the great majority of the states; here, the impact was a relatively discrete piece of legislation. On the other hand, the report on informed consent, *Making Health Care Decisions* (1982), had a more diffuse, though no less important, impact in advancing the ideal that physicians and patients share decisions about treatment; here, medical education and the professional ethos for physician–patient relations were affected. *Securing Access to Health Care* (1983b) focused on the ethical problems represented by the more than 20 million Americans who were without health insurance. This report had relatively less immediate impact than many others because massive government expenditures were necessary to solve the problem at a time when the political ideology of the new presidential administration was to reduce, not expand, government social programs. Ten years after it was issued, however, it was clear that this report contributed to the public and political recognition in the United States of the ethical problem of access to healthcare and to understanding the ethical case for government action.

Deciding to Forego Life-Sustaining Treatment (1983a) was almost certainly the commission's most influential report, for several reasons. Following the *Quinlan* decision in 1976, both public and professional attention to this area steadily increased. In addition, new and more widely disseminated life-sustaining medical technology meant that both professionals and the public had had more personal experience with these difficult decisions; individual professionals, healthcare institutions, and the public were uncertain about what was ethically acceptable and desirable practice in this area. Finally, implementation of the commission's recommendations did not require major new government expenditures. The commission's recommendations centered on patients' or their surrogates' rights to weigh the benefits and burdens of any available treatment, including the alternative of no treatment, according to the patient's values, and to accept or refuse treatment. The report criticized and offered alternative language for some distinctions that until then had had an important influence on the bioethics literature and on practice, such as the differences between not starting and stopping a life-sustaining treatment and between ordinary and extraordinary treatment.

The report filled a vacuum: Hospitals, courts, and others sorely needed guidance about ethically acceptable practice. The fact that this report, like the others, was issued by a presidential commission gave its recommendations an unmatched authoritativeness.

NATIONAL BIOETHICS ADVISORY COMMISSION. After a lengthy hiatus in which the United States lacked any national bioethics commission, in 1996 President Bill Clinton established the National Bioethics Advisory Commission (NBAC). Its initial work plan was interrupted by the cloning of the sheep Dolly and the president's request for a report within ninety days on the ethical, social, and legal issues of cloning. This illustrates one role that public commissions sometimes play: responding in a rapid, but measured and reasoned, way to developments in biotechnology that raise serious ethical concerns. The commission recommended that there be a moratorium on any reproductive cloning, largely based on concerns about safety, to allow time for a public debate and a later revisiting of the issue.

A later report of NBAC addressed a different but related issue—embryonic stem cell research. This was another instance of using a public commission to address an extremely controversial issue in the hopes of achieving a more reasoned debate of the issues and a position that might gain some consensus among parties with widely differing views. One focus of the NBAC report was whether federal funding of this research should be permitted. The commission sought a compromise position by making a distinction in the sources of the stem cells and recommended permitting that funding when the cells were derived from cadaveric tissue or from embryos left over from in vitro fertilization (IVF), but rejected funding of research using cells derived from embryos created for the purposes of research by IVF or by means of somatic cell nuclear transfer. While some found the compromise position appealing, it failed to create any consensus that could guide public policy, in particular on public funding of this research. It was another illustration, along with an earlier fetal tissue study and a failed attempt to establish a national bioethics commission in the late 1980s that foundered on disputes about abortion, of the difficulty of using public commissions to address deeply controversial issues, especially in the United States those that involve the moral status of embryos and fetuses.

As had the earlier U.S. public commissions, NBAC also produced several reports on ethical issues in research, including research with mentally impaired subjects, research in developing countries, and a study of the overall regulatory process of research. This work reflected continuing concern with protecting human subjects in research as well as new concerns such as the potential for exploitation of subjects in the increasingly common research being done in developing countries by investigators from the developed world.

PRESIDENT'S COUNCIL ON BIOETHICS. The charter of NBAC expired in October 2001, and in November 2001 President George W. Bush appointed the President's Council on Bioethics. Through early 2003, the council had produced only one report, *Human Cloning and Human Dignity: An Ethical Inquiry* (2002), which featured special attention to the stem cell research debate. Interestingly, in the case of therapeutic cloning and stem cell research, the council was charged to advise the president on an issue on which he had already taken a formal position, which illustrates the political tensions that these public bodies can sometimes face. There was also considerable controversy about whether the membership of the council was overly slanted in a particular political and ideological direction.

OTHER PUBLIC OR QUASI-PUBLIC BODIES. In the United States, besides the national bioethics commissions, a number of other public or quasi-public bodies have also have entered these frays. Several states, including New Jersey and New York, established bioethics commissions. In addition, many government bodies and commissions with a broader medical or health policy agenda have had one or more bioethicists among their members and have included bioethics issues as a part of their broader concerns. For example, the Task Force on Organ Transplantation of the HHS addressed ethical issues in the procurement and distribution of scarce organs for transplantation, although the ethical issues were not the main focus of its work. The Institute of Medicine within the National Academy of Sciences has done many studies on and issued reports concerning a wide array of bioethics issues as well as broader health and public policy issues that have bioethical components. Furthermore, many other government organizations and studies whose main focus is not ethical issues typically now include some discussion of the ethical aspects of their work.

A striking example of the extent to which bioethics in the United States has become an accepted part of the public realm is the Human Genome Project. This $15 billion, fifteen-year project to map and sequence the complete human genome or genetic code gave the ethical implications of government-sponsored research an unprecedented role. At the time the project was being debated in Congress, there was considerable concern about its ethical, social, and legal ramifications. James Watson, the first director of the National Center for Human Genome Research (now known as the National Human Genome Research Institute) at the National Institutes of Health, committed the center to spending at least 3 percent of its total budget on research into and public and professional education concerning these legal and bioethical issues, and in fact it has ended up spending more. The genome project's Ethical, Legal and Social Implications (ELSI) Research Program has supported a wide range of studies and projects aimed at the general public as well as the academic, research, and public-policy communities.

A last important manifestation of public-policy bodies in bioethics in the United States has been the formation of grassroots citizen groups in a number of states to address bioethics issues. Such groups have often treated issues of health policy, especially how to set priorities among healthcare services with a view to allocating limited funds in government health insurance programs, such as Medicaid. The widely publicized prioritization of healthcare services in the state Medicaid program in Oregon made use of such citizen groups.

International Activity

The United States is hardly alone in turning to government bodies to address issues of bioethics. Indeed, while the United States had no national government bioethics commissions between 1983 and 1996, countries throughout the world established them during and after this period. Nearly every country in northern and western Europe, as well as a number of eastern European countries, now has a national bioethics commission. Such commissions also exist in a number of countries in the Americas and in Asia and Oceania.

These national bioethics commissions have varied greatly—in their form and membership, in the scope of issues addressed, and in their general effectiveness. For example, the Danish Council of Ethics, established by the Danish Parliament in 1988, has followed a populist model, with largely lay members, and has pursued broad educational efforts. In France, the National Consultative Ethics Committee for Health and Life Sciences has followed a more elite model with scholarly and professional members, high public and professional prestige, and more direct attempts to determine government policy. In Great Britain, government-sponsored groups have addressed ethical policy issues in reports comparable in scope and detail with those of the U.S. commissions. The Nuffield Council on Bioethics in Great Britain has established expert panels that have produced major reports of high quality on a wide range of subjects including genetic screening, use of human tissue, mental disorders and genetics, genetically modified crops, stem cell therapy, research in developing countries, patenting DNA, and behavior genetics.

Although there is no international bioethics commission as such, both the United Nations (U.N.), through two of its agencies, and the Council of Europe have created bodies that have been active in bioethics. UNESCO has an International Bioethics Committee that has addressed many bioethics issues and that developed the Universal Declaration on the Human Genome and Human Rights (1997), following up the earlier general U.N. Universal Declaration of Human Rights. The World Health Organization has been active on such issues as resource allocation and genetics, with special emphasis on developing countries. In 1982 the International Association of Bioethics was formed to foster international interchange among scholars and practitioners in bioethics. Most non-U.S. efforts, however, have been at a national level so that they can reflect a particular society's historical, political, legal, and cultural traditions.

Membership and Authority Issues

The use of governmental bodies to address public policy in bioethics raises political and ethical questions of membership, function, decision-making methods, and the authority of their recommendations. With regard to membership, there has often been an attempt to balance two concerns: first, that members have relevant expertise on the issues the body will address and that the body be representative of the relevant professions and disciplines; second, that members represent their communities in such areas as gender, minority status, and political affiliation. Statutes establishing these bodies often mandate the areas from which members must be drawn.

The membership question is related to the proper function of these bodies and the authority of their recommendations. If these bodies were to provide only the highest-level expertise on the issues of concern, the case for representativeness would be weak, though even then the question of who had expertise in bioethics, and the nature of their expertise, would be more contentious than in most areas of scientific medicine. That has not generally been their sole function, however. They have been viewed as combining such expertise with the role of addressing what public policy should be in a particular area. This latter role is by its very nature a more political role, requiring representation of groups that have a substantial stake or interest in the policy question at issue, both on ethical grounds and because the group's recommendations must be able to be "sold" in the political arena.

The difficulty of using governmental bodies to address deeply divisive ethical and political issues is illustrated in the United States by the task force established to address the use of fetal tissue in research. Its recommendations to permit limited use of fetal tissue essentially were ignored in the late 1980s by the first Bush administration because the use of fetal tissue was so closely related to the politically contentious issue of abortion. "Right to life" groups feared any use of fetal tissue could increase or appear to condone abortions. The attempt by the U.S. Congress in the late 1980s to establish a biomedical ethics advisory committee to its Biomedical Ethics Board also failed in large part because of political struggles over abortion.

Representativeness in membership is desirable to ensure that concerns and points of view of significant groups are taken account of for pragmatic reasons, so those groups will support instead of block acceptance and implementation of the recommendations, and for ethical reasons, so those most affected by the recommended policies have some input into what the policies will be. At the same time, powerful professional groups, such as physicians, as well as corporate interests, such as pharmaceutical firms, often have a substantial stake in the policy outcomes. When those interest groups have important or dominant roles within bioethics commissions, they can shape and control the debates, the policy alternatives considered, and the recommendations that emerge. Thus, in the membership of public-policy bioethics bodies, as well as in the policy process more broadly, representation for affected groups must be balanced with preventing powerful professional groups from controlling and distorting the policy process.

For several reasons, the authority of the recommendations of these public-policy bioethics bodies is more problematic than those of analogous scientific bodies. First, the nature and even the existence of expertise in ethics generally, and bioethics in particular, is contested to a greater extent than in scientific medicine. Many people believe that ethical claims express attitudes or feelings and cannot be shown in principle, much less in practice, to be true or false in the manner that claims about empirical matters of fact can be. By contrast, a consensus conference on the appropriate treatment of pulmonary hypertension or breast cancer may be controversial and involve ethical or value issues, but it is usually thought that expertise in the medical aspects of these treatment issues is not problematic to the extent that bioethics expertise is.

Second, appeals to authority are widely acknowledged to be out of place in ethical reasoning—it is the strength of the arguments, not who makes them, that should be persuasive. Because public bodies such as the President's Commission or NBAC typically lack any enforcement powers for their recommendations, their impact ultimately should, and does, lie in their ability to persuade others who do have the authority to pass legislation, render court decisions, and

make institutional policies, of the wisdom of their recommendations. This has led many such bodies to see their task as articulating and advancing an emerging consensus on the issues addressed. The President's Commission put great efforts into reaching consensus and had only one dissent, from a single commissioner, in all of its reports. Moreover, all such bodies will give some weight to arriving at consensus, and as in the more overtly political process, reaching consensus sometimes requires that ethically problematic but politically necessary compromises be made, especially regarding policy recommendations.

Some would argue that the main purpose of such bodies is to sharply delineate the ethical issues, conflicts, and choices. The President's Council for Bioethics, for example, sees its role as providing a deep exploration and delineation of the issues, but not blurring or sidestepping them in the interests of compromise and consensus. Pragmatic or political compromise, according to this view, should be left to the overtly political process. In this way the ethics body can speak more unequivocally to the ethical issues and not compromise or cut and trim the ethical arguments where it is politically expedient to do so. On the other hand, this approach may make the body less effective than it might otherwise be in influencing policy.

Another issue that has received some attention concerning these public bodies is the methodology they do or should employ in their deliberations and in arriving at policy positions. In their 1988 book, *The Abuse of Casuistry,* Albert R. Jonsen and Stephen E. Toulmin argued that when members of the National Commission addressed concrete cases, they were generally able to arrive at consensus, even when they disagreed strongly on the more general moral principles or theories that underlay their consensus. Jonsen and Toulmin contrasted the experience of the National Commission with what is sometimes called principlism, in which bioethics, and applied or practical ethics more generally, are seen as beginning with moral principles or theories that are applied in a relatively mechanical, deductive fashion to particular cases or policy choices.

Because providing justification for concrete moral judgments involves appeal to moral principles or reasons of often substantial generality, public-policy bodies such as bioethics commissions should, and in fact often do, work back and forth between concrete cases and more general moral principles. The aim should be to develop a position on the particular ethical and policy issue that is backed by the most plausible, coherent reasons. This can often be a great challenge when political pressures to reach a publicly acceptable compromise conflict with the policy backed by the best ethical reasons.

Conclusion

Bioethics issues have come to receive prominent attention in public policy, and bioethics scholarship has strongly influenced public policy in healthcare. At the same time, public policy in the form of legal decisions and public-policy bodies deeply influenced the development of both the field and scholarship of bioethics during the last decades of the twentieth century. As bioethics comes to focus more on broader issues of health policy in coming years, this mutual interaction and influence between public policy and bioethics can only be expected to increase.

DAN W. BROCK (1995)
REVISED BY AUTHOR

SEE ALSO: *Communitarianism and Bioethics; Consensus, Role and Authority of; Death, Definition and Determination of; Embryo and Fetus, Embryonic Stem Cell Research; Environmental Policy and Law; Ethics, Social and Political Theories; Fertility Control, Legal and Regulatory Issues; Health Policy in International Perspective; Health Policy in the United States; Informed Consent; Injury and Injury Control; Law and Bioethics; Law and Morality; Maternal-Fetal Relationship: Legal and Regulatory Issues; Medical Ethics, History of the Americas: United States in the Twentieth Century; Organ and Tissue Procurement; Patients' Rights; Privacy in Healthcare; Public Health Law; Research Policy; Social Medicine*

BIBLIOGRAPHY

Beauchamp, Tom L., and Childress, James F. 2001 (1979, 1983, 1989, 1994). *Principles of Biomedical Ethics,* 5th edition. New York: Oxford University Press.

Beecher, Henry K. 1966. "Ethics and Clinical Research." *New England Journal of Medicine* 74(24): 1354–1360.

Brody, Baruch A., ed. 1990. "The Role of Philosophy in Public Policy and Bioethics." Special issue of *Journal of Philosophy and Medicine* 15(4).

"Commissioning Morality: A Critique of the President's Commission for the Study of Ethical Problems in Medicine and Biomedical and Behavioral Research." 1984. *Cardozo Law Review* 6(2): 223–355.

Glover, Jonathan. 1989. *Ethics of New Reproductive Technologies: The Glover Report to the European Commission.* De Kalb: Northern Illinois University Press.

Gray, Bradford H., ed. 1986. *For-Profit Enterprise in Health Care.* Washington, D.C.: National Academy Press.

Jennings, Bruce. 1988. "A Grassroots Movement in Bioethics." *Hastings Center Report* 18(3): S1–S16.

Jonsen, Albert R., and Toulmin, Stephen E. 1988. *The Abuse of Casuistry: A History of Moral Reasoning.* Berkeley: University of California Press.

Quinlan, In re. 70 N.J. 10, 355 A.2d 647 (1976).

Rothman, David J. 1991. *Strangers at the Bedside: A History of How Law and Bioethics Transformed Medical Decision Making.* New York: Basic.

U.S. National Bioethics Advisory Commission. 1997. *Cloning Human Beings.* Rockville, MD: Author.

U.S. National Bioethics Advisory Commission. 2001. *Ethical and Policy Issues in International Research: Clinical Trials in Developing Countries.* Bethesda, MD: Author.

U.S. National Bioethics Advisory Commission. 2001. *Ethical and Policy Issues in Research Involving Human Participants.* Bethesda, MD: Author.

U.S. National Commission for the Protection of Human Subjects of Biomedical and Behavioral Research. 1978a. *The Belmont Report: Ethical Principles and Guidelines for the Protection of Human Subjects of Research.* Washington, D.C.: U. S. Government Printing Office.

U.S. National Commission for the Protection of Human Subjects of Biomedical and Behavioral Research. 1978b. *Research Involving Those Institutionalized as Mentally Infirm: Report and Recommendations.* Washington, D.C.: U.S. Department of Health, Education, and Welfare.

U.S. National Institutes of Health. Advisory Committee to the Director. 1988. *Human Fetal Tissue Transplantation Research Panel: Report of the Advisory Committee,* vol. 1. Bethesda, MD: Author.

U.S. President's Commission for the Study of Ethical Problems in Medicine and Biomedical and Behavioral Research. 1981. *Defining Death: A Report on the Medical, Legal, and Ethical Issues in the Determination of Death.* Washington, D.C.: U. S. Government Printing Office.

U.S. President's Commission for the Study of Ethical Problems in Medicine and Biomedical and Behavioral Research. 1982. *Making Health Care Decisions: A Report on the Ethical and Legal Implications of Informed Consent in the Patient–Practitioner Relationship.* Washington, D.C.: U. S. Government Printing Office.

U.S. President's Commission for the Study of Ethical Problems in Medicine and Biomedical and Behavioral Research. 1983a. *Deciding to Forego Life-Sustaining Treatment: A Report on the Ethical, Medical, and Legal Issues in Treatment Decisions.* Washington, D.C.: U. S. Government Printing Office.

U.S. President's Commission for the Study of Ethical Problems in Medicine and Biomedical and Behavioral Research. 1983b. *Securing Access to Health Care: A Report on the Ethical Implications of Differences in the Availability of Health Services.* Washington, D.C.: U. S. Government Printing Office.

U.S. President's Council on Bioethics. 2002. *Human Cloning and Human Dignity: An Ethical Inquiry.* Washington, D.C.: Author.

U.S. Task Force on Organ Transplantation. 1986. *Organ Transplantation: Issues and Recommendations.* Rockville, MD: U.S. Department of Health and Human Services, Office of Organ Transplantation.

INTERNET RESOURCES

Nuffield Council on Bioethics. 2003. Available from <http://www.nuffieldbioethics.org>.

United Nations Educational, Scientific and Cultural Organization. 1997. "The Universal Declaration on the Human Genome and Human Rights." Available from <http://www.unesco.org/ibc/index.html>.

R

RACE AND RACISM

• • •

In the biomedical sciences of the United States and in their wider cultural context, ideas about race and gender play a prominent but unacknowledged role. Despite their apparent universality, these concepts vary over time and place. Different beliefs about them and their social consequences are found across cultures past and present. Both are, in fact, cultural constructions, one or another culture's folk theories of human biological variation. The great variability found in racial and gender notions is indicative of their local cultural construction.

Biological and behavioral assertions concerning race are without empirical validity. After decades of research, largely in anthropology, the social and cultural bases of racial conceptions have become clear (American Anthropological Association; American Association of Physical Anthropologists). Race is a folk-culture concept. While many, perhaps most, cultures of the world do not hold racial theories, such theories are important to consider in discussions of biomedicine and biomedical ethics, especially in the United States. Here, we find that admittedly folk ideas of race and ethnicity serve as the formal basis for government practice, policy and research (Office of Management and Budget). Given the demonstrable negative social, psychological, and health results of the perpetuation of the invidious distinctions represented by racial (and gender) conceptions, and the antipathy generated by their stereotypes, the continued use of such identities in biomedical work can be said to represent serious ethical, as well as biomedical research, problems.

Historical Constructions of Race

Race is one of a number of popular cultural conceptions about human variability. The Western concept was developed in its present scientific and related lay versions largely in the nineteenth century (Barkan; Gossett; Naroll and Naroll; Stocking). At its most abstract level, race is an explanation for observed human variation; people differ in appearance because they belong to different races. Behavior is also implicated; people behave differently because they belong to different races. Racism is a set of negative beliefs held by individuals or groups with respect to a population thought to be biologically distinct. Such beliefs about fundamental biological differences came late to the Western world, but not as a result of scientific progress.

The ancients—whether the civilizations of Nubia and Egypt or the later Minoan, Mesopotamian, Greek, and Roman civilizations—held no beliefs about essential human biological or racial differences. There was recognition that people differed in appearance, language, custom, and even ethics (MacIntyre), but such differences were not considered reflections of immutable, biological differences among humans. Nor could there have existed assertions that biology determined behavior, for most of these civilizations were composed of a variety of physical and cultural types in various stages of assimilation to a titular ethnic identity (e.g., Sherwin-White). Were this not the case, the ancient empires could not have expanded their numbers through the recruitment of physically and culturally different peoples, for they would have thought them fundamentally different and nonassimilable.

An important step in the development of the notion of race is to be found in the work of the Swedish botanist and taxonomist Carolus Linnaeus (1707–1778). Linnaeus built upon earlier notions of *species,* distinct groups of living things that cannot interbreed. Linnaeus proposed a classification comprising six human *groups*; he did not use the term *race*. These human groups were understood as neither pure nor (biologically) stable; they were not represented as distinct species. Such an assertion would have been contradicted at the time by considerable evidence of interbreeding of Europeans and other groups. Such empirical evidence was later ignored in the West.

The French naturalist and founder of invertebrate paleontology George Louis Buffon (1707–1788) introduced the term *race* into the biological literature in 1749. The term then did not refer to distinct human groups with separate origins or biologies (Montagu). Buffon's and Linnaeus's early reflections on human difference regarded such differences, correctly, as representing variations of a single species.

In the eighteenth and nineteenth centuries, English and German philosophy and science began the construction of ideas of fundamental, incommensurate biological differences dividing human groups (Barkan; Boas; Gould). While evolutionist views of monogenesis (a theory of a single origin of all humans) replaced polygenesis (a theory of multiple, separate origins) and creationist views (those based on religious beliefs and not on investigations of the natural world) in Europe, nineteenth-century theories were largely alike in expressing racist sentiments, though the sentiments were not recognized as such. Triumphant nineteenth-century evolutionism fitted well in racist science.

Monogenecists assigned to non-Europeans fates of early separation from a "main" line of Europeans. JeanBaptiste Lamarck (1744–1829) suggested that differences among human groups around the world were to be attributed to the inheritance of acquired characteristics. He implicated the role of the environment in evolutionary change, although he misconstrued the mechanism of biological change.

Non-Europeans, and many eastern and southern Europeans, were believed to have a common origin by many western European scholars, but were seen as less evolved. Some were said to be little different than nonhuman primates (Barkan; Stocking). And some ethnic groups of western Europe created racial alliances. English historians of the nineteenth century repeatedly referred to the "rational and freedom-loving" character of the English as racial traits of the Anglo-Saxon, believed to be a branch of the "German race" (Gossett). As with the Nazi *race science* of the next century, the notion of the German race excluded most people commonly regarded in the United States as belonging to a "white race" (e.g., the French and other circum-Mediterranean people, Celtic ethnics, the Slavic people) as well as people from what are commonly regarded as other

"races" in U.S. ideology—Asians, Africans, and Native Americans.

In England, Sir Francis Galton (1822–1911), the father of statistical manipulation, lent both ideas and methods to racial theories. He coined the term *eugenics,* and conceived of this new "science" as a program of "racial" improvement. The idea of group biological improvement was carried to horrendous extremes by Nazi "hygienists." Galton's work on head size and intelligence lent credence to later racist work in the United States as well, such as that of physician Robert Bean of Virginia. His work, in 1906, purportedly showed that parts of the brain were of different sizes in "Whites and Negroes" (in Gould). He also claimed to have found measurable differences in males and females and between higher and lower classes. His interpretations and biased readings, soon disproved (Gould), showed the affinity of the ideas of racism, sexism, and elitism in the United States that are also apparent in English science.

Sir Cyril Burt, dean of twentieth-century educational psychology in England, studied twins during the first half of the twentieth century. He purported to show that twins raised apart had the same IQ. It appears he sought scientific proof for the English folk notion that nature determined human abilities such as intelligence. As a consequence, his views were widely received for decades and influenced the establishment of national examinations. The examinations were used to limit the educational opportunities of millions of young people in Britain. In the 1970s, it was discovered that the late scientist had, in fact, fabricated most of his data. He had also fabricated his long-time research assistants, who supposedly collected most of the data, as well as his coauthors (Gould). The advocates of nature over nurture suffered a heavy blow when this key body of literature was discredited.

In the United States, a multicultural society usually referred to as *multiracial,* Burt's elitist arguments were converted to racist (and sexist) theories by his students, psychologists such as Hans Jurgen Eysenck and Jensen (Gould), as well as others (Fausto-Sterling). Research aimed at showing that African-Americans and other "minorities" were intrinsically less intelligent than the generic "White race." Within each group, moreover, women were said to be less capable than men. Many flaws appear in this sort of research. One of the major problems is the fact that social labels, such as White and Black, were used to make genetic arguments; the arguments were flimsy because they regularly excluded from consideration profound differences in the social and educational experience of the members of the various social categories. This was done in order to arrive at (prejudged) conclusions of inborn racial differences.

A similar idea concerning mental illness was developed in German psychiatry in the mid-1800s. The leader of nineteenth-century German psychiatry, Wilhelm Griesinger, adopted a biological definition of mental disorders. His dictum was that "mind diseases are brain diseases" (Gilman). The idea that mental illness was based in biology and not social environment was actually borrowed from German philosophy, which in turn had taken the idea from popular German culture. Griesinger passed on this popular prejudice in his psychiatric science to a follower, Emile Kraepelin. Kraepelin became the twentieth century's father of biological psychiatry and the creator of a racially based "comparative psychiatry" (Gaines, 1992a; Gilman). This influential figure made the case for the biological basis of major mental diseases such as schizophrenia. His ideas were greatly influential on Nazi and contemporary U.S. biological psychiatry (Barkan; Gaines, 1992c; Gilman).

The Nazi "race science" of the 1930s reverted to nineteenth-century polygenesis to explain differences among racial groups and to assert its group's alleged superiority (Montagu). Some Germans were likewise seen as unfit; they were the disabled, the mentally ill, and the homosexual. In contemporary German society, popular and medical beliefs still express the model of mental illness that considers the mentally ill to be biologically different from "normal" people (Townsend).

As is evident, both English and German cultures exhibit biological theories of human difference. A brief historical look suggests that the ideas of these two cultures are related. In both systems, differences are held to be intrinsic and groups are hierarchically ranked, allegedly in terms of abilities. In the relatively isolated society of England, the Germanic notion of inherent differences and similarities based upon shared "blood" was doubtless introduced by invading Germanic tribes in the fifth century. The idea remained but was applied to internal social differences within England. This focus transformed the theory of difference based upon blood into the English notion of "breeding" that was and is applied to members of the British (which includes the Celtic peoples) social system. It produced Britain's rigid class systems wherein abilities are said to be differentially inherited by those differing in breeding. This conception of inborn qualities then serves to justify the respective social positions of society's members.

The Critique of Scientific Racism

Evolutionists explained the increasing knowledge of human diversity in biological terms (Barkan; Gossett). The allegedly different developmental levels of various societies were said to indicate inferior inborn abilities in the societies' people compared with the usual apex of evolution found in (western) Europe. Eastern Europe, not a direct heir to the Renaissance, has been considered marginal in much of western European thought and totally alien and inferior in Germanic thought. History tells us, however, that Europe was the last of the world's areas to develop the hallmarks of civilization, hallmarks largely borrowed from others who were later alleged to be less evolved than (western) Europeans.

ANTHROPOLOGICAL ARGUMENTS. Racist evolutionist ideas, and many not evolutionist, permeated much of medicine, psychology, biology, and other sciences in Europe and the United States at the beginning of the twentieth century. Among the first to lead a concentrated and protracted attack on scientific racism was Franz Boas (1858–1942). A German immigrant, Boas was the foremost anthropologist of his time and the founder of U.S. anthropology. Among many other things, Boas's research demonstrated the plasticity of the human form and the overlap in measurements (anthropometry) of anatomical features previously asserted to be unique to specific racial groups. These findings flatly contradicted the conceptions of races as stable, unchanging, and distinct physical types. Time has continued to enhance our understanding of the enormous plasticity of human biology, a biology so changeable that it has produced all the variations in the human form found in the world in less than 180,000 years.

Boas himself demonstrated how rapidly biology can change, as well as the nonempirical basis of racial differences, by showing that very different anthropometric readings could be obtained from the children of immigrants to the United States when compared with their parents. The cause was the change in environmental factors, especially nutrition. These measurements indicated, according to the current, specific racial measurement norms, that people in the same family appeared to belong to completely different racial groups (Boas).

Boas also advanced fatal arguments against notions of the relatedness of race to behavior. He showed that so-called races did not exhibit distinct religious, linguistic, or general cultural patterns. People of a variety of races spoke the same language and practiced the same religion. And members of the same race spoke different languages, held different religious beliefs, and otherwise exhibited distinct cultures. Race could not be shown to determine even major forms of human behavior (Boas; Stocking). Many of the positions advanced by Boas remain the most powerful antiracist arguments. It is remarkable that he began his assault on scientific racism before 1910, a time when blatantly racist statements were common in science and in the White House (see Brandt, 1985).

Evolutionary schemes were soon generally recognized as based on biased conjecture. There were no empirical bases for the evolutionary stages of Karl Marx, Herbert Spencer, Edward Tylor, or any of the other evolutionary theorists. Boas replaced evolutionist theorizing with the study of the historical diffusion of cultural traits. Historical diffusionism based its arguments on empirical evidence from all the branches of anthropology, physical anthropology, linguistics, archaeology, and sociocultural anthropology as well as from history. Such evidence was used to demonstrate that the current cultural (or physical) features or organization of any group were a result of contact and borrowing from other groups it had encountered. Of less influence in cultural change were innovation and creativity. Cultural arrangements, then, had more to do with a particular history of contact than with innate abilities related to alleged evolutionary stages. This understanding replaced a notion of the evolution of a single human general culture with an understanding of particular cultures' histories.

Evolutionists rank people and cultures from low to high, worst to best. Implicit in evolutionist thinking is the idea of progress, the idea that things are changing for the better. Evolution and progress are unrelated in fact and must be kept separate. Evolutionary change is simply descent with modification; there is no implication of improvement or superiority of later social or biological forms over earlier ones.

But evolutionists depicted some groups, such as Africans, as being near the apes because the groups were perceived as different. They were said to resemble nonhuman primates, such as chimpanzees and apes, who were described as having thick lips, curly hair, and dark skin. This representation has persisted despite the fact that nonhuman primates actually have straight hair covering their rather white skin and are totally lacking lips. That is, nonhuman primates exhibit precisely the characteristics claimed by Europeans as indicative of their own racial superiority.

While racism is still common, though less so than earlier in the twentieth century in the United States, evolutionist notions containing the idea of progress persist. A counter to these ideas is one of Boas's most enduring contributions: his articulation of the notion of *cultural relativism,* which is not a theory but a descriptive reaction to wide experience with other cultures. While evolutionists ranked people and cultures, anthropologists after Boas came to see them in relative terms; cultures were not better or worse than one another, they were simply different. One

could not judge a culture using values from another; cultures must be evaluated using internal, not external, criteria. Relativism has become a central tenet of anthropology, the science of culture.

Biomedical sciences often evidence not the relativism of Boas but the hierarchical evaluative thinking indicative of evolutionism. An implicit ranking system appeared in medicine and persists in notions of defects afflicting groups of people. Historians of medicine show that this idea was disseminated by medicine's association of specific illness states with specific ethnic groups (called races) and/or genders (Chesler; Gilman; Pernick). This was but one of many techniques for the pathologization of often fictitious differences.

Difference from an implicit standard, that is, Anglo, male, adult (Gaines, 1992a; Gilman), in medical and psychiatric thought has been represented as problematic, dangerous, exceptional, pathological, defective, weak, vulnerable, and/or requiring "special" treatment (Gaines, 1992a; Osborne and Feit). Ultimately, the idea communicated is that culturally defined "others"—in the United States, non-European ethnics, women, and children—are simply, and inherently, "not normal" (Ehrenreich and English; Gilman).

One significant problem with the theories about natural racial groups is the fact that the precise number of them has never been agreed upon. Throughout the last century and a half, enumerations of groups said to constitute races fluctuated from author to author. Indeed, the number of racial groups is still changing. A recent example is the creation, starting in the early 1980s, of a Hispanic race.

The dynamics of the numbers of races should not be surprising given that the boundaries created to distinguish among the various groups have no empirical bases. Such discriminations are everywhere the arbitrary choice of an author (Gould; UNESCO; Stocking). The lack of fixed criteria for differentiation is reflected in the changes over time in racial labels of individuals in modern health statistical records (Hahn), in local and personal history (Domínguez), and in the ever-changing number of races, a number that varies somewhere between one race and three hundred. The correct number is one.

THE HETEROGENEITY OF RACE. Analyses of biogenetic differences of human groups lead to the recognition of a great variety of characteristics, most of which are shared in various proportions. Local configurations of traits (height, color, etc.) produce a huge number of distinguishable groups. On the African continent, there are about one thousand biologically distinguishable groups, as opposed to races

(Hiernaux). Human groups are not divisible into groups that exhibit unique, nonoverlapping physiological characteristics. Differences in biology are always local differences that are characteristic of a local inbreeding population. What is seen as normal human biology also changes from culture to culture (see Kuriyama, in Leslie and Young). Just as the cultural elements exhibited by individuals of ethnic groups vary, so does the biology of members of so-called races.

The central problem for racial classifications is that there exist no intrinsically significant human features. Cultures have selected specific features as worthy of concern and hence as criteria of inclusion or exclusion. The selection of any one trait—such as skin, hair, or eye color, body hair, height, weight, religion, or place of birth—as a criterion of group exclusion or inclusion is, by definition, arbitrary. The selected characteristics represent historical attributions of meaning in local cultural contexts, not the expression of universal human nature or physical characteristics.

Racial Theories in the United States

Most observers in the United States, whether lay or scientific, believe that observation of racial differences and racial antipathy has existed since time immemorial, being an understandable outcome of the encounter of dissimilar social groups. However, this is understandable only in a specific cultural context and is not an accurate rendering of the history of cultural contact.

The deleterious effect of racism on perception and cognition is obvious if the ancestry of U.S. racial groups is examined. Misrepresentations appear in scientific research as well as the popular media. The two—research and media—engage in a kind of cultural conversation that confirms the reality of race. An objective look at the ancestry of members of the major groups in the United States reveals race as a fatal conceptual problem in public health and medical research.

In the United States, most people labeled by self and others as Native Americans are biologically part European; in many cases, they are largely so. Many such individuals also have West African ancestry. Virtually all American "blacks," or African-Americans, are biologically part European. In many if not most cases, more of their ancestors came from Europe than from West Africa. Quite commonly, African-Americans also have Native American ancestry (Blu; Domínguez; Gaines, "Medical/Psychiatric Knowledge," in Gaines, 1992a; Hallowell; Naroll and Naroll; Watts).

All classificatory whites claiming multigenerational descent in the South can be shown to have West African ancestry and, very likely, Native American ancestry (Domínguez;

Hallowell; Naroll and Naroll). This is not surprising since most of the colonists who settled in the U.S. South were single males. The relatively few unmarried females were generally of lower status and in long-term bond service. Without Native American and African women, European males in the South could not have had offspring. In the move westward into what was northern Mexico, where the Spanish had settled with Native Americans a century before the English came to the East Coast, one finds again that those "Americans" who went were primarily males from the South and the East. For this reason, the descendants of these early settlers in the West (settlers who were themselves illegal immigrants because this was northern Mexico) are today of mixed ancestry, although this is not publicly known.

Another distortion relates directly to Latinos, Mexicans, and other groups of "Hispanics." Latinos are descendants of western European, Native American, and West African peoples. This mixture is what the term *la raza* means: a "race" born of a mixture of elements. Because many Mexicans are actually Indians or partly so, the difference between Native Americans (many of whom are Spanish-speaking) and Hispanics is often only nationality, a matter of sociolegal definition and not biology. In other instances, Hispanics have no Native American ancestry but do have West African along with their western European ancestry. In many Latino groups (such as those of Venezuela and Puerto Rico), West African ancestry is virtually universal.

Despite the very definition of Latino as people of mixed cultural and biological ancestry, this language group has been homogenized in the scientific literature and, in the 1980s, became a discrete biological group, a "race" (Gaines, "Medical/Psychiatric Knowledge," in Gaines, 1992a; Hahn). In reality, the groups seen as discrete in the United States— white, African-American, Native American, and Latino— are not at all biologically distinct. Indeed, individuals in any of the categories may embody the same mixture of ancestors as do individuals in the others. The difference in the group to which one is assigned depends not on biology but on local context and social history. These groups represent social categories that are unstable and without common biogenetic content.

VARIABLE RACIAL CRITERIA. In considering the referents of the term *race,* no fixed criterion exists even within the United States. Many nonbiological criteria are used to identify races. The term is applied, for example, to people from a region or geographical direction, one usually designated from the perspective of Europe (e.g., Asians/Orientals). Another referent of this cultural term *race* is a specific continental location (e.g., African, [Native] American). A new basis for a racial group has also emerged quite recently—language. Hispanic, a new racial identity in the United States, may be attributed on the basis only of a surname; here language is biologized.

Putative skin color is commonly used as a marker of race, for example, white, red, black, brown, yellow. This use of color-as-race continues despite the fact that Asians run the gamut in complexion from white to black, as in southern India. The same range of skin color is found among people labeled black or white in the United States. The lack of real color "lines" produces cases of people who are black but look white or the reverse, as well as many other oddities. In such instances, it is social history (i.e., knowledge of ancestry) that produces assignment to an allegedly biological category.

A final criterion of race in the United States is religion. Judaism is employed to demarcate an allegedly biologically distinct group. But it is clear that Jews conform to the local physiological characteristics of the communities in which they reside (e.g., Germany, Poland, Russia, England, Scandinavia, Spain, France). The Jews in the United States represent a (fictional) biological group created by religious intolerance.

If a cultural approach has some predictive value, one can anticipate that the antipathy of U.S. people toward Arabs in the 1980s and 1990s will likely result in the social construction of yet another historically unknown race—Muslims. (The British have used the term *Wogs*.) Some indication of this process may be seen in the descriptions of the 1990s conflict in the former Yugoslavia. The U.S. media described the conflict as between "Muslims, Serbs, and Croats," although the Muslims were themselves either Serbs or Croats whose ancestors converted to Islam.

Because racism clearly influences cognition, perception, and affect (emotion), it could well appear in psychiatric classifications as a specific disorder. Rather than a condition of professional psychiatric concern, racism and its twin, sexism, instead appear as significant implicit elements in psychiatric (mis)diagnosis and (mis)treatment (Adebimpe; Chesler; Good).

The erroneous views of race found in the United States encode several distinct ideas: (1) a fixed number of distinct biological populations, or races, exist in nature; (2) races have distinctive physical, mental, and/or behavioral characteristics; (3) racial characteristics (physical and behavioral) are naturally reproduced over time; and (4) specific group characteristics—physical, mental, and often moral—are hierarchically ranked, that is, some groups are superior to others (Boas; Gould; Stocking; Montagu). These assumptions, however, are not the only extant racial views of human difference.

Cultural Systems of Racial Classification Beyond the United States

Some writers have argued that capitalism, with a need for cheap labor and for justifying expropriation of land and resources, provided the political context and motivation that drove science to create a defensible basis in biology for immoral acts such as slavery and genocide (Rex and Mason). Certainly, Europeans' encounters with Native Americans and imported West Africans affected their constructions of human difference (Gossett). However, it appears more likely that racial views are a form of *ethnobiology*, a cultural classificatory theory about the nature of human variability (Gaines, 1992a), because some racial ideologies predate capitalism. As well, various capitalist countries exhibit distinctive notions of race. Their differing views have resulted in very different treatment of those designated as belonging to different races.

RACE IN EUROPE. Both English and German science and society produced biological constructions of affinity and difference (Gaines, 1992a). Those who are alike share a common "blood" in Germany and "breeding" in England. Those of the same blood constitute a "race." This German belief is a kind of biological essentialism. It is a much more exclusive notion of race than that found in the United States. It is in reality a kind of ancient kinship theory, a theory of a coherent, related descent group (Gaines, 1992a) that later merged with evolutionist ideas. As such, it is much narrower than U.S. notions. In contemporary Germany, the cultural system of group membership based upon descent from a common ancestor continues. It determines social identity as well as citizenship and suitability to hold political office, for non-Germans cannot hold office or become citizens.

The same system of social classification is found in Alsace, the culturally Germanic northeastern province of France. The biological German system exists alongside a very different, French cultural system that determines ethnic identity by other means. It accords in-group identity to those sharing French civilization and culture. Membership is primarily based on language, not appearance or place of birth (Gaines, 1992a). The term *race* in France thus refers to people who share a particular language and civilization. Both can be acquired, but the latter only by means of the former. Anyone can become French; being French is a linguistic existential state, not a biological one as in the case of the German system.

The so-called racist groups of France may be seen as *culturalists*; their targets are not races but culturally distinct groups, such as unassimilated Muslims. French-speaking sub-Saharan Africans are not targets of the French racism.

North Africans have been historically white even though their complexions run the gamut from black to pale. The conflicts in France thus cannot be based upon race, though they are reported as such in the U.S. media where cultural differences are always interpreted as "racial differences."

RACE IN JAPAN AND SOUTH AFRICA. In Japan, a modern, industrial, and scientific society, a conception of human races exists that differs from that of the United States. Japanese sciences hold, and offer evidence to support, that the Japanese are a race distinct from Koreans, Chinese, the indigenous Ainu people, and the outcast Eta group (DeVos and Wagatsuma). In contrast, U.S. science and society hold that all these people from the East constitute a single biological race, along with South Asians, Indonesians, Filipinos, and others. These people do not evidence a common language, culture, or physical appearance, so the U.S. cultural system converts a geographical designation of people, borrowed from Europe, into an "Asian race."

In South Africa, there exists yet another system that classifies "racial groups." There, before the official collapse of apartheid, a sociolegal system was in place that distinguished four groups: Black, White, Asian, and Coloured. All people with ancestry in more than one of the first three groups were categorized as Coloured. Chinese were Asian, but Japanese were White. Each group historically has had different rights and privileges (see Schwartz, in Gaines, 1992a). All have equal status, at least legally, in the new South Africa.

In the United States, unlike South Africa, science and society ignore mixed ancestry and label individuals as wholly belonging to the least prestigious group of his or her parents, that is, to one exclusive category or another. In medical research, epidemiological studies, and clinical practice, people of mixed ancestry—that is, most Americans—are treated as if they had no ancestry except (West) African, Native American, Asian, or European. Designations are assumed to refer to homogeneous, distinct biological groups. If "admixture" is noted, researchers tend to ignore European ancestry and focus on genetic "vulnerabilities" deriving only from the subject's putative "minority" ancestry (Duster; Gaines, 1985; Wailoo).

In the United States, virtually all people called black or African-American, a term coined by anthropologist Melville Herskovits, would be classified in South Africa as Coloured because of their mixed ancestry (West African, western European, Native American). Indeed, all U.S. residents who claim long lines of U.S. antecedents would be likewise classified because they too have mixed ancestry. The same would hold true for most Native Americans and Latinos.

Ironically then, the major U.S. racial groups, those with major antipathies and conflicts enduring over centuries based on their racial differences, all would be classified in South Africa as belonging to the same racial group—Coloured.

Race as a Key Variable in Biomedical Research and Practice

The ideas of race enumerated above underlie almost all medical and psychiatric research in the United States that pertains to group differences other than age or sex (Gaines, 1992a; Hahn; Robbins and Regier; Osborne and Feit). Remarkably, these beliefs concerning the existence or homogeneity of human populations called "races" have not the slightest scientific (or logical) basis; no empirical evidence has ever existed for the differentiation of humanity into broad racial groups (Gould; Montagu; UNESCO, 1969). In reality, thousands of biologically distinct human groups exist (Hiernaux, 1970; Montagu; Naroll and Naroll; Watts).

Assertions of the biological bases of differences among races are used to justify caste systems; that is, the results of oppression, discrimination, and poverty are commonly used to justify further discrimination and prejudice (Boas; DeVos and Wagatsuma; Naroll and Naroll; Thomas and Sillen). As is shown below, medical research, theory, and practice often play this same role in U.S. society and thereby serve as "scientific" justification for the persistence of popular conceptions of racial difference and of racism (Brandt, 1985; Gilman; Duster).

Racial groups are mental constructs. As mental constructs they cannot evidence medical conditions. Yet "one of the most common methodological blunders in scientific studies of the significance of racial differences in the United States is the tacit acceptance of this phantasmic notion of race as the basis for establishing research samples" (Harris, 1968, p. 264). Given this, it can be noted that a folk medicine, or *ethnomedicine,* is largely a creation of cultural beliefs. Its practices serve to reinforce and even justify those beliefs. Such is precisely the nature of medical research on group differences in the United States. This supportive role may be seen in research on afflictions said to appear only in certain populations.

THE MYTH OF RACE-SPECIFIC DISEASES. In biology or psychology, research science is used to reach conclusions that are in fact a priori assumptions; "prejudice not … documentation dictates conclusions" (Gould, p. 80). In today's medical and scientific community, expressed ideas concerning ethnic and gender inferiority are largely implicit.

They are replaced in the medical literature by vague assertions such as vulnerability, susceptibility, tendency, increased risk, and difference. One aspect of this discourse that constructs and maintains racial difference concerns "race-specific diseases." Since it is believed that races are distinct groups with their own biologies, it stands to reason that they would exhibit particular diseases. Sickle-cell anemia is a case in point.

At the beginning of the twentieth century, sickle-cell anemia was found originally through laboratory analysis of the blood of five patients—two European-Americans, two *mulattos* (in the parlance of the time, persons of mixed European and West African ancestry, but very largely the former), and one Negro (who doubtless was also part European). The findings were reported in the medical literature, however, as a condition found only in Negroes (Wailoo). In fact, this condition has existed in most world populations including the Mediterranean, Middle Eastern, Indian, Filipino, and South American. Instructively, the condition is not found among people in eastern, southern, or central Africa. Rather, it is found largely in West Africa, the ancestral area of most people in the Americas with African ancestry. Clearly, the condition is not a "racial disease" but rather a characteristic of some local populations.

Tay-Sachs disease is said to be a Jewish disease. In fact, it is a disorder found in a specific local population of the eastern Mediterranean from which some Jews, as well as Arabs, came. Jews not from this area, and not descended from people who were, have no risk of developing the disorder. The same is true of the so-called Portuguese disease, a degenerative, fatal neurological disease said to afflict Portuguese people. The afflicted are in reality descended from a single person (one Joseph) who carried the gene causing the disease. It is purely by chance that the antecedent person was Portuguese. Unrelated Portuguese are not at risk for developing the disease. In Tay-Sachs and the Portuguese diseases, specific sites of affliction are generalized to all in the racial category of the afflicted. "Local biologies" (Gaines, 1992a) are ignored in favor of "racial" ones.

The medical assertion that certain diseases are peculiar to specific races is without merit. The fiction is maintained through a number of techniques. Findings in a single person of a racial group are regularly generalized to all members of that putative group (Brandt, 1978; Wailoo); a part is made to stand for a whole. For example, a clinical finding that Indians in Britain required lower therapeutic levels of certain psychotropic medications became the basis for research comparing "Asians" and "Caucasians" (Lin et al., 1990; Lin et al., 1986; Mendoza et al.).

Tendencies discerned in research are commonly reinterpreted to suggest significant differences in research on hypertensive medications; "diuretics are best for 'blacks' and beta-blockers for 'whites.'" Since members in neither group have common ancestry in the United States, such stereotypes can limit diagnosis of problems to groups "known" to be afflicted; others are then overlooked, misdiagnosed, or considered to be exceptions. As such, they do not challenge the stereotype, though logically such exceptions should call into question the very notion of racial distinctiveness.

Despite the absence of any scientific basis, the idea of race represents the basic population variable, aside from age and sex, on which inquiries focus and in terms of which results are interpreted and recommendations made. The huge body of literature on race-specific problems and racial comparisons are actually of unknown scientific value, though they represent a rich corpus for cultural study.

As long as medical science continues in its archaic racial folk beliefs, its claims to objective, acultural, and disinterested status in the health field are seriously compromised. Because these and gender beliefs are purely popular, modern medical sciences appear as cultural medicines, ethnomedicines, albeit professional ones (Gaines, 1992c; Hahn and Gaines). The validity of racial conceptions has been challenged and its use compromised. The continued use of racial conceptions in biomedical research and practice looms as a central conceptual and methodological problem in the biomedical sciences.

CONSEQUENCES OF RACIAL BELIEFS. Common to intentional and unintentional discriminatory motivations is the unstated theory that ancestry in nonwhite groups "taints" the individual, not only determining identity but also causing disease. This is the implicit pathologization of perceived "difference" typical in research on high blood pressure and diabetes as well as a variety of other conditions (Cowie et al.; Harris, 1991; Jones and Rice). Affliction is attributed to the fact that the individuals are "minority," by which is meant biologically different and therefore "defective."

Considering the study of diabetes in African-Americans more closely, it is found that while no risk factors and very few cases of diabetes exist in West Africa, individuals classified as African-Americans are still commonly said to be at "high risk" for developing the disease because of their "racial or ethnic ancestry." The presence of diabetes in these populations has other probable causes that are normally overlooked in research. They are (1) the European genetic background of the African-Americans; (2) poverty and related poor nutrition caused by discrimination; and (3) the high animal-fat content of the dominant northern European diet.

Racial thinking leads researchers to ignore oppression, racism, and discrimination—all of which can implicate the researchers themselves—as well as other cultural and biological factors. Research is confined to allegedly biological problems existing as defects within the afflicted. The real biogenetic makeup of individuals goes unanalyzed while their social identity is blamed for their illness.

Research on the treatments of choice and treatment recommendations in U.S. biomedicine demonstrates that medical and psychiatric diagnoses and therapeutic choices are often made on the basis of patients' social identity, be it race, class, or gender rather than objective need (Brandt, 1985; Ehrenreich and English; Gilman; Good; Lindenbaum and Lock; Osborne and Feit). Historically, this includes the differential use of anesthesia; the poor didn't need it but the wealthy did, as they were more delicate! (Pernick).

The form of intervention in psychiatry, pharmacotherapy, and psychotherapy is today heavily dependent on racial and/or sexual stereotypes rather than on empirical psychiatric signs or symptoms (Katz; Gaines, 1982, 1992a, 1992c; Littlewood). Blacks and Hispanics are often seen as belonging to that group of patients termed *psychologically unsophisticated* or *not psychologically minded* (e.g., Leff; MacKinnon and Michels; Sudack). Psychopharmacotherapy is seen as more "appropriate" for such patients than forms of "talk" therapy.

It should be recalled that U.S. psychiatry in the nineteenth century "found" that psychiatric disorders afflicted black slaves who otherwise "unaccountably" ran away from their masters. This is a historical version of a biological psychiatry and posits that all conditions are biological and will ultimately yield to somatic interventions. Environment, in this view, can be discounted or its consideration delayed until suspected "biological components" can be studied.

In medical research, behavior is also related to race. Medical researchers often choose research topics that implicate behaviors judged as immoral or incautious when dealing with minority populations, for example, number of sex partners, unwed mothers, and drug addiction (Gaines, 1985; Osborne and Feit). In this way, medical research also becomes moral research and supports blame-the-victim thinking.

In the psychiatric literature, neo-evolutionist racial theories lurk behind some assertions. Certain groups, such as the English, are said to be more evolved and psychologically normal (see Leff). In this view, somatization is allegedly less evolved and is characteristic of less developed "traditional" or "primitive" societies. The position inserts a cultural view of emotion and thought into a not-too-implicit neo-evolutionist scheme.

In the West, emotions are believed to be natural, universal, and distinct from cognition. But anthropological research has shown that specific emotions are not universal nor are they naturally distinct from cognitive or bodily states and functions (see Good et al., Lutz, Obeyesekere, Schieffelin, in Kleinman and Good). While highly valued in a very few cultures, psychologization of distress is not "natural," but rather a learned, shared, and transmitted cultural approach (Kleinman). Psychologization is not found in many areas of Europe itself, for example, the Mediterranean and eastern Europe (Gaines, 1992c; Gaines and Farmer; see Good et al. in Kleinman and Good), or in China, Japan, or India (Kleinman and Good; Leslie and Young).

Research on racial differences provides the scientific bases for the maintenance of popular and scientific racial ideology in the United States. This ideology clearly leads to differential evaluation of social actors in medical and nonmedical contexts. As such, biomedical practices can be said to contribute to the social problems caused by racism. These problems include unequal access and poor medical outcomes (Good). The use of racial categories in biomedical research and practice, then, may be seen to breach the medical profession's own primary ethical injunction "to do no harm."

GENES, RACE, AND VIOLENCE. Biomedicine conceives of its domain as the discovery and manipulation of nature (see Gordon, in Lock and Gordon). Its wider culture perceives nature as something to be dominated and controlled (Pike). Ideas of nature, as well as those of difference and inferiority that are encoded in racial and gender identities, greatly affect practice and research in U.S. biomedical sciences. Classes of people believed to be closer to nature are seen as requiring control and guidance, even domination. Such people—among them women, children, non-Anglo or non-Germanic European ethnics (e.g., French, Italian, Spanish, Celtic, and Slavic people), Africans and their descendants, Native Americans, Hispanics, Pacific Islanders—are, in the United States, rather widely believed to be emotional, and therefore dangerous, unpredictable, and wild. Comments about "natural abilities" (intuitive, musical, irrational, fierce, shrewd) or characteristics of particular groups indicate their closeness to nature; they, like animals, are thought to be dominated by instinct and irrationality, not by "reason," a European cultural and masculine virtue (Chesler; Fausto-Sterling; Kleinman and Good; Pike).

The imputation of wildness, impulsiveness, and irrationality is doubtless a culturally constituted defensive projection of aggression that actually exists in the dominant group (Gilman; Pike). It is used to justify control, domination, and even extermination, as with Africans and Native

Americans in the United States and non-German ethnics and the disabled in World War II Germany.

A similar logic appears in contemporary U.S. society. Urban violence, born of repression, discrimination, violence, and poverty, is recast as "genetic predispositions to violence or criminality" in individuals and the groups to which they are ascribed, especially after periods of civil unrest. However, rather obvious examples of genetic predispositions toward criminality and violence in the dominant group are regularly ignored as are centuries of clear provocations of African-Americans.

If researchers were indeed interested in a dispassionate evaluation of genetic components of violence and criminality, it would be appropriate to study people descended from generations of individuals all of whom have committed crimes of a serious nature. In the United States, such a population would be the many immigrants from Russia or Germany, as well as their offspring. Another group of subjects would be the descendants of slave traders and owners. Mass murderers and serial killers in the United States and Europe are virtually always white; their relatives would be suitable subjects of biological research on white criminality. These data might suggest some genetic basis for the inheritance of violent tendencies, if one were to think in racial terms. But researchers on violence and its causes regularly ignore such evidence. It appears that violence and criminality are possible genetic predispositions only when they appear in individuals belonging to specific low-status racial groups.

RACE AND CLINICAL STUDIES. That racial groups are considered unequally in U.S. biomedical science and society is clearly demonstrated by the infamous and tragic Tuskegee syphilis study. In 1932, the U.S. Public Health Service (PHS) began a prospective study of syphilis infection among four hundred rural Alabamans who were black male sharecroppers. The researchers asserted that the study could be a "natural experiment" because it was assumed (for racist reasons) that "such people" were all infected and would not seek treatment for their condition (Brandt, 1978). For these reasons, the PHS argued that it could observe the natural history of syphilis infection in these black men. As it happened, the subjects, who had been unknowingly selected, began to seek treatment almost immediately.

Rather than provide healthcare, the PHS initiated a vast conspiracy to prevent the subjects from receiving care from any source. It conspired with local and state health officials, clinics and hospitals, and the U.S. Army, in which some of the men had enlisted, to prevent disclosure to the subjects of their diagnosis and to prevent treatment of their affliction.

Despite the fact that the natural experimental premise was invalidated in short order, this horrendous project continued over four decades until 1972, when public outcries finally stopped it. Until that time, however, the study was often reported in the medical literature without raising ethical concerns about informed consent, the sometimes fatal use of these human subjects, or the conspiracy to prevent them from receiving efficacious treatments (Brandt, 1978, 1985).

Aside from specific research projects that indicate differential concern for specific groups in the United States, "minorities" in day-to-day medical settings are often underdiagnosed for problems that could be treated (e.g., heart disease) and overdiagnosed for others. For example, blacks are regularly misdiagnosed with schizophrenia. These misdiagnoses lead to confinement and inappropriate pharmacological regimens. Loss of freedom and improper use of powerful psychotropic medications may themselves lead to chronicity in the illnesses that are left untreated, illnesses that led the patient to the attention of health professionals in the first place (see Adebimpe; Mukherjee et al.; Bell and Mehta; Good). This is one means by which medicine creates chronicity of particular disorders as well as increases in the reported incidence of these disorders in a specific population. The circular logic is completed by the subsequent tendency to diagnose in an individual a disorder that is reported as "common" in members of his or her racial or ethnic group.

It is important for a full understanding of the role of racial classifications in the biomedical field to see it as part of a cultural system. This allows for the recognition of both the clearly concerned altruistic practitioners and researchers and the profoundly troubling aspects of racial thought in biomedical practices. In this view, the problems of racial thinking may be seen to arise frequently from the use of popular racial notions by force of tradition—tradition in the Weberian sense, wherein it is one source of authority for human action (Weber). The use of racial categories is thus not necessarily racist.

Conclusions

The U.S. version of human biology is a folk biology that assumes that social categories—"races"—are reflections of nature rather than culture. As a result, biomedical work, as well as public healthcare, is conducted and interpreted in these terms. In clinical practice in U.S. medicine, every patient record begins with three basic bits of information thought to be of critical importance: age, race, and gender (e.g., "A thirty-seven-year-old black female presented with

...". This is a significant part of the discourse of medicine that reconfirms the cultural conceptions that race, age, and sex are natural and empirical realities that make a difference.

Specific forms of communalism, such as racism and sexism, are intrinsic to U.S. society. As a result, they are fundamentally part of its medical institutions, because U.S. medicine is a reflection of the culture that created it. Culturally specific prejudice makes U.S. biomedicine an expression of a particular culture and its history. That culture has held and still expresses empirically problematic and ultimately unethical conceptualizations of human variation. However, neither contemporary medicine nor society remains monocultural; different ethnic and gender voices are being heard advocating what may be seen as more cultural and therefore humane and equal medical-research concerns and treatment. In many scientific fields, the lessons learned from the Nazi atrocities—as well as the inclusion of Jews, African-Americans, and women into collegial relations— has helped to reduce scientific racism and sexism since the 1950s (Barkan). Trends of pluralism begun then continue and expand.

Modern biomedical thought in the United States appears to lag in its understanding of the bases of human differences. The basis is culture, not biology. Even though racial terms are now often exchanged for ethnic ones, the problems persist in biomedicine and related sciences. Ethnicity has a cultural referent, and race has a putatively biological one. The two terms are incommensurate and cannot be used interchangeably.

Intentionally or unintentionally, biomedicine conserves, employs, and disseminates racial and gender-biased conceptions in its theory and practice. Such actions may be seen to derive both from habit and from nefarious intent. Comparisons are at the heart of science. U.S. science, along with U.S. popular society, has always thought that comparisons of black versus white or other races are the more or less "natural" ones to make in a "multiracial" society. Some others yet seek to show one group's superiority over others.

Biomedical enterprises will surely be subject to increasing ethical and practical criticism in the future "both from without and within its cultural tradition by those it fails to serve and those it serves to fail" (Gaines, 1992c). The growing understanding of the cultural biases of the professional medicines (and sciences) of the world suggests that medicines, like their particular medical ethics, reflect local cultural realities. A pluralistic medicine is needed in a multicultural country such as the United States. In such a country, a single medical voice may easily lead to, if not generate, bioethical conflicts. A medicine without cultural understandings, unreflective of its own cultural foundations, is inadequate, and an inadequate medicine cannot be of great help in a multicultural society.

ATWOOD D. GAINES (1995)
BIBLIOGRAPHY REVISED

SEE ALSO: *Bioethics, African-American Perspectives; Biology, Philosophy of; Eugenics; Feminism; Genetic Discrimination; Genetics and Racial Minorities; Genetics and Human Self-Understanding; Holocaust; Human Dignity; Human Nature; Mental Illness: Conceptions of Mental Illness; Minorities as Research Subjects; Psychiatry, Abuses of; Sexism; Women, Historical and Cross-Cultural Perspectives*

BIBLIOGRAPHY

Adebimpe, Victor R. 1981. "Overview: White Norms and Psychiatric Diagnosis of Black Patients." *American Journal of Psychiatry* 138(3): 279–285.

American Association of Physical Anthropologist (AAPA). 1996. "AAPA Statement on Biological Aspects of Race." *American Journal of Physcial Anthropology* 101: 569–570.

Asma, Stephen T. 1995. "Metaphors of Race: Theoretical Presuppositions Behind Racism." *American Philosophical Quarterly* 32(1): 13–29.

Babbit, Susan E., and Campbell, Sue, eds. 1999. *Racism and Philosophy*. Ithaca, NY: Cornell University Press.

Barkan, Elazar. 1992. *The Retreat of Scientific Racism: Changing Concepts of Race in Britain and the United States Between the World Wars*. Cambridge, Eng.: Cambridge University Press.

Bell, Carl C., and Mehta, Harshad. 1980. "The Misdiagnosis of Black Patients with Manic Depressive Illness." *Journal of the National Medical Association* 72(2): 141–145.

Bernasconi, Robert, and Lott, Tommy Lee, eds. 2000. *The Idea of Race*. Indianapolis, IN: Hackett Publishing Co.

Blu, Karen I. 1980. *The Lumbee Problem: The Making of an American Indian People*. Cambridge, Eng.: Cambridge University Press.

Boas, Franz. 1940. *Race, Language and Culture*. New York: Free Press.

Brandt, Allan M. 1978. "Racism and Research: The Case of the Tuskegee Syphilis Study." *Hastings Center Report* 8(6): 21–29.

Brandt, Allan M. 1985. *No Magic Bullet: A Social History of Venereal Disease in the United States Since 1880*. Oxford: Oxford University Press.

Boxill, Bernard, ed. 2001. *Race and Racism*. New York: Oxford University Press.

Chesler, Phyllis. 1972. *Women and Madness*. San Diego: Harcourt Brace Jovanovich.

Cowie, Catherine C.; Port, Friedrich K.; Wolfe, Robert A.; Savage, Peter J.; Moll, Patricia P.; and Hawthorne, Victor M. 1989. "Disparities in Incidence of Diabetic End Stage Renal

Disease According to Race and Type of Diabetes." *New England Journal of Medicine* 321(16): 1074–1079.

DeVos, George A., and Wagatsuma, Hiroshi. 1966. *Japan's Invisible Race: Caste in Culture and Personality.* Berkeley: University of California Press.

Domínguez, Virginia R. 1986. *White by Definition: Social Classification in Creole Louisiana.* New Brunswick, NJ: Rutgers University Press.

Duster, Troy. 1990. *Backdoor to Eugenics.* New York: Routledge.

Eckersley, Robyn. 1998. "Beyond Human Racism." *Environmental Values* 7(2): 165–182.

Ehrenreich, Barbara, and English, Deirdre. 1973. *Complaints and Disorders: The Sexual Politics of Sickness.* Old Westbury, NY: Feminist Press.

Fausto-Sterling, Anne. 1992. *Myths of Gender: Biological Theories About Women and Men,* 2nd edition. New York: Basic Books.

Gaines, Atwood D. 1985. "Alcohol: Cultural Conceptions and Social Behavior Among Urban 'Blacks.'" In *The American Experience with Alcohol: Contrasting Cultural Perspectives,* pp. 171–197, ed. Linda A. Bennett and Genevieve M. Ames. New York: Plenum.

Gaines, Atwood D. 1992a. "From DSM-I to III-R: Voices of Self, Mastery and the Other: A Cultural Constructivist Reading of U.S. Psychiatric Classification." *Social Science and Medicine* 35(1): 3–24.

Gaines, Atwood D. 1992b. "Medical/Psychiatric Knowledge in France and the United States: Culture and Sickness in History and Biology." In *Ethnopsychiatry: The Cultural Construction of Professional and Folk Psychiatries,* pp. 171–201, ed. Atwood D. Gaines. Albany: State University of New York Press.

Gaines, Atwood D., and Farmer, Paul. 1986. "Visible Saints." *Culture, Medicine and Psychiatry* 10(3): 295–330.

Gaines, Atwood D., ed. 1992c. *Ethnopsychiatry: The Cultural Construction of Professional and Folk Psychiatries.* Albany: State University of New York Press.

Garcia, J. L. 1999. "A Philosophical Analysis and the Moral Concept of Racism." *Philosophy and Social Criticism* 25(5): 1–32.

Gilman, Sander L. 1985. "Difference and Pathology: Stereotypes of Sexuality, Race, and Madness." Ithaca, NY: Cornell University Press.

Good, Byron J. 1993. "Culture, Diagnosis and Comorbidity." *Culture, Medicine and Psychiatry* 16(4): 427–446.

Gossett, Thomas F. 1965. *Race: The History of an Idea in America.* New York: Schocken.

Gould, Stephen Jay. 1981. *The Mismeasure of Man.* New York: W. W. Norton.

Hahn, Robert A. 1992. "The State of Federal Health Statistics on Racial and Ethnic Groups." *Journal of the American Medical Association* 267(2): 268–273.

Hahn, Robert A., and Gaines, Atwood D., eds. 1985. *Physicians of Western Medicine: Anthropological Approaches to Theory and Practice.* Dordrecht, Netherlands: D. Reidel.

Hallowell, A. Irving. 1976. "American Indians, White and Black: The Phenomenon of Transculturalization." In *Contributions to Anthropology: Selected Papers of A. Irving Hallowell,* pp. 498–529. Chicago: University of Chicago Press.

Harris, Marvin. 1968. "Race." In *International Encyclopedia of the Social Sciences,* vol. 9, pp. 263–269, ed. David L. Sills. New York: Macmillan.

Harris, Marvin. 1991. "Epidemiological Correlates of NIDDM in Hispanics, Whites, and Blacks in the U.S. Population." *Diabetes Care* 14(7): 639–648.

Hiernaux, Jean. 1970. "The Concept of Race and the Taxonomy of Mankind." In *The Concept of Race,* pp. 29–44, ed. Ashley Montagu. New York: Free Press.

Holloway, Karla F. C. 1996. *Codes of Conduct: Race, Ethics and the Color of Our Character.* Piscataway, NJ: Rutgers University Press.

Jones, Woodrow, and Rice, Mitchell R., eds. 1987. *Health Care Issues in Black America: Policies, Problems, and Prospects.* New York: Greenwood.

Kleinman, Arthur. 1988. *Rethinking Psychiatry: From Cultural Category to Personal Experience.* New York: Free Press.

Kleinman, Arthur, and Good, Byron, J., eds. 1985. *Culture and Depression: Studies in the Anthropology and Cross-Cultural Psychiatry of Affect and Disorder.* Berkeley: University of California Press.

Lang, Berel. 2000. *Race and Racism in Theory and Practice.* Totowa, NJ: Rowman and Littlefield.

Leff, Julian P. 1981. *Psychiatry Around the Globe: A Transcultural View.* New York: Marcel Dekker.

Leslie, Charles M., and Young, Allan, eds. 1993. *Paths to Asian Medical Knowledge.* Berkeley: University of California Press.

Lin, Keh-Ming; Poland, Russell E.; and Chen, C. 1990. "Ethnicity and Psychopharmacology: Recent Findings and Future Research Directions." In *Family, Culture and Psychobiology,* ed. Eliot Sorel. New York: Legas.

Lin, Keh-Ming; Poland, Russell E.; and Lesser, Ira M. 1986. "Ethnicity and Psychopharmacology." *Culture, Medicine and Psychiatry* 10(2): 151–165.

Lindenbaum, Shirley, and Lock, Margaret M., eds. 1993. *Knowledge, Power and Practice: The Anthropology of Medicine and Everyday Life.* Berkeley: University of California Press.

Littlewood, Roland. 1982. *Aliens and Alienists: Ethnic Minorities and Psychiatry.* Harmondsworth, Eng.: Penguin.

Lock, Margaret M., and Gordon, Deborah R., eds. 1988. *Biomedicine Examined.* Dordrecht, Netherlands: Kluwer.

MacIntyre, Alasdair C. 1966. *A Short History of Ethics.* New York: Macmillan.

MacKinnon, Roger A., and Michels, Robert. 1971. *The Psychiatric Interview in Clinical Practice.* Philadelphia: W. B. Saunders.

Mendoza, Ricardo; Smith, Michael W.; Poland, Russell E.; Lin, Keh-Ming; and Strickland, Tony L. 1992. "Ethnic Psychopharmacology: The Hispanic and Native American Perspective." *Psychopharmacology Bulletin* 27(4): 449–461.

Montagu, Ashley. 1964. *Man's Most Dangerous Myth: The Fallacy of Race,* 4th edition, rev. Cleveland: World.

Mukherjee, Sukdeb; Shukla, Sashi; Woodle, Joanne; Rosen, Arnold M.; and Olarte, Silvia. 1983. "The Misdiagnosis of Schizophrenia in Bipolar Patients: A Multiethnic Comparison." *American Journal of Psychiatry* 140(12): 1571–1574.

Naroll, Raoul, and Naroll, Frada, eds. 1973. *Main Currents in Cultural Anthropology.* New York: Appleton-Century-Crofts.

Office of Management and Budget (US) (OMB). 1997. *Race and Ethnic Standards for Federal Statistics and Administrative Reporting.* Washington, D.C.: U.S. Government Printing Office.

Osborne, Newton G., and Feit, Marvin D. 1992. "The Use of Race in Medical Research." *Journal of the American Medical Association* 267(2): 275–279.

Pernick, Martin S. 1985. *A Calculus of Suffering: Pain, Professionalism, and Anesthesia in Nineteenth-Century America.* New York: Columbia University Press.

Pike, Fredrick B. 1992. *The United States and Latin America: Myths and Stereotypes of Civilization and Nature.* Austin: University of Texas Press.

Rex, John, and Mason, David J., eds. 1988. *Theories of Race and Ethnic Relations.* Cambridge, Eng.: Cambridge University Press.

Robins, Lee N., and Regier, Darrel A., eds. 1991. *Psychiatric Disorders in America: The Epidemiologic Catchment Area Study.* New York: Free Press.

Schmid, W. Thomas. 1996. "The Definition of Racism." *Journal of Applied Philosophy* 13(1): 31–40.

Sherwin-White, Adrian Nicholas. 1967. *Racial Prejudice in Imperial Rome.* Cambridge, Eng.: Cambridge University Press.

Stocking, George W. 1968. *Race, Culture and Evolution: Essays in the History of Anthropology.* New York: Free Press.

Sudak, Howard S., ed. 1985. *Clinical Psychiatry.* St. Louis, MO: W. H. Green.

Thomas, Alexander, and Sillen, Samuel. 1972. *Racism and Psychiatry: A Comparison of Germany and America.* Secaucus, NJ: Citadel.

Townsend, John Marshall. 1978. *Cultural Conceptions and Mental Illness.* Chicago: University of Chicago Press.

UNESCO. 1969. *Race and Science.L* New York: Columbia University Press.

Wailoo, Keith. 1991. "'A Disease sui generis': The Origins of Sickle-Cell Anemia and the Emergence of Modern Clinical Research, 1904–1924." *Bulletin of the History of Medicine* 65(2): 185–208.

Ward, Julie K. and Lott, Tommy Lee, eds. 2002. *Philosophers on Race: Critical Essays.* Williston, VT: Blackwell Publishers.

Watts, Elizabeth S. 1981. "The Biological Race Concept and Diseases of Modern Man." In *Biocultural Aspects of Disease,* pp. 3–23, ed. Henry Rothschild and Charles F. Chapman. New York: Academic Press.

Weber, Max. 1978. *Economy and Society,* vol. 1, ed. Guenther Roth and Claus Wittich. Berkeley: University of California Press.

INTERNET RESOURCE

American Anthropological Association. 1998. American Anthropological Association Statement on "Race." Available from <www.aaanet.org/stmts/racepp.htm>.

REHABILITATION MEDICINE

• • •

Rehabilitation medicine encompasses medical, psychosocial, and vocational interventions provided to persons who have experienced some type of functional impairment. Individuals receiving rehabilitation services may have been born with a disabling condition, such as cerebral palsy, spina bifida, muscular dystrophy, or mental retardation; or they may have acquired disability from stroke, spinal cord injury, polio, amputation, cardiovascular disease, acquired immune deficiency syndrome (AIDS), or traumatic brain injury. They may receive rehabilitation treatments at a traditional acute-care hospital, at a hospital specializing in rehabilitation, or at a post-acute facility, sometimes called a *transitional* or *independent living* facility. Increasingly, individuals receive rehabilitation services in their homes through home health agencies or visiting nurses (DeLisa).

Consumers of rehabilitation medicine, especially if their disabilities are acquired rather than congenital, invariably experience intense feelings of anger, rage, helplessness, and worthlessness (Gunther, 1971). Ethical problems arise from the way disability disrupts one's capacity to make autonomous choices and decisions and to develop and sustain meaningful social relationships. The transformation of a self that experiences profound alienation resulting from a disability to a self that can productively engage the world is the ultimate challenge of rehabilitation and prompts many of its ethical considerations.

Certain aspects of contemporary rehabilitation medicine derive from treatment strategies, dating back to the 1920s, for managing job-related injuries. A series of developments associated with World War II, however, shaped rehabilitation medicine as it is known today. Widespread use of penicillin resulted in the survival of seriously injured soldiers. The resultant crowding of nursing homes and chronic-care facilities created an imperative to return wartime casualties either to the front or to meaningful civilian life. President Franklin Roosevelt, himself no stranger to rehabilitation, wrote to Secretary of War Henry Stimson in

1944 that "No overseas casualty [shall] be discharged from the armed forces until he [sic] has received the maximum benefit of hospitalization and convalescent facilities, which must include physical and psychological rehabilitation, vocational guidance, prevocational training and resocialization." Toward the war's end, financier Bernard Baruch and physicians who included Howard Rusk and Henry Kessler established Veterans Administration hospitals that would translate the war experience of rehabilitation into civilian life. Their vision evolved into the comprehensive multidisciplinary approach of rehabilitation that is known today (Berkowitz).

Admission to a rehabilitation facility, typically a few weeks or months after acute hospitalization, anticipates that the individual is medically stable and not at serious risk of a life-threatening episode. Most important, patients admitted to rehabilitation facilities are deemed to have sufficient capacity and "rehabilitation potential" to engage in various therapeutic programs aimed at restoring as much functional ability as possible (Purtilo, 1992). Absence of rehabilitation potential may result in the individual's admission to a long-term-care facility.

Contemporary rehabilitation interventions focus on reducing the disabling effects of physical impairments (e.g., poor motor control, loss of sensorimotor skills, muscle weakness, loss of sensation, paralysis, loss of bowel and bladder control); cognitive impairments (e.g., poor concentration, memory, attention, insight, information processing, problem solving); or behavioral impairments (e.g., emotional disorganization, poor emotional expression, inability to engage in goal-directed behavior, poor interpersonal skills). Because the patient's impairments often appear in combinations or clusters, rehabilitation medicine involves an array of specialized therapies and services to assist patients in overcoming their often multiple functional limitations (Keith).

In acute rehabilitation hospitals, treatments are typically provided by a specially designated team of professionals that, depending on the nature and extent of the patient's impairments, may include a physiatrist (a physician who specializes in physical medicine and rehabilitation), a rehabilitation nurse, a physical therapist, an occupational therapist, a specialist in communicative disorders, a recreational therapist, a psychologist, a social-service specialist, a spiritual adviser, an orthotistprosthetist, a vocational rehabilitation counselor, and perhaps a rehabilitation engineer (Lyth). Length of stay for rehabilitation patients varies according to medical need and the extent of health insurance. Stroke patients commonly spend two to six weeks in acute rehabilitation (Parfenchuck et al.); persons with serious brain injury may spend one to four months (Cope and Hall); and persons

with spinal cord injury may spend three to five months (Apple).

Bioethical Issues

Because the scope of rehabilitation medicine is so broad, and because other entries will focus on bioethical aspects of disability that either follow from or are independent of an individual's formal stay in an in-patient rehabilitation facility, this entry will discuss certain bioethical aspects of rehabilitation medicine as they derive from the provider-patient relationship. Examining how rehabilitation relationships form and evolve illuminates how bioethical ideals such as autonomy, nonmaleficence, beneficence, and justice occur in the context of treating persons with serious disability. The provider-patient models whose bioethical ramifications will be discussed below are the contractual, paternal, educational, and empowering models.

THE CONTRACTUAL MODEL. The contractual model usually refers to the clinician and the patient developing a mutual understanding and accord on the nature of and need for treatment, its probable benefits and risks, and so forth. Informed consent is central in such discussions; the provider of services assumes certain contractual responsibilities to inform and secure consent to treat the patient, while the patient's consent implies an agreement to the conditions of treatment, including reasonable compliance with the treatment program, remunerating the provider, and so on (Caplan et al.).

The rehabilitation patient's engagement in treatment is not passive, as it would be in an acute, surgical scenario. Active and eventually self-directed, it focuses on learning and performing a variety of functional tasks, such as walking, dressing, toileting, and bathing. Nevertheless, the contractual model in acute rehabilitation is immediately qualified by the fact that many rehabilitation patients have sustained organic impairments that substantially interfere with their cognitive ability to make autonomous decisions. Some patients may not be able to concentrate on, understand, evaluate, or process information well enough to make choices and decisions congruent with their welfare. Or the patient may be psychologically devastated by the onset of disability and unwilling to participate in therapy. Certain rehabilitation patients may experience serious cognitive disorganization accompanied by frightened, anxious feelings and regression to childlike levels of behavior, especially with respect to managing their feelings and impulses (Rosenthal).

Although rehabilitation is defined as elective treatment, many patients do not elect it at all. The onset of a disability like stroke, spinal cord injury, or brain injury can be so abrupt and severe that many rehabilitation patients begin to comprehend the nature and extent of their disability only *after* they have been medically stabilized and referred to the rehabilitation environment. There the patient, confronted with the functional challenges that the disability has imposed, may begin to try to make sense out of what has happened and to deal with the fact that some of his or her life expectations may have to be modified. To the extent that patients are cognitively or psychologically unable to manage these situations, their capacity to make autonomous choices is problematic (Purtilo, 1988). Furthermore, the individual who is discharged directly from an acute hospital to a rehabilitation facility, and only then begins to realize his or her circumstances, has not voluntarily assumed the promissory role that is implicit in the contractual model. To view such a patient's subsequent resistance to or noncompliance with the rehabilitation effort as a violation of a contractual agreement overlooks the fact that the patient may never have reflected on or consented to rehabilitation in the first place.

In sum, the contractual model's presumption of an autonomous self who can voluntarily and insightfully contemplate, assume, and fulfill a variety of promises and obligations is hardly congruent with the reality of the acute rehabilitation environment for many patients. From what has been implied above, a more probable model of care, at least in the early stages of recovery from a neurological event, is the one that will be examined next: the paternalistic model.

THE PATERNALISTIC MODEL. Paternalism has been defined as "the interference with a person's liberty of action justified by reasons referring exclusively to the welfare, good, happiness, needs, interests or values of the person being coerced" (Dworkin, p. 65). Once the prevailing model in provider-patient relationships, paternalism has since 1970 come under increasing fire, both from the patient-rights' movement and in the literature of bioethics. Compelling legal justifications for paternalism now condone overriding a patient's decision only when the decision would pose serious harm to the patient or to identifiable others (Jonsen et al.). In acute rehabilitation, justified paternalism is usually predicated on the patient's impaired cognition or psychological disorganization. As Arthur Caplan observed, "If it is true that time is essential in allowing patients to accommodate to the reality of severe impairment, then this would seem … at least for some patients in some settings, to allow for the presence of paternalistic medical care" (1988, p. 315).

Paternalism in acute rehabilitation frequently appears when patients resist complying with their therapeutic program. Patients may object to the time at which they must rise in the morning to begin therapy, the nature and intensity of their therapies, their diet, the kinds of medications they require, the aesthetics of their hospital room, the personalities of other patients in their room, the date of discharge, or the discharge site. Alternatively, some rehabilitation patients will insist on engaging in activities that pose harm to them, such as trying to walk unassisted despite poor balance or muscle weakness.

Paternalistic interventions in certain instances—such as refusing to comply with a clinically depressed, suicidal patient's request for privacy—are easily justified. Paternalism cannot serve as the preferred provider-patient relationship, however, for at least three reasons. First, justifying a paternalistic intervention in rehabilitation on the basis of a patient's cognitive or psychological impairment requires an objective determination of that impairment. If the rehabilitation patient exhibits profoundly impaired memory, extreme confusion, or very poor judgment, he or she has a doubtful claim to self-determination. Yet providers may disagree on which of the patient's decisions are sufficiently problematic to justify a paternalistic decision. Richard Wanlass and his colleagues showed that rehabilitation clinicians do not consistently or reliably apply the labels "mild," "moderate," and "severe" to cognitively impaired patients; Vivian Auerbach and John Banja found that considerable discrepancy exists among physicians, mental-health professionals, and lawyers in distinguishing competent from incompetent decisions made by persons with traumatic brain injury; and Bruce Caplan noted a marked disparity between patient and provider ratings of the patient's mood. In cases of considerable professional disagreement about a patient's "competence" to make decisions or the severity of a patient's cognitive impairment or mood disorder, it is not possible to justify overriding the patient's decision *on those bases.*

A second reason for rejecting a thoroughgoing paternalism in rehabilitation is that providers with paternalistic attitudes risk misinterpreting resistance to therapy as "noncompliant" or "unmanageable." Whatever their therapeutic value, such attitudes and behaviors may indicate the provider's need to be in control (McKnight). When patients resist the provider's ministrations, the provider may become angry or exhibit behaviors destructive to the therapeutic relationship (Gunther, 1987). What may appear to be noncompliant patient behaviors may in fact be the patient's attempt to assert himself or herself, an attempt that perhaps ought to be applauded as an expression of the patient's striving for independence rather than discouraged as inappropriate behavior.

A third reason for rejecting paternalism is that it ultimately runs counter to the rehabilitation ideal of independence. If the goal of rehabilitation is to help the person's movement toward functional independence, then patients ought to begin learning how to assume control of their lives in the rehabilitation environment. Consequently, the rehabilitationist who excludes the patient's input or interest in defining goals and making decisions is stifling the very behavior and attitude he or she is supposed to be cultivating. Indeed, because a profound change in one's bodily image and functional capacity can so seriously affect one's self-image and identity, the ultimate goal of rehabilitation may well be to bring patients to accept themselves as persons with disability and empower them with the necessary will and information to engage the world on somewhat new terms (Banja).

THE EDUCATIONAL MODEL. Empowerment depends in part on various kinds of information the patient will need to function as autonomously as possible. Newly disabled persons require information on and training in managing their activities of daily living (e.g., bathing, grooming, feeding, toileting, and so on); they may also need to learn about creative recreational opportunities, financial planning, social skills training, problem solving, accessing community resources, sexual enjoyment, using community transportation, assertiveness, and perhaps vocational planning or training. Patients should also learn about their rights as rehabilitation consumers before and after rehabilitation discharge: that they have the right to request reasonable changes in the personnel of their teams; that disclosures of otherwise confidential information may occur, for example, to family members or third-party payers; how rehabilitation termination is decided and what evidence is used to determine the nature and length of the rehabilitation; and how they are protected by legislation, such as the Americans with Disabilities Act (Caplan et al.).

Providing this information responds to the same ethical principles requiring that information be imparted to an individual about to undergo surgery. In the latter case, information is treatment-specific, while in the former, the information addresses a host of functional issues. But whereas consent to surgical procedures pertains only to the intervention at issue, consent to rehabilitation reflects a disabled person's willingness to manage his or her life. If no effort is made to stimulate the rehabilitation patient's will to use that information or to be autonomous, then the rehabilitation effort may ultimately fail. Rehabilitation providers not only must convey important information but also must seek to deepen the patient's appreciation of its value and encourage the patient to use it.

THE EMPOWERMENT MODEL. Able-bodied persons frequently confess to being uncomfortable around and having

negative feelings toward individuals with disability. Persons with disability are therefore often isolated, deprived, discriminated against, and generally assigned to dependent roles. Ironically, even public programs presumed to assist persons with disability toward autonomy and independence sometimes foster dependency (McKnight). Persons who receive services from such programs frequently complain of feeling dehumanized, subservient, devalued, and ostracized. Studies of the psychodynamic aspects of relationships among program personnel and clients suggest that program staff may develop a narcissistic feeling of authority from these relationships that is threatened by their clients' acting independently (Mullins). Consequently, it is not surprising that such programs may be perceived by clients as unhealthy.

According to the empowerment model, which is moored in principles of social justice, the goal of rehabilitation is to facilitate the rehabilitation consumer's access to social goods. Necessary elements of this access involve social attitudes and measures that aim at equalizing opportunity. Because persons with disability face limitations on normal functioning, justice theorists like Norman Daniels (1985) argue that a society ought to assume certain duties to make up for the fact that an unequal distribution of disabilities among citizens unfairly handicaps the disabled person's attempts to satisfy his or her life needs. Legislation such as the Americans with Disabilities Act, which calls for reforms in hiring practices, barrier-free architecture, handicapped-accessible public transportation, and the implementation of communication devices in business operations for employees who are speech- or hearing-impaired, is highly responsive to the goal of empowerment.

The robust sense of autonomy explicit in the empowerment model transcends clinical objectives that stop at restoring functional ability. In seeking to enhance the individual's power to control his or her life, the empowerment model aims at liberating the individual's self by respecting and advocating the individual's right to his or her choices, preferences, and decisions. From a therapeutic standpoint, therefore, the provider may have to honor the patient's preferences even if they contradict the therapist's, allow the patient to take reasonable decision-making risks, and be prepared to assist when the patient fails. Most important, the therapist must provide the patient with the tools necessary to seize, maintain, and enjoy control of his or her life.

Because many rehabilitation patients are depressed and despondent over the onset of their disability, various empowering models or strategies have been formulated by mental-health professionals (O'Hara and Harrell). A key ethical challenge for the therapist is determining when patients are reasonably ready or "competent" to gainsay therapeutic recommendations, or when patients can "reasonably" assume the risks inherent in the enjoyment of their moral and constitutional liberties and freedoms (Purtilo, 1988).

Meeting this kind of challenge requires an acute sensitivity on the therapist's part in judging when certain types of paternalistic interventions are warranted versus when patients may assume control and responsibility. While the empowerment model may not object to vesting decision-making authority in the provider at the beginning of rehabilitation, in ideal cases that power is increasingly channeled to the consumer as rehabilitation discharge nears. The goal is for patients to realize their right to engage the world on their terms and to enjoy the self-esteem and dignity of risk that derives from doing so (O'Hara and Harrell).

Familial and Social Obligations

Families play a critical role during the rehabilitation process, not only supporting their loved ones but also learning how to accommodate their needs after rehabilitation discharge. The nature and extent of familial duty that occurs by virtue of a member's becoming disabled is nevertheless problematic. Overwhelmed by the financial and personal toll that caring for someone with serious disability poses, families may feel that the burdens imposed on them by the individual's care needs are unreasonable. If the family defaults, does an individual's misfortune in sustaining a disability impose special obligations on society? The extent to which the disabled person's family assumes the responsibilities of care depends on the family's love, sense of values, and willingness to sacrifice, rather than on legal or constitutional mandates (Callahan). If both family and society repudiate a duty to care for the person with disability, then the rehabilitation itself is jeopardized.

The future of allocating rehabilitation services requires a moral consensus about what disability within human life means and whether and to what extent society has a duty to accommodate the needs of persons with disability. Because such a consensus about disability does not yet exist in contemporary American society, rehabilitation medicine is available largely on the basis of the ability to pay (Brody). Shrinking financial resources may preclude the provision of rehabilitation resources to those who desperately need but cannot afford them. Although condoning such a situation in an egalitarian society seems ethically repugnant (Purtilo, 1992), a marked reluctance, if not downright hostility, exists toward imposing social obligations—such as increased tax revenues—to improve care for persons with disabilities. In the face of moral arguments that the burdens resulting from disability should be lightened by spreading them as widely and equitably as possible, libertarians counter that because "I am not my brother's keeper," others' disability and its rehabilitation are not their concern (Will).

To the extent, however, that able-bodied persons accept the idea of valid social roles for persons with disabilities, social stigmas that have interfered with the latter's participation in mainstream American life may diminish. The implementation of the Americans with Disabilities Act may facilitate this change in attitude because it insists that greater opportunities be made available for persons with disability to enter the economic mainstream of American life. Furthermore, demographic projections indicate an astonishing rate of growth among elderly persons in the United States, many of whom will require rehabilitation services at some point in their lives. To the extent that they can influence the political will, access to rehabilitation resources may expand rather than shrink through legislative enactments.

If moral arguments are not sufficient to justify the allocation of rehabilitation services, certain purely material considerations might compel an examination of the merits of rehabilitation medicine. Extensive research indicates that the social costs of disability without rehabilitation are staggering (Brooks; Davidoff et al.). Reimbursement for rehabilitation services might be straightforward and noncontroversial, then, simply because of its cost-effectiveness.

Appeals to self-interest may also sustain an interest in rehabilitation's merit. As medical technology and improved lifestyle choices result in increased longevity, the need for rehabilitation services will doubtless increase. To the extent that living longer increases the probability of a disabling neurological or musculoskeletal impairment, Americans might seek to protect their own access to rehabilitation services by advocating an entitlement to such access for everyone else.

In any case, rehabilitation's objective of securing independence for its consumers fits admirably into an egalitarian culture's sociopolitical aspirations. Independence for persons with disability is the same thing as independence for the able-bodied: the ability to enjoy life as a chooser of ends and to participate in a just and democratic society. Much to its credit, and perhaps more than any other medical specialty, the ethos of rehabilitation medicine embodies these cherished ideals of individual freedom and liberty.

JOHN D. BANJA (1995)
BIBLIOGRAPHY REVISED

SEE ALSO: *Autonomy; Beneficence; Care; Chronic Illness and Chronic Care; Competence; Disability; Family and Family Medicine; Healthcare Resources, Allocation of: Microallocation; Informed Consent; Life, Quality of; Long-Term Care; Professional-Patient Relationship; Teams, Healthcare*

BIBLIOGRAPHY

Apple, David F., Jr. 1992. "Spinal Cord Injury." In *Rehabilitation Medicine: Contemporary Clinical Perspectives*, pp. 149–171, ed. Gerald F. Fletcher, John Banja, Brigitta Jann, and Steven Wolf. Philadelphia: Lea & Febiger.

Auerbach, Vivian S., and Banja, John D. 1993. "Competency Determinations." In *Medical-Psychiatric Practice*, vol. 2, pp. 515–535, ed. Alan Stoudemire and Barry S. Fogel. Washington, D.C.: American Psychiatric Press.

Banja, John. 1992. "Ethics in Rehabilitation." In *Rehabilitation Medicine: Contemporary Clinical Perspectives*, pp. 269–298, ed. Gerald F. Fletcher, John Banja, Brigitta Jann, and Steven Wolf. Philadelphia: Lea & Febiger.

Berkowitz, Edward D. 1981. "The Federal Government and the Emergence of Rehabilitation Medicine." *Historian* 43(4): 530–545.

Brody, Baruch A. 1988. "Justice in the Allocation of Public Resources to Disabled Citizens." *Archives of Physical Medicine and Rehabilitation* 69(5): 333–336.

Brooks, Neil. 1991. "The Effectiveness of Post-Acute Rehabilitation." *Brain Injury* 5(2): 103–109.

Callahan, Daniel. 1988. "Families as Caregivers: The Limits of Morality." *Archives of Physical Medicine and Rehabilitation* 69(5): 323–328.

Caplan, Arthur L. 1988. "Informed Consent and Provider-Patient Relationships in Rehabilitation Medicine." *Archives of Physical Medicine and Rehabilitation* 69(5): 312–317.

Caplan, Arthur L.; Callahan, Daniel; and Haas, Janet. 1987. "Ethical and Policy Issues in Rehabilitation Medicine." *Hastings Center Report* 17(4)(spec. suppl.): 1–20.

Caplan, Bruce. 1983. "Staff and Patient Perception of Patient Mood." *Rehabilitation Psychology* 28(2): 67–77.

Carse, Alisa L., and Nelson, Hilde Lindemann. 1996. "Rehabilitating Care." *Kennedy Institute of Ethics Journal* 6(1): 19–35.

Cope, D. Nathan, and Hall, Karyl. 1982. "Head Injury Rehabilitation: Benefit of Early Intervention." *Archives of Physical Medicine and Rehabilitation* 63(9): 433–437.

Daniels, Norman. 1985. *Just Health Care.* New York: Cambridge University Press.

Davidoff, Gary N.; Keren, Ofer; Ring, Haim; and Solzi, Pablo. 1991. "Acute Stroke Patients: Long-Term Effects of Rehabilitation and Maintenance of Gains." *Archives of Physical Medicine and Rehabilitation* 72(11): 869–873.

DeLisa, Joel A., ed. 1988. *Rehabilitation Medicine: Principles and Practice.* Philadelphia: Lippincott.

Dworkin, Gerald. 1972. "Paternalism." *Monist* 56(1): 64–84.

Gunther, Meyer S. 1971. "Psychiatric Consultation in a Rehabilitation Hospital: A Regression Hypothesis." *Comprehensive Psychiatry* 12(6): 572–585.

Gunther, Meyer S. 1987. "Catastrophic Illness and the Caregivers: Real Burdens and Solutions with Respect to the Role of the Behavioral Sciences." In *Rehabilitation Psychology Desk Reference,* pp. 219–243, ed. Bruce Caplan. Rockville, MD: Aspen.

Jonsen, Albert R.; Siegler, Mark; and Winslade, William J. 1992. *Clinical Ethics: A Practical Approach to Ethical Decisions in Clinical Medicine,* 3rd edition, pp. 40–65. New York: McGraw-Hill.

Keith, Robert A. 1991. "The Comprehensive Treatment Team in Rehabilitation." *Archives of Physical Medicine and Rehabilitation* 72(5): 269–274.

Kuczewski, Mark G., and Pinkus, Rosa Lynn B. 1999. *An Ethics Casebook for Hospitals: Practical Approaches to Everyday Cases.* Washington, D.C.: Georgetown University Press.

Lyth, Janalee Reineke. 1992. "Models of the Team Approach." In *Rehabilitation Medicine: Contemporary Clinical Perspectives,* pp. 225–242, ed. Gerald F. Fletcher, John Banja, Brigitte Jann, and Steven Wolf. Philadelphia: Lea & Febiger.

Martone, Marilyn. 2001. "Decisionmaking Issues in the Rehabilitation Process." *Hastings Center Report* 31(2): 36–41.

McKnight, John L. 1989. "Do No Harm: Policy Options That Meet Human Needs." *Social Policy* 20(1): 5–14.

Mullins, Larry L. 1989. "Hate Revisited: Power, Envy, and Greed in the Rehabilitation Setting." *Archives of Physical Medicine and Rehabilitation* 70(10): 740–744.

O'Hara, Christiane C., and Harrell, Minnie. 1991. *Rehabilitation with Brain Injury Survivors: An Empowerment Approach.* Gaithersburg, MD: Aspen.

Parfenchuck, Thomas A.; Parziale, John R.; Liberman, Joan R.; Butcher, Robert P.; and Ahern, David K. 1990. "The Evolution of an Acute Care Hospital Unit to a DRG-Exempt Rehabilitation Unit: A Preliminary Communication." *American Journal of Physical Medicine and Rehabilitation* 69(11): 11–15.

Purtilo, Ruth B. 1988. "Ethical Issues in Teamwork: The Context of Rehabilitation." *Archives of Physical Medicine and Rehabilitation* 69(5): 318–322.

Purtilo, Ruth B. 1992. "'Whom to Treat First, and How Much Is Enough?' Ethical Dilemmas That Physical Therapists Confront As They Compare Individual Patients' Needs for Treatment." *International Journal of Technology Assessment in Health Care* 8(1): 26–34.

Rosenthal, Mitchell. 1987. "Traumatic Head Injury: Neurobehavioral Consequences." In *Rehabilitation Psychology Desk Reference,* pp. 37–63, ed. Bruce Caplan. Rockville, MD: Aspen.

Scott, Ronald W. 1998. *Professional Ethics: A Guide for Rehabilitation Professionals.* St Louis, MO: Mosby Yearbook.

Somers, Martha Freeman. 2001. *Spinal Cord Injury: Functional Rehabilitation,* 2nd edition. Englewood Cliffs, NJ: Prentice Hall.

Thorson, Nancy A., ed. 2002. *Clinical Pathways for Medical Rehabilitation.* New York: Aspen Publishers.

Wanlass, Richard L.; Reutter, Susan L.; and Kline, Amy E. 1992. "Communication Among Rehabilitation Staff: 'Mild,' 'Moderate,' or 'Severe' Deficits?" *Archives of Physical Medicine and Rehabilitation* 73(5): 477–481.

Will, George F. 1986. "For the Handicapped, Rights but No Welcome." *Hastings Center Report* 16(3): 5–8.

REPRODUCTIVE TECHNOLOGIES

• • •

I. INTRODUCTION

The development of effective and imaginative approaches to the management of human infertility has focused public attention on the techniques themselves and on their ethical and legal implications. Although differing widely in their complexity, these methods have one characteristic in common: the separation of human reproduction from the act of coitus. An understanding of these reproductive technologies is essential to an overall consideration of the ethical issues surrounding them.

Artificial Insemination

Artificial insemination involves the mechanical placement of spermatozoa into the female reproductive tract. Inseminations are separated into two broad categories: those using the semen of the husband or designated partner (AIH) and those employing semen of a third party, or donor insemination (DI). Because the ethical and moral issues surrounding AIH and DI take on different dimensions, each will be considered separately.

AIH constitutes effective treatment when, for whatever reason, the male partner is unable to ejaculate within the vagina. Some males are unable to ejaculate during coitus but can ejaculate through masturbation or the use of vibratory stimuli. Certain anatomical abnormalities result in faulty semen placement. Hypospadias, a penile abnormality in which the opening of the urethra is located a distance from the tip of the glans penis, causes the ejaculate to be deposited at the periphery of the vagina even when the penis is well

within. Retrograde ejaculation is a condition usually caused by a complication of prostatic surgery resulting in the formation of a channel that causes the ejaculate to be directed away from the penis and retrograded into the bladder. After ejaculation, semen for artificial insemination can be recovered from the bladder by catheterization.

Normal vaginal intercourse may be precluded by congenital or acquired vaginal abnormalities. In rare cases, the vagina is constricted as the result of in utero exposure to the hormone diethylstilbestrol (DES) or possibly by past trauma. Psychological problems in the male or female or both may interfere with normal coital exchange.

In recent years, AIH has been recommended when the semen displays deficiencies in numbers of sperm or their ability to move. Laboratory techniques have been developed to separate and concentrate the most active spermatozoa. These are then introduced into the uterine cavity, closer to the site of fertilization. Intrauterine insemination has been successful in cases of male infertility and in couples with unexplained infertility (Guzick et al.).

TECHNIQUES OF OBTAINING SEMEN. Semen for use in artificial insemination is usually obtained by masturbation. An alternate possibility is intercourse using a plastic condom. Coitus interruptus is not recommended, as the first portion of the ejaculate, which contains the majority of active, motile spermatozoa, is sometimes lost. In cases of obstruction of the vas deferens, which serves as the conduit for spermatozoa, spermatozoa can be obtained surgically from the epididymis, the storage depot for spermatozoa. Specimens so retrieved have been used successfully for in vitro fertilization.

TIMING OF THE INSEMINATION. Placement of spermatozoa should be timed to coincide with the twelve hours immediately preceding ovulation. Approximately twenty-four hours before ovulation, increased levels of luteinizing hormone can be detected in the urine, using a color indicator to predict ovulation. The day-to-day development of the egg-containing ovarian follicle can be monitored with pelvic ultrasound. To enhance the accuracy of ovulation timing still further while causing the release of additional eggs for fertilization, the use of human gonadotropins to induce ovulation has become increasingly popular.

INSEMINATION AND SEX SELECTION. Insemination has also been used with limited success for sex selection. Laboratory methods have been suggested to separate the X-chromosome-bearing (female-producing) from the Y-chromosome-bearing (male-producing) spermatozoa. Success rates in the production of male offspring in the 80 percent range are claimed (van Kooij and van Oost). Such techniques are useful in animal husbandry but do not yield a consistently satisfactory success rate in humans. Sex selection would be useful to avoid a sex-linked genetic disease. Sex preselection based solely on preference for a boy or a girl has much wider social implications.

DONOR INSEMINATION. Donor insemination was mentioned as a method of treating infertility in the nineteenth century. As DI has become more widely used, the legal climate has become more favorable and the status of the offspring much less uncertain. With this has come awareness of the importance of careful counseling and the use of appropriate permission forms. There has not yet been a case in U.S. law in which the anonymous sperm donor has been assigned parental responsibility.

The clinical indications for donor insemination are related mainly to deficiencies in the semen. The most clearcut cases are those in which the male partner suffers from azoospermia (absence of spermatozoa). Indications have been extended to include those in whom some spermatozoa are present but the quality of the specimen is poor. Known hereditary disorders in the male partner, such as Huntington's disease, Tay-Sachs disease, or hemophilia, are also indications for DI.

In vitro fertilization (IVF) has widened the possibility of conception with severely deficient semen. Donor insemination is sometimes used in IVF when there is failure of fertilization using the male partner's specimen.

EVALUATION OF THE COUPLE FOR DONOR INSEMINATION. A couple considering donor insemination should be thoroughly counseled. If either partner has reservations, it is wise to accept these at face value and encourage consideration of other options, including adoption. The man's fertility should be thoroughly evaluated, and efforts made to correct any abnormalities. The woman also should be thoroughly evaluated for factors that might contribute to infertility. Both partners are usually required to review and sign a detailed informed-consent form.

SELECTION AND SCREENING OF DONORS. Unless he expresses willingness to be identified, the donor is anonymous. Occasionally there is a request that a close relative (usually a brother or even a father) be used. In such cases, the couple should be encouraged to consider carefully the potential for future familial conflicts. Analysis of donor semen should meet the normal standards for fertility (ASRM, 2002). The donor should be in excellent health and be screened for any family history of genetic disorders. Serologic tests for syphilis and serum hepatitis B antigen are obtained

initially and after six months. The genitalia are cultured for gonorrhea and chlamydia. An initial screening for the AIDS virus antibodies is performed and repeated after six months because the antibody test for AIDS may not turn positive until several months after infection. Most centers now use frozen semen exclusively. If a donor is providing repeated specimens, periodic reevaluation of his health status is essential. Clinics should maintain records of pregnancies and set a limit on the number of pregnancies any one donor may produce. To decrease the possibility of consanguinity (procreation between close relatives, such as siblings or first cousins) in a given population, an arbitrary limit of ten or fewer pregnancies is recommended.

It is important to maintain confidential donor records, including all of the information on the screening procedures, so that it is available in the future in case it is needed for medical reasons.

TECHNIQUE OF INSEMINATION. The standard insemination involves placing the specimen, thawed if it has been frozen, into the cervical canal by means of a small, flexible tube (cannula). As the vaginal speculum is removed, the remainder of the specimen is placed in the vagina, at the outer cervical canal. The patient remains supine for twenty minutes or so. The specimen may be held in place with a cervical cap, which is removed four to six hours after insemination. For intrauterine insemination, a plastic cannula is passed through the opening of the cervix into the uterine cavity, where the concentrated, pretreated (i.e., washed) spermatozoa are deposited.

CRYOPRESERVATION OF SEMEN. Since the first successful insemination with freeze-stored semen in 1953, this technique has had a significant impact on clinical practice. In the 1970s, formal semen banks were established, largely to address the needs for long-term preservation of the specimens of men who had undergone vasectomy. Semen also is preserved prior to chemotherapy or radiation, which might result in sterility. Although there is no formal reporting system, information accumulated over the years has failed to uncover an increased incidence of genetic defects among the offspring resulting from insemination with cryopreserved semen.

The response of spermatozoa to cryopreservation is unpredictable and varies on an individual basis. Some specimens freeze well and others do not. The pregnancy rate is lower overall with frozen semen. The only reliable way to determine whether a specimen is suitable for cryopreservation is to cryopreserve it, thaw it, and evaluate the impact of the procedure on the quality of sperm motility. Specimens are usually stored in individual straws or small vials so that fractions may be thawed while the remainder is preserved for future use. The Ethics Committee of the American Society for Reproductive Medicine (formerly the American Fertility Society, AFS) has determined that cryopreservation of human semen is ethically and medically acceptable (ASRM, 2002). Most programs use only cryopreserved semen for donor insemination.

In Vitro Fertilization

In vitro fertilization and embryo transfer (IVF-ET) is increasingly common in infertility practice. Initially used exclusively in women with damaged fallopian tubes, the indications for IVF-ET have been extended to include male factor infertility and cases in which no cause for the infertility can be uncovered. Much as artificial insemination separates procreation from the coital act, in vitro fertilization separates fertilization from the normal maternal environment, allowing the initial phases of development to occur outside the reproductive tract, followed by transfer of the embryo into the uterus. The first successful in vitro fertilization was carried out in a normally ovulating woman whose tubes had been surgically removed. A single egg (ovum, oocyte) was obtained by aspiration at the time of laparoscopy. The procedure required general anesthesia and involved placing a telescope through the umbilicus for visualization of the pelvic structures. The oocyte was fertilized in vitro and transferred to the uterus after two days.

In later developments, the ovaries were stimulated with human urinary gonadotropins to induce development of several follicles, each containing an ovum, in a given cycle. This approach is now standard. Follicular development is followed by means of blood estrogen levels, and the size of the growing follicles is measured by ultrasound. When the follicles are judged ready for ovulation, a second hormone, human chorionic gonadotropin, is administered to induce ovulation. This causes further development of the follicles and the maturing of oocytes within them. The oocytes complete their first division in a process referred to as meiosis, releasing half their complement of chromosomes in a small, round structure, the first polar body. The maternal chromosomes are now ready for the second meiotic division, which occurs after the ovum has been penetrated by the spermatozoa. Within two to three hours of the expected time of ovulation, the oocytes are aspirated from their follicles.

In the early phases of IVF development, this was carried out with the aid of the laparoscope. The oocytes were obtained by needle aspiration. Today, ova are obtained by ultrasound-guided transvaginal aspiration. This procedure can be done without general anesthesia, and the overall approach to in vitro fertilization is greatly simplified.

Another major clinical problem in the early phases of IVF development was that occasionally a patient would ovulate before the oocytes could be obtained, and the cycle would have to be canceled. Analogues of the gonadotropin-releasing hormone are now used to prevent this. These analogues are capable of blocking the release of the patient's pituitary gonadotropins, and the ovaries can be brought under the complete control of exogenously administered hormones. The number of follicles that develop varies from patient to patient, and even in the same patient from one cycle to the next. By and large, the aim is to obtain as many oocytes as possible in a given treatment cycle, especially if the couple has selected cryopreservation as a possible option.

IVF treatment is both physically and emotionally demanding. Several visits for hormone determinations and ultrasound are required. Ovum recovery, although relatively safe, is not without complications. Rarely ovarian infection occurs, which can further compromise the fertility status of the patient. This point is particularly pertinent when oocytes are being obtained for donation.

A freshly ejaculated semen specimen is obtained for insemination. The ova are placed in individual containers and mixed with spermatozoa that have been prepared by separating them from the semen and incubating them in a solution designed to enhance their fertilizability. The inseminated ova are cultured for approximately twenty-four hours and then inspected for evidence of fertilization.

Much has been learned about human fertilization through in vitro fertilization. When it is removed from the woman's body, the ovum is surrounded by layers of small, loosely packed cells, the cumulus oophorus. An inner layer of more densely arranged cells, the corona radiata, immediately surrounds the oocyte. These cells interface with the zona pellucida, a translucent protein shell that immediately surrounds the egg. Penetration past these barriers is accomplished through a sequence of interactions between spermatozoa and the ovum and its layers (Kopf and Gerton). When the spermatozoon reaches the zona pellucida, a series of chemical communications occurs. These condition the spermatozoon so that it can penetrate through the zona pellucida. Once past the zona, the spermatozoon attaches to the egg membrane and is then incorporated into the egg cytoplasm, the tail along with the head. The head is then transformed into a pronucleus. The second polar body is released and the nucleus of the egg is transformed into a pronucleus. The pronuclei then join and the chromosomes are intermingled in preparation for the first cell division. Twenty-four hours after insemination, there are two pronuclei and two polar bodies. This constitutes evidence that the penetration has been successful and fertilization is in process. After three days, the embryo has developed to the eight-to sixteen-cell stage and is ready for transfer into the uterus. Transfer is sometimes delayed until day five or six to allow growth to the blastocyst stage.

EMBRYO TRANSFER. The dividing embryos are incorporated into the end of a catheter that is then passed through the cervical opening into the uterine cavity, where they are discharged. The pregnancy rate is progressively improved if more than one embryo is transferred. If more than three are transferred, there is a greatly increased possibility of multiple pregnancy. Twins are not usually a problem, but triplets or more greatly increase the possibility of fetal loss. Therefore, in many IVF programs no more than two fertilized oocytes are transferred in women under age thirty-five and three in the older group. The availability of cryopreservation has made such decisions easier.

Moral Status of the Embryo

The issue of when meaningful human life begins is pivotal in any discussion of IVF. The fertilization process is a complex series of events. The spermatozoon must be exposed to the environment of the female reproductive tract for a period of time before it acquires the ability to penetrate the layers surrounding the recently ovulated oocyte. This process, referred to as *capacitation,* takes between one and two hours in the human. It is reproduced in vitro in the fluids used for sperm preparation. The series of events involving penetration through the zona pellucida requires complex chemical communication between sperm and egg. After the spermatozoon has penetrated into the cytoplasm, completion of fertilization, although increasingly probable, is not assured.

The events that follow, including the formation and subsequent fusion of the pronuclei, occupy more than twenty-four hours. In the natural sequence of events, the conceptus remains in the fallopian tube for approximately three days. At the eight-to-sixteen-cell stage, it is transported into the uterus. There it develops into a fluid-filled structure, the blastocyst, that attaches to the uterine lining, or endometrium, on the sixth to seventh day after fertilization. The blastocyst is incorporated into the endometrium and invades blood vessels. Development occurs rapidly thereafter, but it is not until the fourteenth day that it develops unique characteristics. This coincides with the formation of the primitive streak, a linear region that can be identified on the early embryonic disk; it signals the beginning of the development of a distinct category of cells. Until this point, there is the potential for division into identical twins. Each of the individual cells in the early conceptus has the potential to develop into a complete adult. On or about day five or six,

specialized cells, the trophoblasts, are formed. They provide the point of attachment for the placenta and are essential to the nourishment of the growing embryo. The Ethics Committee of the American Society for Reproductive Medicine applies the term *pre-embryo* to the conceptus through the first two weeks of gestation (AFS). It takes the position that the moral status of the pre-embryo is different from that of either the unfertilized eggs and spermatozoa or the later stages in embryonic development.

Cryopreservation of Pre-embryos

Techniques for freeze-preserving pre-embryos have contributed to the success of human in vitro fertilization and embryo transfer. The incidence of multiple pregnancy, which increases dramatically if more than two to three pre-embryos are transferred, can be reduced with the availability of cryopreservation. Pre-embryos not transferred during the treatment cycle can be used in subsequent spontaneous ovulation cycles. When pregnancy occurs in the initial treatment cycle and pre-embryos have been cryopreserved, a number of future options must be considered. These issues should be reviewed and decisions made before the pre-embryos are frozen. Patients whose response to stimulation clearly indicates that more than three oocytes will be recovered should consider the freezing option well in advance of ovum recovery. Those who for whatever reason, including deeply felt moral reservations, choose not to cryopreserve may wish to have sperm added to no more than three oocytes and have all of the fertilized specimens transferred. Remaining ova can be disposed of in their unfertilized state. Another alternative short of cryopreservation is to fertilize all available ova and select only the best of the resulting pre-embryos, as determined by their appearance and rate of cell division, for replacement, discarding the remainder.

The standard consent form should contain a detailed description of the possibilities to consider if a decision is made to cryopreserve human pre-embryos. As far as is known, cryopreservation of human pre-embryos is not associated with adverse fetal effects. Generally it is agreed that the pre-embryos will be frozen and stored for use in subsequent cycles. Unforeseen situations can occur, such as failure of equipment, although backup freezer systems and liquid-nitrogen holding facilities are usually available in the event of such an occurrence.

In most major centers, the disposition of unused frozen pre-embryos is reviewed in advance of cryopreservation. Handling of these pre-embryos is subject to the couple's joint disposition. They agree that if one partner is unwilling or unable to assume responsibility for the fertilized eggs, the responsibility reverts to the other partner. If that person is not willing or able to assume ownership, the hospital or clinic usually reserves the right to dispose of the pre-embryos in accordance with policies in existence at the time.

Micromanipulation of Oocytes and Embryos In Vitro

Instruments have been developed to allow manipulation of gametes and pre-embryos under magnification. These techniques of micromanipulation have been used extensively in laboratory mammals. More recently they have been applied to human eggs, spermatozoa, and pre-embryos. When the oocyte is not penetrated by spermatozoa that are otherwise apparently normal, micromanipulation can be used to insert a spermatozoon mechanically through the zona pellucida directly into the oocyte itself, a technique known as intracytoplasmic sperm insertion (ICSI). In males with a congenitally obstructed vas deferens, sperm may be recovered directly from the epididymis and used for ICSI. Pregnancies that would otherwise be impossible can occur as a result of these procedures. Because abnormalities in the semen and vas obstruction may be associated with genetic risk factors, these should be considered before proceeding with ICSI (Dohle et al.).

Micromanipulation has been extended to pre-embryos. It has been suggested that the second polar body, the cell that is released from the ovum at the time it is penetrated by the spermatozoon, be removed for chromosome analysis in an effort to determine whether the embryo is genetically normal. This approach could be used in couples at risk of genetic abnormalities and would avoid the onus of a decision to terminate the pregnancy later on. Individual cells have been removed from the embryo for analysis without apparent harm (Tarin and Handyside). Other possibilities may eventually emerge, including the removal and storage of individual cells as clones of the embryo that is transferred. Some of these approaches have not yet attained clinical practicality, but they raise moral, ethical, and legal issues that it would be wise to address now.

Gamete Intrafallopian Tube Transfer

The procedure referred to as gamete intrafallopian tube transfer (GIFT) involves the transfer of freshly recovered ova and conditioned spermatozoa into the fallopian tubes. Thus, fertilization actually occurs in vivo. GIFT is not applicable to all infertility patients. Those with damaged or absent fallopian tubes are obviously not candidates. GIFT has been recommended for couples with unexplained infertility and women with extratubal disease, such as pelvic adhesions or endometriosis. Although fertilization occurs within the fallopian tube, GIFT is certainly assisted reproductive technology and is clearly separated from the coital act. When more than four ova are recovered at the time of a GIFT procedure, one or more are usually fertilized in vitro and cryopreserved for transfer in subsequent cycles. Transfer of the ova and spermatozoa into the fallopian tubes is usually carried out by means of laparoscopy. The success rate following GIFT is now surpassed by that of in vitro fertilization (SART/ASRM). In most centers, GIFT is now largely supplanted by IVF.

Surrogate Gestational Mothers

Human in vitro fertilization has opened the possibility that the resulting pre-embryos can be transferred to a woman other than the woman providing the oocytes. The second woman, referred to variously as a surrogate carrier, a womb mother, a placental mother, or a surrogate gestational mother, provides the gestational but not the genetic component of that pregnancy. Usually arrangements are made for the couple whose egg and sperm produced the embryo to adopt the newborn.

In another type of surrogacy, a husband's spermatozoa are used to inseminate a woman other than his wife. This surrogate mother carries the gestation to term. Agreement is reached before the procedure is carried out that the contracting couple will have custody of the resulting child.

In everyday infertility practice, there are circumstances that seem to justify these procedures. Consider a woman who was born without a uterus but with normal, functioning ovaries. Her husband is normally fertile. The patient's sister had a tubal sterilization after three pregnancies and is healthy in every way. The patient's sister's husband is entirely in agreement with the patient's sister's desire to act as a gestational surrogate mother. Oocytes are obtained from the patient, they are fertilized with her husband's spermatozoa, and the pre-embryos are transferred to her sister's uterus. In this situation we are virtually 100 percent confident that the pregnancy resulted from the procedure and is not an accidental result of coitus between the surrogate and her husband. The offspring is the genetic product of the husband and wife and has no direct genetic relationship to the patient's sister.

Other cases involve the use of a surrogate mother who contributes 50 percent of the chromosomal makeup of the offspring; this represents a more complex situation. The birth mother, who clearly is genetically related to the offspring, will be giving up her newborn child (hers in terms of both birth process and genetics). Indications for the use of a surrogate gestational mother include any condition in which there are functioning ovaries but an absent or nonfunctioning uterus. The uterus may be congenitally absent or may have been removed because of disease; it may be nonfunctional as a result of in utero DES exposure. A surrogate carrier may also be considered if pregnancy is ill-advised for reasons of maternal health. Another issue concerns responsibility for the child in the event that the child is abnormal or damaged as a result of premature birth or birth trauma. There are also issues of the health status and behavior of the surrogate gestational mother during pregnancy. One must consider the impact of drugs or alcohol and the possibility of transmission of diseases. Finally, there is the matter of payment to the surrogate gestational mother. The possibility for exploitation certainly exists.

Oocyte Donation

The clinical indications for the use of donor ova usually are rather straightforward. They include premature menopause and the inability of the wife to produce genetically normal oocytes. On the surface, the ethical issues surrounding the use of donor oocytes should be no different from those involved in the use of donor semen. They are compounded, however, by the risks involved in obtaining oocytes compared with obtaining a semen specimen. For example, ovarian infection could occur following ovum retrieval, which could result in permanent sterility (Tureck et al.). In addition to the cost of the procedures, which is usually borne by the couple requiring the oocytes, there is also the question of payment to the donor for her time, pain, and suffering.

In contrast to spermatozoa, oocytes are difficult to cryopreserve; hence, menstrual cycle coordination between the recipient and the donor is required. Alternatively, donor oocytes may be fertilized with the husband's sperm, and the pre-embryos cryopreserved for future transfer. Sources of donor oocytes include the excess eggs from patients undergoing IVF, oocytes obtained incidental to an operative procedure such as a sterilization, or a specific donation by a relative or close friend. Increasingly, the source of the eggs is a paid "volunteer" (ASRM Ethics Committee). The availability of this technology allows pregnancy in women who are well past the ordinary childbearing age (Sauer, Paulson, and Lobo).

In an effort to improve oocyte quality, cytoplasmic transfer between human oocytes, that is, ooplasm donation, has been attempted. The procedure involves aspirating cytoplasm, the portion of the egg surrounding but not including the nucleus, from a donor egg and injecting it into a recipient egg. Recipient oocytes were deemed to be of poor quality or were recovered from women in their late reproductive years or who previously had a failed IVF cycle. Not unlike some of the early approaches to IVF, the procedure was carried out with minimal basic research background, although in limited studies the technique was found not to impair successful fertilization and cell division in the mouse. Unfortunately, children born as a result of this technique have now exhibited traces of mitochondrial DNA from the donor egg. This foreign cytoplasmic DNA may result in untoward consequences in the future and, defects that are transmitted might be heritable and therefore could be observed in the next generation. Until and unless the safety and efficiency of this approach is established in suitable animal models, this effort to rejuvenate deficient oocytes must be approached with extreme caution.

Conclusion

The techniques employed in what is known as the *new assisted reproductive technologies* are varied and challenging. They range in complexity from seemingly straightforward artificial insemination to micromanipulation of ova, spermatozoa, and pre-embryos—and perhaps, in the future, to treatment of genetic disease by gene insertion in vitro. Just as the techniques vary, so do the ethical issues surrounding them. In no other field is there a greater opportunity for interaction among the physician-scientist, ethicist, moral theologian, social scientist, and legal scholar.

LUIGI MASTROIANNI, JR. (1995)
REVISED BY AUTHOR

SEE ALSO: *Abortion; Adoption; Christianity, Bioethics in; Cloning; Embryo and Fetus; Fetal Research; Genetic Testing and Screening: Reproductive Genetic Testing; Maternal-Fetal Relationship; Moral Status; Transhumanism and Posthumanism; Women, Contemporary Issues of;* and other *Reproductive Technologies* subentries

BIBLIOGRAPHY

American Fertility Society (AFS). Ethics Committee. 1986. "Ethical Considerations of New Reproductive Technology." *Fertility and Sterility* 46(suppl. 1).

American Society for Reproductive Medicine (ASRM). 2002. "2002 Guidelines for Gamete and Embryo Donation." *Fertility and Sterility* 77(6, suppl. 5): S1–S18.

American Society for Reproductive Medicine (ASRM). Ethics Committee. 2000. "Financial Incentives in Recruitment of Oocyte Donors." *Fertility and Sterility* 74(2): 216–220.

Cohen, J.; Scott, R.; Schimmel, T.; et al. 1997. "Birth of Infant after Transfer of Anucleate Donor Oocyte Cytoplasm into Recipient Eggs." *Lancet* 350: 186–187.

Dohle, G. R.; Halley, D. J.; Van Hemel, J. O.; et al. 2002. "Genetic Risk Factors in Infertile Men with Severe Oligozoospermia and Azoospermia." *Human Reproduction* 17: 13–26.

Guzick, D. S.; Carson, S. A.; Coutifaris, C.; et al. 1999. "Efficacy of Superovulation and Intrauterine Insemination in the Treatment of Infertility." *New England Journal of Medicine* 340: 177–183.

Hawes, S. M.; Sapienza, C.; and Latham, K. E. 2002. "Ooplasmic Donation in Humans: The Potential for Epigenic Modifications." *Human Reproduction* 17: 850–852.

Kopf, Gregory S., and Gerton, George L. 1990. "The Mammalian Sperm Acrosome and the Acrosome Reaction." In *The Biology and Chemistry of Mammalian Fertilization,* ed. Paul M. Wasserman. Boca Raton, FL: CRC Press.

Sauer, Mark V.; Paulson, Richard J.; and Lobo, Rogerio A. 1990. "A Preliminary Report on Oocyte Donation Extending Reproductive Potential to Women over 40." *New England Journal of Medicine* 323(17): 1157–1160.

Sauer, Mark V.; Paulson, Richard J.; and Lobo; Rogerio A. 1993. "Pregnancy after Age 50: Application of Oocyte Donation to Women after Natural Menopause." *Lancet* 341(8841): 321–323.

Society for Assisted Reproductive Technology (SART) and the American Society for Reproductive Medicine (ASRM). 2002. "Assisted Reproductive Technology in the United States and Canada: 1998 Results from the American Society for Reproductive Medicine/Society for Assisted Reproductive Technology Registry." *Fertility and Sterility* 77(1): 18–30.

Tarin, Juan J., and Handyside, Alan H. 1993. "Embryo Biopsy Strategies for Preimplantation Diagnosis." *Fertility and Sterility* 59(5): 943–952.

Tureck, Richard W.; Garcia, Celso-Ramon; Blasco, Luis; et al. 1993. "Perioperative Complication Arising after Transvaginal Oocyte Retrieval." *Obstetrics and Gynecology* 81(4): 590–593.

Van Kooij, Roelof J., and van Oost, Bernard A. 1992. "Determination of Sex Ratio for Spermatozoa with a Deoxyribonucleic Acid-Probe and Quinacrine Staining: A Comparison." *Fertility and Sterility* 58(2): 384–386.

Van Steirteghem, A.; Joris, H.; Liu, J.; et al. 1993. "Assisted Fertilization by Subzonal Insemination and Intracytoplasmic Sperm Injection." In *Gamete and Embryo Quality: The Proceedings of the Fourth Organon Round Table Conference, Thessaloniki, Greece, 24–25 June 1993,* ed. Luigi Mastroianni Jr., H. J. T. Coelingh Bennick, S. Suzuki, et al. Carnforth, UK: Parthenon.

II. SEX SELECTION

Sex selection or sex selection techniques usually refer to methods that can be used to help ensure that children are of a specific sex.

Traditional and Scientific Techniques

INFANTICIDE. The simplest, most effective and most morally problematic form of sex selection is infanticide. Before the development of modern techniques the only way to determine the sex of offspring was to kill infants of the undesired sex after birth. This method has been practiced in many areas and at many times in human history.

While some people argue that infanticide can be morally acceptable (Tooley), such support is usually in cases where the individual would have a life that was not worth living. It is implausible to suppose that sex alone could ever be a condition that makes a life not worth living. Therefore even if we accept that there can be justified instances of infanticide we are not committed to permitting infanticide for the purposes of selecting sex.

PRENATAL DIAGNOSIS AND ABORTION. The first genetic testing technologies emerged in the 1950s. They provided the possibility of determining the sex of the fetus in utero (Bubeck).

The development of ultrasound during the 1970s further opened up the possibilities for determining the sex of offspring. It enabled parents to determine the sex of their child in utero and then abort the fetus if it was not of the desired sex. This practice is prevalent in India, China and other countries where a high value is placed upon the first child being male.

PREIMPLANTATION GENETIC DIAGNOSIS AND EMBRYO SELECTION. Preimplantation Genetic Diagnosis (PGD) was developed primarily so that embryos could be tested for genetic abnormalities before implantation. While the intention was to provide a technique for avoiding genetic diseases, it can also be used for determining the sex of the embryo. While PGD does not involve aborting a fetus growing in utero, it can involve discarding unwanted embryos. Some legislative bodies draw a distinction between techniques that are requested for medical as opposed to nonmedical reasons (see The Ethics Committee of the American Society of Reproductive Medicine). The implication is that a technique may be acceptable for a medical reason (PGD for avoiding genetic disease) but unacceptable for nonmedical reasons (PGD for determining the sex of the child). PGD is, next to infanticide, the most effective method of sex selection with an effectiveness of nearly 100 percent.

SPERM SORTING. Rather than determining the sex of a child after it has become an embryo or fetus, sperm sorting techniques attempt to ensure that sperm is sorted by whether they are X chromosome bearing (female) or Y chromosome bearing (male). If this is done successfully then the sperm can be used in artificial insemination or in vitro fertilization (IVF) to help ensure that any resulting child will be of the desired sex.

Sperm swim up or swim through techniques have been in development for some time but have not proved to be effective. More recently greater success rates have been achieved using flow cytometry. Recent figures on the effectiveness of this technique rate have evaluated it as 88 percent effective for determining X chromosome bearing sperm and 73 percent effective for determining Y chromosome bearing sperm. (Microsort.com)

Successful sperm sorting techniques have a number of advantages over other sex selection methods. They are less expensive in that, instead of invasive and potentially harmful techniques such as ultrasound and abortion or PGD and IVF, they involve relatively noninvasive Assisted Insemination. For those who believe that there is something morally significant about aborting a fetus or discarding unwanted embryos, sperm sorting is morally less problematic than PGD or selective abortion.

While these techniques are not likely to become very cheap in the foreseeable future they are already at a cost that could be born by most parents wanting to access this service. For those needing selection services in order to prevent a genetic disease that is carried by the X or Y chromosome, the techniques provide an attractive alternative to other forms of treatment.

Motives for Determining the Sex of the Child

There are a number of reasons why people might want to determine the sex of their child. These reasons range widely in the ethical difficulties that they present.

SOCIAL VERSUS MEDICAL REASONS. At the least problematic end of the spectrum is the intention to determine the sex of offspring so as to avoid the transmission of sex-linked disease. Sperm sorting for this reason is, arguably, morally unproblematic. PGD might also be justifiably used for this reason. Even ultrasound followed by abortion has a morally strong case to support it. However the greatest demand for these technologies comes from those who want to determine the sex of a child for so-called *social reasons.*

SOCIAL REASONS. Social reasons are reasons for wanting sex selection that do not aim at avoiding disease. John

Robertson (2001) thinks that there are two different types of social reason, which, together, constitute the most significant demand for sex selection services. First, there are those who want a child of a particular sex because they already have a number of children of one sex or because they are only having two children and have a preference for one of each sex. A second group is those who have a strong preference for their first child being of a particular sex. The first scenario is often referred to as a *family balancing* reason and is often viewed as less morally problematic than valuing male children more highly.

Ethical Issues Raised by These Technologies

It is vital that the ethical issues raised by sex selection techniques are carefully considered because they are, essentially, techniques that select for particular genes.

Because couples or individuals, typically, request these techniques, the historical worries about eugenics have tended not to be raised in this context. However in contexts where there is a widely held view about the relative worth of a specific sex whether sex selection is a form of eugenics is much less clear. It is because of considerations such as these that Mary Anne Warren coined the term *Gendercide* for the systematic way in which female embryos, fetuses and children are killed and neglected in some parts of the world.

PROCREATIVE AUTONOMY. The main argument for open access to sex selection services is the interest that individuals have in exercising their reproductive autonomy. One key advocate of extending reproductive autonomy to sex selection is Robertson (1994) who borrows from English philosopher and economist John Stuart Mill's (1806–1873) harm principle. Mill theorized that the only reason a society has for restricting the liberty of individuals is if the exercise of that liberty would result in physical harm to others. A key freedom in western democracies is the liberty to make choices about procreation. The level of harm that is required for us to interfere with procreative autonomy is ordinarily very high. Even if there were some harms to others that result from the use of sex selection technologies, they would not be as serious as the harm that would be required to constrain this important liberty. Therefore we should not restrict access to sex selection services.

A second important defense of autonomy comes from German philosopher Immanuel Kant (1724–1804). He argued that persons must always be treated as ends in themselves and never as a means only. There are a number of reasons upon which Kant based his opinion but very significant among them is the status of human beings as project pursuers. It is the ability of persons to pursue projects that bestows value upon these projects. The wish to have children is an important component of the life projects of many people. Not only do people wish to have children they can also desire that those children be of a specific sex. Thus blocking access to sex selection services is a severe limitation upon the interests of individuals who want a child of a specific sex.

Restricting access to sex selection technologies may frustrate more than just the desire to have a child of specific sex. Robertson (2001) argues that in cases where the sex of a child will be the deciding factor in whether that child is born, selection techniques are necessary for parents to exercise their reproductive autonomy.

RESPECTING CHILDREN AS PERSONS.

While Kantian considerations about how we should treat persons can count in favor of sex selection technologies, the same considerations can also be used to argue against them. When parents wish to use sex selection services they do so because they have a preference about what kind of child they want to have. If they use a sex selection technology and have a child the child's sex has been determined to satisfy an end of the parents and the child has been used as an instrument to bring about this end.

There are a number of responses to this argument. A child is either male or female and all sex selection does is to remove the randomness from the natural process. Children are born a specific sex and removing the randomness from this process does not violate them. A possible counter to this argument is to insist that children have the right to an *open future* (Feinberg). An open future means that a child has the right to its own liberties or conceptions of the good that are not intentionally limited by decisions and preferences of others. In the context of sex selection this would derive to the right to have one's sex determined by a random process. In other words, while most of us know that our sex resulted from no human action, persons whose sex has been selected will know that they are a specific gender because of a parental preference.

A second response is to think carefully about what the Kantian theory demands. Kant requires us to treat persons as ends in themselves and never as a means only. In actuality, it would be impossible to never use other persons as a means because it implies that employing the assistance of another to achieve any end negates the personhood of that other. Kantian theory directs us to only use persons for our own ends when this does not violate their status as persons. So while it may be that parents who use sex selection techniques are using their children as a means it is not obvious that this

in consistent with respecting their children as persons. Furthermore it is not clear that "wanting to have a child of a specific sex" for your own reasons is any different from *wanting to have a child* for your own reasons.

SEX-RATIO IMBALANCES.

A major objection to the widespread introduction of sex selection is that it might result in a significant imbalance of male to female sex ratios. A preference about the value of having male children or a male first child could result in many more male babies being born.

In the Western world there is little reason to be concerned about sex ratio imbalances. Research in the United States and the United Kingdom on the preferences of those requesting sex selection services indicates that there was a slight preference for girls over boys (Lui and Rose). A majority of people wishing to access these services in the West do so for family balancing reasons.

However there are good reasons for worrying about sex ratio balance in parts of the world where male children are more highly valued.

IMPLICATIONS OF SEX SELECTION FOR COUNTRIES OR CULTURES WHERE SONS ARE VALUED MORE HIGHLY.

In some parts of the world there is a significant imbalance in the sex ratios. By comparing the sex ratio of North America and Europe to that of Asia and North Africa there are more than 50 million fewer women in China than there should be. When the sub-Saharan ratio is used (where beliefs about the relative importance of women are more similar to Europe and America) there are 44 million in China, 37 million in India and over 100 million world-wide fewer women than there should be (Sen).

The differences in sex ratios are not due solely to sex selection; they are also a result of factors such as poor diet, limited access to healthcare and other environmental factors.

There is every reason to suppose that the introduction of new sex selection services will increase this imbalance. In 1993 ultrasound machines constituted 20 percent of the total Indian market in medical technology (Miller). Sperm sorting technologies could potentially become readily affordable and they are likely to result in an increase in the number of male babies born.

A society having a balanced sex ratio can be considered to be a public good. It is an indicator that there is equity between the sexes in terms of access to healthcare, education, nutrition and wealth. Barbara Miller has suggested that in India sex ratio imbalances correlate with high levels of intersocietal warfare, the frequency of violence, and violence towards women.

THE IMPLICATIONS FOR WOMEN OF A BAN ON SEX SELECTION. While there is a likelihood that better access to sex selection services in India and China will increase the selection of male offspring, it is important to bear in mind the implications of banning access to these technologies. Without access to pre-conception methods of sex selection women may be forced or coerced into aborting fetuses if they are female. There is also the likelihood that some female neonates will be neglected when that child might have been preconception selected as male. The arguments are counterbalanced to some extent by the fact that the increased use of these technologies might make it easier for these practices to continue and will do little to rectify the value system which makes them possible.

IS THE MOTIVATION SEXIST? OR ARE SOME REASONS MORALLY ACCEPTABLE? On one level it is hard to deny that sex selection is sexist because it is a practice that involves acting on a preference to have a child of a determinate sex. This implies that having a child of a particular sex is in some way better, according to the person with that preference. If a person did not believe that having a child of a specific sex would be better, they would have no reason for wanting a child of a specific sex.

The problem with this analysis is that it implies that any preference that has sex as a distinguishing feature is sexist. This is absurd because it implies that a heterosexual woman who has a preference for cohabitating with a man is sexist. Sexism is the making of morally relevant discriminations on the basis of morally irrelevant features. On this view if parents want to have a female child because they already have a male child and will only have two children, their preference is not sexist; the preference is not based upon believing that there is anything inherently more valuable about male children.

While there are some reasons for wanting to select the sex of a child that are sexist and therefore morally unacceptable, whether society should stop people from acting upon these reasons is another question.

Some justifications people give for their actions are so immoral that we might consider them *illegitimate* reasons—or reasons that are immoral to the extent that a liberal democracy does not need to respect their legitimacy. Profoundly sexist beliefs fall into the class of reasons that we might consider to be illegitimate.

However if a couple wishes to select the sex of their child for sexist reasons it is unclear whether allowing them access to sex selection services will make things any worse or perpetuate sexism. Failing to allow the couple access to these services may not do anything to change their beliefs about the relative worth of male and female children.

GROWING TECHNOLOGIZATION OF REPRODUCTION. Sex selection technologies are part of the growing trend towards the technologization of reproduction. Reproduction used to occur only naturally and within the context of a family unit. Care and concern in parenting has always been the province of traditional family units and technologization of reproduction might be a threat to this important human institution.

While the values that surround nurturing our children are of great value and ought not be placed at risk, it is unfair to single out sex selection technologies. If the growing technologization of reproduction is a serious problem then the response ought to be to place restrictions on all new reproductive technologies.

That there is a broad spectrum of technologization of reproductive services must be considered. At one end are the relatively low-tech practices of artificial insemination and at the other technologies such as PGD. Sex selection by sperm sorting is closer to the low-tech end of the spectrum and therefore does not have the same potential to technologize reproduction as do technologies like PGD.

INAPPROPRIATE USE OF MEDICAL TECHNOLOGY. Sex selection for social reasons is not a healthcare need. We can plausibly think of infertility as constituting a healthcare need because it is a deviation from a capacity that people of childbearing age usually have. But the capacity to determine sex is over and above normal human capacity. Sex selection is more like cosmetic surgery or other services that can be provided by physicians. Given that there are morally problematic reasons for wanting these services, reproductive specialists need to consider whether this is an appropriate use of their resources and expertise (see Dresser). The concern regarding the appropriate use of medical resources can be partially addressed if sex selection services are privately funded and do not result in any person not receiving treatment for a medical condition. However the issue of whether sex selection services are something that the medical profession ought to be using its knowledge and skill to provide is more difficult to resolve.

THE WELFARE OF THE SEX SELECTED CHILD. A major objection to sex selection technologies is that they may result in harm to children. There are a number of ways in which harm may result.

First, if a sex selection technique is used and fails, the child that results may be neglected or be psychologically harmed by the knowledge that he or she is not the sex that the parents wanted. This consideration can be also be used as an argument for sex selection technologies. If a child will be harmed if he or she is not of the desired sex, then it is better to ensure that the parents have a child of the sex that they want.

Second, if parents have strong views about the way in which children of a certain sex ought to be raised, a child of the undesired sex may be born into an overly restrictive environment.

Third, sex selection techniques can carry risks to the child that may result. At this point in time there is no evidence to suggest that there are harms to children born after sperm sorting interventions. PGD may carry some risks to resulting children. When PGD is used to predict disease the benefit may offset the risk of the technique, but when it is used in selecting sex, determining the value of the benefit in relation to the risk is more problematic.

Sex selection techniques present a broad range of ethical issues. Many objections can be turned into arguments for sex selection. However, some reasons for wanting sex selection are undoubtedly unethical. Moreover, the consequences of sex selection may justify regulation, if not prohibition.

JOHN MCMILLAN

SEE ALSO: *Abortion; Adoption; Christianity, Bioethics in; Cloning; Embryo and Fetus; Family and Family Medicine; Feminism; Fetal Research; Genetic Counseling; Genetic Testing and Screening: Reproductive Genetic Testing; Judaism, Bioethics in; Maternal-Fetal Relationship; Moral Status; Population Ethics; Sexism; Transhumanism and Posthumanism; Women, Contemporary Issues of; and other Reproductive Technologies subentries*

BIBLIOGRAPHY

Bubeck, Diemut. 2002. "Sex Selection: The Feminist Response." In *A Companion to Genethics,* ed. Justine Burley and John Harris. Oxford: Blackwell Publishers Limited.

Buchanan, Allen; Brock, Dan; Daniels, Norman; et al. 2000. *From Chance to Choice: Genetics and Justice.* Cambridge, Eng.: Cambridge University Press.

Dresser, Rebecca. 2001. "Cosmetic Reproductive Services and Professional Integrity." *American Journal of Bioethics* 1(1): 11–12.

Ethics Committee of the American Society of Reproductive Medicine. 1999. "Sex Selection and Preimplanatation Genetic Diagnosis." *Fertility Sterility* 72: 595–598.

Feinberg, Joel. 1980. "The Child's Right to an Open Future." In *Whose Child? Children's Rights, Parental Authority and State Power,* ed. W. Aiken and H. LaFollette. Totowa, NJ: Rowman and Littlefield.

Kant, Immanuel. 1997 (1785). *Groundwork of the Metaphysics of Morals,* tr. and ed. Mary Gregor. Cambridge, Eng.: Cambridge University Press.

Lui, P., and Rose, G. 1995. "Social Aspects of > 800 Couples Coming Forward for Gender Selection of their Children." *Human Reproduction* 10: 968–971.

Mill, John Stuart. 1991 (1859). *On Liberty and Other Essays,* ed. John Gray. Oxford: Oxford University Press.

Miller, Barbara. 1997. *The Endangered Sex: Neglect of Female Children in Rural North India.* Oxford: Oxford University Press.

Robertson, John. 1994. *Children of Choice: Freedom and the New Reproductive Technologies.* Princeton, NJ: Princeton University Press.

Robertson, John. 2001. "Preconception Gender Selection." *American Journal of Bioethics* 1(1): 2–9.

Savulescu, Julian. 2001. "In Defense of Selection for Nondisease Genes." *American Journal of Bioethics* 1(1): 16–19.

Sen, Amartya. 1995. "Gender Inequality and Theories of Justice" In *Women, Culture and Development: A Study of Human Capabilities,* ed. Martha Nussbaum and Jonathan Glover. New York: Oxford University Press.

Steinbock, Bonnie. 2002. "Sex Selection: Not Obviously Wrong." *Hastings Center Report* 32(1): 23–28.

Tooley, Michael. 1983. *Abortion and Infanticide.* Oxford: Clarendon Press.

Warren, Mary Anne. 1985. *Gendercide.* Totowa, NJ: Rowman and Littlefield Publishing.

INTERNET RESOURCE

Genetics and IVF Institute. 2003. "MicroSort Current Results." Available from <Microsort.com>.

III. FERTILITY DRUGS

The diagnosis and treatment of infertility in humans is a complex matter. The trend has been to regard infertility as a problem that a couple faces, not an issue that rests with the man or the woman alone. Infertility is generally defined as the inability to achieve a pregnancy after one year of unprotected intercourse (Office of Technology and Assessment). There are a number of approaches to the treatment of infertility, one of which is the use of fertility drugs. Some aspects of these drugs, however, are ethically troublesome or controversial.

The causes of infertility in men are much less understood than the causes in women. Historically, the inability to become pregnant and have a healthy child has been viewed

TABLE 1

Summary of Drugs Used to Stimulate Ovulation

Drug Name	Use	Side Effects
Clomiphene citrate	Mildest drug used to induce ovulation	Headaches, blurred vision Hot flashes Enlarged ovaries Abdominal discomfort Rarely, ovarian hyperstimulation syndrome Dry, thick cervical mucus Luteal phase defect Slightly increased risk of miscarriage Increased risk of multiple births Increased ovarian cancer risk?
Pituitary gonadotropins (FSH and LH)	Strongest drugs used to induce ovulation	Redness/swelling at injection site Mood swings, depression Enlarged ovaries Abdominal distention/pain Ovarian hyperstimulation syndrome (may be severe) Increased risk of ectopic pregnancy Increased risk of miscarriage Increased risk of prematurity Increased risk of multiple births Increased ovarian cancer risk?
Human chorionic gonadotropin (hCG)	Spurs release of oocytes	False positive pregnancy test if given late in cycle
Gonadotropin-releasing hormone (GnRH)	Induces ovulation in cases of certain hormone deficiencies	Redness, swelling at catheter site Headaches, nausea Slight risk of ovarian hyperstimulation syndrome Slight risk of multiple births
GnRH analogs	Disrupts normal cycling to allow greater control over ovarian stimulation	Hot flashes Vaginal dryness, painful intercourse Insomnia, mood swings Bone loss (with lengthy use)

SOURCE: Table reprinted with permission from The New York State Task Force on Life and the Law, Assisted Reproduction, 1998, pp. 43–44.

as a woman's problem, and initial attempts to treat infertility were (and often still are) aimed at the woman—even in the absence of the most basic assessments of the presence of viable sperm in the man. In a 1998 report, the American Society for Reproductive Medicine, the main professional association for infertility specialists in the United States, stated that: "Prior to embarking on a course of induction of ovulation with exogenous gonadotropins (originating outside of the ovaries or testes), other fertility factors should be defined and treated as required. Screening tests for these factors should include at least one semen analysis and a hysterosalpingogram (radiography of the uterus and

oviducts using a contrast medium) or laparoscopy and hysteroscopy" (p. 2).

Given that one of the earliest and most basic elements in the initiation of a pregnancy is the formation of an embryo as a result of fertilization of an oocyte (egg) in a woman, infertility problems are often traced to ovulatory problems—that is, any biological or structural impairments in the ability to ovulate or release one or more oocytes during the menstrual cycle. Implantation, the process of attachment of the early embryo to the uterine wall, is also a crucial step in the development of a pregnancy, but implantation problems are not well understood, and thus not treated with drug therapy.

There are a number of reasons why a clinician might want to provoke increased ovulatory activity in the female (at her request), including: (1) to increase the likelihood that fertilization will take place naturally, or *in vivo* (in the body of the woman), as a result of usual intercourse or artificial insemination; and (2) to aspirate (remove by suction) oocytes from the woman for donation to another infertile woman, for research, or for attempts to create embryos via *in vitro* fertilization (IVF) for donation, research, or transfer back to the uterus for possible implantation, pregnancy, and birth (National Advisory Board on Ethics in Reproduction).

A Brief History of Fertility Drug Development

Drug therapy to treat infertility in women started in the 1930s, when the relationship between the normal menstrual cycle and ovarian and pituitary function began to be understood. It was discovered that "the pituitary gonadotropin follicle stimulating hormone (FSH) and luteinizing hormone (LH) stimulate follicle growth in the ovary producing estrogen, and this influenced endometrial growth in the uterus" (Leibowitz and Hoffman, p. 203). This led to scientific efforts to obtain gonadotropin extracts. Serum from pregnant mares was the source of the first manufactured gonadotropin (PMG, or pregnant mare gonadotropin), an approach that was eventually abandoned because of the threat of allergic response in humans injected with animal protein (Lunenfeld). Human menopausal gonadotropins (HMGs) were developed in the 1950s using extracts from postmenopausal women.

Since the 1960s, a series of drugs have been discovered, synthesized, and developed to promote or provoke ovulatory activity in women. These drugs are generally labeled *fertility drugs,* and the basic types are reviewed in Table 1. Fertility drugs for men are those that promote and enhance ejaculatory activity (e.g., Viagra), although there are no drug remedies for oligospermia (low sperm count) and azoospermia (no sperm in the semen). More recently, for women, naturally occurring agents to stimulate fertility are being replaced by synthetic agents that are highly purified and designed to reduce side effects.

Economic Considerations

There are economic considerations involved in the use of fertility drugs because, in most U.S. states, patients must pay for these drugs themselves (in the absence of third party reimbursement). In fact, it has often been suggested that cost influences the choice of infertility treatment. Drug therapy alone may cost as much as 3,000, which is still considerably cheaper than cycles of *in vitro* fertilization, which, as of 2002, costs between $8,000 and $10,000 per cycle (Jain et. al.). In addition, there are global economic issues that influence the delivery of this care. Drugs to treat infertility have historically been considerably cheaper in Mexico, for example, and individuals or couples may travel outside of the United States to have their prescriptions filled at a lower cost (Kutteh).

Risks and Ethical Issues

There are two distinct steps in drug regimens to stimulate ovulation. The first step is to promote the actual development of oocytes within the ovarian follicles. The second is to administer drugs that provoke the release of oocytes for purposes of retrieval or natural transit through the fallopian tube. The hazards associated with drug use for this purpose include: (1) the likelihood that a large number of follicles may form and rupture at once, which increases the chances that a number of oocytes may be fertilized, resulting in a multiple birth; and (2) the likelihood that ovulation in large numbers will increase the chances of an ectopic pregnancy (a pregnancy that takes place outside of the uterus, often in the fallopian tube). Ectopic pregnancies are life threatening and considered an adverse event in pregnancy management or infertility treatment. Even in a controlled situation, ovarian stimulation entails both known and theoretical risks.

Ovarian hyperstimulation syndrome (OHSS) is a potential complication of ovarian stimulation with exogenous gonadotropins. OHSS can be classified as mild, moderate, or severe (ASRM, 1998). The pathophysiology of this syndrome is not well understood, but it seems to be caused by "increased capillary permeability, which allows major fluid shifts from the intravascular compartment to the extravascular space within the follicle and ovary" (Gianaroli et al., p. 175). Physical symptoms that OHSS might be occurring include: a weight gain of one to two pounds or more daily after human chorionic gonadotropin (hGC) has been administered, severe abdominal pain, nausea, vomiting, or diarrhea (Leibowitz and Hoffman, p. 208). In addition, a concentration of red blood cells can lead to thromboembolic events, electrolyte imbalance, oliguria (low production of urine), shock, or death in 1 percent of women (Miller and Hoffman). It is important to note that ovarian stimulation is sometimes provided by physicians who are not infertility specialists (Dresser), and thus may not have the depth of expertise to judge the dosage of these powerful drugs. They may also not have a sonogram available to view developing follicles.

There has been considerable controversy about a possible relationship between cancer and infertility treatment. However, according to *Pharmacotherapy, A Pathophysiologic Approach* (2002), by Joseph Dipiro et al., "an association between fertility agents and the risk of breast and ovarian cancers has not been confirmed and more studies are needed to clarify any link between infertility treatment and ovarian cancer." (p. 1440).

Multiple Births

At first glance, a multiple birth might be regarded as a welcome event by those who are seeking to remedy the problem of infertility and build their families. Multiple births have been a consistent outcome of infertility treatment using drugs to induce ovulation, and also as a result of *in vitro* fertilization. An increase in the incidence of twins, triplets, and higher multiple births over that observed in the normal pregnant population has been a steady feature of IVF since the birth of the first IVF baby, Louise Brown, in 1978. It has been observed that many infertile couples are delighted on learning that they will be the parents of twins, partly because they can have two children without having to undergo infertility treatment twice. But there are hazards associated with multiple gestation and births, especially when the pregnancy results in the birth of super-multiples (quadruplets or above). The primary hazard associated with multiple gestation and birth is premature birth. The low birthweight of premature babies poses a significant risk to these infants.

The incidence of triplet or higher-order multiples has gone up from 29 per 100,000 live births in 1971 to 174 per 100,000 live births in 1997 (U.S. Centers for Disease Control, 2000). Of these, it is believed that approximately 20 percent are spontaneously conceived, with the remaining 80 percent evenly split between conception by ovarian stimulation and conception by other assisted-reproductive technologies (ARTs). A more recent study of state-specific use of assisted reproductive technologies in 1996 and 1998 indicates that the use of ART is increasing in most states, and that more than half of the infants born as a result are multiple births (U.S. Centers for Disease Control, 2002).

Except in the case of spontaneous twinning, high order multiple births can be minimized in the course of infertility treatment. If a clinician notes that in a given cycle a large number of follicles are maturing, the woman or the couple can be so advised and skip intercourse until the next cycle. Another possibility is to transfer only a small number of embryos back to the uterus for possible implantation in the process of IVF. The United Kingdom, for example, limits the number of transferred embryos to two (Human Fertilisation and Embryology Authority).

Clincally and ethically, the most controversial strategy for avoiding multiple births is reducing the number of fetuses in utero after the pregnancy is underway, which provides more space for a smaller number of fetuses to grow and develop. Although reducing the number of fetuses in utero is not objectionable to some, it can be particularly traumatic for a couple who have been trying to conceive to then be faced with the choice of whether or not to remove some of the fetuses. From a clinical standpoint, multifetal-pregnancy reduction poses serious risks, including the loss of the entire pregnancy. The risk of pregnancy loss increases with the number of fetuses (Alexander; Evans). It is therefore preferable to avoid or prevent the development of a high-order multiple pregnancy in the first place through transfer of only a small number of embryos via IVF, or through the careful monitoring of maturing follicles occurring as a result of ovulation induction (White and Leuthner).

In conclusion, the overriding ethical objective in the use of fertility drugs is to facilitate fertility without causing harm. From a clinical standpoint, this is a balancing act based on careful physical assessment of the couple (and primarily the woman) involved. Ethical practice in this area also involves careful counseling to ensure that the risks are understood and that careful choices are made. The goal of achieving pregnancy and birth must be balanced against the likely health and well-being of children who are born, as well as the ongoing physical and emotional health of the woman and family. To this end, fertility drugs cannot be used carelessly, and pregnancy and number of births alone, particularly in the case of supermultiples, cannot be the sole objectives.

GLADYS B. WHITE

SEE ALSO: *Abortion; Adoption; Christianity, Bioethics in; Cloning; Embryo and Fetus; Feminism; Fetal Research; Genetic Counseling; Genetic Testing and Screening: Reproductive Genetic Testing; Islam, Bioethics in; Judaism, Bioethics in; Maternal-Fetal Relationship; Moral Status; Population Ethics; Sexism; Transhumanism and Posthumanism; Women, Contemporary Issues of; and other Reproductive Technologies subentries*

BIBLIOGRAPHY

Alexander, J. M.; Hammond, K. R.; and Steinkampf, M. P. 1996. "Multifetal Reduction of High-Order Multiple Pregnancy: Comparison of Obstetrical Outcome with Nonreduced Twin Gestations," *Fertility and Sterility* 66: 1–12.

American Society for Reproductive Medicine. 1995. *Ovulation Drugs: A Guide for Patients.* Birmingham, AL: Author.

American Society for Reproductive Medicine. 1998. *Induction of Ovarian Follicle Development and Ovulation with Exogenous Gonadotropins, A Practice Committee Report.* Birmingham, AL: Author.

Dipiro, Joseph I.; Talbert, Robert L.; Yee, Gary C.; et al. 2002. *Pharmacotherapy, A Pathophysiologic Approach,* 5th edition. New York: McGraw-Hill.

Dresser, Rebecca. 2000. "Regulating Assisted Reproduction," *Hastings Center Report* 30(6): 26–27.

Evans, Mark I. 1998. "What are the Ethical and Technical Problems Associated with Multifetal Pregnancy Reduction?" *Clinical Obstetrics and Gynecology* 4: 47–54.

Gianaroli, L.; Ferraretti, A. P.; and Fiorentino, A. 1996. "The Ovarian Hyperstimulation Syndrome." *Reproductive Medicine Review* 5(3): 169–184.

Human Fertilisation and Embryology Authority. 1995. *Annual Report.* London: Author.

Jain, Tarun; Harlow, Bernard L.; and Hornstein, Mark D. 2002. "Insurance Coverage and Outcomes of In Vitro Fertilization." *New England Journal of Medicine* 347(9): 661–666.

Leibowitz, Deborah, and Hoffman, Janet. 2000. "Fertility Drug Therapies: Past, Present, and Future." *Journal of Obstetrical, Gynecological, and Neonatal Nursing* 29(2): 201–210.

Lunenfeld, B. 1993. "Induction of Ovulation with Gonadotropins: Past, Present, and Future," In *Pioneers in In Vitro Fertilization,* ed. A. Aberda, R. Gn, and H. Vermer. New York: Parthenon.

Miller, M., and Hoffman, D. 1990. "Ovulation Induction," In *Principles and Practice of Endocrinology and Metabolism,* ed. K. L. Becker. Phildelphia: Lippincott.

National Advisory Board on Ethics in Reproduction. 1996. "Report and Recommendations on Oocyte Donation by the National Advisory Board on Ethics in Reproduction." In *New Ways of Making Babies, The Case of Egg Donation.* Bloomington: Indiana University Press.

New York State Task Force on Life and the Law. 1998. *Assisted Reproductive Technologies, Analysis and Recommendations for Public Policy.* New York: Author.

Office of Technology Assessment of the U.S. Congress. 1988. *Infertility: Medical and Social Choices.* Washington, D.C.: U.S. Government Printing Office.

Seibel, M., and Crockin, S. L., eds. 1996. *Family Building through Egg and Sperm Donation: Medical, Legal and Ethical Issues.* Sudbury, MA: Jones and Bartlett.

U.S. Centers for Disease Control and Prevention. 2000. "Contribution of Assisted Reproductive Technology and Ovulation-Inducing Drugs to Triplet and Higher Order Multiple Births—United States, 1980–1997." *Morbidity and Mortality Weekly Report* 49(24): 535–538.

U.S. Centers for Disease Control and Prevention. 2002. "Use of Assisted Reproductive Technology—United States, 1996 and 1998." *Morbidity and Mortality Weekly Report* 51(05): 97–101.

White, G. B., and Leuthner, S. R. 2001. "Infertility Treatment and Neonatal Care: The Ethical Obligation to Transcend Specialty Practice in the Interest of Reducing Multiple Births." *Journal of Clinical Ethics* 12(3): 223–230.

IV. LEGAL AND REGULATORY ISSUES

Reproductive freedom is not a simple concept. Encompassing far more than abortion, it also includes the choice of whether and with whom to procreate, how many times to procreate, and by what means. It includes the choice of the social context (e.g., marital, communal, or solitary) in which the reproduction takes place and, to some extent, the characteristics of the children people will have (gender, presence or absence of certain disease). It is grounded, for some moral philosophers, in self-determination, individual welfare, and equality of expectation and opportunity (Brock).

Noncoital reproduction, that is, reproduction achieved despite the absence of sexual intercourse, allows single, homosexual, and infertile people to start and rear families. Often, it entails such controversial techniques as extracorporeal maintenance of an embryo, screening and storage of gametes, or the reproductive assistance of men and women who do not plan to maintain a relationship with the child they help to conceive or gestate.

Thus, new reproductive technologies enable individuals to exercise more reproductive choices. This, in turn, invites exploration of the depths of cultural relativism and the meaning of genetic linkage; the preference for the heterosexual couple as the paradigm for family life; the role of the state as the regulator versus facilitator of individual aspirations; and the role of the state and the professional as the gatekeeper to the technologies that permit people to circumvent infertility or conventional forms of procreation.

Under U.S. law, states can outlaw or regulate certain aspects of reproductive technologies. Areas for possible state intervention include protection of the extracorporeal embryo; protection of patients (and their resulting children) who seek to use reproductive technologies; regulation of contract (i.e., *surrogate*) motherhood; definition of family forms and familial relationships in light of gamete transfers and use of contract birth mothers; and limitation on commercialization of the techniques. But the extent to which states can ban or regulate noncoital reproduction depends on the extent to which procreation is protected by state and federal constitutions, and the extent to which ancillary practices, such as payment for gametes or services of a contract mother, are viewed as part of the act of procreation or as independent acts of commercial negotiation.

In the United States, the more zealously procreation is guarded by constitutional guarantees and the more broadly the definition of procreation is drawn, the more compelling and narrowly drawn must be state efforts to restrict use of noncoital procreation. Those restrictions, when they exist, will be manifested in both common law and statutory law, usually with regard to the fields of contracts, property, or family law. Because the details of such law vary tremendously from state to state, this article focuses primarily on the overarching constitutional issues that limit state policymaking and lawmaking in this field, and compares national responses.

Is There an Affirmative Right to Procreate?

The right to procreate, that is, the right to bear or beget a child, appears to be one of the rights implied by the U.S. Constitution. It is grounded in both individual liberty (*Skinner v. Oklahoma*, 1942) and the integrity of the family unit (*Meyer v. Nebraska*, 1923), and is viewed as a "fundamental right" (*Griswold v. Connecticut*, 1965), one that is essential to notions of liberty and justice (*Eisenstadt v. Baird*, 1972).

The U.S. Supreme court has not explicitly considered whether there is a positive right to procreate—that is, whether every individual has a right to actually bear or beget a child and thereby has a claim on the community for necessary assistance in this endeavor. It has, however, considered a wide range of related issues, including the right of a state to interfere with procreative ability by forcible sterilization (*Skinner v. Oklahoma*, 1942), the right of individuals to prevent conception or to terminate a pregnancy (*Roe v. Wade*, 1973; *Webster v. Reproductive Services*, 1989; *Planned Parenthood v. Casey*, 1992), and the right of individuals to rear children in nontraditional family groups (*Moore v. City of East Cleveland, Ohio*, 1977).

Since the 1942 *Skinner* decision, lower courts have accepted the notion that states may not forcibly sterilize selected individuals unless such a policy can withstand strict constitutional scrutiny. The basis for requiring this level of scrutiny is the assertion that the "right to have offspring," like the right to marry, is a "fundamental," "basic liberty." Further, the *Skinner* and *Eisenstadt* decisions arguably hold that the right to use contraception or to be free of unwarranted sterilization is an aspect of individual, rather than marital, privacy. As stated in *Eisenstadt*: "If the right to privacy means anything, it is the right of the individual, married or single, to be free of unwarranted government intrusion into matters so fundamentally affecting a person as the decision to bear or beget a child" (*Eisenstadt v. Baird*, 1972).

But the right to privacy is no longer the primary justification for abortion rights, or, by extension, reproductive rights. The 1992 *Planned Parenthood v. Casey* decision specifically based its opinion on "liberty" (rather than privacy) rights, and concluded that abortion remains protected from state efforts to prohibit abortion. The emphasis on "liberty" language changes the focus of abortion rights from one of limitations on governmental power (as discussed in "privacy"-based decisions) to one of individual control of one's person. The opinion attempts to explain why abortion is an essential "liberty" for women because it permits control of one's body and one's personal destiny.

Justice Antonin Scalia's dissent mocks this attempt. After reciting the list of phrases used elsewhere by his colleagues, such as "a person's most basic decision," "a most personal and intimate choice," "originat[ing] within the zone of conscience and belief," "too intimate and personal for state interference," Scalia complains that "the same adjectives can be applied to many forms of conduct that this Court … has held are not entitled to constitutional protection—because, like abortion, they are forms of conduct that have long been criminalized in American society. Those adjectives might be applied, for example, to homosexual sodomy, polygamy, adult incest, and suicide" (p. 785).

Scalia's dissent highlights the potentially far-reaching implications of what the plurality has written regarding the fundamental importance of controlling one's fertility. The *Casey* plurality opinion lays out an argument for reexamining the 1879 *Reynolds v. U.S.* decision (upholding the power of the state to outlaw polygamous marriage) and the 1986 *Bowers v. Hardwick* decision (upholding the power of the state to criminalize homosexual behavior), a task critical to determining if states can restrict noncoital reproduction to married couples. It also lays the groundwork for cases sure to arise concerning prenatal diagnosis, sex selection, cloning, and (ultimately) parthenogenesis.

What Can States Do To Regulate Reproductive Technologies?

Even assuming that constitutional protection for procreation remains grounded in a fundamental rights analysis, possibilities remain for areas of state regulation of who may use noncoital reproduction and how they may proceed. First, many aspects of noncoital reproduction arguably do not amount to *procreation*, and therefore are more amenable to state control. Donor gametes and surrogacy do not permit an infertile person to procreate; rather, they allow fertile persons to reproduce without partners or to bypass the infertility of their partners.

Artificial insemination by donor (AID), for example, can be used by single or lesbian women who want to become pregnant but who find the thought of sexual intercourse with a man distasteful. Almost half the states in the United States have statutory language governing AID that appears to ignore the possibility of such a use, leaving the legal status of the donor-father unclear (U.S. Congress, Office of Technology Assessment [OTA], 1988b). Canada and France have also had national commissions recommend that single and lesbian women be barred from using donor insemination in order to conceive (Liu; McLean). Because such women could physically procreate without donor insemination, albeit with great discomfort, it can be argued that such restrictions do not impinge upon a fundamental right to procreate and are therefore potentially tolerable.

Of course, the restrictions would still be subject to challenges based on the unequal treatment of single or lesbian women as compared with the married, heterosexual population. AID for a married couple in which the husband is infertile is also nothing more than a medical alternative to the social solution of adultery; the AID itself does not enable the infertile man to procreate. Nevertheless, in Canada, France, and much of the United States, this form of AID is viewed as therapeutic, seemingly because the *unit* of infertility (i.e., the *patient*) is seen as a monogamous, married, heterosexual couple, not as an unmarried individual.

In typical surrogacy arrangements, in which the husband is fertile and the wife infertile, the surrogacy arrangement, like AID, does not permit the infertile wife to procreate, nor is the fertile husband unable to procreate without resorting to surrogacy. Rather, surrogacy allows the husband to procreate without committing adultery and with some assurance, as in the AID scenario, that the couple will be able to retain exclusive custody of the resulting child. As with AID, such a use of contract motherhood is viewed as therapeutic by many. While even this use of surrogacy has engendered opposition ranging from criminalization to mere unenforceability in countries such as Australia, Canada, England, and France, and in some portions of the United States, it has never encountered the same degree of approbation as the so-called surrogacy of convenience, in which a rearing mother finds it useful to hire someone else to carry the child (Liu; McLean).

Indeed, much of the debate surrounding the most famous surrogacy case in the United States, *Baby M* (1988), focused on whether the rearing mother had declined to become pregnant due to career concerns and undue worry about her health, or rather due to legitimate concern that pregnancy would seriously worsen her multiple sclerosis. This debate exemplifies the increased willingness of the American public to regulate or ban surrogacy when it is not

perceived as a cure for a medical problem such as infertility, a sentiment reflected in the constitutional analysis that permits greater state regulation where the right to procreate is not directly implicated.

Egg donation to a woman who cannot ovulate but who can carry to term does not technically allow the recipient to procreate, as she will not *reproduce* in the genetic sense. But it does allow her to experience pregnancy and childbirth, which for women are intimately associated with genetic procreation. In terms of both biological significance (gestation is, of course, a biological activity) and emotional impact, this would seem to be close to procreation, even in its more narrow definition. Thus, it is difficult to categorize this activity in terms of whether it allows an infertile person to *procreate*.

Despite this fact, there is considerable hesitation about permitting egg donation. Whereas sperm donation is widely accepted, egg donation entails significantly more medical discomfort and even risk on the part of the donor. This in turn raises the specter, at least in the United States, of increased payments for the donation. For some, such payments represent an undue incentive to undergo medical risks, as well as an unacceptable commercialization of human gametes. Nevertheless, at least in California, there is a thriving egg donation practice.

Even those aspects of noncoital reproduction that clearly involve procreation can be regulated or banned, if there is a sufficiently compelling state interest. It is true that artificial insemination by husband (AIH), and in vitro fertilization (IVF) using a couple's own gametes (whether or not a contract mother is hired to carry the child to term), permit an otherwise infertile man or woman to procreate genetically. By bypassing the fallopian tube defect or permitting intrauterine insemination of the husband's concentrated semen, these techniques actually help infertile individuals to participate in the act of reproduction. But a compelling state interest in the protection of embryos and fetuses, for example, could justify significant restraints on even AIH and IVF.

Is There a Compelling State *Interest* in Embryos and Fetuses?

The most likely claim for a compelling state purpose to outlaw or regulate IVF is that of protection for the extracorporeal embryo, whether or not accompanied by a contract with a gestational surrogate.

The *Webster v. Reproductive Services* (1989) and *Planned Parenthood v. Casey* (1992) decisions indicate that the U.S. Supreme Court is now quite tolerant of symbolic legislative statements concerning the sanctity of embryonic life and of significant restrictions on the exercise of constitutionally protected rights, such as abortion, in the name of protecting these early life forms. It seems likely that the court would uphold state statutes, such as the one in Louisiana that regulates management of extracorporeal embryos. Such restrictions may include prohibiting nontherapeutic experimentation on the embryo, embryo discard, and unnecessary creation of *surplus* embryos for the purpose of experimentation. It might also attempt to regulate transfer of embryos. By declaring that life begins at conception, as was done in the Missouri statute upheld in Webster, and by equating the rights of embryos to the rights of children, states could demand that embryo transfers be viewed as adoptions.

This was the approach taken by the trial court in the case of *Davis v. Davis* (1992), a Tennessee divorce case that struggled with determining the legal status of several frozen embryos that were left over from unsuccessful IVF treatments and became the subject of a divorce dispute. Characterizing the question as one of child custody, and viewing the embryos as children, the trial court then awarded custody to the parent whose actions would be in the best interests of the embryos. By assuming that embryos have "interests," and then defining one of those interests as an interest in being born, the trial court awarded the embryos to the wife, who intended to have them implanted in her womb in the hope of bringing them to term.

By contrast, the appellate court backed away from the characterization of the embryos as *children* and the resulting "best interests" analysis. Without ever explicitly calling the embryos property, the court proceeded to treat them as property held jointly by the couple, and thereby concluded that disposition of the embryos must be by agreement because each party had an equal property interest in them.

The Tennessee Supreme Court reviewed available models for disposition of the embryos when unanticipated contingencies arise. Those models range from a rule requiring, at one extreme, that all embryos be used by the gamete-providers or be donated for uterine transfer (such as is required under an as yet unchallenged Louisiana statute), and, at the other extreme, that any unused embryos be automatically discarded. The Tennessee Supreme Court, when it considered the *Davis* case, was aware of the *Planned Parenthood v. Casey* (1992) decision, which reiterated the *Roe* (1973) holding that a state may express an "interest" in a fetus. Unfortunately, like *Roe, Planned Parenthood v. Casey* fails to identify what this interest might be or why it arises, leaving the *Davis* court with little guidance on how to extend the state interest argument to nonabortion settings.

Numerous commentators have struggled to identify this state interest (Joyce; Tooley). Many begin with the premise that a sufficiently detailed biological understanding of embryo potential will yield an answer:

> [E]very living individual being with the natural potential, as a whole, for knowing, willing, desiring, and relating to others in a self-reflective way is a person. But the human zygote is a living individual (or more than one such individual) with the natural potential, as a whole, to act in these ways. Therefore the human zygote is an actual person with great potential.... (Joyce, p. 169)

But others argue that the genetic blueprint of a person cannot be entitled to the same moral standing as that of the person himself or herself, because any inherent "right" to live is premised on the idea that it is in the "interest" of the entity to continue existing (Tooley). Where, as with a zygote, there is no self-concept, there can be no "interest" in continuing to exist, no "desire" to continue to exist, and therefore no "right" to continue to exist.

Such an argument refutes the *Davis* trial court's treatment of the frozen embryos as children with an interest in being brought to term. But the appellate court's assumption that they must therefore be treated as property is equally unjustified. Society may choose nonetheless to grant rights to the zygote or fetus, for any number of reasons, if such steps do not unduly impinge on another liberty recognized by society, such as the liberty of men and women to control their reproductive futures.

In fact, Justice John Paul Stevens takes on this issue in his concurring opinion in *Planned Parenthood v. Casey*:

> Identifying the State's interests—which the States rarely articulate with any precision—makes clear that the interest in protecting potential life is not grounded in the Constitution. It is, instead, an indirect interest supported by both humanitarian and pragmatic concerns. Many of our citizens believe that any abortion reflects an unacceptable disrespect for potential human life and that the performance of more than a million abortions each year is intolerable; many find third-trimester abortions performed when the fetus is approaching personhood particularly offensive. The State has a legitimate interest in minimizing such offense.... These are the kinds of concerns that comprise the State's interest in potential human life. (*Planned Parenthood v. Casey*, 1992, 120 L. Ed. 2d 674 at p. 739)

Struggling with the task of expressing a state interest in embryonic life without unduly impinging upon the reproductive rights of adult men and women, the Tennessee Supreme Court in the *Davis* case concluded that embryos are neither children nor property, but occupy an intermediate status based on their potential for development. This, in turn, would not convey a right to be born under either state or federal constitutional law but would demand some protections. These include implantation where possible, freedom from unnecessary creation or destruction, and dignified management.

The Tennessee court's characterization of an intermediate status for embryos is the most intriguing part of the opinion, as it did not present a coherent theory of that status and its implications. There are, of course, models of intermediate property status. Animals, for example, are treated as property with no "right to life," but at the same time are protected from cruel and painful treatment by their owners. Works of art may be owned, but "moral rights" possessed by the artist in some jurisdictions prohibit defacing or destroying the art. Land may be owned subject to numerous restrictions on use that would permanently destroy some publicly valued attribute. Which, if any, of these models describes the intermediate status held by the embryos? And on what basis? This is indeed the key question left totally unanswered by the Tennessee court. As it stands, though the opinion gives some narrow, nearly regulatory guidance to IVF clinics, it offers little to those wondering in general whether other restraints on embryo creation and management are in order.

Other countries have struggled with the same dilemma. Most often, as in England and Australia, the compromise solution is chosen, in which limited experimentation is permitted on unavoidably abandoned embryos. Deliberate creation of embryos for the purpose of experimentation is frowned upon. Occasionally a stricter view is adopted, as in Germany, where embryo experimentation is simply banned. Generally, however, where embryos are to be created in order to permit implantation and gestation, even extracorporeal maintenance or embryo freezing is tolerated (U.S. Congress, OTA, 1988b; Liu; McLean).

What is the State Interest in the Children Conceived Noncoitally?

Related to state interest in the protection of extracorporeal embryos is its interest in protecting the children born following noncoital conception. This takes its most frequent form in suggestions for limiting use of these technologies to married couples, on the theory that being born into a single-parent home is harmful to a child. On this basis, almost two-thirds of physicians surveyed in 1987 and a number of states either explicitly or implicitly deny artificial insemination services to unmarried women (U.S. Congress, OTA, 1988a, 1988b).

While some may deplore this practice, the fact that unmarried persons are not considered a "suspect" class in constitutional jurisprudence (i.e., they are not considered a class in need of special protection from discriminatory legislation because they are fully able to use the political system to protect their interests), means that such discriminatory practices are largely immune to constitutional challenge as an abridgment of their right to equal protection of the laws. Unless procreation, and specifically the use of artificial insemination, is viewed as a fundamental right, such persons will be limited to challenges under state and federal civil rights statutes in their pursuit of equal access to these technologies.

To the extent that the right to procreate implies a right to create a family, constitutional law from the nineteenth century remains unchallenged in its support for criminalization of family forms, such as polygamy, that fly in the face of Western European tradition. While there have been twentieth-century cases in support of broadening the definition of *family,* there has not yet been any case in which the right to marry is extended beyond a heterosexual couple. Thus, whatever the right to privacy entails, it does not appear to guarantee the right to form familial relationships that achieve the same legal recognition as that bestowed by marriage.

Generally, current interpretations of constitutional law appear to support the assertion that for married couples there is a right to privacy embedded in the wording and history of the constitution and that such privacy extends to reproductive decision making free from unwarranted governmental intrusion. While case law suggests that individuals are entitled to this privacy in equal measure, judicial hostility to claims of a right by homosexuals to marry or engage in sexual activity (*Bowers v. Hardwick,* 1986), by minors to have unrestricted access to abortion (*Hodgeson v. Minnesota,* 1990), and by physicians to give full information concerning abortion (*Rust v. Sullivan,* 1991) suggest limitations on Supreme Court extension of this right.

Indeed, much of the state activity concerning contract motherhood has been directed at protecting the children conceived through these arrangements. In the event a surrogate changes her mind, a custody dispute can break out between the birth mother and the genetic father. Reluctant to extend parental status to the adopting mother without terminating the parental status of the birth mother, but also determined to see the child placed in the safest home, courts have been in a quandary. Most often the solution has been to refuse to use the contract as the basis for a custody decision, and instead to rely on traditional family notions of child welfare. Next, courts have generally refused to terminate the birth mother's status as a presumptive legal parent. But despite these findings, most courts also award custody to the genetic father and his wife, as it is this couple who is usually better able financially and socially to convince the court that they can provide a secure home for the baby (U.S. Congress, OTA, 1988b; McLean).

Other Concerns Regarding Contract Motherhood

Another state interest in surrogacy stems from the fact that the contracts typically entail promises by the contract mother to refrain from certain behaviors such as drinking, smoking, or the use of illicit drugs, as well as affirmative promises to follow prescribed prenatal care regimes and to undergo prenatal testing for fetal health. Enforcing such contract promises raises constitutional issues, requiring a relinquishment of significant autonomy on the part of the contract mother. This is particularly true with regard to promises to follow prescribed medical care, which may entail submission to invasive tests and even surgery, in the case of cesarean sections.

Surrogacy also raises the specter that the hiring couple might gain what amounts to a property interest in the body of the contract mother. This is particularly true where gestational surrogacy is employed, and the child the contract mother is carrying is genetically related to the hiring parents but not to her. At least one court has been known to issue a "prenatal adoption" order, in which the hiring husband and wife were declared the legal parents of the fetus still within the gestational mother's body (*Smith v. Jones,* 1988). In such a case, the hiring parents would have a legally recognized interest in the development of the fetus. Indeed, as parents they might have a legal duty to protect the fetus from harm, as has been confirmed by cases that hold pregnant women criminally liable for behaviors that threaten fetal health. How to protect fetuses while not compromising the physical integrity and legal autonomy of the gestational mother poses a significant constitutional challenge.

Gestational surrogacy also raises fundamental questions about the definition of parenthood, particularly of motherhood. While the law has consistently given preference to biological parents over nonbiological parents, with specific exceptions carved out for adoption and AID, it has never before been forced to consider the definition of *biological.* As of the mid-1990s, only one state has considered the problem. In California, a dispute developed between a couple (the Calverts) whose gametes had been used to conceive a child who was subsequently brought to term by a hired gestational contract mother named Anna Johnson. The trial and appellate courts both concluded that the genetic relationship, which defines "natural" parent for men, would define the "natural" parent for women. The two lower courts

specifically rejected the notion that gestation is a biological relationship formed by the indisputable fusing of maternal and fetal well-being during the nine months of pregnancy that could equally well form the basis for defining the "natural" mother.

California's lower court decisions in *Johnson v. Calvert* (1991), stating that a gestational mother is no more than a foster parent to her own child, are almost without precedent worldwide. Only Israel, bound by unique aspects of religious identity law, has adopted a genetic definition of motherhood. Every other country that has examined the problem—including the United Kingdom, Germany, Switzerland, Bulgaria, and even South Africa with its race-conscious legal structure—has concluded that the woman who gives birth is the child's mother.

The California Supreme Court's 1993 opinion on *Johnson v. Calvert* declined to find either the genetic or the gestational mother to be the definitive "natural" parent. Instead, it chose to view either relationship as a presumptive form of natural parenthood. Then it specifically declined the invitation to have the law reflect what had actually happened, that is, the birth of a child with two biological mothers, one gestational and the other genetic. Agreeing that acknowledging more than one natural mother would be, as the trial court stated, a "recipe for crazymaking," the California Supreme Court said that whichever of the two biologically related women had been the intended mother would then be declared the "natural" mother. It continued by stating that in the event that the gestational and genetic mothers are not the same person, and that the intended mother is neither the genetic nor gestational parent, she would nonetheless be considered the "natural" mother. Thus the court avoided what is at base the most interesting question raised by the use of reproductive technologies: the possibility of declaring more than one woman to be a "natural" parent of a child. To do so, of course, would require escaping the confines of the heterosexual couple as the paradigm for a family and acknowledging that some people become parents by virtue of genetic connection, others by gestational connection, and still others by contract—whether a marital contract with a genetic or gestational parent, or a reproductive technology contract that creates relationships with children conceived with donor gametes or carried to term by contract mothers.

What is the State Interest in Access to Quality Services?

A final and overarching area of state interest lies in consumer access and protection. Only a handful of states have legislation mandating insurance coverage for the most expensive of these technologies, IVF. Those states, including Arkansas, Hawaii, Maryland, Massachusetts, Texas, and Wisconsin, have responded to political pressure from organized medicine as well as from infertility support groups. But no state has yet asserted that insurance coverage is required by virtue of the fact that procreation is a fundamental right that may, for some people, be exercised only when using an expensive technology. Indeed, in the context of abortion services, the Supreme Court has made clear that states may forbid Medicaid or other public funding of such services, although they are clearly linked to the exercise of a fundamental right. In fact, the *Webster* decision upheld a state prohibition on the use of public facilities for abortion services, even when no public funds are used.

Where IVF and other reproductive technology services are being provided, however, the state may well choose to regulate them for the sake of protecting patients from unscrupulous practices. These may include misleading advertising, inadequate facilities, insufficiently trained personnel, and negligent screening of gamete donors for genetic and infectious diseases that might be transmitted to recipients. Even in the exercise of a fundamental right, the state may enforce regulations designed to protect the patient.

Another consumer issue involves the regulation of commercialization of reproductive technologies. Although sperm donation has continued apace in countries where no payment is permitted, most commentators agree that the availability of donor gametes and contract mothers in the United States would be severely reduced if commercialization were prohibited. Nonetheless, even when viewing access to reproductive technologies as an exercise of freedom to procreate, several state courts have concluded that there is ample state authority to prohibit commercialization (*Doe v. Kelley,* 1981; *Baby M,* 1988). The basis for this conclusion can vary. One line of argument, focusing on surrogacy, characterizes it either as baby-selling or the sale of parental rights, both of which traditionally have been forbidden despite significant libertarian arguments in favor of free markets for both. These prohibitions on selling children or parental rights would easily extend to prohibitions on the sale of embryos, if embryos are characterized as children. Prohibitions on the sale of semen and ova probably could be justified on the same basis as the current prohibitions on organ sales, despite the same line of libertarian arguments.

Other arguments in favor of prohibiting commercialization focus on the effect such activities have on public morals, on the creation of property interests in the bodies of others, and on the fear that the creation of an industry surrounding the sale of gametes, embryos, and reproductive services will create a class of professional breeders. A 1987 survey of surrogacy brokers by the OTA revealed significant

discrepancies in economic and educational backgrounds of those who hire contract mothers and those who work as contract mothers (U.S. Congress, OTA, 1988a), leading to the conclusion that the two groups would be unlikely to wield equal bargaining power during the preconception contract negotiations or during postbirth custody disputes.

All of these arguments would probably fail if subjected to the strict scrutiny brought to bear on state interference with a fundamental right. But the reluctance of U.S. courts to view commercialization of reproductive services as an expression of procreative freedom reduces the degree of scrutiny to which state restrictions are subjected. Any rational state purpose will suffice if the restriction interferes with a privilege rather than a fundamental right.

Conclusion

The legal and regulatory issues surrounding reproductive technologies concern the ability of a government to ban or restrict noncoital reproduction because it may harm embryos, children, consumers, or public morals. Where governments choose not to ban the practice, they may wish to regulate it, for example, by limiting what types of prospective parents may use it, which adults will be related to the resulting children, and what kinds of ancillary practices—such as research or commercialization—will be permitted. In the United States, the details of such regulation are a function of state legislation and the resolution of novel cases by the courts. But the federal Constitution places significant limits on how far such legislation or judicial lawmaking may interfere with the opportunity of individuals to exercise procreative choice.

R. ALTA CHARO (1995)
BIBLIOGRAPHY REVISED

SEE ALSO: *Abortion; Adoption; Cloning; Embryo and Fetus; Feminism; Fetal Research; Genetic Counseling; Genetic Testing and Screening: Reproductive Genetic Testing; Healthcare Resources, Allocation of: Microallocation; Law and Bioethics; Maternal-Fetal Relationship; Moral Status; Population Ethics; Sexism; Transhumanism and Posthumanism; Women, Contemporary Issues of;* and other *Reproductive Technologies* subentries

BIBLIOGRAPHY

Andrews, Lori B. 1999. *The Clone Age: Adventures in the New World of Reproductive Technology.* New York: Henry Holt and Company.

Baby M, In re. 109 N.J. 396, 537 A.2d 1227. (1988).

Bonnicksen, Andrea L. 1995. "Ethical and Policy Issues in Human Embryo Twinning." *Cambridge Quarterly of Healthcare Ethics* 4(3): 268–284.

Bowers v. Hardwick. 106 S. Ct. 2841 (1986).

Brock, Dan W. 1992. "Fertility, Contraception, and Reproductive Freedom." Presented at the Meeting on Women, Equality, and Reproductive Technology, United Nations University, World Institute for Development and Economic Research, Helsinki, Finland, August 2–6.

Callahan, Joan, ed. 1995. *Reproduction, Ethics, and the Law: Feminist Perspectives.* Bloomington: Indiana University Press.

Capron, Alexander Morgan. 1987. "So Quick Bright Things Come to Confusion." *American Journal of Law and Medicine* 13(2–3): 169–187.

Charo, R. Alta. 1990. "Legislative Alternatives for Surrogate Mothering." *Journal of Law, Medicine, and Health Care* 17(1): 93–114.

Davis v. Davis. 842 S.W.2d 588. Tenn. (1992).

De Melo-Martin, Inmaculada. 1998. *Making Babies: Biomedical Technologies, Reproductive Ethics, and Public Policy.* New York: Kluwer Academic Publishers.

Doe v. Kelley. 106 Mich. App. 169 (1981).

Eisenstadt v. Baird. 92 S. Ct. 1029 (1972).

Griswold v. Connecticut. 381 U.S. 479, 483 (1965).

Guilhem, Dirce. 2001. "New Reproductive Technologies, Ethics and Legislation in Brazil: A Delayed Debate." *Bioethics* 15(3): 218–230.

Hanna, Kathi E., ed. 1991. *Biomedical Politics.* Washington, D.C.: National Academy Press.

Harris, John, and Holm, Soren, eds. 2000. *The Future of Human Reproduction: Ethics, Choice, and Regulation (Issues in Biomedical Ethics).* New York: Oxford University Press.

Hill, John L. 1991. "What Does It Mean to be a 'Parent'? The Claims of Biology as the Basis for Parental Rights." *New York University Law Review* 66(2): 353–420.

Hodgeson v. Minnesota. 110 S. Ct. 2926 (1990).

Johnson v. Calvert. 1991. 851 P.2d 776 (Cal. Sup. Ct.); 12 Cal.App.4th 977 (1993).

Joyce, Robert E. 1988. "Personhood and the Conception Event." In *What Is a Person?* pp. 199–211, ed. Michael F. Goodman. Clifton, NJ: Humana.

Knoppers, Bartha M., and LeBris, Sonia. 1991. "Recent Advances in Medically Assisted Conception: Legal, Ethical and Social Issues." *American Journal of Law and Medicine* 17(4): 329–361.

Lippman, Abby. 1991. "Prenatal Genetic Testing and Screening: Constructing Needs and Reinforcing Inequities." *American Journal of Law and Medicine* 17(1–2): 15–50.

Liu, Athena. 1991. *Artificial Reproduction and Reproductive Rights.* Brookfield, VT: Dartmouth.

McLean, Sheila, ed. 1992. *Law Reform and Human Reproduction.* Brookfield, VT: Dartmouth.

Meyer v. Nebraska. 262 U.S. 390, 401, 402 (1923).

Moore v. City of East Cleveland, Ohio. 431 U.S. 494 (1977).

Murphy, Timothy F. 1995. "Sperm Harvesting and Postmortem Fatherhood." *Bioethics* 9(5): 380–398.

Overall, Christine. 1987. *Ethics and Human Reproduction: A Feminist Analysis.* Boston: Allen & Unwin.

Planned Parenthood v. Casey. 112 S. Ct. 2791 (1992).

Reynolds v. United States. 98 U.S. 113 (1879).

Robertson, John A. 1989. "Technology and Motherhood: Legal and Ethical Issues in Human Egg Donation." *Case Western Reserve Law Review* 39(1): 1–38.

Robertson, John A. 1990. "In the Beginning: The Legal Status of Early Embryos." *Virginia Law Review* 76(3): 437–517.

Roe v. Wade. 410 U.S. 113 (1973).

Rust v. Sullivan. 111 S. Ct. 1759 (1991).

Schultz, Marjorie Maguire. 1990. "Reproductive Technology and Intent-Based Parenthood: An Opportunity for Gender Neutrality." *Wisconsin Law Review* 1990(2): 297–398.

Seibel, MacHelle M., and Crockin, Susan L., eds. 1996. *Family Building Through Egg and Sperm Donation: Medical, Legal, and Ethical Issues.* Boston, MA: Jones and Bartlett.

Skinner v. Oklahoma ex rel. Williamson. 62 S. Ct. 1110 (1942).

Smith & Smith v. Jones & Jones. 85–532014 DZ, Detroit, Mich. 3rd Cir. (1986).

Spoerl, Joseph S. 2000. "Making Laws on Making Babies: Ethics, Public Policy, and Reproductive Technology." *American Journal of Jurisprudence* 45: 93–115.

Steinbock, Bonnie. 1997. *Life Before Birth: The Moral and Legal Status of Embryos and Fetuses.* New York: Oxford University Press.

Sutton, Agneta. 1996. "The British Law on Assisted Reproduction: A Liberal Law by Comparison with Many Other European Laws." *Ethics and Medicine* 12(2): 41–45.

Tooley, Michael. 1984. "In Defense of Abortion and Infanticide." In *The Problem of Abortion,* 2nd edition, pp. 120–134, ed. Joel Feinberg. Belmont, CA: Wadsworth.

U.S. Congress. Office of Technology Assessment (OTA). 1988a. *Artificial Insemination: Practice in the U.S.: Summary of a 1987 Survey.* Washington, D.C.: Author.

U.S. Congress. Office of Technology Assessment (OTA). 1988b. *Infertility: Medical and Social Choices.* Washington, D.C.: Author.

Wagner, William J. 1990. "The Contractual Reallocation of Procreative Resources and Parental Rights: The Natural Endowment Critique." *Case Western Reserve Law Review* 41(1): 1–202.

Webster v. Reproductive Services. 109 S. Ct. 3040(1989).

Yoon, Mimi. 1990. "The Uniform Status of Children of Assisted Conception Act: Does It Protect the Best Interests of the Child in a Surrogate Arrangement?" *American Journal of Law and Medicine* 16(4): 525–553.

V. GAMETE DONATION

Gamete donation is a procedure that enables those who wish to have children, but who cannot produce or use their own gametes (sperm or eggs), to use gametes provided by others in attempts to procreate. Those at risk of transmitting serious genetic disease to their children and those without a sexual partner (of the opposite sex) may also use the gametes of others to attempt to have children. Sperm donation is carried out by inserting sperm provided by a donor directly into a woman's reproductive tract. Egg (oocyte) donation involves merging eggs extracted from a donor with sperm in a laboratory dish by (*in vitro* fertilization [IVF]) and transferring some of the resulting embryos to a woman's uterus.

While the use of gamete donation has stimulated amazement and curiosity, it has also created significant ethical and public-policy questions. Concerns have been raised about whether this practice might radically alter understandings of marriage, procreation, and parenthood; whether it objectifies and commodifies gamete donors and the offspring who emerge from such procedures; and whether it harms donors, recipients, or the resulting children. There is also a rising concern about whether the procedures associated with gamete donation should be subject to greater oversight and regulation. Egg donation, in particular, is poised to expand in novel directions that will raise ethical and public-policy issues never before considered.

The use of the term *donation* in connection with the provision of gametes is seen as self-contradictory by some, since sperm and egg donors in many instances do not donate their gametes, but are financially remunerated for them. However, since this term is in common usage and is understood to cover both unpaid and paid suppliers, its use will be retained here.

The History of Gamete Donation

Pregnancy following sperm donation was mentioned in Western literature as early as 1790, when the Scottish surgeon John Hunter was said to have artificially inseminated a woman in London. J. Marion Sims, a New York doctor, is believed to have carried out the first sperm insemination in the United States in 1866. The practice was usually kept secret, however, because it was considered shameful and unnatural to introduce the sperm of a man other than her husband into the body of a woman. The first confirmed case of sperm donation took place in the United States in 1884, when William Pancoast, a physician in Philadelphia, inseminated a woman using sperm from a medical student. In 1953, scientists demonstrated that human sperm could be frozen and thawed for insemination

to produce a normal child, paving the way for the first commercial sperm bank, which was opened in 1970 in Minnesota. By 1993 it was estimated that more than 80,000 women were undergoing the procedure each year, resulting in approximately 30,000 pregnancies annually.

Oocyte donation was first reported in 1983 in Australia. Since then, use of this procedure has grown rapidly. In 1987 it was reported to be available at 17 programs in the United States; in 1993 there were 135 known programs, and in 1998 this number had doubled to 260 programs. In 1998, a total of 5,273 egg-donation cycles were initiated, with 4,783 transfers of donated eggs to recipients, for a delivery rate per transfer of 41.2 percent (Society for Assisted Reproductive Technology).

The Practice of Sperm Donation

Sperm donation is usually performed in a medical setting by a physician using sperm acquired from an anonymous donor. It is also practiced in private contexts by those who do not want professional supervision, although this is considered extremely unsafe as the donor has not been screened for infectious diseases that might affect the woman or the resulting child. This private practice employs sperm from a known or anonymous donor using common household implements. There are three major sources of sperm: large sperm banks that ship frozen specimens nationwide, regional sperm banks with a more local distribution area, and pools of donors retained by individual practitioners.

As long as physicians could use friends, colleagues, and informal networks to acquire sperm, supply was not a problem. When these sources became insufficient in the 1980s, medical students were given a modest financial incentive to *donate* sperm. Payment represented closure of the transaction, and donor anonymity was guaranteed (Daniels). Donors today are primarily young single males students who are found by word of mouth and through advertising in college and local newspapers, in magazines, and on the Internet. Sperm banks attempt to recruit a pool of donors exhibiting a variety of physical, mental, and ethnic characteristics. Donors are matched with recipients on the basis of physical and other features as far as possible, while a few sperm banks specialize, offering sperm from donors of high academic or athletic ability.

Practice guidelines of the American Society of Reproductive Medicine (ASRM; formerly the American Fertility Society) recommend that sperm donors undergo medical screening that includes testing for infectious and sexually transmitted diseases. Until the 1980s most insemination with donated sperm was performed with fresh sperm, which were only sometimes tested for venereal disease. That changed dramatically in 1988 when the Centers for Disease Control, concerned about the transmission of AIDS, called for donors to be tested for HIV antibodies at the time of donation and again after their sperm had been frozen for six months before their gametes could be used. This rule was designed to reduce the risk of transmitting HIV through sperm from infected donors who did not have detectable antibodies at the time of donation. Practitioners now only use frozen sperm.

Meanwhile, according to ASRM recommendations, the recipient is also screened medically and tested for cystic fibrosis carrier status. Her partner is clinically evaluated and tested for HIV antibodies, and both are to be offered psychological counseling.

In the United States, sperm donors are paid for their time and expenses, with payment in 1998 ranging from $35 to $50 per unit. The Human Fertilisation and Embryology Authority (HFEA) of the United Kingdom currently allows a fee of U.S.$23 per donation, but it is moving toward completely phasing out payments to gamete donors. Sperm donors are not paid in New Zealand, Sweden, and France.

The Practice of Egg Donation

Egg donation is a more complex, onerous, and risky procedure than sperm donation—both for donor and recipient. Both must follow drug regimens to stimulate the production of multiple eggs and the donor must undergo an intrusive egg-recovery procedure. Consequently, egg donation is necessarily offered under medical auspices through *in vitro* fertilization (IVF) programs affiliated with academic medical centers, community hospitals, and private practices.

Egg donors must undergo the same drug regimens and egg-recovery procedures as women who undergo IVF. An average of thirteen eggs is collected from each donor, and up to twenty-five eggs have been reported extracted at one time. These eggs are fertilized with sperm *in vitro*. Some of the resulting embryos are then inserted into the uterus of the recipient, who has been injected with drugs to prepare her uterus to accept embryos. The remaining embryos may be frozen for later use by the recipient, donated to medical research, donated to others, or discarded.

Egg donation involves medical risks to the donor of varying degrees of severity. As a consequence of the use of fertility drugs, 1 percent of donors experience ovarian hyperstimulation syndrome (OHSS), which can lead to kidney or liver failure, cardiorespiratory dysfunction, or stroke, among other effects. In addition, 10 to 20 percent of

donors experience moderately severe hyperstimulation syndrome, while approximately one-third are affected by milder forms of this syndrome. According to some studies, there is an association between the use of ovulation-stimulating drugs and ovarian cancer. Laparoscopy, which is used to extract eggs from donors, also carries minor risks. Even when there are no complications, the procedure is highly uncomfortable and time-consuming. Recipients of donated eggs, studies suggest, are at increased risk of pregnancy-related complications such as preeclampsia, diabetes mellitus, and anemia, as well as HIV infection.

When egg donation began, it was usual to acquire eggs from anonymous donors who were undergoing IVF and were willing to part with spare eggs. As the practice grew in the late 1980s, and as more donors were needed, infertility specialists sought eggs from known donors who were relatives or friends of recipients and were willing to contribute eggs out of a spirit of altruism. To meet the ever-increasing demand for eggs, they then moved to married women under thirty-five years of age who were not known to the recipient couple, and who had already had as many children as they wanted. Such women, it was reasoned, had exhibited that they were fertile and they were less likely than childless women to attempt to claim the resulting children in the future. Some of these women received financial compensation. Gradually, practitioners realized that they achieved better results using the eggs of young women and began to advertise for college women to serve as donors, for these women were presumed to be healthy, fertile, and in need of extra funds. Donated eggs are now derived primarily from healthy young women who are specifically recruited for this purpose, followed by relatives or friends of the prospective parents, and lastly from infertility patients undergoing IVF who agree to donate extra eggs to others.

Guidelines of the ASRM and the national advisory board on ethics in reproduction (NABER), a private body that is independent of practitioners and that has developed standards for egg donation, recommend medical screening of recipients and psychological evaluation of both recipients and their partners. They also call for medical screening of donors and a genetic evaluation based largely on the donor's stated medical history. Whether HIV antibodies might be transmitted by the donor to the recipient cannot be resolved in egg donation by direct testing of eggs because donated eggs cannot currently be frozen and quarantined for the 180 days required for retesting for HIV antibodies. However, recipients of donated eggs can have the resulting embryos frozen and used six months later if the egg donor tests negative for HIV antibodies at that time. The disadvantage of this is that freezing embryos lessens the chances of successful embryo implantation. Psychological counseling is also recommended for the donor and her partner by both the ASRM and NABER.

Clinics in the United States vary greatly in how much information they offer to recipients about donors. At many programs, matches are made by physicians and nurses on the model of anonymous sperm donation. Recipients are informed about the donor's physical characteristics and given some additional nonidentifying information, and donors usually learn nothing about the recipients. At some centers, brokers recruit and screen donors for a fee. Recipient couples choose an anonymous donor from a list of candidates provided by these brokers. At still other centers, information is provided to donors and recipients about one another and they are urged to meet, a practice known as *open donation* that echoes a growing trend toward *open adoption*.

The cost of egg donation combined with *in vitro* fertilization in the United States rose from about $9,000 per attempt in 1991 to about $20,000 in 2001 (not including donor payment). Donors in the United States are reported to have been paid amounts ranging from $1,500 to $10,000. Some are said to have been offered $50,000 and $100,000. Egg donors in England are currently paid the equivalent of $23 and, as with sperm donation, such payments are to be phased out.

Ethical Issues

Ethical issues raised by the practice of gamete donation tend to fall into two major categories. There are those that focus on underlying conceptual questions, such as whether gamete donation is, in principle, ethically acceptable, and whether this procedure might radically alter understandings of procreation, marriage, and parenthood. Other questions are more oriented toward the consequences of gamete donation, such as its safety; its possible psychological import for donors, recipients, and children; and whether adequate informed consent has been obtained.

Procreation and the Marital Relationship

The use of gamete donation has sparked powerful philosophical differences that center on two features of procreation that many deem essential: it is exclusive and it is embodied. There was a public uproar in 1909 when it was revealed that sperm donation had been carried out by a physician some twenty-five years earlier, and the practice was condemned as a form of mechanical adultery. Some secular and religious critics voice similar concerns today, holding that the use of reproductive materials provided by individuals outside the marital relationship intrudes upon the exclusive union between spouses that is normative in marriage, and is therefore wrong. "There is, generally, strong rabbinic opinion that AID [artificial insemination by donor] should be condemned as 'an act of hideousness' or 'an abomination' or 'human stud farming'" (Rosner, p. 133). Such critics of third-party gamete donation believe that procreative acts that take place in a context other than marital fidelity are diminished and distorted. However, other commentators, including some within the Jewish tradition, accept gamete donation, maintaining that the exclusive relationship between husband and wife remains unchanged when gametes from a third party are used to achieve fertilization (Mackler). Thus, some members of a Church of England working party declared that this procedure is ethically acceptable because "there is no offence against the married partner, there is no breaking of the relationship of physical fidelity, and there is no relationship with a person outside of marriage" (Church of England, p. 57).

The other feature of procreation of special concern to critics of gamete donation, that it is embodied, is undeniably set aside in gamete donation—no act of sexual union takes place between those who will be the rearing parents of the resulting child. Many natural-law theorists hold that it is wrong to replace sexual intercourse with methods of assisted reproduction, particularly when they involve third parties, for to do so wrongly separates the procreative and unitive or loving ends of sexual intercourse. The Roman Catholic Church, in particular, rejects gamete donation because it is thought to erode the unity of body and spirit in the procreative process (Congregation for the Doctrine of the Faith). The Protestant theologian Paul Ramsey (1913–1988) once declared that an ethic that regards "procreation as an aspect of biological nature to be subjected merely to the requirements of *technical* control while saying that the unitive purpose is the free, human, personal end of the matter pays disrespect to the nature of human parenthood" (p. 33). The use of gametes derived from third parties outside a marriage is prohibited in Islamic law, as this risks inadvertent consanguinity ("being of the same blood") dilutes the purity of the family line, and could create confusion about the identity of a child's genetic parents and about a child's heritage (Serour).

Proponents of gamete donation respond that to insist on physical union between man and woman in procreation is to derive ethical norms too simply and narrowly from the usual physical structure of human reproduction. Furthermore, it is to ignore that the use of donated gametes can uphold, rather than violate, the loving dimension of the relation between marital partners and lead to responsible parenthood (Lauritzen, pp. 9–12). It is sufficient that love and procreation are held together within the marital relationship as a whole.

Feminist scholars, in particular, have expressed concern about the metaphorical disembodiment that gamete donation can entail for women. Some of those who have donated gametes maintain that they are not treated as whole persons, but are divided into unrelated parts, each of which is subjected to manipulation in order to produce a child. A woman's body can thus be treated as "a field to be seeded, ploughed, and ultimately harvested for the fruit of the womb" (Raymond, pp. 61–62). Supporters of gamete donation and assisted reproduction respond that neither current ethical analysis nor public policy views women as "fetal containers" (Robertson, pp. 192, 228–229). While they acknowledge that the legitimate needs and interests of women must be recognized, they argue that new technologies such as gamete donation expand the freedom of women and assure them a large measure of control over their reproductive lives.

Parenthood and Family Relationships

Those who challenge the use of donated gametes argue that in a world where the rearing mother or father is no longer the biological source of gametes, there is no obvious answer to the question who are the "real" parents of the child. They argue that the use of third-party gametes thus vitiates lines of kinship and descent that situate individuals within particular and extended familial relationships (Meilaender). Further, when gamete donation is used to enable single women to have babies with donor sperm, and when postmenopausal women to give birth to children using donated eggs, traditional notions of the family are confounded (Cahill).

A second line of argument presented by these critics is that those who engender a biological relationship to a child, as do gamete donors, bear responsibility for the well-being of children who result. It is wrong, they maintain, for men and women to provide their gametes to couples and then leave without concern for the child who emerges. (O'Donovan). Some argue forcefully that sperm donation, in particular, institutionalizes the socially problematic phenomenon of paternal abandonment (Callahan).

Those in the opposite camp respond that while the biological connection is important to parenthood, it is not essential. In adoption, for example, the biological relationship between parent and child is sundered, and yet the practice is well accepted. It is also acceptable, therefore, to allow such separation in gamete donation. If those using gamete donation will provide a stable and caring environment in which the welfare of the child is a central focus, as is presumptively the case in adoption, there is no reason to adjudge gamete donation wrong. In this view, nurturing is of greater significance to parenthood than biological rootedness. Thus, while proponents recognize that gamete donation challenges traditional understandings of the family, they accept this as reflecting contemporary social realities (Robertson, pp. 121–122). Critics respond that this procedure is distinct from adoption, for it amounts to intentional preconception abandonment of future children by donors, as opposed to giving up already born biological children out of necessity (Cahill). Moreover, they maintain that the biological connection of children with their parents and extended family is a significant factor affecting their sense of self that ought not be disregarded.

The use of gamete donation to enable older women to have children has come under special scrutiny, not only because it raises issues of safety for mature women and the children they might bring into the world, but also because of concerns about its impact on the family. Some commentators maintain that egg donation is making biological limitations of aging irrelevant, and this, in turn, is confounding traditional notions of the family as women old enough to be grandmothers give birth to babies. Yet others observe that men have been known to father children in their mature years without criticism, and that there is no reason that the same should not be true of women. Older parents, they argue, may stretch the usual concept of the family, but they do not destroy it. Even so, the risks of egg donation and pregnancy for older women and their children can be serious. NABER and the New York State Task Force on Life and the Law recommend caution about the use of egg donation in women of relatively advanced reproductive age, maintaining that the risks to the woman and the best interests of resulting children must be considered.

Secrecy and Anonymity

Whether it is wrong to keep the use of gamete donation secret has become a pressing ethical, social, and psychological issue. Secrecy in gamete donation is said to place a lie at the center of family life, and therefore to be destructive. Studies show that any lifetime secrets impose a burden on the family members and have a detrimental psychological and social impact on the resulting children. The risk of unexpected disclosure of the circumstances of a child's conception hangs over the family that has concealed this information. Some psychologists maintain that it is important to the healthy development of children that they know their biological origins (Baran and PanNor; Nachtigall). They believe that disclosure of the participation of a gamete donor in the conception of a child improves, rather than weakens, family relationships. Moreover, in a world in which genetic information is of increasing importance, children who do not know of a source of some of their genes are denied information that might be important to their health. The primary reason for concealing this information is that the children who spring from gamete donation might be stigmatized as different. Such stigmatization is decreasing, however, in a world in which families are more often composed of members of varying biological origins.

If secrecy were abjured in families, it would be necessary either that rearing parents and the resulting children at maturity know the identity of their gamete donor, or else have a certain amount of information about him or her that could lead to identification if all involved are amenable to this. Yet identifying donors has been controversial. Perhaps the oldest argument against doing so is that potential donors would be fearful of having a child born with the assistance of their gametes later appear at the front door, or that they might be held responsible for the support of such a child. Many donors would therefore decide against donating, which would diminish the pool of available donors. In addition, recipients fear that donors would seek them out and either claim the children or attach themselves to the children (Cohen, 1996). This is of particular concern when relatives are gamete donors. Coercion within families could surface, as could bad feelings if donation were followed by an adverse outcome.

For such reasons, the identity of those who donate gametes is generally not revealed to recipients. The Ethics Committee of the American Fertility Society formally embraced the principle of anonymity of sperm donors in 1994 in order to encourage men to donate and to safeguard them from unwittingly becoming responsible for the support of the resulting children.

Enthusiasm for maintaining anonymity, however, appears to be diminishing. Surveys indicate that donors are increasingly willing to be contacted after a child born of their gametes turns eighteen if they have assurance that they will have no financial or familial obligation to the child. NABER has proposed that egg donation centers move toward a policy of offering both known and confidential donors to those seeking eggs, and that donors be required to provide information about their medical history and genetic health. Children born of donated gametes would be given access to this information at the age of eighteen, if they so requested, and donors would have the option of providing either relevant identifying or nonidentifying information to them. NABER has also recommended that a centrally coordinated network of registries be established in the United States that would keep records about donors in either identifiable or coded form, depending on the choice of the donor (National Advisory Board on Ethics in Reproduction, pp. 290–291, 300).

Commodification of Procreation and Children

There is growing concern that egg donation, in particular, is being left adrift amidst a stream of commerce, and that procreation is being commodified. The current marketing of egg donation, critics contend, relegates human beings to the status of commercial objects and their gametes to that of products. Some see the current practice of paying significant sums to egg donors as coming uncomfortably close to baby buying, and they maintain that this flies in the face of the accepted view of children as individuals endowed with an underlying dignity. Several commentators observe that gametes, as the means of making new life possible, are not negligible body products that ought to be bought and sold in the open market (Lauritzen; Radin; Cohen, 1999; Shanley). Moreover, they argue, to offer large sums of money to egg donors amounts to a form of undue inducement that can vitiate the voluntary decision of donors to donate eggs. Some feminists argue that poor women, in particular, should not be enticed to turn their reproductive capacities into a commodity.

Defenders of paying women for their eggs outright maintain that women have the right to sell "products" of their bodies if they so choose. State intervention to prohibit the sale of eggs, in their view, would violate the individual liberty interests of such women. Moreover, prohibiting payment to donors would only compound the problems of those who are less well off by depriving them of a source of income (Harris). It is not the sale of human eggs that is wrong, in their view, but the fact that a bidding war for them has emerged with no industry-wide standards that set a fair price. The most prudent social policy would be to regulate the market for human eggs to ensure that egg donors receive appropriate pay for their time and endeavors. (Resnik).

Several review groups that have addressed this question advocate financially reimbursing gamete donors only for their time and inconvenience. Their primary justification for this approach is that it upholds human dignity and avoids undue inducement of women to donate their eggs. It is fair and reasonable, they maintain, to compensate donors for their expenses, travel, lost wages, and, to some extent, the risks that they incur in going through the donation procedure (National Advisory Board on Ethics in Reproduction, 1996; New York State Task Force on Life and the Law,

1998; Ethics Committee of the American Society of Reproductive Medicine, 2000). The ASRM suggests that appropriate compensation for egg donors would amount to $5,000, and that amounts up to $10,000 might be justifiable. It is inappropriate to offer larger amounts to potential egg donors, the society holds.

Oversight

Some legal commentators maintain that individuals have a constitutionally protected right to reproduce, a right that extends from coital reproduction to such methods of assisted reproduction as gamete donation. The use of gamete donation should thus be a matter of individual decision, and the state should play only a limited regulatory role to ensure safety and prohibit uses that would substantially harm others (Andrews; Ethics Committee of the American Fertility Society, 1994, p. S13; Robertson, pp. 41, 119–123). Others agree that individuals have a right to reproduce coitally that lies in a sphere protected from most state intrusion, but they reject the view that methods of assisted reproduction clearly fall under the aegis of this right. They are concerned about the use of gamete donation without sufficient regard for the interests and health of donors, recipients, and the resulting children. Some have therefore recommended that there be national standards and a federal regulatory system governing this and other forms of assisted reproduction (Rao; Massie; Cohen, 1997).

Yet no federal laws govern the procedures of gamete donation in the United States, and no review of novel assisted-reproductive techniques is required by federal regulation. IVF clinics that practice gamete donation are not required to set up institutional review boards or to review innovative treatments under the regulations of the Department of Health and Human Services. The Clinical Laboratory Improvement Amendments of 1988 covers only the laboratory analysis of sperm for purposes of quality control. The Food and Drug Administration requires registration, but not licensure, of sperm banks, although it has indicated that plans to develop guidelines for screening donated sperm to prevent transmission of communicable diseases. Under the Fertility Clinic Success Rate and Certification Act of 1992, data regarding clinic-specific pregnancy and delivery success rates for assisted-reproductive procedures, including oocyte donation, are collected and published by the Centers for Disease Control along with various professional societies (Society for Assisted Reproductive Technology). This produces useful information, but does not regulate procedures of gamete donation. Thus, there is a dearth of federal oversight of the methods and materials used for sperm and egg donation.

There is some state law regulating sperm donation but the vast majority of states do not require sperm banks to be licensed. There is almost no state law regarding egg donation. Judicial holdings in this area have been limited and have focused on deciding who should serve as the rearing parents of children born of gamete donation. In the private sector, a voluntary association of tissue providers, the American Association of Tissue Banks, has developed detailed standards for sperm donor screening, the ASRM has published practice guidelines for egg and sperm donation, and NABER has developed recommendations for egg donation. However, these guidelines do not have the force of law and offer no mechanism for surveillance or enforcement.

Commentators and review groups observe that in a market-driven environment that has been blighted by occasional scandals and misrepresentations, there is a compelling need to provide oversight of the use of gamete donation and other methods of assisted reproduction in the United States (Annas; ISLAT Working Group; National Advisory Board on Ethics in Reproduction; Cohen, 2002; New York State Task Force on Life and the Law). NABER, in 1996, called for a national regulatory body to license and monitor the quality of services of infertility centers and proposed that in the interim a task force composed of practitioners, outside experts from various disciplines, and lay persons should develop uniform intercenter policies to inform and safeguard donors, recipients, and resulting children (National Advisory Board). It also recommended numerous changes in professional guidelines and standards, as well as state and federal law. In addition, in 1998, the New York State Task Force on Life and the Law identified major problems in the provision of gamete donation and drafted guidelines and model consent forms to improve information given to donors and recipients. It, too, offered detailed recommendations for changes in professional standards that would provide some degree of uniformity in practice, and it proposed changes in state law to protect those involved in gamete donation and the children born of these procedures. Also in 1998, the ISLAT (Institute for Science, Law and Technology) Working Group recommended a federal law that would set a minimum standard for the provision of assisted-reproductive technologies and urged that noncompliance should result in criminal or civil liability. Few of these proposals have been adopted.

There are now at least twenty legal jurisdictions around the world that have enacted legislation regarding the uses of the new reproductive technologies. Countries that allow gamete donation combine the prohibition of certain procedures with licensing requirements to limit who may perform reproductive procedures. The use of eggs from donors, for instance, is prohibited by law in Germany, Norway, Sweden, Switzerland, and Japan. Countries that have adopted uniform standards for the infertility industry, such as the United Kingdom and Australia, began by appointing a commission or committee to study the issues and make legislative recommendations, and they then acted upon those recommendations.

Future Directions

Demand for donated eggs will increase in the future, not only to accommodate ever greater numbers of couples and individuals seeking to have children, but also to bolster new areas of research. Investigative programs, such as those in basic human embryology, embryonic stem cells, cloning, and cryopreservation of human eggs, will require large quantities of human eggs before they can proceed. Other sources of human eggs, in addition to living donors, are therefore under investigation for both clinical and research uses.

Researchers have begun to delve into the possibility of using fetal eggs, derived from aborted fetuses and matured *in vitro*, for clinical egg donation programs. Some have prophesied that this could lead to the development of *egg farms,* in which some of the thousands of eggs in a young woman's ovaries that would otherwise fall by the wayside could be salvaged to increase the number of eggs available for personal use or the use of others (Gosden, p. 152). It is not yet known whether the early female eggs, which normally are subject to a high degree of degeneration, can develop into mature eggs capable of giving rise to a normal fetus after fertilization. Moreover, an aborted fetus could be the carrier of a metabolic or genetic disorder that could manifest itself in the resulting child. If such eggs were used to overcome infertility, this would raise concern about the psychological well-being of the resulting children, who might experience harm either from being told that their genetic mother was an aborted fetus or from not being told of this. Since there is currently no compelling need to use fetal oocytes, the ASRM has recommended that this avenue of investigation not be pursued (Ethics Committee of the American Society of Reproductive Medicine, 1997, pp. 6S–7S).

Frozen, stored ovaries are another possible source of human eggs for clinical use. A slice of ovary contains thousands of immature eggs, and ovarian tissue could be removed during surgery for ovarian cyst or endometriosis, or during prophylactic surgery for ovarian cancer. Freezing and storing ovarian tissue currently appears more promising than freezing mature eggs. Moreover, storage of ovarian tissue is relatively easy. This is an experimental procedure that is under development and, consequently, there has been little comment about its safety or its import for the interests of the resulting children.

Because women are currently the sole source of eggs that can be used to create human embryos, and because there is a paucity of eggs for research, women will increasingly be called upon to provide eggs for investigative purposes. This raises significant ethical questions. Women asked to contribute eggs to stem-cell research or research cloning, for instance, would receive neither health benefits to themselves nor the satisfaction of assisting in the birth of a child to others (Baylis). Their primary motivations for undergoing egg donation procedures in such cases would either be the satisfaction of assisting medical science or the prospect of financial reward. If such research were carried out in the public sector under current federal guidelines for stem-cell research that had been extended beyond current restrictions on the sources of such lines, women would be barred from receiving financial compensation for their endeavors and risks in donating eggs. They would provide eggs solely to assist medical research. Thus they would constitute human subjects participating in nontherapeutic investigations that expose them to more than minimal risk, and the Common Rule requiring full, written, informed consent would apply. However, it is clear, commentators have observed, that the common rule for informed consent is currently not being adhered to in either federally or privately funded research when deriving eggs from women to create embryos from which stem cell lines are developed. Therefore, they argue that to protect the voluntary choice and health of women, fully informed consent should be rigorously sought in the future from women whose eggs are used in scientific research, no matter who provides those eggs or what the source of funding for that research.

CYNTHIA B. COHEN

SEE ALSO: *Abortion; Adoption; Cloning; Embryo and Fetus; Feminism; Fetal Research; Genetic Counseling; Genetic Testing and Screening: Reproductive Genetic Testing; Healthcare Resources, Allocation of: Microallocation; Law and Bioethics; Maternal-Fetal Relationship; Moral Status; Population Ethics; Sexism; Transhumanism and Posthumanism; Women, Contemporary Issues of;* and other *Reproductive Technologies* subentries

BIBLIOGRAPHY

American Society for Reproductive Medicine. 2002. "2002 Guidelines for Gamete and Embryo Donation: A Practice Report." *Fertility and Sterility* 77(6), suppl. 5: S1–S8.

Andrews, Lori B. 1989. "Control and Competition: Laws Governing Extracorporeal Generative Materials." *Journal of Medicine and Philosophy* 14(5): 541–560.

Annas, George J. 1998. "The Shadowlands: Secrets, Lies, and Assisted Reproduction." *New England Journal of Medicine* 339(13): 935–939.

Baran, Annette, and Pannor, Reuben. 1989. *Lethal Secrets: The Shocking Consequences and Unsolved Problems of Artificial Insemination.* New York: Warner.

Baylis, Françoise. 2000. "Our Cells/Ourselves: Creating Embryos for Stem Cell Research." *Women's Health Issues* 10(3): 140–145.

Cahill, Lisa Sowle. 1996. "Moral Concerns about Institutionalized Gamete Donation." In *New Ways of Making Babies: The Case of Egg Donation,* ed. Cynthia B. Cohen. Bloomington: Indiana University Press.

Callahan, Daniel. 1992. "Bioethics and Fatherhood." *Utah Law Review* 3: 735–746.

Church of England, Board of Social Responsibility. 1996. *Personal Origins,* 2nd edition. London: Church House.

Cohen, Cynthia B. 1996. "Parents Anonymous." In *New Ways of Making Babies: The Case of Egg Donation,* ed. Cynthia B. Cohen. Bloomington: Indiana University Press.

Cohen, Cynthia B. 1997. "Unmanaged Care: The Need to Regulate New Reproductive Technologies in the United States." *Bioethics* 11(3, 4): 348–365.

Cohen, Cynthia B. 1999. "Selling Bits and Pieces of Humans to Make Babies: 'The Gift of the Magi' Revisited." *Journal of Medicine and Philosophy* 24(3): 88–306.

Cohen, Cynthia B. 2002. "Creating Tomorrow's Children: The Right to Reproduce, Public Policy, and Germ-Line Interventions." In *Designing Our Descendants: The Promise and Perils of Genetic Modifications,* ed. Audrey R. Chapman and Mark S. Frankel. Baltimore: Johns Hopkins University Press.

Congregation for the Doctrine of the Faith. 1987. "Instruction on Respect for Human Life in Its Origin and on the Dignity of Procreation." *Origins* 16: 697–707.

Daniels, K. R. 2000. "To Give or Sell Human Gametes—the Interplay between Pragmatics, Policy, and Ethics." *Journal of Medical Ethics* 26: 206–211.

Ethics Committee of the American Fertility Society. 1994. "Ethical Considerations of Assisted Reproductive Technologies." *Fertility and Sterility* 62 (suppl. 1): 1S–104S.

Ethics Committee of the American Society for Reproductive Medicine. 1997. "Ethical Considerations of Assisted Reproductive Technologies," *Fertility and Sterility* 67(5), suppl. 1: 1S–9S.

Ethics Committee of the American Society for Reproductive Medicine. 2000. "Financial Incentives in Recruitment of Oocyte Donors." *Fertility and Sterility* 74(2): 216–220.

Gosden, Roger. 1999. *Designing Babies: The Brave New World of Reproductive Technology.* New York: W.W. Freeman.

Hard, A. D. 1909. "Artificial Impregnation." *Medical World* 27: 163.

Harris, John. 1992. *Wonderwoman and Superman: The Ethics of Human Biotechnology.* Oxford: Oxford University Press.

Institute for Science, Law and Technology (ISLAT) Working Group. 1998. "ART into Science: Regulation of Fertility Techniques." *Science* 281: 651–652.

Lauritzen Paul. 1993. *Pursuing Parenthood: Ethical Issues in Assisted Reproduction.* Bloomington: Indiana University Press.

Mackler, Aaron L. 2001. "Is There a Unique Jewish Bioethics of Human Reproduction?" *Annual of the Society of Christian Ethics* 21: 319–323.

Massie, Ann Mclean. 1995. "Regulating Choice: A Constitutional Law Response to Professor John A. Robertson's Children of Choice." *Washington and Lee Law Review* 52(1): 135–171.

Meilaender, Gilbert. 1995. *Body, Soul, and Bioethics.* Notre Dame, IN: University of Notre Dame Press.

Nachtigall, R. D.; Tschann, J. M.; Quiroga, S. S.; et al. 1997. "Stigma, Disclosure, and Family Functioning among Parents of Children Conceived through Donor Insemination." *Fertility and Sterility* 68: 83–89.

National Advisory Board on Ethics in Reproduction. 1996. "Report and Recommendations on Oocyte Donation." In *New Ways of Making Babies: The Case of Egg Donation,* ed. Cynthia B. Cohen, Bloomington: Indiana University Press.

New York State Task Force on Life and the Law. 1998. "Gamete and Embryo Donation." In *Assisted Reproductive Technologies: Analysis and Recommendations for Public Policy.* Albany: New York State Department of Health.

O'Donovan, Oliver. 1984. *Begotten or Made?* New York: Oxford University Press.

Radin, Margaret Jane. 1996. *Contested Commodities: The Trouble with Trade in Sex, Children, Body Parts, and Other Things.* Cambridge, MA: Harvard University Press.

Ramsey, Paul. 1970. *Fabricated Man. The Ethics of Genetic Control.* New Haven, CT: Yale University Press.

Rao, Radhika. 1995. "Constitutional Misconceptions." *University of Michigan Law Review* 93: 1473–1496.

Raymond, Janice. 1987. "Fetalists and Feminists: They Are Not the Same." In *Made to Order: The Myth of Reproductive and Genetic Progress,* ed. Patricia Spallone and Deborah Lynn Steinberg Oxford: Pergamon Press.

Resnik, David B. 2001. "Regulating the Market for Human Eggs." *Bioethics* 15(1): 1–25.

Robertson, John A. 1994. *Children of Choice: Freedom and the New Reproductive Technologies.* Princeton, NJ: Princeton University Press.

Rosner, Fred. 2001. *Biomedical Ethics and Jewish Law.* Hoboken, NJ: KTAV Publishing.

Serour, G. I. 1993. "Bioethics in Artificial Reproduction in the Muslim World." *Bioethics* 7: 207–215.

Shanley, Mary Lyndon. 2002. "Collaboration and Commodification in Assisted Procreation: Reflections on an Open Market and Anonymous Donation in Human Sperm and Eggs," *Law and Society Review* 36: 257–283.

Society for Assisted Reproductive Technology, and American Society for Reproductive Medicine. 2002. "Assisted Reproductive Technology in the United States: 1998 Results Generated from the American Society for Reproductive Medicine/Society for Assisted Reproductive Technology Registry." *Fertility and Sterility* 77(1): 18–31.

Trounson, A. J.; Leeton, J.; Besanko, M.; et al. 1983. "Pregnancy Established in an Infertile Patient after Transfer of a Donated Embryo Fertilised *In Vitro*." *British Medical Journal* 286: 835–838.

VI. CONTRACT PREGNANCY

Contract pregnancy, often also called *surrogate motherhood*, consists of a complex set of practices in which women employ their distinctive reproductive powers to give birth to children on the understanding that others will take on the responsibilities and prerogatives involved in the rearing of the children. The controversies surrounding such practices extend even to issues of labeling. Women who provide their ova as well as their abilities to gestate and deliver babies to this enterprise are sometimes referred to as *full surrogates,* as contrasted with *partial surrogates,* who gestate and give birth to children conceived in vitro, typically with the gametes of the commissioning man or couple. For reasons of clarity, the phrase *genetic-gestational* is used in this entry to refer to those women who have agreed to provide both their gametes and their wombs; *gestational* alone indicates those women whose role is to sustain and deliver a child to whom they are not genetically related. More significantly, some writers have argued that referring to women who have carried a fetus to term and delivered a child as *surrogates* slights their status as mothers, and prejudices the discussion of disputes concerning parental status between the birthgiver and the commissioning party in favor of the couple or individual who secured the birthgiver's services. For this reason the term *contract pregnancy,* coined by Laura Purdy, is adopted here, although it should be noted that not all such arrangements are explicitly contractual. The understandings under which women act may well be highly formal arrangements, brokered by intermediaries and involving payment, but they may also be quite informal, with no intermediaries or compensation.

Apart from matters of nomenclature, controversies concerning contract pregnancy have, in practice, revolved around disputes concerning the enforceability of agreements when one (or more) of the parties involved has undergone a change of heart, namely: contract birthgivers who find themselves no longer willing to relinquish custody of the children they have borne, or commissioning parties who have changed their minds about wanting to parent the child born of the arrangement they initiated. In theory, the chief disagreement concerns the conditions that confer parental responsibility—that is, how the elements of gestation, genetics, desire, and intention should be weighed when their customary connections have been purposefully sundered. Other disagreements arise over whether women or children are harmed or wronged by contract pregnancy, whether contract pregnancy involves the commodification of children or of the parent–child relationship, and whether desires on the part of adults to rear children to whom they are in some way biologically related ought to be honored in light of the needs of existing children who lack parents. It has also been suggested that contract pregnancy offers important reproductive options to people who have not previously enjoyed them—women who have undergone hysterectomies and gay men, for example—and that by expanding the ways in which families can grow (and, in principle, the ways in which people can be related to each other), contract pregnancy can add important value to human lives.

Disputes about Motherhood

The incidence of contract pregnancy is not centrally monitored, but empirical studies by Helena Ragone (1994) suggest that most such arrangements prove satisfactory, at least to the adults who are centrally involved. Nevertheless, three prominent court cases exemplify the deeply unsettling controversies that can arise when the strands of motherhood are pulled apart and the affected parties disagree about how to weave them together again. The first two cases discussed below involve a dispute between the commissioning parties and the birthgivers, in a genetic-gestational contract pregnancy and a gestational pregnancy, respectively; the third case involves a disagreement between the man and the woman who constituted the commissioning party.

IN THE MATTER OF BABY M. Contract pregnancy became a matter of public concern as a result of the *Baby M* case, probably the most notorious of contract pregnancy disputes. A 1985 agreement between Mary Beth Whitehead and David Stern, providing that Whitehead should, for financial considerations, conceive, bear, and then surrender their child to the sole custody of Stern, led to the birth of Melissa Stern. The contract was voided on appeal to the New Jersey Supreme Court in 1988, after a drawn-out dispute between Whitehead and the Sterns that featured Whitehead fleeing with the child from New Jersey to Florida. Whitehead was recognized as the child's legal mother, contracts of the sort in question being found contrary to New Jersey public policy and law. Custody, however, was awarded to Stern and his wife, Elizabeth Stern, on a determination that the "best interests of the child" would thus be served. Whitehead was granted visitation rights.

JOHNSON V. CALVERT. Anna Johnson agreed to be implanted with an embryo created from the gametes of Crispina and Mark Calvert on the understanding that the Calverts would rear the ensuing child. In September 1990, before the birth of the child, Johnson challenged the contract. The Supreme Court of California upheld the lower court's ruling in favor of the Calverts, on the grounds that while both "genetic consanguinity" and giving birth are legally recognized means of establishing a mother–child relationship, "when the two means do not coincide in one woman, she who intended to procreate the child—that is, she who intended to bring about the birth of a child that she intended to raise as her own—is the natural mother under California law." Johnson's visitation rights were terminated.

IN RE MARRIAGE OF BUZZANCA. Luanne and John Buzzanca arranged for an unnamed woman to gestate an embryo donated by third parties and agreed to rear the resulting child. Just prior to the child's birth, John Buzzanca filed for divorce, maintaining that he had no parental responsibilities to Jaycee, the child to be carried to term on his estranged wife's behalf. The trial court, accepting the stipulation that the birthgiver was not Jaycee's mother and reasoning that the Buzzancas' lack of a genetic tie to the child ruled them out as well, concluded that Jaycee "had no lawful parents." The appeals court disagreed, ruling in a 1998 decision that "the intent to parent as expressed in the surrogacy contract" established Luanne and John as Jaycee's legal mother and father, and finding John Buzzanca responsible for her support.

Three Analytical Clusters

These cases illustrate various forms of disputes about who counts as a parent, and in virtue of what considerations. Given the deep significance for many people of biological connections to their children, bioethicists have been quite concerned to resolve these matters, and a variety of approaches have been explored. These approaches may be grouped under three headings, according to whose interests are deemed most crucial. The first cluster centers on the *adult parties* involved as competent makers of contracts. These analyses address themselves with the features the contracts should have in order to avoid moral and practical problems. The second cluster focuses especially on the position of *women* in these arrangements, with particular attention to the woman who accepts the commission. These approaches portray women as operating in what is in general a hostile social environment and are skeptical that women's interests will be reliably served or protected by contract pregnancy. The third cluster centers particularly on the claims that the *children* born of these arrangements should be able to make against their parents, drawing on the notion that children have a moral stake in how the responsibilities of the adults who brought them into being are assigned.

Contracts and Commodification

A clearly argued version of the first model provided in a 1988 article by Bonnie Steinbock, contends that there is no sufficient reason to outlaw contract pregnancy or hold such contracts unenforceable. Steinbock maintains that these arrangements ought to be seen as a prenatal version of adoption. Among the safeguards she proposes is that a birthgiver ought to be allowed an opportunity after giving birth to change her mind about surrendering custody of the child to the commissioning party, just as a new mother is allowed to reconsider whether she will give up her child for adoption.

The most significant challenge to contract pregnancy, as Steinbock sees it—the concern that such practices involve a mother's relinquishing her standing as a parent for money—could be obviated by mandating that any payment be for "risk, sacrifice and discomfort" (Steinbock, p. 49) involved in pregnancy, and hence would be made even if the pregnancy ended in a stillbirth. Should the mother change her mind about giving up her child, she would not, however, be entitled to any remuneration for those sacrifices.

With commodification thus deflected as a criticism of contract pregnancy, none of the other concerns Steinbock surveys—for example, potential emotional damage to the mother or the child as a result of their involvement in these arrangements—strike her as sufficient to justify state action against the practice. While the possibility that some women will undergo a change of heart cannot be dismissed, it would be intolerably paternalistic for the state to refuse to allow women to make contractual agreements they believe to be in their own best interests because of concerns that they were too prone to mistake what those interests are. Nor is there any reason to believe that any distress suffered by children would be so intense as to make it reasonable for them to wish that they had never been born via these arrangements (which, of course, are the only possible arrangements that would have led to the birth of precisely those children).

Steinbock does not explicitly discuss gestational contract pregnancy, so it is not clear whether such cases would be understood along the lines of her prenatal adoption model, nor whether gestational birthgivers who change their minds would be able to retain any claim to parental standing they might have, losing merely the money that had been agreed upon. This suggests one difficulty with an approach to contract pregnancy that attempts to adapt standing models of assigning parental rights and duties, such as adoption, to resolve contractual disputes. It seems unlikely that any account of contract pregnancy that does not explicitly grapple with what it is that makes a woman a mother in the first place (in the sense of conferring parental responsibilities and prerogatives upon her) will be altogether satisfactory.

Nor is it clear just how a contract pregnancy that includes substantial economic transactions can be insulated from the concern that what is bought and sold is the baby, rather than the gestational services. Steinbock insists that payment be made even in cases in which the pregnant woman loses the child, thereby underscoring the claim that the money is not a quid pro quo for the infant. In a 1990 article, however, Elizabeth S. Anderson argues that commercial surrogacy devalues children insofar as it regards maternal connections to children as commodities to be exchanged and trivializes a woman's own evolving perspective on her pregnancy by providing her with fiscal incentives for severing whatever emotional links to the child she may develop. If the argument that any payment is solely for inconvenience and risk were to stand against Anderson's points, it would seem that the payment should be made regardless of whether the birthgiver is willing to relinquish her parental relationship to the child. She has, after all, faced risk and inconvenience to bring into the world a child to whom the contracting party has a parental relation. That such an arrangement would severely diminish the attractiveness of the contract pregnancy in the first place strongly suggests that the payment cannot be regarded as mere compensation for the birthgiver's trouble. The whole point of the arrangement is that the child should be given up at birth, rather than becoming a part of the birthgiver's family. So it seems that the would-be parents are paying for more than the birthgiver's inconvenience and risk. Their incentive for paying rests on the assurance that they will have custody of the born child.

Women, Exploitation, and Altruism

The issue of turning children or parental relationships into commodities is a serious challenge to the moral and legal propriety of contract pregnancy. Janice Raymond, however, points out in a 1990 article that even when money does not change hands—an arrangement she calls "altruistic surrogacy"—coercive forces are present in society in general and in families in particular that can influence women to act against their own better judgment and interests. Her argument thus serves as a significant instance of the second, woman-focused model of analysis. While the point has often been made that women who are potential contract birthgivers are likely to be less socially powerful than the men or couples who seek to reproduce through their agency, Raymond focuses on expectations of feminine—and particularly

maternal—altruism that cut across class distinctions and are in her view among the most powerful of the forces that oppress women. While not denying that "women can give freely," Raymond insists on the sociological complexity of "gift giving," arguing in particular that the connections between altruism and femininity can distort individual choice and reinforce unjust patterns of social status. She ties these cautions about altruism to a broader criticism of contract pregnancy. The practice depicts women as "reproductive conduits," "incidental incubator(s) detached from the total fabric of social, affective and moral meanings associated with procreation" (Raymond, p. 11).

Do concerns of this kind constitute reasons to forbid or restrict women's freedom to enter into such contracts as a matter of law? This depends in part on whether women are able to resist coercive or manipulative pressures that may well be more present in altruistic than commercial contexts, and whether altruistic forms of surrogacy can be conceptualized in ways that do not support, and in fact undermine, objectionable connections between women and altruism. By the same token, whether contract birthgivers are mere "reproductive conduits" may hinge on whether contract pregnancy can be absorbed into the social, affective, and moral fabric to which Raymond alludes—perhaps by revaluing brightening and motherhood in ways that are themselves less prone to reinforce women's subordination. While such refiguring of social meanings seem latent possibilities within the practice of contract pregnancy, it is unclear whether or to what extent they are being realized in individual cases. Nevertheless, Elizabeth F. S. Roberts's ethnographic research, published in 1998, suggests that at least some contract birthgivers are indeed engaged in forging their own, new understandings of what it is to bear a child. These understandings may in turn help destabilize traditional understandings of family and motherhood that have been oppressive for women.

Children and Parenthood

Focusing on the moral role of children in contract pregnancy arrangements, James Lindemann Nelson and Hilde Lindemann Nelson have argued that parental responsibilities arise from parents' causal relation to their children. Because parents have brought about their children's existence, and because their children's existence is initially one of vulnerability and dependence, parents are responsible for their children's well-being. If they cannot fulfill their responsibility, they may give up the child for adoption, but they may not deliberately create a situation in which they put it out of their power to look after their children. Their responsibility cannot be relinquished solely as a matter of agreements between adults that are prompted by their own interests. Nelson and Nelson further argue that because biological ties with children are seen as precisely the justification for such practices as contract pregnancy, it is only fair to assume that children too will have an interest in relationships with those to whom they are connected by ties of biology.

As with Steinbock's position, the implications of this position for cases of gestational surrogacy are unclear, and the situation might seem to be even more murky in cases where the commissioning couple are neither the genetic nor the gestational parents, as in *Buzzanca*. What kind of causal involvement with the child's emergence into the world is sufficient to establish at least a presumptive set of moral responsibilities? Further, the position at least leaves open the question why a person whose causal involvement is sufficient to ground such responsibilities cannot discharge them simply by taking steps to ascertain that the parties to whom she will relinquish her responsibilities are likely to be good parents. Regarding this latter question, a distinction between prediction and performance might be invoked. The acts of another can only be predicted, but one can exercise substantial amounts of control over one's own performance. May one divest oneself of the ability to see to it that the needs of a child for whom one is responsible will reliably be met? What constitutes a good enough reason to relinquish one's moral responsibilities to one's offspring? Setting aside concerns about commodification, concerns about exploitation of women, and concerns about the deep distress occasioned by a change of mind, it remains to be asked whether an altruistically motivated interest in helping others to procreate is sufficient to initiate human reproduction with the intent not to participate in raising the resulting children. Two further questions remain as well: Is it justifiable to ask someone else to put herself at the personal and moral risk involved with contract pregnancy in order to have or expand a family? Is it important that biologically linked children could not otherwise be brought into the family?

Reassembling Motherhood

Insofar as questions of this sort can be answered empirically, there seems reason to believe that contract pregnancy has afforded a way for infertile people longing to have children of their own to meet women who are gratified by the opportunity to help them realize their goal. That this process sometimes backfires rather spectacularly, as in the *Baby M, Johnson v. Calvert*, and *Buzzanca* cases, would not seem a decisive reason to regard the process as immoral or so flawed as to outlaw it. The enterprise is attended by moral risks, however, even in the majority of cases in which everyone

walks away feeling satisfied. Giving birth by contract cuts the connections among the genetic, gestational, and intentional elements that constitute motherhood, yet there is no settled, reflective consensus regarding what kind of comparative priority such elements should have when they are sundered. The popularity of such contracts certainly puts force behind a particular answer to the priority question—it strongly privileges the intentional. Given that a rollback toward an answer more influenced by genetic or gestational elements is unlikely in the absence of a showing of serious harm, those concerned about contract pregnancy might consider how the moral risks of this practice might be minimized, and how such pregnancies might achieve moral gains that go beyond the gratification of private impulses.

JAMES LINDEMANN NELSON
HILDE LINDEMANN NELSON

SEE ALSO: *Abortion; Adoption; Cloning; Conflict of Interest; Contractarianism and Bioethics; Embryo and Fetus; Feminism; Fetal Research; Genetic Counseling; Genetic Testing and Screening: Reproductive Genetic Testing; Healthcare Resources, Allocation of: Microallocation; Law and Bioethics; Maternal-Fetal Relationship; Moral Status; Population Ethics; Public Policy and Bioethics; Sexism; Transhumanism and Posthumanism; Women, Contemporary Issues of;* and other *Reproductive Technologies* subentries

BIBLIOGRAPHY

Anderson, Elizabeth S. 1990. "Is Women's Labor a Commodity?" *Philosophy and Public Affairs* 19(1): 71–87.

Andrews, Lori. 1989. *Between Strangers: Surrogate Mothers, Expectant Fathers, and Brave New Babies.* New York: HarperCollins.

Annas, George J. 1988. "Death without Dignity for Commercial Surrogacy: The Case of Baby M." *Hastings Center Report* 18(2): 21–24.

Baby M, In the Matter of. 537 A.2d 1227. (1988).

Baker, Brenda M. 1996. "A Case for Permitting Altruistic Surrogacy." *Hypatia* 11(2): 34–48.

Buzzanca, In re Marriage of. 61 Cal. App. 4th 1410, 72 Cal. Rptr. 2d 280 (1998).

Hartouni, Valerie. 1994. "Breached Birth: Reflections on Race, Gender, and Reproductive Discourse in the 1980s." *Configurations* 2(1): 73–88.

Johnson v. Calvert. 5 Cal. 4th 84; 851 P.2d 776 (1993).

Macklin, Ruth. 1994. *Surrogates and Other Mothers: The Debates over Assisted Reproduction.* Philadelphia: Temple University Press.

Nelson, Hilde Lindemann, and Nelson, James Lindemann. 1988. "Cutting Motherhood in Two: Some Suspicions concerning Surrogacy." *Hypatia* 4(3): 85–94.

Purdy, Laura. 1989. "Surrogate Mothering: Exploitation or Empowerment?" *Bioethics* 3(1): 18–34.

Purdy, Laura. 1996. *Reproducing Persons: Issues in Feminist Bioethics.* Ithaca, NY: Cornell University Press.

Radin, Margaret Jane. 1996. *Contested Commodities.* Cambridge, MA: Harvard University Press.

Ragone, Helena. 1994. *Surrogate Motherhood: Conceptions in the Heart.* Boulder, CO: Westview Press.

Raymond, Janice. 1990. "Reproductive Gifts and Gift-Giving: The Altruistic Woman." *Hastings Center Report* 20(4): 7–11.

Roberts, Elizabeth F. S. 1998. "'Native' Narratives of Connectedness: Surrogate Motherhood and Technology." In *Cyborg Babies: From Techno-Sex to Techno-Tots,* ed. Robbie Davis-Floyd and Joe Dumit. New York: Routledge.

Satz, Debra. 1992. "Markets in Women's Reproductive Labor." *Philosophy and Public Affairs* 21(2): 107–131.

Steinbock, Bonnie. 1988. "Surrogate Motherhood as Prenatal Adoption." *Journal of Law, Medicine, and Health Care* 16(1): 45–50.

VII. SPERM, OVA, AND EMBRYOS

The technical ability to freeze sperm, embryos, and eventually ova for long periods and then thaw them without destroying their biologic potential offers several new reproductive options for both fertile and infertile individuals. It makes the donation of eggs, sperm, or embryos to treat infertility a more efficient and safe procedure. It also allows individuals and couples to preserve sperm, eggs, and embryos to protect against future reductions in gametic viability due to age, disease, or occupational exposure, and permits posthumous reproduction to occur.

As with any technological deviation from the natural mode of conception, these techniques raise both medical questions of safety and efficacy and ethical, legal, and social questions about prohibition, restriction, or regulation of these practices. Once cryopreservation is medically established as safe and effective, its ethical, legal, and social acceptability depends on a general acceptance of noncoital and assisted means of reproduction, with specific issues relating to the particular technique in question.

Sperm

Cryopreservation of sperm is now well established medically and socially as a commercial enterprise. Sperm banking occurs as an aspect of infertility practice, or as an option for men who foresee damage to their gametes as a result of disease or occupational exposure. In the former case, a commercial sperm bank recruits sperm providers, screens them medically and socially, and usually pays them a fee for their sperm (technically they are vendors rather than donors of sperm though the latter word is commonly used to describe their role). The sperm is then distributed to doctors or others who practice artificial insemination with donor sperm, who in turn resell or distribute it to recipients.

A main legal and ethical issue with regard to this practice is the duty of the sperm bank to screen sperm donors and their sperm for infectious diseases, including the human immunodeficiency virus (HIV). Guidelines of the American Fertility Society, the main professional organization of physicians treating infertility, now recommend that donated sperm be screened for HIV diseases. Because there may be a six-month gap before HIV transmission shows up on antibody screening tests, screening requires that the donated sperm be quarantined for six months so that a second test can be performed on a sample to ensure that it is not HIV-infected. Failure to screen in this way is unethical and could make the sperm bank legally liable for transmission of HIV to recipients and offspring.

There are no laws that restrict to whom sperm banks may sell their sperm, and in the United States, the buying and selling of sperm is not generally covered by federal or state laws against selling organs, though several European countries prohibit the practice. Thus a bank could sell sperm to a single woman or representative organizations for use in inseminating single women. Despite fears that a bank or physician who provides sperm to an unmarried woman could be held liable for financial support of a child born as a result, no such legal liability has yet been imposed. While some persons find artificial insemination of single women to be unethical, and the practice is prohibited in some countries, it can allow women who otherwise could not bear children to reproduce, and unmarried women who are committed to reproduction in this way have been shown to be able childrearers.

Commercial sperm banks also provide service to individuals or couples who wish to store sperm for later use because of treatment of disease, occupational exposure, or fear of later impotence. Because no legislation specifically applies to this practice, its legal status would depend upon basic contract law. The depositor would be entitled to keep the sperm in the bank and retrieve it under conditions specified in the contract of deposit. Thus sperm could be released to the depositor or to his designee posthumously, if that is envisaged, and the bank would perhaps have no obligation to maintain the sperm past a specified time if failure to pay storage charges should occur. Clear specification of rights and duties in the original contract is essential. While posthumous release of stored sperm to the appropriate designee could lead to the birth of a child without a rearing father, this situation is similar to the insemination of an unmarried woman and should be treated similarly.

Whether a child born posthumously will be able to share in a deceased's estate is a matter of state inheritance law that does not affect the ethical, legal, or social acceptability of the practice.

The bank would, of course, have a legal duty to return the correct sperm to the depositor. At least one case has arisen in which the bank returned the wrong sperm, which led to the birth of a child who was not of the same race as the depositor. In such instances, suits for damages are likely to be successful. An important issue will concern damages, because there is no way to establish that in fact the lost gametes would have implanted and produced a child. In addition, some states regulate the operation of sperm banks as medical or clinical laboratories to protect the health and safety of consumers of their services.

Many of the issues that arise with commercial sperm banks would also apply to physicians who recruit sperm donors directly. They too would have ethical and legal duties of reasonable care to assure that donors have been tested for genetic and infectious disease. They would also be free to inseminate single women and use sperm posthumously, if that is the clear intention of the parties.

Ova

The ability to freeze and then successfully thaw ova has not yet been developed, due to the larger size of the ovum and the great amount of fluid in it. Once this ability is developed, egg banking will occur.

Frozen ova have less ethical significance than frozen embryos. Once the technical ability to freeze and thaw ova safely is developed, they will play an important role in enabling women to initiate pregnancies through in vitro fertilization (IVF), which involves hormonal stimulation of the ovaries to produce ova, often many more than are needed for fertilization at that time; freezing the extra ova will minimize the need for additional cycles of egg retrieval. Rather than inseminate all eggs retrieved in a cycle of IVF treatment, many couples will prefer to freeze extra eggs, which can then be thawed and inseminated for later attempts at pregnancy. Cryopreservation of ova, rather than embryos, may thus become the preferred method of storage.

Once ova freezing and banking begins, the same issues that currently arise with cryopreservation of sperm will occur. Commercial ova banks, which may be associated with sperm and embryo banks or exist independently, will be established. No doubt such banks will both buy or procure eggs from women and then resell them to doctors and couples in need of an egg donation. The main issues will then concern what the precise arrangement is between the

donor and the bank concerning subsequent use, whether the bank will be responsible for genetic and infectious disease screening, and whether the bank will be responsible for any rearing costs of offspring.

With eggs that have been frozen for subsequent use in initiating pregnancy in an infertile couple, the agreement between the woman or couple and the storage facility will be of paramount importance. The depositor of the eggs will be the owner and will control release or discard of cryopreserved ova within the limits of the storage facility's policies. Thus the contract between the depositor and the facility would largely control deposits of eggs prior to disease treatment or occupational exposure or to use then or at a later time. As long as the depositor has paid storage charges, she would be entitled to have the eggs stored, to expect reasonable care to be taken in their maintenance, and to have the eggs released, transferred, or discarded as directed. Posthumous release and use of stored eggs should be as acceptable as posthumous release and use of stored sperm. As with sperm banking, failure of payment could lead to the bank taking the eggs out of storage, but it would not be entitled to transfer them to other persons in lieu of payment unless there were a specific agreement to that effect. Professional or even legislative regulation of ova banking to ensure standards of health and safety can also be expected.

Embryos

Cryopreservation of embryos (sometimes referred to as preimplantation embryos or *pre-embryos*) is now a well-established adjunct to IVF programs. Standard IVF treatment often produces more eggs than can be safely fertilized and placed in the uterus at one time. Rather than fertilize only the number of eggs that could be safely transferred or fertilize all retrieved eggs and discard the surplus, cryopreservation allows all eggs to be fertilized, a safe number such as two or three placed in the uterus, and the rest frozen for later use. At a later time, the frozen embryos can be thawed and placed in the uterus, donated to others, or discarded. Although the success rate is not as great as with fresh embryos, the pregnancy rate of both fresh and frozen embryos from a single egg-retrieval cycle is 15 to 20 percent greater than the rate from use of fresh embryos alone. Until the ability to freeze and thaw ova is developed, the excess eggs retrieved in a cycle of IVF treatment are likely to be inseminated and then cryopreserved for use during a later cycle.

The main issues that arise with cryopreservation of embryos concern the ethical and legal status of embryos and the locus of dispositional authority over frozen embryos. While some persons have argued that embryos are persons or moral subjects with all the rights of persons, and others claim that embryos are merely tissue with no special status or rights, a wide ethical and legal consensus in the United States, Europe, and Australia views embryos as "deserving of special respect, though not the respect due persons." As a result, embryos may be created, frozen, donated, and even discarded or used in research when there is a valid need to treat infertility or pursue a legitimate scientific goal and rules concerning consent of the gamete providers and institutional review board approval have been followed.

With regard to dispositional authority over frozen embryos, it is now well established that the couple providing the gametes has dispositional authority within the limits of state law and the conditions of storage set by the IVF program or storage facility. If they agree to have embryos created from their gametes cryopreserved, they are *owners* of the embryos and may decide on any disposition of frozen embryos that their agreement with the storage facility and applicable statutes permit.

Since the frozen gametes are the joint property of the persons providing the gametes, their joint consent is needed for disposition until they relinquish or transfer their dispositional authority to others. To maximize their control over embryos and to introduce administrative efficiency into the operation of embryo banking, they should also give written directions at the time of storage for disposition of frozen embryos in the future if the providers have died, divorced, are unavailable for decision, or are unable to agree between themselves on disposition.

In such cases, the IVF program or embryo bank should be able to rely on this prior agreement in decisions concerning stored embryos. This will give advance control to the parties and clear directions to the bank and minimize costly disputes about what to do with stored embryos. Although no court has yet been faced with a case directly involving a disputed contract, there have been cases recognizing the right of the depositing couple to remove their frozen embryo from a bank against the bank's wishes. There is also legal authority recognizing the validity of such advance contracts for disposition in case disputes arise.

The *Davis v. Davis* case (1992) illustrates the wisdom of giving effect to the prior agreement. A couple had frozen seven embryos pursuant to their efforts to have children via IVF. They subsequently decided to divorce but could not agree on disposition of the frozen embryos. The husband opposed thawing them and using them to start pregnancy, while the wife insisted that she or another person have them placed in her. The Tennessee Supreme Court finally resolved this issue by ruling that an agreement between the parties for disposition in the case of divorce would have been

binding, and that in the absence of such an agreement, the relative burdens and benefits of a particular solution must be examined. In that case if the party wishing to retain the embryos had other means of obtaining embryos, such as by going through IVF again with a new partner, that party's wish to have children could still be satisfied without foisting unwanted parenthood on the party who wished that the embryos not be used. On the other hand, if there was no other way for that party to be reasonably able to produce embryos, so that the existing embryos were the last resort or chance to have offspring, then they should be entitled to use them. In that case, fairness would require that the objecting party not have to provide child support. In the facts presented to it, the court ruled in favor of the husband, who did not want frozen embryos implanted after divorce, because the wife had alternative ways to reproduce.

Ethical and legal codes for assisted reproduction in other countries have not yet addressed the problem that arose in the *Davis* case. A country could take the position that all embryos must be preserved, or that provision of gametes for IVF is a commitment to have all resulting embryos placed in the uterus. However, the American preference to have the parties control disposition in the case of divorce or disposition by prior agreement might also be recognized, for it maximizes the procreative liberty of the parties directly involved.

The authority of the gamete providers over the disposition of frozen embryos can be limited by law or the policies of the banks or facilities where frozen embryos are stored. For example, some European countries (Spain and Germany) prohibit embryo discard and research, while others (Great Britain, for example) limit the period of storage to a maximum of ten years or the reproductive life of the woman, whichever is longer. While U.S. legislation on these issues is largely absent, the Ethics Committee of the American Fertility Society (1986) has recommended a similar maximum period of storage, and individual embryo banks and programs for religious or administrative reasons have imposed limitations on dispositions that involve discard, donation, or release of frozen embryos to other programs. As long as the storage facility makes clear its restrictions on disposition of frozen embryos, it may impose these restrictions on couples who request storage of embryos at that facility.

Conclusion

Cryopreservation of sperm, ova, and embryos offers individuals options to extend or enhance their reproductive ability and should presumptively be recognized as adjuncts of their procreative liberty. If this view is accepted, principles of informed consent and contract will inform and regulate most of the transactions and activities that occur with cryopreserved gametes and embryos. In some cases legislation to protect the parties' wishes and ensure the health and viability of stored gametes and embryos may also be desirable.

JOHN A. ROBERTSON (1995)
BIBLIOGRAPHY REVISED

SEE ALSO: *Abortion; Adoption; Cloning; Embryo and Fetus; Feminism; Fetal Research; Genetic Counseling; Genetic Testing and Screening: Reproductive Genetic Testing; Healthcare Resources, Allocation of: Microallocation; Law and Bioethics; Maternal-Fetal Relationship; Moral Status; Organ And Tissue Procurement: Ethical and Legal Issues Regarding Living Donors; Population Ethics; Sexism; Transhumanism and Posthumanism; Women, Contemporary Issues of;* and other *Reproductive Technologies* subentries

BIBLIOGRAPHY

Becker, Gay. 2000. *The Elusive Embryo: How Men and Women Approach New Reproductive Technologies.* Berkeley: University of California Press.

Davis v. Davis. 842 S.W.2d 588 (Tenn. 1992).

Ethics Committee. American Fertility Society. 1986. "Ethical Considerations of the New Reproductive Technologies." *Fertility and Sterility* 46(3) (suppl. 1): 1S–94S.

Murphy, Timothy F. 1995. "Sperm Harvesting and Postmortem Fatherhood." *Bioethics* 9(5): 380–398.

Robertson, John A. 1986. "Embryos, Families, and Procreative Liberty: The Legal Structure of the New Reproduction." *Southern California Law Review* 59(4): 939–1041.

Robertson, John A. 1990. "In the Beginning: The Legal Status of Early Embryos." *Virginia Law Review* 76(3): 437–517.

Steinbock, Bonnie. 1997. *Life Before Birth: The Moral and Legal Status of Embryos and Fetuses.* New York: Oxford University Press.

U.S. Congress. Office of Technology Assessment. 1988. *Infertility: Medical and Social Choices.* Washington, D.C.: Author.

U.S. Department of Health, Education and Welfare. Ethics Advisory Board. 1979. *HEW Support of Research Involving Human In Vitro Fertilization and Embryo Transfer.* Fed. Register 35, 033.

Van Der Ploeg, Irma. 2001. *Prosthetic Bodies: The Construction of the Fetus and the Couple As Patients in Reproductive Technologies.* New York: Kluwer Academic Press.

VIII. ETHICAL ISSUES

The introduction of in vitro fertilization (IVF) in 1978 sparked anew an intense ethical debate about the use of innovative reproductive technologies that had raged a decade earlier. Questions were raised about whether these technologies would harm children and parents and alter people's understanding of the meaning of procreation, family, and parenthood. Gradually the controversy subsided as healthy children were born from these procedures; committees in at least eight countries issued statements indicating that they considered the use of IVF ethically acceptable in principle (Walters). Arguably, one reason for this readiness to embrace IVF and other new reproductive techniques was that they enabled couples to create offspring in a way that seemed an extension of the natural way of procreating. Although IVF involved joining sperm and ovum in a glass dish, the resulting embryo, once implanted, went through a natural period of gestation that culminated in the birth of a child. A second reason was that these technologies, with the exception of artificial insemination by donor, allowed people to have children who were genetically their own. Louise Brown, the first child created through IVF, resulted from the union of the gametes of her biological parents. Third, the children born of these new means of reproduction were born into traditionally structured families. These techniques were assumed to have been developed for use by married couples who, with the new baby, would form what was ordinarily defined as a nuclear family.

In the 1990s, these rationales for accepting novel reproductive technologies are being challenged by medical advances and a changing social environment. Human intervention in the procreative process has become more frequent, more complex, and more highly technological. Oocytes can be removed surgically from one woman and, after fertilization, transferred to another in the procedure of oocyte donation. Women can lend their wombs to others for the incubation of children who have no genetic connection to such "surrogates." Embryos created in vitro can be cryopreserved and stored for use in future years by their genetic parents or by others. Consequently, it is difficult to argue that such innovative measures are mere extensions of the natural way of reproducing. Parthenogenesis (stimulating an unfertilized egg to develop and produce offspring by mechanical or chemical means), cloning (deriving genetically identical organisms from a single cell or very early embryo), and ectogenesis (maintaining the fetus completely outside the body) are on the horizon. Furthermore, third, fourth, and fifth parties, such as oocyte donors, surrogate mothers, and (some suggest) even fetuses and cadavers, are joining sperm donors to assist those who are childless to have offspring. New forms of assisted reproduction are increasingly being used to create children who are not tied to those who will raise them by biological or hereditary links. Finally, these technologies are no longer used almost exclusively to create traditional nuclear families. Unmarried heterosexual and homosexual couples and single women and men now have greater access to them. Such scientific and social changes give new emphasis to the older unresolved ethical questions about the uses of these technologies and raise new questions. Ethical questions raised by the use of the new reproductive technologies The initial ethical question created by these technologies is whether they ought to be used at all. Different religious traditions vary tremendously in their judgments about the licitness of the use of these novel techniques. The Roman Catholic church declared the use of new reproductive technologies morally unacceptable (Catholic Church) because they separate the procreative, life-giving aspects of human intercourse from the unitive, lovemaking aspects, and these, according to Catholic teachings, are morally inseparable in every sexual act. The creation of a child should involve the convergence of the spiritual and physical love of the parents; fertilization outside the body is "deprived of the meanings and the values which are expressed in the language of the body and in the union of human persons" (Catholic Church, p. 28).

Certain other religious groups, such as the Lutheran, Anglican, Jewish, Eastern Orthodox, and Islamic, view some of these methods as ethically acceptable because God has encouraged human procreation (Lutheran Church; Episcopal Church; Feldman; Harakas; Rahman). According to these bodies, it is sufficient that love and procreation are held together within the whole marital relationship; each act of sexual intercourse need not be open to the possibility of conception. Still other religious groups hold that there is no necessary moral connection between conjugal sexual intercourse and openness to procreation, and consequently they accept the use of the new reproductive technologies with few qualifications (Smith; Simmons; General Conference). In Hindu thought, for instance, although there is no authoritative teaching on this subject, the mythologies of ancestors appear to allow IVF, oocyte donation, embryo implantation, and surrogacy (Desai).

Feminists, too, are split about the use of the new reproductive technologies. Some argue that these novel methods define and limit women in ways that demean them, for example, as "fetal containers." They maintain that the desire of many women, both fertile and infertile, for children is, in large part, socially constructed (Bartholet, 1992; Williams). The cultural imperative to have children drives infertile women to undergo physically, emotionally, and financially costly treatment. They are thrust into the hands of a predominantly male medical establishment that uses women as "living laboratories" whose body parts they manipulate without regard to the consequences (Rowland).

Male experts sever what was once a continuous process of gestation and childbirth for women into discrete parts, thereby fragmenting motherhood (Corea).

In contrast, other feminists argue that the new reproductive technologies enhance the status of women by providing them with an increased range of options. By circumventing infertility and providing women with alternative means of reproducing, these technologies extend reproductive choices and freedoms (Jaggar; Andrews; Macklin, 1994). In their view, the charge that surrogacy exploits women is paternalistic because it questions women's ability to know their own interests and to make informed, voluntary, and competent decisions (Macklin, 1990); women have the ability and right to control their bodies and to make autonomous choices about their participation in such practices, these feminists argue.

Some people recommend adoption over the use of the new reproductive technologies because they view the latter as physically and emotionally debilitating and unlikely to succeed, whereas adoption, while not easy, provides a home and family for children in need (Bartholet, 1993). Yet adoption is a second choice for many infertile couples because of its perceived drawbacks. These include the declining number of healthy children available for adoption, the long and emotionally draining wait, the expense, and the difficult and often frustrating system with which adoptive parents must deal (Lauritzen). Although the use of assisted reproduction presents some of the same problems as adoption, it offers what some infertile couples consider distinct advantages: It allows them to have children who are genetically related to at least one of them and (except in the case of surrogacy) makes the experience of pregnancy and birth available to the woman. The desire to reproduce through lines of kinship and to connect to future generations exerts a powerful influence, as does the hope of experiencing the range of fulfilling events associated with pregnancy and childbirth (Overall).

Individual Choice, Substantial Harm, and Community Values

A central issue in the debate about the use of reproductive technologies concerns the scope that should be given to individual discretion over their use. Some philosophical commentators, emphasizing personal autonomy, enunciate a broad moral right to reproduce by means of these technologies (Bayles; Brock). They borrow from legal discussions of the right to reproduce, which some legal theorists take to include the liberty to use methods of assisted reproduction (Robertson, 1986; Elias and Annas, 1987). To limit individual choice about noncoital means of reproduction, the state must show that the use of specific reproductive technologies threatens substantial harm to participants and the children born to them (Robertson, 1988). The philosophers influenced by such legal positions maintain that individuals have great leeway in their choice of whether to procreate, with whom, and by what means. They have a right to enter into contractual arrangements giving them access to these technologies and to utilize third parties in their reproductive efforts. Those who take this approach concede that substantial adverse effects on others, particularly the children, would justify restricting individual use of assisted reproduction.

Since the primary reason for accepting these innovative methods is to bring children into the world, a major consideration in assessing them is whether or not they harm these children. Critics contend that these techniques may cause social and psychological problems to the resulting children because of confusion they engender over divided biological parentage and the social stigmatization to which they may be subjected (Callahan, 1988). John Robertson responds that this criticism is logically incoherent. When the alternative is nonexistence, he argues, it is better for the children to have been born—even though they may experience some harm from the means used to bring them into the world—than never to have existed at all (Robertson, 1986). In most cases, the difficulties they face are not so great as to render life a complete loss.

There are several problems with this influential response. One is that it justifies allowing almost any harm to occur to children born as a result of the use of these techniques in that it can almost always be said they are better off alive. Moreover, this argument presupposes that these children are waiting in a world of nonexistence to be summoned into existence and that they would be harmed by not being born. Since children do not exist at all prior to their arrival in this world, there are no children who could be harmed by not being born. When we say that it is better for a child to have been born, we do not compare that child's current existence with a previous one. Instead, we make an after-the-fact judgment that life is a good for an already existing child, even though that child may have suffered some harm from the technology used to bring him or her into the world. Critics of the use of the new reproductive technologies, however, make a before-the-fact judgment about children who do not exist, but who might. They maintain that it would be wrong to bring children into the world if they would suffer certain substantial harms as a result of the methods by which they are created. This is a logically coherent claim that justifies considering whether the new reproductive technologies severely damage children born as a result of their use.

The criterion of avoiding substantial harm, while valid, may provide inadequate ethical constraints on various ways of employing the new reproductive arrangements. The criterion is derived from a position that especially prizes individuality, liberty, and autonomy—quite possibly at the cost of values that are served by the building of families and communities, and by accounting for the common good (Cahill). Taking respect for individual freedom as the primary value, according to Allen Verhey, runs the danger of reducing the value of persons to their capacities for rational choice and denying the significance of the communities that shape them. People are not just autonomous individuals, they are also members of communities, some of which are not of their own choosing. Freedom is insufficient for an account of the good life in the family. Thus, it may be morally legitimate to recommend limits to individual choice about assisted reproductive techniques, not only to protect the children born of these methods but also to uphold basic community values. What is at issue, he suggests, is what kind of society we are and want to become (Verhey).

Ethical Issues Related to the Introduction of Third Parties

The introduction of third parties into procreative acts, according to some critics, imperils the very character of society by threatening the nuclear family, the basic building block of U.S. society (Callahan, 1988). Religious commentators and groups, in particular, have expressed concern about the effect of the use of gamete donors and surrogates on the relation between married couples within the nuclear family. Richard McCormick, a Roman Catholic theologian, argues that when procreation takes place in a context other than marriage (as when single women use artificial insemination by donor, for example) and another's body is used to achieve conception (as in the case of surrogacy, for example), total dedication to one's spouse is made more difficult; in Roman Catholic terminology, it also violates "the marriage covenant wherein exclusive, nontransferable, inalienable rights to each other's person and generative acts are exchanged" (Ethics Committee, 1986, p. 82).

In Islamic law, artificial insemination by donor is rejected on grounds that the use of the sperm of a man other than the marriage partner confuses lineage and might also constitute a form of adultery because a third party enters into the procreative aspect of the marital relation. The practice is highly controversial in the Jewish religion because (1) some consider it a form of adultery; (2) some take the resulting child to be illegitimate; and (3) if the donor is unknown, the practice might eventually result in incestuous marriage between siblings. Most other religious groups that have commented on surrogacy also reject it because it depersonalizes motherhood and risks subjecting surrogates and procreation itself to commercial exploitation. Such practices will lead people to regard children as products who, in Oliver O'Donovan's terms, are "made" rather than "begotten."

Those who wish to counter concerns about adultery distinguish between adultery and the use of a gamete or womb contributed by a third party to assist a married couple to have a child. A necessary element of adultery, they contend, is sexual intercourse; neither gamete donation nor surrogacy involves sexual contact between the recipient and the donor. Moreover, unlike adultery, no element of unfaithfulness need inhere in participation in gamete donation. Indeed, a couple may participate in gamete donation just because they have a strong commitment to their marriage, rather than out of disdain for it (Lauritzen). When only one parent can contribute genetically to the procreation of a child, but both can nourish and nurture a child, this argument runs, it is ethically acceptable for them to have a child by means of third-party collaboration.

The use of third parties in the provision of the new reproductive technologies leads to confused notions of parentage, critics note, since it severs the connection between the conceptive, gestational, and rearing components of parenthood. It can be difficult to predict who will be declared the rearing parent in different reproductive scenarios, despite the fact that they embrace the same set of facts. For instance, in IVF followed by embryo transfer, the woman who gestates an embryo provided by someone else is considered the mother of the resulting child, but in artificial insemination by donor she is not. Those who respond to this criticism, in attempting to develop a consistent ethical basis for awarding the accolade of parenthood, give priority either to the interests of the children born of these technologies or to those of their adult progenitors.

Those who view the interests of the children as of prime importance argue that genetic connections should constrain the freedom to choose parental status in that biological kinship relations are important to children's development and self-identity (Callahan, 1988). Purposefully to break the link between procreation and rearing, these commentators maintain, harms children born of these procedures because it obscures their identity within a family lineage. Indeed, it has been argued that the biological relationship between gamete donors and the children who result from their contributions carries an obligation for donors to support and nurture those children (Callahan, 1992). Respondents observe that it is not considered wrong to separate the genetic and rearing components of parenthood in such well-established arrangements as adoption, stepparenting, blended families, and extended kin relationships. This precedent suggests that, although the genetic relation may be important, it is not essential to parenthood.

Caring for and raising a child are of greater significance for parenthood than providing the genetic material or gestational environment, according to this view. Consequently, the rearing parent should have moral priority over the genetic parent in the interests of the child (Lauritzen). Others focus on the interests of the parents when the choice is between the genetic and the gestational mother, and they contend that the gestational mother should prevail because of her greater physical and emotional contribution and the risks of childbearing (Elias and Annas, 1986).

Parents who are not the biological progenitors of the children they raise and those who provide them with gametes often fear social stigmatization. This raises the question of whether anonymity and secrecy should be used to envelop all who participate in the use of the new reproductive technologies for their own protection. Anonymity has to do with concealing the identity of the donor; secrecy has to do with concealing the fact that recipients have participated in gamete donation. The practice of artificial insemination by donor has historically been carried out in secrecy with anonymous donors to protect family and donor privacy; oocyte donation, which began with openness about the identity of donors, is moving in that direction as well. The major argument against this development takes the interests of the children as primary and contends that since the personal and social identity of children is dependent on their biological origins, they ought to know about their genetic parents (National Bioethics Consultative Committee). Several countries that accept this argument have adopted regulations allowing children, when they reach maturity, to gain access to whatever information is available about donors who contributed to their birth.

Technologies of assisted reproduction, especially those involving third parties, facilitate the creation of models of family that depart significantly from the traditional nuclear family. As single persons, homosexual couples, and unmarried heterosexual couples increasingly gain access to these technologies, both religious and secular bodies express concern about weakening mutual commitment within the family and about the welfare of the resulting children. Sherman Elias and George Annas observe that "it seems disingenuous to argue on the one hand that the primary justification for noncoital reproduction is the anguish an infertile married couple suffers because of the inability to have a 'traditional family,' and then use the breakup of the traditional family unit itself as the primary justification for unmarried individuals to have access to these techniques" (1986, p. 67). The Warnock Report, developed by a commission of inquiry into the use of artificial means of reproduction in Great Britain in 1984, concluded that "the interests of the child dictate that it should be born into a home where there is a loving, stable, heterosexual relationship and that, therefore, the deliberate creation of a child for a woman who is not a partner in such a relationship is morally wrong" (p. 11).

Some psychologists claim that children who grow up in these nontraditional families will suffer psychological and social damage because they will lack role models of both genders and may consequently develop an impaired view of sexuality and procreation (McGuire and Alexander). Moreover, they argue, two parents are better able than one to cope with the demands of childrearing. Other studies have been used to vindicate the opposite conclusions (McGuire and Alexander). Since few studies have been carried out on the consequences for children of atypical family arrangements that emerge when the new reproductive technologies are employed, it is difficult to provide any clear evidence to support or undermine these opposing contentions. A further concern voiced is that using new reproductive technologies to assist single people and homosexual couples to have children involves a misuse of medical capabilities because these methods are not being employed to overcome a medical problem but to circumvent biological limits to parenthood.

To others, however, the use of new methods of assisted reproduction by single people and homosexual couples mirrors the reality that U.S. society has begun to move away from the nuclear family (Glover). They see the inclusion of homosexual parents within the meaning of family as a move toward greater equality in a society in which those who are homosexual suffer from prejudice and discrimination. If single people and homosexual couples can offer to a child an environment that is compatible with a good start in life, the *Glover Report to the European Commission* maintains, they ought to have access to these techniques, but it is appropriate for those providing them to make some inquiries before proceeding (Glover). The Royal Commission on New Reproductive Technologies of Canada approved of allowing infertility clinics to provide single heterosexual and lesbian women access to donor insemination on grounds that no reliable evidence could be found that the environment in families formed by these gamete recipients is any better or any worse for the children than in families formed by heterosexual couples (Canada, Royal Commission on New Reproductive Technologies).

Ethical Issues Related to Commodification

A concern of special ethical significance is that the introduction of third parties into some of the new reproductive techniques carries with it the danger of commodification of human beings, their bodies, and their bodily products. Giving payment of any sort to surrogates and gamete donors, some argue, risks making them and the children produced with their assistance fungible objects of market exchange, alienating them from their personhood in a way that diminishes the value of human beings (Radin). Third parties who assist others to reproduce should be viewed as donors of a priceless gift for which they ought to be repaid in gratitude, but not in money.

Others argue that persons have a right to do what they choose with their bodies and that when they choose to be paid, their reimbursement should be commensurate with their services (Robertson, 1988). The value of respect for persons is not diminished by using surrogates and gamete donors for the reproductive purposes of others if those third parties are fully informed about the procedure in which they participate and are not coerced into participating—even when they are paid (Harris). There is a presumption on all sides that third parties should not be specifically compensated for their gametes, wombs, or babies. Several groups that have considered the matter, though, such as the Warnock Committee in Great Britain (Warnock) and the Waller Committee in Australia (Victoria), allow third-party payment for out-of-pocket and medical expenses. The American Fertility Society goes further when it maintains that gamete donors should be paid for their direct and indirect expenses, inconvenience, time, risk, and discomfort (Ethics Committee, 1990). It would be unfair and exploitive not to pay donors for their time and effort, John Robertson argues (1988).

Offering large amounts of money to third parties incommensurate with the degree of effort and service that these persons provide may diminish the voluntariness of their choice to participate in assisted reproduction, particularly when they have limited financial means. There is concern that a new economic underclass might develop that would earn its living by providing body parts and products for the reproductive purposes of those who are better off economically. This would violate the principle of distributive justice, which requires that society's benefits and burdens be parceled out equitably among different groups (Macklin, 1994). However, if poor women and men have voluntarily and knowingly accepted their role in these reproductive projects, it could be seen as unjustifiably paternalistic to deny them the opportunity to earn money. The possibility of exploitation of the poor must be weighed "against a possible step toward their liberation through economic gain" from a new source of income connected to innovative methods of reproduction (Radin).

Ethical Issues Related to the Uses of Embryos, Fetuses, and Cadavers

When the process of fertilization is external, the embryo becomes accessible to many forms of intervention. During the brief extracorporeal, in vitro period, embryos can be frozen, treated, implanted, experimented on, discarded, or donated. Theoretically, embryos that result from IVF could be cryopreserved for generations, so that a woman could give birth to her genetic uncle, siblings could be born to different sets of parents, or one sibling could be born to another. A 1993 experiment in which human embryos were split reawakened concerns about these sorts of possibilities, which had remained dormant since a mid-1970s controversy about cloning human beings (National Advisory Board). (Cloning, either by transplanting the nucleus from a differentiated cell into an unfertilized egg from which the nucleus has been removed or by splitting an embryo at an early stage when its cells are still undifferentiated, results in individuals who are genetically identical to the original from which they are cloned.)

Advocates of embryo splitting view it as a way of obtaining greater numbers of embryos for implantation in order to enhance the chances of pregnancy for those who are infertile (Robertson, 1994). Critics claim that cloning in any form negates what we view as valuable about human beings, their individuality and uniqueness. It risks treating children as fungible products to be manipulated at will, rather than as unique, self-determining individuals. These critics maintain that twinning that occurs in nature is an unavoidable accident that does not involve manipulation of one child-to-be to produce a duplicate (McCormick, 1994). Defenders of cloning respond that the similarity of identical twins does not diminish their uniqueness or their sense of selfhood. In any case, cloned individuals would not be identical in that the genome does not fully determine a person's identity. Environmental factors, such as family upbringing and the historical context, weigh heavily in influencing the expression of genes (National Advisory Board).

It is the potential for abuse of cloning that disturbs most critics. The possibility of cryopreserving cloned embryos suggests the option of implanting cloned embryos and bringing them to term should their already-born twin need a tissue or organ transplant. In another scenario, embryos derived from parents who are likely to produce "ideal specimens" would be cloned and sold on a "black market." Critics condemn such potential applications of cloning because they diminish the value of embryos and of human beings by treating them as objects available for any use by others (National Advisory Board). They are concerned that the deep desire of the infertile for children, in combination with scientific zeal and market forces, will create strong pressure to clone embryos without a view to the ethical considerations involved. In 1993 scientists in the United Kingdom announced the possibility of using for infertility treatment eggs and ovaries taken from aborted fetuses (Carroll and Gosden). The eggs could be fertilized in vitro and then transferred into infertile women who lack viable eggs; the ovaries could be transplanted directly into women to mature and produce eggs.

This would help meet the shortage of oocytes for those who lack their own. Such uses of aborted fetuses, however, are highly contentious and strike some as grotesque. Many who object to abortion on ethical grounds maintain that this procedure, like other forms of fetal tissue use, would encourage the practice. Moreover, it seems self-contradictory for a woman to consent to abortion and at the same time consent to become a grandmother. Children created by this procedure, it could be argued, would know little about their genetic heritage or about their mother, other than that she was a dead fetus, and would therefore be at risk of both psychological and social harm.

Female cadavers provide another potential source of oocytes for those who are infertile. It has been proposed that women consider donating their ovaries for use by others after their death, much as individuals donate organs such as kidneys and livers (Seibel). It may soon be possible to collect immature eggs from cadavers, mature and fertilize them in vitro, and then transfer them into infertile women. This procedure would have an advantage over the use of eggs from aborted fetuses in that the recipient would be able to learn the medical and genetic history of the adult donor. An argument for this practice is that it would allow the continuation of the family's biological heritage and serve to console the grieving family because some aspect of their deceased relative will have been preserved. Postmortem recovery of eggs would be done with the consent of the donor and would therefore respect individual rights and allow freedom of choice for individuals and their close relatives.

This proposal is grounded in an analogy between organ and gamete donation. Yet gamete donation is different in that it involves the provision of an essential factor for bringing a child into existence; it is not life-saving but life-giving. The interests of the resulting children, consequently, provide a major consideration to be taken into account in determining whether such procedures ought to be pursued. The difficulty noted earlier in connection with the introduction of third parties arises in this instance as well.

Children develop their identity and self-understanding, in part, through their relationships with their biological parents. Consequently, they might face serious psychological and social harm if one of their biological parents were a cadaver. Indeed, this concern amounts to a central social concern as well, in that the prospect of using gametes derived from the newly dead in order to create children endangers our perception of the respect due to the dead human body and our view of procreation as ideally grounded in an interpersonal relationship between living persons.

Ethical Issues Related to Access and Justice

Although those able to procreate naturally can decide whether and when to do so, the choice to reproduce among those who need medical assistance to do so is more limited. In part, this is because they enter a healthcare system in which providers have responsibilities both to candidates for infertility treatment and to the resulting child, because they are assisting in the creation of a new human being. Although physicians have a special obligation to respect the autonomy and freedom of those who are candidates for treatment, they are not obligated to provide them with all treatments that they request (Chervenak and McCullough). As one of several groups of gatekeepers of the new reproductive technologies, some physicians use a medicalindications criterion to bar access to these technologies to some patients, as when, for example, the physical risk of pregnancy is too great. Yet many physicians find that they cannot easily separate medical indications from indications that are psychological, social, and ethical. Questions requiring judgments that go beyond those that are strictly medical arise in many situations. These questions include possible treatment for candidates who wish to create "designer babies" of a certain sex, intelligence, and/or race; couples who want to use a surrogate mother for frivolous reasons related to personal convenience; infertile single women who request access to both oocyte and sperm donation in lieu of adoption; women of advanced reproductive age who want to have children despite the risk to their own health; and couples who appear severely dysfunctional and prone to violence and child abuse. Physicians are not usually trained to address ethical questions that arise in such situations. Because physicians have personal and professional biases and are part of a largely unregulated and profitable infertility industry, it might be appropriate to assign the gatekeeper role to a specially trained group of professionals who are not physicians. Another possibility is to utilize guidelines for the use of the new reproductive technologies prepared by physician professional associations, institutional ethics committees, private-sector ethics boards, public ethics commissions, and state and national regulatory agencies; such guidelines should address not only medical but social, psychological, and ethical issues (Cohen, 1994; Fletcher).

Public-policymakers and private healthcare insurance regulators also affect who gains access to the new reproductive technologies. If they define infertility treatment as a response to a disease rather than to a social need, a case for financial support of the new reproductive technologies can be made. Because infertility is a physical condition that impairs normal function, many commentators regard it as something like a disease, the victims of which are in need of help from medical science (Overall). However, it can also be argued that since reproductive technologies do not correct the condition causing infertility, they do not constitute medical treatment for a disease. Yet many well-accepted treatments do not correct the underlying condition but only its symptoms or disabilities. Given the importance to many people of having a biological child and the fact that normal functioning allows this, the claim has been made that infertility should be treated as a disease on a par with other physical impairments. Historically, the *barren* woman or man has not been accorded sympathy; the availability of infertility treatment might disarm similar current discriminatory attitudes toward those who are infertile.

Even if infertility were defined as a disease, however, this would not indicate that its treatment would be ethically mandatory. The U.S. healthcare system does not have infinite resources and cannot provide everyone with every desired or desirable health service. Should the new reproductive technologies be subject to more severe criteria for funding than are set for other medical techniques? Because infertility is a physical dysfunction with significant effects on the life plans of those it affects, it can be contended that a just society should include reproductive technologies among the range of treatments covered. The opposing argument is that the costs of such treatment and its relatively low likelihood of success do not justify its inclusion.

A related issue arises from the fact that only a limited range of people—those with greater financial resources—benefit from the new reproductive technologies. Access depends on economic factors, culture, race, and social class. Those in the United States who are poor have little access to specialty services such as infertility clinics because public and private insurers provide limited coverage. If poor people participate at all in the use of these technologies, they do so as surrogates or occasionally as oocyte donors. Thus, the use of new reproductive technologies has potential for creating further unjust schisms in our society between rich and poor and between one subculture and another. As long as IVF services and gametes are in short supply, questions will arise about how to select candidates from among those who seek access to the new methods of assisted reproduction. Those persons who are infertile or who carry a serious genetic disease may have a greater first claim than those who are not infertile but who wish to use these methods to select the features of their children or as a matter of personal convenience.

This is because the need of the former is a more basic need, directly related to the goal of remedying a difficulty in normal species functioning. A more refined set of rationing priorities would take account of such factors as the number of children an individual or a couple already has; whether they have a support system in place to assist them to care for a child adequately; and the greater medical risk to certain recipients of treatment, such as women of advanced reproductive age. These considerations would be grounded in the interests of the potential children and of their would-be parents, as well as in the need to distribute the number of children among couples in an equitable way.

Conclusion

Behind many of the ethical issues raised by the new reproductive technologies lie difficult questions about the importance of genetic parenthood, the nuclear family, and the welfare of children, as well as the role that society should play in overseeing the creation of its citizens. Perplexity about how to resolve these questions is due, in part, to the speed with which these technologies are being developed. There is a growing concern that they are being created too rapidly, before the old technologies, such as artificial insemination, have been integrated into the ethical and social fabric. As the rate of reproductive change accelerates, the ability to provide ethical safeguards for the creation and use of the new reproductive technologies diminishes. This may be the most persuasive reason to provide some form of direction and regulation of the new reproductive technologies that incorporates defensible ethical limits to their use.

CYNTHIA B. COHEN (1995)
BIBLIOGRAPHY REVISED

SEE ALSO: *Abortion; Adoption; Cloning; Embryo and Fetus; Eugenics; Feminism; Fetal Research; Fertility Control; Genetic Counseling; Genetic Testing and Screening: Reproductive Genetic Testing; Healthcare Resources, Allocation of: Microallocation; Law and Bioethics; Maternal-Fetal Relationship; Moral Status; Organ and Tissue Procurement: Ethical and Legal Issues Regarding Living Donors; Population Ethics; Sexism; Transhumanism and Posthumanism; Women, Contemporary Issues of;* and other *Reproductive Technologies* subentries

BIBLIOGRAPHY

Andrews, Lori. 1984. *New Conceptions: A Consumers' Guide to the Newest Infertility Treatments.* New York: St. Martin's Press.

Bartholet, Elizabeth. 1992. "In Vitro Fertilization: The Construction of Infertility and of Parenting." In *Issues in Reproductive Technology I: An Anthology,* pp. 253–260, ed. Helen Bequaert Holmes. New York: Garland.

Bartholet, Elizabeth. 1993. *Family Bonds, Adoption and the Politics of Parenting.* Boston: Houghton Mifflin.

Bayles, Michael D. 1984. *Reproductive Ethics.* Englewood Cliffs, NJ: Prentice-Hall.

Brock, Dan W. 1994. "Reproductive Freedom: Its Nature, Bases, and Limits." In *Health Care Ethics: Critical Issues,* pp. 43–61, ed. John F. Monagle and David C. Thomasma. Gaithersburg, MD: Aspen.

Cahill, Lisa Sowle. 1990. "The Ethics of Surrogate Motherhood: Biology, Freedom, and Moral Obligation." In *Surrogate Motherhood: Politics and Privacy,* pp. 151–164, ed. Larry O. Gostin. Bloomington: Indiana University Press.

Callahan, Daniel. 1992. "Bioethics and Fatherhood." *Utah Law Review* 1992: 735–746.

Callahan, Joan, ed. 1995. *Reproduction, Ethics, and the Law: Feminist Perspectives.* Bloomington: Indiana University Press.

Callahan, Sidney. 1988. "The Ethical Challenge of the New Reproductive Technology." In *Medical Ethics: A Guide for Health Care Professionals,* pp. 26–37, ed. John F. Monagle and David C. Thomasma. Rockville, MD: Aspen.

Canada. Royal Commission on New Reproductive Technologies. 1993. *Proceed with Care: Final Report of the Royal Commission on New Reproductive Technologies.* 2 vols. Ottawa, Canada: Author. See especially Vol. 2.

Carroll, John, and Gosden, Roger G. 1993. "Transplantation of Frozen-Thawed Mouse Primordial Follicles." *Human Reproduction* 8(8):1163–1167.

Catholic Church. Congregation for the Doctrine of the Faith. 1987. *Instruction on Respect for Human Life in Its Origin and on the Dignity of Procreation: Replies to Certain Questions of the Day.* Washington, D.C.: United States Catholic Conference.

Cohen, Cynthia B. 1994. "In Search of a Variety of Bioethics Forums." *Politics and the Life Sciences* 13(1): 82–84.

Cohen, Cynthia B. 1996. "'Give Me Children or I Shall Die!': New Reproductive Technologies and Harm to Children." *Hastings Center Report* 26(2): 19–27.

Corea, Gena. 1985. *The Mother Machine: Reproductive Technologies from Artificial Insemination to Artificial Wombs.* New York: Harper & Row.

Davis, Dena S. 2002. *Genetic Dilemmas: Reproductive Technologies, Parental Choices and Children's Futures (Reflective Bioethics).* London: Routledge.

De Jonge, Christopher J., and Barratt, Christopher L. R., eds. 2002. *Assisted Reproductive Technologies: Current Accomplishments and New Horizons.* New York: Cambridge University Press.

Desai, Prakash N. 1989. *Health and Medicine in the Hindu Tradition: Continuity and Cohesion.* New York: Crossroad.

Edwards, Jeanette. 2000. *Born and Bred: Idioms of Kinship and New Reproductive Technologies in England (Oxford Studies in Social and Cultural Anthropology).* New York: Oxford University Press.

Elias, Sherman, and Annas, George J. 1986. "Social Policy Considerations in Noncoital Reproduction." *Journal of the American Medical Association* 225(1): 62–68.

Elias, Sherman, and Annas, George J. 1987. "Reproductive Liberty." In *Reproductive Genetics and the Law,* pp. 143–167. Chicago: Year Book Medical.

Episcopal Church. General Convention. 1982. *Journal of the General Convention of the Protestant Episcopal Church in the United States of America.* New York: Author. See Res. A067, Sec. C158.

Ethics Committee. American Fertility Society. 1978. "Reproductive Technologies: Ethical Issues." In *Encyclopedia of Bioethics,* vol. 4, pp. 1454–1464, ed. Warren T. Reich. New York: Macmillan and Free Press.

Ethics Committee. American Fertility Society. 1990. "Ethical Considerations of the New Reproductive Technologies." *Fertility and Sterility,* 53(6), Supplement 2:1S–104S.

Feldman, David M. 1986. *Health and Medicine in the Jewish Tradition: L'hayyim—to Life.* New York: Crossroad.

Fletcher, John. 1994. "On Restoring Public Bioethics." *Politics and the Life Sciences* 13(1): 84–86.

General Conference. Mennonite Church. 1985. *Human Sexuality in the Christian Life: A Working Document for Study and Dialogue.* Scottdale, PA: Faith and Life Press and Mennonite Publishing House.

Glover, Jonathan. 1989. *Ethics of New Reproductive Technologies: The Glover Report to the European Commission.* De Kalb: Northern Illinois University Press.

Harakas, Stanley Samuel. 1990. *Health and Medicine in the Eastern Orthodox Tradition: Faith, Liturgy, and Wholeness.* New York: Crossroad.

Harris, John. 1992. *Wonderwoman and Superman: The Ethics of Human Technology.* Oxford: Oxford University Press.

Harris, John and Holm, Soren, eds. 2000. *The Future of Human Reproduction: Ethics, Choice, and Regulation (Issues in Biomedical Ethics).* New York: Oxford University Press.

Jaggar, Alison M. 1983. *Feminist Politics and Human Nature.* Totowa, NJ: Rowman & Allanheld.

Lauritzen, Paul. 1993. *Pursuing Parenthood: Ethical Issues in Assisted Reproduction.* Bloomington: Indiana University Press.

LeMoncheck, Linda. 1996. "Philosophy, Gender Politics, and In Vitro Fertilization: A Feminist Ethics of Reproductive Healthcare." *Journal of Clinical Ethics* 7(2): 160–176.

Lutheran Church. Missouri Synod. Commission on Theology and Church Relations. Social Concerns Committee. 1981. *Human Sexuality: A Theological Perspective.* St. Louis, MO: Concordia.

Macklin, Ruth. 1990. "Is There Anything Wrong with Surrogate Motherhood? An Ethical Analysis." In *Surrogate Motherhood: Politics and Privacy,* pp. 136–150, ed. Larry O. Gostin. Bloomington: Indiana University Press.

Macklin, Ruth. 1994. "Surrogates and Other Mothers: The Debates over Assisted Reproduction." Philadelphia: Temple University Press.

Macklin, Ruth. 1995. "Reproductive Technologies in Developing Countries." *Bioethics* 9(3–4): 276–282.

McCormick, Richard A. 1986. "Ethical Considerations of the New Reproductive Technologies." *Fertility and Sterility* 46(3), supplement 1: 82.

McCormick, Richard A. 1994. "Blastomere Separation: Some Concerns." *Hastings Center Report* 24(2): 664–667.

McGee, Glenn. 2000. *The Perfect Baby: Parenthood in the New World of Cloning and Genetics.* Totowa, NJ: Rowman and Littlefield.

McGuire, Maureen, and Alexander, Nancy J. 1985. "Artificial Insemination of Single Women." *Fertility and Sterility* 43(2): 182–184.

National Advisory Board on Ethics in Reproduction. 1994. "Report on Human Cloning Through Embryo Splitting: An Amber Light." *Kennedy Institute of Ethics Journal* 4(3): 251–282.

National Bioethics Consultative Committee (Australia). 1989. *Reproductive Technology: Record Keeping and Access to Information: Birth Certificates and Birth Records of Offspring Born as a Result of Gamete Donation. Final Report to Australian Health Ministers.* Canberra, Australia: Author.

O'Donovan, Oliver. 1984. *Begotten or Made?* Oxford: Clarendon Press.

Overall, Christine. 1987. *Ethics and Human Reproduction: A Feminist Analysis.* Boston: Allen & Unwin.

Purdy, Laura M. 1996. *Reproducing Persons: Issues in Feminist Bioethics.* Ithaca, NY: Cornell University Press.

Radin, Margaret Jane. 1987. "Market-Inalienability." *Harvard Law Review* 100(8): 1849–1937.

Rahman, Fazlur. 1987. *Health and Medicine in the Islamic Tradition: Change and Identity.* New York: Crossroad.

Robertson, John A. 1986. "Embryos, Families, and Procreative Liberty: The Legal Structure of the New Reproduction." *Southern California Law Review* 59(4): 939–1041.

Robertson, John A. 1988. "Technology and Motherhood: Legal and Ethical Issues in Human Egg Donation." *Case Western Reserve Law Review* 39(1): 1–38.

Robertson, John A. 1994. "The Question of Human Cloning." *Hastings Center Report* 24(2): 6–14.

Rowland, Robyn. 1992. *Living Laboratories. Women and Reproductive Technologies.* Bloomington: Indiana University Press.

Sherwin, Susan. 1995. "The Ethics of Babymaking." *Hastings Center Report* 25(2): 34–37.

Simmons, Paul D. 1983. *Birth and Death: Bioethical Decision-Making.* Philadelphia: Westminster.

Smith, Harmon L. 1970. *Ethics and the New Medicine.* Nashville, TN: Abingdon Press.

U.S. Department of Health, Education and Welfare. Ethics Advisory Board. 1979. *HEW Support of Research Involving Human in Vitro Fertilization and Embryo Transfer: Report and Conclusions.* Washington, D.C.: Author.

Verhey, Allen. 1989. "On Having Children and Caring for Them: Becoming and Being Parents." In *Christian Faith, Health, and Medical Practice,* pp. 178–183, ed. Hessel Bouma III, Douglas Diekema, Edward Langerak, Theodore Rottman, and Allen Verhey. Grand Rapids, MI: W. B. Eerdmans.

Victoria. Committee to Consider the Social, Ethical, and Legal Issues Arising from in Vitro Fertilization. 1984. *Report on the Disposition of Embryos Produced by in Vitro Fertilization.* Melbourne, Australia: Author. Chaired by Louis Waller.

Walters, LeRoy. 1987. "Ethics and the New Reproductive Technologies: An International Review of Committee Statements." *Hastings Center Report* 17(3) (spec. suppl.): 3–9.

Warnock, Mary. 1985. *A Question of Life: The Warnock Report on Human Fertilisation and Embryology.* Oxford: Basil Blackwell.

Williams, Linda S. 1992. "Biology or Society? Parenthood Motivation in a Sample of Canadian Women Seeking in Vitro Fertilization." In *Issues in Reproductive Technology I: An Anthropology,* pp. 261–274, ed. Helen Bequaert Holmes. New York: Garland.

IX. IN VITRO FERTILIZATION AND EMBRYO TRANSFER

In in vitro fertilization (IVF), a woman's ovaries are stimulated with fertility drugs to produce multiple eggs. The physician monitors the woman's response by examining urine samples, blood samples, and ultrasound imaging. After giving her an injection to control the timing of the egg release, the physician retrieves the eggs in one of two ways. In a laparoscopy, done under general anesthesia, the surgeon aspirates the woman's eggs through a hollow needle inserted into the abdomen, guided by a narrow optical instrument called a laparoscope. In the more recently developed transvaginal aspiration, done with local anesthesia, the physician inserts the needle through the woman's vagina, guided by ultrasound.

After they are retrieved, the eggs are placed in separate glass dishes and combined with prepared spermatozoa from the woman's partner or a donor. The dishes are placed for twelve to eighteen hours in an incubator designed to mimic the temperature and conditions of the body. If a single spermatozoon penetrates an egg, IVF has occurred.

A fertilized egg subdivides into cells over a period of forty-eight to seventy-two hours. Microscopic in size, it is generally called a pre-embryo or an embryo after it has divided into two or more cells. When the embryos have divided into four to sixteen cells, they are placed in a hollow needle (catheter) that is inserted into the woman's vagina. The embryo or embryos are released into the woman's uterus in the procedure known as embryo transfer. Implantation in the uterine wall, if it takes place, will occur within days after transfer; a pregnancy is detectable about two weeks after the transfer.

In established IVF clinics, the odds that a continuing pregnancy and birth will occur after embryo transfer are 20 to 30 percent. Because problems can arise at all stages of IVF, such as the inability to retrieve eggs or secure fertilization, the odds are less if they are calculated from the time fertility drugs are first given. Data from several national registries indicate a delivery rate of 9 to 13 percent if calculated from the starting point of hormonal stimulation (Cohen, 1991). The birthrates tend to cluster among clinics, so that some clinics account for a large percentage of the total births while others have few or no deliveries (Medical Research International). Tens of thousands of embryo transfers are carried out each year internationally, and thousands of babies have been born. Clinicians reported over 12,000 deliveries following IVF in one five-year period (1985–1990), and in one country (the United States) alone (Medical Research International).

Present and Future Variations

The first birth following IVF occurred in England in 1978 (Steptoe and Edwards). The technique was originally designed to circumvent blocked or damaged fallopian tubes in women trying to become pregnant. During the late 1970s and early 1980s, physicians combined the male partner's sperm and the female partner's eggs and transferred the embryos shortly after fertilization. If the couple had a large number of embryos, physicians either transferred all at once, which created the risk of a multiple pregnancy, or disposed of extra embryos, which wasted the embryos and was morally problematic.

The start of embryo freezing in the early 1980s has given physicians greater control over the number of embryos transferred at once. Two to four embryos are transferred in the first IVF cycle and the remaining embryos, if any, are frozen for later thawing and transfer. Embryo freezing saves the woman from the hormonal stimulation of repeated start-up IVF cycles, and it allows embryo transfer when the woman's body has returned to a more natural state. By enabling the transfer of a small number of embryos at once, it reduces the odds of a multiple pregnancy and the subsequent risk this poses to the woman and the fetuses. Controlled transfer of embryos is arguably less morally problematic than the selective abortion of fetuses in a large multiple pregnancy. The birth of the first infant to have been frozen as an embryo took place in Australia in 1984. Embryo freezing is now a routine option in IVF.

Another variation that has increased the flexibility of IVF is the use of donated sperm, eggs, and embryos to circumvent fertility problems such as low sperm count in the male partner, lack of ovulation in the female partner, or lack of fertilization with the couple's own eggs and sperm, or to help couples at high risk avoid passing on a serious genetic disorder to their children. Sperm and embryo donation are more straightforward than egg donation, which is complicated by the need to synchronize the menstrual cycles of the donor and recipient. Women are either paid for their services in donating eggs or they donate in the course of their own medical treatment. In addition, some women donate eggs for their sisters or other close relatives. Donation of eggs or sperm raises questions about, among other things, confidentiality of medical records, the child's sense of identity, and the psychological well-being of the donor.

The embryos in IVF can be transferred to a surrogate if the genetic mother does not have a uterus or cannot carry a child to term for other reasons. Although the surrogate is usually unrelated, there have been instances of embryo transfer to the sister or even the mother of a woman who cannot carry a fetus to term. In the latter case, the surrogate is the child's gestational mother and genetic grandmother.

Sperm microinjection is another technique used in connection with IVF. If the male partner has low sperm count or poor sperm quality, a healthy spermatozoon can be manually inserted into the egg with special microinstruments. This alternative to sperm donation allows the transfer of embryos genetically related to the couple. This and other microsurgical procedures remain experimental and infrequent.

Another procedure for IVF is the examination of sperm, eggs, and embryos for chromosomal and genetic abnormalities. Preimplantation diagnosis has been conducted on an experimental basis in the United States, Britain, and other European countries. It is being developed for couples at high risk for passing to their children a genetic disorder such as cystic fibrosis or Tay-Sachs disease but who will not terminate a pregnancy and are therefore not candidates for prenatal screening.

Preimplantation diagnosis includes polar-body analysis (analyzing the DNA of the first polar body of the human egg), trophectoderm biopsy (examining extra-embryonic cells surrounding the inner cell mass), and embryo biopsy (removing a single cell from a four- or eight-cell embryo). It also includes chromosomal analysis to select only female embryos for transfer to couples who are at high risk for passing on a sex-linked disease, such as hemophilia, to male children. Pregnancies and births have been reported following embryo biopsy and sex preselection. Many variables remain to be worked out in preimplantation diagnosis, and physicians urge caution before expanding it in the IVF setting (Trounson). Correcting genetic flaws after they have

been diagnosed is a distant, though foreseeable, possibility (Verlinksy et al.).

Ethical Issues in IVF

A recurring and unresolved issue in IVF involves the status of the embryo (McCormick). The Ethics Advisory Board, set up by the U.S. Department of Health, Education and Welfare, and later disbanded without its recommendations' being acted on, issued a report in 1979 stating that "The human embryo is entitled to profound respect, but this respect does not necessarily encompass the full legal and moral rights attributed to persons" (U.S. Department of Health, Education and Welfare, p. 107). The Warnock Commission issued a report in Britain in 1984 that also accorded the embryo a "special status," though not the same status "as a living child or adult" (Warnock).

The notion that the embryo is an entity with a special status deserving special respect is contested by those who regard the embryo as fully a human being from the moment of conception. An instruction issued by the Vatican concluded that the "human being must be respected—as a person—from the very first instant of his existence" (Catholic Church; Shannon and Cahill). The unique genetic makeup of the embryo, among other things, is given as evidence of its individuality.

Beliefs about the embryo's status are central to conclusions about what in IVF is permissible and what is not. Some observers who regard the embryo as a human being believe IVF is ethically acceptable provided all embryos are transferred and given a chance to survive. Others believe external fertilization is always immoral. If the embryo is regarded as a human being, it has "full human rights," including the right not to be experimented upon without its consent (Ramsey, 1972a, 1972b). Even if one regards IVF as no longer experimental, the conclusion of immorality still extends to IVF's variations, which begin as experimental procedures posing the risk of higher-than-normal embryo loss.

If, on the other hand, the embryo is regarded as only potentially a human, fewer ethical strictures on IVF techniques apply. The Ethics Advisory Board concluded that IVF was ethically acceptable for married couples and that research on human embryos was acceptable provided the research was designed to establish IVF safety, would yield "important scientific information," complied with federal laws protecting research subjects, and proceeded only with the consent of tissue donors. No research was to take place beyond the fourteenth day after fertilization. After fourteen days, the embryo begins to develop an embryonic disk or "primitive streak" and is no longer capable of spontaneous twinning, which means it is on the way to becoming a single individual.

IVF has been criticized as a fundamentally dehumanizing technique that takes place in a laboratory, involves the scientist as a third party, is geared to the production of human beings, and is aimed at conquering nature and producing a "quality" child (Kass). The language of IVF and its business and marketing overtones contribute to a situation in which tissues and children are treated as commodities to be produced and in which intimacy is devalued (Lauritzen). The Vatican instruction concluded that IVF is unnatural because the sperm are secured by masturbation and the union takes place outside the body. Tissue donation is especially illicit, as it is "contrary to the unity of marriage, [and] to the dignity of the spouses" (Catholic Church).

Some feminists have expanded on this theme by criticizing laboratory conception as an intervention that divides reproduction—once a continuous process taking place naturally within the woman's body—into discrete and impersonal parts subject to a male-dominated medical profession (Arditti et al.). They argue that in IVF, women are perennial research subjects in an unending set of techniques that have significant emotional costs (Williams); that IVF benefits men and compromises women; and that it curtails women's autonomy and magnifies gender-based power differences in society (Wikler). Other feminists support IVF if it is bounded by feminist ethics and if it builds women's control over reproduction rather than taking it away (Sherwin).

IVF's variations challenge notions of the family, the interests of the potential child, the distribution of societal resources, and the rights of prospective parents. Tissue donation from relatives creates new biological if not legal relationships—for example, when a sister donates an egg to a sister for IVF or a brother donates sperm for his brother's IVF attempt. Embryo freezing creates the prospect of some embryos being stored indefinitely or transferred in a later generation, possibly endangering the resulting child's sense of identity. It also sets the stage for custody disputes and conflicts over the disposition of unwanted embryos (*Davis v. Davis,* 1992).

Embryo diagnosis for genetic defects raises safety questions for the embryo and potential child. Conceivably, it will lead to screening for many genetic problems and not just the life-threatening disorders envisioned now. On the one hand, discarding embryos after tests reveal a genetic abnormality might be less morally contentious than aborting pregnancies, at least for those who believe the embryo has a lesser status than a fetus. On the other hand, discarding "defective" embryos may blunt societal sensibilities and invite

fertile couples into the costly and uncertain IVF procedure. The ability to preselect embryos according to sex raises concerns that the technique will be used for nonmedical reasons to give couples a child of their preferred gender, which may be male (Wertz and Fletcher).

IVF is highly selective in the people it can help. An expensive procedure covered by few insurance companies, it is available primarily to affluent couples. Critics question the wisdom of directing scarce resources to an elective and costly procedure with low odds of success (Callahan). Others advise paying more attention to preventing infertility in the first place (Blank). Aggressive marketing of IVF, including marketing that distorts success rates to make them seem greater than they actually are, arguably creates needs by making couples feel they ought to try IVF because it is there to try and by interfering with alternatives such as adoption or stopping efforts to conceive.

Concerns about the support of IVF and embryo research have been integrated into formal policy in a number of countries (Knoppers and LeBris). For example, the British Human Embryology and Fertilisation Act of 1990 created a licensing authority to conduct on-site visits to clinics in which human embryos are manipulated, review research proposals, and ensure that quality control is maintained in the laboratories (Morgan and Lee). A restrictive law in Germany, by contrast, makes criminal a range of techniques not therapeutic for the embryo, including sex preselection for nonmedical reasons ("German Embryo Protection Act"). Among the international documents relating to embryo manipulations are a recommendation from the Parliamentary Assembly of the Council of Europe that the Council of Ministers provide a "framework of principles" governing embryo and fetal research ("Parliamentary Assembly"), and a set of principles relating to IVF and its variations ("Council of Europe").

Fifteen states in the United States mention embryos in their statutes, but legislators passed most laws with abortion and fetuses in mind rather than IVF and embryos. Some of these laws would presumably make embryo research illegal, but their constitutionality has not been tested (Robertson). In 1989 the U.S. Supreme Court reviewed Missouri's abortion statute but declined to address the constitutionality of the statute's preamble that "the life of each human being begins at conception" (*Webster v. Reproductive Health Services*). This definition of personhood appears to contradict the Court's abortion rulings, but by leaving it untouched, the Court left the embryo's legal status unclear.

Several states have passed laws mandating insurance coverage for IVF under certain conditions (U.S. Congress,

Office of Technology Assessment). The federal government does not fund proposals involving human embryos; by law, research must be reviewed by an ethics board ("Protection of Human Subjects"), but no board has replaced the Ethics Advisory Board, which was disbanded in 1979. This has led to a de facto funding moratorium.

Conclusion

Prior to and in the years following the first successful use of IVF, critics argued that it challenged the sanctity of marriage and family, posed the threat of psychological and physical harm to unborn children, involved the immoral destruction of human embryos, made women experimental pawns in research in which men asserted control over reproduction, and introduced the senseless creation of people in an era of overpopulation. It was also said to admit no clear stopping point, use scarce medical resources, and amount to an elective technique that did not cure infertility.

Supporters argued that IVF would spare couples the psychological trauma of infertility, meet the needs of tens of thousands of women with blocked fallopian tubes, lead to knowledge that would help ensure healthy children, and preserve the family by bringing children to couples who truly want them. They responded to criticism by saying IVF was no more unnatural than cesarean births, should not be diminished merely because it did not cure infertility, posed no apparent risks to children, and was not immoral, in that embryos were only potential human beings.

Today, basic IVF has shifted from experimental to standard medical practice. It is widely available, is regarded as safe, and is the only viable way women with blocked fallopian tubes can conceive a baby genetically related to them. New technical additions ensure, however, that external fertilization will remain at center stage in the ongoing bioethics debate over reproductive technologies.

The lasting unanswered questions relate to the high value placed on genetic parenthood, equitable access to techniques across race and class, the impact of laboratory conception on women's control over reproduction, and whether priority ought to be placed on conception in a time when discussions are directed to ways of reducing the gap in medical services available to richer and poorer citizens.

Perhaps most significant, however, is the matter of the limits to be placed on reproductive technologies. It appears that the scope of refinements is nearly endless. Should substantive and procedural limits be placed by government on any of IVF's variations? If so, which, and why? Understanding the reasons for placing limits is as important as understanding the reasons laboratory conception is pursued with such intensity in the first place.

ANDREA L. BONNICKSEN (1995)
BIBLIOGRAPHY REVISED

SEE ALSO: *Abortion; Adoption; Cloning; Embryo and Fetus; Feminism; Fetal Research; Genetic Counseling; Genetic Testing and Screening: Reproductive Genetic Testing; Healthcare Resources, Allocation of: Microallocation; Law and Bioethics; Maternal-Fetal Relationship; Moral Status; Population Ethics; Sexism; Transhumanism and Posthumanism; Women, Contemporary Issues of;* and other *Reproductive Technologies* subentries

BIBLIOGRAPHY

Arditti, Rita; Klein, Renate Duelli; and Minden, Shelly, eds. 1984. *Test-Tube Women: What Future for Motherhood?* London: Pandora Press.

Blank, Robert H. 1988. *Rationing Medicine.* New York: Columbia University Press.

Callahan, Daniel. 1990. *What Kind of Life: The Limits of Medical Progress.* New York: Simon & Schuster.

Catholic Church. Congregation for the Doctrine of the Faith. 1987. *Instruction on Respect for Human Life in Its Origin and on the Dignity of Procreation: Replies to Certain Questions of the Day.* Doctrinal statement of the Vatican (March 10). Vatican City: Author.

Cohen, Cynthia B. 1996. "'Give Me Children or I Shall Die!': New Reproductive Technologies and Harm to Children." *Hastings Center Report* 26(2): 19–27.

Cohen, Jean. 1991. "The Efficiency and Efficacy of IVF and GIFT." *Human Reproduction* 6(5): 613–618.

"Council of Europe Publishes Principles in the Field of Human Artificial Procreation." 1989. *International Digest of Health Legislation* 40(4): 907–912.

Davis v. Davis. 18 Fam.L.Rptr. 2029 Tenn. (1992).

Dyson, Anthony. 1995. *The Ethics of IVF (Ethics, Our Choices).* Harrisburg, PA: Morehouse Publishing.

"German Embryo Protection Act (October 24, 1990)" (Gesetz zum Schutz von Embryonen [Embryonenschutzgesetz—ESchG]). 1991. *Human Reproduction* 6(4): 605–606.

Hildt, Elisabeth, and Mieth, Dietmar, eds. 1998. In *Vitro Fertilisation in the 1990s: Towards Medical, Social, and Ethical Evaluation.* London: Ashgate.

Kass, Leon. 1985. *Toward a More Natural Science: Biology and Human Affairs.* New York: Free Press.

Knoppers, Bartha M., and LeBris, Sonia. 1991. "Recent Advances in Medically Assisted Conception: Legal, Ethical and Social Issues." *American Journal of Law and Medicine* 27(4): 329–361.

Lauritzen, Paul. 1990. "What Price Parenthood?" *Hastings Center Report* 29(2): 38–46.

LeMoncheck, Linda. 1996. "Philosophy, Gender Politics, and In Vitro Fertilization: A Feminist Ethics of Reproductive Healthcare." *Journal of Clinical Ethics* 7(2): 160–176.

Leuthner, Steven R., and White, Gladys B. 2001. "Infertility Treatment and Neonatal Care: The Ethical Obligation to Transcend Specialty Practice in the Interest of Reducing Multiple Births." *Journal of Clinical Ethics* 12(3): 223–230.

McCormick, Richard A. 1991. "Who or What Is the Preembryo?" *Kennedy Institute of Ethics Journal* 1(1): 1–15.

Medical Research International, Society for Assisted Reproductive Technology (SART), and American Fertility Society. 1992. "In Vitro Fertilization-Embryo Transfer (IVF-ET) in the United States: 1990 Results from the IVF-ET Registry." *Fertility and Sterility* 57(1): 15–24.

Morgan, Derek, and Lee, Robert G. 1991. *Blackstone's Guide to the Human Fertilisation and Embryology Act, 1990.* London: Blackstone Press.

Parks, Jennifer A. "On the Use of IVF by Post-Menopausal Women." *Hypatia* 14(1): 77–96.

"Parliamentary Assembly of Council of Europe Adopts Recommendation on Use of Human Embryos and Foetuses for Research Purposes." 1989. *International Digest of Health Legislation* 40(2): 485–491.

"Protection of Human Subjects: Fetuses, Pregnant Women, and In Vitro Fertilization." 1975. Federal Register 40:150 (8 Aug.) pp. 33525–33552. Codified in 45 C.F.R. 46, especially section 204(d).

Ramsey, Paul. 1972a. "Shall We 'Reproduce'? I. The Medical Ethics of In Vitro Fertilization." *Journal of the American Medical AssociationL* 220(10): 1346–1350.

Ramsey, Paul. 1972b. "Shall We 'Reproduce'? II. Rejoinders and Future Forecast." *Journal of the American Medical Association* 220(11): 1480–1485.

Robertson, John A. 1992. "Ethical and Legal Issues in Preimplantation Genetic Screening." *Fertility and Sterility* 57(1): 1–11.

Shannon, Thomas, A., and Cahill, Lisa Sowle. 1988. *Religion and Artificial Reproduction: An Inquiry into the Vatican "Instruction on Respect for Human Life in Its Origin and on the Dignity of Human Reproduction."* New York: Crossroad.

Sherwin, Susan. 1989. "Feminist Ethics and New Reproductive Technologies." In *The Future of Human Reproduction,* pp. 259–271, ed. Christine Overall. Toronto: Women's Press.

Spoerl, Joseph S. 1999. "In Vitro Fertilization and the Ethics of Procreation." *Ethics and Medicine* 15(1): 10–14.

Steptoe, Patrick C., and Edwards, Robert G. 1978. "Birth After the Reimplantation of a Human Embryo." *Lancet* 2(8085): 366.

Trounson, Alan L. 1992. "Preimplantation Genetic Diagnosis—Counting Chickens Before They Hatch?" *Human Reproduction* 7(5): 583–584.

U.S. Congress. Office of Technology Assessment. 1988. *Infertility: Medical and Social Choices.* OTA–BA–358. Washington, D.C.: U.S. Government Printing Office.

U.S. Department of Health, Education and Welfare. Ethics Advisory Board. 1979. *Report and Conclusions: HEW Support of Research Involving Human In Vitro Fertilization and Embryo Transfer.* Washington, D.C.: U.S. Government Printing Office.

Verlinsky, Yury; Pergament, Eugene; and Strom, Charles. 1990. "The Preimplantation Genetic Diagnosis of Genetic Diseases." *Journal of in Vitro Fertilization and Embryo Transfer* 7(1): 1–5.

Warnock, Mary. 1985. *A Question of Life: The Warnock Report on Human Fertilisation and Embryology.* Oxford: Basil Blackwell.

Webster v. Reproductive Health Services. 492 U.S. 490 1989.

Wertz, Dorothy C., and Fletcher, John C. 1989. "Fatal Knowledge? Prenatal Diagnosis and Sex Selection." *Hastings Center Report* 19(3): 21–27.

Wikler, Norma Juliet. 1986. "Society's Response to the New Reproductive Technologies: The Feminist Perspectives." *Southern California Law Review* 59(5): 1043–1057.

Williams, Linda S. 1989. "No Relief Until the End: The Physical and Emotional Costs of In Vitro Fertilization." In *The Future of Human Reproduction,* pp. 120–138, ed. Christine Overall. Toronto: Women's Press.

REPROGENETICS

SEE *Gene Therapy; Genetics and Human Behavior; Genetic Testing and Screening*

RESEARCH ETHICS COMMITTEES

• • •

The World Medical Association's Declaration of Helsinki (2000) and the Council for International Organizations of Medical Sciences' *International Ethical Guidelines for Biomedical Research Involving Human Subjects* (hereafter, CIOMS *International Ethical Guidelines*) (2002) establish as the international standard for biomedical research involving human subjects this requirement: "All proposals to conduct research involving human subjects must be submitted for review of their scientific merit and ethical acceptability to one or more scientific review and ethical review committees.... The investigator must obtain their approval or clearance before undertaking the research" (CIOMS, Guideline 2). In most of the world this committee is called the research ethics committee (REC). In the United States, federal law assigns to the committee the name institutional review board (IRB), and the authority and responsibility for approving or disapproving proposals to conduct research involving human subjects ("IRB Review of Research").

History

The Nuremberg Code (1949) and the original Declaration of Helsinki (1964) made no mention of committee review; these documents placed on the investigator all responsibility for safeguarding the rights and welfare of research subjects. The first mention of committee review in an international document was in the Tokyo revision of the Declaration of Helsinki (1975).

In the United States, the first federal document requiring committee review was issued on November 17, 1953. Titled "Group Consideration for Clinical Research Procedures Deviating from Accepted Medical Practice or Involving Unusual Hazard," its guidelines applied only to research conducted at the newly opened Clinical Center at the National Institutes of Health (Lipsett, Fletcher, and Secundy). Very little is known about peer review in other institutions in the 1950s other than that it existed in at least some medical schools. In 1961 and again in 1962, questionnaires were sent to departments of medicine at U.S. universities. Approximately one-third of those responding reported that they had committees, and one-quarter either had or were developing procedural documents (Curran).

On February 8, 1966, the surgeon general of the U.S. Public Health Service (USPHS) issued the first federal policy statement requiring research institutions to establish the committees that subsequently came to be known as RECs (Curran). This policy required recipients of USPHS grants in support of research involving human subjects to specify that

> the grantee institution will provide prior review of the judgment of the principal investigator or program director by a committee of his institutional associates. This review shall assure an independent determination: (1) Of the rights and welfare of the … individuals involved, (2) Of the appropriateness of the methods used to secure informed consent, and (3) Of the risks and potential medical benefits of the investigation.

The evolution of the federal government's charges to the committee and of its recognition of the need for diversity of committee membership was reflected in several revisions of its policy between 1966 and 1969 (Veatch; Levine, 1986); these will be further discussed below.

Purpose

The purpose of the REC is to ensure that research involving human subjects is designed to conform to relevant ethical standards. Historically, the REC's primary focus was on safeguarding the rights and welfare of individual research subjects, concentrating on the plans for informed consent and the assessment of risks and anticipated benefits. In 1978 the National Commission for the Protection of Human Subjects of Biomedical and Behavioral Research (hereafter, National Commission) added a requirement that the REC ensure equitableness in the selection of research subjects (Levine, 1986). The National Commission was concerned primarily with protecting vulnerable subjects from bearing a disproportionately large share of the burdens of research. Subsequently, as participation in some types of research became perceived as a benefit, RECs also assumed responsibility for ensuring disadvantaged persons equitable access to such benefits (Levine, 1994).

A source of continuing controversy is whether the REC has an obligation to approve or disapprove the scientific design of research protocols (Levine, 1986). Those who argue that they do or should have such an obligation point out that the leading ethical codes establish a requirement for good scientific design. Moreover, these observers argue, the REC's obligation to determine that risks to subjects are reasonable in relation to anticipated benefits necessarily relies on a prior determination that the scientific design is adequate, for if it is not, there will be no benefits and any risk must be considered unreasonable.

Opponents to assigning such an obligation to the REC, while conceding these two points, argue that the REC is not designed to make expert judgments about the adequacy of scientific design. RECs are generally competent to appraise the value of the science—what the Nuremberg Code calls "the humanitarian importance of the problem to be solved"— but not the validity of the methods or the results (Freedman; Veatch). In general, responsibility for assessment of scientific validity is, and ought to be, delegated to committees designed to have such competence—such as scientific review committees either within the institution or at funding agencies such as the National Institutes of Health (Levine, 1986; IOM).

Membership

The surgeon general's 1966 memo called for prior review by "a committee of [the investigator's] associates," what was commonly called "peer review." As of 1968, 73 percent of committees were limited in membership to immediate peer groups: scientists and physicians (Curran).

On May 1, 1969, USPHS guidelines were revised to indicate that a committee constituted exclusively of biomedical scientists would be inadequate to perform the functions now expected of it: "The membership should possess … competencies necessary in the judgment as to the acceptability of the research in terms of institutional regulations, relevant law, standards of professional practice and community acceptance."

Regulations of the U.S. Department of Health and Human Services (DHHS), first promulgated in 1974 and since revised several times, maintain the spirit of the 1969 policy and in addition require gender diversity; at least one nonscientist (e.g., lawyer, ethicist, member of the clergy); and at least one member who is not affiliated with the institution (commonly and incorrectly called a "community representative"). Persons having conflicting interests are to be excluded; this concern is also reflected in the CIOMS *International Ethical Guidelines'* requirement for "review committees independent of the research team."

According to Robert M. Veatch (1975), the REC is an intermediate case between two models of the review committee: The "interdisciplinary professional review model," made up of diverse professionals such as doctors, lawyers, scientists, and clergy, brings professional expertise to the review process, while the "jury model … reflects the common sense of the reasonable person." In the jury model "expertise relevant to the case at hand is not only not necessary, it often disqualifies one from serving on the jury" (Veatch, p. 31). Veatch conceded that in order to perform all of its functions, the REC requires both professional and jury skills. He argued, however, that the presence of professionals makes it more difficult for the REC to be responsive to the informational needs of the reasonable person or to be adept at anticipating community acceptance.

John A. Robertson (1979) recommended correcting the "structural bias" of professional domination by introducing a "subject surrogate," an expert advocate for the subjects' interests. DHHS regulations require that if an REC "regularly reviews research that involves a vulnerable category of subjects … consideration shall be given to the inclusion of … [persons who know] about and [are] experienced in working with these subjects" (IRB Membership). For research involving prisoners, the regulations require that at least one member of the REC be either a prisoner or a prisoner representative. There is unresolved controversy over whether persons with AIDS should be appointed to serve on all RECs that review research in the field of HIV infection (Levine, Dubler, and Levine).

In the United States the Institute of Medicine (IOM) endorsed the recommendation of the National Bioethics Advisory Commission (NBAC) that "at least 25 percent of [the IRB's] membership should be reserved for unaffiliated [with the institution] members and those who can provide nonscientific perspectives" (IOM, p. 96). The IOM further expressed its support for the current trends in the United States to enhance the education of REC members and to certify them as competent by independent agencies.

Locale

In the United States the first RECs were established in the institutions where research was conducted. The 1966 surgeon general's policy statement required a committee of "institutional associates." In 1971 the Food and Drug Administration (FDA) promulgated regulations that required committee review only when regulated research was conducted in institutions; hence their name, institutional review committee. Regulations proposed in 1973 by the Department of Health, Education, and Welfare, forerunner of DHHS, also reflected a local setting in their term "organizational review board." In 1974 the National Research Act established a statutory requirement for review by a committee to which it assigned the name "institutional review board," a compromise between the two names then extant.

RECs are required to comply with federal regulations when reviewing activities involving FDA-regulated "test articles," such as investigational drugs and devices, and when reviewing research supported by federal funds. Moreover, all institutions that receive federal research grants and contracts are required to file "statements of assurance" of compliance with federal regulations. In these assurances virtually all institutions voluntarily promise to apply the principles of federal regulations to all research they conduct, regardless of the source of funding (Levine, 1986; IOM).

These points notwithstanding, each REC has a decidedly local character. Most have local names, such as "human investigation committee" or "committee for the protection of human subjects." Each is appointed by its own institution, and each makes its own interpretation of the requirements of federal regulations. For example, at one university, medical students are forbidden to serve as research subjects, whereas at another, involvement of medical students as research subjects is sometimes required as a condition of approval (Levine, 1986).

In its 1978 report, the National Commission recommended that RECs should be "located in institutions where research … is conducted. Compared to the possible alternatives of a regional or national review … local committees have the advantage of greater familiarity with the actual conditions" (U.S. National Commission, pp. 1–2). The

National Commission envisioned the local REC as an ally of the investigator in safeguarding the rights and welfare of research subjects, as well as a contributor to the education of both the research community and the public.

The FDA's change in regulations in 1981 to require REC review of all regulated research, regardless of where it was done, created a problem for the many physicians who were conducting investigations in their private offices; many of these physicians had no ready access to RECs. In response, private corporations developed noninstitutional review boards (NRBs) (Herman). Although there are reasons to question the validity of reviews by NRBs, they appear to be performing satisfactorily (Levine and Lasagna).

In 1986 the FDA began to waive the requirement for local REC review of some protocols designed to evaluate, or to make available for therapeutic purposes, investigational new drugs, particularly those intended for the treatment of HIV infection. In such cases RECs were offered the option of accepting review by a national committee as fulfilling the regulatory requirement for REC review. Such practices have caused some commentators to question the strength of the government's commitment to the principle of local review (Levine and Lasagna).

Internationally, there is much less commitment to the importance of local review. The CIOMS *International Ethical Guidelines* require REC approval for all research involving human subjects and recognize the validity of review at "the institutional, local, regional or national, and in some cases, at the international level." In many European countries, RECs are regional (McNeill).

Several commentators have expressed concern that in the United States the local institution has too much power in protection of human research subjects. Robertson, for example, warned about "the danger ... that research institutions will use [RECs] to protect themselves and researchers rather than subjects" (1979); others point to the close associations between RECs and risk-management offices in many institutions as evidence that RECs are being used in this manner.

Criticisms

Before 1962, "a general skepticism toward the development of ethical guidelines, codes, or sets of procedures concerning the conduct of research" prevailed in the medical research community (Curran, p. 408). In the 1970s several biomedical scientists were harshly critical of the REC system, claiming that it tended to stifle creativity and impede progress (Levine, 1986); survey research, however, showed that only 25 percent of biomedical researchers agreed with

the statement that "The review ... is an unwarranted intrusion on the investigator's autonomy—at least to some extent" (U.S. National Commission, p. 75). Behavioral and social scientists were considerably less accepting of review, claiming that their research activities were much less likely than those of the biomedical scientist to harm subjects. Some argued that because all they did was talk with subjects, review was an unconstitutional constraint on their freedom of speech (Levine, 1986). With the passage of time, most social and behavioral scientists have recognized the value of the REC's review of work in their fields; they have protested, however, that much of the review of social and behavioral research is unsatisfactory because RECs, in general, tend to inappropriately apply rules and procedures that were designed for the "biomedical model" (IOM).

According to Peter C. Williams (1984), RECs do an inadequate job of ensuring that risks will be reasonable in relation to anticipated benefits. This is inevitable for three reasons:

1. Federal regulations on this standard are written in vague language, in contrast to the clearer direction provided for protecting subjects' rights. Moreover, because the regulations permit consideration of the long-range effects of applying knowledge as benefits but not as risks, they create a bias in favor of approval.

2. The membership of the committee, dominated as it is by professionals, is likely to place a higher value than laypersons would on the benefit of developing new knowledge.

3. Groups confronted with choices involving risks may be either more or less cautious or "risk aversive" than the average of individuals within the group; this is known as the *risky shift* or *group polarization phenomenon*. Williams (1984) and Veatch (1975) have argued that in the context of RECs, the groups are likely to be more tolerant of higher levels of risk than would be the individuals who comprise the groups.

Several commentators have proposed that RECs could enhance their effectiveness by sending members to the sites of the actual conduct of research to verify compliance with protocol requirements (Robertson, 1979) or to supervise consent negotiations (Robertson, 1982). Others respond that while such activities should be done when there are reasons to suspect problems in specific protocols, routine monitoring activities might be detrimental to the successful functioning of the committee by eroding its support within the institution (Levine, 1986). The Institute of Medicine concurs with the NBAC's proposal that the REC should engage in routine monitoring of the actual conduct of research, concentrating its efforts on research projects that present to subjects relatively high levels of risks (IOM).

Evaluation

Critics of the REC system claim that there is little or no objective evidence that REC review prevents the conduct of inadequate research. For example, a national survey of RECs revealed that the rate of rejection of protocols is less than 1 in 1,000 (National Commission). Supporters of the system respond that the actual rejection rate is much higher if one includes protocols withdrawn because investigators refuse to modify them as required by RECs. Moreover, rejection rates may be a poor indicator of the REC's quality; protocols may be improved in anticipation of the REC's requirements, and investigators, fearing rejection, may decide not to submit proposals they think might be rejected.

It is very difficult to evaluate the REC's performance objectively; satisfactory subjective evaluations can be made only by experienced REC members and administrators (Levine, 1986). In his excellent theoretical analysis of RECs, published in 1981, Jerry L. Mashaw concluded:

> If [the REC] is to do its core job well, we must live with its inevitable incompetence at other tasks. Moreover, we must also live with the rather vague regulatory standards and with the continuing inability of the federal funding agencies to know for sure whether [RECs] are functioning effectively. If we would have wise judges and paternalistic [skilled in protecting subjects' rights and welfare interests] professionals, we can neither specifically direct nor objectively evaluate their behavior. (Mashaw, p. 22)

ROBERT J. LEVINE (1995)
REVISED BY AUTHOR

SEE ALSO: *Aging and the Aged: Healthcare and Research Issues; AIDS: Healthcare and Research Issues; Autoexperimentation; Children: Healthcare and Research Issues; Commercialism in Scientific Research; Conflict of Interest; Embryo and Fetus: Embryo Research; Empirical Methods in Bioethics; Genetics and Human Behavior: Scientific and Research Issues; Holocaust; Infants: Public Policy and Legal Issues; Informed Consent: Consent Issues in Human Research; Mentally Ill and Mentally Disabled Persons: Research Issues; Military Personnel as Research Subjects; Minorities as Research Subjects; Pediatrics, Overview of Ethical Issues in; Prisoners as Research Subjects; Race and Racism; Research, Human: Historical Aspects; Research Methodology; Research, Multinational; Research Policy; Research, Unethical; Responsibility; Scientific Publishing; Sexism; Students as Research Subjects; Virtue and Character*

BIBLIOGRAPHY

Council for International Organizations of Medical Sciences (CIOMS), in collaboration with the World Health Organization. 2002. *International Ethical Guidelines for Biomedical Research Involving Human Subjects.* Geneva, Switzerland: Author.

Curran, William J. 1970. "Governmental Regulation of the Use of Human Subjects in Medical Research: The Approach of Two Federal Agencies." In *Experimentation with Human Subjects,* ed. Paul A. Freund. New York: George Braziller.

Freedman, Benjamin. 1987. "Scientific Value and Validity as Ethical Requirements for Research: A Proposed Explication." *IRB: A Review of Human Subjects Research* 9(6): 7–10.

Herman, Samuel S. 1989. "A Noninstitutional Review Board Comes of Age." *IRB: A Review of Human Subjects Research* 11(2): 1–6.

Institute of Medicine (IOM). Committee on Assessing the System for Protecting Human Research Participants. 2003. *Responsible Research: A Systems Approach to Protecting Research Participants,* ed. Daniel D. Federman, Kathi E. Hanna, and Laura L. Rodriguez. Washington, D.C.: National Academies Press.

"IRB Membership." 2002. *Code of Federal Regulations* Title 45, Pt. 46.107.

Levine, Carol; Dubler, Nancy N.; and Levine, Robert J. 1991. "Building a New Consensus: Ethical Principles and Policies for Clinical Research on HIV/AIDS." *IRB: A Review of Human Subjects Research* 13(1–2): 1–17.

Levine, Robert J. 1986. *Ethics and Regulation of Clinical Research,* 2nd edition. Baltimore: Urban and Schwarzenberg.

Levine, Robert J. 1994. "The Impact of HIV Infection on Society's Perception of Clinical Trials." *Kennedy Institute of Ethics Journal* 4(2): 93–98.

Levine, Robert J., and Lasagna, Louis. 2000. "Demystifying Central Review Boards: Current Options and Future Directions." *IRB: A Review of Human Subjects Research* 22(6): 1–4.

Lipsett, Mortimer B.; Fletcher, John C.; and Secundy, Marian. 1979. "Research Review at NIH." *Hastings Center Report* 9(1): 18–21.

Mashaw, Jerry L. 1981. "Thinking about Institutional Review Boards." In *Whistleblowing in Biomedical Research: Policies and Procedures for Responding to Reports of Misconduct,* ed. Judith P. Swazey and Stephen R. Scher. U.S. President's Commission for the Study of Ethical Problems in Medicine and Biomedical and Behavioral Research; American Association for the Advancement of Science, Committee on Scientific Freedom and Responsibility; and Medicine in the Public Interest. Washington, D.C.: U.S. Government Printing Office.

McNeill, Paul M. 1989. "Research Ethics Committees in Australia, Europe, and North America." *IRB: A Review of Human Subjects Research* 11(3): 4–7.

Medical Research Council of Canada. 1987. *Guidelines on Research Involving Human Subjects.* Ottawa: Author.

Robertson, John A. 1979. "Ten Ways to Improve IRBs." *Hastings Center Report* 9(1): 29–33.

Robertson, John A. 1982. "Taking Consent Seriously: IRB Intervention in the Consent Process." *IRB: A Review of Human Subjects Research* 4(5): 1–5.

U.S. National Commission for the Protection of Human Subjects of Biomedical and Behavioral Research. 1978. *Report and Recommendations: Institutional Review Boards.* Washington, D.C.: U.S. Government Printing Office.

Veatch, Robert M. 1975. "Human Experimentation Committees: Professional or Representative?" *Hastings Center Report* 5(5): 31–40.

Williams, Peter C. 1984. "Success in Spite of Failure: Why IRBs Falter in Reviewing Risks and Benefits." *IRB: A Review of Human Subjects Research* 6(3): 1–4.

World Medical Association. 1964 (revised 1975, 2000). "Declaration of Helsinki: Ethical Principles for Medical Research Involving Human Subjects." Ferney-Voltaire, France: Author.

RESEARCH, HUMAN: HISTORICAL ASPECTS

• • •

In Western civilization, the idea of human experimentation, of evaluating the efficacy of a new drug or procedure by outcomes, is an ancient one. It is discussed in the writings of Greek and Roman physicians and in Arab medical treatises. Scholars like Avicenna (980–1037) insisted that "the experimentation must be done with the human body, for testing a drug on a lion or a horse might not prove anything about its effect on man" (Bull, p. 221). But records of how often ancient physicians conducted experiments, with what agents, and on which subjects, are very thin. The most frequently cited cases involve testing the efficacy of poisons on condemned prisoners, but the extent to which other human research was carried on remains obscure.

Experimentation was frequent enough to inspire a discussion of the ethical maxims that should guide would-be investigators. Moses Maimonides (1135–1204), the noted Jewish physician and philosopher, instructed colleagues always to treat patients as ends in themselves, not as means for learning new truths. Roger Bacon (1214–1294) excused the inconsistencies in therapeutic practices on the following grounds:

It is exceedingly difficult and dangerous to perform operations on the human body. The operative and practical sciences which do their work on insensate bodies can multiply their experiments till they get rid of deficiency and errors, but a physician cannot do this because of the nobility of the material in which he works; for that body demands that no error be made in operating upon it, and so experience [the experimental method] is so difficult in medicine. (quoted in Bull, p. 222)

Human Experimentation in Early Modern Western History

Human experimentation made its first significant impact on medical practice through the work of the English country physician Edward Jenner (1749–1823). Observing that dairy farmers who had contracted the pox from swine or cows seemed to be immune to the more virulent smallpox, Jenner set out to retrieve material from their pustules, inject the material into another person, and see whether the recipient could then resist challenges from smallpox materials. The procedure promised to be less dangerous than the more standard one of inoculating people with small amounts of smallpox that had been introduced into Europe and America from the Ottoman Empire in the first half of the eighteenth century.

In November 1789, Jenner inoculated his son, then about a year old, with swinepox. When this intervention proved ineffective against a challenge of smallpox, Jenner tried cowpox several months later with another subject. As he recalled: "The more accurately to observe the progress of the infection, I selected a healthy boy, about eight years old, for the purpose of inoculation for the cow-pox. The matter … was inserted … into the arm of the boy by means of two incisions" (Jenner, pp. 164–165). A week later Jenner injected him with smallpox, and noted that he evinced no reaction. The cowpox had rendered him immune to smallpox. One cannot know whether the boy was a willing or unwilling subject or how much he understood of the experiment. But this was not an interaction between strangers. The boy was from the neighborhood, Mr. Jenner was a gentleman of standing, and the experiment did have potential therapeutic benefit for the subject.

For most of the nineteenth century, human experimentation throughout western Europe and the United States was a cottage industry, with individual physicians trying out one or another remedy on neighbors or relatives or on themselves. One German physician, Johann Jorg (1779–1856), swallowed varying doses of seventeen different drugs in order to analyze their effects. Another, Sir James Young Simpson (1811–1870), an Edinburgh obstetrician who was searching for an anesthesia superior to ether, in November 1847 inhaled chloroform and awoke to find himself lying flat on the floor (Howard-Jones). Perhaps the most extraordinary self-experiment was conducted by Werner Forssman. In 1929 he passed a catheter, guided by radiography, into the right ventricle of his heart, thereby demonstrating the feasibility and the safety of the procedure.

The most unusual nineteenth-century human experiment was conducted by the American physician William Beaumont (1785–1853) on Alexis St. Martin. A stomach wound suffered by St. Martin healed in such a way as to leave Beaumont access to the stomach and the opportunity to study the action of gastric juices. To carry on this research, which was very important to the new field of physiology, Beaumont had St. Martin sign an agreement, not so much a consent form as an apprenticeship contract. Under its terms, St. Martin bound himself to "serve, abide, and continue with the said William Beaumont ... [as] his covenant servant," and in return for board, lodging, and $150 a year, he agreed "to assist and promote by all means in his power such philosophical or medical experiments as the said William shall direct or cause to be made on or in the stomach of him" (Beaumont, pp. xii–xiii).

The most brilliant human experiments of the nineteenth century were conducted by Louis Pasteur (1822–1895), who demonstrated an acute sensitivity to the ethics of his investigations. Even as he conducted his animal research to identify an antidote to rabies, he worried about the time when it would be necessary to test the product on a human being. "I have already several cases of dogs immunized after rabic bites," he wrote in 1884. "I take two dogs: I have them bitten by a mad dog. I vaccinate the one and I leave the other without treatment. The latter dies of rabies: the former withstands it." Nevertheless, Pasteur continued, "I have not yet dared to attempt anything on man, in spite of my confidence in the result.... I must wait first till I have got a whole crowd of successful results on animals.... But, however I should multiply my cases of protection of dogs, I think that my hand will shake when I have to go on to man" (Vallery-Radot, pp. 404–405).

The fateful moment came some nine months later when his help was sought by a mother whose nine-year-old son, Joseph Meister, had just been severely bitten by what was probably a mad dog. Pasteur agonized as to whether to carry out what would be the first human trial of his rabies inoculation. He consulted with two medical colleagues, had them examine the boy, and at their urging and on the grounds that "the death of the child appeared inevitable, I resolved, though not without great anxiety, to try the method which had proved consistently successful on the dogs." With great anxiety he administered twelve inoculations to the boy, and only weeks later did he become confident of the efficacy of his approach and the "future health of Joseph Meister" (Vallery-Radot, pp. 414–417).

Claude Bernard (1813–1878), professor of medicine at the College of France, not only conducted ground-breaking research in physiology, but also composed an astute treatise on the methods and ethics of experimentation. "Morals do not forbid making experiments on one's neighbor or one's self," Bernard argued in 1865. Rather, "the principle of medical and surgical morality consists in never performing on man an experiment which might be harmful to him to any extent, even though the result might be highly advantageous to science, i.e., to the health of others." To be sure, Bernard did allow some exceptions; he sanctioned experimentation on dying patients and on criminals about to be executed, on the grounds that "they involve no suffering of harm to the subject of the experiment." But he made clear that scientific progress did not justify violating the well-being of any individual (Bernard, p. 101).

Anglo-American common law recognized both the vital role of human experimentation and the need for physicians to obtain the patient's consent. As one English commentator explained in 1830: "By experiments we are not to be understood as speaking of the wild and dangerous practices of rash and ignorant practitioners ... but of deliberate acts of men from considerable knowledge and undoubted talent, differing from those prescribed by the ordinary rules of practice, for which they have good reason ... to believe will be attended with benefit to the patient, although the novelty of the undertaking does not leave the result altogether free of doubt." The researcher who had the subject's consent was "answerable neither in damages to the individual, nor on a criminal proceeding. But if the practitioner performs his experiment without giving such information to, and obtaining the consent of this patient, he is liable to compensate in damages any injury which may arise from his adopting a new method of treatment" (Howard-Jones, p. 1430). In short, the law distinguished carefully between quackery and innovation, and—provided the investigator had the subject's agreement—research was a legitimate and protected activity.

With the new understanding of germ theory in the 1890s and the growing professionalization of medical training in the next several decades, the amount of human experimentation increased and the intimate link between investigator and subject weakened. Typically, physicians administered a new drug to a group of hospitalized patients and compared their rates of recovery with past rates or with those of other patients who did not have the drug. (Truly random and blinded clinical trials, wherein a variety of patient characteristics were carefully matched and where researchers were kept purposely ignorant of which patient received the new drug, did not come into practice until the 1950s.) Thus, German physicians tested antidiphtheria serum on thirty hospitalized patients and reported that only six died, compared to the previous year at the same hospital when twenty-one of thirty-two patients died (Bull). In Canada, Frederick G. Banting and Charles Best experimented with insulin therapy on diabetic patients who faced imminent death, and interpreted their recovery as clear proof of the treatment's efficacy (Bliss). So too, George R. Minot and William P. Murphy tested the value of liver preparations against pernicious anemia by administering them to forty-five patients in remission and found that they all remained healthy so long as they took the treatment; the normal relapse rate was one-third, and three patients who on their own accord stopped treatment relapsed (Bull). It is doubtful if many of these subjects were fully informed about the nature of the trial or formally consented to participate. They were, however, likely to be willing subjects since they were in acute distress or danger and the research had therapeutic potential.

As medicine became more scientific, some researchers did skirt the boundaries of ethical behavior in experimentation, making medical progress—rather than the subject's welfare—the goal of the research. Probably the most famous experiment in this zone of ambiguity was the yellow-fever work of Walter Reed (1851–1902). When he began his experiments, mosquitoes had been identified as crucial to transmission but their precise role was unclear. To understand more about the process, Reed began a series of human experiments in which, in time-honored tradition, the members of the research team were the first subjects (Bean). It soon became apparent that larger numbers of volunteers were needed and no sooner was the decision reached than a soldier happened by. "You still fooling with mosquitoes?" he asked one of the doctors. "Yes," the doctor replied. "Will you take a bite?" "Sure, I ain't scared of 'em," responded the man. And in this way, "the first indubitable case of yellow fever ... to be produced experimentally" occurred (Bean, pp. 131, 147).

After one fellow investigator, Jesse William Lazear, died of yellow fever from purposeful bites, the other members, including Reed himself, decided "not to tempt fate by trying any more [infections] upon ourselves." Instead, Reed asked American servicemen to volunteer, and some did. He also recruited Spanish workers, drawing up a contract with them: "The undersigned understands perfectly well that in the case of the development of yellow fever in him, that he endangers his life to a certain extent but it being entirely impossible for him to avoid the infection during his stay on this island he prefers to take the chance of contracting it intentionally in the belief that he will receive ... the greatest care and most skillful medical service." Volunteers received $100 in gold, and those who actually contracted yellow fever received a bonus of an additional $100, which, in the event of their

death, went to their heirs (Bean, pp. 134, 147). Although twenty-five volunteers became ill, none died.

Reed's contract was a step along the way to more formal arrangements with human subjects, complete with enticements to undertake a hazardous assignment. But the contract was also misleading, distorting in subtle ways the risks and benefits of the research. Yellow fever was said to endanger life only "to a certain extent"; the likelihood that the disease might prove fatal was unmentioned. And on the other hand, the prospect of otherwise contracting yellow fever was presented as an absolute certainty, an exaggeration that aimed to promote recruitment.

Some human experiments in the pre-World War II period in the United States and elsewhere used incompetent and institutionalized populations for their studies. The Russian physician V. V. Smidovich (publishing in 1901 under the pseudonym Vikentii Veresaev) cited more than a dozen experiments, most of them conducted in Germany, in which unknowing patients were inoculated with microorganisms of syphilis and gonorrhea (Veresaev). George Sternberg, the Surgeon General of the United States in 1895 (and a collaborator of Walter Reed), conducted experiments "upon unvaccinated children in some of the orphan asylums in ... Brooklyn" (Sternberg and Reed, pp. 57–69). Alfred Hess and colleagues deliberately withheld orange juice from infants at the Hebrew Infant Asylum of New York City until they developed symptoms of scurvy (Lederer). In 1937, when Joseph Stokes of the Department of Pediatrics at the University of Pennsylvania School of Medicine sought to analyze the effects of "intramuscular vaccination of human beings ... with active virus of human influenza," he used as his study population the residents of two large state institutions for the retarded (Stokes et al., pp. 237–243). There are also many examples of investigators using prisoners as research subjects. In 1914, for example, Joseph Goldwater and G. H. Wheeler of the U.S. Public Health Service (PHS) conducted experiments to understand the causes of pellagra on convicts in Mississippi prisons.

One of the few instances of an individual investigator being taken to task for the ethics of his research involved Hideyo Noguchi (1876–1928) of the Rockefeller Institute for Medical Research. He was investigating whether a substance he called luetin, an extract from the causative agent of syphilis, could be used to diagnose syphilis; through the cooperation of fifteen New York physicians, he used 400 subjects, most of them inmates in mental hospitals and orphan asylums and patients in public hospitals. Before administering luetin to them, Noguchi and some of the physicians did first test the material on themselves, with no ill effects. But no one, including Noguchi, informed the subjects about the experiment or obtained their permission to do the tests.

Noguchi's work was actively criticized by the most vocal opponents of human experimentation during those years, the antivivisectionists. They were convinced that a disregard for the welfare of animals would inevitably promote a disregard for the welfare of humans. As one of them phrased it: "Are the helpless people in our hospitals and asylums to be treated as so much material for scientific experimentation, irrespective of age or consent?" (Lederer, p. 336). Despite their opposition, such experiments as Noguchi's did not lead to prosecutions, corrective legislation, or formal professional codes. The profession and the wider public were not especially concerned with the issue, perhaps because the practice was still relatively uncommon and mostly affected disadvantaged populations.

Research at War

The transforming event in the conduct of human experimentation in the United States was World War II. Between 1941 and 1945, practically every aspect of American research with human subjects changed. What were once occasional and ad hoc efforts by individual practitioners now became well-coordinated, extensive, federally funded team ventures. At the same time, medical experiments that once had the aim of benefiting their subjects were now frequently superseded by experiments whose aim was to benefit others, specifically soldiers who were vulnerable to the disease. Further, researchers and subjects were far more likely to be strangers to each other, with no sense of shared purpose or objective. Finally, and perhaps most importantly, the common understanding that experimentation required the agreement of the subjects, however casual the request or general the approval, was superseded by a sense of urgency so strong that it paid scant attention to the issue of consent.

In the summer of 1941, President Franklin Roosevelt created the Office of Scientific Research and Development (OSRD) to oversee the work of two parallel committees, one devoted to weapons research, the other—the Committee on Medical Research (CMR)—to combat the health problems that threatened the combat efficiency of American soldiers. Thus began what one participant called "a novel experiment in American medicine, for planned and coordinated medical research had never been essayed on such a scale" (Keefer, p. 62). Over the course of World War II, the CMR recommended some 600 research proposals, many of them involving human subjects, to the OSRD for funding. The OSRD, in turn, contracted with investigators at some 135 universities, hospitals, research institutes, and industrial firms. The accomplishments of the CMR effort required two volumes

to summarize (the title, *Advances in Military Medicine,* did not do justice to the scope of the investigations); and the list of publications that resulted from its grants took up seventy-five pages (Andrus). All told, the CMR expended some $25 million. In fact, the work of the CMR was so important that it supplied not only the organizational model but also the intellectual justification for creating, in the postwar period, the National Institutes of Health.

The CMR's major concerns were dysentery, influenza, malaria, wounds, venereal diseases, and physical hardships (including sleep deprivation and exposure to frigid temperatures). To create effective antidotes required skill, luck, and numerous trials with human subjects, and the CMR oversaw the effort with extraordinary diligence. Dysentery, for example, proliferated under the filth and deprivation endemic to battlefield conditions, and no effective inoculations or antidotes existed. With CMR support, investigators undertook laboratory research and then, requiring sites for testing their therapies, turned to custodial institutions where dysentery was often rampant (OSRD, 1944b). Among the most important subjects for the dysentery research were the residents of the Ohio Soldiers and Sailors Orphanage in Xenia, Ohio; the Dixon, Illinois, institution for the retarded; and the New Jersey State Colony for the Feeble-Minded. The residents were injected with experimental vaccines or potentially therapeutic agents, some of which produced a degree of protection against the bacteria but, as evidenced by fever and soreness, were too toxic for common use.

Probably the most pressing medical problem the CMR faced immediately after Pearl Harbor was malaria, "an enemy even more to be feared than the Japanese" (Andrus, vol. 1, p. xlix). Not only was the disease debilitating and deadly, but the Japanese controlled the supply of quinine, one of the few known effective antidotes. Since malaria was not readily found in the United States, researchers chose to infect residents of state mental hospitals and prisons. A sixty-bed clinical unit was established at the Manteno, Illinois, State Hospital; the subjects were psychotic, backward patients who were purposefully infected with malaria through blood transfusions and then given antimalarial therapies (OSRD, 1944a). With the cooperation of the commissioner of corrections of Illinois and the warden at Stateville Prison (better known as Joliet), one floor of the prison hospital was turned over to the University of Chicago to carry out malaria research and some 500 inmates volunteered to act as subjects. Whether these prisoners were truly capable of consenting to research was not addressed by the researchers, the CMR, or prison officials. Almost all the press commentary was congratulatory, praising the wonderful contributions the inmates were making to the war effort.

In similar fashion, the CMR supported teams that tested anti-influenza preparations on residents of state facilities for the retarded (Pennhurst, Pennsylvania) and the mentally ill (Michigan's Ypsilanti State Hospital). The investigators administered the vaccine to the residents and then, three or six months later, purposefully infected them with influenza (Henle). When a few of the preparations appeared to provide protection, the Office of the Surgeon General of the U.S. Army arranged for the vaccine to be tested by enrollees in the Army Specialized Training Program at eight universities and a ninth unit made up of students from five New York medical and dental colleges.

Because the first widespread use of human subjects in medical research for nontherapeutic purposes occurred under wartime conditions, attention to the consent of the subject appeared less relevant. At a time when the social value attached to consent gave way before the necessity of a military draft and obedience to commanders' orders, medical researchers did not hesitate to use the incompetent as subjects of human experimentation. One part of the war machine conscripted a soldier, another part conscripted a human subject, and the same principles held for both. In effect, wartime promoted teleological as opposed to deontological ethics; "the greatest good for the greatest number" was the most compelling precept to justify sending some men to be killed so that others might live. This same ethic seemed to justify using institutionalized retarded or mentally ill persons in human research.

Human Research and the War Against Disease

The two decades following the close of World War II witnessed an extraordinary expansion of human experimentation in medical research. Long after peace returned, many of the investigators continued to follow wartime rules, this time thinking in terms of the Cold War and the war against disease. The utilitarian justifications that had flourished under conditions of combat and conscription persisted, in disregard of principles of consent and voluntary participation.

The driving force in post-World War II research in the United States was the National Institutes of Health (NIH). Created in 1930 as an outgrowth of the research laboratory of the U.S. Public Health Service, the NIH assumed its extraordinary prominence as the successor agency to the Committee on Medical Research (Swain). In 1945, its appropriations totaled $700,000. By 1955, the figure had climbed to $36 million, and by 1970, $1.5 billion, a sum that allowed it to award some 11,000 grants, about one-third requiring experiments on humans. In expending these funds, the NIH administered an intramural research program at its own Clinical Center, along with an extramural program that funded outside investigators.

The Clinical Center assured its subjects that it put their well-being first. "The welfare of the patient takes precedence over every other consideration" (NIH, 1953a). In 1954, a Clinical Research Committee was established to develop principles and to deal with problems that might arise in research with normal, healthy volunteers. Still, the relationship between investigator and subject was casual to a fault, leaving it up to the investigator to decide what information, if any, was to be shared with the subject. Generally, the researchers did not divulge very much information, fearful that they would discourage patients from participating. No formal policies or procedures applied to researchers working in other institutions on studies supported by NIH funds.

The laxity of procedural protections pointed to the enormous intellectual and emotional investment in research and to the conviction that the laboratory would yield answers to the mysteries of disease. Indeed, this faith was so great that the NIH would not establish guidelines to govern the extramural research it supported. By 1965, the extramural program was the single most important source of research grants for universities and medical schools, by the NIH's own estimate, supporting between 1,500 and 2,000 research projects involving human research. Nevertheless, grant provisions included no stipulations about the ethical conduct of human experimentation and the universities did not fill the gap. In the early 1960s, only nine of fifty-two American departments of medicine had a formal procedure for approving research involving human subjects and only five more indicated that they favored this approach or planned to institute such procedures (Frankel).

One might have expected much greater attention to the ethics of human experimentation in the immediate postwar period in light of the shadow cast by the trial of the German doctors at Nuremberg. The atrocities that the Nazis committed—putting subjects to death by long immersion in subfreezing water, deprivation of oxygen to learn the limits of bodily endurance, or deliberate infection by lethal organisms in order to study the effects of drugs and vaccines—might have sparked a commitment in the United States to a more rigorous regulation of research. (Japanese physicians also conducted experiments on prisoners of war and captive populations, but their research was never subjected to the same judicial scrutiny.) So too, the American research efforts during the war might have raised questions of their own and stimulated closer oversight.

The Nuremberg Code of 1946 itself might have served as a model for American guidelines on research with human subjects. Its provisions certainly were relevant to the medical research conducted in the United States. "The voluntary consent of the human subject is absolutely essential," the code declared. "This means that the person involved should have legal capacity to give consent." By this principle, the mentally disabled and children were not suitable subjects for research—a principle that American researchers did not respect. Moreover, according to the Nuremberg Code, the research subject "should be so situated as to be able to exercise free power of choice" (Germany [Territory Under …], p. 181), which rendered at least questionable the American practice of using prisoners as research subjects. The Nuremberg Code also stated that human subjects "should have sufficient knowledge and comprehension of the elements of the subject matter involved as to make an understanding and enlightened decision" (Germany [Territory Under …], p. 181), thus ruling out the American practice of using the mentally disabled as subjects.

Nevertheless, with a few exceptions, neither the Code nor these specific practices received sustained analysis before the early 1970s. Only a handful of articles in medical or popular journals addressed the relevance of Nuremberg for the ethics of human experimentation in the United States. Perhaps this silence reflected an eagerness to repress the memory of the atrocities. More likely, the events described at Nuremberg were not perceived by most Americans as relevant to their own practices. From their perspective, the Code had nothing to do with science and everything to do with Nazis. The guilty parties were seen less as doctors than as Hitler's henchmen (Proctor).

In the period 1945–1965, several American as well as world medical organizations did produce guidelines for human experimentation that expanded upon the Nuremberg Code. Most of these efforts, however, commanded little attention and had minimal impact on institutional practices whether in Europe or in the United States (Ladimer and Newman). The American Medical Association, for example, framed a research code that called for the voluntary consent of the human subject, but it said nothing about what information the researchers were obliged to share, whether it was ethical to conduct research on incompetent patients, or how the research process should be monitored (Requirements for Experiments on Human Beings). In general, investigators could do as they wished in the laboratory, limited only by what their consciences defined as proper conduct and by broad, generally unsanctioned statements of ethical principle.

The World Medical Association in 1964 issued the Helsinki Declaration, stating general principles for human experimentation, and has revised that document four times.

The declaration is modeled on the Nuremberg Code, requiring qualified investigators and the consent of subjects. The 1975 revision recommended review of research by an independent committee (Annas and Grodin).

How researchers exercised discretion was the subject of a groundbreaking article by Henry Beecher, professor of anesthesia at Harvard Medical School, published in June 1966 in the *New England Journal of Medicine*. His analysis, "Ethics and Clinical Research," contained brief descriptions of twenty-two examples of investigators who risked "the health or the life of their subjects," without informing them of the dangers or obtaining their permission. In one case, investigators purposefully withheld penicillin from servicemen with streptococcal infections in order to study alternative means for preventing complications. The men were totally unaware that they were part of an experiment, let alone at risk of contracting rheumatic fever, which twenty-five of them did. Beecher's conclusion was that "unethical or questionably ethical procedures are not uncommon" among researchers. Although he did not provide footnotes for the examples or name the investigators, he did note that "the troubling practices" came from "leading medical schools, university hospitals, private hospitals, governmental military departments … government institutes (the National Institutes of Health), Veterans Administration Hospitals, and industry" (Beecher).

Two of the cases that Beecher cited were especially important in provoking public indignation over the conduct of human research. One case involved investigators who fed live hepatitis virus to the residents of Willowbrook, a New York State institution for the retarded, in order to study the etiology of the disease and attempt to create a protective vaccine against it. The other case involved physicians injecting live cancer cells into twenty-two elderly and senile hospitalized patients at the Brooklyn Jewish Chronic Disease hospital without telling them that the cells were cancerous, in order to study the body's immunological responses.

Another case that sparked fierce public and political reactions in the early 1970s was the Tuskegee research of the U.S. Public Health Service. Its investigators had been visiting Macon County, Alabama, since the mid-1930s to examine, but not to treat, a group of blacks who were suffering from secondary syphilis. Whatever rationalizations the PHS could muster for not treating blacks in the 1930s, when treatment was of questionable efficacy and very complicated to administer, it could hardly defend instructing draft boards not to conscript the subjects for fear that they might receive treatment in the army. Worse yet, it could not justify its unwillingness to give the subjects a trial of penicillin after 1945 (Jones).

During the 1950s and 1960s, not only individual investigators but government agencies conducted research that often ignored the consent of the subjects and placed some of them at risk. Many of these projects involved the testing of radiation on humans. Part of the motivation was to better understand human physiology; even more important, however, was the aim of bolstering the national defense by learning about the possible impact of radiation on fighting forces. Accordingly, inmates at the Oregon State Prison were subjects in experiments to examine the effects on sperm production of exposing their testicles to X-rays. Although the prisoners were told some of the risks, they were not informed that the radiation might cause cancer. So too, terminally ill patients at the Cincinnati General Hospital underwent whole-body radiation, in research supported by the U.S. Department of Defense, not so much to measure its effects against cancer but to learn about the dangers radiation posed to military personnel. During this period, the Central Intelligence Agency also conducted research on unknowing subjects with drugs and with psychiatric techniques in an effort to improve interrogation and brainwashing methods. It was not until the 1980s that parts of this record became public, and not until 1994 that the full dimensions of these research projects were known.

Regulating Human Experimentation

The cases cited by Beecher and publicized in the press over the period 1966 to 1973 produced critical changes in policy by the leadership of the NIH and the U.S. Food and Drug Administration (FDA). Both agencies were especially sensitive to congressional pressures and feared that criticisms of researchers' conduct could lead to severe budget cuts. They also recognized that the traditional bedrock of research ethics, the belief that investigators were like physicians and should therefore be trusted to protect the well-being of their subjects, did not hold. To the contrary, there was a conflict of interest between investigator and subject: One wanted knowledge, the other wanted cure or well-being.

Under the press of politics and this new recognition, the NIH and the FDA altered their procedures. The fact that authority was centralized in these two agencies, which were at once subordinate to Congress and superordinate to the research community, guaranteed their ability to impose new regulations. Indeed, this fact helps explain why the regulation of human experimentation came first and more extensively to the United States than to other developed countries (Rothman, 1991).

Accordingly, in February 1966, and then in revised form in July 1966, the NIH promulgated through its parent body, the PHS, guidelines covering all federally funded research involving human experimentation. The order of July 1, 1966, decentralized the regulatory apparatus, assigning "responsibility to the institution receiving the grant for obtaining and keeping documentary evidence of informed patient consent." It then mandated "review of the judgment of the investigator by a committee of institutional associates not directly associated with the project." Finally it defined, albeit very broadly, the standards that were to guide the committee: "This review must address itself to the rights and welfare of the individual, the methods used to obtain informed consent, and the risks and potential benefits of the investigation" (Commission on Health Science and Society, pp. 211–212). In this way and for the first time, decisions traditionally left to the conscience of individual physicians came under collective surveillance.

The new set of rules was not as intrusive as some investigators feared, or as protective as some advocates preferred. At its core was the superintendence of the peer review committee, known as the Institutional Review Board (IRB), through which fellow researchers approved the investigator's procedures. With the creation of the IRB, the clinical investigator could no longer decide unilaterally whether the planned intervention was ethical, but had to answer formally to colleagues operating under federal guidelines. The events in and around 1966 accomplished what the Nuremberg trials had not: They moved medical experimentation into the public domain and revealed the consequences of leaving decisions about clinical research exclusively to the individual investigator.

The NIH response focused attention more on the review process than on the process of securing informed consent. Although it recognized the importance of the principle of consent, it remained skeptical about the ultimate feasibility of the procedure. Truly informed consent by the subject seemed impossible to achieve ostensibly because laypeople would not be able to understand the risks and benefits inherent in a complex research protocol. In effect, the NIH leadership was unwilling to abandon altogether the notion that doctors should protect patients and to substitute instead a thoroughgoing commitment to the idea that patients could and should protect themselves. Its goal was to ensure that harm was not done to the subjects, not that subjects were given every opportunity and incentive to express their own wishes (Frankel).

The FDA was also forced to grapple with the problems raised by human experimentation in clinical research. With a self-definition that included a commitment not only to sound scientific research (like the NIH) but to consumer protection as well, the FDA did attempt to expand the prerogatives of the consumer—in this context, the human subject. Rather than emulate the NIH precedent and invigorate peer review, it looked to give new meaning and import to the process of consent.

In the wake of the reactions set off by Beecher's article, the FDA, on August 30, 1966, issued a "Statement on Policy Concerning Consent for the Use of Investigational New Drugs on Humans." Distinguishing between therapeutic and nontherapeutic research, in accord with various international codes like the Helsinki Declaration, it now prohibited all nontherapeutic research unless the subjects gave consent. When the research involved "patients under treatment," and had therapeutic potential, consent was to be obtained except in what the FDA labeled the "exceptional cases," where consent was not feasible or not in the patient's best interest. "Not feasible" meant that the doctor could not communicate with the patient (its example was when the patient was in a coma); and "not in the best interest" meant that consent would "seriously affect the patient's disease status" (its example here was the physician who did not want to divulge a diagnosis of cancer) (Curran, pp. 558–569).

In addition, the FDA, unlike the NIH, spelled out the meaning of consent. To give consent, the person had to have the ability to exercise choice and to have a "fair explanation" of the procedure, including an understanding of the experiment's purpose and duration, "all inconveniences and hazards reasonably to be expected," what a controlled trial was (and the possibility of the use of placebos), and any existing alternative forms of therapy available (Curran, pp. 558–569).

The FDA regulations represented a new stage in the balance of authority between researcher and subject. The blanket insistence on consent for all nontherapeutic research would have prohibited many of the World War II experiments and eliminated most of the cases on Beecher's roll. The FDA's definitions of consent went well beyond the vague NIH stipulations, imparting real significance to the process. To be sure, ambiguities remained. The FDA still confused research and treatment, and its clauses governing therapeutic investigations afforded substantial discretion to the doctor-researcher. But authority tilted away from the individual investigator and leaned, instead, toward colleagues and the human subjects themselves.

The publicity given to the abuses in human experimentation, and the idea that a fundamental conflict of interest characterized the relationship between the researcher and the subject, had an extraordinary impact on those outside of medicine, drawing philosophers, lawyers, and social scientists into a deeper concern about ethical issues in medicine. Human experimentation, for example, sparked the interest in medicine of Princeton University's professor of Christian ethics, Paul Ramsey. Ethical problems in medicine "are by no means technical problems on which only the expert (in this case, the physician) can have an opinion," Ramsey declared, and his first case in point was human experimentation. He worried that the thirst for more information was so great that it could lead investigators to violate the sanctity of the person. To counter the threat, Ramsey had two general strategies. The first was to make medical ethics the subject of public discussion. We can no longer "go on assuming that what can be done has to be done or should be.... These questions are now completely in the public forum, no longer the province of scientific experts alone" (Ramsey, p. 1). Second, and more specifically, Ramsey embraced the idea of consent; consent, in his formulation, was to human experimentation what a system of checks and balances was to executive authority, that is, the necessary limitation on the exercise of power. "Man's capacity to become joint adventurers in a common cause makes the consensual relationship possible; man's propensity to overreach his joint adventurer even in a good cause makes consent necessary.... No man is good enough to experiment upon another without his consent" (Ramsey, pp. 5–7).

Commissioning Ethics

The U.S. Congress soon joined the growing ranks of those concerned with human experimentation and medical ethics. In 1973, it created the National Commission for the Protection of Human Subjects of Biomedical and Behavioral Research, whose charge was to recommend to federal agencies regulations to protect the rights and welfare of subjects of research. The idea for such a commission was first fueled by an awareness of the awesome power of new medical technologies, but it gained congressional passage in the wake of newly uncovered abuses in human experimentation, most notably the Tuskegee syphilis studies.

The U.S. National Commission for the Protection of Human Subjects was composed of eleven members drawn from "the general public and from individuals in the fields of medicine, law, ethics, theology, biological science, physical science, social science, philosophy, humanities, health administration, government, and public affairs." The length of the roster and the stipulation that no more than five of the members could be researchers indicated how determined Congress was to have human experimentation brought under the scrutiny of outsiders. Senator Edward Kennedy, who chaired the hearings that led to the creation of the commission, repeatedly emphasized this point: Policy had to emanate "not just from the medical profession, but from ethicists, the theologians, philosophers, and many other disciplines." A prominent social scientist, Bernard Barber, predicted, altogether accurately, that the commission "would transform a fundamental moral problem from a condition of relative professional neglect and occasional journalistic scandal to a condition of continuing public and professional visibility and legitimacy…. For the proper regulation of the powerful professions of modern society, we need a combination of insiders and outsiders, of professionals and citizens" (Commission on Health Science and Society, part IV, pp. 1264–1265).

Although the National Commission was temporary rather than permanent, and advisory (to the Secretary of Health, Education, and Welfare), without any enforcement powers of its own, most of its recommendations became regulatory law, tightening still further the governance of human experimentation. It endorsed the supervisory role of the IRBs and successfully recommended special protection for research on such vulnerable populations as prisoners, mentally disabled persons, and children. It recommended that an Ethical Advisory Board be established within the Department of Health and Human Services to deal with difficult cases as they arose. This board was inaugurated in 1977 but expired in 1980, leaving a gap in the commission's plan for oversight of research ethics. However, the Office for Protection from Research Risks at NIH exercised vigilance over institutional compliance with research regulations. Finally, the commission issued the Belmont Report, a statement of the ethical principles that should govern research, namely, respect for autonomy, beneficence, and justice. This document not only had an influence on research ethics but on the emerging discipline of bioethics (U.S. National Commission for the Protection of Human Subjects of Biomedical and Behavioral Research).

Conclusion

In the United States, and to a growing degree in other developed countries, many of the earlier practices that had raised such troubling ethical considerations have been resolved. Oversight of research has been accomplished without stifling it, and without violating the prerogatives of research subjects. Almost everyone who has served on IRBs, or who has analyzed the transformation that their presence has secured on medical experimentation, will testify to their salutary impact. To be sure, the formal composition and decentralized character of these bodies seem to invite a kind of back-scratching, mechanistic review of colleagues' protocols, without the kind of adversarial procedures that would reveal every risk in every procedure. Similarly, IRB review of consent forms and procedures rarely takes the concern from the committee room onto the hospital floor to inquire about the full extent of the understanding of subjects who consent to participate. Nevertheless, IRBs do require investigators to

be accountable for the character and severity of risks they are prepared to let others run, knowing that their institutional reputation may be harmed if they minimize or distort it. This responsibility unquestionably has changed investigators' behavior, and social expectations of them. To be sure, abuses may still occur. IRBs must be ready to minimize the amount of risk involved in certain protocols so as to enable researcher-colleagues to pursue their investigations. But they happen considerably less often now that IRB regulation is a fact of life. Scientific progress and ethical behavior turn out to be compatible goals.

DAVID J. ROTHMAN (1995)
BIBLIOGRAPHY REVISED

SEE ALSO: *Aging and the Aged: Healthcare and Research Issues; AIDS: Healthcare and Research Issues; Autoexperimentation; Autonomy; Children: Healthcare and Research Issues; Coercion; Commercialism in Scientific Research; Embryo and Fetus: Embryo Research; Empirical Methods in Bioethics; Freedom and Free Will; Genetics and Human Behavior: Scientific and Research Issues; Holocaust; Infants: Public Policy and Legal Issues; Informed Consent: Consent Issues in Human Research; Mentally Ill and Mentally Disabled Persons: Research Issues; Military Personnel as Research Subjects; Minorities as Research Subjects; Paternalism; Pediatrics, Overview of Ethical Issues in; Public Policy and Bioethics; Prisoners as Research Subjects; Race and Racism; Research, Human: Historical Aspects; Research Methodology; Research, Multinational; Research, Unethical; Responsibility; Scientific Publishing; Sexism; Students as Research Subjects; Virtue and Character;* and other *Research Policy* subentries

BIBLIOGRAPHY

Andrus, Edwin C.; Bronk, D. W.; Carden, G. A., Jr.; et al., eds. 1948. *Advances in Military Medicine Made by American Investigators under CMR Sponsorship.* Boston: Little, Brown.

Annas, George J., and Grodin, Michael A. 1992. *The Nazi Doctors and the Nuremberg Code: Human Rights in Human Experimentation.* New York: Oxford University Press.

Baxby, Derrick. 1981. *Jenner's Smallpox Vaccine: The Riddle of Vaccinia Virus and Its Origin.* London: Heinemann Educational Books.

Bean, William B. 1982. *Walter Reed: A Biography.* Charlottesville: University of Virginia Press.

Beaumont, William. 1980 (1833). *Experiments and Observations on the Gastric Juice and Physiology of Digestion.* Birmingham, AL: Classics of Medicine Library.

Beecher, Henry K. 1966. "Ethical and Clinical Research." *New England Journal of Medicine* 274(24): 1354–1360.

Berg, Kare, and Tranoy, Knut E., eds. 1983. *Proceedings of Symposium on Research Ethics.* New York: Alan Liss.

Bernard, Claude. 1927. *An Introduction to the Study of Experimental Medicine,* tr. Henry Copley Greene. New York: Macmillan.

Bliss, Michael. 1982. *The Discovery of Insulin.* Chicago: University of Chicago Press.

Bull, J. P. 1959. "The Historical Development of Clinical Therapeutic Trials." *Journal of Chronic Diseases* 10(3): 218–248.

Commission on Health Science and Society. 1968. Hearings of 90th Congress, 2nd session.

Curran, William J. 1969. "Governmental Regulation of the Use of Human Subjects in Medical Research: The Approach of Two Federal Agencies." *Daedalus* 98(2): 542–594.

Cushing, Harvey. 1925. *The Life of Sir William Osler.* Oxford: Clarendon Press.

Fox, Renée. 1959. *Experiment Perilous: Physicians and Patients Facing the Unknown.* Glencoe, IL: Free Press.

Frankel, Mark S. 1972. *The Public Health Service Guidelines Governing Research Involving Human Subjects.* Monograph no. 10. Washington, D.C.: Program of Policy Studies in Science and Technology, George Washington University.

Germany (Territory Under Allied Occupation, 1945–1955: U.S. Zone) Military Tribunals. 1947. "Permissible Medical Experiments." In vol. 2 of *Trials of War Criminals Before the Nuremberg Tribunals Under Control Law No. 10,* pp. 181–184. Washington, D.C.: U.S. Government Printing Office.

Henle, Werner; Henle, Gertrude; Hampil, Bettylee; et al. 1946. "Experiments on Vaccination of Human Beings Against Epidemic Influenza." *Journal of Immunology* 53(1): 75–93.

Howard-Jones, Norman. 1982. "Human Experimentation in Historical and Ethical Perspectives." *Social Science Medicine* 16(15): 1429–1448.

Jenner, Edward. 1910 (1798). "Vaccination Against Smallpox." In *Scientific Papers,* pp. 145–220, ed. Charles W. Eliot. New York: P. F. Collier.

Jones, James. 1981. *Bad Blood.* New York: Free Press.

Katz, Jay; Capron, Alexander M.; and Glass, Eleanor Swift. 1972. *Experimentation with Human Beings.* New York: Russell Sage Foundation.

Kaufman, Sharon R. 1997. "The World War II Plutonium Experiments: Contested Stories and Their Lessons for Medical Research and Informed Consent." *Culture, Medicine and Psychiatry* 21: 161–197.

Keefer, Chester S. 1969. "Dr. Richards as Chairman of the Committee on Medical Research." *Annals of Internal Medicine* 71(8): 61–70.

Ladimer, Irving, and Newman, Roger. 1963. *Clinical Investigation in Medicine: Legal, Ethical, and Moral Aspects.* Boston: Law-Medicine Institute of Boston University.

Lederer, Susan. 1985. "Hideyo Noguchi's Luetin Experiment and the Antivivisectionists." *Isis* 76(1): 31–48.

Lederer, Susan. 1992. "Orphans as Guinea Pigs." In *In the Name of the Child: Health and Welfare, 1880–1940,* ed. Roger Cooter. London: Routledge.

McNeil, Paul M. 1993. *The Ethics and Politics of Human Experimentation.* Cambridge, Eng.: Cambridge University Press.

National Institutes of Health. 1953a. *Handbook for Patients at the Clinical Center.* Publication no. 315. Bethesda, MD: Author.

National Institutes of Health. 1953b. *The National Institutes of Health Clinical Center.* Publication no. 316. Washington, D.C.: U.S. Government Printing Office.

Numbers, Ronald L. 1979. "William Beaumont and the Ethics of Experimentation." *Journal of the History of Biology* 12(1): 113–136.

Office of Scientific Research and Development (OSRD). Committee on Medical Research (CMR). 1943. National Archives of the United States, Record Group 227: Contractor Records, S. Mudd, University of Pennsylvania (Contract 120, Final Report), March 3.

Office of Scientific Research and Development (OSRD). Committee on Medical Research (CMR). 1944a. Contractor Records, University of Chicago, Contract 450, Report L2, Responsible Investigator Dr. Alf S. Alving, Bimonthly Progress Report, August 1.

Office of Scientific Research and Development (OSRD). Committee on Medical Research (CMR). 1944b. Contractor Records, University of Pennsylvania, Contract 120, Responsible Investigator Dr. Stuart Mudd, Monthly Progress Report 18, October 3.

Proctor, Robert N. 1988. *Racial Hygiene: Medicine under the Nazis.* Cambridge, MA: Harvard University Press.

Ramsey, Paul. 1970. *The Patient as Person: Explorations in Military Ethics.* New Haven, CT: Yale University Press.

"Requirements for Experiments on Human Beings." 1946. *Journal of the American Medical Association* 132: 1090.

Rothman, David J. 1991. *Strangers at the Bedside.* New York: Basic Books.

Rothman, David J. 2003. "Serving Clio and Client: The Historian as Expert Witness." *Bulletin of the History of Medicine* 77: 25–44.

Sternberg, George M., and Reed, Walter. 1895. "Report on Immunity Against Vaccination Conferred upon the Monkey by the Use of the Serum of the Vaccinated Calf and Monkey." Transactions of the Association of American Physicians 10: 57–69.

Stokes, Joseph, Jr.; Chenoweth, Alice D.; Waltz, Arthur D.; et al. 1937. "Results of Immunization by Means of Active Virus of Human Influenza." *Journal of Clinical Investigation* 16(2): 237–243.

Swain, Donald C. 1962. "The Rise of a Research Empire: NIH, 1930 to 1950." *Science* 138(3546):1233–1237.

United States. Advisory Committee on Human Radiation Experiments. 1996. *Final Report of the Advisory Committee on Human Radiation.* New York: Oxford Press.

U.S. National Commission for the Protection of Human Subjects of Biomedical and Behavioral Research. 1979. *The Belmont Report: Ethical Principles and Guidelines for Protection of Human Subjects of Research.* Washington, D. C.: Author.

Vallery-Radot, René. 1926. *The Life of Pasteur,* tr. Henriette C. Devonshire. New York: Doubleday.

Veresaev, Vikentii V. 1916 (1901). *The Memoirs of a Physician,* tr. Simeon Linden. New York: Knopf.

RESEARCH METHODOLOGY

• • •

I. CONCEPTUAL ISSUES

Research in medicine, in the biomedical sciences, and in science in general is defined as "studious inquiry or examination; *esp*: investigation or experimentation aimed at the discovery and interpretation of facts, revision of accepted theories or laws in the light of new facts, or practical application of such new or revised theories or laws" (Merriam-Webster, p. 992). The U.S. federal government's Common Rule for human-subject investigation (CR) echoes Webster's definition; according to the CR, "*Research* means a systematic investigation, including research development, testing, and evaluation, designed to contribute to generalizable knowledge" (Code of Federal Regulations, sec. 102). Research can refer to investigations that involve intentional manipulation of the objects studied, frequently termed *experimental* studies, as well as those inquiries that collect data generated by naturally occurring events, or *observational* studies. This entry focuses on the burdens and benefits scientific research has on human subjects (or perhaps better, on trial participants) and on society, as well as on laboratory animals. Research methodology comprises those general principles and designs used to describe valid and effective inquiries into nature, which includes humans. Research methodology has philosophical, scientific, and social dimensions.

General Aspects of Research Methodology

Beginning with Plato and Aristotle, philosophers have proposed a number of different though quite general approaches to scientific method. Philosophers René Descartes (1596–1650) and Francis Bacon (1561–1626) wrote on the subject in the seventeenth century, but the study of scientific method received its most systematic treatments in the work of the nineteenth-century philosophers and scientists William Whewell, Stanley Jevons (1835–1882, and John Stuart Mill (1806–1873), who forcefully re-presented the methods of agreement, difference, concomitant variation, and others that continue to influence contemporary philosophers; frequently these are referred to as Mill's Methods. Philosophers of science have continued to stimulate the imagination of practicing scientists. Since the early 1960s, Sir Karl Popper's *falsificationist* approach, T. S. Kuhn's account of revolutionary scientific changes as *paradigm shifts,* and the latter's criticisms of traditional rational and gradualist methodology have been cited in a number of scientific research articles.

Research methodology also involves more specific scientific components, including the analysis of different laboratory methodologies (e.g., molecular approaches and pure culture techniques); the utility of various *animal models* of diseases; and the characterization and assessment of the strengths of distinct study designs, ranging from the report of an individual case to the randomized controlled clinical trial (RCT). These scientific components may involve a considerable amount of sophisticated mathematical and statistical analysis. In this entry, both the philosophical and the scientific dimensions of research methodology will be pursued in the context of questions that they raise for bioethics.

A final major aspect of research methodology is the important *social* dimension of systematic empirical investigations. For the purposes of this entry, the term signifys the ethical, legal, political, and religious aspects of research methodology. More specifically, this rubric treats various moral implications of scientific investigation, including vulnerable or hitherto ignored subject populations (e.g., the disabled and women), from both descriptive and normative perspectives, as well as significant interactions among the philosophical, scientific, and social themes.

The Scope of Research

BIOMEDICAL AND BEHAVIORAL INVESTIGATIONS. Biomedical research (generally understood as also including behavioral research in the psychological and social sciences) covers a broad array of disciplines. The term *biomedical* is itself intended to bridge the gap between the more fundamental, *pure,* or *basic* sciences, such as physiology and biochemistry, and the more *applied* sciences, such as pathology and pharmacology. This interpretation, however, leaves the more *clinical* sciences, such as anesthesiology and medicine, less connected with the meaning of science than is appropriate. Better, perhaps, to follow a more expansive definition as found in *Merriam-Webster's Tenth Collegiate*

Dictionary, which gives as one definition of biomedical: "Of, relating to, or involving biological, medical, and physical science" (Merriam-Webster, p. 115). *Dorland's Medical Dictionary* (28th edition) offers as its preferred meaning "biological and medical" (Dorland, p. 199). In accordance with this expanded characterization of the term, virtually all of the natural, behavioral, and social sciences, as well as engineering, can be conceived of as biomedical sciences if the intent is to place them in the service of advancing generalizable knowledge in the domains of medicine and healthcare.

BASIC SCIENCE AND CLINICAL SCIENCE. A common division is found in the departmental organization in medical schools distinguishing between basic sciences, such as microbiology (but also including more applied sciences such as pharmacology), and the clinical sciences such as medicine and oncology, whose practitioners spend much of their time and effort working with patients. It must not be forgotten that studies employing systems ranging from in vitro (*test tube*) inquiries through research on bacterial viruses to animal-model investigations comprise the bulk of research in the biomedical sciences. Preliminary research on new drug therapies, as well as investigations into human immunodeficiency virus (HIV) pathophysiology, falls into this category. In addition, in recent years there has been heightened awareness of the ethical problems generated by the use of animals in biomedical research, and thus it is appropriate to comment briefly on this basic science dimension of research methodology.

In 1976 an important study investigated the type of research that led to the ten most important advances in the treatment of cardiovascular and pulmonary diseases (Comroe and Dripps). The investigators used a broad definition of *clinically oriented* research; studies involving animals, tissues, or cells (including cell fragments) were included in the definition if the author mentioned a possible clinical application even briefly. In spite of this expansive definition, some 41 percent of key articles involved in the development of these ten clinically relevant advances were not clinically oriented; that is, they reported on basic science research. This finding suggests that supporting only *targeted* or *mission-oriented* research is likely to have adverse effects on clinical research advances.

Another intensive investigation, conducted in 1985 by the National Research Council's Committee on Models for Biomedical Research, examined the nature of research methodology in the biomedical sciences and underscored the intimate and reciprocal relationship between research generally characterized as clinical and research generally characterized as basic. This report introduced the general notion of a

biomatrix, which was defined as a "complex body, or matrix, of interrelated biological knowledge built from studies of many kinds of organisms, biological preparations, and biological processes at various levels" (National Research Council, p. 2). Within such a multidimensional matrix, biomedical research involves *many-many modeling* in which analogous features at various levels of aggregation (e.g., molecules, cells, and organs) are related to each other across various species. The committee suggested that an "investigator considers some problem of interest—a disease process, some normal physiological function, or any other aspect of biology or medicine. The problem is analyzed into its component parts, and for each part and at each level, the matrix of biological knowledge is searched for analogous phenomena.... Although it is possible to view the processes involved in interpreting data in the language of [simple] one-to-one modeling, the investigator is actually modelling back and forth onto the matrix of biological knowledge" (National Research Council, p. 67). The study conducted by Julius Comroe and Robert Dripps, as well as the council's report, thus indicate that clinically relevant advances emerge from research sources beyond those involving human subjects.

Before innovations can be tested on humans, ethical codes and governmental regulation require research involving chemical, cell-fragment, cell, tissue, and intact-animal-model systems. The Nuremberg Code (1947–1948), for example, recommends that human experimentation should be based on the results of animal experimentation. The Declaration of Helsinki (1964, most recently revised in 2000) requires that "medical research involving human subjects must conform to generally accepted scientific principles, be based on a thorough knowledge of the scientific literature, other relevant sources of information, and on adequate laboratory and, where appropriate, animal experimentation" (World Medical Association). These requirements are based on the belief that such inquiries will assist in identifying interventions that are both safer and more effective by the time they are finally applied to human subjects. In the biomedical sciences, including studies involving human subjects, biological diversity and the number of systems that strongly interact in living organisms create considerable complexity. Researchers must often pay special attention to ensuring the (near) identity of the organisms under investigation, except for those differences that are the focus of the scientist's inquiry.

Biomedical investigations involving virtually identical laboratory organisms can yield precise and often nonstatistical results that can then be utilized in more variable human populations. As is discussed in the section below on various study designs, human variability of both genetic and environmental sources will typically require the extensive use of statistical methodologies to uncover generalizable knowledge that is clinically applicable. In more rigidly controllable laboratory experiments—for example, in the rapidly advancing area of molecular genetics—biomedical scientists can often employ the classical methods of experimental inquiry, referred to earlier as Mill's Methods. These methods can be thought of as attempting to discover the causal structure of the world, and in their application scientists endeavor to identify and compensate for possible confounding factors that, if ignored, can lead to mistaken inferences about causes and effects. Thus all natural scientists attempt to compensate for interfering and extraneous factors, frequently by setting up a control comparison or a control group. Such controls are a direct implementation of what Mill termed the *method of difference* and Claude Bernard (1813–1878), the notable nineteenth-century French scientist and methodologist, the *method of comparative experimentation.*

The method of difference may be stated in a form similar to that in which Mill presented it. Suppose that in Case 1 some phenomenon occurs, and in Case 2, that is identical with Case 1 *except for one factor,* the phenomenon does *not* occur. Then the single difference between the two cases is the effect of that phenomenon, or the cause of that phenomenon, or an indispensable part of the cause of that phenomenon. (See Mill, p. 256, for his original language).

Claude Bernard judged that this focus on only one difference was far too stringent and reformulated the experimental idea as his method of comparative experimentation:

> Physiological phenomena are so complex that we could never experiment at all rigorously on living animals if we necessarily had to define all the other changes we might cause in the organism on which we were operating. But fortunately it is enough for us completely to isolate the one phenomenon on which our studies are brought to bear, separating it by means of comparative experimentation from all surrounding complications. Comparative experimentation reaches this goal by adding to a similar organism, used for comparison, all our experimental changes save one, the very one which we intend to disengage. (p. 127–128)

Bernard referred to comparative experimentation as "the true foundation of experimental medicine."

General Ethical Issues Associated with Research on Human Subjects

The principal ethical controversies in biomedical (including behavioral and social) research have emerged from studies involving human subjects. Before discussing the general ethical requirements of studies involving human subjects, however, it is important to describe briefly the often contentious debate about the terms used to distinguish between different kinds of standard medical practice and research, among them *therapeutic research, nontherapeutic research, innovative treatments,* and *experimentation.*

TERMINOLOGICAL CONSIDERATIONS. It is a fundamental tenet of medical ethics that the well-being of human subjects should be protected. This tenet, together with another general ethical principle frequently associated with the name of philosopher Immanuel Kant (1724–1804), to treat oneself or another human being always as an end and never merely or only as a means, requires that a human research subject be expected to obtain some direct benefit from the investigation, or, if not, to waive such benefit on the basis of a free and informed consent. (This Kantian injunction is sometimes characterized as a principle of *respect for persons.*) The need to clarify the therapeutic/nontherapeutic distinction in the light of such principles should be evident.

Thoughtful scholars have generally agreed about the difficulty of drawing a clear distinction between research and accepted practice, but have differed about the usefulness of various terms proposed to assist with this task. Some find the distinction between therapeutic and nontherapeutic experimentation *crucial,* whereas others find it is better phrased as one between beneficial and nonbeneficial experimentation. Tom Beauchamp and James Childress urge caution with the use of the closely related term therapeutic research since "attaching the favorable term *therapeutic* to research can be dangerous, because it suggests *justified intervention* in the care of particular patients and may create a misconception" (p. 320). Robert Levine, an authority on research involving human subjects, contends that the expressions therapeutic research, nontherapeutic research, and experimentation (in human subject contexts) are "unacceptable" and "illogical" (p. 8). The problem arises in part because it is fairly common that a diagnostic and therapeutic plan involve some variation from the textbook norm, and because it is in only rare cases that biomedical research conveys absolutely no benefit on its subjects.

Levine suggests that we employ the term *nonvalidated practices* as a more encompassing term for innovative therapies, acknowledging that it is the uncertainty associated with variation in the outcomes of diagnostic and therapeutic maneuvers that is the principal issue. This suggestion seems to have been accepted in much of the recent literature, though frequently the narrower term *nonvalidated therapy* is also employed. Though no definitive algorithm can be provided that will unambiguously differentiate the various inquiries and activities discussed in the preceding paragraph, the general proposal that appears to emerge from the discussion involves three elements. First, the intent of the investigator is critical in determining whether the intervention (or the withholding of an intervention) is to be characterized as primarily beneficial to the subjects or as contributing to generalizable knowledge. A surgeon employing a novel suturing technique in an attempt to save a patient from bleeding to death does not evidence any intent of beginning a research project to evaluate a new operative technique. Second, the degree of variation from standard practice figures in this determination, and this may depend as well on the degree of possible harm that the intervention entails. Even small variations associated with significant harm are more likely to be seen as nonvalidated in contrast to small variations with minor adverse consequences. For example, a physician may believe that he or she must try a powerful immunosuppressive drug, usually used only in the case of potential organ-transplant rejection, to help a patient suffering with severe rheumatoid arthritis. The dangers associated with such drugs and the departure from their normal use argues that this would be a nonvalidated practice. Finally, there is the element of uncertainty, the degree of likelihood of a particular outcome or set of outcomes. These include both anticipated and unintended effects (side effects). Again, the example just cited of the immunosuppressive drug would be relevant here because of the difficulty of anticipating the effects of powerful drugs on systems as complex as the immune system.

For interventions from which the researcher intends to produce new general knowledge, that represent significant departures from accepted practice, and about which there is reasonable uncertainty regarding consequences, including intended outcomes, it would seem mandatory that the researchers develop a formal research protocol to be assessed by an appropriate institutional review board (IRB). Such a multidimensional *sliding scale,* possibly with thresholds that could be specified in particular areas of clinical investigation, may be the best possible mechanism for determining whether to require IRB review in this complex area.

ETHICAL REQUIREMENTS FOR RESEARCH ON HUMAN SUBJECTS. As noted in the preceding section, general principles requiring free and informed consent and a net balance of benefits over harms for the individual subject (unless this is waived by the subject in the interests of greater social benefits) will be assumed in all research contexts, and the present section will examine additional details regarding these requirements. Furthermore, however, in order both to safeguard research subjects and ensure that the resources used will generate valuable knowledge, a research study must conform to scientifically validated principles of design. To begin with, a prospective research project must be evaluated in terms of the risks of harm—physical, psychological, and social—to the subject(s), as well as in terms of the benefits that are likely to accrue to participants. Only studies in which the expected benefits outweigh the expected harms are morally permissible. Further, there must be no alternative and less risky means for the subject to obtain the anticipated benefits. Subjects must be selected equitably, with special sensitivity to the problems faced by vulnerable populations, such as children, prisoners, pregnant women, mentally disabled persons, or educationally disadvantaged persons. In recent years the practice of *community consultation* has developed, which involves meetings with representatives of the at-large subject community (e.g., HIV-infected individuals) to "assure a suitable balancing of the relevant values [such as respect for persons, individual beneficence and justice] in the design and conduct of a clinical trial" (Levine et al., p. 10).

An investigator must also obtain the legally effective informed consent of the subject or of the subject's legally authorized representative. Such consent must be voluntary and not obtained by coercive measures. The consent must be informed; this means that the investigator must specify the purposes of the research and how long the subject is expected to participate and provide a nontechnical description (in terms readily understandable to the subject) of any procedures to be followed, as well as a designation of procedures considered untested or experimental. The subject must also be provided with a description of any reasonable foreseeable risks or discomforts as well as reasonably anticipated benefits. Alternative procedures or courses of treatment that may be advantageous to the participant must be disclosed. Subjects are also to be provided with a statement about the extent of confidentiality of their records and, for research involving more than minimal risk, an explanation of what, if any, compensation or treatments will be available in the event of injury. According to the CR, subjects must be informed about whom to contact for answers about any questions or injuries that may arise in the course of or as a consequence of the research. They are to be told that their participation is voluntary and that they may refuse to participate or may withdraw from participation without any penalty or loss of benefits to which they would normally be entitled. Should the investigator come to believe in the course of the research that harm to the patient has become likely, the patient should be so informed and withdrawn from the project. The above requirements underscore the point that informed consent should not be conceived of only as a one-time event, but is best construed as an ongoing process involving clinical investigators and trial participants.

In certain types of behavioral and social-science research, investigators have maintained that scientifically valid conclusions can be obtained only if the subjects are kept uninformed or even deliberately deceived about the nature of the research. In a well-known example of this type of research, Stanley Milgram's studies on obedience to authority, subjects were falsely told they were causing pain to another human as part of a learning experiment. A majority of subjects proceeded to escalate the level of fictiously inflicted pain to *agonizing* levels on the instructions of the investigator. Subsequently, when the subjects were informed about this feature of themselves as part of the debriefing, they experienced severe, and in some cases, prolonged anxiety reactions (Milgram, 1963). Milgram defended his study against criticism and reported that most of the subjects had a positive view of their participation (Milgram, 1964).

The ethics of such studies continue to be controversial. Levine notes that he himself chairs an IRB that occasionally approves deceptive studies but generally disapproves of deception (Levine). Various guidelines regarding deceptive research methods have been published, such as those by the American Psychological Association, which can be viewed on their website. In response to many unethical research practices, ranging from Nazi atrocities before and during World War II to well-documented cases in the United States, the U.S. government has mandated a set of formal procedures to ensure compliance with ethical requisites. Institutions involved in research on human subjects are required to have their investigations reviewed and approved by IRBs whose composition, procedures, and record-keeping requirements are well-defined in law and governmental regulations. It should be noted, however, that the determination by a duly constituted IRB of the satisfaction of these ethical requirements does not in all cases resolve all ethical and practical stresses generated by research on human subjects. A number of authors have discerned a deeply rooted dilemma that the physician as healer and the physician as researcher confront in a search for generalizable knowledge employing human subjects. This dilemma has its source partly in the respect-for-persons principle cited above and partly in the ethical principle that the physician should do what is best for his or her patient. The dilemma is also most clearly evident in the context of the RCT but can also arise in less stringent research designs, which it will be necessary to discuss before turning to an account of this troublesome research predicament.

Study Designs

THE SPECTRUM OF STUDY DESIGNS IN BIOMEDICAL AND BEHAVIORAL RESEARCH. Diverse research designs

guide research in the biomedical, behavioral, and clinical sciences. Since this topic can easily become quite technical and mathematically abstruse, this entry presents only a general introduction to this subject. (For specialized information including indications when, and why, one design is preferable to another, see works on clinical epidemiology and monographs devoted to specific research designs, e.g., Feinstein,; Fletcher et al.; Hulley, et al.; Lilienfeld and Lilienfeld; and Sackett et al.)

The chart depicted in Figure 1 can be used as a guide to the various research designs found in clinical research. (This figure is based in part on Lilienfeld and Lilienfeld, p. 192, and in part on Fletcher et al., p. 193.) To these designs should also be added the *case report* and the *case series,* in which a biomedically interesting individual's (or small group of similar individuals's) situation is described. Some writers characterize the case report or case series as another design; others view such a small series as conductible using any of the designs described in the chart below. (The use of small numbers of subjects in any trial design, however, raises concerns that errors of interpretation are likely because of chance events. Problems generated by chance events in biomedical research are analyzed using the tools of mathematical statistics.)

The *interval of data collection* refers to the period of time during which data are collected. If one or more populations are studied over a period of time, the study is described as a *longitudinal* one. Alternatively, we may wish to collect information within one time slice, yielding a *cross-sectional* study. Moving to the next line, the investigator may collect data by looking back in time—for example, inquiring (or reviewing chart records) to learn whether the population was exposed to a specific agent. At least one control group is assembled to provide a comparison, again retrospectively. This *case control* design is the type of approach that Arthur Herbst and his colleagues employed in his pioneering inquiry into the causes of vaginal cancer in daughters of mothers who had been given diethylstilbestrol (DES), a synthetic estrogen believed to help prevent miscarriages, during their pregnancies. The case-control type of study is generally thought to be open to a number of potential errors, termed *biases.* Potentially confounding elements therefore need to be monitored carefully.

If the putative active difference between the comparison groups, such as the administration of a new drug, is intentionally introduced by the investigators, a study is characterized as *experimental.* If the suspected active difference occurs by accident or is chosen by the subjects—for example, a subject's decision to begin cigarette smoking or to

FIGURE 1

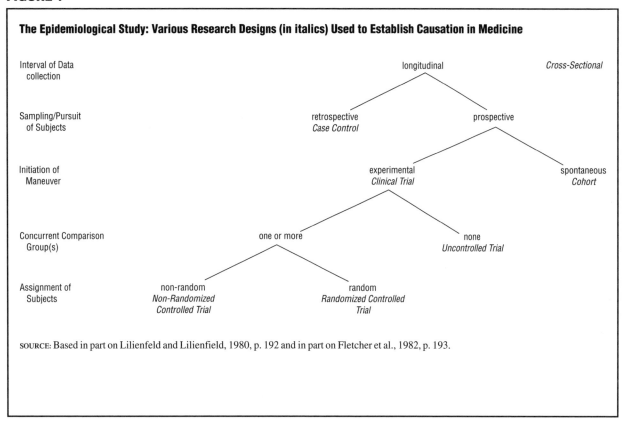

The Epidemiological Study: Various Research Designs (in italics) Used to Establish Causation in Medicine

SOURCE: Based in part on Lilienfeld and Lilienfield, 1980, p. 192 and in part on Fletcher et al., 1982, p. 193.

reduce blood cholesterol by diet—the investigation is termed a *cohort* study. A longitudinal prospective experimental study is a clinical trial, but such trials may or may not involve a comparison control group. Good examples of uncontrolled types of clinical trials are Phase I and Phase II investigations of new drugs, though occasionally a Phase II investigation may involve randomized controls (see Byar et al.). Phase I studies look at the metabolism and toxicity of new drugs, often in normal subjects, and Phase II inquiries test for preliminary efficacy of a drug or a procedure. The terms Phase I and Phase II were introduced in 1977 by the U.S. Food and Drug Administration (FDA). (For details of the procedures by which toxicity and efficacy of interventions are evaluated, see Gilman et al., chapter 68.)

A Phase III investigation is almost always a RCT. Randomization refers to the process of assigning a patient to one rather than another treatment (or to the control group) by the flip of a coin or a more mathematically sophisticated but analogous procedure of using a table of random numbers. The RCT refers to that form of investigation that involves (1) one or more treatment groups and a control group that will typically receive a placebo (an inert substance) or the standard therapy (i.e., the traditionally accepted therapy); (2) randomized assignment of patients to

the two or more groups (possibly after stratification or subgrouping based on known factors that will make a difference) sometimes referred to as *arms* of the trial; and (3) often a single- or double-blind design in which the assignments of the agents or procedures being tested are not known to the patients (single-blind) or possibly also to the treating health professionals (double-blind). (In place of the word *blind*, some accounts use the word *masked*.) In one unusual exception to that rule, the trial of the anti-HIV drug didanosine, or ddI, the whole experimental cohort were given ddI; these subjects were compared with *historical*, or retrospectively identified, control subjects (Waldholz; FDA).

Considerable debate has occurred about the methodological value and the ethical significance of randomization in controlled clinical trials. Various types of studies described above differ in their *strength*, that is, their ability to detect what is actually causing the changes that are being observed. The case series is traditionally the weakest of the research designs; other designs, in order of increasing strength, are the case-controlled study, the cohort study, and the RCT. The principal reason for the increase in design strength is the decrease in the likelihood of bias, or lack of comparability of the matched populations, as one moves from case series through to the RCT.

There are many types of bias, and some of them are quite subtle (Sackett). A major source of bias is selection or susceptibility bias, in which the groups compared have distinctly different outcome probabilities (more specifically, different prognostic likelihoods for the study's endpoint). This type of bias can occur within the study, or it can arise as part of the selection process and affect the generalizability of a study's results. In this type of situation, unrepresentative individuals are selected, and subgroups drawn from the unrepresentative class are then assigned to the arms of the study. An example of this type of bias would occur if only the sickest patients in a study were given the new drug and the better-off patients were assigned standard therapy (or a placebo). Another source of noncomparability is performance bias, in which the interventions in the trial are not reasonably equal. An example would be if the patients receiving the new drug were monitored much more closely and treated for concurrent health problems with no such monitoring and treatment being provided to the control group. A third type of bias is *confounding* bias, in which another, unsuspected causal variable *travels along* with the putative causal variable and actually accounts for the outcome. This could occur in a study to determine the effects of alcohol consumption on lung function, if alcohol drinkers were also much more likely to be smokers and the effect of smoking was not considered by the investigators. Other significant types of bias are detection or measurement bias, where the outcome event is detected differently in the comparison groups—for example, if the test group received MRIs and the control group standard X rays—and transfer bias, in which subject dropouts or reassignments may yield differences in outcome. The arguments for randomization in clinical investigations typically cite the ability of randomized assignment to decrease the likelihood of bias because, many maintain, randomizing will average together, and thus cancel out, factors that are not suspected by the investigators to affect the outcome.

RCTs can generate potential conflicts of interest between the roles of the physician as healer and physician as investigator, including questions about the suitability of placebo controls and its possible resolution using the concept of *clinical equipoise*.

META-ANALYSIS. Human variability, based on both genetics and environment, requires the extensive use of statistical methodologies to uncover generalizable, clinically applicable knowledge. This is in contrast to laboratory investigations in which virtually identical organisms yield cleaner and often *deterministic* results. Besides the variability of the subjects studied, many sources of bias such as the ones described can also lead to incorrect research conclusions.

Under these circumstances, researchers have turned increasingly to a method of clinical trial pooling and interpretation that seems to provide a better means of inferring correct conclusions from repeated clinical investigations. This methodology, known as meta-analysis, uses a set of formal statistical techniques to aggregate a group of separate but similar studies. In contrast to the widely employed scientific practice of summing up such studies qualitatively in a review article, meta-analysis purports to fulfill this summarizing function quantitatively and thus more precisely and objectively. Meta-analysis has been practiced for many years in a variety of scientific disciplines, from physics to the biomedical and the behavioral sciences, but only since the early 1980s has it had a major impact in the clinical arena, particularly in the areas of cardiovascular disease and obstetrics and gynecology (Chalmers et al., 1989; Mann).

Simple introductions as well as accessible authoritative accounts of the methodology are available. (See Mann, for an introduction, and Friedman et al, pp. 310–316, for a more comprehensive overview.) The technique remains controversial even as its use in biomedicine escalates exponentially.

EVIDENCE-BASED MEDICINE. Many of the issues reviewed above coalesce in what is termed *evidence-based medicine* (EBM), which is both a critical methodological approach as well as a kind of social movement. EBM had its origins in the 1980s discipline of clinical epidemiology, and developed rapidly in Canada, the United Kingdom, and then the United States and other countries in the 1990s. Initially EBM saw itself as representing a kind of Kuhnian paradigm shift, urging the replacement of the received view of medical evidence—seen as a combination of clinical expertise and basic science—with evidence based mainly on rigorously evaluated empirical clinical trials. (Haynes). More recently, EBM advocates have taken a more nuanced position on this replacement view though the distinction is still evident in EBMs databases (Haynes). EBM provides evaluations and clinician guidance through its literature, various websites, and electronically available systematic reviews including the Cochrane collaboration. EBM provides grades of recommendation from A (excellent) to D (poor) based on studies's empirical strengths following a detailed assessment protocol based on five *levels* of study types, several of which have sublevels. The levels range from the best (a systematic review with homogenous RCTs as the main element) to the worst (expert opinion without explicit critical appraisal, or essentially based on physiology, whether bench research or general principles). The specifics of these grades, the levels on which they are based, and the definitions of the concepts involved (such as *homogeneity*) can be obtained at <http://minerva.minervation.com/cebm/>. EBM has not gone uncriticized, both from without and within the movement. One of its founders, Brian Haynes, laments the fact that EBM itself has not, and probably ethically cannot, be subject to its own highest standards of evaluation: a series of homogeneous RCTs in which EBM is utilized as an intervention but is not employed in the control groups of patients (Haynes).

Conclusion

This entry has reviewed a number of conceptual issues associated with current research methodology in the biomedical sciences. It contains a review of research in the basic sciences, such as biochemistry and microbiology, but has concentrated on the clinical sciences, such as medicine, oncology, and virology, since it is in the latter that ethical issues affecting human subjects arise. Scientific research on humans takes place in the context of a complex web of ethical and legal requirements, and the interplay between methodological and ethical/legal components of research has been examined. Ethical and regulatory principles (primarily as affecting U.S. research) have been presented, and several conceptual issues regarding scientific inquiry have been outlined, including different types of research designs. This entry is limited to an introduction to these issues, which become very technical in their details; references to further reading have been provided.

Although scientific methodology has a venerable history, many current issues are of much more recent vintage. In point of fact, the RCT is essentially a post-World War II invention, and the discipline of meta-analysis is a creature of the late 1980s and 1990s. New issues will continue to arise as better methodologies and improved safeguards for human subjects are sought, and the reader is urged to consult on-line bibliographic services, such as the bioethics database at the U.S. National Library of Medicine, in addition to references provided in this entry, to keep up to date with a continuously evolving subject.

KENNETH F. SCHAFFNER (1995)
REVISED BY AUTHOR

SEE ALSO: *Aging and the Aged: Healthcare and Research Issues; AIDS: Healthcare and Research Issues; Autoexperimentation; Autonomy; Children: Healthcare and Research Issues; Commercialism in Scientific Research; Embryo and Fetus: Embryo Research; Empirical Methods in Bioethics; Genetics and Human Behavior: Scientific and Research Issues; Holocaust; Infants: Public Policy and Legal Issues; Informed Consent: Consent Issues in Human Research;*

Mentally Ill and Mentally Disabled Persons: Research Issues; Military Personnel as Research Subjects; Minorities as Research Subjects; Pediatrics, Overview of Ethical Issues in; Prisoners as Research Subjects; Race and Racism; Research, Human, Historical Aspects; Research, Multinational; Research Policy; Research, Unethical; Responsibility; Scientific Publishing; Sexism; Students as Research Subjects; Virtue and Character; and other *Research Methodology* subentries

BIBLIOGRAPHY

Beauchamp, Tom L., and Childress, James F. 2001. *Principles of Biomedical Ethics,* 5th edition. New York: Oxford University Press.

Bernard, Claude. 1865 (reprint 1957). *An Introduction to the Study of Experimental Medicine,* tr. Henry C. Green. New York: Dover.

Byar, David P.; Schoenfeld, David A.; Green, Sylvan B.; et al. 1990. "Design Consideration for AIDS Trials." *New England Journal of Medicine* 323(19): 1343–1348.

Chalmers, Jain; Enkin, Murray; Keirse, Mark; and Enkin, Eleanor, eds. 1989. *Effective Care in Pregnancy and Childbirth.* New York: Oxford University Press.

Chalmers, Thomas C.; Block, Jerome; and Lee, Stephanie. 1972. "Controlled Studies in Clinical Cancer Research." *New England Journal of Medicine* 287(2): 75–78.

Code of Federal Regulations. 1993. 45 CFR 46 (Protection of Human Subjects).

Comroe, Julius H., Jr., and Dripps, Robert D. 1976. "Scientific Basis for the Support of Biomedical Science." *Science* 192(4235): 105–111.

Dorland, W. A. Newman. 1994. *Dorland's Illustrated Medical Dictionary,* 28th edition. Philadelphia: W. B. Saunders.

Federal Register. 1991. Federal Policy for the Protection of Human Subjects. 56(117): 28013–28028.

Feinstein, Alvin R. 1986. *Clinical Epidemiology: The Architecture of Clinical Research.* Philadelphia: W. B. Saunders.

Fletcher, Robert H.; Fletcher, Suzanne W.; and Wagner, Edward H. 1982. *Clinical Epidemiology: The Essentials.* Philadelphia: Williams & Wilkins.

Freireich, Emil, and Gehan, Edmund. 1979. "The Limitations of the Randomized Clinical Trial." In *Methods of Cancer Research:* vol. 17 *Cancer Drug Development—Part B,* eds. Vincent T. De Vita and Harris Busch. New York: Academic Press.

Friedman, Lawrence M.; Furberg, Curt D.; and DeMets, David L. 1998. *Fundamentals of Clinical Trials,* 3rd edition. New York: Springer.

Goodman, Louis S., and Gilman, Alfred G., eds. 1980. *Goodman and Gilman's The Pharmacological Basis of Therapeutics,* 6th edition. New York: Macmillan.

Haynes, R. Brian. 2002. "What Kind Of Evidence Is It That Evidence-Based Medicine Advocates Want Health Care Providers And Consumers To Pay Attention To?" *BMC Health Services Research* 2(1): 3-X.

Herbst, Arthur L.; Uhlfelder, Howard; and Poskanzer, David C. 1971. "Adenocarcinoma of the Vagina: Association of Maternal Stilbestrol Therapy with Tumor Appearance in Young Women." *New England Journal of Medicine* 284(16): 878–881.

Hulley, Stephen B.; Cummings, Steven R.; and Browner, Warren S., eds. 1988. *Designing Clinical Research: An Epidemiologic Approach.* Baltimore: Williams & Wilkins.

Levine, Carol; Dubler, Nancy N.; and Levine, Robert J. 1991. "Building a New Consensus: Ethical Principles and Policies for Clinical Research on HIV/AIDS." *IRB* 13(1–2): 1–17.

Levine, Robert J. 1986. *Ethics and Regulation of Clinical Research,* 2nd edition. New Haven, CT.: Yale University Press.

Lilienfeld, Abraham M., and Lilienfeld, David E. 1980. *Foundations of Epidemiology.* New York: Oxford University Press.

Mann, Charles. 1990. "Meta-Analysis in the Breech." *Science* 249: 476–480.

Milgram, Stanley. 1963. "Behavioral Study of Obedience." *Journal of Abnormal Psychology* 67(4): 371–378.

Milgram, Stanley. 1964. "Issues in the Study of Obedience: A Reply to Baumrind." *American Psychologist* 19(11): 848–852.

Merriam-Webster's Collegiate Dictionary, 10th edition. 2002. Springfield, MA: Merriam-Webster.

Mill, John Stuart. 1843 (reprint 1959). *A System of Logic.* London: Longmans, Green and Co.

National Research Council's Committee on Models for Biomedical Research. 1985. *A New Perspective.* Washington, D.C.: National Academy Press.

Sackett, David L. 1979. "Bias in Analytic Research." *Journal of Chronic Diseases* 32(1–2): 51–63.

Sackett, David L.; Haynes, R. Brian; Straus, Sharon E.; et al. 2000. *Evidence Based Medicine.* Orlando, FL: Harcourt Health Sciences.

U.S. Food and Drug Administration. 1977. *General Considerations for the Clinical Evaluation of Drugs,* DHEW Publication No. (FDA) 77–3040. Washington, D.C.: U.S. Government Printing Office.

U.S. Food and Drug Administration. 1991. "Summary Minutes of Antiviral Drugs Advisory Committee," July 18/19, Meeting #6, Bethesda Holiday Inn, Bethesda, MD. Available from FDA on request.

U.S. President's Commission for the Study of Ethical Problems in Medicine and Biomedical and Behavioral Research. 1983. *IRB Guidebook.* Washington, D.C.: U. S. Government Printing Office.

Waldholz, Michael. "Bristol-Meyers Guides AIDS Drug Through a Marketing Minefield." *Wall Street Journal,* October 10, 1992, p. A1.

INTERNET RESOUCES

American Psychological Association. "Ethical Principals of Psychologists and Code of Conduct 2002." Available from <www.apa.org/ethics/code2002.html>.

U.S. National Library of Medicine. 2003. Available from <www.nlm.nih.gov>.

World Medical Association. 2003. "Declaration of Helsinki." Available from <http://www.wma.net/e/policy/17-c_e.html>.

II. CLINICAL TRIALS

In the last half of the twentieth century, clinical trial methodology fundamentally transformed the nature of biomedical research. During this period, investigators developed ways to avoid certain biases in research design and to adapt methods of statistical analysis to empirical research. The story of biomedical research's progressive sophistication, however, does not begin in clinics or hospitals, but in a cornfield. Ronald A. Fisher (1890–1962), the famous British statistician, biologist, and geneticist, devised methods for testing hypotheses on how to improve crops (Gigerenzer et al.). By dividing fields into two or more groups, making them as similar as possible in composition and treatment, Fisher hoped to isolate the effects of one feature on the individuals studied. For example, would a fertilizer given to some of the corn improve yield? The resulting differences between groups could then be expressed as probabilities about whether outcomes were due to chance or their different treatment. By studying more individuals for longer periods, confidence levels increase that variations between group outcomes were due to their different treatment.

In the late 1940s, Fisher and others began to adapt and refine these pioneering principles for use with human research, and in 1948 clinical trial methodology was systematically launched into medicine with the testing of streptomycin to treat tuberculosis (Concato, Shah, and Horwitz). Since that time, investigators have used clinical trial methods to evaluate virtually everything affecting patients, including: therapies, diagnostic techniques, prevention of illnesses, vaccines, counseling, health delivery systems, and even the benefits of classical music, pets, and humor on health. In one study, for example, people were divided into large groups; some got a daily aspirin and others a placebo (an inert substance). This helped ensure that groups were treated alike even down to the number of pills that they were given. The group receiving aspirin suffered fewer heart attacks (Steering Committee). Like methods developed in agricultural research, the goal of clinical trial methodology is to compose and treat groups as similarly as possible except for the one feature under study. Investigators attempt to identify other features that are likely to affect outcomes and stratify or distribute individuals with those features equally between groups. For example, the healthiest individuals (whether people, pigs, or parsnips) should be stratified equally among the groups because health often affects outcomes.

To help further ensure that groups are similar, investigators generally use another method, randomization (nonhuman choice), such as, charts of random numbers, to assign individuals to groups. For example, suppose that investigators want to study the influence of caffeine upon alertness. They know other things affect alertness, such as people's interest in the subject or their intelligence, and the investigators try to stratify people with these variables equally between groups. But the investigators also know that many additional features affect alertness, such as people's sleeping, eating, or television-watching habits. Unable to identify all such variables or distribute people with similar features equally between groups, the investigators try to minimize the impact of these "nuisance" variables and achieve uniform groups through randomization. Even simple random methods, such as flipping a coin to determine group assignments, help ensure that people with distinctive features that could affect results do not cluster in one group. The larger the groups, the more likely that randomization will produce similar groups. The goal of randomization is to combat bias in group assignments by distributing individual characteristics whose effects are unknown equally among the study arms to minimize their influence. In human studies, randomized clinical trials (RCTs) use random assignment to eliminate, through equal distribution, the effects of variables such as nutritional habits, beliefs, attitudes, behavior, ancestry, and education in correlating the variable under investigation with its observed effects. Nonrandomized trials generally seem second best because of the risk of bias in the formation of the groups.

Investigators use other methods in addition to randomization and stratification to make groups similar and to eliminate bias. In single-blind studies, subjects do not know their group assignment, thereby minimizing the effects of their beliefs and expectations about the different modes of treatment. For unbiased results, the subjects should be treated so similarly that they cannot know which treatment they receive. Investigators' subconscious beliefs, preferences, or attitudes may also affect how they take care of individuals or evaluate outcomes. Believing one medicine works best, for example, may affect their estimates of how individuals respond. To combat such biases, investigators may use double-blind designs in which the group assignments are kept from subjects, their clinicians and investigators until after the trial so that clinicians' or investigators' own views will not contaminate the study's results.

Impartial studies can expose bias, prejudice, the flaws of common wisdom, the errors of standard practice, and the harms or benefits of established treatments. For example, in the 1940s and early 1950s doctors believed that giving copious amounts of oxygen to premature infants prevented death and brain damage. By 1953 this common wisdom was being challenged by clinical trials, and by 1954 the link between the lavish use of oxygen and blindness from retrolental fibroplasia was clearly established (Silverman). Other studies uncovered previously unforeseen adverse drug reactions. For example, systematic testing of commonly used antibiotics showed that premature infants receiving sulfisoxazole (gantrisin) had a much higher incidence of death and retardation than other groups. Further investigation revealed that premature infants could not metabolize and detoxify bilirubin, thus causing kernicterus, or neurological damage to the brain (Behrman and Vaughan).

Clinical trials also account for many treatment advances. In three decades of continual evaluation of alternative therapies through clinical trials, childhood leukemia went from a uniformly fatal disease to an often-curable illness. RCTs also demonstrated that coronary artery bypass surgery was ineffective for many of the diseases for which it had been widely used.

In a controlled clinical trial (CCT), investigators compare the outcomes for patients getting one treatment with those who do not. This allows investigators to separate the treatment's effects from other influences. The U.S. Department of Health and Human Services (HHS) cites five kinds of control groups distinguished, in part, upon whether the comparison involves a historical control group (in which patients' outcomes are compared with records from past patients) or a concurrent control group (in which patients' outcomes are compared with patients currently being treated):

1. placebo concurrent control;
2. dose comparison, concurrent control;
3. no treatment concurrent control;
4. active treatment concurrent control; and
5. historical control.

Investigators often regard the double-blind RCT with a concurrent control group getting a placebo as the "gold standard" because it offers the greatest assurances that differences between groups have not been distorted by people's different diagnosis criteria, treatments, observations, measurements, or expectations (Ellenberg and Temple; Temple and Ellenberg).

Gaining General Acceptance: An Example Involving Breast Cancer

Enrolling patients in clinical trials involved fundamental shifts in how to think about patient–doctor relationships. Consequently, it was one thing to work out a good methodology and another to find clinicians and patients willing to participate in CCTs. For example, by 1968, 70 percent of women with breast cancer had radical mastectomy, which entails removing the breast, lymph nodes, and chest wall muscles on the affected side. Many clinicians believed this gave women their best chance of a "cure" (defined as surviving five years or longer), at no real loss, because in their view, the breast of an older woman was entirely expendable (Lerner). Beginning in the 1970s, these views changed gradually, but many clinicians clung to these beliefs into the 1990s, long after information gained from a series of RCTs showed radical mastectomy as unnecessarily mutilating and disabling. Ultimately, these trials established that removal of only the tumor or the breast, with or without radiation therapy, resulted in survival comparable to that achieved with the radical mastectomy (Fisher). Follow-up studies done twenty-five years later confirmed that there is no advantage to the more mutilating surgery (Fisher et al.).

Getting clinicians to agree to participate and women to enroll in CCTs or RCTs in the 1970s and 1980s was a crucial step to discrediting radical mastectomies. Investigators had to persuade skeptical physicians who believed that the radical mastectomy was necessary to give their patients the best chance of survival. Many clinicians asserted that they had a "therapeutic obligation" or duty to pick what they viewed as the best therapy for their patients. Some were so convinced radical mastectomy was best that they did not inform women of other options, let alone enroll them in RCTs; others did not want to communicate the uncertainties about which therapies were best or feared that informed consent would destroy trust in the doctor–patient relationship (Taylor, Margolese, and Soskolne).

Such paternalistic attitudes increasingly troubled both investigators (how did clinicians know what was best?) and women (do they not have a say about what is best for them?). Women were learning about the controversies over treatment options swirling in the medical literature at the same time that informed-consent policy took root. Consequently, investigators and clinicians had to make room for good informed consent and choice. In response, therapeutic research became an increasingly cooperative venture among doctors, patients, and investigators (Kopelman, 1994; Fisher).

Increasingly, patients and clinicians saw the advantages of participation in multi-institutional research using the same protocols. These large trials proved to have many research advantages, because they can involve many patients and get results quickly, and because they can help neutralize biases that result from distinctive groups of people who use certain institutions. In addition, large trials can even result in improved care for all groups and better fulfillment of consent requirements. This is because these cooperative studies are often designed by experts and include quality-control provisions. In addition, they are also reviewed for approval by many agencies. Moreover, expert panelists review data and stop the trials if early results show clear advantages to some assignments.

By the 1990s, great progress in treating cancer resulted, in part, from doctors' willingness to enroll patients in clinical trials and patients' willingness to participate. Patients often acted from altruism to help the next generation of patients, just as the last generation had helped them. Clinical trials, by this time, were also seen as a way to get good care, leading many people to be eager to enroll and disappointed if they were excluded. Largely gone were the sweeping general denunciations of the 1970s and 1980s when critics claimed an inherent incompatibility existed between these research methods on the one hand and doctors' duties to protect patients, patient's rights and welfare, and good patient–doctor relationships on the other (Fried; Gifford; Marquis; Wikler).

An Imperfect Consensus with Enduring Issues

For clinical trials to be morally acceptable, a consensus exists that they must meet the following conditions:

1. The study is important.
2. Patients or their representatives give informed consent including knowledge of all alternatives, of their right to withdraw at any time, and of clinicians' and investigators' conflicts of interest.
3. Physicians and investigators place the well-being of the patients ahead of research interests.
4. The study has gained appropriate approval from institutional review boards or research ethics committees.
5. A data safety monitoring panel will end studies if it is demonstrated that one or more of the study arms prove better than others and will report significant new findings to doctors or patients.
6. The uncertainty principle or null hypothesis is justified, meaning that the arms of the study are "equally good."

Before a trial begins, then, investigators must do a comprehensive review of the literature to show that all treatments being given and compared have a therapeutic success rate that is acceptably high for all arms, and that it is uncertain whether any one of the treatments being tested is better than any of the others. In addition, it must be shown that no study arm provides what is known to be inferior care (HHS; Beauchamp and Childress; Concato, Shah, and Horwitz; Emanuel, Wendler, and Grady; WMA).

Serious questions exist about implementing these assumptions. Patients have legitimate preferences about how they want to be treated, and doctors have responsibilities to try to give patients the best care to meet their individual needs, goals, and desires. Controlled trials restrict people's choices and limit the ways therapies can be adapted for them by the methodologies of stratification, randomization, inflexible interventions, eligibility requirements, and single-blind or double-blind study designs. Some of these concerns are discussed below.

PHYSICIANS' ROLES AS CLINICIANS AND AS SCIENTISTS. When physicians enroll patients in clinical trials, they help patients collectively by gaining knowledge but may lose flexibility in tailoring treatments for individual patients. This can create a conflict between doctors' roles as scientists dedicated to conducting the best studies to gain knowledge, and as healers dedicated to adapting treatments to each patient's needs, goals, and values. To address this potential conflict, most agree that physicians should not enroll a patient in a clinical trial if they have reason to believe a patient might, thereby, obtain inferior care (Byar et al.; Chalmers, Block, and Lee; Kopelman, 1986; WMA; Ellenberg; Levine, Dubler, and Levine; Shaw and Chalmers; Zelen, 1990; Emanuel, Wendler, and Grady).

Although agreement exists that doctors should not enroll patients in studies in which they get inferior care, substantive disagreements remain about when arms of studies are considered equally good. One controversy concerns what values to employ in deciding if treatments are "equally good." Investigators tend to measure equality among treatments in terms of easily quantified outcomes such as survival after cancer treatments or reduction of blood pressure. Patients and some clinicians, however, also consider how treatments affect the quality of patients' lives and whether patients think the treatment makes them feel better (Levine, Dubler, and Levine). Views, therefore, about what treatments are equally good differ when people regard different things as relevant benefits and burdens. Hence nausea, hair loss, sexual impotence, weakness, extra costs, inconvenience, or more hospital visits may be more important outcomes from a patient's perspective than from an investigator's perspective in determining when treatments are equally good.

Another controversy that involves how to use the uncertainty principle may be called "the problem of clinician preference," or, should conscientious clinicians with any preference at all for one treatment arm enroll their patients in a clinical trial? Some argue that clinicians have a duty to provide what they believe to be the best available care for patients; consequently, as long as physicians have any preference about which treatment is best for their patients, they should not enroll their patients in clinical trials (Fried; Gifford; Waldenstrom). It is rare that clinicians have no preference whatsoever about what is best for their patients, especially for the treatment of serious illnesses where the outcomes, conveniences, risks, and possible benefits are different. Moreover, if asked, patients will often have preferences even if the clinicians do not, and this could break the tie for doctors. Consequently, these critics find trials, especially RCTs, generally unethical.

In his 1987 article, "Equipoise and the Ethics of Clinical Research," philosopher Benjamin Freedman tried to solve the problem of clinician preference by distinguishing between "theoretical equipoise" and "clinical equipoise." Theoretical equipoise is an epistemic (cognitive) state in which the evidence is exactly balanced, meaning that treatments are of equal value. Clinical equipoise, in contrast, is that state in which the community of expert clinicians is undecided as to the preferred treatment for the given population as determined by the study's eligibility criteria; the study should be designed to disturb clinical equipoise and to terminate when it is achieved. Freedman argued that clinical equipoise is a better way to understand that treatments are equally useful for a particular group and, thus, that the uncertainty principle has been reached. To decide equipoise, then, the focus should not be on the treatment that the particular clinician prefers, but on what the community of clinicians believes to be equally good treatments for some condition given their respective benefits and burdens. A clinician may have a preference for one treatment but respect colleagues with different views. Thus, as the trial begins, treatments (including any placebo arm) must be in clinical equipoise, or be regarded as having equal merit by the community of experts in treating some condition for a certain group. Disagreements should be expected in a rapidly advancing field such as medicine, and it is these disagreements that help explain why trials are important. Exceptions are sometimes made to this policy of requirement equipose if there is no more than minimal risk of harm to the subjects, such as testing the efficacy of nose drops in the common cold.

This solution presupposes agreement or justification about who should be in the community of expert clinicians deciding which treatments are equally good and whether their views adequately represent those of the potential patients. Disputes arise over this, however (Kopelman, 1994). Some people disvalue the views of any but the most acclaimed clinical investigators. Others contend that many perspectives, including those of investigators, clinicians, and patient advocates, represent patients' sometimes differing values. Increasingly, clinical trials are moving out of the academic centers and into private doctors' offices. Clinicians often find such arrangements professionally fulfilling, but they can also be financially lucrative when drug companies, who typically sponsor these studies, offer monetary incentives to enroll patients. In contrast to academic medical centers, little oversight or accountability exists in private offices, argued Jason E. Klein and Alan R. Fleischman in 2002; but more opportunity exists for patients to misunderstand that they are being enrolled in research programs not necessarily designed for their benefit. Klein and Fleischman argued that financial incentives to clinicians should be limited, patients should have an independent resource to answer their questions, and doctors should be required to disclose potential conflicts of interest. Arguably, in both the academic and private practice settings where there are genuine risks, the treating physician should not be the investigator.

STARTING TRIALS. Disagreements can erupt about the overall benefits of the new treatments or investigational new drugs when compared with standard care or to a placebo. To justify the time, energy, risks, and expense of testing a new therapy for some condition by means of a CCT or RCT, investigators must produce preliminary evidence of its safety, efficacy, and proper dose. Some knowledgeable people are likely to be more impressed with these findings than others, especially for serious diseases with no established treatments (Levine, Dubler, and Levine). Consequently, they disagree about if or when trials should begin. In addition, resources are limited so not all good studies can be funded. These funding choices depend not only upon the merits of the study but also on political and social interests because funding for studies is limited and often comes from tax revenues.

PLACEBO-CONTROLLED RCTS. One of the most persistent controversies concerns the use of the placebo arm in a controlled trial. A placebo is used because people's beliefs and expectations can influence how they react. Suppose there are two groups, and persons in one group get a red pill with specific activity. People sometimes react to getting pills. If one group gets a red pill, and if the two groups are being treated exactly the same, then arguably, the other group should also get a red pill, although without the same active preparation. The red pill might be a sugar pill. As noted, placebo-controlled RCTs are widely regarded as the gold standard for assessing the safety and efficacy of therapies.

A knotty problem exists over whether placebos should be used when there is a proven and effective treatment. Defenders of the use of a placebo arm in such cases cite its enormous methodological advantages in evaluating treatments and justify its use as long as subjects are not made worse off (Varmus and Satcher; Temple and Ellenberg). In one case, for example, investigators wanted to study the safety and efficacy of mood disorder medications adopted

long ago without rigorous testing. Some of these drugs have a good track record of abating serious symptoms including suicidal ideation. Disputes arose over whether these drugs should be tested against a placebo because beliefs and expectations affect mood disorders. A distinguished panel of experts could not reach consensus and concluded: "Research is needed on the ethical conduct of studies to limit risks of medication-free intervals and facilitate poststudy treatment. Patients must fully understand the risks and lack of individualized treatment involved in research" (Charney et al., p. 262). Yet obtaining consent for what can be risky studies from such patients may also be problematic because their illnesses often disturb their thought processes.

Perhaps the most contentious debate so far concerned using placebo-controlled trials to study perinatal transmission of HIV/AIDS when a proven and effective therapy existed (Angell; Temple and Ellenberg; Ellenberg and Temple; Lurie and Wolfe). The funding was from rich countries where, because proven and effective therapies were the standard of care, the studies could not be done. Some argued these studies were immoral because the stakes were life and death (Angell; Lurie and Wolfe); others said that the studies were needed and that these poor people were made no worse off by being given local standards of care (Temple and Ellenberg; Ellenberg and Temple; Varmus and Satcher). They maintained this was the most efficient way to obtain urgently needed information to fight the HIV/AIDS epidemic.

In 2000 the influential World Medical Association (WMA) took a stand. It issued a new draft of the Declaration of Helsinki stating that placebos should not be used if there was a proven and accepted treatment. This put the declaration on a collision course with the U.S. Food and Drug Administration (FDA), which often requires the use of placebo despite the existence of a proven and accepted treatment. Defenders also point out that if placebos are not permitted, trials may have to be a great deal larger and therefore more costly.

One possible middle ground is to consider the harm of not having the treatment. If there is only a minor risk of harm, such as minor discomfort or inconvenience to being denied the proven and effective treatment, then studies might be permitted. As potential harms to those on the placebo arm increase, it should become more difficult to approve the study, even with consent from subjects or their representatives.

An entirely different set of concerns exists, challenging the placebo as the gold standard. In their 2001 article, "Is the Placebo Powerless?" Asbjorn Hrobjartsson and Peter Gotzsche questioned whether the placebo is really as powerful as claimed. The placebo itself, they pointed out, was adopted without testing. They conducted a meta-analysis comparing placebo with no treatment arms, finding that in many cases, there was no difference between them at all. They wrote, "We found little difference in general that placebos have powerful clinical affects. Although placebos had no significant affects on objective or binary outcomes, they had possible small benefits in studies with continuous subjective outcomes and for treatments of pain. Outside the setting of clinical trials, there is no justification for the use of placebos" (Hrobjartsson and Gotzsche, p. 1594). In a 2000 article, John Concato and colleagues also raised doubts about the ascendancy of the placebo-controlled RCT when compared to all other methods. They argued that even observational studies can, when carefully done, control bias as well as an RCT.

Kenneth J. Rothman and Karin B. Michaels, in a 1994 article titled "The Continuing Unethical Use of Placebo Controls," concluded that the FDA's insistence upon viewing the placebo as the gold standard not only has moral problems but also is essentially a political decision. The FDA scientists argued that the placebo-controlled studies make it easier to show statistical significance with smaller numbers of subjects; but larger studies would reduce statistical variability. Unfortunately, this is expensive. Concato and colleagues also objected, stating that it is the drug companies that benefit from the FDA policy of fostering small CCTs and RCTs given that such studies are less costly; it is the patients who bear the burdens of this policy because they are denied proven and effective treatments.

Yet another challenge to the use of placebos as the gold standard comes from those who study complementary and alternative medicines (CAMs). RCTs and CCTs try to eliminate nuisance variables, and they include in this category people's different hopes and beliefs. There is little doubt, however, that these are powerful forces in people's lives. Some argue that research that eliminates hope and belief has limited utility, just because mental attitude is so powerful. In 2002 Kenneth J. Schaffner argued that the study of CAMs "...might lead us to question"

> a standard research design methodology that priorities randomized clinical trials and objective measures of health ... and think about the arguments of [the American philosopher Thomas] Kuhn and the disunity of science proponents, and about varying local methodologies ... [with their] different evidential standards ... CAM can help make us realize both that the influence of the belief systems may have powerful effects on health and that discerning these effects may require a realization of these Procrustean standards. (Schaffner 2002, p. 12)

ENDING TRIALS. The goal of a study is to learn whether different treatments are equally good for certain conditions. But justification for claiming to know something is a matter of degree, and there can be substantial disagreements about where to draw the line for the purpose of saying that it is known that treatments are or are not equally good. Investigators should adopt rules about when to stop at the outset of a study. Although investigators generally do not release preliminary data, there are some exceptions. A data safety monitoring panel is often charged with monitoring the data and deciding if trials should be ended early because people in one arm of the study are doing far worse than others. For example, azidothymidine (AZT) was first tested against a placebo in a double-blind RCT to see if it helped patients with AIDS. Doctors and nurses believed they knew from the abatement of symptoms, which patients were getting AZT and which were getting a placebo. After several months, 16 of the 137 patients in the placebo arm died, whereas only 1 of the 145 patients receiving AZT died. The trial was ended and all received AZT (Beauchamp and Childress).

Deciding when to stop a trial is not an entirely scientific choice but is also a moral decision. Investigators, panels, and journal editors typically require a probability of at most 0.05 (five chances in a hundred) that the observed results between groups occurred by chance, as a ground for holding that *sufficient evidence* exists to say they *know* that the groups are different. Although the 0.05 standard is a reasonable and well-established convention, it should not be misunderstood. As Daniel Wikler (1981) and Loretta M. Kopelman (1986, 1994) have argued, it is at best a moral trade-off between continuing the study so long that some people receive obviously suboptimal care and stopping so early that some people are harmed because insufficiently verified treatments are adopted or discredited. Some will draw that line differently, especially when treatments are tested for serious illnesses with few other means of treatment, as in AIDS research (Kopelman, 1994).

INFORMED CONSENT AND RESEARCH INTEGRITY. For people to enroll in studies, they or their guardians must give informed consent, meaning authorization that is competent, adequately informed, and voluntary. Assuming that people are competent to give consent and do so voluntarily, what do they need to know to give informed consent for clinical studies?

Generally they must be told about the study's nature, purpose, duration, procedures, and foreseeable risks and benefits. Moreover, they need to know about any alternative treatments, inconveniences, additional costs, and extra procedures or hospitalizations resulting from enrollment. They must also be told of their right to withdraw from the study at any time should they agree to participate (U.S. 45 CFR 46.116). If the study design includes different groups, randomization, or placebos, for example, prospective subjects need to be informed. Consent for therapy or research requires giving people all information that a reasonable person would want to know in order to make a choice.

These widely recognized consent requirements create tensions in relation to the research goals of clinical trials. For example, suppose in testing treatments, one study arm uses surgery with medical management resulting in a faster recovery if there are no complications, and the other study arm uses medical management alone, with fewer risks but a slower recovery. If distinctive groups have special preferences, such as the elderly preferring medical management and the young surgery, then the study of the different treatment results could be biased through self-selection.

Thus, there is a difficulty that may be called "the problem of subject preference": How can people's preferences be accommodated while preserving the scientific integrity of the CCT or RCT? Some criticize regulations on informed-consent doctrine as unrealistic, too individualistic, and shortsighted because they give too much weight to individual choice and make it hard to conduct good studies (Tobias; Zelen, 1979, 1990). Physicians and healthcare professionals, they argue, have a duty to take proper care of patients but are not typically required to educate them about these technical and complex matters; patients should get good treatment given by conscientious professionals, but patients do not need to know how, when, or why investigators evaluate their treatments. Most patients cannot understand the investigation's complexities, they argue, and would be harmed by learning of the uncertainties about what care is best or that they are being studied. Investigators should be free to design the best possible trials consistent with good care, they argue, and the current understanding of patients' rights disrupts clinical trials, thereby slowing medical progress. If people have only the right to good care and not the right to refuse to be enrolled in a study, it would be easier for investigators to conduct research and minimize problems of bias introduced by people's preferences. For example, Marvin Zelen devised schemas in which patients give their consent for a treatment without knowing that the treatment was selected by a random method and/or that they are in a study; other designs prerandomize people to group assignments before consent is sought (Zelen, 1979, 1990).

Such paternalism, in general, and Zelen's designs in particular, has garnered legal and moral criticism (Ellenberg, 1984, 1992; Kopelman, 1986, 1994). It not only denies people self-determination, but, without pertinent information, people do not have means to protect their own well-being. The doctrine of informed consent developed because many patients and activists wanted impartial information and participation in choices about their care, especially when they will be serving as research subjects. For example, statistician Susan S. Ellenberg criticized Zelen's prerandomization schemas in which patients are assigned to groups before consent is sought. She argued that this threatens impartiality in gaining consent, risking that the informational sessions will be shaped to enhance the benefits and minimize the risks of each individual assignment (Ellenberg, 1984, 1992).

On the other hand, others are skeptical that most subjects give genuine informed consent to research (Tobias; Wikler; Zelen, 1979). Most patients, they claim, do not understand the benefits or burdens of their treatment options, let alone the scientifically rigorous methodology used in testing. A related criticism is that investigators do not tell the patients, and most patients do not understand, that at some point in the trial it may become increasingly apparent that some groups are getting suboptimal care (Wikler). Investigators, they argue, put medical advances ahead of subject-patient rights and welfare because those rights typically violate physicians' duties to their patients (Fried; Gifford; Marquis; Wikler). Some support for this view comes from a study that George Annas reports was conducted by the FDA, which carried out spot checks on 1,000 investigations; the FDA found that investigators did not seek informed consent in 213 studies, did not follow their approved research protocol in 364 investigations, and failed to report adverse reactions for 140 test subjects. Unfortunately, the FDA results square with others, reports Annas (Annas).

In contrast to these two positions implying that one must choose between good trials and good informed consent, other commentators argue that clinical trials, including RCTs, can be cooperative ventures between patients and investigators (Freedman; Kopelman 1986, 1994; Levine, Dubler, and Levine; Levine, 1986). They believe that investigators and patients should work together with candor, respect, and trust about the goals and means of the research, and view consent as an on-going process. They maintain that with proper consent some studies (but not all) are morally justifiable. Subjects may *have* to be regarded as partners in a cooperative venture, however, if investigators expect people to enroll and cooperate. People can defeat trials if they do not identify with the investigators' goals. In one case, investigators were testing whether patients infected with HIV who were not yet showing symptoms of AIDS would benefit from AZT. At the end of the trial, researchers estimated that 9 percent of the patients in the placebo arm had been taking AZT. If more patients in the placebo group had secretly taken AZT, investigators might have judged a beneficial drug ineffective and refused to release it for this use (Merigan). These patients, facing a life-threatening disease, found a way to get the drug they believed useful and inadvertently jeopardized a clinical trial and the welfare of future patients. Poor cooperation results when the subjects fail to identify with the goals of the study, do not understand its importance, or are asked to risk too much in terms of health and convenience (Spilker).

PROTECTION OR ACCESS. During the period from the 1970s to the early twenty-first century, patients and physicians have gone from being wary of participating in CCTs and RCTs to seeking access to them. Studies were increasingly seen as opportunities for good care rather than as dangerous projects from which vulnerable people should be protected (Dresser; Kopelman, 1994). For example, AZT, the first effective drug to treat AIDS, was initially tested for safety and efficacy against a placebo in a double-blind RCT, as has been mentioned. Until the early 1990s, many biomedical research study populations excluded people of color, women, and children in order to "protect" what were considered to be these more vulnerable populations. Advocates argued that this was unfair because enrollment in trials often provides people the only or best available access to adequate or promising care. For example, children with AIDS initially could not get AZT because only adults could be enrolled in studies. Even after some studies showed that AZT was beneficial for treatment of adults, regulations initially forbade its prescription for children because it had not been tested with them (Pizzo). Moreover, a study excluding people of color, females, and children focuses upon a narrow range of the patient population (adult white males), making it uncertain whether the results of a study apply to other groups. There may be differences among groups; if there are, variations might be due to nature, nurture, or a combination of both. A study on depression, for example, conducted exclusively with white men, leaves uncertainty as to whether the results would be the same for other groups who have different social standing, burdens, genes, or physiologies.

More flexible eligibility requirements, advocates argue, would give all groups access to new treatments and would also yield results that more accurately reflect the entire patient population. Opponents respond that this would tend to make it harder to ensure that groups are comparable unless they have more subjects in the group. This would, of course, make the studies more costly. Despite these objections, policies were adopted to address unequal access and to revise eligibility criteria that excluded groups simply to save money and hold down the cost of trials, especially when studies were supported by tax dollars.

Patient-advocacy groups also demanded more access to preliminary information about the safety and efficacy of different modes of care. They wanted less secrecy regarding early trends, especially in cases in which patients have few treatment options for serious diseases. Many patients with severe or chronic diseases, or their families, have learned to follow closely relevant research, and they want greater access to promising new treatments.

These proposals generated a variety of responses (Byar et al.; Levine, Dubler, and Levine; Merigan; Schaffner, 1986; "Expanded Availability," 1990). For example, programs now make some investigational new treatments more available by means of expanded access or a "parallel track" ("Expanded Availability"). In the past, there was a single way, or *track*, for patients to get certain investigational new treatments, namely, participating in the study as a subject. Some people were excluded because they lived too far from the study site(s) or because of age, gender, or prognosis (Dresser; Kopelman, 1994). New programs expanded access or offered a parallel track to make it possible for some patients who are not subjects to have investigational new treatments. Patients with HIV-related diseases, for example, can sometimes obtain investigational new treatments even though they are not enrolled as trial subjects. Some investigators recommend this approach when there are no therapeutic alternatives, when the investigational new treatments are being tested, when there is some evidence of their efficacy, when there are no unreasonable risks for the patient, and when the patient cannot participate in the clinical trial (Byar et al.). This solution presupposes that there is agreement about who should make these verdicts. Community representation on panels that make these decisions may be reassuring to groups advocating more openness.

These and other proposals allow greater flexibility but also may make it harder to conduct and interpret the results (Ellenberg; Merigan). For example, if patients can get the investigational new treatment without enrolling in a clinical trial, some may refuse to participate in the study. Thus, even if these proposed changes are adopted, tensions still exist between individual and collective interests in conducting trials.

Conclusion

The CCT and RCT methodologies are powerful ways to combat the effects of bias. By using these methods, bias can be minimized, but it can never be entirely eradicated. People's beliefs, hopes, duties, prejudices, values, or interests can create biases in their choices about what studies to fund, when to begin and end studies, what measures will be used, how groups are established, and how results are interpreted.

When people consider the adoption of procedures such as copious amounts of oxygen for premature infants (later found to cause blindness), a high premium is placed on protection of the public from someone's idea of *promising* new treatments; when they think of drugs that have proved to help sustain or improve people's lives, however, a high premium is placed on early access. Who should decide the optimal degree of testing or protection needed in order to establish the safety and efficacy of drugs before they are available? This question of access versus protection is a social and moral decision, not just a scientific matter. It is not unlike the decision about how much inspection of foods or buildings is necessary in order to protect the public. When the stakes are high, as in fatal or chronically degenerative diseases with no promising treatments, the disputes about when to begin or end trials are sometimes a tangle of scientific, moral, social, political, statistical, and medical problems.

LORETTA M. KOPELMAN (1995)
REVISED BY AUTHOR

SEE ALSO: *Aging and the Aged: Healthcare and Research Issues; AIDS: Healthcare and Research Issues; Autoexperimentation; Children: Healthcare and Research Issues; Commercialism in Scientific Research; Embryo and Fetus: Embryo Research; Empirical Methods in Bioethics; Genetics and Human Behavior: Scientific and Research Issues; Holocaust; Infants: Public Policy and Legal Issues; Informed Consent: Consent Issues in Human Research; Mentally Ill and Mentally Disabled Persons: Research Issues; Military Personnel as Research Subjects; Minorities as Research Subjects; Pediatrics, Overview of Ethical Issues in; Prisoners as Research Subjects; Race and Racism; Research, Human: Historical Aspects; Research, Multinational; Research Policy; Research, Unethical; Responsibility; Scientific Publishing; Sexism; Students as Research Subjects; Virtue and Character;* and other *Research Methodology* subentries

BIBLIOGRAPHY

Angell, Marcia. 1997. "The Ethics of Clinical Research in the Third World." *New England Journal of Medicine* 337(12): 847–849.

Annas, George J. 1999. "Regs Ignored in Research." *National Law Journal,* 15 November, p. A20.

Beauchamp, Tom L., and Childress, James F. 1989, 2001. *Principles of Biomedical Ethics,* 3rd and 5th editions. New York: Oxford University Press.

Behrman, Richard E., and Vaughan, Victor C., III. 1987. *Nelson Textbook of Pediatrics,* 13th edition. Philadelphia: Saunders.

Byar, David P.; Schoenfeld, David A.; Green, Sylvan B.; et al.1990. "Design Considerations for AIDS Trials." *New England Journal of Medicine* 323(19): 1343–1348.

Chalmers, Thomas C.; Block, Jerome B.; and Lee, Stephanie. 1972. "Controlled Studies in Clinical Cancer Research." *New England Journal of Medicine* 287(2): 75–78.

Charney, Dennis S.; Nemeroff, Charles B.; Lewis, Lydia; et al. 2002. "National Depressive and Manic-Depressive Association Consensus Statement on the Use of Placebo in Clinical Trials of Mood Disorders." *Archives of General Psychiatry* 59(3): 262–270.

Concato, John; Shah, Nirav; and Horwitz, Ralph I. 2000. "Randomized, Controlled Trials, Observation Studies, and the Hierarchy of Research Designs." *New England Journal of Medicine* 342(25): 1887–1892.

Dresser, Rebecca. 1992. "Wanted: Single, White Male for Medical Research." *Hastings Center Report* 22(1): 24–29.

Ellenberg, Susan S. 1984. "Randomization Designs in Comparative Clinical Trials." *New England Journal of Medicine* 310(21): 1404–1408.

Ellenberg, Susan S. 1992. "Randomized Consent Designs for Clinical Trials: An Update." *Statistics in Medicine* 11(1): 131–132.

Ellenberg, Susan S., and Temple, Robert. 2000. "Placebo-Controlled Trials and Active-Control Trials in the Evaluation of New Treatments," Part 2: "Practical Issues and Specific Cases." *Annals of Internal Medicine* 133(6): 464–470.

Emanuel, Ezekiel J.; Wendler, David; and Grady, Christine. 2000. "What Makes Clinical Research Ethical?" *Journal of the American Medical Association* 283(20): 2701–2710.

"Expanded Availability of Investigational New Drugs through a Parallel Track Mechanism for People with AIDS and HIV-Related Disease." 1990. *Federal Register* 55, no. 98 (May 21): 20,856–20,860.

Fisher, Bernard. 1992. "Justification for Lumpectomy in the Treatment of Breast Cancer: A Commentary on the Underutilization of That Procedure." *Journal of the American Medical Women's Association* 47(5): 169–173.

Fisher, Bernard; Jeong, Jong-Hyeon; Anderson, Stewart; et al. 2002. "Twenty-five-Year Follow-up of a Randomized Trial Comparing Radical Mastectomy, Total Mastectomy, and Total Mastectomy Followed by Irradiation." *New England Journal of Medicine* 347(8): 567–575.

Freedman, Benjamin. 1987. "Equipoise and the Ethics of Clinical Research." *New England Journal of Medicine* 317(3): 141–145.

Fried, Charles. 1974. *Medical Experimentation: Personal Integrity and Social Policy.* New York: American Elsevier.

Gifford, Fred. 1986. "The Conflict between Randomized Clinical Trials and the Therapeutic Obligation." *Journal of Medicine and Philosophy* 11(4): 347–366.

Gigerenzer, Gerd; Swijtink, Zeno; Porter, Theodore; et al., eds. 1989. *The Empire of Chance: How Probability Changed Science and Everyday Life.* Cambridge, Eng.: Cambridge University Press.

Hrobjartsson, Asbjorn, and Gotzsche, Peter. 2001. "Is the Placebo Powerless? An Analysis of Clinical Trials Comparing Placebo with No Treatment." *New England Journal of Medicine* 344(21): 1594–1602.

Klein, Jason E., and Fleischman, Alan R. 2002. "The Private Practicing Physician-Investigator: Ethical Implications of Clinical Research in the Office Setting." *Hastings Center Report* 32(4): 22–26.

Kopelman, Loretta M. 1986. "Consent and Randomized Clinical Trials: Are There Moral or Design Problems?" *Journal of Medicine and Philosophy* 11(4): 317–345.

Kopelman, Loretta M. 1994. "How AIDS Activists Are Changing Research." In *Health Care Ethics: Critical Issues,* eds. John F. Monagle and David C. Thomasma. Gaithersburg, MD: Aspen.

Lerner, Barron H. 2001. *The Breast Cancer Wars: Hope, Fear, and the Pursuit of a Cure in Twentieth-Century America.* New York: Oxford University Press.

Levine, Carol; Dubler, Nancy N.; and Levine, Robert J. 1991. "Building a New Consensus: Ethical Principles and Policies for Clinical Research on HIV/AIDS." *IRB: A Review of Human Subjects Research* 13(1–2): 1–17.

Levine, Robert J. 1986. *Ethics and Regulation of Clinical Research,* 2nd edition. Baltimore, MD: Urban and Schwarzenberg.

Lurie, Peter, and Wolfe, Sidney M. 1997. "Unethical Trials of Interventions to Reduce Perinatal Transmission of the Human Immunodeficiency Virus in Developing Countries." *New England Journal of Medicine* 337(12): 853–856.

Marquis, Don. 1986. "An Argument That All Prerandomized Clinical Trials Are Unethical." *Journal of Medicine and Philosophy* 11(4): 367–383.

Merigan, Thomas C. 1990. "You Can Teach an Old Dog New Tricks: How AIDS Trials Are Pioneering New Strategies." *New England Journal of Medicine* 323(19): 1341–1343.

Pizzo, Philip A. 1990. "Pediatric AIDS: Problems within Problems." *Journal of Infectious Diseases* 161(2): 316–325.

Rothman, Kenneth J., and Michels, Karin B. 1994. "The Continuing Unethical Use of Placebo Controls." *New England Journal of Medicine* 331(6): 394–398.

Schaffner, Kenneth F. 1986. "Ethical Problems in Clinical Trials." *Journal of Medicine and Philosophy* 11(4): 297–315.

Schaffner, Kenneth F. 2002. "Assessment of Efficacy in Biomedicine: The Turn toward Methodological Pluralism." In *The Role of Complementary and Alternative Medicine: Accommodating Pluralism,* edited by Daniel Callahan. Washington, D.C.: Georgetown University Press.

Shaw, Lawrence W., and Chalmers, Thomas C. 1970. "Ethics in Cooperative Trials." *Annals of the New York Academy of Sciences* 169(2): 487–495.

Silverman, William A. 1980. *Retrolental Fibroplasia: A Modern Parable.* New York: Grune and Stratton.

Spilker, Bert. 1992. "Methods of Assessing and Improving Patient Compliance and Clinical Trials." *IRB: A Review of Human Subjects Research* 14(3): 1–6.

Steering Committee of the Physicians' Health Study Research Group. 1989. "Final Report on the Aspirin Component of the Ongoing Physicians' Health Study." *New England Journal of Medicine* 321(3): 129–135.

Taylor, Kathryn M.; Margolese, Richard G.; and Soskolne, Colin L. 1984. "Physicians' Reasons for Not Entering Eligible Patients in a Randomized Clinical Trial of Surgery for Breast Cancer." *New England Journal of Medicine* 310(21): 1363–1367.

Temple, Robert, and Ellenberg, Susan S. 2000. "Placebo-Controlled Trials and Active-Control Trials in the Evaluation of New Treatments," Part 1: "Ethical and Scientific Issues." *Annals of Internal Medicine* 133(6): 455–463.

Tobias, Jeffrey Stuart. 1988. "Informed Consent and Controlled Trials." *Lancet* 1988, vol. 2(8621): 1194.

Varmus, Harold, and Satcher, David. 1997. "Ethical Complexities of Conducting Research in Developing Countries." *New England Journal of Medicine* 337(14): 1003–1005.

Waldenstrom, Jan. 1983. "The Ethics of Randomization." In *Research Ethics,* edited by Kare Berg and Knut Erik Tranoy. New York: Alan R. Liss.

Wikler, Daniel. 1981. "Ethical Considerations in Randomized Clinical Trials." *Seminars in Oncology* 8(4): 437–441.

World Medical Association (WMA). 1996, revised 2000. "Declaration of Helsinki: Ethical Principles for Medical Research Involving Human Subjects." Ferney-Voltaire, France: Author.

Zelen, Marvin. 1979. "A New Design for Randomized Clinical Trials." *New England Journal of Medicine* 300(22): 1242–1245.

Zelen, Marvin. 1990. "Randomized Consent Designs for Clinical Trials: An Update." *Statistics in Medicine* 9(6): 645–656.

INTERNET RESOURCE

U. S. "Protection of Human Subjects." 1993. *Code of Federal Regulations.* Title 45, pt. 46. Available from <http://ohrp.osophs.dhhs.gov/humansubjects/guidance/45cfr46.htm>.

III. SUBJECTS

Selecting individuals to participate in research involves not only scientific decisions about appropriate entry criteria but also ethical decisions about the distribution of benefits and burdens. In *The Belmont Report* (1979), the U.S. National Commission for the Protection of Human Subjects of Biomedical and Behavioral Research cited three ethical principles as the foundation of research ethics. The first, respect for persons, and the second, beneficence, have been analyzed more often and in greater depth than the third, justice. Investigators, regulators, and institutional review boards (IRBs) are accustomed to applying the principle of beneficence by examining the risk-benefit ratio and applying the principle of respect for persons by examining informed consent. But the third principle—the selection of subjects as a matter of justice—has often been considered last and in only one of its aspects, the protection of vulnerable groups from exploitation as subjects.

This situation is changing as persons and groups previously excluded from research on grounds of vulnerability seek access to what they perceive as research benefits, primarily the opportunity to try new drugs for serious and life-threatening illnesses. However, the concept of vulnerability is itself coming under greater scrutiny as being ill-defined and too broad. In his 2001 paper, *Vulnerability in Research Subjects,* Kenneth Kipnis proposed a new taxonomy of vulnerability, which he defined as limitations on the ability to provide informed consent. He outlined six types of vulnerability, based on characteristics of the individual or society:

1. cognitive: the ability to understand information and make decisions;
2. juridic: being under the legal authority of someone such as a prison warden;
3. deferential: customary obedience to medical or other authority;
4. medical: having an illness for which there is no treatment;
5. allocational: poverty or educational deprivation; and
6. infrastructure: limits of the research setting to carry out the protocol.

According to the U.S. National Commission, justice is relevant to the selection of subjects at two levels: the social and the individual. At the individual level, "researchers [should] exhibit fairness: thus, they should not offer potentially beneficial research only to some patients who are in their favor or select only 'undesirable' persons for risky research" (U.S. National Commission, p. 7). At the social level, "distinctions [should] be drawn between classes of subjects that ought, and ought not, to participate in any particular kind of research, based on the ability of members of that class to bear burdens and on the appropriateness of placing further burdens on already burdened persons" (U.S. National Commission, p. 7). Specifically, on the grounds of social justice, classes of subjects should be ranked (e.g., adults before children) and some classes of potential subjects (e.g., prisoners and the institutionalized mentally infirm) should be selected only under certain conditions and should perhaps not be selected at all.

Very few philosophers or other scholars have proposed standards by which to establish priorities in the selection of subjects. Hans Jonas (1970) proposed a "descending order of permissibility" for the "conscription" of subjects. In his view, researchers themselves should be the first to test a new therapy, in that they can best understand the risks and benefits. Believing that very sick or dying patients are particularly vulnerable to researchers' invitations, Jonas opposed using them in research not directly related to their care.

Another approach has been to assert an obligation to participate in biomedical research. Arthur L. Caplan (1984) argued that research is a form of voluntary social cooperation that generates obligations of fairness and reciprocity. If a competent individual voluntarily seeks care in a hospital or institution that conducts biomedical research, he or she benefits from research and should share in its costs (i.e., participate). This obligation is a general one, not an obligation to volunteer for the first available trial or any particular trial.

Selecting the Least Vulnerable

Underlying these different views is the assumption that research is risky or at least burdensome. If this is true, subjects should be selected in a way that protects those whose social, demographic, or economic characteristics make them particularly vulnerable to coercion and exploitation. Volunteering for research is seen as either a duty to be discharged or an altruistic act to be applauded. This emphasis on protecting vulnerable persons is understandable given the signal event in the modern history of clinical research ethics—the cruel and often fatal experiments performed on unconsenting prisoners by Nazi doctors in World War II (Caplan, 1992). Public opinion in the United States also was shaped by the revelations of unethical experiments such as the Tuskegee Syphilis Study of poor black sharecroppers (Jones), the Willowbrook hepatitis B studies at an institution for mentally retarded children (Rothman, 1982), and the Jewish Chronic Disease Hospital studies in which live cancer cells were injected into uninformed elderly patients (Katz, Capron, and Glass). The most influential single article was one by Henry Knowles Beecher, a respected anesthesiologist, published in the *New England Journal of Medicine* in 1966; it described a series of studies at major research institutions that placed subjects at risk and in which the researchers failed to obtain informed consent (Rothman, 1991).

The view of research as inherently risky and of research subjects as inherently needing protection began to change in the early 1980s, but the pendulum may be swinging back to a more cautious view in the light of rare but highly publicized deaths of research subjects. In September 1999 Jesse Gelsinger, eighteen years old, died in a gene transfer. Ellen Roche and Hoiyan Wan, both young "normal, healthy volunteers," died in trials at Johns Hopkins University and the University of Rochester, respectively (Steinbrook, 2002a, 2002b). Research studies at several prominent medical centers were shut down temporarily after deficiencies in their procedures were identified.

The actual risk in most research studies is generally considered to be quite low, but there are no recent data. The

U.S. President's Commission for the Study of Ethical Problems in Medicine and Biomedical and Behavioral Research (1982) asked three large research institutions to summarize their experience with research-related injuries. Each group found a very low incidence of adverse effects. In one institution, out of more than 8,000 subjects involved in 157 protocols, only three adverse effects were reported, including two headaches after spinal taps. The definition of "adverse effect" is vague, however, especially among sick people, and it is possible that many adverse effects are not reported because they are deemed unrelated to the research study.

Sharing the Benefits of Research

The benefits side of the equation has assumed greater weight in individual decision making. Patients and advocacy groups are demanding more autonomy and less paternalism in the selection of subjects. Desperately ill patients forcefully argue that they are willing to trade a higher level of risk for the potential benefits of promising new procedures, devices, or drugs. Advocates for women and children point out that the typical exclusion or underrepresentation of these populations in clinical trials means that the drugs, when approved, will be prescribed for them with little direct data about dosage, efficacy, or side effects. These trends have been spurred by the vigorous, sometimes confrontational, efforts of persons with acquired immunodeficiency syndrome (AIDS). This advocacy also has stressed the inclusion of groups with poor access to trials, mainly women and minorities (C. Levine, 1988, 1993).

Increased emphasis on women's health issues has provided some information on subject recruitment. Examining the inclusion of women in clinical trials, the U.S. General Accounting Office reviewed the practices of the National Institutes of Health (NIH) and the Food and Drug Administration (FDA) (Nadel; U.S. General Accounting Office, 1992). In both instances women were found to be underrepresented. The FDA review found that women were represented in every clinical trial of the fifty-three drugs approved by the FDA in the previous three and a half years. For more than 60 percent of the drugs, however, the proportion of women in the trial was less than the proportion of women with the relevant disease. Women were particularly underrepresented in trials of cardiovascular drugs, even though cardiovascular disease is the leading cause of death in women.

In arguing for wider inclusion criteria in clinical trials, patient advocates and some clinicians have noted that in the interest of good medical care, drugs should be tested on the populations that will use them. This belief runs counter to the more traditional research view of subject selection, which focuses on testing drugs in a small, homogeneous population in order to detect differences in efficacy and side effects as rapidly as possible.

Even with broadened inclusion criteria, not all patients who want access to promising new agents can be enrolled in clinical trials because they fail to meet the inclusion criteria, they live too far from a research center, or the trials are already closed. Several other mechanisms have been developed, such as the "parallel track," in which qualified patients who cannot enroll in clinical trials may obtain a promising drug through their physician ("Expanded Availability," 1992). Community-based research, especially in cancer and AIDS, also has made clinical trials more accessible to patients.

The NIH has formalized the movement toward broader selection of subjects by mandating that its research grant recipients include appropriate numbers of women and minorities (Kirschstein). The 1993 NIH Revitalization Act (Pub. L. 103–43) extended the revised NIH policy by requiring the NIH director to ensure that women and members of minority groups are included in each federally funded project. The director may waive the requirement if the inclusion is inappropriate for health reasons, the purpose of the research, or any other circumstance. Cost, however, is not considered a permissible reason to fail to include women and members of minority groups.

This trend has limits, however. The inclusion of pregnant women in clinical trials is still controversial unless the trial is specifically designed to benefit the fetus, such as trials to prevent maternal–fetal transmission of the human immunodeficiency virus (HIV), which is associated with AIDS. Some of the objections to including pregnant women rely on ethical concerns about, for example, placing a fetus, who cannot consent, at risk. Most of the concerns are based on fears of legal liability should the fetus be born with an injury that might be attributed to the investigational drug. Other subject groups for which protection is still deemed essential include children (Levine, 1991), prisoners, and mentally ill persons. Still other groups sometimes cited as vulnerable include elderly people, military personnel, pharmaceutical company employees, and medical students. Although for these individuals some conditions and some protocols might be coercive, in general they can make choices voluntarily. Special procedures have been set up in some instances to ensure voluntariness (see, e.g., Winter, on the U.S. Department of Defense).

From the societal perspective, equitable selection of subjects means that the groups bearing the burdens of research should also share in its benefits. Opponents of research in prisons argue that the fruits of the research—newly approved drugs—are rarely available in that setting. Similarly, although many drug trials have been carried out in Third World countries, these nations are often so poor or so lacking in healthcare services that they cannot afford to provide the tested drugs to their citizens.

More recently, representatives of Third World countries and of poorly served communities in the United States have been demanding a greater role in the distribution of benefits (Lurie et al.; U.S. National Commission on AIDS; Thomas and Quinn). Their agreement to participate in clinical drug trials is sometimes conditioned on a promise from trial sponsors to provide something of benefit to the population—the drug, if it proves efficacious, or the health infrastructure needed to deliver the therapy. Efficacy trials for vaccines, which require thousands of subjects, cannot be conducted without the goodwill and participation of a community's leaders. Community consultation, in which investigators and community spokespersons collaborate on the design and implementation of a trial, is becoming a frequent strategy for ensuring that the concerns of the pool of potential subjects and their representatives are addressed.

Recognizing the importance of social justice in the distribution of burdens and benefits, the Council for International Organizations of Medical Sciences (CIOMS) guidelines for international research state:

Before undertaking research in a population or community with limited resources, the sponsor and the investigator must make every effort to ensure that:

- the research is responsive to the health needs and the priorities of the population or community in which it is to be carried out; and

- any intervention or product developed, or knowledge generated, will be made reasonably available for the benefit of that population or community. (CIOMS, p. 19)

Principal 19 of the World Medical Association's most recent restatement of the Declaration of Helsinki (1964, revised 2000) states: "Medical research is only justified if there is a reasonable likelihood that the populations in which the research is carried out stand to benefit from the results of the research."

The equitable selection of subjects now includes an assessment of both the need for protecting vulnerable individuals and groups and the importance of allowing them maximum choice in making the ultimate decision to participate. In the future, even more emphasis will be placed on the equitable distribution of the benefits of research.

CAROL LEVINE
THOMAS W. OGLETREE (1995)
BIBLIOGRAPHY REVISED

SEE ALSO: *Aging and the Aged: Healthcare and Research Issues; AIDS: Healthcare and Research Issues; Autoexperimentation; Autonomy; Children: Healthcare and Research Issues; Coercion; Commercialism in Scientific Research; Embryo and Fetus: Embryo Research; Empirical Methods in Bioethics; Freedom and Free Will; Genetics and Human Behavior: Scientific and Research Issues; Holocaust; Infants: Public Policy and Legal Issues; Informed Consent: Consent Issues in Human Research; Mentally Ill and Mentally Disabled Persons: Research Issues; Military Personnel as Research Subjects; Minorities as Research Subjects; Paternalism; Pediatrics, Overview of Ethical Issues in; Public Policy and Bioethics; Prisoners as Research Subjects; Race and Racism; Research, Human: Historical Aspects; Research Methodology; Research, Multinational; Research, Unethical; Responsibility; Scientific Publishing; Sexism; Students as Research Subjects; Virtue and Character;* and other *Research Policy* subentries

BIBLIOGRAPHY

Beecher, Henry K. 1966. "Ethics and Clinical Research." *New England Journal of Medicine* 274(24): 1354–1360.

Caplan, Arthur L. 1984. "Is There a Duty to Serve as a Subject in Biomedical Research?" *IRB: A Review of Human Subjects Research* 6(5): 1–5.

Caplan, Arthur L., ed. 1992. *When Medicine Went Mad: Bioethics and the Holocaust.* Totowa, NJ: Humana.

Council for International Organizations of Medical Sciences (CIOMS), in collaboration with the World Health Organization. 2002. *International Ethical Guidelines for Biomedical Research Involving Human Subjects.* Geneva, Switzerland: Author.

"Expanded Availability of Investigational New Drugs through a Parallel Track Mechanism for People with AIDS and Other HIV-Related Disease." 1992. *Federal Register* 57(73): 13250–13259.

Jonas, Hans. 1970. "Philosophical Reflections on Experimenting with Human Subjects." In *Experimentation with Human Subjects,* ed. Paul A. Freund. New York: George Braziller.

Jones, James H. 1993. *Bad Blood: The Tuskegee Syphilis Experiment,* new and expanded edition. New York: Free Press.

Katz, Jay; Capron, Alexander M.; and Glass, Eleanor Swift, eds. 1972. *Experimentation with Human Beings: The Authority of the Investigator, Subject, Professions, and State in the Human Experimentation Process.* New York: Russell Sage Foundation.

Kipnis, Kenneth. 2001. *Vulnerability in Research Subjects: A Bioethical Taxonomy.* Bethesda, MD: National Bioethics Advisory Commission.

Kirschstein, Ruth L. 1991. "Research on Women's Health." *American Journal of Public Health* 81(3): 291–293.

Levine, Carol. 1988. "Has AIDS Changed the Ethics of Human Subjects Research?" *Law, Medicine, and Health Care* 16(3–4): 167–173.

Levine, Carol. 1991. "Children in HIV/AIDS Clinical Trials: Still Vulnerable after All These Years." *Law, Medicine, and Health Care* 19(3–4): 231–237.

Levine, Carol. 1993. "Women as Research Subjects: New Priorities, New Questions." In *Emerging Issues in Biomedical Policy: An Annual Review,* ed. Robert H. Blank and Andrea L. Bonnicksen. New York: Columbia University Press.

Levine, Robert J. 1984. "What Kinds of Subjects Can Understand This Protocol?" *IRB: A Review of Human Subjects Research* 6(5): 6–8.

Levine, Robert J. 1988. *Ethics and Regulation of Clinical Research,* 2nd edition. New Haven, CT: Yale University Press.

Lurie, Peter; Bishaw, Makonnen; Chesney, Margaret A.; et al. 1994. "Ethical, Behavioral, and Social Aspects of HIV Vaccine Trials in Developing Countries." *Journal of the American Medical Association* 271(4): 295–301.

Nadel, Mark V. 1990. "National Institutes of Health: Problems Implementing Policy on Women in Study Populations. Statement of Mark V. Nadel, Associate Director, National and Public Health Issues, Human Resources Division, before the Subcommittee on Health and the Environment, Committee on Energy and Commerce, House of Representatives." GAO/T-HRD-90-38. Washington, D.C.: U.S. General Accounting Office.

National Institutes of Health Revitalization Act. 1993. U.S. Public Law 103-43.

Rothman, David J. 1982. "Were Tuskegee and Willowbrook 'Studies in Nature'?" *Hastings Center Report* 12(2): 5–7.

Rothman, David J. 1991. *Strangers at the Bedside: A History of How Law and Bioethics Transformed Medical Decision Making.* New York: Basic.

Steinbrook, Robert. 2002a. "Protecting Research Subjects: The Crisis at Johns Hopkins." *New England Journal of Medicine* 346(10): 716–720.

Steinbrook, Robert. 2002b. "Improving Protection for Research Subjects." *New England Journal of Medicine* 346(18): 1425–1430.

Thomas, Stephen B., and Quinn, Sandra Crouse. 1991. "The Tuskegee Syphilis Study, 1932 to 1972: Implications for HIV Education and AIDS Risk Education Programs in the Black Community." *American Journal of Public Health* 81(11): 1498–1504.

U.S. General Accounting Office. 1992. "Women's Health: FDA Needs to Ensure More Study of Gender Differences in Prescription Drug Testing: Report to Congressional Requesters." GAO/HRD-93-17. Washington, D.C.: Author.

U.S. National Commission for the Protection of Human Subjects of Biomedical and Behavioral Research. 1979. *The Belmont Report: Ethical Principles and Guidelines for the Protection of Human Subjects of Research.* Washington, D.C.: U.S. Government Printing Office.

U.S. National Commission on AIDS. 1992. *The Challenge of HIV/AIDS in Communities of Color,* ed. Linda C. Humphrey and Frances Porcher. Washington, D.C.: Author.

U.S. President's Commission for the Study of Ethical Problems in Medicine and Biomedical and Behavioral Research. 1982. *Compensating for Research Injuries: A Report on the Ethical and Legal Implications of Programs to Redress Injuries Caused by Biomedical and Behavioral Research.* Washington, D.C.: Author.

Winter, Philip E. 1984. "Human Subject Research Review in the Department of Defense." *IRB: A Review of Human Subjects Research* 6(3): 9–10.

World Medical Association (WMA). 1964 (revised 2000). "Declaration of Helsinki: Ethical Principles for Medical Research Involving Human Subjects." Ferney-Voltaire, France: Author.

RESEARCH, MULTINATIONAL

• • •

The term *multinational research* refers to biomedical, epidemiological, or social science research that involves investigators and subjects from more than one nation. The type of multinational research that has raised the most ethical concerns is that in which the investigators or sponsors are from an industrialized country and the research is conducted in a developing country (the "host" country). Two chief ethical concerns have dominated this type of research in the past. The first concern is that research subjects in the host country might be vulnerable by virtue of their low educational level or lack of familiarity with modern scientific concepts and, therefore, open to exploitation in some manner. The second concern is that the cultural norms and practices in the industrialized and host countries may differ, leading to the question of which to adhere to when such norms and practices conflict.

More recently, a third ethical concern has become prominent: the level of care and treatment provided to research subjects during a clinical trial. Should it be identical to what subjects in the industrialized, sponsoring country would receive in a similar trial? Or can a lower level of care be justified based on affordability and a less well-developed infrastructure in resource-poor countries? These latter questions have been prompted primarily by HIV/AIDS research conducted in countries in Africa and Asia. A fourth concern has also risen to prominence in recent years: What, if anything, is owed to trial participants, to the community, or to the host country as a whole when a biomedical research project results in a successful product?

Two trends bring concern about biomedical research ethics in a multinational context to the fore. The first is a vast increase in the number of studies conducted in developing countries and sponsored by the pharmaceutical industry or by governmental agencies of industrialized countries (Brennan; U.S. Department of Health and Human Services). The second trend is the growing gap in the burden of disease between industrialized and developing countries, a result in part of the AIDS epidemic but also stemming from the lack of affordable treatments for diseases such as malaria and tuberculosis in resource-poor countries (Michaud, Murray, and Bloom).

Although the chief ethical concerns of the past continue to require vigilance in the ethical review and conduct of multinational research, the two more recent concerns have generated considerable controversy. A clinical trial conducted in Thailand and other developing countries, aimed at finding an affordable and appropriate treatment to prevent the transmission of HIV/AIDS from pregnant women to their infants, led to fierce debates in leading medical and bioethics journals (Angell; Lurie and Wolfe; Varmus and Satcher; Annas and Grodin, 1998; Crouch and Arras; Lie; Schüklenk). The controversy went beyond the debates in academic journals, leading eventually to a prolonged process to revise two of the leading international ethical guidelines for research: the World Medical Association's Declaration of Helsinki and the *International Ethical Guidelines for Biomedical Research Involving Human Subjects,* prepared by the Council for International Organizations of Medical Sciences (CIOMS) in conjunction with the World Health Organization.

International Research Guidelines and Recommendations

The first international code of ethics for research involving human subjects, the Nuremberg Code, was drafted in 1947 at the Nuremberg Doctors' Trial in response to the atrocities committed by physicians in Nazi Germany in experiments they conducted on inmates of concentration camps (Annas and Grodin, 1992). The purpose of the code was both to acknowledge the importance of research involving human beings and to provide a set of universally applicable rules for protecting human subjects of research from violations of their rights and welfare. The first principle of the Nuremberg Code is: "The voluntary consent of the human subject is absolutely essential." This requires that the subject "be able to exercise free power of choice, without ... any element of force, fraud, deceit, duress ... or coercion; and should have sufficient knowledge and comprehension of the elements of the subject matter involved as to enable him to make an understanding and enlightened decision." Other principles in the Nuremberg Code require that the proposed research be meaningful and essential, that it be based on prior animal experiments, and that it "avoid all unnecessary physical and mental suffering and injury."

The Declaration of Helsinki, first promulgated by the World Medical Association (WMA) in 1964, with relatively minor revisions in 1975, 1983, 1989, and 1996, adapted and expanded the principles of the Nuremberg Code to apply more readily to clinical research in the medical setting. Until the revision in 2000, the Declaration of Helsinki did not address the special features of research sponsored by industrialized countries and carried out in developing countries. However, the controversy that surrounded the trial to test an affordable drug to prevent maternal-to-child transmission of HIV/AIDS produced a subsequent, related controversy over a provision in the Declaration of Helsinki itself.

Critics of the HIV/AIDS trial in developing countries argued that the trial design was unethical because some of the pregnant women were given a placebo, an inactive substance, thereby withholding from them a treatment proven to be effective in reducing the transmission of HIV/AIDS in the United States. These critics also contended that the trial violated the following provision in the Declaration of Helsinki: "In any medical study, every patient—including those of a control group, if any—should be assured of the best proven diagnostic and therapeutic method. This does not exclude the use of inert placebo in studies where no proven diagnostic or therapeutic method exists" (WMA, II, 3). Whereas critics of the placebo-controlled trials cited the Declaration of Helsinki in support of their contention that the trials were unethical (Lurie and Wolfe), defenders of the trials argued that the Declaration of Helsinki was in need of revision (Levine).

The WMA embarked on a process to revise the declaration, a process that took place over a two-year period and was itself fraught with controversy. In an effort to make the process transparent and democratic, the WMA posted a draft of the revised version on its web site and invited comments. As a consequence of many comments that found the draft unsatisfactory primarily because it weakened the provision requiring that a control group be given "the best proven diagnostic and therapeutic method," the WMA appointed a new drafting committee whose members reinstated the original requirement in slightly different words: "The benefits, risks, burdens and effectiveness of a new method should be tested against those of the best current prophylactic, diagnostic, and therapeutic methods. This does not exclude the use of placebo, or no treatment, in studies where no proven prophylactic, diagnostic or therapeutic method exists" (WMA, paragraph 29).

The newly revised draft was posted on the WMA web site, once again with an invitation for comments. In October 2000 the WMA adopted the second revised version at its meeting in Edinburgh, Scotland. But that did not end the controversy. A substantial number of influential spokespersons from the research community, the pharmaceutical industry, and U.S. federal agencies that sponsor research objected that adherence to this provision would prevent important research from going forward that could benefit developing countries. In an attempt to compromise between these opposing factions, the WMA issued the following clarification in 2001:

> The WMA is concerned that paragraph 29 of the revised Declaration of Helsinki (October 2000) has led to diverse interpretations and possible confusion. It hereby reaffirms its position that extreme care must be taken in making use of a placebo-controlled trial and that in general this methodology should only be used in the absence of existing proven therapy. However, a placebo-controlled trial may be ethically acceptable, even if proven therapy is available, under the following circumstances:
>
> - Where for compelling and scientifically sound methodological reasons its use is necessary to determine the efficacy or safety of a prophylactic, diagnostic or therapeutic method; or
> - Where a prophylactic, diagnostic, or therapeutic method is being investigated for a minor condition and the patients who receive placebo will not be subject to any additional risk of serious or irreversible harm….

This clarification did not lay the controversy to rest. Defenders of placebo-controlled trials conducted in developing countries would cite what they consider "compelling and scientifically sound methodological reasons" for using placebo controls. Critics of such trials would then question whether the reasons provided were scientifically compelling and would propose instead a trial design comparing the experimental treatment with a treatment currently and widely used in the industrialized country sponsoring the research. The debate appears intractable, with each side comprising researchers, bioethicists, governmental spokespersons, and others from both developing and industrialized countries.

The same controversial clinical trials that prompted revision of the Declaration of Helsinki created a need to undertake a review and revision of the CIOMS *International Ethical Guidelines,* which were first published in 1993. In part because the CIOMS guidelines were promulgated with the purpose of applying the standards of the Declaration of Helsinki in developing countries, but also because the rapidly increasing amount of multinational research called for a reassessment of the 1993 guidelines, a multistage process was undertaken for the CIOMS revisions.

Predictably, the same debate that arose among defenders and opponents of placebo-controlled trials in the revision of the Declaration of Helsinki surfaced among drafters, members of an appointed steering committee, and commentators who responded to a posting of drafts on the CIOMS web site. The controversial guideline that emerged from this process departs significantly from the strict requirement in the Declaration of Helsinki; it permits clinical trials "in which the comparator is other than the best current intervention, such as placebo or no treatment or a local remedy" (CIOMS, Guideline 11). The justification for withholding the best current intervention is that it "cannot be used as comparator because its use as comparator would not yield scientifically reliable results that would be relevant to the health needs of the study population" (CIOMS, Guideline 11). Critics of this position argue that it is unethical to use placebos when doing so can lead to serious or irreversible harm to subjects in the control group.

Other studies of multinational research were launched at about the same time. The U.S. National Bioethics Advisory Commission (NBAC) launched an international project and in 2001 issued a final report, *Ethical and Policy Issues in International Research.* This report contains a recommendation on the same controversial point:

> Researchers and sponsors should design clinical trials that provide members of any control group with an established effective treatment, whether or not such treatment is available in the host country. Any study that would not provide the control group with an established effective treatment should include a justification for using an alternative design. Ethics review committees must assess the justification provided, including the risks to participants, and the overall ethical acceptability of the research design. (NBAC, Recommendation 2.2)

This recommendation sets up a strong presumption to provide an "established effective treatment" to the control group. But it also contains an escape hatch, allowing the proposal of an alternative trial design, which must be approved by an ethics review committee.

The Nuffield Council on Bioethics in the United Kingdom issued a report on multinational research one year after publication of the NBAC report. The Nuffield report's recommendation on level of care provided to a control group is also less stringent than the requirements in the 2000 Declaration of Helsinki:

> Wherever appropriate, participants in the control group should be offered a universal standard of care for the disease being studied. Where it is not appropriate to offer a universal standard of care, the minimum standard of care that should be offered to the control group is the best intervention available for that disease as part of the national public health system. (Nuffield Council, paragraph 7.29)

This unresolved controversy about what should be provided to a control group gives rise to a series of philosophical questions about ethical guidelines: When reasonable people disagree on key provisions, what should be done? Should the controversy be resolved in favor of the position held by the majority? Should it be resolved in favor of the more influential party to the dispute? Or should there be no guideline at all on points of major contention among reasonable persons of good will? On the one hand, if a published ethical guideline is systematically violated, it leads to disrespect for or cynicism about the guidelines as a whole. This is the contention of critics of the paragraph in the Declaration of Helsinki requiring that a control group receive "the best current treatment." On the other hand, if a guideline is published and held by some to be exploitative of research subjects in developing countries, it creates a general skepticism concerning the ethical conduct of multinational research. This is the view of defenders of the paragraph requiring the "best current treatment" for the control group in studies in developing countries.

Understanding the Controversy

Opponents on both sides of this controversy are committed to finding appropriate and affordable diagnostic, prophylactic, and therapeutic methods for populations in developing countries. Both sides believe that to be ethical, research must be responsive to the health needs of the population where the research is conducted. That is where their agreement ends.

The chief difference between the two sides from an ethical perspective concerns the obligation to research subjects enrolled in a clinical trial. A study with the identical design of the maternal-to-child transmission study carried out in Thailand could not have been conducted in the United States for both moral and practical reasons. Morally, women outside the trial in the United States had access to an effective treatment, so they would be made worse off if they

participated in the trial. Practically, many would obtain the effective treatment from other sources, undermining the study. In contrast, women in the trials in developing countries had limited or no access to a preventive treatment for their infants outside the trial, so those in the placebo group would not be made worse off by participating in the trial. Defenders of the placebo controls contended that women in the control group received the "standard of care" in their country. Critics argued that they could have been provided with the effective treatment, which could then have been compared to the experimental treatment.

As the Thai studies demonstrate, what appears to be a straightforward debate about obligations to research subjects in a clinical trial turns in part into a debate over research methodology. Defenders of the placebo-controlled trials argue that the research question to be addressed is: "In cases where there is no standard treatment whatsoever, is the experimental treatment better than nothing?" To answer that question, the only appropriate research design is one that uses a placebo control. Moreover, some test placebo against standard treatments in the United States because they can make the case that the treatment may not be any better than placebo and it is important to find that out. Critics of these placebo-controlled trials argue that a different research question is meaningful and could be addressed: "Is the experimental drug as good, or almost as good, as the best current treatment used in the United States?" The first group argues that an answer to the latter question is not responsive to the needs of the developing country. The second group replies that given a large enough number of subjects, the use of appropriate statistical tools, and a research design comparing the experimental and the proven treatments, a research question relevant to the developing country can be formulated and answered.

Thus a resolution to this ethical controversy turns, in part, on a methodological issue in the design and conduct of clinical trials. Because researchers and methodologists can be found on both sides of the debate, there is little hope that this type of controversy can be resolved by rational means unless the risks of harm are low.

Providing Posttrial Benefits in Developing Countries

The 2000 version of the Declaration of Helsinki added two new provisions that were not included in the revision issued only four years earlier. These new paragraphs reflect the widely acknowledged fact that much past research conducted in developing countries failed to produce subsequent benefits to the populations of the countries in which the research was carried out; the benefits of biomedical research typically accrued to the populations in industrialized countries. This imbalance violates the principle of distributive justice, which calls for an equitable distribution of the benefits and burdens of research. Paragraph 19 of the declaration addresses this point: "Medical research is only justified if there is a reasonable likelihood that the populations in which the research is carried out stand to benefit from the results of the research." And paragraph 30 states: "At the conclusion of the study, every patient entered into the study should be assured of access to the best proven prophylactic, diagnostic and therapeutic methods identified by the study."

Both of these newly added provisions are a response to criticisms that have been leveled against past research sponsored by industrialized countries or industry in which any resulting benefits of the research have accrued to the sponsoring country but not to the population from which the research subjects were drawn. Paragraph 19 of the 2000 declaration seeks to ensure that research is not carried out on inhabitants of developing countries solely for the benefit of inhabitants of wealthy, industrialized countries. Paragraph 30 seeks to ensure that the sponsoring country or industry does not simply pull out when the study is concluded, abandoning research subjects who still need a treatment that has been demonstrated to be effective.

Although these situations might very well occur when research is conducted wholly within an industrialized country, the lack of access to affordable treatments outside a research study is much more prevalent in resource-poor countries. This has been especially true of medications to treat HIV/AIDS. By the year 2000, virtually all pregnant women in the United States had access to effective treatments to prevent HIV transmission to their infants, but those treatments remained out of reach for most inhabitants of most developing countries (Joint United Nations Programme on HIV/AIDS, 2002). Effective treatments to prevent progression of HIV infection into symptomatic AIDS is also available to large numbers of people in industrialized countries, but here again, only a small minority of people in developing countries can afford the cost of these drugs, which remain too expensive for purchase by the ministries of health, as well. (Brazil has been an exception, as the government made a commitment to provide treatments for HIV/AIDS to its entire infected population.)

The requirement that research be responsive to the health needs of the population of the country in which the research is conducted has been a feature of the CIOMS guidelines, which were promulgated specifically with developing countries in mind. The 2002 revision of the guidelines reiterates a requirement in the 1993 version that the research be responsive to the health needs and priorities of the community in which it is carried out. The 2002 revision goes considerably further than the 1993 version by elevating a key provision to the status of a guideline instead of being relegated to the commentary under a guideline:

Guideline 10: Research in populations and communities with limited resources

Before undertaking research in a population or community with limited resources, the sponsor and the investigator must make every effort to ensure that:

- the research is responsive to the health needs and the priorities of the population or community in which it is to be carried out; and
- any intervention or product developed, or knowledge generated, will be made reasonably available for the benefit of that population or community.

Although the term *reasonably available* has been criticized as being too vague, the guideline nevertheless establishes a presumption for sponsoring countries or industry to seek to ensure access to successful products developed in the course of research conducted in developing countries. The reports of both the NBAC and the Nuffield Council on Bioethics address this issue, but their recommendations permit a failure to ensure access if researchers provide sufficient justification to a research ethics committee.

Preventing Exploitation

The ongoing controversy over what should be provided to a control group and the acceptability of placebo controls, along with the question of posttrial obligations to research subjects, the community, and the country in which the research takes place, have overtaken the main ethical concerns of the past regarding multinational research. Yet those past concerns have not disappeared. The need to prevent exploitation of research subjects is an ethical requirement everywhere, but it becomes more problematic in settings where subjects are illiterate or semiliterate, and where they are unfamiliar with the concepts of modern science as well as the purpose and conduct of biomedical research. Two mechanisms exist to aid in protecting research subjects from violations of their rights and welfare: prior ethical review of research protocols by an independent committee; and an adequate process for obtaining voluntary, informed consent from individual subjects. Problem exist with regard to the effectiveness of both of these mechanisms in developing countries.

PRIOR ETHICAL REVIEW. The first and most obvious shortcoming is the absence of ethical review committees in many developing countries and in the institutions within those countries (such committees are termed institutional review boards [IRBs] in the United States, research ethics boards [REBs] in Canada, and other names elsewhere). Even where such committees exist, they may be newly established and therefore inexperienced. Even committees that are not recently established may lack adequate education and training for their members. Or they may be staffed with researchers or institutional officials who have a conflict of interest regarding the research to be reviewed. In the poorest countries, institutions lack the resources to make photocopies of the protocols to be reviewed by all the members, and time spent on committee work means loss of income from clinical work for which they would otherwise be paid.

Recent guidelines and reports acknowledge these shortcomings and propose that they be remedied through efforts to build capacity for local or national ethical review in developing countries. For example, a guidance document issued by the Joint United Nations Programme on HIV/AIDS (UNAIDS) contains the following point, titled "Capacity building": "Strategies should be implemented to build capacity in host countries and communities so that they can practise meaningful self-determination in vaccine development, can ensure the scientific and ethical conduct of vaccine development, and can function as equal partners with sponsors and others in a collaborative process" (UNAIDS, p. 15). Although the guideline specifically addresses vaccine research, a similar point appears in many other documents.

The revised version of the CIOMS guidelines issued in 2002 elevates to the level of a guideline the obligation of sponsors of research to engage in building capacity for ethical review (in the 1993 CIOMS guidelines, the obligation appeared under a commentary):

Guideline 20: Strengthening capacity for ethical and scientific review and biomedical research

Many countries lack the capacity to assess or ensure the scientific quality or ethical acceptability of biomedical research proposed or carried out in their jurisdictions. In externally sponsored collaborative research, sponsors and investigators have an ethical obligation to ensure that biomedical research projects for which they are responsible in such countries contribute effectively to national or local capacity to design and conduct biomedical research, and to provide scientific and ethical review and monitoring of such research.

The obligation of sponsoring countries and agencies to build capacity for ethical review of research is included as a recommendation in both the NBAC and Nuffield reports. The NBAC report states:

Recommendation 5.7: Where applicable, U.S. sponsors and researchers should assist in building the capacity of ethics review committees in developing countries to conduct scientific and ethical review of international collaborative research.

INFORMED CONSENT. The second mechanism designed to prevent exploitation of research subjects is the requirement for voluntary, informed consent from each prospective research subject. All ethical guidelines for research include this requirement, which can pose special problems in multinational research in countries in which customs, traditions, and even the concept of a person vary considerably from those that predominate in the North America and Europe. In some developing countries a substantial portion of the population is illiterate or semiliterate. It is clear that the practice of requiring written, signed consent documents when the research subjects are illiterate is inappropriate. For semiliterate subjects, a written consent document may be appropriate, especially because family members whom the subject may wish to involve in the consent process may be literate.

It is important to distinguish between the requirement that a written document be provided to a prospective subject and the requirement that the subject sign the document. In some countries, the meaning of signing a document is quite different from what it is in North America or Western Europe. Even when the need for individual, informed consent is fully accepted, if the country has a history of oppressive regimes, or if people are fearful, based on their experience, that a signed document might be used against them in some manner, it is appropriate for the research ethics committee to waive the requirement of a signature on a consent document (NBAC).

One challenge for researchers who conduct clinical trials in developing countries is how to deal with practices that depart from the requirements of informed consent in the United States and other industrialized countries. These practices include withholding diagnoses from patients who become research subjects (Sugarman et al.; Kass and Hyder) and not disclosing key elements that comply with the substantive ethical standard of informed consent, such as the use of placebo controls, the process of randomizing subjects into different groups in a clinical trial, and the expected efficacy (or lack of efficacy) of a method being tested (Sugarman et al.). Even if the custom of routinely withholding complete information from patients with certain diseases might be defended in ordinary medical practice, it poses a severe challenge to the need to adhere strictly to the ethical standard of disclosure required for research involving human subjects. Potential subjects cannot make an informed decision to participate without knowing that they may not receive a proven treatment that will benefit them. To enroll individuals who are not provided with these key items of information deviates from the substantive ethical standard of disclosure required for adequate informed consent.

A different problem arises when research subjects are unacquainted with the concepts and methods of modern science or biomedical research. These problems are addressed in NBAC's 2001 report, *Ethical and Policy Issues in International Research,* which contains several recommendations on informed consent. Recommendation 3.2 urges researchers to seek creative ways of presenting information, for example, by means of analogies readily understood by the population:

> Researchers should develop culturally appropriate ways to disclose information that is necessary for adherence to the substantive ethical standard of informed consent, with particular attention to disclosures relating to diagnosis and risk, research design, and possible post-trial benefits. Researchers should describe in their protocols and justify to the ethics review committee(s) the procedures they plan to use for disclosing such information to participants. (NBAC, p. 40)

It is not sufficient simply to present the information. An important component of the process is determining whether the prospective subjects adequately understand what they have been told. To this end, NBAC has two recommendations:

> Recommendation 3.4: Researchers should develop procedures to ensure that potential participants do, in fact, understand the information provided in the consent process and should describe those procedures in their research protocols.

and

> Recommendation 3.5: Researchers should consult with community representatives to develop innovative and effective means to communicate all necessary information in a manner that is understandable to potential participants. When community representatives will not be involved, the protocol presented to the ethics review committee should justify why such involvement is not possible or relevant. (NBAC, p. 42)

Some have considered it problematic in cross-cultural contexts to require that informed consent be obtained from each individual recruited as a research subject. This has been described as "philosophically and practically difficult" (Christakis and Levine, p. 1783). The problem is characterized as one in which some cultures lack the individualistic concept of a person to which the Western world adheres, so the question of how to apply the respect for persons principle becomes problematic. Debate on this point is illustrated in the following two positions.

The first holds that researchers should adhere to local customs and traditions regarding individual informed consent, and that it is ethical imperialism to insist on Western requirements in other cultures (Newton). The second maintains the opposite view that individual informed consent is a requirement that should not be eliminated or altered: "We see no convincing arguments for a general policy of dispensing with, or substantially modifying, the researcher's obligation to obtain first-person consent in biomedical research conducted in Africa" (IJsselmuiden and Faden, p. 883).

The Nuffield Council on Bioethics report addresses the tension between respect for culture and respect for persons:

> [W]e cannot avoid the responsibility of taking a view when the two aspects of respect—respect for culture and respect for persons—come into conflict with one another. We are of the view that the fundamental principle of respect for persons requires that participants who have the capacity to consent to research should never be subjected to research without such consent. (Nuffield Council, paragraph 6.22)

Those who would subordinate the respect for persons principle to other considerations have not identified a competing ethical principle that deserves a higher ranking. The unstated assumption that respect for cultural tradition may outrank respect for persons construes respect for cultural tradition as an ethical principle on a par with the following three widely acknowledged principles: respect for persons, beneficence, and justice (National Commission). Although an ethical obligation to be culturally sensitive should be honored, a limit is reached when a cultural practice violates an internationally accepted principle of research ethics.

A different sort of problem arises when it is necessary to obtain permission from a community leader or tribal chief in order to enter the community to embark on research. That requirement has to be respected, but it is no different, in principle, from the need in Western culture to obtain permission from the head of a workplace or a school principal to enter the premises to conduct research. Permission from a tribal chief or village leader may be required but should not serve as a substitute for individual informed consent obtained from each potential subject. The NBAC report contains the following recommendation:

> Where culture or custom requires that permission of a community representative be granted before researchers may approach potential research participants, researchers should be sensitive to such local requirements. However, in no case may permission from a community representative or council replace the requirement of a competent individual's voluntary informed consent. (NBAC, p. 43)

Considerably more problematic is the need to obtain individual informed consent from women in cultures in which the husband or father of an adult woman normally grants permission for her participation in activities outside the home. NBAC's recommendation on this point calls for a presumption to treat men and woman equally in the informed-consent process but allows for a loophole:

> Researchers should use the same procedures in the informed-consent process for women and men. However, ethics review committees may accept a consent process in which a woman's individual consent to participate in research is supplemented by permission from a man if all of the following conditions are met:
>
> a. it would be impossible to conduct the research without obtaining such supplemental permission; and
>
> b. failure to conduct this research could deny its potential benefits to women in the host country; and
>
> c. measures to respect the woman's autonomy to consent to research are undertaken to the greatest extent possible.
>
> In no case may a competent adult woman be enrolled in research solely upon the consent of another person; her individual consent is always required. (NBAC, p. 45)

Here, as in other recommendations, NBAC leaves the ultimate decision on controversial matters to the discretion of the ethics review committee. The Nuffield Council's recommendation on this point is also somewhat flexible.

Unlike the NBAC and Nuffield recommendations, the CIOMS 2002 guidelines do not permit a departure from the need to obtain individual informed consent from the woman only. The commentary under Guideline 16 states:

> [O]nly the informed consent of the woman herself is required for her participation. In no case should

the permission of a spouse or partner replace the requirement of individual informed consent. If women wish to consult with their husbands or partners or seek voluntarily to obtain their permission before deciding to enroll in research, that is not only ethically permissible but in some contexts highly desirable. A strict requirement of authorization of spouse or partner, however, violates the substantive principle of respect for persons.

In this, as in other areas of multinational research, what some people take to be ethical imperialism, others consider proper adherence to universally applicable ethical standards.

INDUCEMENTS. In avoiding exploitation when research is conducted in developing countries, there are two important considerations: whether inducements are offered for participation and whether such inducements are undue, that is, so attractive as to diminish voluntariness on the part of subjects who are invited to enroll. When medical treatment is an inevitable part or accompaniment of clinical research, this may provide a strong inducement to enrollment for people without access to medical care. The Nuffield Council report noted that this need not amount to exploitation. The report stated, however, that "when participants are ill and do not have alternative ways of receiving treatment, the possibility for exploitation is greater" (Nuffield Council, paragraph 6.29). The report urged that special care should be taken in determining the type and amount of additional healthcare that may be offered to participants as an inducement.

The NBAC report addresses this concern, distinguishing between, on the one hand, an inducement that may exist because participants receive beneficial clinical care and, on the other hand, the different circumstance that arises out of the "therapeutic misconception"—the belief that the purpose of a clinical trial is to benefit the individual patient rather than to gather data for the purpose of contributing to scientific knowledge. This misconception is widespread even among research subjects in industrialized countries and may be considerably greater in developing countries where people are unfamiliar with scientific research and view medical researchers as healers in whom they place great trust. The NBAC report recommends the following: "Researchers working in developing countries should indicate in their research protocols how they would minimize the likelihood that potential participants will believe mistakenly that the purpose of the research is solely to administer treatment rather than to contribute to scientific knowledge" (NBAC, p. 48).

Guideline 7 of the 2002 CIOMS document permits both monetary payments to subjects as an inducement to participate in research and the provision of free medical services. CIOMS cautions that the monetary payments should not be so great or the medical services so extensive that they induce people to participate against their better judgment. Any payments or provision of medical services should be approved by an ethical review committee.

Crossing National Boundaries: Ethical Standards and Procedural Variations

Different views exist regarding how conflicts between Western cultural conceptions and norms and those of non-Western cultures should be resolved. This raises the question of how ethical standards should be arrived at and whose standards should be adopted. The 1993 CIOMS guidelines included in Guideline 15 a provision intended to prevent exploitation, titled "Obligations of sponsoring and host countries" in externally sponsored research. This guideline required scientific and ethical review of proposed research "according to the standards of the country of the sponsoring agency, and the ethical standards applied should be no less exacting than they would be in the case of research carried out in that country." This provision prompted the criticism that the guidelines reflected a "Western bias" because of "the assumption that the circumstances … in the developed world are the norm. Thus, the developed world is envisioned as more advanced, not only technologically but also morally" (Christakis and Levine, p. 1781).

This criticism is not shared by the many developing countries that by 2002 had enacted laws or adopted ethical guidelines governing research (NBAC). Most provisions in these regulations and guidelines replicate the CIOMS guidelines and the Declaration of Helsinki. All require that informed consent be obtained from each individual research subject, yet, as outlined in these regulations and guidelines, certain procedures for obtaining consent may diverge from the requirement for written, signed informed-consent forms that is included in the U.S. regulations.

Guidelines issued by the Medical Research Council of South Africa in 1993 include two rules regarding informed consent: (1) research subjects should know that they are taking part in research; and (2) research involving subjects should be carried out only with their consent. Yet these guidelines also say: "It can be proper for research involving less than minimal risk and which is easily comprehended to proceed on the basis of oral consent given after an oral description of what is involved." Similarly, the guidelines issued in 2000 by the Indian Council of Medical Research require that informed consent be obtained from each individual subject. But the guidelines also say that the nature and form of the consent may depend on a number of different factors.

The NBAC international report (2001) makes a useful distinction between substantive and procedural ethical requirement in research. Substantive ethical requirements are those embodied in the fundamental principles of bioethics stated in the *Belmont Report:* respect for persons, beneficence, and justice (National Commission). These substantive requirements are the ones that constitute ethical *standards,* and they should be applied universally. Examples are the requirement to obtain informed consent individually from each adult participant and the need to disclose complete information about the research maneuvers to be performed and the expected risks of those interventions. Procedural requirements, on the other hand, may vary according to cultural and other differences in multinational research. Examples include the requirement that informed-consent documents be signed, and the composition of ethical review committees and their rules of procedure. Attention to the distinction between substantive and procedural ethical requirements shows that the same ethical standards can be applied across national borders, while permitting differences in specific procedures in order to respect cultural variations.

Ethical codes and international guidelines are not likely to resolve all questions or conflicts that may arise in proposing, reviewing, and conducting multinational research. Any differences in judgments made by two or more committees that review a research protocol will have to be negotiated. On some points, codes and guidelines may be insufficiently specific. In other respects, provisions in codes or guidelines that address the same point may vary in minor or even major respects. An example of an unresolved conflict is the difference in existing guidelines and recommendations on the use of placebo controls and the level of care and treatment to be provided to research subjects during and after a clinical trial. As long as unresolved differences remain among parties committed to conducting such research according to the highest ethical standards, it is open to question whether ethical codes or guidelines should attempt to settle the conflict by imposing an unequivocal rule.

RUTH MACKLIN

SEE ALSO: *AIDS: Healthcare and Research Issues; Anthropology and Bioethics; Epidemics; Human Rights; Informed Consent: Consent Issues in Human Research; International Health; Patenting Organisms and Basic Research; Pharmaceutical Industry; Placebo; Research, Human: Historical Aspects; Research Policy; Scientific Publishing*

BIBLIOGRAPHY

Angell, Marcia. 1997. "The Ethics of Clinical Research in the Third World." *New England Journal of Medicine* 337(12): 847–849.

Annas, George J., and Grodin, Michael A. 1998. "Human Rights and Maternal-Fetal HIV Transmission Prevention Trials in Africa." *American Journal of Public Health* 88(4): 560–563.

Annas, George J., and Grodin, Michael A., eds. 1992. *The Nazi Doctors and the Nuremberg Code.* New York: Oxford University Press.

Brennan, Troyen A. 1999. "Proposed Revisions to the Declaration of Helsinki: Will They Weaken the Ethical Principles Underlying Human Research?" *New England Journal of Medicine* 341(7): 527–531.

Christakis, Nicholas A., and Levine, Robert J. 1995. "Multinational Research." In *Encyclopedia of Bioethics,* 2nd edition, ed. Warren T. Reich. New York: Macmillan/Simon and Schuster.

Council for International Organizations of Medical Sciences (CIOMS), in collaboration with the World Health Organization. 1993 (revised 2002). *International Ethical Guidelines for Biomedical Research Involving Human Subjects.* Geneva, Switzerland: Author.

Crouch, Robert A., and Arras, John D. 1998. "AZT Trials and Tribulations." *Hastings Center Report* 28(6): 26–34.

Grady, Christine. 1998. "Science in the Service of Healing." *Hastings Center Report* 28(6): 34–38.

IJsselmuiden, Carel B., and Faden, Ruth R. 1992. "Images in Clinical Medicine." *New England Journal of Medicine* 326(12): 830–834.

Indian Council of Medical Research. 2000. *Ethical Guidelines for Biomedical Research on Human Subjects.* New Delhi: Author.

Joint United Nations Programme on HIV/AIDS (UNAIDS). 2000. *Ethical Considerations in HIV Preventive Vaccine Research: UNAIDS Guidance Document.* Geneva, Switzerland: Author.

Joint United Nations Programme on HIV/AIDS (UNAIDS). 2002. *Report on the Global HIV/AIDS Epidemic.* Geneva, Switzerland: Author.

Kass, Nancy, and Hyder, Adnan A. 2001. "Attitudes and Experiences of U.S. and Developing Country Investigators Regarding U.S. Human Subjects Regulations." In *Ethical and Policy Issues in International Research: Clinical Trials in Developing Countries,* by National Bioethics Advisory Commission. Bethesda, MD: National Bioethics Advisory Commission.

Levine, Robert J. 1999. "The Need to Revise the Declaration of Helsinki." *New England Journal of Medicine* 341(7): 531–534.

Lie, Reidar K. 1998. "Ethics of Placebo-Controlled Trials in Developing Nations." *Bioethics* 12(4): 307–311.

Lurie, Peter, and Wolfe, Sidney. 1997. "Unethical Trials of Interventions to Reduce Perinatal Transmission of the Human Immunodeficiency Virus in Developing Countries." *New England Journal of Medicine* 337(12): 853–856.

Marshall, Patricia. 2001. "The Relevance of Culture for Informed Consent in U.S.-Funded International Health Research." In *Ethical and Policy Issues in International Research: Clinical Trials in Developing Countries,* by National Bioethics Advisory Commission. Bethesda, MD: National Bioethics Advisory Commission.

Michaud, Catherine M.; Murray, Christopher J. L.; and Bloom, Barry R. 2001. "Burden of Disease: Implications for Future Research." *Journal of the American Medical Association* 285(5): 535–539.

Newton, Lisa. 1990. "Ethical Imperialism and Informed Consent." *IRB: A Review of Human Subjects Research* 12(3): 10–11.

Nuffield Council on Bioethics. 2002. *The Ethics of Research Related to Healthcare in Developing Countries.* London: Author.

Schüklenk, Udo. 1998. "Unethical Perinatal HIV Transmission Trials Establish Bad Precedent." *Bioethics* 12(4): 312–319.

Sugarman, Jeremy; Popkin, Benjamin; Fortney, Judith; et al. 2001. "International Perspectives on Protecting Human Research Subjects." In *Ethical and Policy Issues in International Research: Clinical Trials in Developing Countries,* by National Bioethics Advisory Commission. Bethesda, MD: National Bioethics Advisory Commission.

U.S. Department of Health and Human Services. Office of Inspector General. 2001. "The Globalization of Clinical Trials: A Growing Challenge in Protecting Human Subjects." Washington, D.C.: Author.

U.S. National Bioethics Advisory Commission (NBAC). 2001. *Ethical and Policy Issues in International Research: Clinical Trials in Developing Countries.* Bethesda, MD: Author.

U.S. National Commission for the Protection of Human Subjects of Biomedical and Behavioral Research. 1979. *The Belmont Report: Ethical Principles and Guidelines for the Protection of Human Subjects of Research.* Washington, D.C.: U.S. Government Printing Office.

Varmus, Harold, and Satcher, David. 1997. "Ethical Complexities of Conducting Research in Developing Countries." *New England Journal of Medicine* 337(14): 1003–1005.

World Medical Association (WMA). 1996 (revised 2000). "Declaration of Helsinki: Ethical Principles for Medical Research Involving Human Subjects." Ferney-Voltaire, France: Author.

INTERNET RESOURCES

Council for International Organizations of Medical Sciences (CIOMS), in collaboration with the World Health Organization. 2002. *International Ethical Guidelines for Biomedical Research Involving Human Subjects,* revised edition. Available from <http://www.cioms.ch>.

Indian Council of Medical Research. 2000. *Ethical Guidelines for Biomedical Research on Human Subjects.* Available from <http://icmr.nic.in/ethical.pdf>.

Joint United Nations Programme on HIV/AIDS (UNAIDS). 2000. *Ethical Considerations in HIV Preventive Vaccine Research: UNAIDS Guidance Document.* Available from <http://www.unaids.org/publications/documents/vaccines/>.

Nuffield Council on Bioethics. 2002. "The Ethics of Research Related to Healthcare in Developing Countries." Available from <http://www.nuffieldbioethics.org/developingcountries/>.

South Africa. Medical Research Council. 1993. "Guidelines on Ethics for Medical Research," revised edition. Available from <http://www.mrc.ac.za/ethics/consent.htm>.

U.S. Department of Health and Human Services. Office of Inspector General. 2001. "The Globalization of Clinical Trials: A Growing Challenge in Protecting Human Subjects." Available from <http://oig.hhs.gov/oei/>.

U.S. National Bioethics Advisory Commission (NBAC). 2001. *Ethical and Policy Issues in International Research: Clinical Trials in Developing Countries.* Available from <http://bioethics.georgetown.edu/nbac/pubs.html>.

World Medical Association (WMA). 2000. "Declaration of Helsinki: Ethical Principles for Medical Research Involving Human Subjects." Available from <http://www.wma.net/e/policy/17-c_e.html>.

RESEARCH POLICY

• • •

I. General Background

II. Risk and Vulnerable Groups

III. Subjects

I. GENERAL BACKGROUND

Since the 1960s the challenges of human research have received increasing attention and have caused a great deal of concern. In 1966 Professor Henry Beecher captured the attention and aroused the ire of the academic research community in the United States with the disclosure of what he considered unethical research practices at some premier research facilities. Beecher initiated a cycle of disclosure and reaction that has characterized the country's approach to ensuring the well-being of participants in research for more than four decades (Papworth).

Early Criticisms of Research Procedures

Beecher's article came at a time when public investment in research and development, particularly in biomedicine and technology, was growing at an unprecedented rate and the prospects for medicine and the future of biotechnology appeared limitless. The boom in private, corporate-sponsored clinical trials had not yet materialized but was not beyond people's imagination. The disturbing events at the Jewish Chronic Diseases Hospital in New York (Katz), in which a physician scientist injected live cancer cells into unwitting recipients, had been noted by Dr. James Shannon, at that time the director of the National Institutes of Health.

Prompted by that disclosure, in 1966 Shannon moved to require for the first time a mechanism for peer review of proposed scientific research by individuals that was concerned primarily with the well-being and safety of research subjects. However, much of the scientific community remained oblivious or insensitive to the apparent disregard for the safety and the rights of subjects in the research practices of that period. For the first time the scientific community began to realize that scientists could not be allowed on their own to determine how they would conduct experimental studies on other human beings.

The First Cycle of Regulations

Beecher's article and the monumental work subsequently published by Jay Katz just as the U.S. Public Health Service syphilis study in rural Alabama came to light (Tuskegee Syphilis Study Ad Hoc Advisory Panel) evoked strong emotional reactions among scientists, the public, and government regulators. That scientists working for the government could intentionally, for research purposes, allow poor African-American men to live with untreated syphilis for thirty years after the discovery of safe, effective treatment was appalling. Studies of the transmission of hepatitis in institutionalized children at the Willowbrook School (see Katz) underscored the need for special societal and legal protections of those incapable of protecting their own interests, including children. Many people called for new government regulations to protect the safety of research subjects, and the government responded. Within two years Congress passed the National Research Act of 1974, establishing the National Commission for the Protection of Human Subjects in Biomedical and Behavioral Research and laying a course for regulatory action. The act required the U.S. Department of Health, Education and Welfare, the predecessor of the Department of Health and Human Services (DHHS), to codify its policy for the protection of human subjects in the form of regulations.

Almost immediately the perception of scientists and physicians who worked in human research was altered. Activities that once were held in the highest esteem, conducted by individuals who were trusted and respected as much as anyone in society, suddenly were cast in an unflattering light as potential sources of injury and harm from which individuals needed protection despite the potential benefit to humankind of those activities.

The National Commission for the Protection of Human Subjects in Biomedical and Behavioral Research, which conducted its deliberations over a period of several years before it was disbanded in the late 1970s, attempted to define a set of fundamental ethical principles underlying the responsible conduct of human research first for the general population and subsequently for special populations that were deemed to need special protections, notably children, prisoners, pregnant women, and fetuses. The Commission also recognized the special challenges posed by research involving individuals with mental illnesses and impaired decision-making capability, many of whom were institutionalized at the time of the its discussions.

The Commission did not state a preference for any particular philosophy or ideology, although traditional Western values of individual autonomy and justice were reflected prominently in its Belmont Report. The justification of human experimentation and the attendant exposure of individuals to uncertain risks for little or no direct benefit, but for the benefit of science and society is fundamentally utilitarian. At the time of the Commission's work, feminism, consumerism, and communitarian ethics were not yet part of mainstream thinking and thus were not reflected prominently in the debate. The lack of universality of ethical principles across cultures may limit the generalizability of the Commission's recommendations.

Today most parties to the human research process in the U.S. are at least aware of the commission's Belmont Report and are able to name the principles of respect for persons, beneficence, and justice discussed therein (National Commission for the Protection of Human Subjects in Biomedical and Behavioral Research 1979), but this is a relatively recent development resulting primarily from the requirements imposed by the National Institutes of Health (NIH) that all individuals who participate in human research receive *training* in research ethics and regulatory requirements (National Institutes of Health). The fact that members of the research community would seek training in the responsible conduct of human research only as a condition of receiving funding from a federal agency is an unfortunate commentary on the way in which the research community establishes priorities. This pattern of behavior is what many critics and scholars of the human research process have come to expect and has not been lost on legislators.

The bioethicist Carol Levine once said that human research ethics were "born in scandal and reared in protectionism." That quip often is repeated because it resonates with current perceptions of reality. That statement captures the continuing cycle of disclosure and reaction that has characterized regulatory activities at the federal level, beginning with the amendment of the Public Health Service Act in 1974 and the subsequent promulgation of revised

regulations by the DHHS for the protection of human subjects in 1981 (Code of Federal Regulations, Title 45, Part 46).

Although frequently cited as a framework for the ethical conduct of human research, those regulations do not constitute a set of ethical principles. The regulations are a set of rules established under the Public Health Service Act that attempt to operationalize the ethical principles set forth in the Belmont Report. They establish the minimum necessary requirements for implementing and maintaining a system for the protection of human subjects in research, including formal requirements for the establishment and operations of institutional review boards and the processes for obtaining and documenting informed consent, as recommended by the National Commission in 1978.

The DHHS expended considerable effort in crafting those regulations so that they would allow enough flexibility to encompass the wide variety of biomedical, behavioral, and social research it supported. The regulations reflected a well-intended effort to ensure that the ethical principles delineated in the Belmont Report would be applied in a uniform and appropriate manner by all recipients of federal research funds. Unfortunately, the DHHS was unable to establish a uniform set of regulations governing the oversight of all human research under its jurisdiction, most notably excluding privately sponsored clinical trials of new drugs, devices, and biologics performed under the regulatory authority of the U.S. Food and Drug Administration (FDA), which operates under a separate statutory authority, the Food Drug and Cosmetic Act of 1972. Those studies are covered by separate regulations (Code of Federal Regulations, Title 21, Parts 50 and 56) that are substantially similar to but more narrowly focused on clinical investigation than are the Public Health Service regulations. The lack of a uniform oversight process and standards has probably contributed to inconsistent and ineffective implementation and noncompliance with the regulations. This situation has been and is likely to continue to be a source of confusion and frustration to individual investigators, sponsors, institutions, and review boards that attempt in good faith to comply with the requirements of the often overlapping regulations and oversight processes that apply to their activities.

The Common Rule

The situation in the DHHS is compounded in other federal agencies. In 1991 sixteen agencies adopted 45 CFR 46 Subpart A, the main body of the DHHS's regulations, as signatories to the common Federal Policy on Protection of Human Subjects in Biomedical and Behavioral Research, informally known as the Common Rule. Many of those agencies, including the National Bioethics Advisory Commission (2001c), had noted previously that it had taken a full decade for some of the federal agencies to sign on to those important regulations, yet not all federal agencies have done that, including some that engage in or support human research. Those that have adopted the Common Rule do not always agree fully on the interpretation and application of the regulations and some continue to impose specific additional regulatory and administrative requirements of their own. Thus, research entities and individuals have been left to reconcile the differences as best they can, often with little specific guidance, support, and cooperation from the various federal agencies involved in the support and oversight of human research activities.

Both investigators and institutions, including their review boards, have complained that the complexity and inflexibility of the regulations have made it difficult for them to comply. Although these are contributing factors, there are more likely explanations for the widespread noncompliance discovered when the former Office for Protection from Research Risks (OPRR) began a series of not-for-cause site visits to major research institutions across the country in the late 1990s. The 1998 reports from the Office of Inspector General offered insight into the nature of the problems in the system by noting that institutional review boards "review too much too quickly, with too little expertise" (p. 5). The report also notes the inadequacy of resources provided to support their work.

Problems in the Implementation of the Regulations

Apparently, while implementing the requirements of the regulations, institutions that received research support failed to invest adequately in robust programs for the protection of human subjects despite dramatic growth in their research budgets and their assurances to the government that they would do so.

At most of those institutions funds to support programs for human research protection were allocated to so-called indirect costs as an administrative activity. Within the indirect cost pool the allocation for administration and facilities costs had been capped by the federal Office for Management and Budget (OMB) at 26 percent of the direct costs of research after some institutions had been discovered using those funds for unallowable expenses. As healthcare reform began to affect the flow of clinical revenues that could be used to subsidize research activities, funding for programs for human research protection were marginalized further and in many cases minimized. The overriding goal seemed to be to achieve regulatory compliance at the lowest possible cost. Accordingly, many institutions relied heavily on volunteers (or "conscripts") and part-time personnel, many of whom had little or no formal training in research ethics or regulatory affairs, to fulfill those important responsibilities.

Although it is easy to lay the blame for this situation on the research institutions, that would be unfair. From the outset research institutions, which did not ask for those regulations, considered the required implementation of programs for human research protection an unfunded or at least underfunded federal mandate. The dramatic growth in corporate-sponsored clinical trials that rely heavily on those programs, which was only beginning when the regulations first were adopted, may warrant the consideration of a mechanism through which industry can offset the associated costs at arm's length from the review and approval process as part of a comprehensive funding scheme for human research oversight.

However, without knowledge of the actual costs associated with implementing and maintaining effective programs for the protection of human research subjects, the allocation of appropriate funding for those programs is unlikely if not impossible. Few credible attempts have been made to measure those variables since the 1970s. The little information that is available regarding those costs reflects at best an estimate of what was being expended to support programs of questionable efficacy. Because there is no well-established approach to measuring efficacy, it is unlikely that a rational formula for supporting those programs will emerge in the near future despite the pressing need to develop one.

Public and Private Reports

The current state of dissatisfaction and anxiety that affects almost everyone in the human research enterprise is not a new phenomenon. Almost immediately after the adoption of the DHHS's regulations for the protection of human subjects in 1981, the first of what was to become a long series of reports on the challenges of human studies was issued in 1982 by the President's Commission for the Study of Ethical Problems in Medicine and Biomedical and Behavioral Research. In the same year a report was issued by the Council for International Organizations of Medical Sciences (CIOMS). That report was followed in 1993 by the report of the President's Advisory Committee on Human Radiation Experiments, several reports from the National Bioethics Advisory Commission (1998, 1999, 2001a, b, and c), the General Accounting Office (1996, 2000, 2001), the Office of Inspector General of the DHHS (1998–2001), the recently disbanded National Human Research Protections

Advisory Committee (2001), and the Institute of Medicine (1994, 2002). Many private organizations have issued reports or guidelines, including the Association of American Universities (2001), the Association of American Medical Colleges (2001), the American Association of University Professors (2001), the American Academy of Pharmaceutical Physicians (2001), the American Medical Association (2000), the American Society for Gene Therapy (2000), the American Society of Clinical Oncology (2002), and the Association of Clinical Research Professionals (2001).

This array of reports covers ethics, regulatory affairs, financial relationships, conflicts of interests, and the responsible conduct of research. Generally, all the reports recognize and emphasize the dependence of human research on the willingness of individuals to participate voluntarily as subjects, acknowledging the key role that trust plays in the relationship between investigators and subjects. They acknowledge the fact that past and present events have undermined that sense of trust and that steps must be taken to rebuild and maintain it. They all offer recommendations, most of which are consistent or at least compatible, yet most observers agree that little progress has been made since the 1970s in implementing those recommendations apart from the adoption of the regulations and the implementation of institutional review boards and informed consent as the "twin pillars" of protection for human subjects. Some people think that those recommendations afford more of an impediment to research than effective protections for human subjects. Many are perplexed that it seems so hard for the scientific community and the government to do what is morally and legally appropriate when doing so is clearly in the interest of science and society.

The Ethical Issues in Human Research

There is no simple solution to this problem, which involves a complex interplay of ethics, economics, and expediency in a system affected by people, politics, and profits. The most fundamental issue is the moral dilemma inherent in human research: In all cases of human experimentation individuals are subject to risks for the benefit of science and society. Human research is an endeavor that exploits some individuals for a greater good, but that exploitation is considered acceptable and even justifiable as long as participation is voluntary and informed and the research is conducted within the well-established ethical framework of respect for persons, beneficence, and justice.

Human research entails a dynamic tension between the interests of those who do research and the interests of those on whom research is done. Can science and society justifiably place their own interests above the interests, rights, and well-being of research subjects? More correctly, should the interests of science and society prevail over those of individual subjects? Even if one identified compelling circumstances in which it would be ethically permissible to do that, those cases probably would be rare. However, it is tempting and easy to allow the pursuit of knowledge, the lure of fame and fortune, advantage in the marketplace, and the chance of academic promotion to color one's judgment and influence one's conduct.

The events the past three decades in which subjects have been harmed and misconduct revealed have shown that not all scientists, institutions, and sponsors are immune to temptation. Breaches of responsible conduct may go unnoticed and unreported, but when they are serious and are discovered and criticized, they evoke a host of reactions, including sorrow, anger, indignation, and defensiveness. The consequences of those breaches are far-reaching and long-lasting, leaving no party untouched. The corrective actions that follow may provide long-term benefits but are painful and costly in both human and financial terms.

The Deaths of Jesse Gelsinger and Ellen Roche

No two cases more aptly illustrate these points than the deaths of Jesse Gelsinger at the University of Pennsylvania in 1999 and Ellen Roche at Johns Hopkins University Medical Center in 2001. Gelsinger, suffering from a genetic metablioc disorder, died in a gene-transfer study just days after receiving an infusion of a corrected gene attached to a virus intended to introduce the new gene into his liver cells. Roche was a normal healthy young woman participating in a study of the mechanisms of airway responsiveness, a study that required inhalation of a chemical that blocked certain pathways of nerve transmission. The second case has been described (Steinbrook) and analyzed (Kreiger and De Pasquale) extensively. The death of Jesse Gelsinger was a critical event because it catalyzed a coalescence of will in the government and public to face the problems of human research directly, particularly the potential impact of financial relationships and conflicts of interests on the well-being of research participants (Shalala).

The Roche case eventually may have an even more far-reaching impact. It is particularly relevant because it involves a failure to protect research participants adequately not only at the level of an individual study but also at the level of an institutional system as judged not only by government regulators but also by an external evaluating committee of peers selected by the institution. In this case attention was focused not just on an individual's untimely death, the failings of a single investigator, the shortcomings of an institutional review board, and a deficient institutional system for the protection of human subjects: The focus ultimately became the culture of the institution and more generally the culture of science as it relates to the responsible conduct of human research. The message here is the need to move beyond a culture of compliance to a culture of conscience in science (Koski, 2003a).

Resistance to Change

Since the Renaissance the pursuit of knowledge through science has been regarded as a noble profession. Recognizing the importance of the pursuit of truth in science, one might expect scientists to be intolerant of those among them who fail to respect truth or undermine the integrity of science. However, in this regard perception and reality sometimes diverge. Statements of ethical principles and codes of conduct have done much to guide the scientific community, along with the medical profession, in the pursuit of truth, but some members of those professions betray the truth. When a profession is willing to tolerate rather than hold accountable those whose behavior violates the principles and traditions of the profession, the credibility of the principles on which the profession is established are undermined. *Pseudoaccountability,* a term coined by a Jerome Kasirer, results in a profession that traverses the road of good intentions but does not arrive at its destination.

Accounts of Beecher's efforts to publish in the medical literature his concerns about the ethics of research studies conducted in the early 1960s suggest that that was not an easy task. Initial rejections finally gave way to an agreement with the editor of the *New England Journal of Medicine* to publish the paper only after Beecher agreed to limit the number of cases to a small fraction of those about which he was concerned and to withhold identification of the investigators and their institutions. As a respected physician, scientist, and professor at Harvard Medical School Beecher demonstrated courage and integrity in attempting to bring those issues before his peers, but many in the scientific community did not receive his paper enthusiastically.

One can only wonder how human research might be different today if the scientific community at that time had responded with a concerted effort to achieve a higher standard of conduct, promoted integrity with an expectation that all who engage in research involving other human beings would act in accordance with the highest ethical standards, and shown a willingness to hold accountable those who did not live up to those standards. If the scientific community rather than the government had taken action to ensure the well-being of research participants not because it was required to do so by regulations but out of concern for the integrity of science, the continuing pursuit of knowledge, and an earnest desire and commitment to prevent harm to fellow human beings while honoring the rights of others, there might not be regulations on the books requiring them to do so.

Laws and regulations are one way in which a society attempts to influence the behaviors of its citizens. Regulations may be used to prescribe certain actions and prohibit others. However, regulations can be a double-edged sword.

In a 2003 article published in the *Emory Law Journal* Robert Gatter discusses the normative and expressive functions of the law in the context of regulations that address continuing concerns about financial conflicts of interest in human research. Many laws are not directed toward criminal activity, but seek to establish a recognized norm of conduct, and to do so by expressing the normative message through regulations and guidance. The regulations for the protection of human subjects in research are analogous to those involving financial conflict in that they are intended to establish a norm of conduct for investigators and institutions through the expression and application of the ethical principles delineated in the Belmont Report. Laws, however, do not always achieve their desired goals, particularly if the regulated community is resistant to acceptance of the normative standard and the implementation or enforcement provisions make it unlikely that noncompliance will be discovered or punished. As Gatter points out, regulations can evoke "juridification," by which those who are subject to regulations try to find ways to avoid or circumvent them rather than embrace them. Although scientists and physicians may be no less hostile to regulation of their activities than are others, one might expect them to more readily accept such regulation in light of their codes of professional conduct that already express values compatible with those embodied in the regulations.

Since the 1970s researchers have worked within a regulatory framework in which the regulated parties too frequently have viewed the requirements of the regulations as unnecessarily complicated, costly, and onerous administrative impediments to their research activities. That viewpoint, which seems to contrast markedly with the values that society traditionally associates with scientists and the pursuit of knowledge, may reflect changes in the culture of science that occurred in the second half of twentieth century or may indicate significant juridification, to use Gatter's terminology, of the human research community in response to the imposition of regulations by the government in response to a limited number of high-profile breaches of responsible conduct.

There is no question that the American system for the responsible conduct of human research and the protection of human subjects is undergoing dramatic change. It may be far more difficult to effect cultural change that requires behavioral changes consistent with acceptance of fundamental values than it is to overcome and reverse the juridification that has occurred in response to failures in the normative and expressive functions of the applicable law and regulations.

New Initiatives

The death of Jesse Gelsinger launched a new cycle of reform in human research and the protection of the human subjects. Although the initial calls were for more stringent regulations and penalties, the DHHS, with strong leadership from the former secretary, Donna Shalala, has taken a different course. In June 2000 the department established a new Office for Human Research Protections (OHRP), replacing the Office for Protection for Research Risks. The new office was placed within the office of the secretary to give it the visibility and autonomy necessary to lead a major remodeling effort to improve the performance and effectiveness of the national system for the protection of human subjects in research. The strategy and approach taken by the DHHS were outlined in September 2000 in testimony delivered before the House Oversight Committee on Veterans Affairs (Koski, 2000).

Those initiatives mark a shift from a reactive, compliance-focused approach to the oversight of human research toward a proactive model focused on the prevention of harm. Recognizing the widely varying and sometimes idiosyncratic behavior of local institutional review boards, the new approach emphasizes education and support as the umbrella under which activities aimed at improving performance are conducted (Figure 1). The goal of current efforts is to move from an approach focused on achieving regulatory compliance to one that attempts to achieve excellence and trust. In this model activities to ensure the well-being of research participants are conducted in two primary domains: the compliance domain and the performance domain. The compliance domain includes both for-cause investigations and not-for-cause evaluations. Both types of compliance oversight activities are intended to ensure accountability and

fall generally into the class of quality control and quality assurance processes. In this model the identification of deficiencies should be focused on system failures in an attempt to strengthen processes rather than use punishment or sanctions except in cases of gross negligence or willful disregard for regulatory requirements, thus avoiding the counterproductive impact of a reactive, juridifying approach to regulatory enforcement. Traditionally, these activities have been conducted primarily by government oversight agencies or parties acting on their behalf. Activities within the performance domain generally are classified as quality improvement activities, including continuous quality improvement, largely in the form of consultation and feedback on actual performance. Objective validation processes such as accreditation of institutions or programs and professional certification of individuals provide empirical evidence of proficiency and recognition of excellence. Education and support are overarching activities that work to improve the effectiveness and efficiency of the system. Realization of positive results and appropriate validation of excellence provide incentives to shift resources toward the performance domain. Ultimately, prevention of harm to human participants through responsible conduct builds trust and promotes public confidence in the research process, enhancing voluntary participation in research. Those activities are focused on improving, measuring, and validating the performance of the system in its entirety, utilizing proven continuous quality improvement methods to achieve those goals (Institute of Medicine, 2002).

In the past the government generally waited until it received a complaint from an outside source or a report from one of the institutions under its regulatory authority to initiate an investigation into the circumstances of an event. Those for-cause investigations, many of which were conducted through correspondence alone, were the mainstay of the OPRR's oversight activities. The bulk of its resources were dedicated to review, negotiation, and approval of assurances, documents submitted by entities receiving federal support for research to satisfy regulatory requirements that such a document be filed as a condition of receiving support. Too often those were empty assurances, paper commitments insufficiently backed by substantive actions and resources.

The creation of the OHRP added significant new resources to the office and a reorganization plan that redirected those resources toward enhanced educational programs and the development and implementation of a new quality improvement program through which the office provides consultation and support for institutions that seek to improve their programs for human research protection.

FIGURE 1

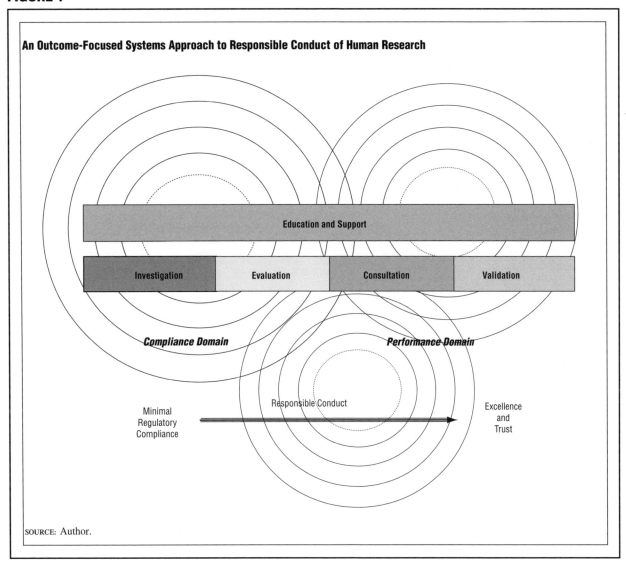

An Outcome-Focused Systems Approach to Responsible Conduct of Human Research

SOURCE: Author.

To a large extent that redistribution of resources was made possible by a dramatic simplification of the assurance process. Rather than continue the long-standing practice of negotiating and processing multiple types of assurances and interagency agreements, the office adopted a single standardized federal assurance that could be utilized by all participating federal agencies and was consistent with the original intent of the Common Rule. Significant progress is being made toward establishing a more effective system for the protection of human subjects in research (Koski, 2003b) despite the fact that the regulations adopted since the 1970s remain essentially unchanged. In large measure this progress is a direct result of a renewed willingness in the research community to adopt a more proactive, responsible approach toward the conduct of its activities. Whether this progress continues will be a principal determinant of the nature and

scope of future regulatory actions in the area of human research.

GREG KOSKI

SEE ALSO: *Aging and the Aged: Healthcare and Research Issues; AIDS: Healthcare and Research Issues; Autoexperimentation; Autonomy; Children: Healthcare and Research Issues; Commercialism in Scientific Research; Embryo and Fetus: Embryo Research; Empirical Methods in Bioethics; Genetics and Human Behavior: Scientific and Research Issues; Holocaust; Infants: Public Policy and Legal Issues; Informed Consent: Consent Issues in Human Research; Law and Bioethics; Mentally Ill and Mentally Disabled Persons: Research Issues; Military Personnel as Research Subjects; Minorities as Research Subjects; Paternalism; Pediatrics,*

Overview of Ethical Issues in; Public Policy and Bioethics; Prisoners as Research Subjects; Race and Racism; Research, Human: Historical Aspects; Research Methodology; Research, Multinational; Research, Unethical; Responsibility; Scientific Publishing; Sexism; Students as Research Subjects; Virtue and Character; and other *Research Policy* subentries

BIBLIOGRAPHY

Advisory Committee on Human Radiation Experiments. 1995. *Final Report: Advisory Committee on Human Radiation Experiments.* Washington, D.C.: U.S. Government Printing Office.

American Association of University Professors. 2001. "Protecting Human Beings: Institutional Review Boards and Social Science Research." *Academe* 87(3): 55–67.

American Medical Association, Council on Ethical and Judicial Affairs. 2000. *Code of Medical Ethics: Current Opinions.* Chicago: Author.

Association of American Medical Colleges. 2001. *Protecting Human Subjects, Preserving Trust, Promoting Progress—Policy Guidelines for the Oversight of Individual Financial Interests in Human Subjects Research.* Washington, D.C.: Author.

Association of American Universities, Task Force on Research Accountability. 2001. *Report on Individual and Institutional Financial Conflicts of Interest.* Washington, D.C.: Author.

Beecher, Henry K. 1966. "Ethics and Clinical Research." *New England Journal of Medicine* 274(24): 1354–1360.

Council for International Organizations of Medical Sciences. 1993. *International Ethical Guidelines for Biomedical Research Involving Human Subjects.* Geneva: Author.

Gatter, R. 2003. "Walking the Talk of Trust in Human Subjects Research: The Challenge of Regulating Financial Conflicts of Interest." *Emory Law Journal* 52(1): 327–402.

General Accounting Office. 1996. *Scientific Research: Continued Vigilance Critical to Protecting Human Subjects.* Report No. GAO/HEHS–96–72. Washington, D.C.: Author.

General Accounting Office. 2000. *VA Research: Protections for Human Subjects Need to Be Strengthened.* Report No. GAO/HEHS–00–15. Washington, D.C.: Author.

General Accounting Office. 2001. *Biomedical Research: HHS Direction Needed to Address Financial Conflicts of Interest.* Report No. GAO/HEHS–02–89. Washington, D.C.: Author.

Institute of Medicine. 2001. *Preserving Public Trust: Accreditation and Human Research Participant Protection Programs.* Washington, D.C.: National Academy Press.

Institute of Medicine. 2002. *Responsible Research: A Systems Approach to Protecting Research Participants.* Washington, D.C.: National Academy Press.

Kassirer, Jerome. 2001. "Pseudoaccountability." *Annals of Internal Medicine* 134: 587–590.

Katz, Jay. 1972. *Experimentation on Human Beings.* New York: Russell Sage Foundation.

Koski, G. 1999. "Resolving Beecher's Paradox: Getting Beyond IRB Reform." *Accountability in Research* 7: 213–225.

Koski, G. 2003a. "Research, Regulations and Responsibility: Confronting the Compliance Myth." *Emory Law Journal* 52(1): 403–416.

Kreiger, D., and DePasquale, S. 2002. "Trials and Tribulations." *Johns Hopkins Magazine* 54(1): 28–41.

National Bioethics Advisory Commission. 1998. *Research Involving Persons with Mental Disorders That May Affect Decisionmaking Capacity.* Rockville, MD: Author.

National Bioethics Advisory Commission. 1999. *Research Involving Biological Materials: Ethical Issues and Policy Guidance.* vol. 1. Rockville, MD: Author.

National Bioethics Advisory Commission. 2001a. *Ethical and Policy Issues in International Research: Clinical Trials in Developing Countries.* Rockville, MD: Author.

National Bioethics Advisory Commission. 2001b. *Ethical and Policy Issues in Research Involving Human Participants.* vol. 1. Bethesda, MD: Author.

National Bioethics Advisory Commission. 2001c. "Federal Agency Survey on Policies and Procedures for the Protection of Human Subjects in Research." In *Ethical and Policy Issues in Research Involving Human Participants.* vol. 2: *Commissioned Papers and Staff Analysis.* Bethesda, MD: Author.

National Commission for the Protection of Human Subjects in Biomedical and Behavioral Research. 1978. *Report and Recommendations: Institutional Review Boards.* Washington, D.C.: U.S. Government Printing Office.

National Commission for the Protection of Human Subjects in Biomedical and Behavioral Research. 1979. *The Belmont Report: Ethical Principles and Guidelines for the Protection of Human Subjects of Research.* Washington, D.C.: U.S. Government Printing Office.

Office of Inspector General, U.S. Department of Health and Human Services. 1998. *Institutional Review Boards: A Time for Reform.* Report No. OEI–01–97–0193. Washington, D.C.: Author and U.S. Government Printing Office.

Papworth, M. 1990. "Human Guinea Pigs—A History." *British Medical Journal* 301: 1456–1460.

President's Commission for the Study of Ethical Problems in Medicine and Biomedical Research. 1983. *Implementing Human Research Regulations.* Washington, D.C.: U.S. Government Printing Office.

Shalala, Donna. 2000. "Protecting Research Subjects—What Must Be Done." *New England Journal of Medicine* 343(11): 808–810.

Steinbrook, R. 2001. "Protecting Research Subjects—The Crisis at Johns Hopkins." *New England Journal of Medicine* 346: 716–720.

World Medical Association. 2000. *Declaration of Helsinki: Principles for Medical Research Involving Human Subjects,* rev. edition. Ferney-Voltaire, France: World Medical Association.

INTERNET RESOURCES

Koski, G. 2000. Statement of Greg Koski, PhD, MD, Director of the Office for Human Research Protection, Office of the

Secretary, Department of Health and Human Services, for the Hearing on Human Subjects Protections before the Subcommittee on Oversight and Investigations, Committee on Veterans Affairs, United States House of Representatives, September 28, 2000, Washington, D.C. Available from <http://ohrp.osophs.dhhs.gov/references/tkoski.htm>.

Koski, G. 2003b. Statement of Greg Koski, PhD, MD, Former Director of the Office for Human Research Protection, Office of the Secretary, Department of Health and Human Services, for the Hearing on Human Subjects Protections before the Subcommittee on Oversight and Investigations, Committee on Veterans Affairs, United States House of Representatives, June 18, 2003, Washington, D.C. Available from <http://veterans.house.gov/hearings/schedule108/jun03/6–18-03/gkoski.html>.

National Human Research Protections Advisory Committee. 2001. *NHRPAC Recommendations on HHS's Draft Interim Guidance on Financial Relationships in Clinical Research.* Available from <http://www.dhhs.gov>.

National Institutes of Health. 2000. *Required Education in the Protection of Human Research Participants.* OD–00–39. Available from <http://www.nih.gov>.

Office for Human Research Protections. 2000. *OHRP Compliance Activities: Common Findings and Guidance.* Available from <http://orhp.osophs.dhhs.gov/references/findings.pdf>.

II. RISK AND VULNERABLE GROUPS

There are two groups of people considered to be vulnerable research subjects. First, people lacking capacity to give informed consent are vulnerable because they depend on others to protect them, such as young children and adults impaired by trauma, illness, retardation, or dementia. Second, people who are likely to be coerced or manipulated are vulnerable because fear, ignorance, or pressure may account for their agreement to participate. Institutionalized persons, prisoners, members of the military, students, hospital staff, laboratory assistants, and pharmaceutical personnel are frequently cited as vulnerable to coercion or manipulation (U.S. Public Health Service; CIOMS). In addition, the indigent, uninsured, or desperate may be unduly tempted into study participation that they would otherwise reject by financial remuneration. Insofar as participation of vulnerable subjects is problematic, enrolling them in research protocols often requires special justification and safeguards (CIOMS; "Protection of Human Subjects," 45 C.F.R. 46).

Dilemmas of Inclusion vs. Exclusion

It is important to include all segments of society in research, including vulnerable people, so that everyone benefits from research studies. Yet dangers exist in both too many and in too few protections. When too few protections exist, vulnerable people may be exploited. When too many protections exist, however, it is hard to conduct research with vulnerable populations; consequently there is little information about how to diagnose, treat or understand their conditions. Without good research information, people from these groups become neglected. Doctors must then choose between using only modalities that have been tested on the group in question and risk undertreating these subjects, or using untested interventions and risk adverse effects. There are several ways to address this apparent dilemma, and many guidelines adopt some combination of them.

First, all research guidelines require studies to have a strict review by boards known by various names: institutional review boards (IRBs), research ethics committees (RECs), or ethical review committees (ERCs). These boards have discretion to disapprove or approve studies or to adopt suitable additional protections for studies with all or some vulnerable subjects. These committees should be sensitive to various forms of vulnerability (cognitive, environmental, institutional, deferential, medical, economic and social) and respond with appropriate and situationally-appropriate restrictions. The National Bioethics Advisory Commission (NBAC), which carefully distinguishes these different forms of vulnerability, relies upon review board discretion to protect vulnerable subjects because it is flexible (NBAC). But this option has been undermined by high-profile revelations of poor oversight or compliance by some of these review boards. Moreover, confidence in these boards varies according to people's perceptions of whether they represent the interests of vulnerable populations or are seen as favoring the research enterprise or commercial interests.

Second, others favor another approach with special regulatory requirements that must be met before enrolling some or all vulnerable subjects. Such regulations generally exist for infants, children, pregnant women, and prisoners. But critics argue that expanding regulations for other groups could become unwieldy since many, perhaps even most, people may be perceived as vulnerable in some situations (NBAC). If special regulations existed for all or most groups of people who might be vulnerable, it could become unreasonably difficult to approve or conduct research. Moreover, some competent persons, such as pregnant women, object to special restrictions placed upon their freedom of choice.

Third, some guidelines limit risk when subjects are deemed vulnerable. The Food and Drug Administration (FDA, 1997, 4.8.14) stipulates that, when people cannot give consent for trials that do not directly benefit them, risks must be low and other considerations must be fulfilled (i.e., the study cannot be conducted with consenting subjects, consent is obtained from subjects' legal representatives, IRB approval is gained, the negative impact on the subjects is minimized and low, and the study is not illegal). The Council for International Organizations of Medical Science (CIOMS) limits the risk of harm to vulnerable subjects to a "minimal risk," unless the study offers direct benefit to subjects; in some cases a minor increase over minimal risk is permitted in order to study vulnerable people's disorders or conditions. Critics argue that this policy unreasonably restricts people's choices and opportunities, especially when the vulnerable people are competent adults. As noted, NBAC objects to this proliferation of regulations and maintains that once review boards put safeguards in place, vulnerable subjects should be enrolled in studies on the same basis as other subjects.

While these research approaches suggest some similar ways to protect vulnerable people, the moral and policy issues differ greatly for those who are not legally competent and those who are. NBAC describes these two groups' vulnerability as "intrinsic" and "situational," respectively, and CIOMS refers to them as "absolute" and "relative." Yet this language is misleading. First, many children and legally incompetent adults have the capacity to participate in some tasks but not others, so they are neither "absolutely" nor "intrinsically" incompetent; if they have the capacity to assent, which refers to their permission and is a notion different from legal consent, it generally should be sought for research participation. Second, it is misleading to call people either absolutely or intrinsically incapacitated when, for many members of these groups, capacity fluctuates or it grows, as it does for most for children. Third, legally competent persons may view additional protections and restrictions as unjustified paternalism that places obstacles in their path to gain participation in research on the same basis as others; they deny that their situation or relations make them vulnerable. Because the issues are so different for the two groups, their policy options are discussed separately.

Competent Adults Vulnerable to Coercion and Manipulation

There has been some consensus, at least in theory, about how to protect the rights and welfare of competent adults who are vulnerable to coercion or manipulation. First, since the right to consent is grounded in its utility, fairness, and the right of self-determination, studies should be reviewed to ensure that consent is voluntary and that the risks of research are not unfairly distributed to vulnerable groups (CIOMS; "Protection of Human Subjects," 45 C.F.R. 46). This evaluation should be conducted by IRBs, RECs, or ERCs.

Review boards bear a heavy responsibility in recognizing when competent persons may be vulnerable and need additional protection as research subjects. The views of reviewers, however, may differ from those of the potential subjects. One remedy is to assemble a group of prospective subjects and conduct a group consultation to learn their views.

Second, most review boards, investigators, and bioethicists agree that the greater the vulnerability and risk to competent adults, the more specific protections should be adopted; where it is difficult to supervise the voluntariness of vulnerable people's consent, it may be necessary to adopt special regulatory protection. For example, because prisoners live in settings that are inherently coercive and because of past abuses, most guidelines provide additional protections for this population (CIOMS; U.S. "Protection of Human Subjects," 45 C.F.R. 46 Subpart C). In general, research guidelines limit the risk of harm to prisoners to a minimal risk unless the study offers direct benefit to the prisoner subjects (individually or as a class) and requires demonstrated utility, special safeguards, experts' approval, and authorization from the U.S. Secretary of Health and Human Services. In some cases a minor increase over minimal risk is permitted to study their disorders or conditions. These restrictions make biomedical research with prisoners difficult to justify, because there are no diseases unique to them as a class. Given their extraordinary living conditions, however, social or behavioral studies might gain approval.

A third area of general agreement about protecting vulnerable competent adults from coercion or manipulation concerns the importance of avoiding interference with people's self-determination or unjustified paternalism. There is less consensus, however, on how to do this. Competent people may resent paternalistic restrictions of their liberties because someone views them as potentially vulnerable. People may deeply object to being denied options open to others, such as innovative or subsidized care for their illnesses in research programs. Impoverished people, including students, may willingly volunteer for risky studies that pay well. They may argue that if firefighters or fighter pilots receive high pay for taking risks, civilians, too, should have the choice to obtain high pay for taking research risks. They may object to the views of some that payment, other than expenses and tokens, constitutes undue influence and should be prohibited (CIOMS).

DISPUTES ABOUT INCLUDING WOMEN. Perhaps the greatest sustained debate has been over limiting the research options for women of childbearing years or women who are pregnant. One dilemma, as noted, is that if some group is excluded from studies, then it is hard to provide good treatment options for them. Pregnant women have diseases and conditions that need study for their own sakes as well as for the sake of their fetuses. At issue is who makes the decision, the woman herself or others.

In many but not all guidelines, women of childbearing years and especially pregnant woman are listed as "vulnerable" and sometimes denied opportunities open to others. In its instructions to the IRB, for example, the U.S. federal regulations state that: "When some or all of the subjects are likely to be vulnerable to coercion or undue influence such as children, prisoners, pregnant women, mentally disabled persons, or economically or educationally disadvantaged persons, additional safeguards have been included in the study to protect the rights and welfare of these subjects" (U.S. "Protection of Human Subjects," 45 CFR 46.111[b]). The U.S. Public Health Service's "Consultation on International Collaborative Human Immunodeficiency Virus" also includes pregnant and nursing women on their list of possibly vulnerable groups. The goal of these guidelines is to protect the fetuses, newborns, and pregnant and nursing women from research risk. Such policies are controversial since there is no uniform agreement about how to rank duties to protect the women and her fetus and duties to also honor women's rights of self-determination.

Many regulations view pregnant women and those of childbearing years as "vulnerable" and favor more regulatory protections, even if they restrict women's options. These restrictions include limiting the array of studies in which they can participate to those designed to benefit them or their fetus, or those having low risk and requiring their husbands' consent as well as their own. In the United States, for example, research with pregnant women designed to benefit the fetus requires the consent of the father (unless he is unavailable, incompetent, or incapacitated, or the pregnancy resulted from rape or incest). (U.S. CFR 45 46.203 [e]).

Pregnant women's illnesses need to be studied, and it is not in their interests if regulations make this difficult. For example, without research pregnant women are denied the benefits of learning about how drugs affect them as a group. Second, participation in research may be a woman's only or best means to gain access to subsidized care or to investigational drugs or therapy, so restrictions deny them options or direct benefit that are available to others. It may be an unfair denial of benefits to rule that women cannot be considered as subjects. Third, it seems unfair that men of reproductive age are not similarly excluded from drug studies; yet many drugs cause changes in male germ cells that are mutagenic.

A consensus is developing that where there is a conflict between the health needs of the mother and that of the fetus, the mother should be at liberty to resolve the conflict herself

(CIOMS; U.S. 45 C.F.R. 46 Subpart B). Restrictions to protect the fetus sometimes rest upon poorly founded assumptions about what might cause harm to the fetus. Informed consent from any woman, however, presupposes that she is informed of the likely harms or benefits, including those that effect her fetus. Pregnancy and nursing make women neither incapable of consent, like children, nor vulnerable to coercion or manipulation, like students and prisoners.

CIOMS does not automatically include women as vulnerable subjects, separating guidelines for vulnerable groups and those for women. It states that vulnerable subjects are those "incapable of protecting their own interests … they may have insufficient power, intelligence, education, resources, or other needed attributes to protect their own interests" (CIOMS, Guideline 13). For vulnerable persons or groups, CIOMS limits the risk of harm to a minimal risk unless the study offers direct benefit to them; in some cases a minor increase over minimal risk is permitted to study vulnerable people's disorders or conditions. In Guideline 16, CIOMS states, "Investigators, sponsors or ethical review committees should not exclude women of reproductive age from biomedical research. The potential for becoming pregnant during a study should not, in itself, be used as a reason for precluding or limiting participation." In CIOMS's commentary on these guidelines, the committee notes that the general presumption should be to include women and that past practices of excluding them is unjust, but that "it must be acknowledged that in some parts of the world women are vulnerable to neglect or harm because of …social conditioning to submit to authority…." CIOMS also takes a stand on seeking consent from husbands: "In research involving women of reproductive age, whether pregnant or non-pregnant, only the informed consent of the woman herself is required for her participation. In no case should the permission of a spouse or partner replace the requirement of individual informed consent … A strict requirement of authorization of spouse or partner, however, violates the substantive principle of respect for persons." Thus, CIOMS favors women's rights of self-determination and their needs to have drugs and other interventions tested on them. NBAC agrees, and even goes beyond CIOMS, arguing that once review boards put safeguards in place, women and other potentially vulnerable subjects should be enrolled in studies on the same basis as other subjects.

Thus, when vulnerable people are competent, disagreements abound concerning what specific restrictions on their choices are fair, promote their well-being, and respect their self-determination. Too little protection risks their exploitation; too much protection risks unjustified paternalism.

Before limiting the liberty of competent people, reviewers and researchers should use community consultation with members of the potentially vulnerable group to consider if they want such protection, if the probability and magnitude of harm warrants constraints, and if the restrictions are the least invasive to secure their well-being.

People Lacking Capacity to Give Consent

As with the competent people, the ethical basis for research policy with persons lacking capacity to give informed consent concerns promoting their self-determination, fair treatment, and well-being. There are four important policy options that were adopted in the twentieth century, and each offers different approaches to ranking what is fair, most protective of incompetent people's well-being, and most respectful of whatever self-determination they have or may develop. These four policies represent different regulative ideals because they rank these primary values differently, and because they offer different authority principles (stating who decides) and guidance principles (substantive directions about how decisions should be made). The remaining discussion will focus on these options.

THE "SURROGATE" OR "LIBERTARIAN" SOLUTION. The oldest policy adopts no special regulatory protection for people lacking the capacity to consent, and allows the same sort of research with them as with other subjects, if their legal guardians consent. Since guardians have the authority to choose the mode of care, religion, and schooling for their dependents, then, according to this view, guardians should determine whether their charges participate in research.

Critics argue that guardians have no authority to volunteer another for studies that are hazardous or that do not hold out benefit for them (Ramsey; Levine; Kopelman, 1989). Guardians have authority insofar as they promote the well-being of those under their care and prevent, remove, or minimize harms to them. They have discretion about how to do this. In nonresearch settings guardians can allow their children or wards to participate in dangerous activities, such as football, presumably because in their judgement there are also direct benefits to them. This differs from volunteering them for risky research, however, when there are no direct benefits to compensate for the risks and where others benefit from that information. Volunteering to put oneself in harm's way to gain knowledge may be morally admirable. But volunteering to put another in harm's way is not admirable, and violates the guardian's protective role. Critics argue that allowing guardians to enroll their charges in potentially harmful experiments wrongs the charges, sets a

dangerous precedent, and has a brutalizing effect upon society.

THE "NO CONSENT-NO RESEARCH" OR "NUREMBERG" SOLUTION. Another policy forbids enrolling people as research subjects without their consent. This view is maintained in the first international research statement, the Nuremberg Code. Its first principle states, "The voluntary consent of the human subject is absolutely essential." It goes on to define consent—in a way that has become fairly standard—as requiring legal capacity, free choice, and understanding of "the nature, duration, and purpose of the experiment; the methods and means by which it is conducted; all inconveniences and hazards reasonably to be expected; any effects upon his health or person which may possibly come from participation in the research" (Germany Military Tribunals).

Composed at the end of World War II, the Nuremberg Code stands as an international response to the horrible, involuntary medical studies done by Nazi physicians in which many unwilling subjects and prisoners were killed or permanently maimed (Proctor). It is uncertain if it was intended as a comprehensive code for research (McCormick). If it is taken as a general policy, however, subjects who lack capacity to give informed consent cannot serve as research subjects.

Critics argue that this policy would cripple evidenced-based medicine for people who cannot give consent, turning them into "therapeutic orphans" (Shirkey; McCormick; Levine). Children, retarded persons, and those incapacitated by mental illness have unique medical problems; thus, studies with normal adult volunteers may be inapplicable. Normal adults cannot serve as subjects in studies comparing treatments for schizophrenia, bipolar illness, or lung disease in premature infants. To test the safety and efficacy of many standard, innovative, or investigational treatments for distinctive groups, and give them due consideration, some members of the groups have to be subjects in controlled testing.

THE "NO CONSENT-ONLY THERAPY" SOLUTION. A third policy permits persons who lack the capacity to give informed consent to be enrolled as research subjects if the studies are therapeutic and offer at least as much direct benefit to subjects as other alternatives, and if guardians consent. This view was represented in the next major international code for research to follow the Nuremberg Code, the World Medical Assembly's Declaration of Helsinki, written in 1964 and revised in 1975, 1983, and 1989. (The Declaration's 2000 revision abandoned the "no consent-only therapy" stance after many years.)

This policy option distinguishes *clinical* or *therapeutic research* (studies seeking generalizable knowledge and intending to provide medically acceptable therapy for the individual) from *nontherapeutic biomedical research* (studies seeking generalizable knowledge and not intended as therapy to benefit the individual directly). Therapeutic studies attempt to benefit the person through prevention, diagnosis, or treatment of disease. Thus, drawing the line at therapeutic research for people who lack capacity to give informed consent seems to defenders to be a good solution to the problem of when to permit incompetent people to serve as subjects (Ramsey).

One difficulty with this third option concerns the difficulty of classifying studies as therapeutic or nontherapeutic in a way that is not arbitrary or misleading. Therapeutic studies often have features that are not a part of routine therapy, such as extra tests, inflexible research protocols, and additional hospitalizations, or visits to the doctor. If these nontherapeutic features increase costs, risks, or inconvenience to the patient, classifying the study as therapeutic may be arbitrary and misleading. Moreover, this classification can be misleading if people assume therapeutic studies are always safe or beneficial. They may have a "therapeutic misconception" based on such labels. Labeling something as "therapeutic" may mask risk, inconvenience, costs, or nonbeneficial features, creating an inappropriate bias for participation.

A second problem is that it seems unreasonable to prohibit important low-risk research especially when it offers nontherapeutic direct benefits to subjects or allows progress for these groups. Subjects would be neither harmed nor wronged if they gained from the experience, liked participating, and were not at risk of harm. Children may enjoy and learn from participating in nontherapeutic studies in which they are asked to do such things as stack similar blocks or identify animals from sounds they make. Yet these nontherapeutic studies could be important for establishing criteria of normal vision and hearing. Adults who are not legally competent may also enjoy and learn from serving as research subjects in nontherapeutic studies. For example, they might like an outing to a research facility, meeting the investigators or learning about the study. In addition, they can benefit indirectly from nontherapeutic studies.

Because this option rules out even low-risk studies it seriously impedes medical progress for these groups including the formation of standards about children's typical growth and development. Such standards presuppose carefully tested criteria distinguishing people with developmental delays or impairments from those with normal growth and development. Establishing such norms requires collecting and analyzing data on the growth and development of large numbers of healthy children. Such safe but important research, however, is forbidden under this policy because it is not therapeutic. Even though these studies establishing norms for growth and development are safe, they are nontherapeutic because they are designed not to benefit the subjects directly but to gain generalizable knowledge. If children stack blocks at play, it is not research; if people test views about how they stack blocks, it is research but may be no more burdensome to the child. Thus, when nontherapeutic studies are needed to promote the well-being of incompetent people as a *group,* and involve little or no risk of harm or inconvenience to them, it is hard to understand how critics can make the case that the subjects are always harmed or wronged by participation.

This option also prohibits epidemiological studies and the investigation of the natural history of disease when there are no therapies. These are among the most important methods for collecting information, so this policy is flawed.

The initial justification for excluding persons who lack the capacity to give informed consent from nontherapeutic research was to honor their rights and protect their welfare. Safe, nontherapeutic research, however, seems neither unfair nor a violation of the rights or welfare of people who lack the capacity to give consent. Failing to do safe but important studies might be unfair and violate their rights and welfare, since it fails to consider all their needs. The Declaration of Helsinki (2000) now permits nontherapeutic studies with guardians' consent and if other subjects cannot be used; no upper level of risk is given unlike the next option.

THE "RISK-BENEFIT" OR "U.S. FEDERAL REGULATION" SOLUTION. A fourth approach allows research on procedures or interventions with incompetent persons when the research holds out direct benefit to them or does not place them at unwarranted risk of harm, discomfort, or inconvenience. Defenders of the fourth option should clarify what risk is unwarranted. This policy uses risk assessment to set priorities between the social utility of encouraging studies and the protection of people's rights of self-determination and well-being. To try to set priorities between the social utility of such studies and respect and protection of incompetent people, this option stipulates that the greater the risk, the more rigorous and elaborate the procedural protection and consent requirements. The U.S. federal regulations (U.S. "Protection of Human Subjects," 45 CFR 46 Subpart D) reflect this fourth policy option in the codes for research with children adopted and those proposed (in 1978 but never adopted) for institutionalized people with mental impairment or retardation. The Council for International Organizations of Medical Science has adopted a similar standard (CIOMS). Under this fourth option, therapy is one of the intended direct benefits that should be taken into account in a risk analysis. Whenever possible, the incompetent persons should give their assent to participate. Assent means affirmative agreement, not just lack of objection.

There are advantages to focusing directly upon the likely benefits and harms of procedures or interventions being studied. First, there are benefits other than therapy that may play a role in deciding if it is reasonable to serve as a subject. A safe, nontherapeutic study that increases a child's understanding of a sibling's chronic illness, for example, might have important lessons about empathy for the child. Those giving consent need to know, of course, the nature and magnitude of the intended benefits (such as education or therapy) or risks of harms associated with the study. Second, calling something "therapeutic" can create the unwarranted idea that participating in the study is in a person's best interest. Risk assessment can reveal hazards, inconveniences, and costs in therapeutic studies that some reasonable people would prefer to avoid.

Using a likely-harms-to-benefits calculation, the U.S. regulations specify four categories of research for children (U.S. "Protection of Human Subjects," 45 CFR 46 Subpart D). IRBs can approve research that they judge to be in the first three categories, and all three generally require the child's assent, if possible, parental approval, and other safeguards such as minimizing risks of harm, having competent investigators and suitable background studies. The first category permits studies with no greater than a minimal risk; the second allows studies with higher risks as long as they are likely to have at least as much direct benefit to subjects as other available therapies; the third category allows research involving a minor increase over minimal risk and no likelihood of direct benefit to each individual subjects, if it is likely to yield vitally important knowledge about the children's disorder or condition. U.S. policy is unique in allowing studies having more than a minor increase over a minimal risk and that do not hold out benefit for the subjects but approval is needed from the federal government. As in the case of the guidelines for prisoners cited earlier, procedural safeguards increase with risk.

There are no final guidelines in the United States for research on those institutionalized as mentally infirm, but there is a proposal about how to treat those institutionalized with impairments like mental illness, senility, psychosis, mental retardation, or emotional disturbances (U.S. Department of Health, Education and Welfare, 1978a, 1978b). It is similar to that proposed for children, except that it allows incompetent adults more authority to decline to participate in studies. The consent or assent of those institutionalized

with such impairments must be sought. Those who refuse may not be enrolled in any study that does not hold out direct benefit, without authorization from the courts. CIOMS has a policy that permits enrolling incompetent adults if the study has no more than a minimal risk, others cannot be subjects, the consent of the person or the permission of a responsible family member is obtained, and the research goal is to study the person's disorder or to benefit them.

Unfortunately, this fourth, popular policy option has difficulties. Key terms are either undefined or have vague definitions, permitting broad interpretations about what risks of harm are warranted and what constitutes a benefit. For example, the pivotal concepts of "minimal risk" and "a minor increase over a minimal risk" are problematic (Kopelman, 1989; 2000). The regulations state "'minimal risks' means that the probability and magnitude of harm or discomfort anticipated in the proposed research are not greater in and of themselves than those ordinarily encountered in daily life or during the performance of routine physical or psychological examinations or tests" (U.S. "Protection of Human Subjects," 45 CFR 46 102 I). Many other countries and organizations have adopted a similar definition (Kopelman, 2000).

The first part of the definition is vague because daily risks include dangers from drive-by shootings, playing in traffic, flying in airplanes, terrorists attacks, and weapons of mass destruction. Can one know the nature, probability, and magnitude of these "everyday" hazards well enough to serve as a baseline to estimate research risk? And if one can, what reason exists for regarding them as a morally justifiable baseline? It seems easier to determine whether asking a four-year-old to stack blocks is a minimal-risk study than to determine the nature, probability, and magnitude of whatever risks people normally encounter in their daily lives. Moreover, it is unclear if it is the "everyday risks" refer to those some encounter (called the relative standard) or all of us encounter (called the absolute standard). It is also unclear why everyday risks should be a proper baseline to determine that research risk is minimal. Some people have terrible risks in their daily life, but it would seem unfair to use that to justify higher-risk studies for them than for other people.

The second disjunctive of the definition seems to set a standard for physical interventions that have a minimal risk, especially if it is understood as referring to the routine examinations of healthy persons. The test is whether the risk in the research activity is like that of a routine examination. Accordingly, review boards may not approve *as minimal risk* research such procedures as X rays, bronchoscopy, spinal taps, or cardiac catheterization because they are not part of routine examinations, at least for healthy persons. Review boards, however, can approve studies that have a minor increase over minimal risk, and some of these procedures have been approved as having a minor increase over a minimal risk if their goal is to study a child's "disorder or condition." The terms "minor increase over minimal risk" and "condition" are undefined and vague with no definition for the crucial upper limit of risk that can be approved by review boards, considerable variation exists in how they are understood (NBAC; Kopelman, 2000; 2002).

Finally, this definition of "minimal risk" offers little guidance about how to assess *psychosocial risks* such as invasion of privacy, breach of confidentiality, labeling, and stigmatization. In routine visits, doctors and nurses ordinarily encounter discussions of family abuse, sexual orientation, and diagnoses that could affect reputations or the ability to get jobs or insurance.

Without clear standards for risk assessment, how effective are these guidelines? A 1981 survey of pediatric department chairs and pediatric research directors (Janofsky and Starfield) found considerable differences of opinion about whether procedures such as venipuncture, arterial puncture, and gastric and intestinal intubation are hazardous. For example, most regarded arterial puncture to have a "greater than minimal risk"; but between 8 and 24 percent thought it had less than a minimal risk, depending on the child's age. An editorial in the *Journal of Pediatrics* found such variation "cause for concern" and said that better standards of risk assessment are needed (Lascari). Two decades later, similar concerns remain (NBAC; Kopelman, 2000, 2002).

In short, this fourth policy is vague and open to very different interpretations. For example, in 1992 the National Institutes of Health appointed a nine-member review board to assess whether a study of the safety and efficacy of synthetic growth hormone (hGH) was in compliance with federal research guidelines. Eighty children whose adult height was projected to be at or below the first percentile would participate with their parents' consent. The children would receive injections three times a week for four to seven years (600 to 1,100 injections), half getting hGH and, for comparison, the other half receiving salt water, an ineffective placebo. Neither the doctors, the parents, nor the children would know who got water and who got the growth hormone. Each year all the children would come to the National Institutes of Health to undergo a variety of tests, including physicals, X rays, nude photographs, and psychological evaluations. Of the nine panelists, a majority held there was a minor increase over minimal risk, but this risk was offset by the health benefits of being in the study. Two others judged there was no benefit to offset the risks, inconvenience, and discomfort to those getting water rather

than hGH, but the study was important enough to be justified. One panelist (this author) argued that a study of a terrible disease might justify these risks for the group getting hundreds of water injections; but shortness is no disease, and so the risk is unwarranted.

If there is any consensus that the fourth approach represented by the U.S. rules and others is the best way to set priorities between the need to protect the rights and welfare of people who lack the capacity to give informed consent with the need to encourage research, it may mask different understandings of what constitutes an acceptable risk of likely-harms-to-benefits ratio. There is a lively debate in the literature about how to clarify these thresholds and, not surprisingly, some favor more restrictive definitions than others (NBAC; Kopelman, 2002).

Conclusion

IRBs, ERCs, and RECs should continue to play an important role in protecting vulnerable subjects while making it possible to continue important research, but there are sharp differences about whether additional regulatory protections are needed (NBAC). Without safeguards, vulnerable subjects risk exploitation. Excessive restrictions, however, have dangers as well. They can thwart the advance of knowledge needed to improve medical care for the groups they seek to protect. Where potential subjects are capable of giving legal consent but are vulnerable to pressure or manipulation, their consent should be monitored to see if it is coerced or manipulated, and regulations should be sought only when they can be justified. There is general agreement that competent adults should serve as research subjects whenever possible, and that when people who lack capacity to give consent are enrolled as subjects in biomedical research, the study should be related to their healthcare needs. The guardian's consent should be obtained; and, if possible, the assent or permission of the person lacking capacity to consent should also be sought. Since there are difficulties with each of the four policies regarding subjects lacking capacity to give informed consent, IRBs, ERCs, and RECs will have to consider issues of utility, fairness, and protection without entirely satisfactory guidance.

LORETTA M. KOPELMAN (1995)
REVISED BY AUTHOR

SEE ALSO: *Aging and the Aged: Healthcare and Research Issues; AIDS: Healthcare and Research Issues; Autoexperimentation; Autonomy; Children: Healthcare and Research Issues; Coercion; Commercialism in Scientific Research; Embryo* and Fetus: Embryo Research; Empirical Methods in Bioethics; Freedom and Free Will; Genetics and Human Behavior: Scientific and Research Issues; Holocaust; Infants: Public Policy and Legal Issues; Informed Consent: Consent Issues in Human Research; Mentally Ill and Mentally Disabled Persons: Research Issues; Military Personnel as Research Subjects; Minorities as Research Subjects; Paternalism; Pediatrics, Overview of Ethical Issues in; Public Policy and Bioethics; Prisoners as Research Subjects; Race and Racism; Research, Human: Historical Aspects; Research Methodology; Research, Multinational; Research, Unethical; Responsibility; Scientific Publishing; Sexism; Students as Research Subjects; Virtue and Character; and other Research Policy subentries

BIBLIOGRAPHY

Council for International Organizations of Medical Science (CIOMS). 2002. International Ethical Guidelines for Biomedical Research Involving Human Subjects. Geneva: Author.

Germany (Territory Under Allied Occupation, 1945–1955: U.S. Zone) Military Tribunals. 1947. "Permissible Medical Experiments." In Volume 2 of Trials of War Criminals Before the Nuremberg Tribunals Under Control Law No. 10. Washington, D.C.: U.S. Government Printing Office.

Janofsky, Jeffrey, and Starfield, Barbara. 1981. "Assessment of Risk in Research on Children." Journal of Pediatrics 98(5): 842–846.

Kopelman, Loretta M. 1989. "When Is the Risk Minimal Enough for Children to Be Research Subjects?" In Children and Health Care: Moral and Social Issues, edited by Loretta M. Kopelman and John C. Moskop. Dordrecht, Netherlands: Kluwer.

Kopelman, Loretta M. 2000. "Children as Research Subjects: A Dilemma." The Journal of Medicine and Philosophy 25(6): 745–764.

Kopelman, Loretta M. 2002. "Pediatric Research Regulations Under Legal Scrutiny: Grimes Narrows Their Interpretation." Journal of Law, Medicine & Ethics 30: 38–49.

Levine, Robert J. 1986. Ethics and Regulation of Clinical Research, 2nd edition. Baltimore: Urban & Schwarzenberg.

McCormick, Richard A. 1974. "Proxy Consent in the Experimental Situation." Perspectives in Biology and Medicine 18(1): 2–20.

National Institutes of Health, Human Growth Hormone Protocol Review Committee. 1992. Report of the NIH Human Growth Hormone Protocol Review Committee. Bethesda, MD: Author.

Proctor, Robert. 1988. Racial Hygiene: Medicine Under the Nazis. Cambridge, MA: Harvard University Press.

Ramsey, Paul. 1970. The Patient as Person: Explorations in Medical Ethics. New Haven, CT: Yale University Press.

Shirkey, Harry C. 1968. "Therapeutic Orphans." Journal of Pediatrics 72(1): 119–120.

U.S. Code of Federal Regulations Title 21—Food and Drug Administration Title 21 "ICH (International Conference on Harmonization Guideline) for Good Clinical Practice" as adopted by the FDA, published in the Federal Register May 9, 1997.

U.S. Department of Health, Education, and Welfare; National Commission for the Protection of Human Subjects of Biomedical and Behavioral Research. 1978a. Research Involving Those Institutionalized as Mentally Infirm: Report and Recommendations. Washington, D.C.: Author.

U.S. Department of Health, Education, and Welfare; National Commission for the Protection of Human Subjects of Biomedical and Behavioral Research. 1978b. Appendix to Report and Recommendations, Research Involving Those Institutionalized as Mentally Infirm. Washington, D.C.: Author.

U.S. Protection Human Subjects, 45 Code of Federal Regulations 46.

U.S. Public Health Service. 1991. "Consultation on International Collaborative Human Immunodeficiency Virus (HIV) Research." Law, Medicine and Health Care 19(3–4): 259–263.

World Medical Assembly. 1989. "The Declaration of Helsinki: Recommendations Guiding Medical Doctors and Biomedical Research Involving Human Subjects." Law, Medicine, and Health Care 19(3–4): 264–265. (Adopted by the 18th World Medical Assembly, Helsinki, Finland, in 1964; amended in 1975, 1983, 1989, and 2001.)

INTERNET RESOURCE

National Bioethics Advisory Commission (NBAC). 2001. Ethical and Policy Issues in Research Involving Human Participants Volume I: Report and Recommendations. Bethesda, MD: Author. Available from <http://georgetown.edu/research/nrcbl/nbac/pubs.html>.

III. SUBJECTS

Selecting individuals to participate in research involves not only scientific decisions about appropriate entry criteria but also ethical decisions about the distribution of benefits and burdens. The U.S. National Commission on the Protection of Human Subjects of Biomedical and Behavioral Research (U.S. National Commission) cited three ethical principles as the foundation of research ethics. The first, respect for persons, and the second, beneficence, have been analyzed more often and in greater depth than the third, justice. Investigators, regulators, and institutional review boards (IRBs) are accustomed to applying the principle of beneficence by examining the risk-benefit ratio and applying the principle of respect for persons by examining informed consent. But the third principle—the selection of subjects as a matter of justice—has often been considered last and in only one of its aspects, the protection of vulnerable groups from exploitation as subjects. This situation is changing as persons and groups previously excluded from research on grounds of vulnerability seek access to what they perceive as research benefits, primarily the opportunity to try new drugs for serious and life-threatening illnesses.

According to the U.S. National Commission, justice is relevant to the selection of subjects at two levels: the social and the individual. At the individual level, "researchers [should] exhibit fairness: thus, they should not offer potentially beneficial research only to some patients who are in their favor or select only 'undesirable' persons for risky research" (p. 7). At the social level, "distinctions [should] be drawn between classes of subjects that ought, and ought not, to participate in any particular kind of research, based on the ability of members of that class to bear burdens and on the appropriateness of placing further burdens on already burdened persons" (U.S. National Commission, p. 7). Specifically, on the grounds of social justice, classes of subjects should be ranked (e.g., adults before children) and some classes of potential subjects (e.g., prisoners and the institutionalized mentally infirm) should be selected only under certain conditions and perhaps not at all.

Very few philosophers or other scholars have proposed standards by which to establish priorities in the selection of subjects. Hans Jonas proposed a "descending order of permissibility" for the "conscription" of subjects. In his view, researchers themselves should be the first to test a new therapy, in that they can best understand the risks and benefits. Believing that very sick or dying patients are particularly vulnerable to researchers' invitations, Jonas opposed using them in research not directly related to their care.

Another approach has been to assert an obligation to participate in biomedical research. Arthur Caplan (1984) argued that research is a form of voluntary social cooperation that generates obligations of fairness and reciprocity. If a competent individual voluntarily seeks care in a hospital or institution that conducts biomedical research, he or she benefits from research and should share in its costs (i.e., participate). This obligation is a general one, not an obligation to volunteer for the first available trial or any particular trial.

Selecting the Least Vulnerable

Underlying these different views is the assumption that research is risky or at least burdensome. If this is true, subjects should be selected in a way that protects those whose social, demographic, or economic characteristics make them particularly vulnerable to coercion and exploitation. Volunteering for research is seen as either a duty to be discharged or an altruistic act to be applauded. This emphasis on protecting vulnerable persons is understandable, given the signal event in the modern history of clinical research ethics—the cruel and often fatal experiments performed on unconsenting prisoners by Nazi doctors in World War II (Caplan, 1992). Public opinion in the United States also was shaped by the revelations of unethical experiments such as the Tuskegee Syphilis Study of poor black sharecroppers (Jones), the Willowbrook hepatitis B studies at an institution for mentally retarded children (Rothman, 1982), and the Jewish Chronic Disease Hospital studies in which live cancer cells were injected into uninformed elderly patients (Katz et al.). The most influential single article was one by Henry Knowles Beecher, a respected anesthesiologist, in the *New England Journal of Medicine;* it described a series of studies at major research institutions that placed subjects at risk and failed to obtain informed consent (Beecher; Rothman, 1991).

The view of research as inherently risky and of research subjects as inherently needing protection began to change in the early 1980s. Why? First, consider research at the level of individuals. The empirical question of the actual risk in most research studies has been answered: quite low. The U.S. President's Commission for the Study of Ethical Problems in Biomedical and Behavioral Research asked three large research institutions to summarize their experience with research-related injuries (U.S. President's Commission). Each group found a very low incidence of adverse effects. In one institution, out of more than 8,000 subjects involved in 157 protocols, only three adverse effects were reported, including two headaches after spinal taps. Some of these reassuring results may be due to the vigilance of IRBs and investigators in reducing the likelihood of risk in designing and implementing studies. While risk is always an element that subjects should consider when deciding whether to enter a study, it is often no longer the paramount issue.

Sharing the Benefits of Research

Even more important, the benefits side of the equation has assumed greater weight in individual decision making. Patients and advocacy groups are demanding more autonomy and less paternalism in the selection of subjects. Desperately ill patients forcefully argue that they are willing to trade a higher level of risk for the potential benefits of promising new procedures, devices, or drugs. Advocates for women and children point out that the typical exclusion or underrepresentation of these populations in clinical trials means that the drugs, when approved, will be prescribed for them with little direct data about dosage, efficacy, or side effects. These trends have been spurred by the vigorous, sometimes confrontational, efforts of persons with the acquired immunodeficiency syndrome (AIDS). This advocacy also has stressed the inclusion of groups with poor access to trials, mainly women and minorities (C. Levine, 1988, 1993). Increased emphasis on women's health issues has provided some information on subject recruitment. Examining the inclusion of women in clinical trials, the U.S. General Accounting Office reviewed the practices of the National Institutes of Health (NIH) and the Food and Drug Administration (FDA) (Nadel; U.S. General Accounting Office). In both instances women were found to be underrepresented. The FDA review found that women were represented in every clinical trial of the fifty-three drugs approved by the FDA in the previous three and a half years. However, for more than 60 percent of the drugs, the proportion of women in the trial was less than the proportion of women with the relevant disease. Women were particularly underrepresented in trials of cardiovascular drugs, even though cardiovascular disease is the leading cause of death in women.

In arguing for wider inclusion criteria in clinical trials, patient advocates and some clinicians have noted that in the interest of good medical care, drugs should be tested on the populations that will use them. This belief runs counter to the more traditional research view of subject selection, which focuses on testing drugs in a small, homogeneous population in order to detect differences in efficacy and side effects as rapidly as possible.

Even with broadened inclusion criteria, not all patients who want access to promising new agents can be enrolled in clinical trials because they fail to meet the inclusion criteria, they live too far from a research center, or the trials are already closed. Several other mechanisms have been developed, such as the "parallel track," in which qualified patients who cannot enroll in clinical trials may obtain a promising drug through their physician ("Expanded Availability"). Community-based research, especially in cancer and AIDS, also has made clinical trials more accessible to patients.

The NIH has formalized the movement toward broader selection of subjects by mandating that its research grant recipients include appropriate numbers of women and minorities (Kirschstein). The 1993 NIH Revitalization Act (P.L. 103–43) extended the revised NIH policy by requiring the NIH director to ensure that women and members of minority groups are included in each federally funded project. The director may waive the requirement if the inclusion is inappropriate for health reasons, the purpose of the research, or any other circumstance. Cost, however, is not a permissible reason to fail to include women and members of minority groups.

This trend has limits, however. The inclusion of pregnant women in clinical trials is still controversial unless the trial is specifically designed to benefit the fetus, such as trials to prevent maternal-fetal transmission of the human immunodeficiency virus (HIV), which is associated with AIDS. Some of the objections to including pregnant women rely on ethical concerns about, for example, placing at risk a fetus, who cannot consent. Most of the concerns are based on fears of legal liability should the fetus be born with an injury that might be attributed to the investigational drug. Other subject groups for which protection is still deemed essential include children (Levine, 1991) and prisoners and mentally ill persons. Still other groups sometimes cited as vulnerable include elderly people, military personnel, pharmaceutical company employees, and medical students. Although some conditions and some protocols might be coercive, in general these individuals can make choices voluntarily. Special procedures have been set up in some instances to ensure voluntariness (see, e.g., Winter, on the U.S. Department of Defense).

From the societal perspective, equitable selection of subjects means that the groups bearing the burdens of research should also share in its benefits. Opponents of research in prisons argue that the fruits of the research— newly approved drugs—are rarely available in that setting. Similarly, although many drug trials have been carried out in Third World countries, these nations are often so poor or so lacking in healthcare services that they cannot afford to provide the tested drugs to their citizens.

More recently, representatives of Third World countries and of poorly served communities in the United States have been demanding a greater role in the distribution of benefits (Lurie et al.; National Commission on AIDS; Thomas and Quinn). Their agreement to participate in clinical drug trials is sometimes conditioned on a promise from trial sponsors to provide something of benefit to the population—the drug, if it proves efficacious, or the health infrastructure needed to deliver the therapy. Efficacy trials for vaccines, which require thousands of subjects, cannot be conducted without the goodwill and participation of a community's leaders. Community consultation, in which investigators and community spokespersons collaborate on the design and implementation of a trial, is becoming a frequent strategy for ensuring that the concerns of the pool of potential subjects and their representatives are addressed.

Recognizing the importance of social justice in the distribution of burdens and benefits, the World Health Organization (WHO) and the Council for International Organizations of Medical Sciences (CIOMS) guidelines for international research state:

Before undertaking research involving subjects in underdeveloped communities, whether in developed or developing countries, the investigator must ensure that:

- persons in underdeveloped communities ordinarily will not be involved in research that might equally well be carried out in developed communities;
- the research is relevant to the health needs and responsive to the priorities of the community. (WHO-CIOMS)

The commentary on this guideline states: "If any product is to be developed, such as a new therapeutic agent, clear understandings should be reached about whether and how the product, once developed, will be made available to members of the community in which the research was conducted" (WHO-CIOMS, pp. 38–39).

The equitable selection of subjects now includes an assessment of both the need for protecting vulnerable individuals and groups and the importance of allowing them maximum choice in making the ultimate decision to participate. In the future, even more emphasis will be placed on the equitable distribution of the benefits of research.

CAROL LEVINE (1995)
REVISED BY AUTHOR

SEE ALSO: *Aging and the Aged: Healthcare and Research Issues; AIDS: Healthcare and Research Issues; Autoexperimentation; Children: Healthcare and Research Issues; Commercialism in Scientific Research; Embryo and Fetus: Embryo Research; Empirical Methods in Bioethics; Genetics and Human Behavior: Scientific and Research Issues; Holocaust; Infants: Public Policy and Legal Issues; Informed Consent: Consent Issues in Human Research; Mentally Ill and Mentally Disabled Persons: Research Issues; Military Personnel as Research Subjects; Minorities as Research Subjects; Pediatrics, Overview of Ethical Issues in; Prisoners as Research Subjects; Race and Racism; Research, Human: Historical Aspects; Research, Multinational; Research Policy; Research, Unethical; Responsibility; Scientific Publishing; Sexism; Students as Research Subjects; Virtue and Character;* other *Research Methodology* subentries

BIBLIOGRAPHY

Annas, George J., and Grodin, Michael A. eds. 1995. *The Nazi Doctors and the Nuremberg Code: Human Rights in Human Experimentation.* New York: Oxford University Press.

Appelbaum, Paul S. 1996. "Examining the Ethics of Human Subjects Research." *Kennedy Institute of Ethics Journal* 6(3): 283–287.

Beecher, Henry K. 1966. "Ethics and Clinical Research." *New England Journal of Medicine* 274(24): 1354–1360.

Brody, Baruch A. 1998. "The Ethics of Biomedical Research: An International Perspective." New York: Oxford University Press.

Caplan, Arthur L. 1984. "Is There a Duty to Serve as a Subject in Biomedical Research?" *IRB* 6(5): 1–5.

Caplan, Arthur L., ed. 1992. *When Medicine Went Mad: Bioethics and the Holocaust.* Totowa, NJ: Humana.

Chastain, Garvin, and Landrum, R. Eric, eds. 1999. *Protecting Human Subjects: Departmental Subject Pools and Institutional Review Boards.* Washington, D.C.: American Psychological Association.

"Expanded Availability of Investigational New Drugs Through a Parallel Track Mechanism for People with AIDS and Other HIV-Related Disease." 1992. *Federal Register* 57, no. 73 (April 18): 13250–13259.

Foster, Claire. 2001. *The Ethics of Medical Research on Humans.* New York: Cambridge University Press.

Jonas, Hans. 1970. "Philosophical Reflections on Experimenting with Human Subjects." In *Experimentation with Human Subjects,* pp. 1–31, ed. Paul A. Freund. New York: George Braziller.

Jones, James H. 1993. *Bad Blood: The Tuskegee Syphilis Experiment.* New and expanded edition. New York: Free Press.

Kahn, Jeffrey P.; Mastroianni, Anna C.; and Sugarman, Jeremy, eds. 1998. *Beyond Consent: Seeking Justice in Research.* New York: Oxford University Press.

Katz, Jay; Capron, Alexander M.; and Glass, Eleanor Swift, eds. 1972. *Experimentation with Human Beings: The Authority of the Investigator, Subject, Professions, and State in the Human Experimentation Process.* New York: Russell Sage Foundation.

Kirschstein, Ruth L. 1991. "Research on Women's Health." *American Journal of Public Health* 81(3): 291–293.

Kopelman, Loretta M. 2000. "Children as Research Subjects: A Dilemma." *Journal of Medicine and Philosophy* 25(6): 745–764.

Levine, Carol. 1988. "Has AIDS Changed the Ethics of Human Subjects Research?" *Law, Medicine and Health Care* 16(3–4): 167–173.

Levine, Carol. 1991. "Children in HIV/AIDS Clinical Trials: Still Vulnerable After All These Years." *Law, Medicine and Health Care* 19(3–4): 231–237.

Levine, Carol. 1993. "Women as Research Subjects: New Priorities, New Questions." In *Emerging Issues in Biomedical Policy: An Annual Review,* pp. 169–188, ed. Robert H. Blank and Andrea L. Bonnicksen. New York: Columbia University Press.

Levine, Robert J. 1984. "What Kinds of Subjects Can Understand This Protocol?" *IRB* 6(5): 6–8.

Levine, Robert J. 1988. *Ethics and Regulation of Clinical Research,* 2nd edition. New Haven, CT: Yale University Press.

Loue, Sana. 2000. *Textbook of Research Ethics: Theory and Practice.* New York: Plenum Publishers.

Lurie, Peter; Bishaw, Makonnen; Chesney, Margaret A.; et al. 1994. "Ethical, Behavioral, and Social Aspects of HIV Vaccine Trials in Developing Countries." *Journal of the American Medical Association* 271(4): 295–301.

Mastroianni, Anna, and Kahn, Jeffrey. 2001. "Swinging on the Pendulum: Shifting Views of Justice in Human Subjects Research." *Hastings Center Report* 31(3): 21–28.

Moreno, Jonathan D. 2001. "Goodbye to All That: The End of Moderate Protectionism in Human Subjects Research." *Hastings Center Report* 31(3): 9–17.

Nadel, Mark V. 1990. *National Institutes of Health: Problems Implementing Policy on Women in Study Populations. Statement of Mark V. Nadel, Associate Director, National and Public Health Issues, Human Resources Division, Before the Subcommittee on Health and the Environment, Committee on Energy and Commerce, House of Representatives.* GAO/T-HRD-90–38. Washington, D.C.: U.S. General Accounting Office.

National Commission on AIDS. 1992. *The Challenge of HIV/AIDS in Communities of Color,* ed. Linda C. Humphrey and Frances Porcher. Washington, D.C.: Author.

Pincus, Harold Alan; Lieberman, Jeffery A.; and Ferris, Sandy, eds. 1999. *Ethics in Psychiatric Research: A Resource Manual for Human Subjects Protection.* Arlington, VA: American Psychiatric Press.

Resnik, David B. 1998. "The Ethics of HIV Research in Developing Nations." *Bioethics* 12(4): 286–306.

Rothman, David J. 1982. "Were Tuskegee and Willowbrook 'Studies in Nature'?" *Hastings Center Report* 12(2): 5–7.

Rothman, David J. 1991. *Strangers at the Bedside: A History of How Law and Bioethics Transformed Medical Decision Making.* New York: Basic Books.

Sales, Bruce D., and Folkman, Susan, eds. 2000. *Ethics in Research With Human Participants.* Washington, D.C.: American Psychological Association.

Schuklenk, Udo, and Ashcroft, Richard. 2000. "International Research Ethics." *Bioethics* 14(2): 158–172.

Thomas, Stephen B., and Quinn, Sandra Crouse. 1991. "The Tuskegee Syphilis Study, 1932 to 1972: Implications for HIV Education and AIDS Risk Education Programs in the Black Community." *American Journal of Public Health* 81(11): 1498–1504.

U.S. Congress. 1993. "National Institutes of Health Revitalization Amendment." *Public Law* pp. 103–143. Washington, D.C.: Author.

U.S. General Accounting Office. 1992. *Women's Health: FDA Needs to Ensure More Study of Gender Differences in Prescription Drug Testing: Report to Congressional Requesters.* GAO/HRD-93–17. Washington, D.C.: Author.

U.S. National Commission for the Protection of Human Subjects of Biomedical and Behavioral Research. 1979. *The Belmont Report: Ethical Principles and Guidelines for the Protection of Human Subjects of Research.* Washington, D.C.: U.S. Government Printing Office.

U.S. President's Commission for the Study of Ethical Problems in Medicine and Biomedical and Behavioral Research. 1982. *Compensating for Research Injuries: A Report on the Ethical and Legal Implications of Programs to Redress Injuries Caused by Biomedical and Behavioral Research.* Washington, D.C.: Author.

World Health Organization and Council for International Organizations of Medical Sciences (WHO-CIOMS). 1993. "International Ethical Guidelines for Biomedical Research Involving Human Subjects." Geneva, Switzerland: Author.

Winter, Philip E. 1984. "Human Subject Research Review in the Department of Defense." *IRB* 6(3): 9–10.

RESEARCH, UNETHICAL

• • •

Unethical research is a concept inevitably relative to accepted views concerning research's ethical requirements. For Claude Bernard, an early French exponent of the scientific method in medicine who felt that the principle underlying medical morality requires that persons not be harmed, paradigm cases of unethical research are studies that offer their subjects risks that exceed their potential benefits. The Nuremberg Tribunal, by stating in its first principle of ethical research that the subject's free consent is absolutely essential, added as paradigmatic cases of unethical research those studies performed upon unconsenting persons (Germany [Territory Under Allied Occupation, ...]). U.S. regulations that require an equitable selection of research subjects imply that a study that is otherwise ethical (e.g., a study with an acceptable risk-benefit ratio and whose subjects have freely consented) becomes unethical when it unfairly draws its research population from persons disadvantaged by reason of race, religion, or dependency, among others ("Federal Policy").

Examples of Unethical Research

Whichever ethical requirement may be chosen, the history of human research offers grim examples of its violation. During World War II, German researchers performed a large number of experiments in concentration camps and elsewhere. Subject-victims of Nazi research were predominantly Jews, but also included Romanies (Gypsies), prisoners of war, political prisoners, and others (Germany [Territory Under Allied Occupation ...]; Caplan). Nazi experimental atrocities included investigation of quicker and more efficient means of inducing sexual sterilization (including clandestine radiation dosing and unanesthetized male and female castration) and death (an area of study Leo Alexander

[1949] termed "thanatology," which includes studies of techniques for undetectable individual assassination—i.e., murder that mimics natural death—as well as mass murder). Among the best-known cases were the hypothermia experiments, which investigated mechanisms of death by freezing and means of preventing it. These studies, motivated by the loss of German pilots over the North Sea, included immersing prisoners in freezing water and observing freezing's lethal physiological pathways.

Beginning in 1932, the U. S. Public Health Service funded a study of the natural progression of untreated syphilis in black men. Four hundred subject-victims were studied, along with 200 uninfected control subjects. The study, whose first published scientific paper appeared in 1936, continued until a newspaper account of it appeared in 1972. Its subject-victims were uninformed or misinformed about the purpose of the study, as well as its associated interventions. For example, participants were told that painful lumbar punctures were given as treatment, when in fact treatment for syphilis was withheld even after the discovery of penicillin (Brandt; Jones).

Numerous other examples of unethical research may be cited, though they have received far less attention. A New Zealand study on women that began in 1966 and was active for at least ten years had macabre similarities to the Tuskegee study. It concerned the natural history of untreated cervical carcinoma in situ (i.e., cancer that had not spread), and as in Tuskegee, its subject-victims were both uninformed and had treatment withheld for the study's duration (Paul). Parallel to the Nazi studies during World War II were those conducted by Japan. They included experimental attacks with biological weapons on at least eleven Chinese cities, and studies conducted on subject-victims that included efforts to induce gas gangrene by exploding fragmentation bombs near the exposed limbs and buttocks of 3,000 prisoners of war who were housed at a detention center known as Unit 731 (McNeill; Williams and Wallace).

Much unethical research comes to light only many years after its conduct, as is true of unethical military research conducted by the United States during and immediately following World War II. At that time, over 60,000 U.S. servicemen were involuntarily enrolled in studies involving exposure to chemical warfare agents (mustard gas and lewisite); at least 4,000 of them were exposed to high concentrations in field experiments and test chambers (Institute of Medicine).

Information about experiments on human radiation response supported by the U.S. government beginning in 1945 came to public attention in 1993. In one study, conducted from 1945 to 1947, eighteen patients considered to be terminally ill were injected with high doses of plutonium to determine how long it is retained in the human body. Military secrecy surrounding atomic energy precluded informed consent. Rather than telling subject-victims they would receive an injection of radioactive plutonium, the investigators told subjects they would receive a "product." Experiments on intellectually handicapped teenagers in a Massachusetts institution involved feeding the subjects very small amounts of radioactive iron and calcium to study the body's absorption of these materials. While the radiation exposure in these studies was low and unlikely to result in harm, the subject-victims were all incompetent, and their parents, who consented on their behalf, were simply asked by the institution to agree to "nutritional experiments." In reaction to news accounts of these and other studies, orders were issued in 1993 to declassify documents relating to unethical exposure of U.S. service personnel and citizens to radiation from atomic-weapons testing after World War II; in 1994 President Bill Clinton appointed a panel to guide a federal investigation into the radiation studies (Mann).

Several themes emerge from the known examples of unethical research. Such studies are likely to be done using disenfranchised or disadvantaged populations as subjects. In the absence of public outcry, unethical research may continue for many years, despite the fact that readers of the scientific literature in many cases have had access to all the facts they need to expose unethical practice (see Beecher). The larger and more egregious studies are especially likely to have been motivated by national security concerns and funded by the military.

Use of Data from Unethical Research

Very early sources reflect differing views on the permissibility of making medical or other use of information derived from unethical practices. The Babylonian Talmud (Shabbat 67b) states that the prohibition on Amorite practices (pagan sorcery) does not forbid actions done for the sake of healing, and it cites several cases of permitted incantations and sympathetic magic. Robert Burton quotes Paracelsus's *De occulta philosophia* to similar effect: "It matters not whether it be God or the Devil, Angels or unclean Spirits cure him, so that he be eased" (Burton, 1628, p. 7). By contrast, Thomas Aquinas prohibits "inquiring of demons concerning the future." Even if demons should know scientific truths, he writes, it is improper to "enter into fellowship" with them in this way (Aquinas).

A large variety of empirical and ethical arguments have been marshaled to oppose the use of data from unethical research. Empirical arguments, which depend upon the facts of particular cases, question the scientific reliability of such data. For example, Robert Berger, through a close analysis of the Nazi hypothermia data, claims that even by then-current scientific standards, the information is unreliable. He describes incomplete and contradictory data reporting, the absence of a controlling scientific protocol, and the control of the research program by scientifically untrained personnel (including Heinrich Himmler, Commander of the SS). In fact, the principal investigator, Sigmund Rascher, had a previous record of deception and was arrested in 1944 and charged with crimes that included scientific fraud. Some commentators argue that such data may be used, but only when the information is exceptionally reliable and useful. Most or all instances known of data gathered unethically, however, fail to meet this test (see Schafer).

Ethical arguments opposing use of the data are especially numerous. From a consequentialist point of view, unethical studies should be "punished" by "non-use," to discourage future investigators tempted to resort to unethical research practices. Other theories of punishment may be appealed to as well: As a matter of justice, it is argued that unethical investigators should not be rewarded by having the data from their studies used. By expunging the records of unethical research, the society of scientists expresses its solemn condemnation of the methods employed to acquire it; failing to do so would make science complicit with the research studies. Appropriate symbolism may call for the "burial" of this data, as it calls for the burial of the subject-victims from whom the data was derived (see Caplan; Martin; Post).

Rebuttals of these ethical arguments are equally numerous, relying upon the premise that data from unethical research studies may be valuable in principle: Any coincidence between "good science" and "good ethics," these writers argue, is only contingently true. As a practical matter, it is argued, the most serious instances of unethical research could not have been deterred by the punishment of non-use; some of the most heinous research studies were commissioned by governments, especially national security apparatuses. Punishment should be visited upon the investigators who engaged in unethical research; by withholding the use of data, current patients whose care might have been improved by use of that data are made to bear the brunt. Arguments from complicity are rejected because there is no causal connection between the prior acquisition of the data and its current use (the Nazis did not gather information about hypothermia in anticipation of its use by Canadian researchers a generation later); and because the current use of the data, far from being a continuation of the Nazi project, is for humanitarian purposes antithetical to the original Nazi intentions. In that way, the symbolism associated with the use of these data is seen to have a positive, redemptive value,

while retaining the data's possible value to science and society (Freedman; Greene).

The debate about the use of data from unethical studies should distinguish the different ways scientific results can be used. Three different meanings for data use have been suggested: reference to data, for example, by scientific publication or citation, to serve as grounding for a scientific argument; reliance upon data in establishing or validating a practice, scientific or technological (including clinical); and using data as suggestive of further areas for inquiry (Freedman). This last meaning, while the most common in practice, has been the least debated; it is unlikely that data, once disclosed, could fail to be used in this way.

Much debate has centered on the first meaning, use of data through publication or citation. Kristine Moe found that the Nazi hypothermia studies had been referenced at least forty-five times in the medical literature (Moe). The *New England Journal of Medicine,* among other publications, has taken the position that it will not publish studies considered unethical by its editor; moreover, it will allow references to unethical research only in articles that focus on ethical condemnation of the research in question (Ingelfinger). Robert J. Levine has argued that a preferable stance would permit the publication of scientifically sound but ethically questionable research, while requiring the simultaneous publication of editorial discussion of the ethical issues raised (Levine).

Use of data in the second sense, as grounding scientific or ethical practices, was central to a 1988 controversy. While considering air pollution regulations on phosgene, a chemical used in plastics manufacture and a component of pesticides, the U. S. Environmental Protection Agency (EPA) withdrew an analysis that made reference to data derived from Nazi experiments after some EPA scientists circulated a protest letter (Sun). Phosgene was a component of some chemical weapons, and the Nazis had studied the response of French prisoners to various levels of phosgene exposure. EPA officials, while recognizing scientific and technical flaws in the data's collection and reporting, held the data to be useful additions to the existing animal toxicology information. Nazi data is often said not to be generalizable to a normal population because it was derived from prisoners under horrible conditions of privation. However, even this aspect of the data was applicable because the EPA's recommendations were designed to minimize risk to those most physiologically vulnerable. Those opposed to use of the data presented arguments based on both fact and value. The data were said to be valueless because of their omission of consideration of vital variables like sex and weight of subject-victims. In addition, some agency scientists felt that data derived from this source, however valuable, should never be used.

In the majority of cases, the scientific value and impact of unethical research has been modest. Ethically, however, the Nazi, Tuskegee, and other studies have loomed large in raising both public awareness and ethical standards for the conduct of research. Unethical research has found its main use in ethics.

BENJAMIN FREEDMAN (1995)

SEE ALSO: *Animal Welfare and Rights: Ethical Perspectives on the Treatment and Status of Animals; Bias, Research; Bioterrorism; Children: Healthcare and Research Issues; Commercialism in Scientific Research; Competence; Conflict of Interest; Embryo and Fetus: Embryo Research; Embryo and Fetus: Embryonic Stem Cell Research; Harm; Holocaust; Informed Consent: Consent Issues in Research; Mentally Ill and Mentally Disabled Persons: Research Issues; Military Personnel as Research Subjects; Minorities as Research Subjects; Moral Status; Prisoners as Research Subjects; Race and Racism; Research Policy; Sexism; Surrogate Decision-Making; Transhumanism and Posthumanism*

BIBLIOGRAPHY

Alexander, Leo. 1949. "Medical Science Under Dictatorship." *New England Journal of Medicine* 241(2): 39–47.

Aquinas, Thomas. 1947. "Whether It Is Unlawful to Practice the Observance of the Magic Art." In vol. 2 of *Summa Theologica,* pp. 1608–1609 (II–II, q. 96), tr. the Fathers of the English Dominican Province. New York: Benziger Brothers. See especially the reply to "Objection 3."

Beecher, Henry K. 1966. "Ethics and Clinical Research." *New England Journal of Medicine* 274(24): 1354–1360.

Berger, Robert L. 1990. "Nazi Science—The Dachau Hypothermia Experiments." *New England Journal of Medicine* 322(20): 1435–1440.

Bernard, Claude. 1957. *An Introduction to the Study of Experimental Medicine,* tr. Henry Copley Green. New York: Dover. 1957.

Brandt, Allan M. 1978. "Racism and Research: The Case of the Tuskegee Syphilis Study." *Hastings Center Report* 8(6): 21–29.

Burton, Robert. 1961 (1628). *The Anatomy of Melancholy.* London: J. M. Dent.

Caplan, Arthur L., ed. 1992. *When Medicine Went Mad: Bioethics and the Holocaust.* Totowa, NJ: Humana Press.

"Federal Policy for the Protection of Human Subjects; Notices and Rules." 1991. *Federal Register* 56(117)(June 18): 18081–28032.

Freedman, Benjamin. 1992. "Moral Analysis and the Use of Nazi Experimental Results." In *When Medicine Went Mad: Bioethics and the Holocaust,* pp. 141–154, ed. Arthur L. Caplan. Totowa, NJ: Humana Press.

Germany (Territory Under Allied Occupation, 1945–1955: U.S. Zone) Military Tribunals. 1947. "Permissible Medical Experiments." In vol. 2 of *Trials of War Criminals Before the Nuremberg Tribunals Under Control Law,* (10): 181–183. Washington, D.C.: U.S. Government Printing Office.

Greene, Velvl. 1992. "Can Scientists Use Information Derived from the Concentration Camps?" In *When Medicine Went Mad: Bioethics and the Holocaust,* pp. 155–170, ed. Arthur L. Caplan. Totowa, NJ: Humana Press.

Ingelfinger, Franz J. 1973. "Ethics of Experiments on Children." *New England Journal of Medicine* 288(15): 791–792.

Institute of Medicine (U.S.) Committee to Survey the Health Effects of Mustard Gas and Lewisite. 1993. *Veterans at Risk: The Health Effects of Mustard Gas and Lewisite,* ed. Constance M. Pechura and David P. Rall. Washington, D.C.: National Academy Press.

Jones, James H. 1981. *Bad Blood: The Tuskegee Syphilis Experiment.* New York: Free Press.

Levine, Robert J. 1986. *Ethics and Regulation of Clinical Research,* 2nd edition. Baltimore: Urban & Schwarzenberg.

Mann, Charles C. 1994. "Radiation: Balancing the Record." *Science* 263: 470–473.

Martin, Robert M. 1986. "Using Nazi Scientific Data." *Dialogue* 25: 403–411.

McNeill, Paul M. 1993. *The Ethics and Politics of Human Experimentation.* New York: Cambridge University Press.

Moe, Kristine. 1984. "Should the Nazi Research Data Be Cited?" *Hastings Center Report* 14(6): 5–7.

Paul, Charlotte. 1988. "The New Zealand Cervical Cancer Study: Could It Happen Again?" *British Medical Journal* 297(6647): 533–539.

Post, Stephen G. 1988. "Nazi Data and the Rights of Jews." *Journal of Law and Religion* 6(2): 429–433.

Schafer, Arthur. 1986. "On Using Nazi Data: The Case Against." *Dialogue* 25(3): 413–419.

Sun, Marjorie. 1988. "EPA Bars Use of Nazi Data." *Science* 240(4848): 21.

Williams, Peter, and Wallace, David. 1989. *Unit 731: Japan's Secret Biological Warfare in World War II.* New York: Free Press.

RESPONSIBILITY

• • •

Responsibility has emerged as a central ethical category, directing attention to human beings as moral actors. It highlights the importance for ethical understanding of self-conscious moral commitments, discretion in moral judgment, personal strengths necessary to effective action, a wise use of the power and authority of societal offices, and accountability to oneself and to fellow human beings, perhaps also to God, for moral judgment and action. Discussions of responsibility do not displace systematic treatments of moral principles, laws, and rules; neither do they set aside critical studies of values worthy of promotion in human affairs. They recast these inquiries in terms of the personal lives and social roles of human beings.

Themes associated with responsibility have long been prominent in philosophical and religious discourse, though in different conceptual forms. Especially important are accounts of the moral and intellectual virtues, of moral character, and of the obedient or resolute wills of the upright (Aristotle; Aquinas; Calvin; Kant; cf. Cohen). Also relevant are themes elaborated in conceptions of moral law, including natural law; in notions of the orders of nature or creation; in interpretations of divine commandments and ordinances; and in treatments of God's covenant with Israel, or of the Christian idea of a new covenant in Jesus Christ (Aristotle; Aquinas; Brunner; Häring). Contemporary accounts of responsibility weave these classic themes together in ways that take account of modern social realities, and that utilize theories of action provided by the human sciences.

In regard to modern realities, the concept of responsibility corresponds to social complexity, which routinely generates problems with more features than any system of moral rules can encompass. It fits well with advanced technologies and high levels of specialization, where expert knowledge and skill are indispensable to moral judgment. Responsibility takes account of open spaces within democratic and free-market settings for individuals and groups to follow independent initiatives in the pursuit of cherished social goals. It accords with modern social theory, which conceives of social institutions—the state, business enterprises, special-interest associations, even families and religious bodies—as the constructions of autonomous individuals contracting for mutual advantage. Finally, responsibility can accommodate reflections on the moral ambiguities of the social and organizational contexts that structure human activity. In respect to each of these characteristics, themes relating to responsibility take on considerable importance.

The concept of responsibility enjoys prominence, then, because it can draw together a wide range of ethical ideas in a fashion pertinent to contemporary social existence. For some thinkers it serves as the unifying principle of a comprehensive ethical theory (cf. Niebuhr; Jonsen). Responsibility virtually becomes the first principle of ethics, so that the admonition "Be responsible!" conveys all that needs to be said about the moral life (Jonsen; cf. Glatzer). The theoretical task is to unfold the dimensions of responsibility in their bearing on personal and social processes.

The dimensions of responsibility appear both in the personal lives of individuals and in the roles, positions, and offices that order social institutions. All of these dimensions may not be explicit in a particular ethical theory, though most enter into discussion at some point. For religious thinkers, responsibility includes relationship to God, which uncovers a theological basis for ethical understanding.

Duties

At the most elementary level, responsible persons are those who recognize and carry out their duties. Duties define the moral requisites of human social existence: what we normally must do, no matter what else we might hope to accomplish, and what we normally may not do, regardless of our larger objectives. Moral duties can be qualified or set aside only when exceptional steps are necessary to secure the values they are designed to protect. Thus, medical procedures normally may not be performed without a patient's informed consent, even if the patient's life is at risk. However, in a medical emergency, they may be performed without consent, provided the patient is unable to respond and there is no one present with authority to decide on his or her behalf.

Duties are formulated as laws, regulations, and rules, perhaps in conjunction with underlying moral principles. Responsible persons abide by moral principles in their personal lives. They pay special attention to principles and rules linked to their social roles: parent, spouse, physician, research scientist, junior executive at a medical center, senator. They support collective efforts to uphold moral standards that order human activities in institutional contexts (cf. Beauchamp and Childress). For those who are religious, moral duties may derive their ultimate authority from divine purposes.

Tasks

Within the constraints of moral principles and rules, responsibility consists in the reliable performance of assumed or assigned tasks. We may speak of our tasks as our responsibilities. Responsible persons know what needs to be done, they appreciate its significance, they proceed on their own, they get the job done, and they do it well (Jonsen).

Some tasks are broad and open-ended: sustaining a good marriage; bearing and nurturing children; promoting the public good as a citizen, public servant, or professional. Others are specialized, such as the practice of pediatric medicine. Some may be narrowly focused, for example, the execution of insurance claims. Even specialized tasks lack clear limits. When do physicians know enough to be confident that they are providing optimal care for their patients? When have they done enough to promote life, health, and healing? Responsible persons maintain standards of excellence in relation to expectations associated with their social roles. Those who are religious may further connect their tasks with a vocation to serve a wider, divine purpose in all areas of their lives.

General Well-being

In conjunction with explicit moral commitments and role-determined assignments, responsible persons strive for just, fair, and good conditions where they live and work. They seek to bring about and maintain states of affairs that favor human well-being, perhaps the well-being of all creatures. Similarly, they resist and, where possible, seek to change circumstances that do harm to fellow human beings, even to other living creatures. They strive to improve the execution of tasks, and to see that basic moral imperatives are honored in everyday social interactions. Those who are religious may be sustained in their quest for a greater good by their hope in the promises of God.

Thus, a physician's responsibility does not end with patient care or with professional relationships wherein standards of quality care are maintained. It includes a public interest in the healthcare system as a whole, and in its ability to provide appropriate services for all people. More broadly, it embraces the promotion of human health in basic life patterns.

Commitment

Responsibility is about personal commitment. It expresses human care about the moral life (cf. Fingarette). Those who are responsible claim their duties and tasks as their own, as ways of acting that are internal to who they have become and are becoming (Gustafson; cf. Jonsen).

Classic ethical theories dealt with commitment either in terms of moral virtues (Aristotle; Aquinas) or in terms of the resolute will (Calvin; Kant; cf. Novak). Moral virtues are habits, stable ways of acting that accord with the good. They derive their energy from passions that have been *perfected* through disciplined practice, until an actor is disposed to do the good as a kind of *second nature.* In terms of normative content, the central moral virtue is justice, the disposition to grant to each person what he or she is due.

In Judaism and in Reformed Protestant thought, the basic commitment to do the good has been defined not as habit or disposition but as volition, a self-conscious determination to do one's duty in all things. Here the aim is not to shape the passions but to control them. Immanuel Kant gave these latter traditions philosophical form by speaking of the unqualified value of the "good will," that is, the will ever ready to do what the moral law commands (Kant).

Modern psychological theories generally set aside accounts of the self that isolate discrete virtues or particular psychic functions, such as the will. They portray the self as a complex, dynamic process in which a centered unity can be only a relative achievement (cf. Wallwork). Post-Freudian thinkers place special emphasis on the formative power of human relationships in these complex dynamics (cf. Erikson; Winnicott; Kohut; Chodorow). Thus, our moral commitments are integral to the relational bonds that form and sustain us as human beings. We come to understand these commitments through our life stories, including both family stories and the stories of communities to which we belong. It is by means of narrative that we apprehend and claim our moral identities (Taylor; Ricoeur).

Psychological perspectives substantially inform ethical discussions of responsibility (cf. Fingarette; Rouner; Wallwork; Taylor). They render more intelligible seemingly irrational features of human behavior: individuals acting in socially inappropriate ways or in ways that work against their self-conscious purposes (cf. Fingarette). They help us grasp dynamics that leave some persons virtually incapable of consistent care for the good, and hence unable to respond to concrete situations with moral sensitivity. In other instances, persons may profess moral concern, yet find themselves internally torn, deeply ambivalent, or emotionally empty. They lack focused energy to carry out the good they claim to honor.

In classic thought, such cases either revealed bad habits, called vices (Aristotle; Aquinas), or they represented the bondage of the will to sinful inclinations (Augustine; Calvin; Luther; cf. Kant). Modern perspectives introduce notions of pathology to account for this "irresponsible" behavior. They offer neither moral admonition nor judgment but therapy, a supportive relationship wherein a skilled professional helps a patient gain insight into the internal conflicts that impel him or her to destructive behavior. Therapy provides resources for self-discovery that open the way to mature moral concern (cf. Fingarette; Wallwork). Through processes of self-discovery we reconnect with values and relationships that give identity and significance to human life.

Moral commitment involves social roles and offices. Responsible persons incorporate into their personal identities moral principles and values that are linked to positions they occupy. Social roles, like social institutions, are invariably marred by moral ambiguities. They gain their moral import from the fact that despite their ambiguity, they serve a greater good, at least by minimizing harm. Responsible actors seek to advance the moral promise of their offices while resisting their morally questionable tendencies.

Strength

Responsibility presumes that we have the personal strengths and the requisite skills to carry out our duties and to perform our tasks. Classic traditions of moral virtue and volition focus on distinctively moral strengths. In volitional approaches, the pivotal strength is willpower, the determination to control any fears, desires, even natural inclinations, that might distract us from our duty. Those who are religious seek divine support for moral rectitude.

In theories of virtue, moral strength derives from an ability to harness the passions in the service of purposive activity (Aristotle; Aquinas). On the one hand, responsibility requires personal toughness, perseverance, courage. These strengths stem from a natural, organic combativeness that through practice has been shaped into a virtue. If we lack such strength, the pressures, threats, and risks common to social existence will force us to shrink from the proper performance of basic tasks and duties. For example, a physician might remain silent after witnessing a senior colleague's failure to observe minimal professional standards in practice. Although the physician cares about standards, he or she cannot bear the stresses of a formal complaint. Courage equips us to follow through on our commitments, even those that entail danger.

On the other hand, responsibility requires self-control, the ability to restrain our wants, desires, and feelings when they dispose us to betray our commitments. Here, too, we develop self-control or temperance through practice. We learn to shape our wants and desires to accord with the larger good toward which we aspire. Without self-control we are unreliable. Our desires continually override good judgment, perhaps even impelling us to harmful actions (cf. Aristotle; Aquinas).

Because of an attraction to a patient, a psychiatrist violates sexual boundaries that define professional relationships. A research scientist falsifies research data or makes improper use of the findings of others in order to advance his or her career. In the interest of increased income, a specialist in internal medicine proposes medical procedures of dubious merit to a dying patient. Responsibility requires the discipline to restrain our wants for the sake of our moral integrity.

Modern psychological theories deal with similar phenomena, although with greater emphasis on the complex dynamics, including interpersonal relationships, that figure so prominently in our makeup. As a result, moral strengths appear less as matters of personal accomplishment and more as functions of self-formation in relationships. As inherently social beings, we derive both courage and self-control from human bonds that cohere with our moral purposes (cf. Kohut; Chodorow; Rouner; Glatzer).

Personal strengths are not limited to emotional resources or volitional restraints. They embrace intellectual capacities, general and specialized knowledge, competence in oral and written communication, self-confidence, self-esteem, the mastery of skills crucial to typical tasks, physical strength and agility, energy, stamina, and manual dexterity.

We may not associate all of these elements with the moral life, yet they profoundly affect a person's ability to act. The responsible life includes, therefore, a commitment to cultivate native talents and abilities, and to devise ways of mitigating disabilities. Similarly, social responsibility requires policies that enhance human potential for effectiveness: opportunities for education and advanced training; specialized equipment and physical arrangements for persons hampered by "handicapping conditions"; nondiscriminatory practices regarding race, gender, ethnic origin, age, religious identification, and sexual orientation.

Responsibility for personal strengths includes self-care and discipline in holding personal and professional commitments to manageable levels. Mistakes, indiscretions, intemperate and abusive behavior, even addictive and self-destructive patterns, are more likely when we habitually overextend ourselves. Personal strengths are indispensable to the good we are disposed to do. They also allow us to broaden our moral commitments, perhaps to assume leadership in promoting the common good.

Power

The human capacity to act derives from social offices and positions as well as from personal strengths (cf. Brunner; Bonhoeffer). Responsible persons are attentive to power dynamics that operate in their interactions with colleagues, associates, and employees, as well as with patients, clients, customers, and users of services. They resist abuses of power in these interactions and draw upon the resources of their offices to promote justice and the common good. They model fairness and concern for general well-being in their own activities; they commend similar practices by others.

Judgment

Responsibility involves sound judgment about the good to be done in concrete situations. Our ability to judge depends upon stable moral commitments and personal strengths to act on those commitments. It is affected by the perceptions of those to whom we are closely related, and also by interests that structure our business, professional, and political activities. Yet judgment is still a distinct skill, a "practical intellectual virtue" cultivated through practice (Aristotle; Aquinas).

Moral judgment operates in a number of ways, all of which involve the creative imagination and accumulated practical wisdom of morally mature individuals. It consists in the interpretation and application to concrete cases of laws, regulations, and rules that define moral duties (cf. Ramsey). These regulations may be borne by the common culture or the culture of professional practice; they may also be codified in public law or in the operating procedures of complex organizations, such as hospitals. The task is to discern what is at stake in these regulations so that they can appropriately inform particular moral judgments. Interpretation generally leads to a search for principles that disclose what is morally at stake in various regulations, for example, the claim that these regulations protect conditions essential to human existence and well-being.

By their very nature, principles, laws, and rules are abstract. It is not uncommon, therefore, to confront cases that are not adequately covered by existing regulations. Moral judgment may then consist in the construction of new rules that can inform our responses to these problem cases. The new rules may represent reformulations or extensions of familiar standards. They may consist of novel directives derived from elemental moral principles. The goal is to furnish stable guidelines for dealing with an emerging class of cases in the context of changing social circumstances. Bioethics continually confronts such challenges as it responds to enlarged technical capacities within biomedical practice.

Some cases are sufficiently distinct that they are best treated as exceptions to the rules. Moral judgment then entails adapting the rules to take account of variables that define the exception. Through experience, we learn to distinguish genuine exceptions from sets of cases that expose problems with existing rules. For the latter, we must rethink the rules, devising fresh formulations suited to the new cases.

In many life contexts, such as biomedical practice, we regularly deal with so many specific variables that general principles and rules cease to prove helpful as guides to moral judgment. Especially important are cases where conflicting values and disvalues are likely to result from any conceivable course of action, such as the treatment of the terminally ill or experiments with promising medical procedures that invariably have negative side effects. Practical wisdom for handling such cases emerges through experience accumulated in the treatment of similar cases. By evaluating a significant number of cases, we increase our ability to isolate variables pertinent for assessing each new case. This pattern of moral judgment is continuous with classic traditions of casuistry, or case reasoning. Casuistry locates moral judgment in the comparative study of recognizable classes of cases that require human decision and action (cf. Jonsen and Toulmin). Medical centers now institutionalize casuistic thinking through case conferences and regular consultations with specialists and advisers.

Responsiveness

H. Richard Niebuhr dramatizes the social matrix of action. We act in response to actions upon us and in anticipation of further responses to our own actions in ongoing social interactions. In this interactive framework, moral judgment involves responsiveness, self-conscious attempts to draw upon the perceptions and experiences of others in our own deliberations (cf. Gilligan). Responsiveness is best realized in conversation among representative actors in a situation. The conversation is not primarily an occasion for debate, in which the stronger positions defeat the weaker until the most cogent prevails. Its purpose is to facilitate vision. It may confirm widely held judgments, yet it may uncover matters that have been concealed, clarify phenomena that have been obscured, and bring to awareness considerations previously passed over.

Responsiveness begins with the attempt to understand what is going on. It does not presume that the morally important issues in a situation are obvious. Through conversation we surface the pivotal issues and construct ways of portraying them to ourselves and others. Historical studies and social analyses inform these efforts. The account we provide of the situation sets the stage for a consideration of appropriate responses.

Responsive judgments are guided by the notion of what is *fitting*. The fitting action may be largely self-evident once we have grasped what is morally at stake in a situation. Yet it may emerge only gradually, through the thoughtful balancing of multiple variables with their negative and positive features. Moral imagination and discernment are as important to this balancing process as are conceptual precision and logical rigor. The reasoning involved, moreover, is often more akin to weaving a tapestry than to forging a chain. Various strands of thinking supplement, complement, and perhaps clash with one another within a complete configuration. A fitting response is integral to that configuration. It consists of the most promising means of negotiating multiple considerations. For Niebuhr, fitting actions are also responses to God, the center of values that bestows authority on all values.

Responsiveness gains moral urgency from the partial, even distorted, nature of all human viewpoints. Biases rooted in special interests plague our most sincere efforts to promote justice. For example, a white male medical establishment gave lower priority to breast cancer than to prostate cancer. In studying heart disease, it focused on male rather than female subjects. Exalting scientific advances and technical achievements, the U.S. healthcare system institutionalizes almost unlimited care for those with comprehensive health coverage while failing to offer basic care for the poor. Other biases—racial, ethnic, religious—have distorted biomedical practices from time to time. We overcome socially mediated biases by responsiveness to the voices of those previously left out of the conversation.

Responsiveness is not merely a personal trait. It can be incorporated into professional, organizational, and institutional practices. We can create contexts for exchanges of views among peers, colleagues, coworkers, support staff, and volunteers. We can regularly seek information from those who receive medical services: patients, clients, consumers, constituents. Within a particular organization, these exchanges promote collaboration on common projects, facilitate coordination among interrelated activities, and enhance both quality and efficiency in performance. As a dimension of responsibility, responsiveness contributes to good management. Similarly, professionals routinely respond to peer judgments through associations, convocations, conferences, and publications, as well as through regular consultations and case conferences. Ideally, they also elicit the active participation of clients to whom they offer their services.

Responsiveness in moral judgment is especially pertinent to the formation of public policy, such as debates about healthcare reform. These debates begin with attempts to interpret "what is going on" and move to proposals for the "fitting" response (Niebuhr). In the United States, controversial policy issues are rarely resolved by a new public consensus on the proper treatment of pressing social problems. Practical accomplishments require compromise. To gain support for new directions in policy, public actors accommodate the special interests of competing groups. In so doing, they consent to measures that fall short of their larger goals. The search for acceptable compromises is crucial to public responsibility.

Accountability

Responsibility embraces accountability for judgments and actions (cf. Jonsen). Because our actions affect the lives of fellow human beings, we have to answer to others for what we do. We must be able to give an account of our intentions and of their moral bases that is credible within the relevant conversational context, whether it be familial, communal, professional, or public. Responsible persons seek feedback from others because they are conscientious about quality performance. Structures of accountability may be formalized in well-defined review processes, including disciplinary hearings, and civil and criminal actions. Yet they also operate in everyday human interactions.

The morally committed have a strong sense of accountability to self. Conscience names the dynamism whereby we answer to ourselves for our fidelity to our commitments. If we violate our own normative standards, we feel guilt. If others have been disadvantaged or harmed by our actions, we recognize a need to apologize, perhaps to make restitution. In religious contexts, accountability involves answering to God as the source and ground of the moral life. We confess our failures, seek forgiveness, and pray for strength to renew our commitments.

Responsibility includes a readiness to hold others accountable for their actions, in the interest of the common good. It will not suffice to be conscientious only about our own actions. Because substantive moral commitments are requisite to human existence and well-being, we must hold one another accountable to those commitments. Accountability is especially important for professionals, who alone are adequately equipped to assess the performances of peers. Likewise, we are obliged to promote mutual accountability in the organizational and communal contexts in which we normally live and work; this includes support for appropriate disciplinary hearings and criminal proceedings.

The notion of accountability directs us to revisit all of the dimensions of responsibility, though with a focus on our obligation to nurture, model, encourage, cultivate, and teach responsibility to fellow human beings, especially the children, youth, and young adults of a coming generation.

THOMAS W. OGLETREE (1995)

SEE ALSO: *Care; Compassionate Love; Communitarianism and Bioethics; Freedom and Free Will; Holocaust; Lifestyles and Public Health; Paternalism; Profession and Professional Ethics*

BIBLIOGRAPHY

Aquinas, Thomas. 1966. *Treatise on the Virtues,* tr. John A. Oesterle. Notre Dame, IN: University of Notre Dame Press.

Aristotle. 1934. *Nicomachean Ethics,* tr. Harold Rackham. New York: G. P. Putnam.

Augustine. 1953. "On Free Will." In *Augustine: Earlier Writings,* tr. John H. S. Burleigh. Philadelphia: Westminster Press.

Beauchamp, Tom L., and Childress, James F. 1994. *Principles of Biomedical Ethics,* 4th edition. New York: Oxford University Press.

Bonhoeffer, Dietrich. 1955. *Ethics,* tr. Neville H. Smith. New York: Macmillan.

Brunner, Emil. 1937. *The Divine Imperative: A Study in Christian Ethics,* tr. Olive Wyon. London: Lutterworth Press.

Calvin, John. 1957. *Institutes of the Christian Religion,* tr. John Allen. Grand Rapids, MI: Eerdmans.

Chodorow, Nancy. 1978. *The Reproduction of Mothering: Psycho-analysis and the Sociology of Gender.* Berkeley: University of California Press.

Cohen, Hermann. 1972. *Religion of Reason: Out of the Sources of Judaism,* tr. Simon Kaplan. New York: Frederick Ungar.

Erikson, Erik. 1968. *Identity: Youth and Crisis.* New York: Norton.

Fingarette, Herbert. 1967. *On Responsibility.* New York: Basic Books.

Gilligan, Carol. 1982. *In a Different Voice: Psychological Theory and Women's Development.* Cambridge, MA: Harvard University Press.

Glatzer, Nahum N., ed. 1966. *The Way of Response: Martin Buber, Selections from His Writings.* New York: Schocken.

Gustafson, James M. 1975. *Can Ethics Be Christian?* Chicago: University of Chicago Press.

Häring, Bernard. 1961. *The Law of Christ: Moral Theory for Priests and Laity,* 3 vols., tr. Edwin G. Kaiser. Westminster, MD: Newman Press.

Harron, Frank; Burnside, John W.; and Beauchamp, Tom L. 1983. *Health and Human Values.* New Haven, CT: Yale University Press.

Jonsen, Albert R. 1968. *Responsibility in Modern Religious Ethics: A Guide to Making Your Own Decisions.* Washington, D.C.: Corpus Books.

Jonsen, Albert R., and Toulmin, Stephen E. 1988. *The Abuse of Casuistry: A History of Moral Reasoning.* Berkeley: University of California Press.

Kant, Immanuel. 1949. *Fundamental Principles of the Metaphysics of Morals,* tr. Thomas K. Abbott. Indianapolis, ID: Bobbs-Merrill.

Kohut, Heinz. 1977. *The Restoration of the Self.* New York: International Universities Press.

Luther, Martin. 1957. "The Freedom of the Christian, 1520." In *Career of the Reformer: I.* Vol. 31 of *Luther's Works,* tr. W. A. Lambert and rev. Harold J. Grimm. Philadelphia: Muhlenberg Press.

Niebuhr, H. Richard. 1963. *The Responsible Self: An Essay in Christian Moral Philosophy.* New York: Harper & Row.

Novak, David. 1974. *Law and Theology in Judaism.* 2 vols. New York: Ktav.

Ramsey, Paul. 1970. *The Patient as Person: Explorations in Medical Ethics.* New Haven, CT: Yale University Press.

Ricoeur, Paul. 1992. *Oneself as Another,* tr. Kathleen Blamey. Chicago: University of Chicago Press.

Rouner, Leroy S., ed. 1992. *Selves, People, and Persons: What Does It Mean to Be a Self?* Notre Dame, IN: University of Notre Dame Press.

Taylor, Charles. 1991. *The Ethics of Authenticity.* Cambridge, MA: Harvard University Press.

Wallwork, Ernest. 1991. *Psychoanalysis and Ethics.* New Haven, CT: Yale University Press.

Winnicott, Donald W. 1965. *The Maturational Process and the Facilitating Environment.* New York: International Universities Press.

RIGHT TO DIE, POLICY AND LAW

• • •

Prior to World War II, death came naturally or accidentally. There was little that doctors could do to forestall it. With the development and application of a variety of drugs and devices, this slowly began to change in the 1950s and 1960s. In addition to the improved medical capabilities, public attitudes toward the respective roles of physicians and patients in making decisions about whether to deploy medical technology also began to shift. In the 1950s and 1960s, influenced by the civil rights and the consumer rights movements, the public gradually shifted the almost sole responsibility for deciding whether and how to treat patients from physicians' hands to the hands of patients or their families.

The Development of Patient Autonomy

Autonomy—or as it is sometimes referred to, self-determination—is the core value that has driven the development of the right to die, as well as the more fundamental right to refuse medical treatment out of which the right to die has grown. Legal recognition of the right of patients to make decisions about the medical care they do and do not wish to receive has deep historical roots. However, the right to make medical decisions is itself of relatively recent vintage, perhaps because until recently there was not a great deal in the way of medical treatment to choose from and certainly not much that was efficacious. Before the last decades of the twentieth century, there was not so much a right of patients to choose but a right to veto what the doctor proposed.

As medical capability has gradually increased, so have efforts aimed at increasing the role of patients in making decisions about whether and how to employ that capability. Autonomy has had a long struggle to dislodge the long-standing dominance of medical paternalism in the doctor-patient relationship. By the last quarter of the twentieth century, patient autonomy had become the prevalent value in law, public policy, and bioethics. However, there remains a considerable gap between theory and actual clinical practice (Solomon, et al.).

Another important trend that has affected the shift in medical decision making is the role of law in society in general. Prior to the twentieth century, law played a much more limited role in resolving controversies among private citizens and lawsuits by patients against physicians were exceedingly rare. These few lawsuits fell into two groups: claims based on an allegation of negligent medical practice, and claims of nonconsensual treatment amounting to a civil battery. Ultimately, these two themes were merged in the 1950s and 1960s in the development of the concept of informed consent to medical treatment.

Originally, the law of battery played the more significant role. Although mostly thought of as a protection against conduct involving violence against another person (and in fact it does provide such protection), battery provides a legal remedy for an intentional, nonconsensual touching of another person that results in either harm or offense. Out of the law of battery developed a right to refuse medical treatment. The relationship between the two is clear: the converse of the right not to be touched—in a medical context, treated—without consent, is a right to refuse treatment. Viewed from a broader perspective, the law of battery could be seen as creating a right of individual autonomy or self-determination, and certainly there is significant judicial authority to support that view.

Prior to the 1970s, the right to refuse treatment existed more in form than in substance. In clinical medical practice, although it is unlikely that physicians frequently forced treatment on unwilling patients, the instances in which they did were of the sort—emergencies, patients lacking in decision-making capacity—that any legal challenged was unlikely to arise. In most instances, the situation was such that either the patient recovered and in retrospect no longer objected to the treatment or the patient died or was otherwise unable to pursue a legal remedy.

The Era of Passively Hastening Death

The two trends— of medicine's increasing ability to stave off death if not provide complete cure, and the increasing recognition of patient autonomy —collided in the Karen Ann Quinlan case in 1975 (*In re Quinlan*,). It is virtually certain that such collisions occurred before the *Quinlan* case, but none of these clinical cases metamorphosed into legal cases with the attendant public visibility of *Quinlan* (Filene).

Karen Ann Quinlan, a twenty-one-year old woman, stopped breathing and was taken to the hospital by emergency medical personnel. Doctors were able—through a variety of medical means that were not available only a decade earlier—to resuscitate her. She was then placed on a ventilator. Because of prolonged oxygen deprivation before she was resuscitated, Quinlan suffered severe brain damage and was ultimately diagnosed as being in a persistent vegetative state, a condition in which her brain stem was still alive and maintained her so-called vegetative functions (digestion, metabolism, etc.), but in which the remainder of her brain had died and along with it the higher brain functions such as awareness and cognition.

When Quinlan's prognosis became clear to her parents, they concluded that Karen would not want to be kept alive in this twilight state in which her corporeal existence was maintained but in which she could no longer, think, feel, perceive, or have any contact with other people or her environment. Therefore, after seeking additional medical consultation and religious counseling, they requested that her doctors discontinue the ventilator that was keeping her alive, and that she be allowed to die naturally.

The doctors, however, refused. They refused because they believed it was contrary to the ethics of the medical profession to do so. The treating physicians and several of the qualified experts who testified in the case asserted that removal from the respirator would not conform to medical practices, standards, and traditions. The physicians also refused because they were concerned that they could be subject to liability for criminal homicide if they did so. In effect, the doctors issued an invitation to Quinlan's parents to sue, which they accepted by filing an action for a declaratory judgment—not a case seeking monetary damages against the doctor, but a case requesting the court to declare that Karen had the right to have life-sustaining medical treatment removed, which would, it was thought, inevitably lead to her death.

The trial court refused to issue such an order, and the Quinlan family appealed to the New Jersey Supreme Court. Although the court's opinion is confused and important portions of it were superseded by later decisions, it did grapple with a number of fundamental ethical and legal issues in an unprecedented way. It prescribed procedures for making end-of-life decisions that did not routinely require judicial supervision, and it endowed physicians and patients' close family members with substantial discretion to carry out what they believed to be the patients' wishes about forgoing treatment.

The *Quinlan* decision, despite its shortcomings, can be said to be the foundation on which an entire body of law and public policy have been erected concerning end-of-life decision making. This case ushered in what in retrospect should be called the era of passively hastening death because, along with similar cases that followed in its wake for the next fifteen years or more, it established the right of terminally ill and permanently unconscious patients to have their deaths hastened passively, that is by having life-sustaining medical treatment withheld or withdrawn.

The Consensus about Forgoing Life-Sustaining Treatment

The *Quinlan* case was a catalyst to the development of law and policy about the termination of end-of-life medical treatment. It spurred state legislatures to adopt advance directive legislation intended to head off similar litigation. Federal and state commissions were appointed to study and make recommendations on these issues. Other landmark cases were litigated in other states; in the quarter century following *Quinlan,* courts in half the states decided more than one hundred similar cases—and within a decade, a remarkably uniform body of law and policy had emerged.

Each element of this consensus fed the others. Court cases spurred legislative action. Government commissions relied on important court cases and legislation as guidance for their deliberations and recommendations. Further court cases adopted the recommendations of the commissions. Although there are some important exceptions, taken together, these cases, statutes, and commission reports constitute a consistent consensus about how end-of-life decisions should be made.

Although Congress and the United States Supreme Court have played some role in its development, the legal components of this consensus have been almost exclusively state appellate judicial cases and state legislation. By the time the Supreme Court issued its first and only ruling in a case involving the passive hastening of death—the *Cruzan* case in 1990—the consensus was largely developed based on state law. The *Cruzan* ruling did little more than put the Supreme Court's imprimatur on a number of features of the existing consensus.

In the wake of *Cruzan,* Congress enacted the Patient Self-Determination Act (PSDA) in the same year. This law required institutional providers of healthcare to provide patients with information about their decision-making rights—including the right to make an advance directive. However, the Act was entirely procedural in nature; it did not establish any new rights, but only required that patients be told about their already-existing rights under *state* law.

COMPETENT PATIENTS. The centerpiece of the consensus on end-of-life decision making is the unanimous agreement that competent patients have a legal right to refuse treatment. So well established is this right that its existence has been largely assumed by both courts and legislatures. Although no court has ever said that this right is absolute, the manner in which courts increasingly discuss and apply it strongly suggests that they are headed toward that conclusion. In addition to the strong support in law-making institutions, the consensus of the public, of policy makers, of bioethicists, and the healthcare professions also supports a strong right to refuse medical treatment for competent patients.

LEGAL SOURCES OF THE RIGHT. Although in the *Quinlan* decision the New Jersey Supreme Court predicated the right to refuse treatment on a federal constitutional right of privacy, few other courts have based rulings on the right to privacy. It has become clear that this is a particularly weak basis for the right. Later courts have tended to ground the right in the common law—specifically, in the right to be free from unwanted interferences with bodily integrity protected by the law of battery. The United States Supreme Court, when addressing this issue in the *Cruzan* case, stated that the "logic of" a series of earlier cases decided by the Supreme Court suggests that there is a constitutional basis for such a right, but assumed this logic without actually holding that such a right exists. Presumably, this right is grounded in the protection of liberty contained in the Fourteenth Amendment to the United States Constitution, rather than the discredited right of privacy cited in *Quinlan.*

Regardless of the particular constitutional provision in which this right is grounded, the right is one that may only be asserted against individuals or institutions acting as agents of a state or federal governmental entity, and not against private individuals or institutions. Thus, the broadest and firmest legal basis for the right to refuse treatment is state law—state common law, state statutes, and state constitutional provisions—because it usually accords protections against actions taken by private individuals and institutions as well those taken by agents of the state.

HOW ABSOLUTE IS THE RIGHT? It can be said with absolute certainty that no legal right is absolute. In cases predating the *Quinlan* decision—mostly involving the refusal of blood transfusions by members of the Jehovah's Witness religion—judges readily gave lip service to the right to refuse treatment but exhibited an enormous reluctance to match words with deeds, and exhibited a high degree of creativity in evading the full implications of the right. They did so by finding patients incompetent who might not have been, declaring emergencies on flimsy evidence, and insisting that the state had a strong interest in children having two living parents.

With the passage of time, these efforts to evade the full force of a competent patient's strong right to refuse treatment have substantially dissipated if not disappeared. In a series of legal cases beginning in the late 1980s, courts—especially the Florida Supreme Court (*Wons v. Public Health Trust; In re Dubreuil*), but others too—began gradually to enforce a full-blown right to refuse treatment when Jehovah's Witnesses refused blood transfusions. No longer did judges find patients incompetent primarily because they refused treatment, nor find an emergency to exist simply because a physician says the patient would probably die without a blood transfusion. Courts also recognized that parents of minor children have no obligation to avoid risk-taking behavior simply because they are parents of minor children (*Fosmire v Nicoleau*).

This change in attitude is probably accounted for primarily by the fallout from *Quinlan* and cases like it. As courts increasingly strengthened the right of terminally ill or permanently unconscious *incompetent* patients to refuse treatment, it became increasingly difficult, if not impossible, to justify denying that right to fully competent patients. It is significant that although the objection to medical treatment in the Jehovah's Witness cases was based on religious belief, the decisions themselves were generally grounded on a common-law right to refuse treatment applicable to all, regardless of religious belief.

A parallel trend beginning in the mid 1980s involved non-religious refusers of treatment who also were not terminally ill or permanently unconscious. In a handful of cases beginning in the mid-1980s, permanently disabled, competent patients began to raise the question of whether they had a right to refuse life-sustaining medical treatment. In the landmark *Bouvia* case in California, the court held that a woman in her 30s, a victim of cerebral palsy, had a right not to be force fed by medical procedures even if the refusal led to her death (*Bouvia v. Superior Court*). In three cases in Georgia (*State v. McAfee*), Nevada (*McKay v. Bergsted*), and California (*Thor v. Superior Court*), the highest courts in those states held that quadriplegic accident victims who were being kept alive by ventilators had the right to refuse further treatment and thus die. In all four of these cases, if treatment were continued the individuals were

likely, with adequate nursing care, to have a relatively long life expectancy and to remain mentally intact.

Thus, it was not just the patients who were as close to death as they could be while still alive who had the right to refuse treatment and allow nature to take its course, but also patients whose prospects for a meaningful existence were virtually certain.

INCOMPETENT PATIENTS' RIGHT TO REFUSE TREAT-MENT. A core point of the *Quinlan* decision, which has become a cornerstone of the consensus on end-of-life decision making, is that incompetent patients, as well as competent patients, have a right to refuse medical treatment. *Quinlan* and subsequent cases raised two subsidiary issues. The first was whether the termination of life support would raise the prospect of legal liability for criminal homicide on the part of those who terminated treatment. The second was whether or not there were any limits on the right to refuse treatment.

Lack of criminal liability. In the development of the consensus in the courts, in public policy—most notably by the President's Commission for the Study of Ethical Problems in Medicine and Biomedical and Behavioral Research (President's Commission)—and in bioethics, there has been a unanimous assertion that forgoing life-sustaining treatment that results in a patient's death does not constitute a crime as long as there is proper authorization for the termination of treatment, either from the patient, from someone legally authorized to speak for the patient, or from a court.

There are a number of explanations offered in support of this conclusion. One is that when treatment is withheld or withdrawn, there is no *intent* to kill but rather to relieve suffering. Thus there cannot be liability for homicide or aiding suicide because each of these crimes requires intent. Another is that the *cause* of death is not the conduct of the party who withholds or withdraws treatment (or who authorizes the termination), but the patient's underlying illness or injury. It can be asserted that the patient is not killed, but rather is allowed to die when life-sustaining treatment is forgone.

A third explanation is that when life-sustaining treatment is forgone, there is no liability for assisted suicide because the kind of act required for assisting—"affirmative, assertive, proximate, direct conduct such as furnishing a gun, poison, knife or other instrumentality" (*Bouvia v Superior Court*, p. 306)—does not exist. This explanation is less successful if the crime to be charged is homicide because an omission to act when there is a duty to do so, as might be the case when the actor is a physician or other healthcare professional, will support liability for homicide equally well as an act would (*Barber v. Superior Court*).

The fourth explanation given is that there is no criminal liability because the patient is exercising the legal right to refuse treatment. It is clear that this is not an explanation at all but a restatement of the question. Nonetheless, it is probably the best explanation. No liability, either criminal or civil, should arise as a result of a patient's death from forgoing life-sustaining treatment if this occurs in the exercise of a legal right to refuse treatment either by the patient or someone with legal authority to speak on his behalf. To conclude otherwise would be, in effect, to eliminate the right itself.

Limits on incompetents' rights: countervailing state interests. That there is a legal right of incompetent patients to forgo treatment does not mean that there are no limitations on that right. The courts have identified a number of countervailing societal interests that, in theory at least, may be invoked in opposition to the forgoing of treatment. These interests, recited in virtually every legal opinion on forgoing life-sustaining treatment, are:

1. the preservation of life;
2. the prevention of suicide;
3. the protection of third parties;
4. the ethical integrity of the medical profession.

In practice, these societal interests have not been accorded significant weight if the patient is terminally ill or permanently unconscious (or if the patient is competent). As to the preservation of life, the prevailing legal view is that of the New Jersey Supreme Court in *Quinlan*: "the State's interest ... weakens and the individual's right to privacy grows as the degree of bodily invasion increases and the prognosis dims."

The prevention of suicide is not a significant matter because of the virtually unanimous view that the forgoing of life-sustaining treatment is not suicide. However, in instances in which a person is very seriously disabled but not terminally ill or permanently unconscious, some courts are more reluctant to permit the forgoing of life support unless there is clear and convincing evidence of the patient's refusal of treatment in circumstances such as these, prior to losing decision making capacity (*Martin v. Martin*; *In re Edna M.F. v. Eisenberg*; *Wendland v. Wendland*).

As previously mentioned, one of the ways that courts found to circumvent the right of Jehovah's Witnesses to refuse blood transfusions was to invoke the societal interest in the protection of the children of these patients. In the case of minor children, however, the view is beginning to prevail that even though it is desirable for them to have not just one but two living parents, many other children do not, and in any event, to impose medical treatment on an individual in furtherance of this interest is to deny that person the choice of which risks to take, a choice assigned to adults—even those with minor children—in virtually all other circumstances. The interests of other close family members are just too attenuated to prevail in the face of the strong right of individuals to make their own medical choices.

Likewise, the judicial view is virtually unanimous that the forgoing of life-sustaining treatment does not offend the ethical integrity of the healthcare professions because these professions no longer hold the belief, if they ever did, that the sole goal of treatment is cure. In cases where cure is impossible or even highly unlikely, "the prevailing ethical practice seems to be to recognize that the dying are more often in need of comfort than treatment" (*Superintendent of Belchertown State School v. Saikewicz,* p. 426). And, returning to basics, "if the doctrines of informed consent and right of privacy have as their foundations the right to bodily integrity ... and control of one's own fate, then those rights are superior to the institutional considerations" (*Superintendent of Belchertown State School v. Saikewicz,* p. 427).

Decision making procedures for incompetent patients. A central issue in *Quinlan* was the issue of how the right to refuse treatment is to be exercised when the patient is literally incapable of doing so. The two extremes that the court had available were to require that all such decisions be reviewed by a court, or that they take place in the privacy of the doctor-patient-family relationship without any oversight. Rather than choosing either extreme, the court settled on a middle ground: decisions to forgo life-sustaining treatment were ordinarily to be made in the privacy of the clinical setting without judicial involvement. However, to provide some safeguards against inappropriate decisions, the court mandated that the decision receive approval by a multidisciplinary ethics committee. This was a novel approach adopted from a law review article written by a physician just one year earlier (Teel).

One serious difficulty with this approach was the assumption that hospitals had ethics committees when in fact very few did. However, by mandating the use of an ethics committee, the court set in motion a movement for most healthcare institutions to create them. Another problem was the fact that, although the committee was labeled an ethics committee, the role the court assigned to it was to confirm the patient's prognosis, a medical function for which such a multi-disciplinary committee was unsuited. The more fundamental criticism, however, was that ethics committees had no clear moral authority to make or even review decisions about forgoing life-sustaining treatment.

As a consequence of these difficulties, no other court or legislature mandated the use of ethics committees in end-of-life decision making. In the *Saikewicz* case, decided just a year after *Quinlan,* the Massachusetts Supreme Judicial Court required that such decisions always be made by courts, because

> questions of life and death seem to us to require the process of detached but passionate investigation and decision that forms the ideal on which the judicial branch of government was created. Achieving this ideal is our responsibility and that of the lower court, and is not to be entrusted to any other group purporting to represent the "morality and conscience of our society," no matter how highly motivated or impressively constituted. (*Superintendent of Belchertown State School v. Saikewicz,* p. 435)

However, practical—and some philosophical—considerations ultimately won out. No other law-making body concurred in this position and within just two years, the Massachusetts court itself backed away from it. Requiring judicial review of all decisions to forgo life-sustaining treatment is too cumbersome, slow, and time-consuming. More fundamentally, it creates a tremendous intrusion by instruments of the state into the very private process of dying.

Thus, after a very heated debate, a consensus developed that all procedural aspects of the decision making process— the determination of whether or not the patient lacks decision making capacity, the designation of a surrogate decision maker, and any review of the decision about forgoing treatment—should ordinarily be made in the clinical setting. An ethics committee may play a role if the parties choose to have it do so, but it is not legally mandated. And in situations in which there is intractable disagreement among participants in the decision-making process about administering or forgoing treatment, or if there is a serious conflict of interest, the courts are available to adjudicate the issue.

Decision making standards for incompetent patients. One of the central tenets of the consensus concerns the standard by which a surrogate may make a decision for a patient who lacks decision-making capacity. In theory, surrogates could be empowered to exercise complete discretion—to make whatever decision they wish, for whatever reason they wish. Rather than according such unfettered discretion, courts have sought guidance from the values in which medical decision making is grounded, the primary one being autonomy. When competent patients make medical decisions for themselves, they are guided by their own values and goals. On the assumption that decision making for incompetent patients should be similarly guided, the courts have invoked autonomy as the guiding principle for decision making by surrogates as well.

The difficulty, of course, is that when the patient lacks decision-making capacity—and in many instances lacks even rudimentary communication capacity—the patient's values and goals cannot be determined contemporaneously. To honor and implement autonomy, the courts have mandated that surrogates attempt to determine what the patient would have decided if the patient were capable of deciding. Some believe, however, that this is an elusive and ultimately futile search and that for individuals for whom autonomy is lost, decision making must be based on other values (Dresser; Harmon).

The predominant standard that has evolved and been adopted is referred to as the *substituted judgment* standard. It requires the surrogate to determine what the patient would have wanted had the patient actually given thought to the matter—in other words, the patient's *probable* wishes.

A small number of courts (most notably, the New York Court of Appeals) reject the substituted judgment standard altogether and insist that decision making for patients who lack decision-making capacity must be made on the basis of their *actual* wishes, that the evidence adduced to establish their wishes be clear and convincing, and that the statements made by the patient have been uttered under "solemn" circumstances and not merely be casual or offhand remarks, such as those made in reaction to the treatment of another (*In re Westchester County Medical Ctr.* [O'Connor]). Those adhering to this standard are preoccupied by the possibility of an erroneous decision to allow a patient to die—that is, a decision that does not reflect the patient's own wishes—and that in the case of uncertainty, it is better to err on the side of keeping the patient alive.

The opposing view recognizes that prolonging life can entail undesired effects as well, as expressed by U.S. Supreme Court Justice William Brennan in a dissenting opinion in the *Cruzan* case:

> Dying is personal. And it is profound. For many, the thought of an ignoble end, steeped in decay, is abhorrent. A quiet, proud death, bodily integrity intact, is a matter of extreme consequence.... Such conditions are, for many, humiliating to contemplate, as is visiting a prolonged and anguished vigil on one's parents, spouse, and children. A long, drawn-out death can have a debilitating effect on family members.... For some, the idea of being remembered in their persistent vegetative states rather than as they were before their illness or accident may be very disturbing.

Sentiments such as these have motivated other courts and the President's Commission to permit surrogates to forgo life-sustaining treatment in the absence of any information concerning the wishes of the patient, on the basis of the *best interests* standard. These authorities take the position that while autonomy is the predominant value, it is not the only one, and that when autonomy cannot be effectuated because of ignorance of the patient's wishes, the patient's *welfare* must govern instead. In such a case, the surrogate is obligated to do what is best for the patient, which entails a weighing of the benefits of continued treatment against its burdens. If the burdens predominate, the surrogate may authorize the termination of treatment (*Barber v. Superior Court; In re Conroy*).

Family members as surrogates for incompetent patients. An important corollary of the views that decisions about life-sustaining treatment should ordinarily be made in the clinical setting without outside supervision, and that the patient's own views should govern decision making, is the presumption that close family members are the appropriate persons to speak for the patient. When a decision needs to be made whether to administer or forgo life-sustaining medical treatment, physicians should turn to close family members, who have moral and legal authorization to decide for the patient, even if they have not been appointed as guardians by a court or designated by the patient to be their spokesperson. This presumption is based on the belief that close family members best know the patient's actual or probable wishes (substituted judgment) and when they do not are most likely to act for the patient's welfare (best interests).

Advance directives in decision making for incompetent patients. Because of the centrality of the patient's wishes in decision making and the inability to ascertain those wishes in precisely the instances in which that information is most needed, the use of advance directives in end-of-life decision making has taken on a very high degree of importance. An advance directive is a device by which competent individuals make their wishes known about treatment if, at some future time, they should lack decision-making capacity. This is best done through a formal written instrument which either gives instructions about future medical treatment (referred to as a *living will*), appoints another person (*agent* or *proxy*) to make such decisions (referred to as a *health care power of attorney*), or both.

In the wake of the *Quinlan* and similar judicial decisions, it became readily apparent that it would be useful, if not essential, for individuals to have an advance directive. In 1976, the same year that *Quinlan* was decided, California became the first state to enact legislation to provide a firm legal basis to assure the validity of advance directives. For many years, there was some uncertainty about the validity of

an advance directive without such legislation. By the end of the twentieth century, however, every state had enacted some type of advance directive legislation.

Some uncertainty continues to surround the use of advance directives. Advance directive statutes can be very limiting. Perhaps the most restrictive requirement is that before an advance directive becomes effective, the patient must be in a *terminal condition* or *permanently unconscious*. However, some individuals may wish to engage in advance healthcare planning for other conditions that they find particularly troublesome, such as dementia. It is still open to question in law, at least in some states, as to whether such "nonconforming" advance directives are legally enforceable.

The theory of healthcare decision making, based as it is on individual autonomy, would seem to allow individuals to issue instructions—especially instructions to forgo life-sustaining treatment, such as feeding tubes—to cover such situations. However, a highly defensible position, as stated more or less explicitly in the statutes themselves, is that the statutes do not create legal rights to refuse (or consent) to healthcare, but merely provide a mechanism for doing so. The Uniform Health Care Decisions Act, a model law drafted by the National Council of Commissioners on Uniform State Laws, lacks the restrictions found in most advance directive statutes, but must be adopted in an individual state before it has the force of law, and so far it has not been.

Perhaps the largest obstacle to the efficacy of advance directives—to which the previously-mentioned PSDA was seen as a solution—is that most people do not have them, either out of ignorance of what they are or of their importance, or because of an aversion to planning for death, exhibited also by the failure of many people to buy life insurance or write wills.

Forgoing Artificial Nutrition and Hydration

In the *Quinlan* case, the legal question was whether Karen Quinlan could be allowed to die from the withdrawal of the ventilator that was keeping her alive. After the New Jersey Supreme Court answered this question in the affirmative, and her physicians gradually withdrew her ventilatory support, she continued breathing on her own, contrary to the medical assumption on which the case had been decided. Thereafter, she was kept alive by a feeding tube, raising the question of whether her parents could authorize the termination of the feeding tube as well.

Because they did not seek to do so, this question remained unanswered until 1983, when it arose in the California case of *Barber v. Superior Court*. In this case, physicians were subjected to criminal prosecution for the termination of a feeding tube from a patient diagnosed, like Quinlan, as being in a persistent vegetative state. This case, for the first time in a judicial forum, raised the question of whether it is permissible to withhold or withdraw nutrition and hydration. It is also the first of only two criminal prosecutions that have ever occurred for forgoing life-sustaining treatment with the consent of someone legally authorized to make such decisions for the patient.

Opponents of permitting the forgoing of nutrition and hydration usually raise two major objections. First, nutrition and hydration is not a medical procedure but basic sustenance, and thus should not be treated the same as, for example, a ventilator. In this view, one is no more morally entitled to remove nutrition and hydration from an incompetent patient than from a young child who cannot provide itself with nourishment. Perhaps the best legal rejoinder to this claim was issued in the *Cruzan* case by U.S. Supreme Court Justice Sandra Day O'Connor, who addressed the question by declining to answer it. Rather than entering into the debate about whether nutrition and hydration provided by a feeding tube was or was not a form of medical treatment, she observed that regardless of how it is characterized, when provided to an unwilling patient it constitutes a restraint on individual liberty. Since it is certainly contrary to individual autonomy to force feed a competent patient, it is contrary to the individual autonomy of an incompetent patient as well, when the patient's surrogate refuses it based on the patient's previously expressed wishes.

The second objection is that death resulting from the forgoing of nutrition and hydration amounts to killing, rather than letting nature take its course, and is therefore unlawful and immoral. The standard rejoinder to this is that there is no difference between termination of nutrition and hydration and other treatments. When a ventilator is terminated, the patient dies because his injury or illness prevents him from breathing and that is the cause of death. Similarly, feeding tubes are placed in, and only removed from, patients whose injury or illness prevents them from eating in the ordinary way, and thus it is the injury or illness, rather than the actions of the individual who removes the feeding tube, which is the cause of death.

Actively Hastening Death

The distinction between passively and actively hastening death has been central to the development of the consensus about end-of-life decision making. The former is equated with forgoing life-sustaining treatment, which includes both withholding treatment not yet begun and withdrawing treatment that is in progress. Actively hastening death consists of both active euthanasia (sometimes referred to as mercy killing) and assisted suicide. Active euthanasia is the direct ending of a human life, by a lethal injection, for example, whereas assisted suicide is defined as giving another the means by which that person ends his or her own life, such as providing a prescription for a lethal dose of medication which the person then ingests. Both legal and ethical thought have, for the most part, drawn a bright line between passively and actively hastening death, holding the former to be both morally and legally licit and condemning the latter as killing, and thus immoral and illegal.

The reasons for viewing passively hastening death as not constituting a crime were previously discussed. By contrast, when death is actively hastened—whether by the patient with assistance from another (assisted suicide) or directly by another (active euthanasia)—it is usually said that criminal liability cannot be avoided because all of the elements of a crime—act, intent, causation, consequence—are present. In the case of active euthanasia, to wit, the actor commits an *act,* with the *intent* of bringing about the patient's death, which is the *cause* of the patient's *death.*

From a legal, political, and policy perspective, this reasoning has been essential to the development of the consensus. It was simply not possible politically for legislatures or courts to have characterized forgoing life-sustaining treatment as killing and then to have attempted somehow to permit it. It was far simpler and more palatable to the public and to judges themselves to legitimate passively hastening death by denying that it was killing. Similarly, it would simply have been too great a leap from existing mores to legitimate actively hastening death, had any judge or legislator even wished to do so, because it involves practices that traditionally have been viewed as killing, even when done with merciful motives.

With the passage of time and increasing clamor for the legalization of actively hastening death—or at least for the legalization of suicide assisted by a physician—the weaknesses in the reasoning used to distinguish passively and actively hastening death have gradually become more apparent. Nonetheless, with a few exceptions both in the United States and other countries, legal barriers to actively hastening death remain.

Beyond the Consensus: The Legalization of Actively Hastening Death

Although the bright line between passively and actively hastening death is part of the bedrock on which the ethical, legal, and policy consensus about forgoing life-sustaining treatment has been grounded, it has not been immune from challenge. These challenges have come in writings by ethicists, in litigation, and in legislation.

It has occasionally been asserted that a physician is prohibited by law and ethics from undertaking an act that would end a patient's life because it constitutes killing, but is permitted to omit treating a patient because he or she is merely allowing nature to take its course and the patient to die. Both the courts and public policy makers (President's Commission) have been quick to correct this misunderstanding. Certainly taking an affirmative act to end the patient's life, such as giving the patient a lethal injection, is a legal wrong; omitting is also a legal wrong if there is a duty to act, and a physician is under a duty to treat unless excused from doing so by the patient, the patient's surrogate, or a court. Thus the categorical distinction between wrongness of acting and rightness of omitting is fallacious.

The same is true of withholding and withdrawing treatment. It has sometimes been thought that withdrawing treatment is a wrong because it involves an act, but withholding treatment is legally and ethically acceptable because it involves an omission. Again, if there is a duty to act, withholding is a legal wrong, unless properly excused. However, withdrawing treatment, even though it involves an act, is not considered killing because, unlike the administration of a lethal substance to the patient, withdrawing treatment merely allows nature to take its course. On policy grounds, the distinction between withdrawing and withholding is an especially pernicious one, because permitting treatment to be withheld but not withdrawn would discourage physicians from trying to treat some patients thought to be hopelessly ill out of fear that once started, treatment could not later be stopped, even if it were ineffective in reversing the patient's condition.

While the weaknesses in the reasoning that supports passively hastening death but rejects actively hastening death have long been apparent (Rachels), they have been papered over by the courts and justified by policy analysts when this has seemed necessary to achieve what some see as the desirable result of not legitimating actively hastening death. Some recognize the desirability of permitting actively hastening death in individual cases but oppose legalization, preferring to leave it to the private actions of doctors and patients, and to allow the legal system to exercise discretion in not prosecuting those truly merciful cases that come to its attention. The difficulty with this approach is that because the legal outcome for those who provide assistance or engage in mercy killing is so uncertain and so potentially serious, few will be willing to take the chance. Consequently, actively hastened death will not, in fact, be available to those whose conditions may warrant it, or else will be available on an arbitrary basis.

Apart from those who see actively hastening death as killing and condemn all killing as wrong, the primary concern seems to be a practical one. If actively hastening death becomes legally acceptable, there will be no way to draw lines to confine it to those for whom it might be appropriate, on both policy and ethical grounds, and it will become susceptible to widespread abuse through incremental extensions of existing accepted practices. For instance, if physician-assisted suicide becomes legal, what reasoning can confine actively hastening death to those who can self-administer the instrumentality of death? There will be individuals whose claims to actively hastening death are equally high, but who are no longer able to end their own life and thus must have someone end it for them. If actively hastening death is then extended to this group, there will be individuals who lose their decision-making capacity before being able to have their lives ended. Should not, in the name of equity, individuals be allowed to execute an advance directive requesting that their deaths be actively hastened when they are no longer able to do so themselves, and when they meet the conditions specified in the advance directive? And if this becomes permissible, then surely an actively-hastened death will be permissible for individuals whose wishes were never committed to paper but can be intuited by relatives using the substituted judgment standard. And if such evidence is lacking, then perhaps the best interests standard should be applied to permit an actively hastened death as it sometimes is to allow for passively hastened death. While this may not be the bottom of the proverbial slippery slope, it is far enough to demonstrate to many the lack of wisdom of ever stepping onto the slope by legitimating any form of actively-hastened death.

Proponents of taking the first step, however, believe first that it is merely a logical extension of the same process that recognized the legality and ethicality of passively-hastened death. Further, they believe that taking one step, or even more than one, does not necessarily entail a commitment to taking the next step. Experience and policy considerations may suggest limitations even where logic might dictate otherwise. Finally, proponents point to the inequity of permitting the terminally ill who depend on life-sustaining medical treatment to have their lives ended, but not permitting the same merciful release from suffering to the terminally ill who may have an equal claim but who happen not to be dependent on life-sustaining medical treatment.

Legalization of Physician-Assisted Suicide

Events began to overtake logic in the 1990s in the United States. Efforts to legalize physician-assisted suicide through voter initiatives took place in five states; all but one failed to win passage. Oregon voters approved a ballot initiative in 1994, which did not go into effect until 1997 because of efforts to overturn it in the courts and through a second voter initiative. Bills have been introduced into the legislatures of many states to legalize physician-assisted suicide, but none received very much support until 2002 when the Hawaii legislature narrowly defeated such an effort.

Several lawsuits have been filed seeking to declare unconstitutional state laws making assisted suicide a crime. Lower federal courts invalidated such laws in Washington state and New York state, at least when the person seeking assistance in dying was competent and terminally ill, and when the person rendering the assistance was a licensed physician. The two cases, *Washington v. Glucksberg* and *Vacco v. Quill*, were reversed by the United States Supreme Court in 1997. The Court held that there is no federal constitutional right to physician-assisted suicide—that states are constitutionally permitted to make assisted suicide a crime, but it is also constitutionally permissible for a state to legalize physician-assisted suicide, as Oregon had done.

All of the discussion of legalizing actively hastening death in the 1990s took place against the backdrop of the activities of Dr. Jack Kevorkian, a retired physician who publicly announced that he would aid individuals in ending their lives. He publicized many of his cases—totaling well in excess of one hundred until he was imprisoned in 1999. The high visibility of his activities was taken as a defiant invitation to legal authorities to file criminal charges against him on several occasions, but none were successful until he went beyond aiding patients' deaths and administered a lethal substance to a terminally ill man and then gave a videotape of the event to a national television network, where it was publicly broadcast. He was then indicted for murder, tried, and convicted.

Another important component in discussions of legalizing actively hastening death has been the experience with the open practice of active euthanasia in the Netherlands since the early 1970s. Until 2001, voluntary active euthanasia by physicians for competent terminally ill patients has been formally illegal, but actively practiced and not prosecuted by the authorities—if the physician complied with guidelines proposed by the Minister of Justice and the Secretary of Health—and supported by the Royal Dutch Medical Association. In that year, the Netherlands formally legalized voluntary active euthanasia along lines quite similar to the informal practice that had previously prevailed.

Dr. Kevorkian's activities were widely viewed as highly irresponsible by both supporters and opponents of the legalization of actively hastening death. Nonetheless, most admit that his activities—as well as the developments in the Netherlands—did have the consequence of helping to open public debate on this issue. One of the undoubtedly salutary consequences of the public debate has been an acknowledgement and realization that the medical profession has been laggard in providing adequate palliative care—especially pain relief—to terminally ill individuals, and that there has been inadequate education of physicians about these issues. In the view of many, improvements in these areas are not only necessary to relieve the suffering of the dying, but they may also go a long way in derailing the legalization of actively hastening death. Others, however, see these two approaches as complementary, rather than working in opposition to each other.

THE OREGON EXPERIENCE WITH PHYSICIAN-ASSISTED SUICIDE. Physician-assisted suicide was legalized by a voter initiative in Oregon in 1994 and went into effect in November 1997. The law does not actually refer to physician-assisted suicide; the title of the law is the Oregon Death with Dignity Act, but in fact physician-assisted suicide—or, as some prefer to call it, physician aid-in-dying—is the practice that is made legal. The law permits a competent terminally ill patient to have a physician prescribe a lethal dose of medication for the patient to self-administer; it does not permit the physician or anyone else to administer the medication (active euthanasia).

In the first four years of its operation, 140 (2001: 44; 2000: 39; 1999: 33; 1998: 24) people obtained lethal prescriptions from their doctors and 89 (2001: 19; 2000: 27; 1999: 27; 1998: 16) used them to end their lives. The remainder died without using the prescriptions. The death rate for those using a lethal prescription varied between six and nine per ten thousand, which is in the same range as the death rate of individuals who die otherwise. Most patients suffered from cancer. The three most commonly mentioned reasons that patients wanted to end their lives were loss of autonomy, a decreasing ability to participate in activities that made life enjoyable, and losing control of bodily functions. The overwhelming proportion of patients died at home.

Fears that people who would avail themselves of physician-assisted suicide would do so because of lack of alternatives were not borne out by experience. More than three-fourths of patients were also enrolled in a hospice care program, and all had some form of health insurance. Likewise, patients who used physician-assisted suicide were similar in terms of age and race to those who died without using it. Patients who used physician-assisted suicide were also better educated. However, more women died in this manner than men with comparable disease, and those who died in this way were more likely to be divorced and possibly not have as good family support systems (Oregon Department of Human Services).

Opponents of the legalization of physician-assisted suicide in Oregon have mounted several efforts to have the law invalidated. The first was a lawsuit challenging the constitutionality of the law, which delayed its implementation for three years. While this lawsuit was pending, opponents were able to put an initiative to overturn the original legalization on the Oregon ballot in 1997. Although the original approval was by a 51 percent to 49 percent margin, Oregon voters underscored their approval of the physician-assisted suicide legalization by refusing to repeal the law by a 60 percent to 40 percent margin. However, shortly after the law went into effect, the director of the federal Drug Enforcement Administration (DEA) ruled that it was a violation of the federal controlled substances act for doctors to use controlled substances in the implementation of the Oregon law. This was quickly reversed by the U.S. Attorney General Janet Reno. Bills were then introduced in two sessions of Congress to prevent the use of controlled substances in physician-assisted suicide, but neither was enacted. With a change of administration in 2000, Attorney General John Ashcroft reversed the policy of the former Attorney General and banned the use of controlled substances in physician-assisted suicide. A lawsuit was then filed to prevent implementation of the Attorney General's order, and a federal court ruled that the order was illegal and could not be implemented.

Beyond the Consensus: Autonomy Turned Upside Down

Although patient autonomy is the foundation on which the consensus around end-of-life decision making has been built, autonomy has encountered a serious challenge in the form of so-called futility cases. These cases reverse the usual right-to-die cases. In those cases, competent patients or family members have determined that further treatment is unwarranted and challenged physicians who have wanted to continue to provide treatment. In futility cases, physicians and other healthcare professionals conclude that further treatment is unwarranted, but are met by resistance from competent patients—or, more likely, family members of incompetent patients—who insist that treatment be continued. Despite the raft of literature on this subject, there has been very little contribution to resolution of this debate by either courts or legislatures. Most likely, situations of this sort are eventually resolved in the clinical setting either by the patient's death, for the patients involved are usually very critically ill, or by a realization by family members over time that further treatment will not improve the patient's condition.

Future Challenges for Policy Makers, Legislators, and Health Professionals

The consensus about forgoing life-sustaining treatment has become well-accepted in public policy, law, and clinical practice. Despite the fact that half of the states have not yet experienced a major legal case, it does not seem likely that these states will make major changes in the consensus.

The same sort of stability is not likely to exist with respect to actively hastening death. Coming decades are likely to witness continuing challenges to the prohibition on assisted suicide in the courts, in state legislatures, and through ballot initiatives. Acceptance in law is likely to be very gradual, if it occurs at all. However, the influence of the movement to legalize actively hastening death will continue to be felt in improved efforts at providing alternatives in the form of hospice care, palliative care, and the more judicious use of pain relief medications, even if they might hasten death.

ALAN MEISEL

SEE ALSO: *Autonomy; Christianity, Bioethics in; Competence; Conscience, Rights of; Death; Death, Definition and Determination of; Dementia; Harm; Homicide; Informed Consent; Islam, Bioethics in; Judaism, Bioethics in; Law and Bioethics; Law and Morality; Life, Quality of; Medical Ethics, History of Europe, Contemporary Period: The Benelux Countries; Medical Codes and Oaths; Pain and Suffering; Palliative Care and Hospice; Patients' Rights; Professional-Patient Relationship; Suicide; Virtue and Character*

BIBLIOGRAPHY

Barber v. Superior Court. 195 Cal. Rptr. 484 (Ct. App. 1983).

Bouvia v. Superior Court (Glenchur). 225 Cal. Rptr. 297 (Ct. App. 3d 1986).

Conroy, In re. 486 A.2d 1209 (N.J.) (1985).

Cruzan v. Director, Missouri Department of Health. 497 U.S. 261 (1990).

Dresser, Rebecca. 1986. "Life, Death, and Incompetent Patients: Conceptual Infirmities and Hidden Values in the Law." *Arizona Law Review* 28: 373–405.

Dubreuil, In re. 629 So. 2d 819 (Fla.) (1993).

Edna M.F., In re v. Eisenberg. 563 N.W.2d 485 (Wis. 1997).

Filene, Peter G. 1998. *In the Arms of Others: A Cultural History of the Right-to-Die in America.* Chicago: Ivan R. Dee.

Fosmire v. Nicoleau. 551 N.E.2d 77 (N.Y. 1990).

Harmon, Louise. 1990. "Falling Off the Vine: Legal Fictions and the Doctrine of Substituted Judgment." *Yale Law Journal* 100: 1–71.

Martin v. Martin. 538 N.W.2d 399 (Mich. 1995); *cert. denied.* 516 U.S. 1113. (1996).

McKay v. Bergstedt. 801 P.2d 617 (Nev. 1990).

National Council of Commissioners on Uniform State Laws. 2002. "Uniform Health-Care Decisions Act." *Uniform State Laws* 9: §§ 1–19.

President's Commission for the Study of Ethical Problems in Medicine and Biomedical and Behavioral Research. 1983. *Deciding to Forego Life-Sustaining Treatment.* Washington, D.C.: Government Printing Office.

Quinlan, In re. 355 A.2d 647 (N.J.), *cert. denied* 429 U.S. 922. (1976).

Rachels, James. 1975. "Active and Passive Euthanasia." *New England Journal of Medicine* 292: 78–80.

Solomon, Mildred, et al. 1993. "Decisions Near the End of Life: Professional Views on Life-Sustaining Treatments." *American Journal of Public Health* 83: 14–25.

State v. McAfee. 385 S.E.2d 651 (Ga. 1989).

Superintendent of Belchertown State Sch. v. Saikewicz. 370 N.E.2d 417 (Mass. 1977).

Teel, Karen. 1975. "The Physician's Dilemma: A Doctor's View: What The Law Should Be." *Baylor Law Review* 27: 6–9.

Thor v. Superior Court. 855 P.2d 375 (Cal. 1993).

Wendland, In re. 28 P.3d 151 (Cal. 2001).

Westchester County Medical Ctr., In re (O'Connor). 531 N.E.2d 607 (N.Y. 1988).

Wons v. Public Health Trust. 541 So. 2d 96 (Fla. 1989).

INTERNET RESOURCES

Oregon Death with Dignity Act. Oregon Revised Statute 127.800–127.995. Available from <www.ohd.hr.state.or.us/chs/pas/ors.htm>.

Oregon Department of Human Services. 2003. *Oregon's Death with Dignity Act.* Available from <http://www.ohd.hr.state.or.us/chs/pas/pas.htm>.

S

SCIENCE, PHILOSOPHY OF

• • •

Philosophy of science as an autonomous subject is a product of the twentieth century. Its development stemmed from the great intellectual challenges of the quantum and relativity theories, but philosophical issues surrounding such theories as psychoanalysis, evolutionary theory, Marxist and capitalist economics, the ethics of human experimentation, and the enormously increased importance of science as an intellectual endeavor led to a great expansion of the field.

Work within philosophy of science tends to fall into two approaches. The first sees science as a testing ground for traditional philosophical problems. Chief among these traditional problems is this: Can we have any knowledge that is certain and in terms of which all other knowledge in the area can be justified (*foundationalism*), or are all claims to knowledge uncertain (*fallibilism*)? Within the realm of things that can be known by empirical investigation, it would seem that science has the best claim to secure knowledge. Philosophers of science have thus devoted a considerable amount of time to what kinds of scientific methods are effective in producing such reliable knowledge. On the other hand, many philosophers, especially in recent times, have denied that science does actually produce a privileged body of knowledge, and have argued that all scientific knowledge is a product of its historical and social context.

The second approach to philosophy of science focuses on issues that are peculiar to individual sciences. Of particular interest here is the possibility of reducing biology to chemistry or physics, and of reducing some of the social sciences, especially psychology, to biology. If these reductionist projects were to be successful, then issues that currently appear to be peculiarly biological, such as the question of what makes something a living organism, would turn out to be merely a question of degrees of complexity, and not specifically biological at all. In addition, the moral issues that pertain to humans and animals because of their psychological characteristics would be approached very differently if psychological properties were considered to be unreal or merely disguised biological properties. These differences between the sciences are crucial. For example, a great deal of medical research cannot enjoy the unlimited freedom of laboratory experimentation that is characteristic of physics simply because of the ethical constraints its subjects require. Moreover, the variability of its subjects makes universal laws hard to formulate in biology, in distinction to, for example, astronomy.

Predecessors to Contemporary Viewpoints

It was the logical positivists and logical empiricists of the Vienna Circle (1923–1936) and the Berlin school (1928–1933) who succeeded in placing scientific issues near the heart of the philosophical enterprise. (A classic, albeit sententious, presentation of the logical positivists' views can be found in A. J. Ayer's *Language, Truth and Logic,* 1946.) For philosophers such as Moritz Schlick, Rudolf Carnap, Hans Reichenbach, and Carl Hempel, all of whom had a scientific education, the task was to provide a foundation for genuine knowledge, and this foundation was to be as secure as the best science of the time. The logical positivists were squarely within the empiricist tradition, which holds that all genuine knowledge must be reducible in principle to knowledge obtainable by empirical methods, and ultimately to that obtainable through the human sensory apparatus. To this empiricist view they added a deep concern with language resulting from developments in logic in the late nineteenth and early twentieth centuries. Although the most famous manifestation of their approach was the attempt to eliminate metaphysical claims through the verificationist criterion of meaning (which asserts that a sentence is factually significant to a given individual if and only if he knows what observations would lead him to accept that proposition as true or to reject it as false), their true legacy has been the view that it is by means of logical analyses of philosophical concepts that genuine understanding is achieved. It is no exaggeration to say that philosophy of science since 1950 has been primarily engaged in a struggle to decide which elements of the positivist monolith to retain, and what should be the replacement approaches for those parts that have been rejected.

Falsificationism

An important alternative to the positivist program has been the falsificationist approach of Karl Popper. Although his *Logik der Forschung* was published in 1934, its impact was muted until the expanded English translation appeared in 1959 as *The Logic of Scientific Discovery.* Popper set himself the task of providing a criterion that would distinguish between genuine scientific hypotheses and pseudoscientific statements. A key belief driving Popper's work was his view that the traditional problem of induction could not be solved. Most generally, inductive inference involves reasoning from what has been observed to what has not been observed, a characterization that covers inferences from the past to the future, from observed data to the existence of directly unobservable microentities such as prions, and from finite data sets to the universal hypotheses that represent scientific laws and general theories. Justifying inductive inferences was a serious problem for logical positivism, because the verificationist criterion ruled out all universal scientific theories and laws as meaningless, simply because no amount of finite data could conclusively verify these general claims. Popper instead proposed the demarcation criterion that a statement or theory was scientific only if it was falsifiable; that is, it must be possible to state in advance a set of possible observations which, if observed, would result in the statement or theory being rejected. Theories such as astrology and psychoanalysis were, according to Popper, branded as pseudoscientific on the basis of this criterion because they traditionally accommodated themselves to fit any observations whatsoever. To refuse to relinquish a theory in the face of recalcitrant data is a characteristic feature of scientific irrationality. Popper's brand of falsificationism is comprehensive, for it requires that even reports of observations be falsifiable. Thus, in contrast to the

positivists' foundationalism, which is grounded in an empirical base that is certain, falsificationism is a deeply fallibilist position, within which claims to certainty are relinquished at all levels of generality.

Popper was well aware of a point often made by the French philosopher Pierre Duhem: In order to draw out testable predictions from scientific hypotheses, one ordinarily needs to assume the truth of various background assumptions and theories (Duhem). Thus, if the prediction turns out to be false, the force of the falsification could be deflected away from the principal hypothesis onto the background assumptions. Hence the need in the above specification of falsificationism to state *in advance* what would result in the hypothesis being rejected.

Although this strategy removes the force of Duhem's criticism that there are no crucial experiments that can conclusively decide between competing theories, it moves the emphasis away from a method of testing that is based only on logic and empirical data to one where a (human) decision plays a central role, and this introduces a characteristically conventional element into the picture. Falsificationism is primarily a normative methodology, for it prescribes and proscribes courses of action with respect to scientific hypotheses. As historical and sociological studies of science have become increasingly influential, there has been a concomitant emphasis on the need for methodological theories to be descriptively accurate of what scientists do and have done. It is easy to find cases where historically important episodes of science do not fit the falsificationist model, ones where scientists refused to abandon theories in the face of clear counter evidence. The difficult task is to articulate when this furthers broad scientific ends, rather than just narrow personal motives. But to reject falsificationism merely because it is not descriptively accurate of everything done in the name of science would be as misguided as the attempt to turn ethics into a purely descriptive enterprise.

Thomas Kuhn's Work

One of the best known alternatives to the positivist approach is Thomas Kuhn's. Ironically, Kuhn's seminal work *The Structure of Scientific Revolutions* (1996) was originally published in the positivists' *International Encyclopedia of Unified Science* (Kuhn, 1955). Kuhn's strategy was to use the history of science as a proving ground for methodological positions in the philosophy of science. This history, Kuhn claimed, could be divided into two distinct types of periods. There were long stretches of normal science punctuated by brief periods of revolutionary science. To illuminate both kinds of science, Kuhn introduced the concept of a scientific paradigm. This concept, in its mature characterization, consists of four components. First, there are the symbolic generalizations, those fundamental laws and principles of a science that underpin all theoretical work in the field, such as the laws of genetic replication or the principle of natural selection of species. Second is the metaphysical component of the paradigm, within which the fundamental kinds of things constituting the subject matter of the science are specified, such as atomistic or field-theoretic assumptions in physics, or a commitment to specifically mental properties, as opposed to material properties, in psychology. Third, there are the value commitments. These not only concern what constitutes an acceptable piece of evidence in the science, but what the appropriate goals are for a science, and what the ethical standards are to which one should adhere. Thus, double-blind studies will be considered the standard methodology for drug trials. Fourth, there are the exemplars, those quintessential successes that a scientific field can point to as evidence for the fruitfulness of the first three elements, as, for instance, Newtonian mechanics could point to its success in predicting the existence of the planet Neptune.

Normal science, then, is science conducted entirely within the framework of a single paradigm, whereas revolutionary science consists in the development of a competing paradigm and the process of a scientific community's transfer of allegiance to the new paradigm. A seemingly inescapable consequence of paradigm change in periods of revolutionary science, and one that is deeply disturbing to many, is that the process of change is determined by neither rational argument nor empirical evidence. Because a change in paradigm necessarily involves a change in at least one of the four components already described, there will inevitably be fundamental differences of opinion about whether the old or the new component is preferable, and the remaining three components will frequently not provide a large enough common ground to resolve the dispute in an impartial way. In this way, paradigms are, to use Kuhn's term, incommensurable. There is then a deep difference between Kuhn on the one hand and both Popper and the positivists on the other.

Equally important is the distinction between internal and external descriptions of science. Within both the positivists' and Popper's approaches, the way in which science proceeds ought to be appraised only in terms of influences that are purely internal to the science at hand, including the construction of theories, the invention of new experimental apparatus, and the verification or falsification of hypotheses by empirical data. Any interference by nonscientific factors, such as economic considerations, political pressure, and religious prohibitions, are to be condemned as illegitimate influences to be resisted in practice, and ignored in writing the history of the science. In contrast, Kuhn holds that not

only are such influences usually present and causally effective in propelling or impeding the elaboration of a paradigm, but they are frequently important in fixing the values component of a paradigm. Thus, the religious opposition to research on fetal tissue derived from deliberate abortions, the political pressure to direct funds in molecular biology toward acquired immunodeficiency syndrome (AIDS) research, and the decision to allocate significant financial resources to the Human Genome Project are all part of an externalist appraisal of the scientific research concerned. Inseparable from this externalist approach is the shift in emphasis from scientific theories as logical entities whose existence and appraisal are objective matters, and the truth or falsity of which is something to be discovered, to a position where the opinions of a community of scientists are primary, and acceptance of a paradigm is determined by a consensus in that community rather than by the paradigm's truth or falsity. Coupled with the inclusion of externalist factors, this leads naturally toward a focus on the sociology of science, rather than its philosophy as traditionally conceived.

Some further consequences of the Kuhnian approach are worth mentioning. Because of the incommensurability of paradigms, revolutions lead to schisms in the path of science, with a resulting loss of the notion of scientific progress. Comparative judgments of the kind "Paradigm A is superior to Paradigm B" can no longer be made on a uniform scale of comparison, and what remains is technological progress without any necessary concomitant progress toward the truth. Consequently, what has come to be known as the Whig view of the history of science, which sees the development of science as an uninterrupted triumphal march to the peak of contemporary success, has to be abandoned in favor of a contextually sympathetic interpretation of previous theoretical traditions. Finally, if Kuhn is correct, there is no longer anything peculiarly privileged in the scientific enterprise. The development of art, architecture, music, and so forth can all be characterized in terms of paradigms, normal practice, and revolutionary changes, a feature that has not escaped Kuhn's critics.

Contemporary Work in the Field

Perhaps the most important consequence of the collapse of the positivists' domination in the philosophy of science has been the splintering of the field into a number of subsets. One principal division is between those who continue to hold that there are general principles underlying various scientific methods, and those for whom only local, context-specific approaches are feasible. Certain areas of science still seem to be amenable to the first approach. The nature of scientific explanation is a topic of perennial interest, with various causal and unification approaches (Salmon) serving as the chief contenders to replace Carl Hempel's logical model. How scientific hypotheses and theories are confirmed is the subject of another area of research (Achinstein), with computer-assisted diagnostic procedures in medicine forming a small but important proving ground for inference procedures. There is considerable current interest in causal inference, particularly of the kind used in epidemiology (Pearl). Despite these successes, issues related to the autonomy of particular sciences have increasingly come to the fore. The positivists' orientation towards reducing all sciences to physics, at least in principle, has been replaced by a recognition that at least in practice, and perhaps even in principle, this reduction cannot be carried out. There is now a "philosophy of X" for almost every science, from economics to geology. In particular, the philosophy of biology and the philosophy of medicine are well established subfields with their own problems and methods. Accompanying this trend has been a reduced emphasis on grand unifying theories in favor of local models that capture, albeit imperfectly, the structure of specific systems (Humphreys). This latter approach works well for biological models, within which the sheer number and complexity of the influences on a system and the importance of its historical evolution render simple general theories inadequate.

A second primary division is between those for whom normative, objective, and a priori characterizations of science are desirable and attainable, and those who maintain that such characterizations are inevitably descriptively inaccurate and unrevealing of the true nature of science. Within this latter orientation lie contemporary naturalistic and cognitive approaches to philosophical issues. Philosophers using these methods hold that scientific knowledge from areas such as psychology and evolutionary biology shed more light on why certain methods are successful than can more traditional a priori approaches. For example, instead of specifying a priori the inferences that an ideal reasoner should make in deciding which course of action is appropriate in some clinical setting, a naturalist will investigate the heuristics that underlie reasoning used in clinical practice (Gigerenzer, Todd, and ABC Research Group).

Another dispute is between those who hold that many objects of scientific investigation, such as various psychiatric disorders, are social constructions, and those who hold that there is an objective reality that science investigates (Hacking). Much of this work is interesting and legitimate, but the rejection of traditional norms of rationality has led in certain quarters to a denial that science has any claim to superior methods of investigating the world. The so-called "science wars" between those who seek to maintain the epistemological superiority of science and those who wish to undermine it are an extreme, albeit avoidable (Koertge) consequence of this division.

All of the threads described have made formulating a satisfactory account of scientific progress less easy than it was in earlier periods, especially within the philosophy of biology. The piecemeal framework of models, the attacks on both the rationality of scientific appraisal and the objectivity of reality, the autonomy of multiple sciences—all have made a defense of progress towards a unified scientific account of the world more difficult than one might wish. Nevertheless, mere complexity and locality does not preclude science from accurately describing an objective reality in a systematic and rational fashion.

Summary

Philosophy of science and bioethics share a common concern. Each must draw a line between the prescriptive and the descriptive, between what is rational and justified on the one hand, and what is merely popular opinion and prejudice on the other. Both Galileo and Ignaz Semmelweiss were victims of such antiscientific attacks, the first for advocating the correct theory of the solar system, the second for discovering the mode of transmission of childbed fever. It is thus essential to have some clear distinction between fact and opinion, between the rational evaluation of a hypothesis or ethical view and its mere acceptance, between what is ethically justified and the way individuals happen to act. To use a specific example, it is essential to distinguish between what science can do to allow premature babies to survive and how one can evaluate the quality of life they might expect. This, if nothing else, is why the apparently dry and abstract issues of the foundations of knowledge, of internal and external influences on science, and of fact versus convention bear directly upon matters of more immediate concern.

PAUL W. HUMPHREYS (1995)
REVISED BY AUTHOR

SEE ALSO: *Biology, Philosophy of; Research Bias; Research Methodology*

BIBLIOGRAPHY

Achinstein, Peter. 2001. *The Book of Evidence.* New York: Oxford University Press.

Ayer, A. J. 1946. *Language, Truth, and Logic,* 2nd edition. London: Gollancz.

Curd, Martin, and Cover, J.A., eds. 1998. *Philosophy of Science: The Central Issues.* New York: Norton.

Duhem, Pierre. 1906 (reprint 1962). *The Aim and Structure of Physical Theory.* New York: Atheneum.

Gigerenzer, Gerd; Todd, Peter M.; and the ABC Research Group. 1999. *Simple Heuristics That Make Us Smart.* Oxford: Oxford University Press.

Hacking, Ian. 1999. *The Social Construction of What?* Cambridge, MA: Harvard University Press.

Hempel, Carl G. 1966. *Philosophy of Natural Science.* Englewood Cliffs, NJ: Prentice Hall.

Humphreys, Paul. 2003. *Extending Ourselves.* New York: Oxford University Press.

Klee, Robert. 1997. *Introduction to the Philosophy of Science.* New York: Oxford University Press.

Klee, Robert. 1999. *Scientific Inquiry: Readings in the Philosophy of Science.* New York: Oxford University Press.

Koertge, Noretta, ed. 1998. *A House Built on Sand.* Oxford: Oxford University Press.

Kuhn, Thomas S. 1955. *The Structure of Scientific Revolutions,* In *The International Encyclopedia of Unified Science,* vol. 2, no. 2, ed. Otto Neurath. Chicago: University of Chicago Press.

Kuhn, Thomas S. 1996. *The Structure of Scientific Revolutions,* 3rd edition. Chicago: University of Chicago Press.

Pearl, Judea. 2000. *Causation.* Cambridge, Eng.: Cambridge University Press.

Popper, Karl R. 1935. *Logik der Forschung.* Vienna: Julius Springer, tr. Karl Popper, Julius Freed, and Lan Freed (1959) under the title *The Logic of Scientific Discovery.* London: Hutchinson.

Salmon, Wesley C. 1990. *Four Decades of Scientific Explanation.* Minneapolis: University of Minnesota Press.

Van Fraassen, Bas C. 2002. *The Empiricist Stance.* New Haven: Yale University Press.

SCIENTIFIC PUBLISHING

• • •

During the late 1970s and the 1980s, an ethics of scientific publication began to evolve. Competition among scientists for academic rewards and research funds, the continued fragmentation and commercialization of science, and reports of scientific misconduct, as well as increasing governmental and legal interference with the inner workings of the scientific community led many within that community to perceive a need for reforms to guide both the conduct of science and the dissemination of scientific information. Journal editors, universities, professional associations, funding agencies, and governments have taken active roles in debating and setting ethical standards and editorial policies for the dissemination of scientific information. In 1978, a self-appointed group of editors, the International Committee of Medical Journal Editors (ICMJE), representing leading general medical journals, met in Vancouver, British Columbia, to set technical guidelines for the submission of manuscripts. These guidelines, the Uniform Requirements for the Submission of Manuscripts to Biomedical Journals, have evolved to include statements for the ethical conduct of authors, editors, and peer reviewers. While the ICMJE statements set international standards for biomedical publishing, the number of journals that adhere to them is unknown (ICMJE, 1991, 1993b). This entry presents an overview of the major ethical issues in biomedical and scientific publishing.

Editorial and Peer Review

The prestige and influence of biomedical journal publication are closely related to the quality control and selection process that precedes publication. Thus, the essential tasks of medical editing are the selection and improvement of articles submitted for publication. These tasks are generally accomplished through processes of editorial review (evaluation by the journal's editorial staff) and peer review (evaluation by experts in a given field who are considered the authors' "peers"). These two processes may overlap, particularly when an editor is also an expert in a manuscript's topic, but editorial review usually focuses on the appropriateness, clarity, and priority of articles for the journal's readership. Peer reviewers are selected by the editor to assess the quality of an article's scientific and technical content and to offer advice about publication. Since decisions regarding rejection, revision, or acceptance are made solely by the editor, the term *referee* exaggerates a reviewer's advisory role and should be avoided.

Peer review was first used for biomedical publications by the Royal Societies of London and Edinburgh in the eighteenth century, but evolved haphazardly; it was not employed regularly until after World War II (Lock). Two striking aspects of peer review are that it is based almost entirely on uncompensated, voluntary labor and that the peer review system itself has only recently come under scientific scrutiny (Lock; "Guarding the Guardians,"; Rennie and Flanagin, 1994b). Journals follow differing policies about revealing reviewers' identities to authors and authors' identities to reviewers (Lock; "Guarding the Guardians,"; Rennie and Flanagin, 1994b). Some editors believe that disclosure of reviewer identities to authors decreases the potential for bias, while others believe such disclosure leads to less critical reviews. Many biomedical journals do not attempt to remove the identities of authors or their institutions from submitted manuscripts; studies have shown that author identities may be discerned by reviewers from the paper's content or from bibliographic citations, especially in narrow subspecialties (Lock). On the other hand, these same journals do not reveal the identities of peer reviewers to authors. While most editors are impressed by the care and objectivity usually reflected in reviewer comments and recommendations, the anonymous review of papers whose authors are known obviously involves potential for abuse. To maintain integrity in the peer review process, reviewers are expected to disclose any conflicts of interest involved in their review, and editors are expected to be alert to any signs of bias that may interfere with an objective evaluation of the merits of the paper.

Maintaining the confidentiality of an author's work before publication is an important ethical principle in scientific publishing. Most journals inform peer reviewers that the information in unpublished manuscripts is privileged and should be kept confidential, and also require manuscripts to be either returned to the editorial office or destroyed after review. However, maintaining confidentiality depends on an honesty among editors, authors, and reviewers that is nearly impossible to guarantee. Conscious or unconscious intellectual theft by peer reviewers may occur but cannot be measured. Journal editors have a particular responsibility to maintain strict confidentiality about the peer review process, editorial decisions, and all manuscript submissions.

How well do the processes of editorial and peer review work? Many persons involved in publishing recognize the improved quality of articles that have been revised after review, and this has been clearly demonstrated with regard to improvements of study designs and statistical methods ("Guarding the Guardians,"; Rennie and Flanagin, 1994b). Nevertheless, both editorial and peer review are based on human judgments that carry the potential for bias and error.

One form of publication bias is the tendency for papers with statistically significant "positive" results (for example, those showing that a new treatment works better) to be published in favor of papers with statistically nonsignificant "negative" results (for example, those showing that a new treatment does not have any effect or does not work any better than other treatments). Studies have shown that such publication bias exists, but its extent is unknown and controversial ("Guarding the Guardians,"; Rennie and Flanagin, 1992, 1994b). Prepublication bias (the tendency of authors not to submit negative results for publication because the findings are incomplete or nonsignificant or because funding runs out) and postpublication bias (bias in the reception and interpretation of published research data

by researchers, funding agencies, editors, and the media) may be more substantial problems. All of these forms of bias can lead to inappropriate medical policies and treatment decisions, especially with new or controversial therapies. Hence, the evaluation of scientific results should be based on their quality and importance, not on their direction.

Authorship

Despite the fact that university promotion committees evince some shift in the emphasis from the quantity to the quality of publication, academic pressures to publish remain. In many academic circles, achievement is still measured by the length of an individual's bibliography. As a result, authorship of an article published in a peer-reviewed scientific journal carries considerable merit, and consequently, considerable responsibility (Rennie and Flanagin, 1994a).

During the past several decades, the meaning of authorship has become diluted as the number of names appearing in scientific article bylines has grown. Authors have justified lengthy bylines by the increasing specialization of science and the need for collaboration among many subspecialists. But the once-accepted practices of adding the names of a department chair or laboratory chief to the end of bylines (guest authorship), and hiring someone to write up a paper without credit (ghost authorship), have caused many editors to adopt formal policies to curtail inflated bylines (Huth, 1986a, 1986b; Lundberg and Flanagin; Rennie and Flanagin, 1994a) and limit the number of names that can appear in a byline without formal justification.

In 1985, the ICMJE recommended that only those persons who have participated sufficiently to take public responsibility for the work should be authors and that "authorship credit should be based solely on substantial contributions to (a) conception and design, or analysis and interpretation of data; (b) drafting the article or revising it critically for important intellectual content; and (c) final approval of the version to be published" (ICMJE, 1991). Each of these criteria must be met by each person listed in the byline, and the authors must state that they meet these criteria in the cover letter accompanying each submitted manuscript. In the latter half of the 1980s, a number of medical journals, including the *Annals of Internal Medicine* and the *Journal of the American Medical Association* (JAMA), began requiring authors to sign authorship statements based on the ICMJE criteria. Anyone who does not meet these conditions but has contributed or assisted significantly can be recognized in an acknowledgment within the article, if he or she has given written permission to be so named (ICMJE, 1993b).

Group authorship results when investigators from many different institutions or participants in study groups, consensus conferences, or working groups prepare reports of their works. Frequently these groups comprise hundreds of investigators, technicians, and specialists. While it is conceivable that each of these individuals contributed critical time and information to the overall work, it is unlikely that each meets the ICMJE authorship criteria. In these cases, those participants who do meet the authorship criteria can be listed with the name of the study group in the byline. Those participants who do not qualify for authorship are then listed in a group box or in an acknowledgment. If all of the participants do meet the criteria for authorship, then the group name can be listed as the sole byline, with the individuals composing the group named in a separate box or the acknowledgment.

Unlike the definition of authorship, there are no established standards for order of authorship, although a number have been proposed, ranging from alphabetical listings to mathematical formulas for determining individual contribution levels and ranking. Many editors agree that authors should be listed according to how much they contributed, with the author who contributed the most listed first and the author who dontributed least listed last (Huth, 1986a, 1986b; Riesenberg and Lundberg). In addition, a number of publications and indexes limit the number of names to be published in a reference list to three, six, or ten. But there is still no consensus on the order of authorship, mostly because there are no widely accepted objective measures of individual coauthors' contribution levels. Editors recommend that authors determine the order of authorship before writing their papers, or before beginning their study, with an agreement to reevaluate the order later if necessary. Editors also recommend that authors solve disagreements over order among themselves, since the authors are in the best position to determine levels of contribution (Riesenberg and Lundberg; ICMJE, 1991).

Duplicate Publication

Another result of the pressures to publish and a driving force behind the need for ethical standards in scientific publication is the practice of duplicate publication. Also known as multiple, dual, or redundant publication, duplicate publication is the simultaneous or subsequent publication of the same article or major parts of an article—methods, results and data, discussion, conclusions, and graphic or illustrative material—in two or more journals or other media, including electronic journals and databases, without notifying the editors (Huth, 1986a, 1986b; ICMJE, 1993b; Iverson et al.). The types of duplicate publication range from selfplagiarism (publishing two or more identical articles or large parts of an article in different journals without citing each article in the texts and references lists) to "salami slicing" (dividing up different parts of the same study for publication in different journals) to sequential publication (reporting follow-up of the same study with additional subjects but without new results). Word-for-word duplication is uncommon, as duplicators usually attempt to alter or disguise the similarities.

Duplicate publication should be distinguished from secondary publication, in which an article or abbreviated version is subsequently republished, in the same or another language, with the consent of both editors. The secondary article should include a footnote on the title page, informing all readers that the information was published previously, and a complete citation to the primary article. Duplicate publication may violate copyright law, and it is unethical for an author to submit duplicate papers to different journals without notifying the editors. By doing so, authors clutter the literature with redundant information; waste the valuable time and resources of editors, reviewers, and readers; and prevent other authors from publishing their work because of limited journal space. To discourage such practices, many scientific journals state in their instructions for authors that they will only consider papers that have not been previously published or submitted to other journals, and some journals will publish notices of duplicate publication, publicly admonishing those authors who publish duplicate articles in violation of the journal's written policies (Iverson et al.).

Conflicts of Interest

Reflecting the increasing commercialization of science and the public doubts about researchers' once hallowed and rarely questioned integrity, financial conflicts of interest are now recognized as another ethical problem for authors and editors. During the 1980s, the public's trust of the scientific community diminished as a result of a number of public scandals and government investigations of biomedical researchers' ties to drugs with potential public health benefits and high financial rewards for stockholders and manufacturers (Relman; Lundberg and Flanagin; U.S. Congress). These cases have generally involved researchers being biased by their direct but undisclosed financial interests, such as stock ownership and paid consultancies. However, there are several other potential sources of author bias: funds from granting agencies, any research or material support, employment, money paid for expert testimony, and honoraria paid for public speaking.

Recognizing that not all financial interests will bias an author, editors disagree over how to handle these financial interests. Most journals publish an author's source of funding or material support, but that is usually because the funding institution requires that it be published. Some journals require authors to disclose all financial interests relevant to the work reported in their submitted manuscripts. If a manuscript is subsequently accepted for publication, the editors of these journals will determine whether it is necessary to publish such financial interests. In this manner, readers can judge for themselves the author's potential for bias from a financial interest just as they can judge an author's potential for intellectual bias based on his or her previously published works or specialty status (Rennie et al.). In 1990, the *New England Journal of Medicine* instituted a stringent policy prohibiting anyone with relevant financial interests from publishing editorials or review articles in that journal. Critics have argued that such prohibition is scientific censorship.

In 1989, the American Federation for Clinical Research and the Association of American Medical Colleges recommended full disclosure of all relevant financial interests and the possible divestiture of any stock or equity in a company that makes a product the researcher is studying (U.S. Congress). The Editorial Policy Committee of the Council of Biology Editors (CBE) recommends that authors disclose all relevant financial interests to the editors at the time of manuscript submission, and that editors disclose authors' financial interests to reviewers and readers when appropriate (CBE). There is no consensus among editors for the need and extent of such disclosure. In 1993, however, the ICMJE approved a statement that all participants in the peer review and publication process disclose any conflicting interests (ICMJE, 1993a). Some journals with disclosure policies have applied the basic principles of disclosure to everyone in the editorial process, including editors, editorial board members, and in some cases, reviewers (Relman; Rennie et al.).

Fraudulent Publication Resulting from Scientific Misconduct

The publication of a fraudulent article remains the most serious transgression of the ethics of scientific publication. The once generally accepted view that scientific misconduct was rare and committed by a few deviants has been replaced by a view, unsubstantiated, that it is more common and can involve respected scientists from leading institutions. Scientific misconduct has been defined as plagiarism (presenting another's ideas without attribution), fabrication (presenting data or facts that do not exist), falsification (changing or selecting certain data to obtain a desired result, misrepresenting evidence or facts, or misrepresenting authorship), or other serious deviations from accepted practice in the proposing, conducting, or reporting of research (U.S. Department of Health and Human Services). Policy makers have disagreed over the merits of including the phrase *deviations from accepted practice* in the definition. Some argue that the phrase is too vague and thus open to misinterpretation and overuse (Committee on Science); others argue that it must be included to address misconduct that would not technically be considered plagiarism, fabrication, or falsification. Examples of such deviations include misuse or theft of privileged information by a reviewer or editor, submitting a paper listing several coauthors who are unaware that they are named as coauthors, misrepresenting publication status of articles in a bibliography, or failing to perform funded research while filing reports stating that such work has been done (U.S. Department of Health and Human Services).

Variations in the definition of fraud have caused some confusion, but most editors acknowledge a major difference between fraud and unintentional errors. Although unprofessional and in some cases unethical, the following usually are not considered fraudulent: errors in study design or application of methods, inappropriate use or interpretation of statistics, faulty interpretation or overgeneralization of study results, failure to cite relevant literature or studies, duplicate publication or fragmentary reporting of results, prepublication release of information, publication bias, failure to disclose intellectual or financial conflicts of interests, or violations of experimentation rules protecting humans or animals.

Plagiarism is probably more commonly acknowledged, since it is easier to detect and prove. Detecting and proving falsification or fabrication of data in a published article is not so easy, and it carries grave ethical and legal consequences for editors, authors, institutions, and funding agencies. While an editor has a duty to see that questions of fraud are appropriately and confidentially pursued, the Association of American Medical Colleges, the National Academy of Sciences, and the ICMJE recommend that primary responsibility for investigating cases of suspected fraud rests with the author's institution or funding agency (Association of American Medical Colleges; Committee on Science; ICMJE, 1991). If it is determined that a fraudulent paper has been published, the journal should print—in a timely manner—a retraction, written by the author(s) or an appropriate representative of the institution. Since the validity of any previous work by the author of a fraudulent paper cannot be assumed, the editor must ask the institution to verify the validity of any of the author's articles previously published in the journal or to retract them (ICMJE, 1991).

Protecting Patient Rights

The two major issues regarding patient rights in medical publishing are requirements for the ethical conduct of published research and the protection of patient confidentiality. A now well-established principle followed by all credible medical journals is that reports of experimental investigations of human or animal subjects must include a statement that the research project has been approved by an appropriate institutional review board (IRB). For investigators not covered by a formal ethics review board, the report should state that the researchers have followed the principles of the Declaration of Helsinki (World Medical Association), which includes requirements for freely given informed consent and for the review of the research protocol by a committee independent of the investigator and the sponsor. Many journals also require an additional statement of the manner in which informed consent was obtained from human subjects, since informed consent is a central tenet for ethical research.

Many editors now agree that journal publication should protect patient confidentiality. For example, placing a black bar over the eyes in a facial photograph does not effectively disguise identity. Patients may also be identified from detailed case descriptions. In 1991, the ICMJE published expanded guidelines for the protection of patients' right to anonymity (ICMJE, 1991). These guidelines state that identifying information should be avoided unless it is essential for scientific purposes; informed consent should be obtained for the publication of identifying descriptions or photographs; changing patient data should not be used as a way of securing anonymity; and journals should publish editorial policies to preserve patient confidentiality (ICMJE, 1991).

One problematic area regarding patient anonymity is the publication of pedigrees from genetics research, since the family as a whole or individual family members can sometimes be identified from pedigree information. Following the ICMJE guidelines, identifying information should be deleted if possible, but pedigree data should not be altered. Pedigree publication is complicated by the fact that a large number of family members may be involved, not all of whom may have given consent for, or even be aware of, the collection of family data. A requirement for informed consent for publication from each individual member of a large pedigree may be impossible to meet, particularly if family members disagree about publication. Whether some kind of group consent would be ethically permissible, or whether identifiable pedigrees should not be published without the consent of each individual family member, remains an unsettled issue.

Release of Information

Scientific journals play a major role in informing the public, as well as health professionals, about biomedical developments. This function involves a balance between the timely release of information and the adequate evaluation of the quality of the information. Conflicts sometimes occur between scientists, who want rapid dissemination of new or controversial research findings; editors, who as gatekeepers want to make sure that only accurate and valid scientific information is released; and the news media, which compete with each other to be the first to publicize new scientific information. The process of scientific publication after peer review takes time. Some investigators have chosen to short-circuit this traditional process by announcing results at a news conference rather than waiting for a paper to be evaluated by a scientific journal. Advocates for a particular disease (acquired immunodeficiency syndrome [AIDS], for example) have also pressed for faster release of research results. Even if well-intended, such attempts to bypass careful evaluation and publication may result in the dissemination of misinformation (Angell and Kassirer).

In 1969, Franz Ingelfinger, then editor of the *New England Journal of Medicine,* promulgated a policy (subsequently known as the *Ingelfinger rule*) that manuscripts would be considered for publication only if their substance had not been submitted or reported elsewhere. Other journals adopted similar policies to discourage both duplicate publication and the public dissemination of results before peer review and publication. Such policies have been criticized as self-serving on the part of journals, but they usually exempt presentations at scientific meetings (including published abstracts and media coverage from such meetings) and the rare situations when an appropriate public health authority determines that there is an immediate need for dissemination. Some medical journals also ask news media to observe a press embargo for a brief period to allow physician subscribers to read and evaluate information before their patients begin seeing it in the media.

Copyright

Copyright protection covers text and illustrative material—whether in print or electronic (digital) format. U.S. copyright law provides that the creator of a written work, the author, owns all legal rights to that work for his or her life span plus fifty years, unless the author transfers those rights to another party. Two exceptions to individual copyright ownership are works prepared by employees of the U.S. government and works made for hire, in which an individual, either by an employment mandate or by contract, agrees in writing that all work prepared within the scope of employment or contract is the property of the employer or contractor (*Copyright Law of the United States of America*). Different countries have different copyright laws, but the Universal Copyright and Berne Conventions protect works published and distributed in other countries.

Most journals require authors to transfer copyright to their publishers before publication, giving the publisher exclusive rights to the work after publication. Therefore, anyone who wishes to reprint or adapt from an article (in part or whole) must receive written permission to do so from the publisher. However, certain uses of a published work without permission from the owner—such as photocopying for teaching, scholarship, or research purposes—may not be an infringement of copyright under the provisions of "fair use." Fair use can be difficult to justify in court and must take into account the following factors: (1) the purpose of the use, including whether it is educational or commercial; (2) the nature of the copyrighted work; (3) the amount of the copyrighted work to be used; and (4) the effect of use on the potential marketability or value of the copyrighted work (*Copyright Law of the United States of America*).

Rights to Unpublished Data

Unlike rights to copyrighted work, rights to unpublished data are difficult to define, and most ethical dilemmas concern access to rather than ownership of such information. Unpublished scientific data include written and electronic laboratory notes, experimental materials, project records and observations, databases, descriptions of methods and processes, analyses, and illustrative material. Traditionally, unpublished scientific data have been owned by their creators—the scientific investigators—and most scientists believe they have a duty to share data with their peers and, when appropriate, with the public. Any data reported in a published article become the property of the publisher, but rights to relevant, supportive data not reported in a published article (sometimes called raw data) are not transferred to the publisher. Problems arise when investigators, institutions, the government, and the public compete for control of and access to the same data. For example, who should have first rights to publication of research data: the principal investigator, the coinvestigators, or the institution that funded the research? Legally, the investigator controls access to unpublished data, except under the following circumstances: (1) the investigator is an employee of an organization that claims rights to any work conducted by its employees; (2) the investigator is under federal contract or has received a federal grant to perform the work; or (3) a court decides that public interest in the data outweighs the interest of the owner (CBE). Government or industrial sponsorship

of research may impose specific restrictions on data control and sharing, particularly when such data are proprietary or commercial. This area of law will continue to evolve as electronic technology makes data ownership and access more difficult to define and control by narrow standards and laws.

While it is generally agreed that data must be kept in an accessible format for a reasonable period of time, no standard has been universally accepted, because different types of data from different specialties require various modes and spaces for storage, which can be prohibitively expensive. Some institutions have recommended three or five years, and longer periods for data that support publications (Committee on Science). The National Research Council Committee on National Statistics recommends and many journals require that editors have access to data during the peer review process, which means that the data must be maintained until publication (CBE). Some journals require authors to provide data to editors for their evaluation if requested, but this requirement does not have a time limit. Some journals require authors to send their data to national or international storage centers at the time of publication.

Disputes over who has rights to use scientific data have caused ethical dilemmas for editors. For example, what should an editor do with a manuscript from an author that reports an analysis of unpublished data originally collected and analyzed by another author? The ICMJE and the Committee on National Statistics recommend that editors consider such secondary analyses on their scientific merit as long as full credit and appropriate citations are given to the original data collections (ICMJE, 1991; CBE). Other open questions concern the nature of sharing data, which is a vital part of the scientific enterprise. Should there be restrictions on the access, use, and citation of unpublished works by other authors and investigators? Most scientists and editors would argue that such restrictions would stifle scientific exchange. But what about access to unpublished data by those outside the scientific community, such as representatives of the media, the courts, and people with commercial interests? Many of these questions are currently under debate, and whether or not access will be widened or restricted is difficult to predict.

Advertising

Advertisements for pharmaceutical products and medical/laboratory devices provide major financial support for biomedical publications. Advertising income is essential for many large biomedical publications since their costs would not be met by subscription revenue. Whether this situation represents one aspect of the success of the free enterprise system or a major ethical problem for editors is a matter of controversy.

To protect a journal's integrity and credibility, complete separation between advertising and editorial decisions is essential, and advertisers should have no influence on editorial content. Advertisements, including advertorials, should have a distinct appearance or labeling so that readers can readily distinguish them from editorial content, and ads for a product should not be placed adjacent to editorial material dealing with the product or disorders for which it might be used (Rennie). Publication of industry-sponsored journal supplements is problematic, since the supplement's editorial content may be selected or influenced by the sponsor to favor their products, and the review process may not be as rigorous or as independent as it is for the journal's regularly published issues.

The accuracy of advertisements in medical publications is more controversial. The purpose of advertisements is promotional, and studies have shown that the prescribing behavior of physicians is indeed influenced by advertisements. Because of their effect on the health of the public, advertisements for drugs and medical devices are regulated by a government health agency in many countries. In the United States, this responsibility lies with the Food and Drug Administration (FDA), which reviews and approves marketing and *labeling* (the package insert that describes the indications and side effects of a drug) but does not routinely review or approve advertisements prior to their dissemination. However, the FDA does review advertisements after publication and can require companies to withdraw or publicly correct ads that it determines to be inaccurate or misleading.

The standards by which print advertisements should be judged and the method of enforcing standards remain unsettled. Some have recommended the development of multidisciplinary review boards, such as the Canadian Pharmaceutical Advertising Advisory Board, to review and approve medical advertisements before their dissemination.

Enforcement of Ethical Standards

The enforcement of ethical standards in scientific publishing is a responsibility shared among authors, institutions, funding organizations, peer reviewers, and editors. Authors are primarily responsible for upholding the scientific commitment to a search for truth, accepting responsibility and credit for the work that bears their names, and fully disclosing any conflicts of interest. Institutions where research is performed and organizations that fund research share the main responsibility for ensuring that studies are designed and conducted ethically, and also for investigating and

sanctioning allegations of misconduct. Peer reviewers are charged with performing objective and timely appraisals of papers submitted for publication, while maintaining strict confidentiality and disclosing their own conflicts of interest. Editors should exercise sound judgment and objectivity in selecting papers for publication, maintaining vigilance for any ethical problems, and ensuring that authors, reviewers, and institutions fulfill their responsibilities. Clear ethical standards and implementation policies are certainly desirable, and editors have taken the lead in setting standards and policies (U.S. Congress). Yet the ethics of scientific publication is based on trust, and obsessive "policing" of the research community and the publication enterprise could be counterproductive. Persistent emphasis on the importance of maintaining ethical standards in the entire research process, from initial research ideas to their eventual publication, should be an expectation shared by all involved in that process. However, defining and enforcing such standards will be an even greater challenge as the electronic revolution extends the traditional boundaries of authorship and scientific publication.

RICHARD M. GLASS
ANNETTE FLANAGIN (1995)
BIBLIOGRAPHY REVISED

SEE ALSO: *Advertising; Bias, Research; Commercialism in Scientific Research; Conflict of Interest; Research, Unethical*

BIBLIOGRAPHY

Angell, Marcia, and Kassirer, Jerome P. 1991. "The Ingelfinger Rule Revisited." *New England Journal of Medicine* 325(19): 1371–1373.

Association of American Medical Colleges. Ad Hoc Committee on Misconduct and Conflict of Interest in Research. 1992. *Beyond the "Framework": Institutional Considerations in Managing Allegations of Misconduct in Research.* Washington, D.C.: Author.

Committee on Science, Engineering, and Public Policy. Panel on Scientific Responsibility and the Conduct of Research. 1992–. *Responsible Science: Ensuring the Integrity of the Research Process,* vol. I. Washington, D.C.: National Academy Press.

Copyright Law of the United States of America, as Contained in Title 17 of the United States Codes. 1993. Washington, D.C.: U.S. Government Printing Office.

Council of Biology Editors (CBE) Editorial Policy Committee. 1990. *Ethics and Policy in Scientific Publication.* Bethesda, MD: Author.

DeAngelis, Catherine D.; Fontanarosa, Phil B.; and Flanagin, Annette. 2001. "Reporting Financial Conflicts of Interest and Relationships between Investigators and Research Sponsors." *Journal of the American Medical Association* 286(1): 89–91.

Flanagin, Annette. 2000. "Human Rights in the Biomedical Literature: the Social Responsibility of Medical Journals." *Journal of the American Medical Association* 284(5): 618–619.

Fontanarosa, Phil B., and Flanagin, Annette. 2000. "Prepublication Release of Medical Research."*Journal of the American Medical Association* 284(22): 2927–2929.

Fontanarosa, Phil B.; Flanagin, Annette; and DeAngelis, Catherine D. 2000. "The Journal's Policy Regarding Release of Information to the Public." *Journal of the American Medical Association* 284(22): 2929–2931.

Garrett, Jinnie M., and Bird, Stephanie J. 2000. "Ethical Issues in Communicating Science."*Science and Engineering Ethics* 6(4): 435–442.

"Guarding the Guardians: Research on Editorial Peer Review: Selected Proceedings from the First International Congress on Peer Review in Biomedical Publication." 1990. *Journal of the American Medical Association* 263(10): 1317–1441.

Huth, Edward J. 1986a. "Guidelines on Authorship of Medical Papers." *Annals of Internal Medicine* 104(2): 269–274.

Huth, Edward J. 1986b. "Irresponsible Authorship and Wasteful Publication." *Annals of Internal Medicine* 104(2): 257–259.

International Committee of Medical Journal Editors (ICMJE). 1991. "Statements from the International Committee of Medical Journal Editors." *Journal of the American Medical Association* 265(20): 2697–2698.

International Committee of Medical Journal Editors (ICMJE). 1993a. "Conflicts of Interest." *Annals of Internal Medicine* 118(8): 646–647.

International Committee of Medical Journal Editors (ICMJE). 1993b. "Uniform Requirements for Manuscripts Submitted to Biomedical Journals." *Journal of the American Medical Association* 269(17): 2282–2286.

International Congress on Peer Review in Biomedical Publication. 1991. *Peer Review in Scientific Publishing.* Chicago: Council of Biology Editors.

Iverson, Cheryl; Dan, Bruce B.; Glitman, Paula; et al. 1989. *American Medical Association Manual of Style,* 8th edition. Baltimore: Williams & Wilkins.

Jones, Anne Hudson, and McLellan, Faith, eds. 2000. *Ethical Issues in Biomedical Publication.*.Baltimore: Johns Hopkins University Press.

Lock, Stephen. 1986. *A Difficult Balance: Editorial Peer Review in Medicine.* Philadelphia: ISI Press.

Lundberg, George D., and Flanagin, Annette. 1989. "New Requirements for Authors: Signed Statements of Authorship Responsibility and Financial Disclosure." *Journal of the American Medical Association* 262(14): 2003–2004.

Olson, Carin M.; Rennie, Drummond; Cook, Deborah; et al. 2002. "Publication Bias in Editorial Decision Making." *Journal of the American Medical Association* 287(21): 2825–2828.

Relman, Arnold S. 1984. "Dealing with Conflicts of Interest." *New England Journal of Medicine* 310(18): 1182–1183.

Rennie, Drummond. 1991. "Editors and Advertisements: What Responsibility Do Editors Have for the Advertisements in Their Journals?" *Journal of the American Medical Association* 265(18): 2394–2396.

Rennie, Drummond, and Flanagin, Annette. 1992. "Publication Bias: The Triumph of Hope Over Experience." *Journal of the American Medical Association* 267(3): 411–412.

Rennie, Drummond, and Flanagin, Annette. 1994a. "Authorship! Authorship! Guests, Ghosts, Grafters, and the Two-Sided Coin." *Journal of the American Medical Association* 271(6): 469–471.

Rennie, Drummond, and Flanagin, Annette. 1994b. "Selected Proceedings from the Second Internatinal Congress on Peer Review in Biomedical Publication." *Journal of the American Medical Association* 272(2): 91–173.

Rennie, Drummond; Flanagin, Annette; and Glass, Richard M. 1991. "Conflicts of Interest in the Publication of Science." *Journal of the American Medical Association* 266(2): 266–267.

Riesenberg, Don, and Lundberg, George D. 1990. "The Order of Authorship: Who's on First?" *Journal of the American Medical Association* 264(14): 1857.

Smith, Richard. 2001. "Maintaining the Integrity of the Scientific Record."*British Medical Journal* 323(7313): 588.

U.S. Congress. House Committee on Government Operations. 1990. *Are Scientific Misconduct and Conflicts of Interest Hazardous to Our Health?* Washington, D.C.: U.S. Government Printing Office.

U.S. Department of Health and Human Services. Office of the Assistant Secretary for Health. 1991. *First Annual Report: Scientific Misconduct Investigations: Reviewed by the Office of Scientific Integrity Review, March 1989-December 1990.* Washington, D.C.: Author.

World Medical Association. 1990. "Declaration of Helsinki." *Bulletin of the Pan American Health Organization* 24(4): 606–609.

SEXISM

• • •

Sexism is the failure to give equal weight to women's interests. It is the antithesis of feminism, a moral, political, and social movement that seeks justice for women. Sexism is important because it undermines the welfare of one-half of the human population and is a major source of women's oppression.

Each of these terms—interests, justice, welfare, oppression—is theory-laden, suggesting a particular way of understanding the origins and remedies for wrongful sex- and gender-based distinctions. This entry is eclectic but relies primarily on the liberal language of rights and interests.

Women have two kinds of rights, the ones shared with men by virtue of their common humanity, and the ones required by virtue of their differences from men. Sexism fails to recognize these rights by assuming, on the basis of inadequate evidence, that there are morally relevant differences between women and men, or by overlooking morally relevant differences that call for different treatment.

Medical treatment of heart disease in women is an example of both kinds of sexism. On the one hand, ignoring contrary evidence, practitioners have assumed that heart disease is not a women's problem. On the other, they have refused to take seriously the possibility that heart disease might manifest itself differently in women than in men. Consequently, heart disease in women is underdiagnosed, treatments are geared toward men's needs, and women needlessly suffer and die more often than men.

Although sexism can be a result of inattention, or a deliberate policy of subordinating women's interests to those of men or children, it may also result from historically embedded social institutions that naturalize assumptions about gender. A key assumption is that biology determines women's nature, whereas men construct themselves. Woman's inherent function is to nurture children and men. Women therefore do not elicit the respect due to rational persons with legitimate life-plans of their own; their interests are relatively unimportant, and may be subordinated to others with which they come in conflict. The consequences range from abortion, infanticide, and starvation for female Indian children, to more subtle but still significant losses for Western women. Among these are lack of representation in positions of public power and prestige, longer hours of work for less pay, lack of sexual or reproductive freedom, less advanced healthcare, and less leisure, pleasure, and financial and physical security.

No thoughtful person wants to be seen as sexist. But because of widespread negativism about feminism, many people believe that there is neutral territory between the two. However, where women's interests are affected there is either a (feminist) commitment to count them equally or there is a (sexist) discounting of those interests. Neutrality can exist where gender is not at issue or where it is difficult to determine whether sexism is at work.

Oppression, Discrimination, Sexism

Oppression is the systematic and unjust subordination of some people by others. Sexism is a major source of women's oppression. Oppression may be based on superior power, without any attempt at justification. However, it is usually predicated on the alleged inferiority of a class of people, such

as women, the poor, people of color, the elderly, homosexuals, or adherents of certain religions. In principle, recognizing the wrong of one kind of oppression implies recognizing the wrong of other types, but in practice these connections are often ignored.

Because many mainstream thinkers (consciously or unconsciously) accept sexist assumptions, they are unconvinced of women's oppression, and they doubt evidence alleged to support the claim that such oppression exists. Even when the facts (e.g., women's lesser wealth) are undisputed, they are attributed to the consequences of women's inferiority, their autonomous choices, or to social necessity.

Feminists respond by arguing that these defenses are mere rationalizations, and that there are systematic and interlocking patterns of sex and gender relationships that disadvantage women. Sexism leads to the high valuation of qualities associated with men but not women. Also, pervasive patterns of gender socialization affect women's capacities (such as strength or mathematical achievement) and mean that women's choices may not be as autonomous as they seem. Moreover, many of women's disadvantages are rooted in the sexist failure to recognize the special rights that need to be granted because of the differences between women and men. Social and political arrangements allegedly based on necessity are essential only for men's convenience. Relegating women to inferior positions is therefore unjustified, and constitutes oppression.

Discrimination is an effective tool for creating and maintaining oppression. Discrimination can be used descriptively or normatively. Descriptive discrimination among concepts and entities is essential for thought and language. Such distinctions are usually considered to reflect the world, and are thus *natural.* However, categories may depend on choices about what characteristics count for inclusion and so morally significant groupings may instead be constructed (e.g., race). Normatively, discrimination always implies wrongful treatment of members of a group. The constructed nature of some descriptive groupings may facilitate the creation of normative ones. Thus, for example, conceptualizing the class of potentially pregnant women may make it easier to discriminate against them in the workplace or in medical research.

Recognizing Sexism

Sometimes it can be difficult to determine whether a decision or policy is sexist or feminist. For example, selective abortion of female fetuses is often cited as a paradigm case of sexism. But different contexts can render the same act sexist or feminist. Aborting a female because of the belief that boys are superior to girls is sexist; aborting a female to prevent a girl's suffering can be feminist.

In addition, it is important to distinguish between legal and moral contexts. Because motivation is difficult to determine in legal contexts, sexism in law is most successfully rooted out by a focus on disparate impact. Moral investigation, however, can and must delve further into motivation and intention.

Is it sexist to abort female fetuses to ensure that there are both male and female children in a family? If "balance" is a pretext for ensuring the birth of a boy to secure the alleged social benefits only he can provide (e.g., continuation of the family name), then it promotes and maintains a sexist world. But what if the decision to abort is based on the reasonable belief that social pressures generally lead girls and boys to develop somewhat differently (no matter what the family environment), and that raising them is likely to be an equally desirable, but different, experience?

Baseline Assumptions

Evaluating whether assumptions that underlie decisions are sexist can be challenging. For example, it would be sexist to exclude women from drug trials because they are different from men in relevant ways, but not because they are alike in those ways. But which assumption is it reasonable to start with in the absence of knowledge? Assuming that the sexes are alike could be just another instance of taking males as the norm, without paying attention to ways that females might be different. Assuming they are different could be just another instance of the belief that females have more in common with the females of other species than with male humans. A similar quandary arises for race.

Inquiry suggests that women are harmed by their exclusion from clinical trials because such exclusion can result in poorer healthcare. Do cholesterol-lowering drugs or aspirin prevent heart disease in women? Nobody knows because the original research was done in men, and only at the very end of the twentieth century did the relevant studies begin for women.

Digging into the history and culture of medicine reinforces this conclusion. In the past, women were not admitted to most medical schools because they were considered fit only for nursing or midwifery. Harvard University began accepting women only in 1945, when World War II had reduced the number of male applicants; women could not exceed 6 percent of each class until the 1970s. Sue Rosser and Eileen Nechas and Denise Foley were pioneers in documenting obstacles facing women in medicine in the twentieth century. Adriane Fugh-Berman describes a dispiriting range of problems she encountered at a leading medical school. Among them were medical disinterest in women's bodies (breasts were discarded on the first day of anatomy class) and welfare (students were taught that women can have a satisfactory sex life without orgasms). Some professors did not see women students as equals and refused to teach them certain procedures or topics (sexually transmitted diseases). Male students compounded the hostile environment by harassing and threatening with rape the members of a women's study group. A survey of recent literature on problems women encounter in medicine shows that there is still much room for progress.

In 2003 women still experience substantial sexism as consumers of healthcare, as the aforementioned example of heart disease shows. Stereotypes about women's nature (irrational, focused on reproduction) may continue to lead healthcare researchers and providers to sometimes dismiss what women say about their symptoms (e.g., in women with AIDS, or menstrual pain). It may also encourage the development of procedures that put women disproportionately at risk in what should be joint ventures with men (contraception, infertility treatment). More generally, until the end of the twentieth century, researchers emphasized conditions that affect men, ignoring such complaints as dysmenorrhea, incontinence in the elderly, and nutrition in postmenopausal women. At the same time, medicine has also tended to inappropriately medicalize the bodily experiences connected with reproduction: menstruation, pregnancy, childbirth, and menopause. Medicine has also promoted and reinforced the assumption that only women —not men or society at large—are responsible for babies's health.

Is there any evidence to suggest that women's exclusion from research (and the failure to analyze studies they did participate in by sex) is a result of concern for women? No. It appears that women have been excluded either for researchers's convenience or due to concern about harm to possible offspring (or concern about liability for such harm). Men have been assumed to lack hormonal cycles that would confound study results; women however, engender the opposite assumption. But men appear to have their own hormonal cycles, and if women's cycles affect outcomes, being excluded harms the latter. Also, some researchers have had easier access to male populations (the military, prisons). But ease of access does not justify ignorance about the medical care of women. Excluding women because of possible pregnancy accepts the stereotypes that women are ignorant about their bodies, and careless about the welfare of fetuses; the exclusion of women also ignores the evidence that sperm are affected by exposure to toxins. Non-sexist drug trials would thus regard women and men as equally likely to risk harm to offspring. Both would therefore need to be warned against reproduction, and both sexes ought to be trusted to heed those warnings to the same degree. Abandoning women for such sexist reasons is especially unjust when research is publicly funded. It follows that women should be included in experimentation, and that results should be analyzed by sex. Excluding women from health studies could be seen as a feminist position only when there are excellent reasons for believing that to include women would create more harm than good for women as a class.

In conclusion, the concept of sexism points to the ways that women's interests are systematically discounted in comparison with those of men. Sexism is a kind of discrimination that oppresses women as a class. Groundless stereotyped assumptions about women and the unjust failure to take seriously both the ways that women resemble men and the ways that the two sexes differ play a central role in sexism. Women have been seriously harmed by sexism in medicine, and only in the last decades of the twentieth century have the women's health movement and practitioners in the field of women's health begun to rectify this wrong. Bioethics, which, among other tasks, critiques the healthcare system, was itself quite blind to sexism in healthcare until the 1990s; sexism in bioethics remains a serious problem, as overtly feminist bioethics literature is marginal.

LAURA PURDY

SEE ALSO: *Abuse, Interpersonal: Abuse between Domestic Partners; Access to Healthcare; Circumcision, Female Circumcision; Feminism; Fertility Control; Healthcare Delivery; Healthcare Resources, Allocation of; Maternal-Fetal Relationship; Medical Ethics, History of South and East Asia: China, Contemporary China; Medicine, Profession of; Mental Illness: Conceptions of Mental Illness; Metaphor and Analogy; Moral Status; Nursing, Profession of; Paternalism; Population Policies; Professional-Patient Relationship; Race and Racism; Reproductive Technologies; Research Methodology; Research Policy; Sexual Ethics; Sexual Ethics and Professional Standards; Women as Health Professionals; Women, Historical and Cross-Cultural Perspectives*

BIBLIOGRAPHY

Bryson, Valerie. 1992. *Feminist Political Theory: An Introduction.* New York: Paragon House.

Card, Claudia. 1991. *Feminist Ethics.* Lawrence: University Press of Kansas.

Daniels, Cynthia. 1999. "Fathers, Mothers, and Fetal Harm: Rethinking Gender Difference and Reproductive Responsibility." In *Fetal Subjects, Feminist Positions,* ed. Lynn M. Morgan and Meredith W. Michaels. Philadelphia: University of Pennsylvania Press.

Faludi, Susan. 1991. *Backlash: The Undeclared War Against American Women.* New York: Crown.

Frye, Marilyn. 1983. *The Politics of Reality: Essays in Feminist Theory.* Trumansburg, NY: The Crossing Press.

Fugh-Berman, Adriane. "Tales Out of Medical School." *The Nation.* January 20, 1992.

Kramerae, Cheris, and Spender, Dale, eds. 1992. *The Knowledge Explosion: Generations of Feminist Scholarship.* New York: Columbia Teachers Press.

Levin, Michael E. 1987. *Feminism and Freedom.* New Brunswick, NJ: Transaction Books.

Mill, John Stuart. 1869. *The Subjection of Women.* London: Longmans, Green, Reader, and Dyer.

Millett, Kate. 1970. *Sexual Politics.* Garden City, NY: Doubleday.

Morgan, Robin, ed. 1984. *Sisterhood Is Global.* New York: Anchor Books.

Nechas, Eileen, and Foley, Denise. 1994. *Unequal Treatment: What You Don't Know about How Women are Mistreated by the Medical Community.* New York: Simon and Schuster.

Okin, Susan Moller. 1989. *Justice, Gender and the Family.* New York: Basic Books.

Rhode, Deborah L. 1997. *Speaking of Sex: The Denial of Gender Inequality.* Cambridge, MA: Harvard University Press.

Rosser, Sue V. 1994. *Women's Health—Missing from U.S. Medicine.* Bloomington: Indiana University Press.

Valian, Virginia. 1998 *Why So Slow? The Advancement of Women.* Cambridge, MA: MIT Press.

SEXUAL BEHAVIOR, SOCIAL CONTROL OF

• • •

The twentieth century witnessed an explosion of knowledge about the physiology, psychology, and sociology of human sexuality, thanks to the revolution in public acceptability of discourse about sexual conduct and the freeing of scholarly interest that followed the trailblazing works published in the late Victorian era by Richard von Krafft–Ebing (1939 [1886]), Havelock Ellis (1901), and Sigmund Freud (1955a [1895], 1955b [1905]). However, controversy still rages over the basic issue of how sexual behavior is molded, encouraged, and discouraged by social customs and practices. Are males naturally more aggressive in seeking sexual contact than females, or is this a product of social patriarchy? Is homosexuality caused primarily by biological factors, or is it largely caused by social experiences during formative stages of the child's development? Is cultural permissiveness responsible for the dramatic increase in reports of sexual harassment and abuse, or are changing mores encouraging victims to name parents, doctors, and priests who were in the past able to hide their misconduct under a cloak of respectability?

The answers to these questions are not only empirical, they are also ethical and political. Allegedly scientific beliefs about the *naturalness* of certain sexual acts often reflect unacknowledged cultural biases, and thoughts and theories affect the behavior they label, characterize, and implicitly valorize or demean. As feminists and historians such as Michel Foucault (1990) have pointed out, the neutral scientific language of medicine is no guarantor of the moral innocuousness of theories about gender and sexual behavior; to the contrary, claims of scientific objectivity about these topics are apt to be all the more dangerous morally for pretending to be value-free.

Theories of sexual behavior cannot avoid assumptions about power and domination that too frequently perpetuate injustices. Thus, sexologist Alfred Kinsey's claim that males are naturally more aggressive in initiating sex (Kinsey, Pomeroy, and Martin) is not merely the objective scientific statement it purports to be, but a statement that supports the power of men over women in society. Anyone who is concerned about power and justice needs continually to scrutinize and critique so-called scientific claims about human sexuality by attending to how they perpetuate social stereotypes that are not universal and, by assigning more value to the experiences of certain people (e.g., white heterosexual males), help to empower some and disempower others. One would expect social ethicists to be sensitized to these issues, but the most influential recent theorists of justice (e.g., John Rawls, Ronald Dworkin, Robert Nozick, Michael Walzer) scarcely even mention gender justice, much less consider sexual roles a central matter for ethical scrutiny (see Susan Okin's 1989 work). One reason for this neglect is the traditional public/private dichotomy that assigns sexual behavior to a private arena outside the concerns of the social theorist. Employment of this dichotomy in the past to keep cases of domestic rape and child abuse out of American courts, on the grounds that they occur within a zone of privacy protected from public scrutiny, shows that it is scarcely an ethically neutral matter for a social scientist to point out how individuals' sexual lives are influenced by a social ethos that makes such distinctions.

Essentialism and Constructionism

Theories about human sexual behavior in its social context range along a continuum stretching from essentialism (or

naturalism) on the one hand to social construction theory on the other.

Essentialism attributes certain sexual and gender behaviors to the unchanging nature of the human species. According to this perspective, what is natural is *good*; what is social is *artificial* and tends to be *bad* insofar as it inhibits realization of the proper natural end of sexual conduct, be it erotic pleasure or procreation. Thomistic natural-law theory is explicitly essentialist in identifying procreation as the natural end of human sexuality, but modern sexologists assume essentialism in contending that a wide variety of pleasurable erotic acts are no less natural than heterosexual intercourse. Kinsey, for example, uses an essentialist argument when he draws on the sexual behavior of other mammals, "primitive" cultures, and human physiological capacities to contend that masturbation and homosexual acts are natural expressions of sexuality and, hence, irrationally condemned and punished by society. Kinsey also employs essentialist arguments, citing mammalian data, in support of such dubious contentions as that male extramarital coitus is more natural than female extramarital coitus (Kinsey, Pomeroy, Martin et al.; Irvine). American sexologists William Masters and Virginia Johnson assume essentialism in viewing sex exclusively in terms of physiological responses unencumbered by social and psychological factors. It is not an issue for Masters and Johnson that the socialization of Western women has discouraged female sexuality; rather the woman's naturally superior sexual responsiveness to the male, as evidenced by her capacity for multiple orgasms, is what counts for them (Irvine). What is missing in the sexologist's essentialist view of culture as an impediment is any acknowledgement of the multiple ways cultures give meaning to sexual behaviors and structure sexual and gender relationships beyond physiological responses.

According to social constructionists, sexual behavior and gender roles are products of a specific history, culture, and set of social institutions. French social scientist Émile Durkheim succinctly expressed the constructionist emphasis on the primacy of culture over biology when he argued, at the end of the nineteenth century, that if an adolescent did not have cultural concepts to identify sexual desires, he or she might feel a vague urge but not know what it was, much less how to act on it (Durkheim; Wallwork, 1972, 1984). A second main feature of the social constructionist approach involves situating sexual role behavior within the prevailing economic and political system, with its male-dominated hierarchies of status and power. The constructionist perspective encourages exploration of the ways in which widespread cultural beliefs about sexual behavior (and the research projects they inspire) serve to perpetuate a patriarchal vision of human nature, social institutions, gender, and sex roles. Constructionists note with concern that the focus in research has more often than not been on the male sexual experience; Masters and Johnson's research, for example, limits sexuality to genitally-oriented orgasm (Masters and Johnson). Feminist critics Alice Rossi (1973) and Leonore Tiefer (1978) complain that research focusing on genital physiology as the standard of sexual involvement evidences a "phallic fallacy" that implicitly devalues the pregenital or nongenital sexual experiences of women, such as the emotionally intense erotic feelings associated with looking at the beloved or anticipating a reunion with him or her.

The obvious strength of social constructionist theory is that it is able to account for the considerable diversity of sexual behavior and the meanings associated with such behavior cross-culturally, and to link these meanings to other role relationships. The power of society to mold human sexuality is evident in how nonerotic body parts—for example, crushed feet among the Chinese of a former era, the naked foot and even shoes in medieval Europe, and hair—have been eroticized by different peoples at different times (Stoller). The power of social custom is also obvious when one contrasts the negative conception of homosexuality in the Judeo-Christian West with its positive evaluation among Melanesian societies and certain African tribes. Among the Sambia in the New Guinea highlands, boys from prepuberty to their mid-teens are expected to engage in oral-genital sexuality with the older teenage males with whom they live as a prerequisite to becoming heterosexual adult males (Herdt and Stoller). Because Sambians believe semen is essential for males to grow and mature physically, the ingestion of semen is deemed essential to becoming an adult heterosexual male and to fathering children.

Even within the same society, there are fads and fashions of sexual behavior. For instance, since the 1960s there has been a dramatic increase in oral-genital behavior in the United States (Janus and Janus; Walsh). Among contemporary males in the West, premature ejaculation is defined as a dysfunction for which medical treatment is often sought; but in many developing countries males are expected to reach orgasms quickly (in fifteen to twenty seconds in the East Bay society in Melanesia, for example) and those who take a "long time" are ridiculed (Reiss).

But it would be a mistake to assume from the considerable evidence for the importance of the elaborate cultural ideas, stimulants, and norms that surround the biologically limited range of sexual behaviors of which the human body is capable that social constructionists are winning the battle with essentialists. In fact, the nature–nurture pendulum, which swung back and forth several times in the twentieth century, was swinging back again toward the nature pole as the century ended. During the 1980s, 1990s, and 2000s, biological explanations have been on the ascendancy in many scientific circles. Sociobiologists challenge the constructionist assumption that most sexual behavior is determined by culture, arguing instead that certain basic mammalian and primate traits that lie beneath the social surface determine the configuration of human sexual behavior (Wilson). At the same time, the biologizing of psychology is well underway, as physiological models and research strategies are held to offer the best route to understanding traditional subjects of psychological inquiry such as mental illness and sexual orientation.

Interactionist Model

The most plausible position on the essentialism-constructionism debate would appear to be that the biological factors in sexual desire, such as genes and hormones, do not act alone but instead interact with environmental factors, such as visual or auditory erotic stimuli, the significance of which depends in turn upon the individual's subjective erotic sensitivities, identities, fantasies, cognitive schemata, and behavioral patterns. These subjective factors, which lead some people to be excited by depictions of sadomasochistic acts and others not, are themselves influenced by the way a unique individual with certain inherited strengths and vulnerabilities interacts with significant others and specific sociocultural environments during the various psychosexual, ego-social, and cognitive stages of development. Biological factors certainly play a role; for example, testosterone appears to influence the intensity of sexual desire. But biological factors do not invariably cause sexual motives or behavior, for testosterone is itself highly responsive to environmental stimuli. Nurture, psychological development, subjective fantasies and beliefs, erotic stimuli, moral and aesthetic standards, social roles and expectations, and ego strengths and weaknesses all mold the range of the individual's sexual potentialities in certain directions rather than others. This molding is clear from the inability of biologists and sociobiologists, who study determinants that have operated within the species for thousands of years, to explain changes in sexual customs within a single generation or variations in sexual customs that occur in the same gender cross-culturally. Unfortunately, researchers have not yet developed a theoretical model sufficiently complex and nuanced to integrate and assign proper weight to all the multiple factors, including the individual's self-control, that influence human sexual behavior. The sociological point of view adopted here, which falls at the constructivist end of the essentialism-constructionism continuum, remains one among several plausible selective perspectives on social control of sexual behavior. Others are history, anthropology, ethnography, psychoanalysis, and social psychology.

Social Control Requirements

Sexual behavior, defined broadly as any action or reaction involving erotic arousal or genital responses, is viewed by most sociologists as sufficiently problematic to require some degree of social control. One explanation often proffered for this social-control requirement, whether as controlled permission or regulated prohibition, is that at some point in the distant past human beings lost the preformed automatic sexual instincts of the lower animals—that is, the sexual control that is in nature—and came to depend upon culture and social institutions to guide the varied reproductive and nonreproductive behaviors that are considered sexual. The loss of preformed instinctual patterns of sexual behavior, by freeing human beings from the comparatively rigid behavior patterns of other animals, helped to create the great adaptability of the human species to its changing environment. It also meant, with the human female's loss of the periodic estrus of other mammals, that the human female and male were potentially capable of sex at any time. Sexual motives came to pervade virtually all aspects of human life in a way that is uniquely characteristic of the species. At the same time, because the sexual drive differs from instinctual needs like respiration, thirst, and hunger, which must be gratified for the individual organism's survival, sexual desire was modified by subtle psychological and social influences.

Social control of sexual behavior has been necessitated in all social units—from the family to the clan, tribe, local community, and state—in part by the serious threats to social stability and maintenance of group life over time created by the potential for sex on demand all the year round. One such threat is incest, which is inimical to the group's evolutionary survival as well as to the psychological well-being and functioning of those who might be victimized by it. Another serious social consequence of sex on demand is the likelihood of children, which every society has a stake in limiting, assigning to families peacefully, and raising, educating, and training to be law-abiding, productive contributors. Still another consequence of sexual behavior that has required its social control is its potential for either reinforcing or disrupting existing roles and status hierarchies by creating strong new social bonds. Any rape or seduction of young girls or boys, or any adulterous relation, is liable to spark violence or some other disruption of the existing social order.

Societies attempt to handle another crucial consequence of sexual liaisons—the transmission of family and communal property, prestige, and power—by means of legalized sexual union in marriage and the begetting of *legitimate children*. Any dramatic increase in the number of illegitimate children and abandoned wives strains the system of distributing limited economic resources, shifting some of the burden from the family onto the rest of the community. The perpetuation of a society's religious ideals, moral norms, and laws is also intertwined with the monitoring of sexual conduct, since the way sexual conduct is controlled is often paradigmatic of the way the society expects individuals to pursue other moral and spiritual goals (Stone). The well-known sexual asceticism of the Puritan, for instance, was only one part of a lifestyle that affected every aspect of the Puritan's life, just as the idealization of female virginity affects every aspect of the life of the traditional Southern Italian villager (Parsons).

IDEALS AND TABOOS. Social control of sexual behavior is exercised most obviously by widely shared, explicit ideals of sexual behavior that form the basis for taboos against inappropriate conduct. Taboos are backed by social punishments ranging from mild disapproval and loss of status to ostracism, imprisonment, and death. Within Judaism, Christianity, and Islam, the standard-of-standards has been heterosexual intercourse in the context of marriage. Accordingly, masturbation, homosexuality, and extramarital sexuality have been condemned and often severely punished. Among the Greeks during the classical period, pederasty was idealized as the purest form of love, but it was also hedged about by rigid taboos. The accepted sexual relationship was limited to an older free man and a pubescent free boy. Oral and anal intercourse were unacceptable, and if a boy allowed himself to be penetrated anally, he lost his rights to citizenship. For the Greek male, what was important was not whether one's partner was male or female, but whether one was dominant or submissive (Foucault).

SOCIAL ROLES. In addition to the values and norms shared throughout a culture, social control is also maintained by the basic institutions of society, especially the family, religion, schools, medicine, and law. An institution is defined sociologically as a stable cluster of values, norms, statuses, and roles that develop around a basic need of society. An important function of an institution is to socialize developing individuals through inculcation of social roles, which are social actions that take account of social expectations. A person's role is not simply what he or she habitually does (for this may not be socially significant), nor even what he or she is expected to do, if an expectation is only what one might predict from past actions. The role is what is expected of him or her, in the sense of what is approved or required, by, say, fashion, tradition, charismatic authority, or standards of rationality.

Gender roles, which indicate how males and females are expected to behave, significantly influence sexual behavior. In Western culture, the expectation has been that the woman is more passive and receptive, and more attuned to emotional connections, than the male, who is expected to be more aggressive, autonomous, and focused on power. Such gender roles have an effect on sexual conduct, independent of explicit sexual standards. For example, rape is strongly disapproved of in contemporary culture, yet date rape is disturbingly frequent, in part because males are socialized to dominate women in many social situations involving power. Hence, if a male's charm and powers of psychological persuasion fail in a sexual situation, coercion remains as a last resort. Here, as in most sexual acts, erotic desire is only one of several motivations that enter into the behavior. In addition, the need to maintain the male-dominant role identity and the propensity for males in Western societies to turn anger at frustration into aggression and violence are equally powerful motives.

Recently, sociologists have applied *script theory* to sexual behavior in order to account for the more specific patterns that enable participants to make reasonably good guesses about the sequence of events probable in an otherwise loosely structured social situation (Gagnon and Simon; Laumann, Gagnon, Michael, et al.; McKinney and Sprecher). Scripts are mental schemas that enable participants to jointly structure the interaction so that uncertainty is systematically reduced and cooperation enhanced. Sexual scripts enable participants to decode novel situations by reading the meaning of certain actions and to organize the situation into sequences of specifically sexual interactions (e.g., nonverbal courtship behaviors signaling availability, like smiling, gazing, hair flipping, the "opening line," leaning close, and the proverbial invitation to see one's etchings). However, research on conflicts between the sexes in dating and marriage also shows that scripting is far from perfect, that the sexes often miscue each other or are dissatisfied in predictable ways—say, with the male's excessive sexual demands or emotional constriction, or the woman's unresponsiveness or moodiness.

HEALTH CONCERNS. Empirical beliefs—especially medically sanctioned ones—about the consequences of various sexual practices on the individual's health also play a significant role in the social control of sexual behavior. In classical Greece, for example, physicians recommended sexual moderation to prevent the excessive loss of life force in the too-frequent ejaculation of semen. In ancient China, somewhat similar beliefs about the consequences of excessive semen loss led to the cultivation of special techniques of intercourse without ejaculation in order to conserve the *yang* (the positive, light, masculine principle whose interaction with *yin*—the negative, dark, feminine principle—was believed to influence the destiny of creatures and things). And, of course, Western doctors have for centuries warned that masturbation would bring about some dreaded disease, disfigurement, or insanity. By the turn of the twenty-first century, fear of AIDS had dramatically changed sexual behavior, primarily by altering beliefs about the risks of unprotected sexual intercourse (Laumann, et al.). Viagra has altered time-honored myths about impotence, while offering hope for continuing sexual relations into old age. It is one of Foucault's main contentions that medical beliefs, precisely because they are so important to patients, provide physicians with power that historically often has been used to dominate and control unjustly (Foucault).

It is easy to be impressed by the ideals, moral rules, and prudential teachings that are set forth so impressively in explicit doctrine by leading social authorities. But these action guides are not always reinforced by other cultures or even by other institutions in the same cultural context. Complex societies are not systematic cultural ensembles, despite the beliefs of sociological functionalists like Émile Durkheim and Talcott Parsons. Illicit sexual cultures—like red-light districts or the houses of prostitution that flourished in medieval Europe (Ariès and Bejin)—exist side by side with licit sexual cultures, counterbalancing and correcting excessive asceticism, and on some points canceling out the influence of the licit culture. A complex interrelationship often exists between these cultures, so there is often plenty of room for compromises and loopholes. Moreover, the different social-status groups and classes of the same society usually have different sexual cultures. For example, libertine elites concentrated around courts (as in ancient Egypt, classical Greece and Rome, imperial China, India, and Japan) have surrounded themselves with a rich panoply of erotic art, pornographic literature, artificial physical stimuli, toys, and partners not encouraged among lower social ranks (Stone). Consider, too, how Roman Catholic bishops have tolerated the sexual abuse of children and adolescents by priests in flagrant violation of the church's explicit moral teachings (see, for example, the work of the *Boston Globe* Investigative Staff).

Control and Permissiveness

The so-called sexual revolution that occurred in the post–World War II epoch is sometimes viewed—erroneously—as releasing the individual from the constraining pressures of social control. But the new permissiveness is more accurately perceived as substituting new and, in some instances, somewhat different social standards, controls, and permissions for older ones. The most important contemporary cultural standards focus less on the legitimation of sex by marriage and more on the goods of sensual pleasure, intimacy, the autonomy of the parties (violated in the case of rape and harassment), and the basic equality of partners. Some salient features of the sexual revolution are the greater explicit public acknowledgment of sexuality (for example, in films, advertisements, soap operas, talk shows, and advice columns); the availability of cheap and reliable contraception, particularly birth control pills, which have for the first time in history released women from the fear of unwanted pregnancies; the increased availability of erotic stimulants (e.g., adult magazines, pornographic videos, explicit Internet sites); the rise of feminism and correlative decline in social inequality between the sexes; the increased acceptance or tolerance of sexual behaviors that were formerly disapproved, like masturbation, homosexuality, extramarital sexual affairs, and oral-genital sex; and the increase in teenage sexual conduct and at younger ages (Michael, Gagnon, Laumann, et al.; Laumann and Michael). Around the turn of the twenty-first century, there also emerged a recreational ideology, which holds that the purpose of sexual activity is not procreation or even mutual affection, but physical pleasure.

Although these changes reflect a certain permissiveness, there is evidence that men and women today have higher expectations, demands, and worries about their sexual performance (McKinney and Sprecher; Janus and Janus). The liberating views of sexologists have brought in their train new demands for mutual orgasm and standards of erotic performance that not all couples are capable of realizing at all times. Anger about date rape on university campuses and sexual harassment in the workplace has given rise in the United States to explicit policies, sometimes accompanied by detailed lists of *do's* and *don'ts,* designed to make sure there is willing and verbal consent to each individual sexual act, for example, kissing, fondling of breasts, touching of genitals, intercourse. New policies, grievance procedures, and punishments are proliferating to prevent and punish sexual harassment and rape (Gross). Some professional ethics codes (for example, the new Principles and Standards of the American Psychoanalytic Association) prohibit sexual relations of any sort between professionals and clients, even in situations of mutual consent years after the professional relationship has ended, on the grounds that a misuse of professional authority is likely to have coerced the subordinate in the relationship (Dewald and Clark).

The permissiveness associated with the sexual revolution also coexists with the continuation of strong cultural constraints on frank interpersonal communication about sexual behavior that has disturbing implications for preventing unwanted pregnancies and venereal diseases and for containment of the AIDS epidemic. Western society has a long history of prudishness about sexual topics that stretches back several millennia into the biblical period, when writers of the Hebrew Bible and Christian New Testament used euphemisms like "flesh," "loin," "thigh," "side," and "feet" (for penis), "lewdness" (for female genitals), and "one flesh" (for intercourse) in lieu of explicit sexual terms (Baab). Despite the new sexual permissiveness, and research showing that, for example, 9 percent of American school children have initiated sexual intercourse before age thirteen, that 53.1 percent of students in grades nine through twelve have had sexual intercourse, and that 17.8 percent of high school students have had sexual intercourse with four or more sexual partners (Centers for Disease Control), parents continue to find it difficult to talk with their children in a knowledgeable way about sexual behavior. In a 1987 national survey, 69 percent of adult Americans viewed premarital coitus as "always wrong" for fourteen- to sixteen-year-olds (Davis and Smith). Research suggests that many adolescents perceive their parents as not very well informed about sex and as negative, rigid, and conservative in their attitudes toward sexuality (Metts and Cupach). Although adolescents tell researchers they would like to learn more about sex from their parents, their perceptions as well as the reported attitudes of many parents discourage open communication.

The difficulty parents have communicating information about sex is also found among many professionals charged with conveying information about sex to children, such as schoolteachers, clergy, and physicians. Research shows that adolescents learn most of their information about sexuality, such as petting and sexual intercourse, from same-sex peers, who are often ill-informed about contraception or the prevention of sexually transmitted diseases. However, some studies indicate that some sex education programs are able to convey factual information about anatomical and physiological aspects of sexuality, and to influence understanding of the risks of sexual behaviors (Orbuch; Metts and Cupach). Unfortunately, most teenagers remain unprepared for their first sexual encounters. Much remains to be done in communicating information about how to avoid unwanted pregnancies and infection by the human immunodeficiency virus (HIV) that causes AIDS.

Constraints on open discussion of sexual desires and practices is one factor in the high rates of unwanted sexual contact. Research shows that young men remain reluctant to declare their desire for sexual intercourse to a new date, while young women are less than open about their reluctance. Discussion of contraceptive measures is apparently still difficult for couples who have not had coitus, despite the threat of AIDS (Reiss). The culture of sexual permissiveness is thus riddled with constraints on forthright discussion of choosing among alternative sexual options. To help counter these constraints, healthcare professions need improved educational programs on human sexuality, more training in public health, and opportunities to cultivate skills of communicating with patients as knowledgeable allies and responsible agents, not as passive recipients of authoritative information and advice.

A peculiar problem with many attempts to control sexual behavior is that the constraints and repressions designed to foster licit or safe sex often themselves contribute to the flourishing of illicit or unsafe sexual behavior, which becomes all the more alluring, exciting, and frequent precisely because it is prohibited. The firmest social controls of sexual behavior appear to be those that acknowledge the unique value of sexual desires, fantasies, and actions in human life in a spirit of tolerance toward nonharmful illicit wishes and behaviors, even as actual conduct is directed toward goals that are compatible with the best interests of the individuals involved and the groups of which they are a part.

ERNEST WALLWORK (1995)
REVISED BY AUTHOR

SEE ALSO: *Coercion; Confidentiality; Epidemics; Homosexuality; Sexual Ethics; Sexual Ethics and Professional Standards; Sexual Identity; Sexuality, Legal Approaches to; Public Health Law*

BIBLIOGRAPHY

Ariès, Philippe, and Bejin, André, eds. 1985. *Western Sexuality: Practice and Precept in Past and Present Times.* Oxford: Basil Blackwell.

Baab, Otto J. 1962. "Sex, Sexual Behavior." In *The Interpreter's Dictionary of the Bible.* vol. 4, ed. George Arthur Buttrick. New York: Abingdon.

Bezemer, Willeke; Cohen-Kettenis, Peggy; Slob, Koos; and Son-Schoones, Nel Van, eds. 1992. *Sex Matters: Proceedings of the Xth World Congress of Sexology.* Amsterdam: Excerpta Medica.

Boston Globe Investigate Staff. 2002. *Betrayal: The Crisis in the Catholic Church.* Boston: Little, Brown and Company.

Boswell, John. 1980. *Christianity, Social Tolerance, and Homosexuality: Gay People in Western Europe from the Beginning of the Christian Era to the Fourteenth Century.* Chicago: University of Chicago Press.

Centers for Disease Control. 1996. "Youth Risk Behavior Surveillance—United States, 1995." *MMWR* 40 (No. SS-4), 1–86.

Davis, James A., and Smith, Tom W. 1987. *General Social Surveys, 1972–1987: Cumulative Codebook.* Chicago: National Opinion Research Center.

Dewald, Paul A., and Clark, Rita W. 2001. *Ethics Case Book of the American Psychoanalytic Association.* New York: The American Psychoanalytic Association.

Durkheim, Émile. 1893 (reprint 1933). *Emile Durkheim on the Division of Labor in Society,* tr. and ed. George Simpson. New York: Macmillan.

Ellis, H. Havelock. 1901. *Studies in the Psychology of Sex.* 7 vols. Philadelphia: F. A. Davis.

Foucault, Michel. 1990. *The History of Sexuality,* tr. Robert Hurley. New York: Vintage Books.

Freud, Sigmund. 1895 (reprint 1955a). *Studies on Hysteria.* Vol. 2 of *The Standard Edition of the Complete Psychological Works of Sigmund Freud,* tr. James Strachey. London: Hogarth.

Freud, Sigmund. 1905 (reprint 1955b). "Three Essays on the Theory of Sexuality." In *The Standard Edition of the Complete Psychological Works of Sigmund Freud.* Vol. 7, tr. James Strachey. London: Hogarth.

Gagnon, John H., and Simon, William. 1973. *Sexual Conduct: The Social Sources of Human Sexuality.* Chicago: Aldine de Gruyter, Inc.

Gross, Jane. 1993. "Combating Rape on Campus in a Class on Sexual Consent." *New York Times* September 25: A1, A9.

Hayes, Cheryl D., ed. 1987. *Risking the Future: Adolescent Sexuality, Pregnancy and Childbearing.* Washington, D.C.: National Academy Press.

Herdt, Gilbert H. 1981. *Guardians of the Flutes: Idioms of Masculinity.* New York: McGraw-Hill.

Herdt, Gilbert H., and Stoller, Robert J. 1990. *Intimate Communications.* New York: Columbia University Press.

Irvine, Janice M. 1990. *Disorders of Desire: Sex and Gender in Modern American Sexology.* Philadelphia: Temple University Press.

Janus, Samuel S., and Janus, Cynthia L. 1993. *The Janus Report on Sexual Behavior.* New York: Wiley.

Kann, Laura; Anderson, John E.; Holtzman, Deborah; et al. 1991. "HIV-Related Knowledge, Beliefs, and Behaviors Among High School Students in the United States: Results from a National Survey." *Journal of School Health* 61(9): 397–401.

Kinsey, Alfred Charles; Pomeroy, Wardell B.; and Martin, Clyde E. 1948. *Sexual Behavior in the Human Male.* Philadelphia: W. B. Saunders.

Kinsey, Alfred Charles; Pomeroy, Wardell B.; Martin, Clyde E.; and Gebhard, Paul H. 1953. *Sexual Behavior in the Human Female.* New York: Pocket Books.

Klassen, Albert D.; Williams, Colin J.; and Levitt, Eugene E.; eds. 1989. *Sex and Morality in the U.S.: An Empirical Enquiry Under the Auspices of the Kinsey Institute.* Middetown, CT: Wesleyan University Press.

Krafft-Ebing, Richard von. 1886 (reprint 1939). *Psychopathia Sexualis: A Medico-Forensic Study.* New York: Pioneer.

Laumann, Edward O.; Gagnon, John H.; Michael, Robert T.; and Michael, Stuart. 1994. *The Social Organization of Sexuality: Sexual Practices in the United States.* Chicago: University of Chicago Press.

Laumann, Edward O., and Michael, Robert T. 2000. *Sex, Love, and Health in America: Private Choices and Public Policies.* Chicago: University of Chicago Press.

Masters, William H., and Johnson, Virginia. 1966. *Human Sexual Response.* New York: Little, Brown.

McKinney, Kathleen, and Sprecher, Susan, eds. 1989. *Human Sexuality: The Societal and Interpersonal Context.* Norwood, NJ: Ablex.

Metts, Sandra, and Cupach, William R. 1989. "The Role of Communication in Human Sexuality." In *Human Sexuality: The Societal and Interpersonal Context,* ed. Kathleen McKinney and Susan Sprecher. Norwood, NJ: Ablex.

Michael, Robert T.; Gagnon, John H.; Laumann, Edward O.; et al. 1994. *Sex in America: A Definitive Survey.* Boston: Little, Brown.

Okin, Susan Moller. 1989. *Justice, Gender, and the Family.* New York: Basic Books.

Orbuch, Teeri L. 1989. "Human Sexuality Education." In *Human Sexuality: The Societal and Interpersonal Context,* ed. Kathleen McKinney and Susan Sprecher. Norwood, NJ: Ablex.

Parsons, Anne. 1969. *Belief, Magic, and Anomie: Essays in Psychosocial Anthropology.* New York: Free Press.

Reiss, Ira L. 1989. "Society and Sexuality: A Sociological Theory." In *Human Sexuality: The Societal and Interpersonal Context,* ed. Kathleen McKinney and Susan Sprecher. Norwood, NJ: Ablex.

Rossi, Alice S. 1973. "Maternalism, Sexuality, and the New Feminism." In *Contemporary Sexual Behavior: Critical Issues in the 1970s,* ed. Joseph Zubin and John Money. Baltimore, MD: Johns Hopkins University Press.

Stoller, Robert J. 1991. *Porn: Myths for the Twentieth Century.* New Haven, CT: Yale University Press.

Stone, Lawrence. 1985. "The Strange History of Human Sexuality: Sex in the West." *New Republic* July 8: 25–37.

Tiefer, Leonore. 1978. "The Context and Consequences of Contemporary Sex Research: A Feminist Perspective." In *Sex and Behavior: Status and Prospectus,* ed. Thomas E. McGill, Donald A. Dewsbury, and Benjamin D. Sachs. New York: Plenum.

Wallwork, Ernest. 1972. *Durkheim: Morality and Milieu.* Cambridge, MA: Harvard University Press.

Wallwork, Ernest. 1984. "Religion and Social Structure in The Division of Labor." *American Anthropologist* 86(1): 43–64.

Wallwork, Ernest. 1992. *Psychoanalysis and Ethics.* New Haven, CT: Yale University Press.

Walsh, Robert H. 1989. "Premarital Sex Among Teenagers and Young Adults." In *Human Sexuality: The Societal and Interpersonal Context,* ed. Kathleen McKinney and Susan Sprecher. Norwood, NJ: Ablex.

Wilson, Edward Osborne. 1975. *Sociobiology: The New Synthesis.* Cambridge, MA: Harvard University Press.

SEXUAL ETHICS

• • •

Insofar as bioethics is concerned with human bodily health, it has an interest in the way health is influenced by and contributes to sexual functioning. There is a sense, then, in which bioethics includes sexual ethics, or at least some of the key questions of sexual ethics, such as the meaning of human sexuality and the causes and effects of sexual attitudes, orientations, and activities. Concepts of the human person—of desire and obligation, disease and dysfunction, even of justice and purity—can be found overlapping in various bioethical and sexual ethical theories. Like bioethics generally, sexual ethics considers standards for intervention in physical processes, rights of individuals to self-determination, ideals for human flourishing, and the importance of social context for the interpretation and regulation of sexual behavior. Bioethics specifically incorporates issues surrounding contraception and abortion, artificial reproduction, sexually transmitted diseases, sexual paraphilias, gendered roles and sexual conduct of the medical professionals, and sex research, counseling, and therapy. All of these issues are importantly shaped by moral traditions, so that health professionals frequently find themselves called upon to deal with questions of sexual ethics.

Historically, medicine has interacted with philosophy and religion in shaping and rationalizing the sexual ethical norms of a given culture. Medical opinion often simply reflects and conserves the accepted beliefs and mores of a society, but sometimes it is also a force for change. In either case, its influence can be powerful. For example, from the Hippocratic corpus in ancient Greece to the writings of the physician Galen in the second century C.E., medical recommendations regarding sexual discipline echoed and reinforced the ambivalence of Greek and Roman philosophers regarding human sexual activity. Galen's theories retained considerable power all the way into the European Renaissance. The interpretation of syphilis as a disease rather than a divine punishment came in the fifteenth century as the result of medical writings in response to a high incidence of the disease among the socially powerful. In nineteenth century western Europe and North America, medical writers were enormously influential in shaping norms regarding such matters as masturbation (physicians believed it would lead to insanity), homosexuality (newly identified with perversions that medicine must diagnose and treat), contraception (considered unhealthy because it fostered sexual excess and loss of physical power), and gender roles (promoted on the basis of medical assessments of women's capacity for sexual desire). Today sex counseling and therapy communicate, however implicitly, normative ethical assumptions. Indeed, so great has been the influence of the medical profession on moral attitudes toward sexual options that critics warn of the "tyranny of experts," referring not to moral philosophers or religious teachers but to scientists and physicians.

The history of sexual ethics provides a helpful perspective for understanding current ethical questions regarding human sexuality. This article focuses on Western philosophical, scientific-medical, and religious traditions of sexual ethics and on the contemporary issues that trouble the heirs of these traditions. A historical overview of sexual ethics is not without its difficulties, however, as critical studies have shown (Brown; Foucault, 1978; Fout; Plaskow).

First of all, while it is possible to find a recorded history of laws, codes, and other guides to moral action regarding sexual behavior, it is almost impossible to determine what real people actually believed and did in the distant past. Or at least the historical research has barely begun. Second, ethical theory regarding sex (e.g., what is to be valued, what goals are worth pursuing, what reasons justify certain sexual attitudes, activities, and relationships) is predominantly theory formulated by an elite group of men. Women's experiences, beliefs, and values are largely unrecorded and, until recently, have been almost wholly inaccessible. The same is true of men who do not belong to a dominant class. Third, what we do find through historical research is necessarily subject to interpretation. It makes a difference, for example, whether one is looking for historical evaluations of human sexual desire or historical silences about sexual abuse of women. Finally, if one takes seriously the social construction of gender and sexuality, it is not clear that any kind of coherent historical narrative is possible. All of these difficulties notwithstanding, it is possible to survey (with appropriate caution) a Western normative and theoretical history regarding sex and to gain from the richness of varying contemporary interpretations. Central strands of this history can be traced to classical Greek and Roman antiquity, Judaism, and early and later developments in Christianity.

Ancient Greece and Rome

GENERAL ATTITUDES AND PRACTICE. Ancient Greece and Rome shared a general acceptance of sex as a natural part of life. Both were permissive regarding the sexual behavior of men. In Athens, for example, the only clear proscriptions applicable to citizen-class men were in incest, bigamy, and adultery (insofar as it violated the property of another man). The focus of sexual concern in the two cultures was significantly different, however. For the Greeks, adult male love of adolescent boys occupied a great deal of public attention, whereas the Romans focused public concern on heterosexual marriage as the foundation of social life.

Marriage for both Greeks and Romans was monogamous. In Greece, however, no sexual ethic confined sex to marriage. Marriage as the expected pattern for citizen-class individuals was based not on the affective bond between husband and wife but on what were considered natural gender roles regarding procreation and service to the city. Male human nature was generally assumed to be bisexual, and the polyerotic needs of men were taken for granted. Concubinage, male and female prostitution, and the sexual use of slaves were commonly accepted. In practice, much of this was true in ancient Rome as well, even though ideals of marital fidelity became much more important. The development of marriage as a social institution was, however, considered a central achievement of Roman civilization. This included a growing appreciation of the importance of affective ties between wives and husbands.

Greece and Rome were male-dominated societies, and for citizens a gendered double standard prevailed in regard to sexual morality. Both Greek and Roman brides, but not bridegrooms, were expected to be virgins. In Greece, the only women who were given some equal status with men were a special class of artistically and educationally sophisticated prostitutes, the *hetaerae*. Generally women were considered intellectually inferior to men. In addition, Greek husbands and wives were unequal in age (wives were much younger) and in education. Wives had no public life, though they were given the power and responsibility of managing the home. In the Roman household, on the contrary, the husband retained power and could rule with an entirely free hand. Here the ideal of the *patria potestas* reached fulfillment. Mutual fidelity was much praised, but in fact absolute fidelity was required of wives while husbands could consort freely with slaves or prostitutes. Although by the first century C.E., women in Rome had achieved considerable economic and political freedom, they could not practice the sexual freedom traditionally granted to men.

Homosexuality was accepted in both Greek and Roman antiquity. Especially for the Greeks, however, it was less a matter of some men being sexually attracted only to men (or, more likely, boys) than a matter of men generally being attracted to beautiful individuals, whether male or female. Desire was of greater interest, as both possibility and problem, than its object; and desire was not essentially differentiated according to the gender of its object. Greek men were expected to marry, in order to produce an heir. Yet love and friendship, and sometimes sex, between men could be of a higher order than anything possible within marriage (for gender equality obtained between men, despite differences in age). Same-sex relations were not thereby wholly unproblematic, however, as cultural cautions against male passivity attested. Moreover, the ethos tended not to support a positive evaluation of sexual relationships between women. Lesbian relations were often judged negatively because they counted as adultery (since women belonged to their husbands) or because a cultural preoccupation with male sexual desire made sex between women appear unnatural.

In both Greece and Rome, abortion and infanticide were common. Concern about the need to limit population influenced Greek sexual practices at various times, whereas efforts to improve a low birthrate in imperial Rome led to legal incentives to marry and to procreate. Divorce was more readily available in ancient Greece than in Rome, but eventually both cultures provided for it and for the resulting economic needs of divorced women; in Greece, husbands continued to administer their former wives' dowries, while in Rome a woman took her dowry with her.

Scholars today tend to dispute the belief that the last years of the Roman Empire saw a great weakening of sexual norms, a sexual dissipation at the heart of a general moral decline. The favored historical reading is now the opposite: that general suspicion of sexuality grew, and normative restrictions of sexual activity increased. In part, this was the result of the gradual influence of philosophical theories that questioned the value of sexual activity and emphasized the dangers in its consequences.

GREEK AND ROMAN PHILOSOPHICAL APPRAISALS.
Michel Foucault's influential history of Graeco-Roman theory regarding sex identifies two problems that preoccupied philosophers: the natural force of sexual desire, with its consequent tendency to excess, and the power relations involved in the seemingly necessary active/passive roles in sexual activity (Foucault, 1986, 1988). The first problem contributed to the formulation of an ideal of self-mastery within an aesthetics of existence. Self-mastery could be achieved through a regimen that included diet, exercise, and various practices of self-discipline. The second problem yielded criteria for love and sex between men and boys. Active and passive roles were not a problem in adult male relations with women or with slaves, for the inferior passive role was considered natural to women, including wives, and to servants or slaves. This was a problem, however, for citizen-class boys, who must come to be equal with men. The solution, according to some philosophers (e.g., Demosthenes), was to regulate the age of boy lovers and the

circumstances and goals of their liaisons with men. Others (e.g., Plato) preferred transcending and eliminating physical sex in erotic relations between men and boys.

The aspects of Greek and Roman thought about sex that were to have the most influence on subsequent Western theory included a distrust of sexual desire and a judgment of the inferior status of sexual pleasure, along with the inferior status of the body in relation to the soul. While sex was not considered evil, it was considered dangerous—not only in its excess but also in its natural violence (orgasm was sometimes described as a form of epileptic seizure); in its expenditure of virile energy (it was thought to have a weakening effect); and in its association with death (nature's provision for immortality through procreation made sex a reminder of mortality) (Foucault, 1986).

The Pythagoreans in the sixth century B.C.E. advocated purity of the body for the sake of cultivating the soul. The force of their position was felt in the later thinking of Socrates and Plato. Although Plato moved away from a general hostility to bodily pleasure, he made a careful distinction between lower and higher pleasures (in, for example, the *Republic, Phaedo, Symposium,* and *Philebus*): Sexual pleasure was a lower form of pleasure, and self-mastery required domination over its demands. Plato advocated unleashing, not restraining, the power of eros for the sake of uniting the human spirit with the highest truth, goodness, and beauty. Insofar as bodily pleasures could be taken into this pursuit, there was no objection to them. But Plato thought that sexual intercourse diminished the power of eros for the contemplation and love of higher realities and that it even compromised the possibility of tenderness and respect in individual relationships of love (*Phaedrus*).

Aristotle, too, distinguished lower and higher pleasures, placing pleasures of touch at the bottom of the scale, characteristic as they are of the animal part of human nature (*Nicomachean Ethics*). Aristotle, more this-worldly than Plato, advocated moderation rather than transcendence. However, for Aristotle the highest forms of friendship and love, and of happiness in the contemplation of the life of one's friend, seemed to have no room for the incorporation of sexual activity or even for Platonic eros. Aristotle never conceived of the possibility of equality or mutuality in relationships between women and men, and he opposed the design for this that Plato had offered in the *Republic* and *Laws*.

Of all Graeco-Roman philosophies, Stoicism probably had the greatest impact on later developments in Western thought about sex. Musonius Rufus, Epictetus, Seneca, and Marcus Aurelius, for example, taught strong doctrines of the power of the human will to regulate emotion and of the desirability of such regulation for the sake of inner peace. Sexual desire, like the passions of fear and anger, was in itself irrational, disruptive, liable to excess. It needed to be moderated if not eliminated. It ought never to be indulged in for its own sake but only insofar as it served a rational purpose. Procreation was that purpose. Hence, even in marriage sexual intercourse was considered morally good only when engaged in for the sake of procreation.

With the later Stoics came what Foucault calls the "conjugalization" of sexual relations (1988, p. 166). That is, the norm governing sexual activity was now "no sex outside of marriage," derived from what others have called the "procreative" norm. Marriage was considered a natural duty, excused only in special circumstances such as when an individual undertook the responsibilities of life as a philosopher. The good effects of marriage included progeny and the companionship of husband and wife. It became the context for self-control and the fashioning of the virtuous life. Plutarch (in *Dialogue on Love*) took the position that marriage, not homosexual relationships, was the primary locus for erotic love and for friendship.

Overall, the Graeco-Roman legacy to Western sexual ethics holds little of the sexual permissiveness that characterized ancient Greece. The dominant themes carried through to later traditions were skepticism and control. This may have been due to the failure of almost all Greek and Roman thinkers to integrate sexuality into their best insights into human relationships. Whether such an integration is possible in principle has been at least a tacit question for other traditions.

The Jewish Tradition

Earliest Jewish moral codes were simple and without systematic theological underpinnings. Like other ancient Near Eastern legislation, they prescribed marriage laws and prohibited rape, adultery, and certain forms of prostitution. In contrast with neighboring religions, the Jews believed in a God who is beyond sexuality but whose plan for creation makes marriage and fertility holy and the subject of a religious duty (Gen. 2:24). At the heart of Judaism's tradition of sexual morality is a religious injunction to marry. The command to marry holds within it a command to procreate, and it assumes a patriarchal model for marriage and family. These two aspects of the tradition—the duty to procreate and its patriarchal context—account for many of its specific sexual regulations.

While the core of the imperative to marry is the command to procreate, marriage was considered a duty also because it conduced to the holiness of the partners. Holiness referred to more than the channeling of sexual desire,

though it meant that also; it included the companionship and mutual fulfillment of spouses. In fact, monogamous lifelong marriage was considered the ideal context for sexuality, and in time it became the custom and not only an ideal. Yet the command to procreate historically stood in tension with the value given to the marriage relationship. Thus while the laws of *onah,* of marital rights and duties, aimed to make sex a nurturant of love (Lamm), polygamy, concubinage, and divorce and remarriage were long accepted as solutions to a childless marriage. Only in the eleventh century C.E. was polygamy finally banned (much later in the East), and it was only in the twelfth century that Maimonides explicitly condemned concubinage (Novak, 1992).

Judaism has traditionally shown a concern for the "improper emission of seed" (appealing to interpretations of Gen. 38:9). Included in this concern have been proscriptions of masturbation and homosexual acts. The latter in particular have been considered unnatural (Lev. 18:22, 20:13), failing in responsibility for procreation, beneath the dignity of humanly meaningful sexual intercourse, indicative of uncontrolled (and hence morally evil) sexual desire, and a threat to the stability of heterosexual marriage and the patriarchal family. Lesbian relations were not regulated by biblical law, and in rabbinic literature were treated far less seriously than male homosexuality.

Throughout the Jewish tradition there has been a marked difference in the treatment of women's and men's sexuality (Plaskow). In part, this was because of women's subordinate role in the family and in society. The regulation and control of women's sexuality was considered necessary to the stability and the continuity of the family. Premarital sex, extramarital sex, and even rape were legally different for women than for men. In the biblical period, husbands but not wives could initiate divorce (Deut. 24:1–4), although later rabbinic law made it possible for either to do so. Adultery was understood as violating the property rights of a husband and could be punished by the death of both parties. Women's actions and dress were regulated in order to restrict their potential for luring men into illicit sex. The laws of onah required men to respect the sexual needs of their wives; but the laws of *niddah* (menstrual purity) had the symbolic consequence, however unintended, of associating women with defilement.

The perspective on sex, in all the branches of Judaism, has been an enduringly positive one, yet not without ambivalence. The sexual instinct was considered a gift from God, but it could still be called by the rabbis the "evil impulse" (*yetzer hara*) (Plaskow). The tradition was not immune from the suspicion regarding sex that, with the rise of Stoic philosophies and the advent of certain religious movements from the East, permeated all Middle Eastern cultures. Interpretations of the relation between sexuality and the sacred have not been univocal, as evidenced in differences between mainstream Jewish thinking and kabbalistic mysticism. Hence, some issues of sexual ethics have not been resolved once and for all. Contemporary developments in the Jewish tradition include growing pluralism regarding questions of premarital sex, contraception, abortion, gender equality, and homosexuality (Borowitz; Feldman; Plaskow; Biale; Posner). Current conflicts involve the interpretation of traditional values, the analysis of contemporary situations, and the incorporation of hitherto unrepresented perspectives, in particular those of heterosexual women and of gays and lesbians.

Christian Traditions

Like other religious and cultural traditions, the teachings of Christianity regarding sex are complex and subject to multiple influences, and they have changed and developed through succeeding generations. Christianity does not begin with a systematic code of ethics. The teachings of Jesus and his followers, as recorded in the New Testament, provide a central focus for the moral life of Christians in the command to love God and neighbor. Beyond that, the New Testament offers grounds for a sexual ethic that (1) values marriage and procreation on the one hand, and singleness and celibacy on the other; (2) gives as much or more importance to internal attitudes and thoughts as to external actions; and (3) affirms a sacred symbolic meaning for sexual intercourse, yet both subordinates it to other human values and finds in it a possibility for evil. As for unanimity on more specific sexual rules, this is difficult to find in the beginnings of a religion whose founder taught as an itinerant prophet and whose sacred texts were formulated in "the more tense world" of particular disciples, a group of wandering preachers (Brown, pp. 42–43).

EARLY INFLUENCES ON CHRISTIAN UNDERSTANDINGS OF SEX. Christianity emerged in the late Hellenistic age, when even Judaism was influenced by the dualistic anthropologies of Stoic philosophy and Gnostic religions. Unlike the Greek and Roman philosophies of the time, Christianity's main concern was not the art of self-mastery and not the preservation of the city or the empire. Unlike major strands of Judaism at the time, its focus was less on the solidarity and continuity of life in this world than on the continuity between this world and a life to come. Yet early Christian writers were profoundly influenced both by Judaism and by Graeco-Roman philosophy. With Judaism they shared a theistic approach to morality, an affirmation of creation as the context of marriage and procreation, and an ideal of single-hearted love. With the Stoics they shared a

suspicion of bodily passion and a respect for reason as a guide to the moral life. With the Greeks, Romans, and Jews, Christian thinkers assumed and reinforced views of women as inferior to men (despite some signs of commitment to gender equality in the beginnings of Christianity as a movement). As Christianity struggled for its own identity, issues of sexual conduct were important, but there was no immediate agreement on how they should be resolved.

Gnosticism was a series of religious movements that deeply affected formulations of Christian sexual ethics for the first three centuries C.E. (Noonan). For example, some Gnostics taught that marriage was evil or at least useless, primarily because the procreation of children was a vehicle for forces of evil. This belief led to two extreme positions—one in opposition to all sexual intercourse, and hence in favor of celibacy, and the other in favor of any form of sexual intercourse so long as it was not procreative. Neither of these positions prevailed in what became orthodox Christianity.

What did prevail in Christian moral teaching was a doctrine that incorporated an affirmation of sex as good (because part of creation) but seriously flawed (because the force of sexual passion as such cannot be controlled by reason). The Stoic position that sexual intercourse can be brought under the rule of reason not by subduing it but by giving it a rational purpose (procreation) made great sense to early Christian thinkers. The connection made between sexual intercourse and procreation was not the same as the Jewish affirmation of the importance of fecundity, but it was in harmony with it. Christian teaching could thus both affirm procreation as the central rationale for sexual union and advocate celibacy as a praiseworthy option (indeed, the ideal) for Christians who could choose it.

With the adoption of the Stoic norm for sexual intercourse, the direction of Christian sexual ethics was set for centuries to come. A sexual ethic that concerned itself primarily with affirming the good of procreation, and thereby the good of otherwise evil tendencies, was reinforced by the continued appearance of antagonists who played the same role the Gnostics had played. No sooner had Gnosticism begun to wane than, in the third century, Manichaeanism emerged. It was largely in response to Manichaeanism that Saint Augustine formulated his sexual ethic, an ethic that continued and went beyond the Stoic elements incorporated by Clement of Alexandria, Origen, Ambrose, and Jerome.

THE SEXUAL ETHICS OF SAINT AUGUSTINE AND ITS LEGACY. Against the Manichaeans Augustine argued in favor of the goodness of marriage and procreation, though he shared with them a negative view of sexual desire as in itself an evil passion. Because evil was for Augustine, however, a privation of right order (something missing in what was otherwise basically good), he thought at first that it was possible to reorder sexual desire according to right reason, to integrate its meaning into a right and whole love of God and neighbor. This reordering could be done only when sexual intercourse was within heterosexual marriage and for the purpose of procreation (*On the Good of Marriage,* 6). Intercourse within marriage but without a procreative purpose was, according to Augustine, sinful, though not necessarily mortally so. Marriage, on the other hand, had a threefold purpose: not only the good of children but also the goods of fidelity between spouses (as opposed to adultery) and the indissolubility of the union (as opposed to divorce).

In his later writings against the Pelagians (*Marriage and Concupiscence*), Augustine tried to clarify the place of disordered sexual desire in a theology of original sin. Although for Augustine the original sin of Adam and Eve was a sin of the spirit (a sin of prideful disobedience), its effects were most acutely present in the conflict between sexual desire and reasoned love of higher goods. Moreover, this loss of integrity in affectivity was passed from one generation to another through the mode of procreation—sexual intercourse. In this debate Augustine argued that there is some evil in all sexual intercourse, even when it is within marriage and for the sake of procreation. Most of those who followed Augustine disagreed with this, but his basic formulation of a procreative ethic held sway in Christian moral teaching for centuries.

Some early Christian writers (e.g., John Chrysostom) emphasized the Pauline purpose for marriage—marriage as a remedy for incontinence. Such a position hardly served to foster a more optimistic view of sex, but it did offer a possibility for moral goodness in sexual intercourse without a direct relation to procreation. However, from the sixth to the eleventh century, it was Augustine's rationale that was codified in penitentials (manuals for confessors, providing lists of sins and their prescribed penances) with detailed prohibitions against adultery, fornication, oral and anal sex, contraception, and even certain positions for sexual intercourse if they were thought to be departures from the procreative norm. Gratian's great collection of canon law in the twelfth century contained rigorous regulations based on the principle that all sexual activity is evil unless it is between husband and wife and for the sake of procreation. A few voices (e.g., Abelard and John Damascene) maintained that concupiscence (sexual passionate desire) does not make sexual pleasure evil in itself, and that intercourse in marriage can be justified by the simple intention to avoid fornication.

Overall, the Christian tradition in the first half of its history developed a consistently negative view of sex, despite the fact that Augustine and most of those who followed him were neither anti-body nor anti-marriage. The statement that this tradition was negative must be a qualified claim, of course, for it was silent or vacillating on many questions of sexuality (e.g., on the question of homosexuality); and there is little evidence that Christians in general were influenced by the more severe sexual attitudes of their leaders (Boswell). The direction and tone that the early centuries gave to the tradition's future, however, were unmistakable. What these leaders were concerned about was freedom from bondage to desires that seemingly could not in themselves lead to God. In a quest for transformation of the body along with the spirit, even procreation did not appear very important. Hence, regulation of sexual activity and even the importance of the family were often overshadowed by the ideal of celibacy. As Peter Brown's 1988 massive study has shown, sexual renunciation served both eros and unselfish love, and it suited a worldview that broke boundaries with this world without rejecting it as evil.

THE TEACHING OF AQUINAS. Thomas Aquinas wrote in the thirteenth century, when rigorism already prevailed in Christian teaching and church discipline. His remarkable synthesis of Christian theology did not offer much that was innovative in the area of sexual ethics. Yet the clarity of what he brought forward made his contribution significant for the generations that followed. He taught that sexual desire is not intrinsically evil, since no spontaneous bodily or emotional inclination is evil in itself; only when there is an evil moral choice is an action morally evil. Consequent upon original sin, however, there is in human nature a certain loss of order among natural human inclinations. Sexual passion is marked by this disorder, but it is not morally evil except insofar as its disorder is freely chosen.

Aquinas offered two rationales for the procreative norm the tradition had so far affirmed. One was the Augustinian argument that sexual pleasure, in the fallen human person, hinders the best working of the mind. It must be brought into some accord with reason by having an overriding value as its goal. No less an end than procreation can justify it (*Summa theologiae,* I-II.34.1, ad 1). But second, reason does not merely provide a good purpose for sexual pleasure. It discovers this purpose through the anatomy and biological function of sexual organs (*Summa theologiae* II-II.154.11; *Summa contra Gentiles* III.122.4, 5). Hence, the norm of reason in sexual behavior requires not only the conscious intention to procreate but also the accurate and unimpeded (i.e., noncontraceptive) physical process whereby procreation is possible.

From the procreative norm there followed other specific moral rules. Many of them were aimed at the well-being of offspring that could result from sexual intercourse. For example, Aquinas argued against fornication, adultery, and divorce on the grounds that children would be deprived of a good context for their rearing. He considered sexual acts other than heterosexual intercourse to be immoral because they could not be procreative. Aquinas's treatment of marriage contained only hints of new insight regarding the relation of sexual intercourse to marital love. He offered a theory of love that had room for a positive incorporation of sexual union (*Summa theologiae* II-II.26.11), and he suggested that marriage might be the basis of a maximum form of friendship (*Summa contra Gentiles* III.123).

Though what had crystallized in the Middle Ages canonically and theologically would continue to influence Christian moral teaching into the indefinite future, the fifteenth century marked the beginning of significant change. Finding some grounds for opposing the prevailing Augustinian sexual ethic in both Albert the Great and in the general (if not the specifically sexual) ethics of Aquinas, writers (e.g., Denis the Carthusian and Martin LeMaistre) began to talk of the integration of spiritual love and sexual pleasure, and the intrinsic good of sexual pleasure as the opposite of the pain of its lack. This did not reverse the Augustinian tradition, but it weakened it. The effects of these new theories were felt in the controversies of the Reformation.

PROTESTANT TEACHINGS ON SEX. Questions of sexual behavior played an important role in the Protestant Reformation beginning in the sixteenth century. Clerical celibacy, for example, was challenged not just in its scandalous nonobservance but also as a Christian ideal. Marriage and family replaced it among the reformers as the center of sexual gravity in the Christian life. Martin Luther and John Calvin were both deeply influenced by the Augustinian tradition regarding original sin and its consequences for human sexuality. Yet both developed a position on marriage that was not dependent on a procreative ethic. Like most of the Christian tradition, they affirmed marriage and human sexuality as part of the divine plan for creation, and therefore good. But they shared Augustine's pessimistic view of fallen human nature and its disordered sex drive. Luther was convinced, however, that the necessary remedy for disordered desire was marriage (*On the Estate of Marriage*). And so the issue was joined over a key element in Christian sexual ethics. Luther, of course, was not the first to advocate marriage as the cure for unruly sexual desire, but he took on the whole of the tradition in a way that no one else had. He challenged theory and practice, offering not only an alternative justification for marriage but also a view of the human person that demanded marriage for almost all Christians.

According to Luther, sexual pleasure itself in one sense needed no justification. The desire for it was simply a fact of life. It remained, like all the givens in creation, a good so long

as it was channeled through marriage into the meaningful whole of life, which included the good of offspring. What there was in sex that detracted from the knowledge and worship of God was sinful, but it had simply to be forgiven, as did the inevitable sinful elements in all human activity. After 1523, Luther shifted his emphasis from marriage as a "hospital for the incurables" to marriage as a school for character. It was within the secular, nonsacramental institution of marriage and family that individuals learned obedience to God and developed the important human virtues. The structure of the family was hierarchical, husband having authority over wife, parents over children.

Calvin, too, saw marriage as a corrective to otherwise disordered desires. He expanded the notion of marriage as the context for human flourishing by maintaining that the greatest good of marriage and sex was the society that is formed between husband and wife (*Commentary on Genesis*). Calvin was more optimistic than Luther about the possibility of controlling sexual desire, though he, too, believed that whatever fault remained in it was "covered over" by marriage and forgiven by God (*Institutes of the Christian Religion*, 2.8.44). Like earlier writers, he worried that marriage as a remedy for incontinence could nonetheless in itself offer provocation to uncontrolled passion.

As part of their teaching on marriage, Luther and Calvin opposed premarital and extramarital sex and homosexual relations. So concerned was Luther to provide some institutionally tempering form to sexual desire that he once voiced an opinion favoring bigamy over adultery. Both Luther and Calvin were opposed to divorce, though its possibility was admitted in a situation of adultery or impotence.

MODERN ROMAN CATHOLIC DEVELOPMENTS. During and after the Roman Catholic Counterreformation, from the late sixteenth century on, new developments alternated with the reassertion of the Augustinian ethic. The Council of Trent (1545–1563) was the first ecumenical council to address the role of love in marriage, but it also reaffirmed the primacy of procreation and reemphasized the superiority of celibacy. In the seventeenth century, Jansenism, a morally austere and ultimately heretical movement, reacted against what it considered a dangerous lowering of sexual standards and brought back the Augustinian connection between sex, concupiscence, and original sin. Alphonsus Liguori in the eighteenth century gave impetus to a manualist tradition (the development and proliferation of moral manuals designed primarily to assist confessors) that attempted to integrate the Pauline purpose of marriage (as a remedy for incontinence) with the procreative purpose. Nineteenth-century moral manuals focused on "sins of impurity," choices of any sexual pleasure apart from procreative marital intercourse. Then came the twentieth century, with the rise of Catholic theological interest in personalism and the move by the Protestant churches to accept birth control.

In 1930, Pope Pius XI responded to the Anglican approval of contraception by reaffirming the procreative ethic (*Casti connubii*). But he also gave approval to the use of the rhythm method for restricting procreation. Moral theologians began to move cautiously in the direction of allowing sexual intercourse in marriage without a procreative intent and for the purpose of fostering marital union. The change in Roman Catholic moral theology from the 1950s to the 1970s was dramatic. The wedge introduced between procreation and sexual intercourse by the acceptance of the rhythm method joined with new understandings of the totality of the human person to support a radically new concern for sex as an expression and cause of married love. The effects of this theological reflection were striking in the 1965 Second Vatican Council teaching that the love essential to marriage is uniquely expressed and perfected in the act of sexual intercourse (*Gaudium et spes*, 49). Although the Council still held that marriage is by its very nature ordered to the procreation of children, it no longer ranked what the tradition considered the basic ends of marriage, offspring and spousal union, as primary and secondary.

In 1968, Pope Paul VI insisted that contraception is immoral (*Humanae vitae*). Rather than settling the issue for Roman Catholics, however, this occasioned intense conflict. The majority of moral theologians disagreed with the papal teaching, even though a distinction between nonprocreative and antiprocreative behavior mediated the dispute for some. Since then, many of the specific moral rules governing sexuality in the Catholic tradition have come under serious question. Official teachings have sustained past injunctions, though some modifications have been made in order to accommodate pastoral responses to second marriages, homosexual orientation (but not sexual activity), and individual conscience decisions regarding contraception. Among moral theologians there has been serious debate (and by the 1990s, marked pluralism) regarding premarital sex, homosexual acts, remarriage after divorce, infertility therapies, gender roles, and clerical celibacy (Curran and McCormick).

POST-REFORMATION PROTESTANTISM. Twentieth-century Protestant sexual ethics developed even more dramatically than Roman Catholic sexual ethics. After the Reformation, Protestant theologians and church leaders continued to affirm heterosexual marriage as the only acceptable context for sexual activity. Except for the differences regarding celibacy and divorce, sexual norms in Protestantism looked much the same as those in the Catholic tradition. Nineteenth-century Protestantism shared and contributed to the cultural pressures of Victorianism. But in the twentieth century, Protestant thinking was deeply affected by biblical and historical studies that questioned the foundations of Christian sexual ethics, by psychological theories that challenged traditional views, and by the voiced experience of church members.

It is difficult to trace one clear line of development in twentieth-century Protestant sexual ethics, or even as clear a dialectic as may be found in Roman Catholicism. The fact that Protestantism in general was from the beginning less dependent on a procreative ethic allowed it almost unanimously to accept contraception as a means to responsible parenting. Overall, Protestant sexual ethics has moved to integrate an understanding of the human person, male and female, into a theology of marriage that no longer deprecates sexual desire as self-centered and dangerous. It continues to struggle with issues of gendered hierarchy in the family, and with what are often called "alternative lifestyles," such as the cohabitation of unmarried heterosexuals and the sexual partnerships of gays and lesbians. For the most part, the ideal context for sexual intercourse is still seen to be heterosexual marriage, but many Protestant theologians accept premarital sex and homosexual partnerships with general norms of noncoercion, basic equality, and so on. Every mainline Protestant church in the 1990s has task forces working particularly on questions of homosexuality, professional (including clergy) sexual ethics, and sex education. Traditional positions have either changed or are open and conflicted.

Modern Sexology: Philosophical, Medical, Social Scientific

The contemporary shaking of the foundations of Western sexual ethics, religious and secular, is traceable to many factors. These quite obviously include the rapid development of reproductive technologies, none more important than the many forms of contraception. But there have been other factors as well, such as changes in economic structures under capitalism and in social structures following major shifts of population to urban centers. Of important influence, too, has been the rise of the modern women's movement and of movements for gay and lesbian civil rights. Along with these developments, as both cause and effect, there have been significant contributions from disciplines such as history, psychology, anthropology, sociology, and medicine. Philosophy has generally followed these changes, though in the late twentieth century it, too, has contributed to cultural alterations in perspectives on sex.

PHILOSOPHICAL DEVELOPMENTS. As surveyors of the history of philosophy note, philosophers have not paid much attention to sex. They have written a great deal on love but have left sexual behavior largely to religion, poetry, medicine, or the law (Baker and Elliston; Soble). After the Greeks and Romans, and medieval thinkers such as Thomas Aquinas whose work is philosophical as well as theological, there is not much to be found in the field regarding sexuality until the twentieth century. Some exceptions to this are the sparse eighteenth-century writings on sex and gender by David Hume, Jean-Jacques Rousseau, Immanuel Kant, Mary Wollstonecraft, and Johann Gottlieb Fichte, and the nineteenth-century writings of Arthur Schopenhauer, Karl Marx, Friedrich Engels, John Stuart Mill, and Friedrich Nietzsche. Most of these writers reinforced the norm of heterosexual procreative sex within marriage. Hume, for example, in his "Of Polygamy and Divorce" (1742), insisted that all arguments finally lead to a recommendation of "our present European practices with regard to marriage." Rousseau's La Nouvelle Héloïse (1761) deplored the faults of conventional marriage but strongly opposed divorce and marital infidelity. Kant defended traditional sexual mores, although in his Lectures on Ethics (1781) he introduced a justification for marriage not in terms of procreation but of altruistic love, arguing that only a mutual commitment in marriage can save sexual desire from making a sexual partner into a mere means to one's own pleasure. Schopenhauer viewed sexual love as subjectively for pleasure, though objectively for procreation; his strong naturalism paved the way for a more radical theory of sex as an instinct without ethical norms (The Metaphysics of Sexual Love, 1844).

Philosophers in these centuries came down on both sides of the question of gender equality. Fichte, for example, asserted an essentially passive nature for women, who, if they were to be equal with men, would have to renounce their femininity (The Science of Rights, 1796). But Mary Wollstonecraft in her "A Vindication of the Rights of Women" (1792), and Mill in his "The Subjection of Women" (1869), offered strong challenges to the traditional inequality of gender roles in society. Marx and Engels critiqued bourgeois marriage as a relationship of economic domination (e.g., in their The Origin of the Family, Private Property and the State, first published by Engels in 1884). Schopenhauer, reacting to feminist agendas, advocated polygamy on the basis of a theory of male needs and female instrumental response (On Women, 1848). Nietzsche, like Schopenhauer, moved away from traditional ethical norms but also reinforced a view of the solely procreative value of women (Thus Spake Zarathustra, 1892).

Twentieth-century European philosophers attempted to construct new meanings for human sexuality in the light of new philosophical theories of freedom and interpersonal love. Jean-Paul Sartre analyzed sexuality as an ontological paradigm for human conflict (Being and Nothingness, 1943); Maurice Merleau-Ponty tried to challenge this and to go beyond it (The Phenomenology of Perception, 1945); Simone de Beauvoir fueled a feminist movement with a stark and revealing analysis of sexism and its influence on the meaning of both gender and sex (The Second Sex, 1949). With the exception of Bertrand Russell (Marriage and Morals, 1929), it was not until the late 1960s that British and American philosophers began to turn their attention to sexual ethics. Then, however, key essays by analytic philosophers began to appear on issues such as sexual desire, gender, marriage, adultery, homosexuality, abortion, sexual perversion, rape, pornography, and sexual abuse (Baker and Elliston; Shelp; Soble). All of these efforts were profoundly influenced by nineteenth- and twentieth-century contributions from other disciplines.

FREUD AND PSYCHOANALYSIS. The emergence of psychoanalytic theory brought with it new perceptions of the meaning and role of sexuality in the life of individuals. Whatever the final validity of Sigmund Freud's insights, they burst upon the world with a force that all but swept away the foundations of traditional sexual morality. Augustine's and Luther's assertions about the indomitability of sexual desire found support in Freud's theory, but now the power of sexual need was not the result of sin but a natural drive, centrally constitutive of the human personality (Three Essays on the Theory of Sexuality, 1905). Past efforts to order sexuality according to rational purposes could now be understood as repression. After Freud, when sex went awry, it was a matter of psychological illness, not moral evil. Taboos needed demythologizing, and freedom might be attained not through forgiveness but through medical treatment.

Yet psychoanalytic theory raised as many questions as it answered. Freud argued for liberation from sexual taboos and from the hypocrisy and sickness they caused, but he nonetheless maintained the need for sexual restraint. His theory of sublimation called for a discipline and channeling of the sexual instinct if the individual and society were to progress (Civilization and Its Discontents, 1930). The concern for sexual norms therefore remained, and Freud's own recommendations were in many ways quite traditional. But new work had clearly been cut out for thinkers in both secular and religious traditions.

SCIENCE, SOCIAL SCIENCE, AND MEDICINE. Freud was not the only force in nineteenth- and twentieth-century scientific and social thought that shaped changes in Western sexual mores. Biological studies of the human reproductive process offered new perspectives on male and female roles in sex and procreation. Animal research showed that higher forms of animals masturbate, perform sexual acts with members of the same sex, and generally engage in many sexual behaviors that were previously assumed to be unnatural for humans because they were unnatural for animals. Anthropologists found significant variations in the sexual behavior of human cultural groups, so that traditional notions of human nature seemed even more questionable. Surveys of sexual activities in Western society revealed massive discrepancies between accepted sexual norms and actual behavior, undercutting consequential arguments for some of the norms (e.g., the fact that 95% of the male population in the United States engaged in autoerotic acts made it difficult to support a prohibition against masturbation on grounds that it leads to insanity).

Modern sexology, then, has incorporated the work not only of sexual psychology but also of biology, anthropology, ethnology, and sociology—the research and the theories of individuals like Richard von KrafftEbing, Havelock Ellis, Magnus Hirschfield, Alfred Kinsey, Margaret Mead, William Masters, and Virginia Johnson. The results have not all been toward greater liberty in sexual behavior, but they have shared a tendency to secularize and medicalize human sexuality. In theory, sex has become less an ethical or even an aesthetic problem than a health problem. In practice, experts of all kinds—physicians, counselors, psychiatrists, social workers, teachers—provide guidance; and the guidance can at least appear to carry moral weight. An example of the intertwining of science, the medical professions, and morality is clear in the long efforts to define and identify sexual deviance or perversion—from Krafft-Ebing in the nineteenth century to the debates in the American Psychiatric Association in the 1970s and 1980s over the classification of homosexuality as a disease.

LESSONS OF HISTORY. Historians, too, have played an important role in the weakening of traditional sexual ethical norms. The very disclosure that sexual prescriptions have a history has revealed the contingency of their sources and foundations. To see, for example, that a procreative ethic rose as much from Stoic philosophies as from the Bible has allowed many Christians to question its validity. Feminist retrievals of elements in the Western tradition have led to critiques of taboo moralities and a consequent need for reconstruction. In an effort to make sense of present beliefs, historians have searched for the roots and developments of these beliefs, and the result has seldom been a reinforcement of the original rationales (Foucault, 1978; Boswell).

But it is not only the history of ideas that has had an impact on contemporary sexual ethics. It is also the historical excavation of the moral attitudes and actual practices of peoples of the past, and an identification of the shifting centers of influence on the sexual mores of different times and places (D'Emilio and Freedman; Peiss and Simmons; Fout). Sometimes referred to as a history of sexuality rather than a history of theories about sexuality or of institutionalized norms for sexuality, this is a task that is barely under way, and it has strong critics. Yet it has already had an impact on, for example, understandings of homosexuality and what can be called the politics of sex. This kind of history also attempts to provide narratives, describing shifts like the one in the United States from family-centered procreative sexual mores to romantic notions of emotional intimacy to a commercialization of sex and its idealization as the central source of human happiness (D'Emilio and Freedman). The history of sexuality and of sexual ethics, no less than the analysis of contemporary sexual norms, thus becomes subject to interpretation.

Interpretive Theories: Sex, Morality, and History

No one may have been more influential in determining current questions about the history of sexuality and sexual ethics than the French philosopher Michel Foucault. His ideas permeate much of the work of other sexual historians as well as philosophers and theologians. Yet his is not the only formative study in the history of sexual ethics, and his conclusions have provoked both positive and negative responses.

MICHEL FOUCAULT: A HISTORY OF DESIRE. Foucault originally planned to write a history of what he called "the experience of sexuality" in modern Western culture. In the course of his work, he became convinced that what was needed was a history of desire, or of the desiring subject. At the heart of this conviction was the premise that sexuality is not an ahistorical constant. Neither is sex a natural given, a biological referent that simply expresses itself in different experiences of sexuality shaped historically by changing moral norms. Sexuality is, rather, a transfer point for relations of power—between women and men, parents and children, teachers and students, clergy and laity, and so forth. Power in this sense is diffused through a field of multiple "force relations immanent in the sphere in which they operate" (Foucault, 1978, p. 92). In other words, sex is not a "stubborn drive" that requires the control of power. Power produces and constitutes sexual desire much more than it ever represses it. Power determines, shapes, and deploys sexuality, and sexuality determines the meaning of sex (Foucault, 1978).

Foucault denied, then, the "repressive hypothesis" as an explanation of the eighteenth- and nineteenth-century Western experience of sexuality. That is, he denied that the Victorian era had been an era of sexual repression and socially enforced silence about sex. He argued, rather, that it had been a time of an expanding deployment of sexuality and a veritable explosion of discourse about sexuality. The questions that interested him were not "Why are we repressed?" but "Why do we say that we are repressed?" and within this, not "Why was sex associated with sin for such a long time?" but "Why do we burden ourselves today with so much guilt for having made sex a sin?" (Foucault, 1978, pp. 8–9). Since the key to these questions was, Foucault thought, to be found in a study of discourse, he began with an examination of what he considered a Western impulse to discover the "truth" about sex. This, in his view, included a striking Western compulsion to self-examination and self-reporting regarding sexual experience, whether in the discourses of religion, medicine, psychiatry, or criminal justice.

To make sense of the connections between power, sexuality, and truth in the modern period, Foucault revised his project to include a study of the variations on sexual themes in other historical periods. His move to the past began with his thesis that a forerunner of modern discourse on sex was the seventeenth-century Christian ecclesiastical emphasis on confession. To put this in perspective, he undertook studies of pagan antiquity and of Christianity prior to the seventeenth century. Thus, volumes 2 and 3 of his *History of Sexuality* address the sexual mores of the fourth-century B.C.E. Greeks and the first- and second-century C.E. Romans (1990 and 1988, respectively). His unpublished fourth volume (*The Confessions of the Flesh*) examine developments within Christianity. The contrasts (and, as it turned out, the continuities) between the different historical periods shed some light on each period and on the overall Western pursuit of the kind of knowledge that promised power in relation to sex, what Foucault called the scientia sexualis.

Foucault came to the conclusion that the sexual morality of the Greeks and Romans did not differ essentially from Christian sexual morality in terms of specific prescriptions. He rejected the commonly held view that the essential contrast between sexual ethics in antiquity and in early Christianity lies in the permissiveness of Graeco-Roman societies as distinguished from the strict sexual rules of the Christians, or in an ancient positive attitude toward sex as distinguished from a negative Christian assessment. Both traditions, he argued, contained prohibitions against incest, a preference for marital fidelity, a model of male superiority, caution regarding same-sex relations, respect for austerity, a positive regard for sexual abstinence, fears of male loss of

strength through sexual activity, and hopes of access to special truths through sexual discipline. Nor were these basic prescriptions very different from what could be found in post-seventeenth-century Western society.

Yet there were clear discontinuities, even ruptures, between these historical periods. The reasons for moral solicitude regarding sexuality were different. In Foucault's reading, the ancients were concerned with health, beauty, and freedom, while Christians sought purity of heart before God, and bourgeois moderns aimed at their own self-idealization. The Greeks valued self-mastery; Christians struggled for self-understanding; and modern Western individuals scrutinized their feelings in order to secure compliance with standards of normality. Eroticism was channeled toward boys for the Greeks, women for the Christians, and a centrifugal movement in many directions for the Victorian and post-Victorian middle class. The Greeks feared the enslavement of the mind by the body; Christians dreaded the chaotic power of corrupted passion; post-nineteenth century persons feared deviance and its consequent shame. Sexual morality was an aesthetic ideal, a personal choice, for an elite in antiquity; it became a universal ethical obligation under Christianity; and it was exacted as a social requirement under the power of the family and the management of the modern professional.

Foucault's study of the history of sexuality left open a question with which he had become preoccupied: How did contemporary Western culture come to believe that sexuality was the key to individual identity? How did sex become more important than love, and almost more important than life? He exposed the lack of freedom in past constructs of sexuality, and he critiqued past formulations of sexual prescriptions. But his presentation of current strategies for sexual liberation yielded no less skeptical a judgment. It suggested, rather, that however historically relative sexual ethics may be, moral solicitude regarding sexuality is not entirely a mistake.

CATHARINE MACKINNON: A HISTORY OF GENDERED VIOLENCE. Many Western feminists have shared Foucault's convictions that sexuality is socially constructed and the body is a site of power. Like Foucault, they have exposed continuing roles of medicine, education, and psychology in determining post-eighteenth-century sexual mores. With Foucault, they have emphasized discourse as a key to identifying underlying forces that link power, sexuality, and identity. But feminists fault Foucault for not extending his analytics of power to gender. Legal scholar Catharine MacKinnon, for example, opposes a Foucaultian history of desire on the grounds that the unacknowledged desiring subject is male. A history of sexuality that emphasizes sexual desire and change misses the enduring aspects of history—the unrelenting sexual abuse of women. History, then, remains silent regarding sexual exploitation, harassment, battery, and rape. Without attention to these unchanging experiences of women, MacKinnon argues, there can be no accurate analysis of sex and power.

A feminist theory of sexuality, according to MacKinnon, "locates sexuality within a theory of gender inequality" (1989, p. 127). It is a mistake, therefore, to adopt the stance that what sex needs is socially constructed freedom, that all sex can be good—healthy, appropriate, pleasurable, to be approved and expressed—if only it is liberated from ideologies of allowed/not allowed. Since sexuality is socially constructed not by a diffuse multiplicity of powers (in Foucault's sense) but by hegemonic male power, it is culturally determined as violent toward women. Pornography is a means through which this social construction is achieved.

Although not all feminists share MacKinnon's radical critique of historical and contemporary sexual understandings and practices, there is significant agreement that sexuality needs norms, and that past and present norms require gender analysis and critique. From this standpoint, a Foucaultian treatment of male discourse regarding sexuality perpetuates a view of sexuality as eroticized dominance and submission; it fails to expose this conflict as gendered.

EVOLUTIONARY INTERPRETATIONS. Foucault and MacKinnon represent interpretations of the history of sexuality and sexual ethics that deny any progress. They refuse to applaud advances in understandings of sexuality or to sanctify the present as enlightened and free. To some extent, they even reject notions of change in history—Foucault arguing for different, but not causally connected, historical perspectives; and MacKinnon focusing on similarities across time and cultures—indeed, a failure to change. Others, however, have charted an evolutionary process across the Western history of ideas about sex and the moral norms that should govern it. Those who believe that contemporary sexual revolutions have liberated persons and their sexual possibilities belong in this category. So do those who acknowledge the significance of advances in biology and psychology and call for appropriate adjustments in philosophical and theological ethics. Thoughtful commentators do not necessarily conclude that there has been real progress, though they identify evolutionary changes (Green; Shelp; Soble).

Richard Posner belongs to this latter group, offering what he calls an "economic theory of sexuality." That is, he relies heavily on economic analysis both to describe the practice of sex and to evaluate legal and ethical norms in its regard. There are, he argues, three stages in the evolution of sexual morality. These stages correlate with the status of women in a given society (Posner). In the first stage, women's occupation is that of "simple breeder." When this is the case, companionate marriage is an unlikely possibility, and practices that are considered "immoral" are likely to flourish (e.g., prostitution, adultery, homosexual liaisons).

The second stage begins when women's occupations expand to include "child rearer and husband's companion." Here, companionate marriage is a possibility, and because of this, "immoral" practices that endanger it are vehemently condemned. When companionate marriage is idealized as the only possibility for everyone, societies become puritanical in their efforts to promote and protect it. In the third stage, women's roles are enlarged to include "market employment." Marriages will be fewer, but where they exist, they will be companionate. Other forms of sexual relationship, previously considered immoral, no longer appear to be either immoral or abnormal. This stage characterizes some Western societies more than others—notably, according to Posner, contemporary Sweden.

A very different kind of evolutionary theory can be found in the philosopher Paul Ricoeur's 1967 analysis of the symbolism of evil in Western history. In this analysis, the Greco-Hebraic history of the consciousness of evil has three moments or stages: defilement, sin, and guilt. The sense of defilement is a pre-ethical, irrational, quasi-material sense of something that infects by contact. Sin is a sense of betrayal, of rupture in a relationship. And guilt is the subjective side of sin, a consciousness that the breakdown of a relationship is the result of an evil use of freedom. According to Ricoeur, sexual morality has appeared historically paradigmatic of the experience of defilement. This association has not been left behind; there remains in the implicit consciousness of the West an inarticulable but persistent connection between sexuality and evil. The result is that ethical wisdom regarding sexuality has remained far behind other developments in Western ethics, even though there has been a significant demythologizing of sex.

Contemporary Ethical Reconstruction

The turn to history may have relativized much of traditional sexual ethics, but the motivation for the turn is more complicated. Given all the factors that have helped to weaken traditional sexual norms, ethical reflection has been left with very little anchorage. Science and medicine help, but they sometimes add to human suffering experienced in relation to sex. Philosophy and religion find their traditions struggling for relevance, for clarity, for reasonable guidance and more than reasoned inspiration. The turn to history has been an effort to find a truth that continues to be elusive.

And history, like other disciplinary efforts, has probably both helped and heightened the need for the quest.

Contemporary efforts in sexual ethics recognize multiple meanings for human sexuality—pleasure, reproduction, communication, love, conflict, social stability, and so on. Most of those who labor at sexual ethics recognize the need to guide sexual behavior in ways that preserve its potential for good and restrict its potential for evil. Safety, nonviolence, equality, autonomy, mutuality, and truthfulness are generally acknowledged as required for minimal human justice in sexual relationships. Many think that care, responsibility, commitment, love, and fidelity are also required, or at least included as goals. With social construction no longer ignored, the politics of sex has become an ethical matter for persons and societies, institutions and professions. New questions press regarding the ways in which humanity is to reproduce itself and the responsibilities it has for its offspring. In all of this, sexual ethics asks, How is it appropriate—helpful and not harmful, creative and not destructive—to live and to relate to one another as sexual beings?

MARGARET A. FARLEY (1995)
BIBLIOGRAPHY REVISED

SEE ALSO: *Autonomy; Body; Care; Coercion; Compassionate Love; Confidentiality; Emotions; Epidemics; Eugenics; Feminism; Freedom and Free Will; Homosexuality; Natural Law; Sexual Ethics; Sexual Ethics and Professional Standards; Sexual Identity; Sexuality, Legal Approaches to*

BIBLIOGRAPHY

Baker, Robert, and Elliston, Frederick, eds. 1975. *Philosophy & Sex.* Buffalo, NY: Prometheus.

Baker, Robert; Elliston, Frederick A.; and Wininger, Kathleen J., eds. 1998. *Philosophy and Sex.* Prometheus Books.

Biale, David. 1992. *Eros and the Jews: From Biblical Israel to Contemporary America.* New York: Basic Books.

Borowitz, Eugene B. 1969. *Choosing a Sex Ethic: A Jewish Inquiry.* New York: Schocken.

Boswell, John. 1980. *Christianity, Social Tolerance, and Homosexuality.* Chicago: University of Chicago Press.

Brown, Peter. 1988. *The Body and Society: Men, Women, and Sexual Renunciation in Early Christianity.* New York: Columbia University Press.

Curran, Charles E., and McCormick, Richard A. 1993. *Dialogue about Catholic Sexual Teaching.* New York: Paulist Press.

D'Emilio, John, and Freedman, Estelle B. 1988. *Intimate Matters: A History of Sexuality in America.* New York: Harper and Row.

Epstein, Louis M. 1967 (1948). *Sex Laws and Customs in Judaism.* New York: Block. Reprint. New York: KTAV.

Feldman, David M. 1974 (1968). *Marital Relations, Birth Control, and Abortion in Jewish Law.* New York: Schocken Books.

Foucault, Michel. 1978. *The History of Sexuality.* Vol. 1, *An Introduction,* tr. Robert Hurley. New York: Pantheon.

Foucault, Michel. 1986. *The History of Sexuality.* Vol. 2, *The Use of Pleasure,* tr. Robert Hurley. New York: Vintage.

Foucault, Michel. 1988. *The History of Sexuality.* Vol. 3, *The Care of the Self,* tr. Robert Hurley. New York: Vintage.

Fout, John C., ed. 1992. *Forbidden History: The State, Society, and the Regulation of Sexuality in Modern Europe.* Chicago: University of Chicago Press.

Green, Ronald M., ed. 1992. *Religion and Sexual Health: Ethical, Theological, and Clinical Perspectives.* Dordrecht, Netherlands: Kluwer.

Greenberg, David F. 1988. *The Construction of Homosexuality.* Chicago: University of Chicago Press.

Gruen, Lori and Panichas, George E., eds. 1997. *Sex, Morality, and the Law.* London: Routledge.

Lamm, Maurice. 1980. *The Jewish Way in Love and Marriage.* San Francisco: Harper and Row.

Lemoncheck, Linda. 2002. *Loose Women, Lecherous Men: A Feminist Philosophy of Sex.* New York: Oxford University Press on Demand.

MacKinnon, Catharine A. 1989. *Toward a Feminist Theory of the State.* Cambridge, MA: Harvard University Press.

Nelson, James B. 1978. *Embodiment: An Approach to Sexuality and Christian Theology.* Minneapolis, MN: Augsburg.

Noonan, John T., Jr. 1986. *Contraception: A History of Its Treatment by the Catholic Theologians and Cannonists.* Enlarged ed. Cambridge, MA: Harvard University Press.

Novak, David. 1992. "Some Aspects of Sex, Society, and God in Judaism." In *Jewish Social Ethics,* pp. 84–103. New York: Oxford University Press.

Nussbaum, Martha Craven, and Sihvola, Juha, eds. 2002. *The Sleep of Reason: Erotic Experience and Sexual Ethics in Ancient Greece and Rome.* Chicago, IL: University of Chicago Press.

Peiss, Kathy, and Simmons, Christina, eds. (with Robert A. Padgug). 1989. *Passion and Power: Sexuality in History.* Philadelphia: Temple University Press.

Plaskow, Judith. 1990. *Standing Again at Sinai: Judaism from a Feminist Perspective.* San Francisco: Harper San Francisco.

Posner, Richard A. 1992. *Sex and Reason.* Cambridge, MA: Harvard University Press.

Ricoeur, Paul. 1967. *The Symbolism of Evil.* New York: Harper and Row.

Shelp, Earl E., ed. 1987. *Sexuality and Medicine.* 2 vols. Dordrecht, Netherlands: D. Reidel.

Soble, Alan, ed. 1991. *The Philosophy of Sex: Contemporary Readings.* 2nd edition. Savage, MD: Rowman and Littlefield.

Soble, Alan, ed. 2002. *Philosophy of Sex: Contemporary Readings.* 4th edition. Totowa, NJ: Rowman and Littlefield.

Stewart, Robert M., and Stewart, Columba. 1997. *Philosophical Perspectives on Sex and Love.* New York: Oxford University Press.

SEXUAL ETHICS AND PROFESSIONAL STANDARDS

• • •

The Hippocratic oath gives early expression to a general prohibition against professionals taking advantage of the vulnerability of clients or patients and their families to enter into sexual relations: "Whatever house I may visit, I will come for the benefit of the sick, remaining free of all intentional injustice, of all mischief and in particular of sexual relations with both female and male persons, be they free or slaves" (Verhey, p. 72). The prohibition was reiterated for mental-health professionals by Sigmund Freud (Schoener et al.). From these roots grows a general prohibition against professional-client sexual relations, including relations between teacher and student, supervisor and supervised, clergy and parishioner, therapist and client, and physician and patient. In some professions, the taboo has been so strong that sexuality is the problem professionals "don't talk about" (Rassieur) or "the problem with no name" (Davidson).

Yet some famous therapists (e.g., Carl Jung) have been notorious for having sexual relations with their clients (Schoener et al.). Studies of various professions indicate a rate of sexual contact between professionals and clients or patients of between 5 and 11 percent (Schoener et al.; Bonavoglia). The phenomenon has become sufficiently widespread to be called a "national disgrace" (Pope and Bouhoutsos) and an "epidemic" (Rutter).

In the ten years following the publication of *Betrayal* (Freeman and Roy), which described one woman's successful lawsuit over sexual misconduct by a psychiatrist, over $7 million was paid out in legal claims. In the face of revelations of misconduct, professional societies began to insert clear prohibitions into their codes: "sexual intimacies with clients are unethical" (American Psychological Association); "the social worker should under no circumstances engage in sexual activities with clients" (National Association of Social Workers); "sexual relations between analyst and patient are antithetic to treatment and unacceptable under any circumstance" (American Psychoanalytic Association). Even in the controversial field of sex therapy, direct sexual contact

between therapist and client is discouraged; sexual surrogates are used instead (Masters et al.).

Several jurisdictions have enacted laws making it a felony for a psychotherapist (including clergy) to have sexual contact with a client, and at least one holds the therapist's employer liable if the employer knew or should have known of a history of sexual abuse (Bonavoglia; for statutes, see Schoener et al.). Sexual contact is variously defined, but generally includes not only sexual intercourse but also intimate touching and other sexualizing of the relationship.

The prohibition against professional-client sexual contact rests on three foundations: the likelihood of great harm from the sexual contact, the responsibility of the professional to work for the good of the client, and the vulnerability of the client and the power gap between client and professional, which raises questions even in the absence of demonstrable harm.

There is growing consensus that significant harm is done to patients or clients who enter sexual relations with professionals in whom they have vested trust: "[T]he balance of the empirical findings is heavily weighted in the direction of serious harm resulting to almost all patients sexually involved with their therapists" (Pope and Bouhoutsos, p. 63). A few therapists have argued for the beneficial effects of sexual relations between therapist and client (Shepard; Schoener et al.), but their data have been challenged (Pope and Bouhoutsos; Schoener et al.). Studies of women who have had sexual relations with their gynecologists, psychotherapists, and clergy all point to deleterious consequences including loss of trust, poor self-concept, loss of confidence in one's judgment, and difficulty establishing subsequent relationships (Pope and Bouhoutsos). Several commentators have noted the similarities to incest because of the power of the professional and have argued that the consequences are as deleterious as those of incest (e.g., Fortune, 1989). Others note that women who enter relations with therapists often have a history of sexual abuse, and thus are being revictimized (Rutter; Pope and Bouhoutsos).

Sexual contact between professional and client thus subverts the legitimate goal of the profession—the healing or making whole of one who is wounded and vulnerable (Verhey). There is both exploitation of the client for benefit of the professional and a failure to provide the services implied by the professional role.

However, harm and failure to help are not the only ethical issues at stake. Several commentators argue that the power of the professional is morally relevant (Lebacqz; Lebacqz and Barton). Professionals may hold several types of power: Asclepian power—the power of professional training; charismatic power—the power of personal magnetism and authority; social power—the power of the role and its authority (Brody). By contrast, the client lacks the power of the role and of its associated training. In addition, female clients facing male professionals generally lack the social power that men have in a sexist context (Lebacqz; Lebacqz and Barton). Clients are vulnerable.

The vulnerability of clients and the power of professionals mean that professionals can take advantage of clients. Sexual relations between professional and client are therefore an abuse of professional power—an illegitimate use of that power for the professional's own ends instead of for the ends of healing the client (Lebacqz and Barton; Schoener et al.; Rutter; Fortune, 1989).

Moreover, the vulnerability of patients or clients and the power gap between client and professional may compromise the freedom needed to give truly informed consent for sexual intimacies (Pope and Bouhoutsos; Lebacqz and Barton). The psychotherapeutic notion of transference (redirecting childhood feelings toward a new object) suggests a special vulnerability that may literally paralyze patients, making them unable to resist a therapist's advances (Freeman and Roy). Noting special vulnerabilities in the sexual arena, Karen Lebacqz and Ronald Barton (1991) propose that sexual intimacies differ from other acts to which patients, clients, and parishioners might continue to consent.

Some argue that vulnerability does not end when therapy ends and that there should be a prohibition on posttherapy sexual contact (Schoener et al.; Rutter). John C. Gonsiorek and Laura S. Brown proposed that sexual relations posttherapy should never be permitted where there was significant transference or where the client was severely disturbed, but might be permitted after two years with former clients who were not disturbed and showed little transference (Gonsiorek and Brown). Such a proposal raises difficult issues regarding who would make this judgment, but it reflects a clear principle that the base for determining whether sexual relations are permissible is the relative power and vulnerability of professional and client. Sexual contact might not be wrong where the power gap is minimized. Although few codes of professional ethics address the posttherapy issue, in 1993, the American Psychiatric Association explicitly addressed it: "Sexual activity with a current or former patient is unethical" (APA).

In a similar vein, Lebacqz and Barton (1991) argue that romantic or sexual relations might be acceptable under circumstances where the power of professional and client is relatively equal and the relationship is under public scrutiny—for example, when clergy date parishioners with whom they are not involved in a pastoral counseling relationship and members of the church are informed.

All commentators agree, however, that "sexualizing … therapy is a betrayal of a trusting relationship" (Pope and Bouhoutsos, p. 54) and that no sexual relationship should be permitted where there is a counseling or therapeutic relationship involved (Pope and Bouhoutsos; Fortune, 1989; Rutter). The professional-client relationship that involves psychotherapy or particular vulnerability on the part of the client is a "forbidden zone" for sexuality (Rutter).

Professional-client sexual contact must be addressed on institutional, not just personal, levels. Professional societies and supporting organizations such as churches are complicit when they fail to punish offenders, try to cover up the problem, blame the victim, and otherwise minimize the issue (Fortune, 1989; Bonavoglia). Underreporting is a significant issue: 65 percent of therapists in one study had seen clients who were sexually abused by a previous therapist; they judged that abuse harmful in 87 percent of cases but reported it in only 8 percent (Schoener et al.). Peter Rutter acknowledges the reluctance of men to blow the whistle on each other (Rutter). Gary Richard Schoener notes that the professional literature "documents more in the way of inaction than of active and creative study leading toward solutions" (Schoener et al.). Professional misconduct damages the profession and institutions as well as individuals (Fortune, 1989). Lack of internal regulation within the professions has led some U.S. state legislatures (e.g., Minnesota) to pass laws that hold institutions as well as individuals responsible for sexual misconduct of professionals (Lebacqz and Barton).

Underlying social and cultural patterns—sexism, the eroticization of domination, and the maldistribution of power in society—are causal factors (Lebacqz and Barton; Rutter). Since Phyllis Chesler's early feminist exposé of therapy in *Women and Madness* (1972), feminists have paid attention to the ways in which traditional therapy often reinforces passive and self-destructive behaviors for women, including behaviors that would make women likely victims of sexual abuse. Dynamics of sexual contact cannot be understood without recognizing sex-role patterning and power imbalances in the general culture (Schoener et al.; Lebacqz and Barton; Brown and Bohn,). Evidence indicates, for example, that male clients may not experience the sexualizing of relationships to be as harmful as female clients do (Pope and Bouhoutsos). Such gender differences may reflect social patterning of male and female sexuality, in which men gain and women lose power when entering a sexual relationship. There is also evidence that women therapists do not engage in sexual contact with clients as frequently as male therapists do, and that they judge it more harmful (Schoener et al.).

The traditional prohibition against sexual contact between professionals and their clients continues to be reaffirmed in spite of arguments and practices to the contrary. An adequate ethical framework requires attention not only to professional responsibility, harm, and power imbalances but also to institutional structures and to cultural dynamics of sexuality and power.

KAREN LEBACQZ (1995)
BIBLIOGRAPHY REVISED

SEE ALSO: *Coercion; Confidentiality; Epidemics; Medicine, Profession of; Nursing, Profession of; Profession and Professional Ethics; Sexual Behavior, Social Control of; Sexual Ethics; Sexual Identity; Sexuality, Legal Approaches to; Public Health Law*

BIBLIOGRAPHY

American Psychological Association. 1981. *Ethical Principles of Psychologists.* Washington, D.C.: Author.

Bonavoglia, Angela. 1992. "The Sacred Secret." *Ms.*, March-April, pp. 40–45.

Brackenridge, Celia. 2001. *Spoilsports: Understanding and Preventing Sexual Exploitation in Sport (Ethics and Sport).* London: Routledge.

Brody, Howard. 1992. *The Healer's Power.* New Haven, CT: Yale University Press.

Brown, Joanne Carlson, and Bohn, Carole R., eds. 1989. *Christianity, Patriarchy, and Abuse: A Feminist Critique.* New York: Pilgrim Press.

Burgess, Ann W., and Hartman, Carol R., eds. 1986. *Sexual Exploitation of Patients by Health Professionals.* New York: Praeger.

Chesler, Phyllis. 1972. *Women and Madness.* New York: Avon Books.

Crain, Karen A., and Heischmidt, Kenneth A. 1995. "Implementing Business Ethics: Sexual Harassment." *Journal of Business Ethics* 14(4): 299–308.

Crouch, Margaret A. 2002. *Thinking about Sexual Harassment: A Guide for the Perplexed.* New York: Oxford University Press.

Davidson, Virginia. 1977. "Psychiatry's Problem with No Name: Therapist-Patient Sex." *American Journal of Psychoanalysis* 37(1): 43–50.

Francis, Leslie Pickering. 2000. *Sexual Harassment as an Ethical Issue in Academic Life.* Totowa, NJ: Rowman and Littlefield.

Fortune, Marie M. 1983. *Sexual Violence: The Unmentionable Sin.* New York: Pilgrim Press.

Fortune, Marie M. 1989. *Is Nothing Sacred? When Sex Invades the Pastoral Relationship.* San Francisco: Harper and Row.

Freeman, Lucy, and Roy, Julie. 1976. *Betrayal: The True Story of the First Woman to Successfully Sue Her Psychiatrist for Using Sex in the Guise of Therapy.* New York: Stein and Day.

Gabbard, Glen O., ed. 1989. *Sexual Exploitation in Professional Relationships.* Washington, D.C.: American Psychiatric Press.

Gonsiorek, John C., and Brown, Laura S. 1989. "Post Therapy Sexual Relationships with Clients." In *Psychotherapists' Sexual Involvement with Clients: Intervention and Prevention,* ed. Gary Richard Schoerer et al. Minneapolis, MN: Walk-in Counseling Center.

Lebacqz, Karen. 1985. *Professional Ethics: Power and Paradox.* Nashville, TN: Abingdon.

Lebacqz, Karen, and Barton, Ronald G. 1991. *Sex in the Parish.* Louisville, KY: Westminster/John Knox.

Masters, William H.; Johnson, Virginia E.; and Kolodny, Robert C., eds. 1977. *Ethical Issues in Sex Therapy and Research.* Boston: Little, Brown.

McLaren, Angus. 2002. *Sexual Blackmail: A Modern History.* Cambridge, MA: Harvard University Press.

National Association of Social Workers. 1980. *Compilation of Public Policy Statements.* Washington, D.C.: Author.

Plasil, Ellen. 1985. *Therapist: The Shocking Autobiography of a Woman Sexually Exploited by Her Analyst.* New York: St. Martin's/Marek.

Pope, Kenneth S., and Bouhoutsos, Jacqueline C. 1986. *Sexual Intimacy between Therapists and Patients.* New York: Praeger.

Ragsdale, Katherine Hancock, ed. 1996. *Boundary Wars: Intimacy and Distance in Healing Relationships.* Cleveland, OH: Pilgrim Press.

Rassieur, Charles L. 1976. *The Problem Clergymen Don't Talk About.* Philadelphia: Westminster.

Rutter, Peter. 1989. *Sex in the Forbidden Zone.* Los Angeles: Jeremy P. Tarcher.

Sanderson, Barbara E., ed. 1989. *It's Never O.K.: A Handbook for Professionals on Sexual Exploitation by Counselors and Therapists.* St. Paul: Minnesota Department of Corrections.

Schoener, Gary Richard; Milgram, Jeanette Hofstee; Gonsiorek, John C.; Luepker, Ellen T.; and Conroe, Ray M. 1989. *Psychotherapists' Sexual Involvement with Clients: Intervention and Prevention.* Minneapolis, MN.: Walk-in Counseling Center.

Shepard, Martin. 1971. *The Love Treatment: Sexual Intimacy between Patients and Psychotherapists.* New York: Peter H. Wyden.

Verhey, Allen. 1987. "The Doctor's Oath—and a Christian Swearing It." In *On Moral Medicine: Theological Perspectives in Medical Ethics,* pp. 72–82, eds. Stephen E. Lammers and Allen Verhey. Grand Rapids, MI: William B. Eerdmans.

SEXUAL IDENTITY

• • •

Because some terms are deeply embroiled in controversial debates, the task of defining them itself becomes controversial. So it is with the term *sexual identity.* Providing any definition immediately situates the definer within a particular perspective. One important perspective, which has served as the backdrop of much contemporary discussion, claims that the term refers to the distinct biological types of *male* and *female.* This "traditionalist" definition of sexual identity has sometimes been associated with one or more of the following additional positions: that certain specific and "complementary" psychological attributes and social roles, specifically those of *masculinity* and *femininity,* correspond to each of these distinct biological types; that a "natural" sexual attraction exists between these two biological types; that this attraction is most naturally satisfied through the act of intercourse; and that the act of intercourse, while naturally motivated by attraction, should also be motivated by other concerns, most importantly by love and by the desire to have children within the context of marriage.

These claims have been challenged over the last few decades by feminists, by those advocating various forms of sexual liberation, by gays and lesbians, and by scholars. All of these challenges raise questions about what is meant by *sexual identity.* Some of the positions developed in response to the traditionalist set of views have themselves been challenged. For the sake of clarity, one can group the challenges and counterchallenges around the following set of questions:

1. The sex question: Are there really two distinct biological types, *male* and *female*?
2. The gender question: How should one think about the relationship between biology and psychological attributes and forms of behavior?
3. The sexuality question: What constitutes sexual desire? What are the various ways in which it can be characterized?
4. The sexual ethics question: How ought one think about sexual practices? Which, if any, should be condoned, which prohibited, and why?

The Sex Question

Over the past few decades, many have rejected the claim that there exist two sexes without gradations. Some feminists have argued that, biologically, it is more useful to think of many of the physical characteristics associated with sexual difference as manifested across the human species in a range of degrees, rather than as being associated exclusively with either sex. They claim that only a social desire to emphasize difference has caused us to think of such variations in stark, bipolar ways. Thus, for example, though one often thinks of men as physically bigger than women, many individual women are taller, heavier, longer limbed, and so forth, than many men. Similarly, while one tends to think of women and men as possessing very distinctive hormones, in actuality the situation is more complex. For example, the hormones estrogen and androgen are often thought of as the "female" and "male" hormones, respectively, suggesting that women have one and men the other. In reality, both hormones are found in both women and men, and after menopause, women often exhibit a lower ratio of estrogen to androgen than do men of a comparable age (Spanier). These feminists argue that many of the striking differences we see are at least partially the consequence of social pressures exerted on women and men to manifest such differences. Thus women are encouraged to remove body hair and to buy shoes that make their feet look as small as possible.

Some cultural historians claim that the view of men and women as possessing sharply differentiated bodies has developed only within the last few centuries. Thomas Laqueur, for example, points out that prior to the eighteenth century, women's bodies were thought of as less developed versions of men's bodies. In this *one-sex* view, the vagina was not thought of as different from the male penis but, rather, as an inverted form of it. But during the eighteenth century there emerged a view of *the two-sex body,* that is, of female and male bodies being fundamentally different. With this new development, organs that had previously been referred to by the same name were given separate names. Thus, what had previously been *the testicles* now became differentiated into *the testicles* and *the ovaries.* Others that previously had no name were given names, for example, the vagina. Even parts of the body remote from reproductive functions, such as the skeleton and the nervous system, began to be depicted as distinctive for women and men.

Recent research in biology suggests that differentiating the male from the female is no simple task. Various indicators of maleness and femaleness are individually sometimes ambiguous. Even when all of the indicators are clear, they do not necessarily cohere. For example, within contemporary science the standard distinguishing criterion has been taken to be the presence or absence of the Y chromosome. Most people possess two sets of chromosomes, one from each parent; females are understood to be those with two X chromosomes and males those with one X chromosome and one Y chromosome. However, there are problems with any neat application of this criterion. Some individuals inherit only one X chromosome but no Y chromosome. Or a piece of a Y chromosome may become attached to an X chromosome, producing an individual with an XXY pattern.

Even those individuals who possess a standard XX or XY pattern may exhibit characteristics that would incline many not to identify them by their chromosomal pattern. An XY individual may have testes that do not secrete the male hormone testosterone, or may have cells that are not sensitive to testosterone. That person will end up looking more like a female than a male (Lowenstein). There are also XY individuals who look female at birth and are raised as girls, but who develop masculine bodily features at adolescence. There are XX people whose adrenal glands secrete large amounts of male hormones. One consequence is clitoral enlargement, causing them to be taken for boys at birth. As adults they may also possess increased muscle mass and hairiness (Lowenstein). In short, recent scientific research has supported the point that even the biological distinction between male and female is not always clear-cut.

The Gender Question

Until the emergence of the second wave of feminism in the 1960s, the term *gender* was used primarily to indicate differences between female and male forms within language. Differences between women and men were commonly indicated by the term *sex,* as in the phrase "the battle of the sexes." Feminists, however, began to use the term *gender* to refer to what they argued were socially constructed differences between women and men. It was felt that the term *sex,* when applied to differences between women and men, suggested that such differences were biological in origin. A new term was needed to refer to differences that were a product of society.

Studies done within the social sciences pointed to the great differences among societies in expectations of what was appropriate behavior for men and women. For example, the anthropologist Michelle Zimbalist Rosaldo noted that there are some societies where women trade or garden, and others where men do; some where men are prudish or flirtatious, and others where women are (Rosaldo, Lamphere, and Bamberger). Psychologists and other social scientists stressed the importance of socialization in structuring an individual's sense of self. Thus, John Money and Anke Ehrhardt (1972) asserted that when children were assigned a gender at birth that did not match their chromosomal sex, it was most likely that their adult sense of self would conform to their assigned gender rather than to their chromosomal sex.

The term *gender* has been very useful in encouraging a greater recognition of the social construction of differences between women and men. Increasingly, however, scholars have been raising questions about how gender should be understood, and particularly how its relationship to sex should be interpreted. Using the term *sex* to describe biological differences, and *gender* to describe socially constructed ones—what R. W. Connell calls the "two realms model"—ignores the fact that biological distinctions are themselves social constructions, at least in part. That modern biology, for example, interprets the penis as an organ distinct from the vagina is a social construction, more a consequence of changing cultural metaphors than of new scientific evidence (Laqueur). The notion of a "pre-social sexed body" (Heyes) which is identifiable in purely biological terms, then, has lost much of its appeal. As a result, the distinction between gender and sex based on the categories of the social and the biological respectively has also lost its force and theorists are struggling with what Connell calls "an additive conception of sex and gender." As she explains, "our new model begins with the observation that human bodies are active players in social lives. They are neither biological machines producing social effects mechanically, nor blank pages on which cultural messages are written" (Connell, p. 463).

Another problem with emphasizing the difference between sex and gender is that the relationship between psychological traits and biological phenomena is still often understood to be that the former follows from the latter. While *gender* emphasizes that many psychological traits are social constructions, it does not necessarily undermine the view that such traits follow from biological differences. All it adds is that the path from biology to psychology proceeds by way of social construction.

Any model that claims that psychology follows from biology has problems accounting for those individuals whose socialization deviates from the norm. In other words, to the extent that gender is still viewed as tied to sex, there remains the problem of explaining the phenomena of girls who grow up exhibiting "masculine" psychological traits and boys who grow up with a "feminine" sense of self. The most striking examples of such cases are transsexuals, people who experience a dramatic misalignment between their physical features and their internalized sense of self. Such people frequently desire physical restructuring of their bodies to bring the physical and the psychic into alignment.

The term *gender* may still suggest, as did the term *sex,* that people's psychic lives and behavior are necessarily unified, that it is appropriate to talk about a male or a female identity. One suggestion has been that we talk about *gender* be used not to describe individual identity, but to describe acts or performances all humans play out (Butler). Such a model allows one to move the focus of *gender* from the individual to the activity. This type of shift is consistent with an overall tendency on the part of many contemporary scholars to think of gender as a type of social coding that is applied not only to behavior but also to psychic stances and to bodies. A further aspect of this notion of social coding is suggested by Jan Clausen, who describes her experience when she changed from a committed lesbian to a woman involved in a long-term exclusive relationship with a man. Clausen claims that "the notion of sexual identity ... implies some expectation about the future" (pp. 97–98); the inclusive approach—that which covers behavior, psychology and the materiality of the body—thus extends over time as well.

The Sexuality Question

At least since the 1890s in industrialized Western countries, one paradigm of sexuality has been dominant: that which describes genital-to-genital intercourse between one male and one female as "normal," and as "abnormal" or "perverse," sexual practices that fall outside that paradigm. "Perverse" practices in this paradigm include but are not limited to the following: voyeurism; exhibitionism; incest (sex between close relatives); oral sex; anal sex; sex with children (pedophilia); sex involving more than two persons; sex between humans and animals (zoophilia); sex with oneself (masturbation); sex involving the use of visual images (pornography); sex with a corpse (necrophilia); sex involving heightening sexual pleasure by dressing in garments associated with the opposite sex (transvestism); sex associated with the giving or experiencing of pain or humiliation (sadomasochism); sex strongly associated with a particular object or part of the body (fetishism); and sex between members of the same sex (homosexuality).

Homosexuality has, in particular, been the subject of much attention and debate. The stigmatizing label *homosexual* has been used to negatively characterize certain individuals since the late nineteenth century (Weeks, 1989); laws have been enacted against homosexuality and people have been jailed for practicing it (e.g., the English playwright Oscar Wilde). During the twentieth century, medical doctors and other scientific specialists have depicted it as a pathology and, as with other pathologies (but not accepted practices), have searched for causes (Bayer).

Much debate has centered on the question of whether homosexuality is a product of genetic inheritance or some other biological trait, or is a consequence of socialization. During the 1960s and 1970s, homosexual men (who increasingly adopted the label *gay*) and homosexual women (lesbians) began to form political organizations to resist the laws, practices, and beliefs that stigmatized them. They

argued that homosexuality was not a perversion or a pathology to be outlawed or cured, but a difference in preference or *orientation* that should be tolerated within a free and open society. Since the 1960s, the American psychiatric community has moved away from a description of homosexuality as pathology. In December 1973, the board of trustees of the American Psychiatric Association moved to delete the category *homosexuality* as necessarily a pathology from the second edition of the *Diagnostic and Statistical Manual of Psychiatric Disorders,* retaining the term *ego dystonic homosexuality* to cover those not comfortable with their sexual orientation. In yet another revision, any specific reference to homosexuality was removed altogether, but the term *sexual orientation distress* was retained to permit treatment of those disturbed about their sexuality (Bayer).

More recently, there has been a good deal of interest in studying the possible biological origins or causes of homosexuality. There are two major explanatory pictures, both of which have been variously received with skepticism and approval. The first is the anatomical approach, which claims that one can (or should be able to) find structural differences between heterosexuals and homosexuals. Simon LeVay, for instance, published a study in 1991 showing that the interstitial nuclei of the anterior hypothalamus (INAH) of homosexual men was on average significantly smaller than those of heterosexual men (Murphy). Other candidates for anatomical explanations include the anterior commissure and the suprachiasmatic nucleus (Hamer, 1993). None of these studies have been met with unmixed approval. Some criticisms of the anatomical approach include the claim that sexual orientation is far too complex a phenomenon to be mapped to a single (and seemingly simple) physical cause, concern over the size of the sample pools, and even the attempt to "explain" homosexuality at all (Murphy).

The other possible explanatory story is that of the so-called gay gene. In 1993, Dean Hamer and a team of scientists concluded a study of the genetic make-up of gay men and their family members (most importantly brothers who were also gay) and announced that "our data indicate a statistically significant correlation between the inheritance of genetic markers on chromosomal region Xq28 and sexual orientation in a group of homosexual males" (Hamer, Hu, Magnuson, et al., p. 321). This study has also been criticized: for instance, the demographic homogeneity (and size) of the subject pool has led some to question whether the correlation is really genetic or merely environmental (Kaplan). This concern is made even more problematic by the fact that a precise causal connection between the possession of specific genetic markers and homosexual orientation is still lacking (Murphy). Most disturbing about any attempt to establish a biological link to homosexuality, according to some theorists, is the very fact that alternative sexual orientations are *in need of* explanation. In other words, the research itself may imply that there is something abnormal, or indeed perverse, about such orientations and thus, something that needs "curing" (Kaplan).

Other questions have been added to the debate, among them whether homosexuality describes a particular kind of person or, more appropriately, a specific type of activity. Social historians have pointed out that the category "the homosexual" was constructed in the latter part of the nineteenth century to depict a specific type of person, followed shortly by the construction of "the heterosexual" (Katz; Halperin). Prior to the creation of "the homosexual," people who engaged in acts one would label as homosexual were not necessarily seen to require a special label. This is at least partially a consequence of the fact that the sex of one's partner has not always been viewed as an overriding feature of the sex act. For example, within many Native American societies, certain men, "the berdache," took on many of the tasks and characteristics associated with women. These men would have sex with other men. However, what was seen as distinguishing the sexual practices of the berdache was not that they had sex with other men but that they took the passive role in sex. Their male partners were not distinguished from men who had sex only with women (Williams). The same distinction between active and passive (or dominant and submissive) is believed by many to be the primary form of categorization of sexuality in ancient Greece (Stein; Kaplan). For such reasons, Eve Sedgwick has observed that, given the many dimensions along which genital activity can be described, it is quite amazing that the sex of object choice has emerged as central during the twentieth century, and has come to define what is meant by "sexual orientation" (Sedgwick).

The Sexual Ethics Question

Just as matters of individual sexual identity have been oversimplified into a single male-female dichotomy, the many varieties of sexual behavior have often been reduced to a simple distinction between normality and perversion.

The condemnation of homosexuality and other deviant sexual activities and "perversions" leads to a discussion of sexual ethics and to the question of alternative sexual paradigms. A paradigm is an exemplary instance that serves as a standard. A sexual paradigm is an example of sexual activity that is taken as a standard for "normal" sexual behavior. The most obvious sexual paradigm is heterosexual genital-to-genital intercourse, but in order to employ this paradigm as a norm, one needs to specify not only the overt activity but the aims and desires of the participants. Is the

purpose of sexual intercourse, for example, to produce children? Or to produce pleasure? Or to express love? Or to mark a "conquest"? One can further distinguish between minimalist and murky paradigms of sexuality: minimalist accounts tend to define sexuality as a simple, straightforward desire, while murky accounts dig deeper in order to find hidden or unconscious desires. Thomas Nagel, for example, introduces the minimalist notion of "unadorned sexual intercourse," although he adds that such behavior, "unadorned," may well be perverse, and that a typical sexual encounter involves a complex of communicative gestures. Janice Moulton defines sexuality simply as the desire for physical contact, although she then provides a rich discussion of its many associated meanings. Alan Goldman isolates what he calls "plain sex," which he defines as "a desire for contact with another's body," and rejects accounts that try to define sexuality in terms of any further goal or purpose.

On the murky side, there is the lasting legacy of Plato's *Symposium* and its various discussions of eros. In particular, there is Aristophanes' famous tale about the divine fission of individual human beings out of complete wholes, according to which sexual desire is nothing less than the impossible desire to join together with "one's other half" and become "complete once again," and Socrates' much more effete conception of eros as the love of Beauty as such. Two thousand years of Christian theology have attempted both to chastise and to spiritualize sexuality, and the Tantric traditions of India and Tibet have refined sexuality into a spiritual road to enlightenment. In the twentieth century, Sigmund Freud and Carl Jung profoundly deepened conceptions of sexuality, which is, in their accounts, no mere desire but a focus for the darkest and most explosive secrets of the psyche.

THE REPRODUCTIVE PARADIGM. Biologically, sexuality can be defined in terms of a very specific genetic process, although even that has its ambiguities and confusions. This biological definition and its implied reproductive paradigm play an enormous role in contemporary conceptions of sexuality. Whatever embellishments, variations, and alternatives humans and some other vertebrates have evolved or invented, heterosexual intercourse remains something of an "original text" in our sexual hermeneutics. It can be rejected, refuted, even reviled, but it must, first of all, be taken account of.

One might distinguish here, in line with a three-thousand-year-old moral tradition, between an individual's purpose and what one might call *nature's purpose.* Until the end of the nineteenth century, when teleology or the purposiveness of nature was taken seriously, this phrase could be interpreted literally. In the twenty-first century, in the wake of increasingly antiteleological conceptions of evolution, the phrase *nature's purpose* must be taken as, at best, shorthand for a complex set of causal processes that are themselves the result of chance and natural selection. Even so, one might distinguish between the various drives and desires favored by natural selection because they increase the likelihood of a more adaptive genotype (what Richard Dawkins calls "the selfish gene"), and the more or less conscious and sometimes articulate desires of an adult human being. But humans are not, like most creatures, mere sexual pawns of cunning nature. Some teenagers may not know of the various consequences and the significance of sexual activity, but for most adults this knowledge is profound, if not extensive, and sexuality may never be free of those associations. But whether or not this is the hidden purpose of *all* sexual desire and activity, it is clearly the conscious and conscientious choice of *some* sexual activity. Building a family is not, for most people, the only purpose of sexual activity; but by having sexual intercourse, it is possible to have children. Whatever creative alternatives may be dreamed up by medicine, one undeniable aspect of sexuality is, and will be, its traditional role in procreation.

The view that sexuality and sexual desire are really aimed at reproduction, even if the sexual participants desire only to perform a particular activity without thinking of the consequences, tends to lead from the minimalist view of sexuality to various murky views. The self-evident desires are no longer taken at face value, and a deeper biological (or theological) narrative, which may not be self-evident to the participants, comes into play. Thus the psychological consequences of thousands or millions of years of evolution manifest themselves in desires that may seem straightforward. Or, behind seemingly simple sexual desire lurks the secret of God's creation and the biblical injunction to be fruitful and multiply. But what links all the murky views is that sexuality does have a purpose or purposes, however they are to be explained, and these purposes are typically not self-evident. According to the minimalist views, sex is best understood as "plain" or "unembellished"; the murky views, on the other hand, insist that sex so understood is not understood at all.

The target of many, if not most, of the minimalist accounts is the restricted reproduction of the procreative paradigm of sexual activity. For two thousand years, the harsher side of Biblical commentary and the Christian theological tradition has insisted that sex is primarily, if not solely, procreative. In this view, the pleasures and desires associated with sexual activity not only are inessential but also are to be minimized. Emphasizing pleasure to the exclusion of the possibility of reproduction—for example, using contraception or engaging in activity that cannot result in impregnation—is forbidden. Essential to sexuality, in the reproductive paradigm, are male ejaculation, female receptivity, fertility, and conception.

THE PLEASURE PARADIGM. In opposition to the reproductive model, with all of its strict prohibitions and limitations, and its suggestions of deep biological drives and purposes, the attractiveness of what one can call the pleasure paradigm is unmistakable. The availability of improved birth control methods since the 1960s has contributed greatly to its appeal. Sex is for pleasure, and what is desired is pleasure. There is nothing murky about this. Indeed, to many people the pleasure paradigm is self-evident. Accordingly, the restrictions on sexuality that limit and direct it toward heterosexual intercourse drop away, and in effect, anything that feels good is acceptable. Of course, one might well object that pleasure is not in itself sexual, and so one might want to circumscribe pleasures that are sexual from those that are not. But, for the defender of the pleasure paradigm, this requirement comes later. First comes the liberation from the restrictions of the reproductive model. Homosexuality, autosexuality, even bestiality seem to be normal on the pleasure paradigm. Heterosexual intercourse is but one of many activities serving the paradigm, and however many couples may continue to prefer it, it does not have any special claim to normality. According to this paradigm, good sex is that which provides maximum mutual pleasure; bad or mediocre sex is that which fails to satisfy either or both partners.

Once the reproduction model has been rejected, there are no longer the restrictions on either the objects or the obvious aims of sexual activity, but neither is it the case that "anything goes." Homosexuality is no longer a perversion of sex, but rape certainly will be. Almost any sexual activity between consenting adults is acceptable, but forcing sex on a person is not. Sexual activities that will not result in conception are no longer secondary, and sex that is conscientiously prevented from resulting in undesired conception becomes the norm. Masturbation becomes part of the paradigm of acceptable sexuality, even though its lacks the dimension of shared sexual enjoyment. The appeal of the paradigm and the cornerstone of most contemporary sexual ethics is the idea that sex ought to be pleasurable and, within moral but not particularly sexual bounds, unrestricted.

We might call the pleasure paradigm the *Freudian* model of sexuality, in order to pay homage to the person most responsible for its contemporary dominance. Sigmund Freud, in his *Three Contributions to the Theory of Sex,* argued that sexuality should be conceived as enjoyable for its own sake, not as a means to further ends, whether natural or divine. But the centrality of Freud here also suggests that the pleasure paradigm may not be so simple and self-evident as originally suggested: Freud is one of the great contemporary architects of "deep," if not labyrinthine, accounts of the psyche and of sexuality in particular. And so, for him and for us, pleasure and satisfaction are not to be construed so straightforwardly. Pleasure, as Aristotle noted more than two millennia ago, is not just a sensation. It is the "bloom" on successful activity. It accompanies but does not constitute satisfaction. But the difficult question is, Satisfaction of what? And here Freud's theory moves from an apparently minimalist physiological model to an extremely murky deep psychology.

In Freud's early theories, the pleasure paradigm rested on a male-dominated biological foundation, a *discharge* model in which sexual pleasure has its origins in the release of tension (catharsis). But the tensions released in sexual behavior are not merely physiological; they also arise from complexes of ego needs and identifications with various sexual "objects," usually (but not always) other people. Thus Freud distinguished between mere physical gratification and *physical satisfaction.*

The pleasure paradigm, for all of its seeming simplicity, invites murky interpretations. What is it that is enjoyed? What is it that is satisfied? A sensation is not pleasant in itself but in terms of its context, as a love bite on the shoulder by one's lover or a nasty passerby, respectively, makes evident. Indeed, even orgasm is not pleasant in itself, however often that might be fallaciously supposed; an orgasm in an inappropriate context is typically an extremely unpleasant experience. And so the pleasure Freud postulates is no simple release of tension but the satisfaction, often symbolic and indirect, of some of the murkiest of hidden and forbidden desires.

THE METAPHYSICAL PARADIGM. Some of these desires and motives are so profound that they deserve to be called *metaphysical.* Freud's discussion of the Oedipus complex sometimes takes on these ontological overtones, and Jung's various archetype theories surely do. But perhaps the most basic of all metaphysical paradigms of sexuality goes back (at least) to the fable told by Aristophanes in Plato's *Symposium,* and the idea that the gods split what we now call human beings out of complete wholes, with sexual desire being the desire to reunify the divided halves. One need not literally accept the more consciously absurd aspects of the story to appreciate the deep insight captured in the idea of "two out of one" or "merged selves" that Plato's Aristophanes suggested.

Sexual activity is an expression of a profound desire that has very little to do with merely physiological need or satisfaction, and the metaphysical paradigm is, accordingly, very much a part of the contemporary conceptions of romantic love and the idea that two people were "made for each other."

Indeed, despite the prevalence of the pleasure model in much of the current literature, there can be little doubt that much more is usually demanded of sexuality than mere pleasure, even mutual pleasure. People demand *meaningful* relationships. The metaphysical model provides this sense of *meaning.* Pleasure, according to the metaphysical model, is no longer the purpose of sex, although it will surely appear as its accompaniment. But sex without love, no matter how enjoyable, is to be rejected on this paradigm. Even if it is not "perverse" or "immoral," "plain sex" will be meaningless, and the meaning of a relationship is primary in the metaphysical model.

THE COMMUNICATION PARADIGM. Sex is often "meaningful" without love, however, although sometimes those "meanings" are demeaning, as in a sadomasochistic relationship. What is one to say of the many varieties of sexual activity that are aimed neither at reproduction, nor at pure pleasure, nor at expressions of romantic love and togetherness? What of those relationships that seem to thrive on domination and pain? What does it say about current paradigms of love that sadomasochistic relationships are now celebrated and preferred by some of our more avant-garde social visionaries? And what of those many tender encounters that, nonetheless, make no pretenses of love?

To explain such aspects of sexuality, a fourth paradigm is in order: sex as communication, as a physical form of expression of one's emotions and attitudes toward other people. It is a language, for the most part a body language, whose vocabulary consists of touches, gestures, and physical positions. It may be an expression of domination and submission; it may be an expression of respect, fear, tenderness, anger, admiration, worship, concern, or (of course) love. In the 1940s Jean-Paul Sartre defended a truncated version of this model in his classic *Being and Nothingness.* He interpreted all sexuality as the expression of conflict, a war for domination and freedom. But what is communicated in sex is rarely this alone, nor is sex plausibly always an expression of conflict. Nevertheless, Sartre forces us to see something that the defenders of the pleasure and metaphysical paradigms of sex prefer not to see: that sexual relationships, even normal, fully consensual sexual relationships, are not always innocent or loving. Sex is a medium for all sorts of emotions, some of them manipulative and even malicious.

The communication paradigm shifts the emphasis in sexuality from the more physical and sensual aspects of reproduction and pleasure to interpersonal roles and attitudes, and from expressions of love alone to expressions of all emotions and attitudes. Thus Sartre's model is clearly a communication model, but it is, like Sartre's view of emotions in general, too narrow, emphasizing only the more conflict-ridden and competitive interpersonal attitudes— one of which, he thinks, is love. In this view, certain sexual activities are visibly more expressive of domination and submission, or equality and respect, or resentment and fear, or shyness and timidity. According to the communication model, these nonverbal expressions are essential to sexuality, its very purpose and content. This does not mean, however, that other sexual aspects need be excluded. The intention to impregnate a woman, for example, may be an expression of male domination and conquest, as described in several of Norman Mailer's novels. Pleasure is an important aspect of the communication model, but pleasure for its own sake is not: pleasure—both the giving and the receiving of it, as well as the sharing of it—is vital to the communication of many emotions. But pain may be important as well, and inflicting small amounts of pain, as well as enduring moderate discomfort, is familiar as a means of expression in sex. What distinguishes the communication paradigm from the three more traditional ones is its emphasis on expression of interpersonal emotions and attitudes. These expressions are recognized by the other paradigms, but not as essential and primary.

IMPLICATIONS OF THE VARIOUS SEXUAL PARADIGMS. It is evident that the answers to such questions as "What is normal sex?" and "What is perverse?" are immensely complicated. On a strict reproduction paradigm of sexuality, normal sex is whatever minimal genital activity is necessary to promote conception. All else is either irrelevant or immoral. In fact, of course, the reproduction paradigm is usually defended within the moral institution of marriage, and rarely defended without some reference to both love and mutual pleasure. On the pleasure paradigm, by contrast, whatever gives pleasure (to consenting adults) is normal and acceptable. Perversions of this paradigm provide pain instead of pleasure, ignore the pleasure of the other person, or produce pleasure in a manner that is, in the longer run, harmful. On the metaphysical paradigm, normality is sex as an expression of mutual meaningfulness, such as mutual love. On the communication paradigm, what is normal becomes extremely complex, for one must view the emotions being expressed and the entire psyches of the people involved to make any intelligent judgment.

Human sexuality seems particularly appropriate for expressing the tender feelings of love and affection, but there are circumstances under which this is absolutely inappropriate (for example, with children); and all too often sexual activity that claims the expression of love as its aim may actually be an avoidance of intimacy. Indeed, the common context of sexual activity— two people alone, attending only to one another—is particularly conducive to intimate communication. But if we take two-party sex as our paradigm, then multiple-party sex, insofar as it confuses the communication becomes perversion. Moreover, masturbation, while not exactly perverse, would surely be less than wholly sexual, just as talking to oneself is less than a whole conversation. And perhaps, any form of deceit would be perverse, just as lying is a "perversion" of verbal communication.

Conclusion: The Problem of Normality

So long as biological specification and sexual intercourse alone define sexuality, *normality,* as opposed to *perversion,* seems to be easily defined. Males are equipped with certain obvious features, and females are differently equipped with equally obvious sexual features; *normal* sex is intercourse between male and female. But as more is learned about the complexities of chromosome configuration and the biology of sex, the distinction between male and female becomes increasingly difficult. And as soon as one adds the essential concerns of psychology and the many worlds of cultural norms, practices, and paradigms to the unfolding medical complications, the traditional view of *normality* becomes a Pandora's box of problems.

This confusion extends to the task of defining a *normal* model of sexuality. Of the various cases and models considered in this article, not a single one would be accepted as *normal* in every society and by everyone. Moreover, a pure instance of an ideal type or paradigm is probably nowhere to be found; not even the most pious proponent of a religiously oriented reproductive view would deny the desirability of love, pleasure, and emotional expression in sex, nor would the most enthusiastic hedonist deny the desirability of reproduction on at least some occasions, and perhaps of love and communication as well. And when these four paradigms of sexuality are integrated with the matrix of possibilities that are to be found in the various combinations of gender identity and sexual orientation (and, in the most extreme cases, transsexual biological operations), the result is an enormous number of sexual lifestyles, desires, and activities, every one of which would be insisted upon as *normal,* at least according to some people.

How does one decide what is normal and what is not? In one sense, *normal* simply means *statistically predominant,* and there are still many people who would insist that this is a proper definition. But it is clear that, in ethical contexts, *normal* also means *morally correct.* But in an area where most behavior is private, and involves only consenting adults and a great many individual differences, the relevance of statistics is easily challenged. Furthermore, what is statistically predominant in one portion of a population may be relatively rare and considered *perverted* in another. If sexual normality includes subjective preferences and psychological as well as biological considerations, then any definition of sexual normality will give priority to certain preferences and paradigms over others. But which ones? The traditional religious standards? The more modern "anything goes between consenting adults" attitude? The current "local standards" criterion of the courts, which assumes that it can be made clear how large or small a domain—a home, a town, or a state—is "local"?

The problem of normality thus becomes a dilemma. It begins with a built-in ambiguity between the statistically dominant and what ethically ought to be. The first is ascertained easily enough, assuming either truthful informants or extremely intrusive investigators; but the second, the quest for a sexual ethics, arises from within diverse psychological, cultural, and personal settings that presuppose many of the norms and attitudes that are to be investigated.

The result of these complexities should not be the abandonment of a search for ethical norms or the rejection of the concepts of normality and perversion. What emerges instead is an extremely complex matrix of considerations to be taken into account, in which tolerance is a wise approach and mutual understanding is the desirable outcome. In other words, what is needed in the examination of sexual identity is not just a good deal of medicine, biology, social psychology, and anthropology. It is also a good deal of appreciation for diversity and complexity. It is with this appreciation for diversity and complexity that the contemporary quest can proceed.

ROBERT C. SOLOMON
LINDA J. NICHOLSON (1995)
REVISED BY ROBERT C. SOLOMON
JENNIFER K. GREENE

SEE ALSO: *Body; Gender Identity; Genetic Discrimination; Homosexuality; Human Nature; Sexual Ethics*

BIBLIOGRAPHY

Appiah, K. Anthony. 1994. "Identity, Authenticity, Survival: Multicultural Societies and Social Reproduction." In *Multiculturalism,* ed. Amy Gutmann. Princeton, NJ: Princeton University Press.

Baker, Robert, and Elliston, Frederick, eds. 1975. *Philosophy and Sex.* Buffalo, NY: Prometheus.

Bayer, Ronald. 1981 (reprint 1987). *Homosexuality and American Psychiatry: The Politics of Diagnosis.* Princeton, NJ: Princeton University Press.

Bene, Eva. 1965. "On the Genesis of Female Homosexuality." *British Journal of Psychiatry* 111: 815–821.

Bene, Eva. 1965. "On the Genesis of Male Homosexuality: An Attempt at Clarifying the Role of the Parents." *British Journal of Psychiatry* 111: 803–813.

Bieber, Irving; Dain, Harvey J.; Dince, Paul R.; et al. 1962. *Homosexuality: A Psychoanalytic Study.* New York: Basic Books.

Butler, Judith. 1990. *Gender Trouble: Feminism and the Subversion of Identity.* New York: Routledge.

Clausen, Jan. 1999. *Apples and Oranges: My Journey through Sexual Identity.* Boston: Houghton Mifflin Company.

Connell, R.W. 1999. "Making Gendered People: Bodies, Identities, Sexualities." In *Revisioning Gender,* ed. Myra Marx Ferree, Judith Lorber, and Beth B. Hess. Thousand Oaks, CA: Sage Publications.

Dawkins, Richard. 1976. *The Selfish Gene.* New York: Oxford University Press.

Ferree, Myra Marx; Lorber, Judith; and Hess, Beth B., eds. 1999. *Revisioning Gender.* Thousand Oaks, CA: Sage Publications.

Freud, Sigmund. 1962. *Three Contributions to the Theory of Sex.* New York: Dutton.

Gagnon, John H., and Simon, William. 1973. *Sexual Conduct: The Social Sources of Human Sexuality.* Chicago: Aldine.

Goldman, Alan. 1977. "Plain Sex." *Philosophy & Public Affairs* 6(3): 267–287.

Greene, Richard. 1974. *Sexual Identity Conflict in Children and Adults.* New York: Basic Books.

Halperin, David M. 1990. *One Hundred Years of Homosexuality.* New York: Routledge.

Hamer, D.H.; Hu, S.; Magnuson, V.L.; Hu, N.; et al. 1993. "A Linkage Between DNA Markers on the X Chromosome and Male Sexual Orientation." *Science* 261: 321–327.

Hamer, Dean, and Copeland, Peter. 1994. *The Science of Desire: The Search for the Gay Gene and the Biology of Behavior.* New York: Simon & Schuster.

Heyes, Cressida J. 2000. *Line Drawing: Defining Women through Feminist Practice.* Ithaca, NY: Cornell University Press.

Hubbard, Ruth. 1990. *The Politics of Women's Biology.* New Brunswick, NJ: Rutgers University Press.

Jaggar, Alison. 1983. *Feminist Politics and Human Nature.* Totowa, NJ: Rowman and Allanheld.

Kaplan, Jonathan Michael. 2000. *The Limits and Lies of Human Genetic Research: Dangers for Social Policy.* New York: Routledge.

Katz, Jonathan. 1983. *Gay/Lesbian Almanac: A New Documentary.* New York: Harper and Row.

Ketchum, Sara Ann. 1980. "The Good, the Bad and the Perverted: Sexual Paradigms Revisited." In *Philosophy of Sex:*

Contemporary Readings, ed. Alan Soble. Totowa, NJ: Littlefield Adams.

Kinsey, Alfred Charles; Pomeroy, Wardell; and Martin, Clyde E. 1948. *Sexual Behavior in the Human Male.* Philadelphia: W. B. Saunders.

Kohlberg, Lawrence. 1966. "A Cognitive-Developmental Analysis of Children's Sex-Role Concepts and Attitudes." In *The Development of Sex Differences,* ed. Eleanor E. Maccoby. Stanford, CA: Stanford University Press.

Kolodny, Robert C.; Masters, William H.; Hendryx, Julie; and Toro, Gelson. 1971. "Plasma Testosterone and Semen Analysis in Male Homosexuals." *New England Journal of Medicine* 285: 1170–1174.

Laqueur, Thomas. 1990. *Making Sex: Body and Gender from the Greeks to Freud.* Cambridge, MA: Harvard University Press.

Levay, Simon. 1991. "A Difference in Hypothalamic Structure Between Heterosexual and Homosexual Men." *Science* 253: 1034–1037.

Lowenstein, Jerold M. 1987. "The Conundrum of Gender Identification: Two Sexes Are Not Enough." *Pacific Discovery* 40(2): 38–39.

Maccoby, Eleanor Emmons, and Jacklin, Carol Nagy. 1974. *The Psychology of Sex Differences.* Stanford, CA: Stanford University Press.

Mead, Margaret. 1935. *Sex and Temperament in Three Primitive Societies.* New York: William Morrow.

Mischel, Walter. 1970. "Sex-Typing and Socialization." In *Carmichael's Manual of Child Psychology,* vol. 2, 3rd edition, ed. Paul H. Mussen. New York: Wiley.

Money, John, and Ehrhardt, Anke A. 1972. *Man and Woman, Boy and Girl: The Differentiation and Dimorphism of Gender Identity from Conception to Maturity.* Baltimore: Johns Hopkins University Press.

Money, John, and Tucker, Patricia. 1975. *Sexual Signatures: On Being a Man or a Woman.* Boston: Little, Brown.

Money, John; Hampson, Joan G.; and Hampson, John L. 1955. "Hermaphroditism: Recommendations Concerning Assignment of Sex, Change of Sex, and Psychologic Management." *Bulletin of the Johns Hopkins Hospital* 97: 284–300.

Moulton, Janice. 1976. "Sexual Behavior: Another Position." *Journal of Philosophy* 73(16): 537–546.

Murphy, Timothy F. 1997. *Gay Science: The Ethics of Sexual Orientation Research.* New York: Columbia University Press.

Nagel, Thomas. 1969. "Sexual Perversion." *Journal of Philosophy* 66(1): 5–17.

Nicholson, Linda. 1986. *Gender and History: The Limits of Social Theory in the Age of the Family.* New York: Columbia University Press.

Offer, Daniel, and Sabshin, Melvin. 1966. *Normality: Theoretical and Clinical Concepts of Mental Health.* New York: Basic Books.

Offer, Daniel, and Sabshin, Melvin, eds. 1984. *Normality and the Life Cycle: A Critical Integration.* New York: Basic Books.

Rosaldo, Michelle Zimbalist; Lamphere, Louise; and Bamberger, Joan, eds. 1974. *Woman, Culture, and Society.* Stanford, CA: Stanford University Press.

Rose, Robert M.; Bourne, Peter G.; Poe, Richard O.; Mougey, Edward H.; et al. 1969. "Androgen Responses to Stress: II. Excretion of Testosterone, Epitestosterone, Androsterone, and Etiocholanolone During Basic Combat Training and Under Threat of Attack." *Psychosomatic Medicine* 31(5): 418–436.

Sanders, Judith Rose. 1974. "Parental Sex Preference and Expectations of Gender-Appropriate Behavior in Offspring." M.A. thesis, Brooklyn College.

Sartre, Jean-Paul. 1956. *Being and Nothingness: An Essay in Phenomenological Ontology,* tr. Hazel Barnes. New York: Philosophical Library.

Sayers, Janet. 1982. *Biological Politics: Feminist and Anti-Feminist Perspectives.* New York: Tavistock.

Scott, Joan. 1988. *Gender and the Politics of History.* New York: Columbia University Press.

Sears, Robert Richardson; Maccoby, Eleanor E.; and Levin, Harry. 1957. *Patterns of Child Rearing.* Evanston, IL: Row, Peterson.

Sedgwick, Eve. 1990. *Epistemology of the Closet.* Berkeley: University of California Press.

Seidman, Steven. 1992. *Embattled Eros: Sexual Politics and Ethics in Contemporary America.* New York: Routledge.

Solomon, Robert C. 1974. "Sexual Paradigms." *Journal of Philosophy* 71(11): 336–345.

Solomon, Robert C. 1975 (reprint, 1989). "Sex and Perversion." In *From Hegel to Existentialism.* Oxford, UK: Oxford University Press.

Spanier, Bonnie. 1993. *Gender Ideology in Science: Molecular Biology from a Feminist Perspective.* Bloomington: Indiana University Press.

Stein, Edward. 1998. "Essentialism and Constructionism." In *The Philosophy of Biology,* ed. David L. Hull and Michael Ruse. Oxford, UK: Oxford University Press.

Vidal, Gore. 1991. "The Birds and the Bees." *Nation* October 28: 509–511.

Weeks, Jeffrey. 1985. *Sexuality and Its Discontents: Meanings, Myths and Modern Sexualities.* London: Routledge & Kegan Paul.

Weeks, Jeffrey. 1989. "Inverts, Perverts, and Mary-Annes: Male Prostitution and the Regulation of Homosexuality in England in the Nineteenth and Early Twentieth Centuries." In *Hidden from History: Reclaiming the Gay and Lesbian Past,* ed. Martin Duberman, Martha Vicinus, and George Chauncey, Jr. New York: Penguin.

Whitehead, Stephen M., and Barrett, Frank J., eds. 2001. *The Masculinities Reader.* Malden, MA: Blackwell Publishers.

Wilder, Hugh T. 1980. "The Language of Sex and the Sex of Language." In *Philosophy of Sex,* ed. Alan Soble. Totowa, NJ: Littlefield Adams.

Williams, Walter L. 1986. *The Spirit and the Flesh: Sexual Diversity in American Indian Culture.* Boston, MA: Beacon.

SEXUALITY, LEGAL APPROACHES TO

• • •

This entry discusses law's relationship to sexuality from an American perspective, although the framework suggested here may lend itself to application in other cultural contexts.

Sexual Status and Sexual Conduct

From the point of view of American law, sexuality has two dimensions: status and conduct. Sexuality as status, in law as in the culture at large, contains two primary alternatives—heterosexuality and homosexuality—although recent efforts on the part of those claiming bisexual status to make political alliance with gay and lesbian activists may presage increased legal recognition of this third alternative. Sexuality as conduct also has two principle aspects. The first encompasses explicitly sexual acts, of which intercourse is perhaps the paradigmatic example. Law prohibits intercourse, and sometimes other sexual activity, in a wide variety of situations, either when one of the parties has not consented or is unable to consent, or when the intercourse or other activity, although consensual, offends norms of public decency. Child sexual abuse, sexual assault and rape, statutory rape (intercourse with a woman, or in a few states with an individual, who is considered too young to provide meaningful assent), and incest are uniformly prohibited. Prostitution—the buying and selling of sex—is authorized only in Nevada. Sodomy, both homosexual and heterosexual, is unlawful in a large minority of states. Sex before marriage and outside of marriage is still prohibited in some states, although enforcement of these prohibitions is virtually nonexistent because of the disconnect between the law and prevailing cultural attitudes.

Law also regulates sexual intercourse by controlling or limiting postcoital choices. State limits on access to abortion, a hotly contested issue ultimately adjudicated by the U.S. Supreme Court in *Planned Parenthood of Southeastern Pennsylvania v. Casey* (1992), illustrates one such regulatory measure. Similarly, adult use of contraception remains constitutionally protected, while access to particular contraceptive techniques is regulated on health grounds. President Bill Clinton's reversal in 1993 of the first Bush administration's opposition to the introduction of RU-486, a "morning-after pill" and early abortifacient, provides a dramatic example of the interplay between public policies and medicine. Meanwhile, contraceptive freedom has not been extended to minors, and contraception remains regulated in the nation's high schools (Miller, Turner, and Moses).

In other contexts, law precludes procreation as a consequence of intercourse. The eugenics movement in the United States in the 1920s and 1930s produced laws compelling the sterilization of certain classes of criminals and those with mental disabilities or illness. Although no longer enforced, these laws remain on the books in several states and never have been held unconstitutional. Today, most if not all states provide a mechanism by which those legally responsible for sexually active people determined to be mentally incompetent can petition the state to authorize sterilization or contraception.

The second aspect of sexuality as conduct encompasses sexual displays the law views as expressing or arousing sexual receptivity or interest and thereby offending norms of public decency or order. The sexual displays regulated by law vary in character; they include solicitation, public nudity, and provocative dressing, as well as all forms of pornography. In this arena, too, enforcement is by no means uniform, and constitutional freedoms of speech and expression have created uncertainty with regard to the legitimacy of regulation.

Law's Multiple Relationships to Legal Status and Conduct

Law's relationship to sexuality in part constitutes law's account of what is permissible in the sexual arena—which behaviors are to be encouraged and which are to be discouraged. Legislative statutes help establish guidelines for behavior, while judges determine the constitutionality of the statutory law. This relationship between law and sexuality is importantly shaped, however, by the fact that law's authority is actually invoked in sexual matters by public agencies or private parties in only a small fraction of the possible cases.

The gap between the laws as written and as enforced has a variety of origins. For example, sometimes those who might initiate action against a violator do not know that the law offers them protection. Sometimes the enforcement of legal norms governing private sexual behavior is simply impractical; for example, sodomy, unlike public nudity, seldom comes to the attention of law enforcement personnel. Often, police and prosecutors make conscious decisions not to investigate or prosecute certain offenses for a variety of reasons, including the difficulty or the costliness of prosecution, the behavior of the victim, and the nature of the statute that has been broken (e.g., laws against adultery and premarital sexual contact). Or it may be because enforcing officers are dubious of the regulation or its particular application. Many rape prosecutions, especially those involving parties who are not strangers, founder for one or more of these reasons. Those who have argued that specific victims of pornography should be allowed to bring civil actions against pornographers and distributors of pornography base their argument, in part, on the reluctance of public authorities to take appropriate action (MacKinnon, 1987).

Those who urge giving private parties greater responsibility for or authority to initiate legal action must also realize that individuals are often unwilling or unable to invoke the law even when they understand that a law has been violated. For example, the trauma of childhood sexual abuse often results in the repression of memory (Ernsdorff and Loftus, 1993). If the memory ever surfaces, it may be long after the statute of limitations has passed. Potential claimants may be fearful of retribution on the part of the one they accuse; this is often true for sexual-harassment claimants and battered women who charge their abusers with physical and sexual violence. They may be anxious about the financial and emotional costs involved in testifying. They may fear having their credibility challenged or their character impugned and may see participation in the legal system as just another opportunity to be victimized. Finally, claimants in some circumstances may be able to resolve the situation without using the formal legal system.

If the law's relationship to sexuality is influenced by the limited nature of actual legal interventions in sexual matters, it is equally influenced by limited public understanding of the legal norms governing sexuality. How social actors perceive law's application to their own or others' sexual status or conduct may derive from actual individual or institutional knowledge of the law or of enforcement practices; but it may equally derive from impressions gleaned from a limited number of personal experiences or from stories emphasized by the media. Generalizations, often derived from limited information, then guide an individual's interaction with the legal system around sexual matters— setting standards for personal conduct, governing expectations about how the system will respond to legal violations, and providing the initiative for involvement in political efforts to change the law or replace its agents.

Given this multilayered relationship between law and sexuality, it is important to appreciate what law does and does not do, as well as how laws are implemented, what they say, and what people understand the law to be.

The Tools of Regulation

In regulating sexuality, the legal system draws on a variety of cultural authorities and principles. The two principal sources of authority guiding legal regulation of sexuality have been morality and medical science. Morals derive from either secular ethical precepts or religion, both of which are complicated by America's religious diversity and the political struggles over the separation of church and state. But when moral and religious precepts are broadly accepted and secularized within society, they become a legitimate basis for legal intervention. The law justifies its intervention by appealing to the secularized form of the moral mandate: to public decency or public order; to the value of life or the state's practical interest in heterosexual unions; to the "degeneracy" of certain sexual practices. When social consensus around a moral issue begins to erode, the link between particular moral notions and their specific religious underpinnings becomes exposed again, and law's endorsement of one side of the debate can be challenged as an improper conflation of church and state. This challenge to the moral basis of law has been most dramatic in the debates regarding abortion and homosexual marriage.

The issues involved in law's reliance on medical science have a different quality, because the concerns here are perceived to be those of knowledge rather than faith. In areas involving sexuality, medical science has provided the law with an understanding of what is necessary to protect public health and welfare and with guidelines concerning sexual status and conduct. In addressing the fundamental issue of sexual identity, medical science has drawn and redrawn the lines between aspects of sexuality that depend upon genetic programming, aspects that are the product of physical or mental disease or malfunction, and aspects that are the product of willed or chosen conduct. Changes in the medical understanding of homosexuality, for example, have in turn been central to legal debates about regulating homosexual relationships and activity. In the abortion arena, the law has looked to medicine for a scientific ruling about the beginning of human life.

The problems inherent in the relationship between law and medical science have two interrelated sources. First, medical science does not stand still, and the law often lags behind the newest research. Compulsory sterilization laws provide a dramatic example. The genetic "science" on which these laws were based has been discredited, and yet not all such laws have been repealed. Second, medical science is not as value-free as the deferential legal community often assumes; many shifts in the medical understanding of sexuality reflect shifts in values more than they do real advances in knowledge.

What of the legal principles governing the regulation of sexuality? Several of those legitimizing interventions have already been spelled out: maintaining public order, decency, health, and welfare. These laws fall within the traditional *police power* of the state. Another traditional basis for governmental intervention has been to encourage forms of association and sexuality that promote the state's conception of its interests. Matrimony and childbearing and child rearing within matrimonial relationships are the clearest historical examples. Nevertheless, the concepts of public order, decency, health, and welfare, and indeed of the state's interests, are malleable enough to serve the modern vision of social and family life.

The legal principles limiting regulation of sexuality have traditionally been those of privacy and autonomy, especially those forms of autonomy protected by the First Amendment. Both of these principles reflect a constitutional order that sees government as a threat to liberty; both are prepared to accord some cultural space to sexual activity and expression that deviate from widely held cultural norms to guard against the erosion of liberty.

In the shift from the nineteenth-century Victorian vision to the modern vision, the principles of privacy and autonomy have been pressed into service in new contexts while their hold over other arenas has been challenged. The privacy accorded family life was an important bulwark to the patriarchal authority of the male head of household, but it no longer serves to shield family members from charges of sexual abuse. Instead, privacy now provides the foundation for the constitutional protection given to both abortion and contraception, and efforts are being made to have sodomy statutes ruled unconstitutional on similar grounds.

Since the 1970s, the champions of the modern vision of social and family life have invoked the legal principle of equality. Equality has provided a basis for the abolition of old intrafamilial immunities and has supported the exposure of family abuses. Equality has translated the private pain of sexual harassment in the workplace into a public claim of discrimination when the job itself or other workplace privileges are conditioned on consent to sexual activity, or when the harassment creates a hostile working environment (MacKinnon, 1979; *Burlington Industries, Inc. v. Ellerth*, 1998; *Oncale v. Sundowner Offshore Services, Inc.*, 1998).

Equality has also offered a new analysis of pornography. Whereas previous regulation of pornography depended on the "obscenity" that made it offensive to norms of public decency, the new analysis emphasizes the role pornography plays in endorsing and promoting the sexual objectification of women that denies women equal status in society (MacKinnon, 1987, 1993). This characterization more properly represents what is at stake in regulating pornography. By the mid-1990s, however, none of the municipal ordinances based on it had survived constitutional scrutiny. The violation of women's right to be free of discrimination must still be weighed against the First Amendment freedoms of pornographers, distributors, and users; in this balance, pornography opponents have not prevailed. Importantly, women themselves are divided on this issue; many see the proliferation of pornography as enabling a liberating sexuality for women and support the First Amendment protection of pornography, whereas others remain concerned that pornography fosters male dominance and female subjugation (Strossen, 1993).

Finally, equality is frequently offered by advocates as a basis for outlawing differential treatment on the basis of sexual identity and for providing a protected sphere in which gay and lesbian people can enjoy both privacy and autonomy in their experience of their sexuality (Mohr, "Sexual Orientation and the Law"). This argument has made limited headway within the legal system. While most courts continue to uphold state statutes restricting marriage to opposite-sex couples, a few courts have taken positions favorable to same-sex marriage. In its 1999 decision in *Baker v. State of Vermont,* the Vermont Supreme Court held that "the State is constitutionally required to extend to same-sex couples the common benefits and protections that flow from marriage under Vermont law." The court carefully noted that its decision did not entitle same-sex couples to a marriage license but merely ordered the state legislature to either allow same-sex marriage licenses or "establish an alternative legal status to marriage for same-sex couples."

The controversial *Baker* decision has led some legal commentators to wonder about the futures of traditional and same-sex marriage. Some have speculated that if courts find marriage benefits constitutionally required, then they will likely find the title and status of marriage constitutionally required as well, ultimately leading to legalized same-sex marriages (Duncan). While the issue of legalized same-sex marriages remains unresolved, Hawaii's courts, like Vermont's, have taken steps toward legalizing same-sex marriage, finding the state's same-sex marriage ban to be a form of sex discrimination and directing the state legislature to resolve the issue accordingly (*Baehr v. Lewin,* 1993; *Baehr v. Miike,* 1998). The legal developments in Vermont and Hawaii have been controversial nationally in part because many states fear that the U.S. Constitution's full faith and credit clause (found in Article 4) will require them to recognize same-sex marriages, with potential positive and negative consequences for children, parents, families, social structures, and social values (Gushiken).

Conclusion

In matters relating to sexuality, the law attempts to strike a delicate balance between the impetus to regulate and the impetus to stay government's hand, while always remaining aware of shifting cultural values. Issues resolved in the direction of regulation in one era may be revisited and resolved in the direction of abstention in another. In the decades to come, it seems likely that the most contested territory is going to involve, first, the extent to which regulation of sexuality will be directed toward achieving the egalitarian vision of social and family life, freeing women and children from sexual exploitation and abuse, and second, the extent to which law will be persuaded to lift the burden of regulation currently imposed on homosexual conduct and give equal protection to those who claim homosexual status.

CLARE DALTON (1995)
REVISED BY NATHANIEL STEWART

SEE ALSO: *Sexism; Sexual Behavior, Social Control of; Sexual Ethics; Sexual Ethics and Professional Standards; Sexual Identity*

BIBLIOGRAPHY

Baehr v. Lewin. 74 Haw. 530; 852 P.2d 44 (1993).

Baehr v. Miike. 80 HAW. 341; 910 P.2D 112 (1996).

Baker v. State of Vermont. 170 Vt. 194 (1999).

Burlington Industries, Inc. v. Ellerth. 524 U.S. 742; 118 Sup. Ct. 2257 (1998).

Danielsen, Dan, and Engle, Karen, eds. 1994. *After Identity: A Reader in Law and Culture.* New York: Routledge.

Duncan, William C. 2001. "Domestic Partnership Laws in the United States: A Review and Critique." *Brigham Young University Law Review* 2001(3): 961–992.

Dworkin, Ronald. 1993. *Life's Dominion: An Argument about Abortion, Euthanasia, and Individual Freedom.* New York: Knopf.

Editors of the Harvard Law Review. 1990. *Sexual Orientation and the Law.* Cambridge, MA: Harvard University Press.

Ernsdorff, Gary M., and Loftus, Elizabeth F. 1993. "Let Sleeping Memories Lie? Words of Caution about Tolling the Statute of Limitations in Cases of Memory Repression." *Journal of Criminal Law and Criminology* 84 (Spring): 129–174.

Grossberg, Michael. 1985. *Governing the Hearth: Law and the Family in Nineteenth-Century America.* Chapel Hill: University of North Carolina Press.

Gushiken, Brad K. 2000. "The Fine Line between Love and the Law: Hawaii's Attempt to Resolve the Same-Sex Marriage Issue." *Hawaii Law Review, 2000* no. 22 (Spring): 149–184.

Inness, Julie C. 1992. *Privacy, Intimacy, and Isolation.* New York: Oxford University Press.

Law, Sylvia A. 1988. "Homosexuality and the Social Meaning of Gender." *Wisconsin Law Review, 1988,* no. 2: 187–235.

MacKinnon, Catharine A. 1979. *Sexual Harassment of Working Women: A Case of Sex Discrimination.* New Haven, CT: Yale University Press.

MacKinnon, Catharine A. 1987. *Feminism Unmodified: Discourses on Life and Law.* Cambridge, MA: Harvard University Press.

MacKinnon, Catharine A. 1993. *Only Words.* Cambridge, MA: Harvard University Press.

Miller, Heather G.; Turner, Charles F.; and Moses, Lincoln E., eds. 1990. *AIDS: The Second Decade.* Washington, D.C.: National Academy Press.

Mohr, Richard D. 1988. *Gays/Justice: A Study of Ethics, Society, and Law.* New York: Columbia University Press.

Okin, Susan Moller. 1989. *Justice, Gender, and the Family.* New York: Basic.

Olsen, Frances E. 1983. "The Family and the Market: A Study of Ideology and Legal Reform." *Harvard Law Review* 96(7): 1497–1578.

Oncale v. Sundowner Offshore Services, Inc. 523 U.S. 75; 118 Sup. Ct. 998 (1998).

Petchesky, Rosalind P. 1990. *Abortion and Woman's Choice: The State, Sexuality, and Reproductive Freedom,* revised edition. Boston: Northeastern University Press.

Planned Parenthood of Southeastern Pennsylvania v. Casey. 505 U.S. 833; 112 Sup. Ct. 2791 (1992).

Robson, Ruthann. 1992. *Lesbian (Out)law: Survival under the Rule of Law.* Ithaca, NY: Firebrand.

Roe v. Wade. 410 U.S. 113; 93 Sup. Ct. 705 (1973).

"Sexual Orientation and the Law." 1993. Special issue of *Virginia Law Review* 79(7).

Strossen, Nadine. 1993. "A Feminist Critique of 'The' Feminist Critique of Pornography." *Virginia Law Review* 79(5): 1099–1190.

Thorne, Barrie, and Yalom, Marilyn, eds. 1992. *Rethinking the Family: Some Feminist Questions,* rev. edition. Boston: Northeastern University Press.

SIKHISM, BIOETHICS IN

• • •

Origins and Teachings

Sikhism began with Guru Nanak (1469–1539 C.E.), who was born a Hindu in the Punjab, which is still home for the vast majority of Sikhs. The word *Sikh* means *learner* or *disciple,* and today the community numbers approximately 16 million. Nanak was the first of ten personal Gurus. Following the death in 1708 of the tenth Guru, Gobind

Singh, the function of the Guru passed to the scripture and to the community. For this reason the Adi Granth (the Sikh scripture) is particularly venerated by the community.

In the North India of Nanak's day, a popular mode of religion among ordinary people was worship of a God of grace, immanent in all creation and never incarnated as a person or as an idol. This was the Sant Tradition and Nanak provided in his teachings its clearest statement. The presence of God is known through the *nam* (divine Name), mystically manifested in the beauty and order of the world around us, and one's duty is to meditate on the *nam*. This may be done by repeating a particular word or mantra, by singing hymns, or by silently meditating. In so doing one grows ever nearer to God, eventually achieving a condition of perfect union. In this union the cycle of transmigration (movement of the soul, at the death of the body, into a new body) is finally ended.

Those who accepted these teachings from Nanak were the first Sikhs. A line of successor Gurus followed him, the same divine spirit believed to inhabit each of them. The first four successors continued Nanak's teachings concerning the divine Name and, in 1603–1604 Arjan, the fifth Guru, collected their hymns and his own into a scripture, adding to it the works of other members of the Sant Tradition. During the time of the sixth Guru, Hargobind, the community attracted the attention of the Moghuls, at that time the rulers of northern India. By this time the community had grown noticeably large and the Moghuls were becoming suspicious of its increasing numbers. This danger receded, but it returned in the time of the ninth Guru, Tegh Behadur, who was executed by the Moghuls in 1675.

The Foundation of the Khalsa

In 1699 Tegh Bahadur's son and successor, Gobind Singh, inaugurated the Khalsa, a new order loyal Sikhs were summoned to join. Membership in the Khalsa was by an initiation ceremony and by a lifelong vow to maintain certain outward symbols, particularly uncut hair. Emphasis on the centrality of the divine Name was retained, but in place of the strictly inward faith taught by Guru Nanak, the tenth Guru created an organization that proclaimed the identify of his followers to all.

The inauguration of the Khalsa was crucial because it laid down for members an explicit code, or Rahit. Tradition records that the Guru promulgated all that the modern Khalsa observes today. In fact, many of the individual items of the Rahit can be traced to experiences that follow the actual foundation. The essential nature of the Khalsa, however, remains unaffected. Gobind Singh summoned loyal Sikhs to join his Khalsa; the Khalsa Sikh was to be known by certain outward features. These conspicuously included the obligation to bear arms and to retain uncut hair. Men were to add Singh ("Lion") to their name and women were to add Kaur ("Princess").

Ranjit Singh, the Singh Sabha, and Modern History

The eighteenth century, a time of much turbulence in the Punjab, was followed by a settled period during the early nineteenth century. Under Maharaja Ranjit Singh, who became ruler of the central Punjab in 1801, strong government was introduced and during the next twenty-five years, the boundaries were enlarged in three directions. In the southeast, where the British advanced against Ranjit Singh, the border was drawn along the Satluj river, leaving many Sikhs in British territory or in the territory of their client states. Amritsar was not the capital city, but it was confirmed as the principal religious center. Ranjit Singh gilded the two upper storeys of its main temple, converting it into the famous Golden Temple.

His death in 1839 has been interpreted as marking the beginning of a steep decline in Sikh fortunes. In 1849, following two wars, the British annexed the Punjab. In 1873, however, the Singh Sabha (Singh Society) was founded and under its influence, the Sikh community was revived and reshaped. In 1920 the Singh Sabha was taken over by the more radical Akali movement, which was dedicated to the liberation of the gurdwaras (temples). With the partition of India in 1947, the Punjab was divided and the Sikhs in Pakistan moved across to the Indian area. Since then many Sikhs have claimed greater Punjab autonomy. The Indian army assault on the Golden Temple in 1984 led to decade-long demands by many Sikhs for Khalistan, a completely independent state. By 1993, however, these demands had subsided.

The Singh Sabha and the Rahit

The dominant concern of the Singh Sabha reformers was to demonstrate that Sikhs formed an entirely distinct faith and that, in particular, they should not be confused with the Hindus. Special concern focused on the question of how a Sikh should behave. The intention was to show that the ways of the Sikh were emphatically not the ways of the other groups in India.

This required a restatement of the Rahit. According to tradition, Guru Gobind Singh had promulgated the Rahit in all its details, but by the late nineteenth century it had become impossible to determine his words with precision. The Rahit had been recorded for Sikhs in a number of Rahit-namas (Rahit manuals), none of which was entirely satisfactory. Those present at the founding of the Khalsa in 1699 would know what was required of them, and likewise those who associated with the Guru until his death in 1708. Most of the eighteenth century was, however, charged with warfare and persecution, and Sikhs had little time to record the Rahit that had been delivered to them. Ignorant or mischievous people might have corrupted the received Rahit, and the Rahit-namas could only be trusted after a scrupulous hand excised those portions that misled readers and restored those parts that had been lost.

The Singh Sabha leaders made unsuccessful attempts to produce an authentic Rahit-nama. Eventually, however, an acceptable version, Sikh Rahit Maryada, was issued in 1950, and appeals to this written authority are possible. The Sikhs have no clergy and so the publication of an authoritative text was truly significant. The question of orthodoxy, however, remains. Sikh Rahit Maryada represents the Khalsa version of orthodoxy, that is, the insistence on uncut hair; there is no doubt that since the days of the Singh Sabha, this has been the dominant style. There are, however, Sikhs who do not observe this version, preferring to venerate the Gurus and scripture while cutting their hair. They do not observe the Rahit, yet still insist that they are Sikhs. It is here that Sikh identity becomes difficult to define and with it, the whole question of what constitutes Sikhism. The remainder of this article describes Khalsa Sikhism, but it is important to remember that many who call themselves Sikhs are not members of the Khalsa. This applies particularly to Sikhs living outside India.

Khalsa Regulations

Members of the Khalsa are identified by what are called the Five Ks (uncut hair, a comb, a steel wrist-band, a sword or dagger, and shorts). Smoking and intoxicants are firmly banned, the latter largely ignored but the former strictly maintained. Khalsa Sikhs are insistent on the right to carry a sword, a feature that enhances their reputation for violence. This reputation is greatly exaggerated. The Sikh should draw the sword (or use arms) only defensively, only when the cause is just, and only when all other methods have failed.

In Sikhism the key term when discussing ethical and moral issues is *seva* (service). Little guidance is given regarding health, disease, and the environment other than the most general principles. The objective is simply a life of personal righteousness, largely undefined. *Seva* is primarily considered a duty toward the gurdwara, and consists of obligations performed for the Guru on its holy ground. These include

service in the *langar*, the free refectory that all gurdwaras are required to maintain, symbolizing the equality of all people. The concept is, however, further interpreted to mean genuine concern for the needs of others. According to Sikh Rahit Maryada, every Sikh is required to devote his or her entire life to the welfare of others.

In general, Sikhs are directed to see themselves as distinct from other faiths, particularly from all forms of Hindu tradition. This is the case with funerals, which involve a simple rite. Cremation follows death but all who assemble are required to restrict their lamenting. The corpse is dressed in clean garments, complete with the Five Ks, and the ceremony is conducted while hymns are sung. Such practices as laying the corpse on the floor or breaking the skull are sternly forbidden. Specific ethical injunctions are comparatively rare in Sikh Rahit Maryada, although those that are mentioned are clearly intended to be mandatory. The emphasis is, instead, placed on the duty of the individual Sikh to live a worthy life as circumstances of time and place dictate.

With two exceptions, matters of bioethical concern are not spelled out. Sikhs are left to determine them in the light of their religious faith. One exception is that female infanticide is strictly prohibited. This reflects an earlier period in Punjab history. The second exception is that, strictly speaking, initiated Khalsa members should not eat from the same dish as an uninitiated Sikh or one who has renounced the faith. All other issues, such as abortion, birth control, suicide, and euthanasia, are left to the individual or the family to decide.

W. H. MCLEOD (1995)

SEE ALSO: *Death: Eastern Thought; Eugenics and Religious Law: Hinduism and Buddhism; Hinduism, Bioethics in; Jainism, Bioethics in; Medical Ethics, History of South and East Asia: India; Population Ethics, Religious Traditions: Hindu Perspectives*

BIBLIOGRAPHY

Avtar, Singh. 1970. *Ethics of the Sikhs.* Patiala, India: Punjabi University.

Grewal, J. S. 1990. *The Sikhs of the Punjab.* Vol. II.3 of *The New Cambridge History of India.* Cambridge, MA: Cambridge University Press.

Kohli, Surindar Singh. 1975. *Sikh Ethics.* New Delhi: Munshiram Manoharlal.

McLeod, W. H., ed. and tr. 1991. *Textual Sources for the Study of Sikhism.* Chicago: University of Chicago Press.

Oberoi, Harjot. 1994. *The Construction of Religious Boundaries: Culture, Identity, and Diversity in the Sikh Tradition.* Delhi: Oxford University Press.

Rehat Maryada: A Guide to the Sikh Way of Life. 1978. English translation of the Sikh Rahit Maryada. Amritsar: Shiromani Gurdwara Parbandakh Committee.

Sri Guru Granth Sahib in English Translation, 1984–1991. 4 vols. tr. Gurbachan Singh Talib. Patiala, India: Punjabi University.

SMOKING

• • •

From the time when the native peoples of the Americas introduced Europeans to tobacco until the second decade of the twentieth century smoking and other forms of tobacco use focused on questions of production, commerce, and morality rather than on questions of medicine (U.S. Department of Health and Human Services, 1992). The first public policy issues concerning tobacco centered on its role as an important cash crop and a potential source of tax revenue. Medical questions about tobacco use did not materialize because until the 1920s there were no scientific grounds for supposing that smoking endangers the health of smokers. Half a century passed before epidemiologists began to make a case for the dangers of environmental tobacco smoke (ETS) to nonsmokers. Smoking and other forms of tobacco use provide a vivid illustration of how ethical considerations can change over time as scientific evidence and the social, political, and economic dimensions of an issue change.

Scientists began to build the case for the dangers of smoking when A. C. Broders (1920) published an article correlating tobacco use with lip cancer. Subsequent studies repeatedly linked tobacco use, in particular smoking, with a variety of diseases, primarily lung cancer and respiratory diseases. Evidence was derived from epidemiological studies, typically retrospective laboratory studies, and findings at autopsy. In 1957 based on the findings of a federally sponsored study group on smoking and health the U.S. Public Health Service (USPHS) concluded that there was a causal link between smoking and lung cancer (U.S. Department of Health, Education, and Welfare). The USPHS also affirmed a causal link between smoking and numerous other cancers, as well as other diseases in 1964, when Surgeon General Luther Terry issued an advisory report titled *Smoking and Health* (U.S. Department of Health, Education and Welfare).

Since 1964 a wealth of research has demonstrated the deleterious effects of tobacco use on health. Both government and private agencies have been instrumental in publicizing and documenting research findings and their implications, most efficiently through their websites. For example, the Centers for Disease Control and Prevention (CDC) lists all the surgeon general's reports on tobacco and health from 1964 to 2001. These reports summarize the state of research and education on tobacco use at the time of each report. Research articles, tobacco industry documents, tobacco control guideline programs, and educational materials can be accessed through the CDC's site. Other websites—the Agency for Healthcare Research and Quality (AHRQ), the U.S. Department of Health and Human Services (USDHHS), the National Library of Medicine, and the National Institutes of Health (including the National Cancer Institute), as well as private foundations such as the American Cancer Society and the American Lung Association—all provide access to research and educational materials for laypersons and professionals. The importance of tobacco use and exposure as a health risk is demonstrated further in the USDHHS document *Healthy People 2010* (2000a), which cites morbidity and mortality related to tobacco use and ETS as one of the leading indicators of the health of the American people for the next ten years.

Reflection on some of the facts gives one a sense of the ethical and policy problems posed by smoking. Approximately 440,000 deaths in the United States are due to smoking and diseases related to tobacco use (American Lung Association, 2002). Exposure to ETS (also known as passive smoking) increases the risk of cancer in people who have never smoked (Hackshaw et al.). Tobacco use has become a serious pediatric health issue, but in spite of regulation, children and adolescents continue to be able to obtain tobacco products (U.S. Department of Health and Human Services, 2000b). Control of the risks and diseases related to tobacco use has been hampered by continuing efforts by the tobacco industry to promote and market its products without constraints (U.S. Department of Health and Human Services, 2000b; Ong and Glatz).

The negative health effects of tobacco use are widely known and may be widely acknowledged even though individuals may not change their behavior on the basis of that knowledge. The reasons for the lack of behavioral change are many and complex (U.S. Department of Health and Human Services, 2000b). The ethical issues are also complex and have evolved over time and as a result of political and legal factors. Major ethical issues related to smoking and other tobacco use are: (1) the protection of nonsmokers from the effects of ETS; (2) the protection of children from an addictive product; (3) the scientific integrity of tobacco industry research; and (4) corporate integrity in marketing tobacco products.

In the past ethical arguments about smoking focused on issues of autonomy, paternalism, and societal harm. Smoking as an individual choice was juxtaposed against the restriction of individual smoking behavior as a consideration in protecting the individual from himself or herself and protecting society from smokers. Today the moral issues associated with tobacco use have moved away from individual autonomy and individual values because of the recognition of the significant public health implications of smoking. However, the earlier ethical arguments regarding smoking and tobacco use will be reviewed here to gain a historical perspective.

Ethics and Restrictive Policies: Autonomy, Paternalism, and Societal Harm

Before the harmful effects of ETS were demonstrated, the health risks of smoking suggested that at least some restrictive policies designed to protect smokers from themselves could be ethically justified. Knowledge of the risks that smokers impose on nonsmokers could support public policies designed to keep smokers from exposing nonsmokers to ETS or imposing on nonsmokers the medical costs of smoking. In addition to these two considerations the promotion of health has served as a third impetus for a restrictive policy. For example, in 1992 the Joint Commission on the Accreditation of Health Care Organizations (JCAHO), the chief hospital accreditation agency in the United States, required hospitals to forbid smoking within their premises by 1994 as a condition of accreditation (Center for Disease Control Chronology of Significant Developments). Robert Goodin (1989) used these considerations to develop a vigorous case for a public policy aimed at a total ban on smoking. Today bans on smoking in public places are common and often complement state tobacco control programs that have been shown to be effective, at least in one instance, in reducing the mortality from heart disease attributed to smoking (Fichtenberg and Glantz).

Restrictive social policies that attempt to protect an individual from harming himself or herself have been viewed as paternalistic. At least since John Stuart Mill's (1859) *On Liberty* antipaternalistic sentiment has been widespread in the English-speaking philosophical community, with Joel Feinberg being one of its leading contemporary voices. Feinberg has emphatically rejected legal paternalism, the doctrine that "[i]t is always a good reason in support of a prohibition that it is necessary to prevent harm (physical, psychological, or economic) to the actor himself" (Feinberg,

p. xvii). Despite an absence of consensus on what constitutes a competent choice, factors such as coercion, ignorance, mental impairment, and addiction serve as grounds for challenging the competence of a choice. The rejection of restrictive smoking policies on the basis of their paternalistic nature and curtailment of individual autonomy thus was considered a viable moral argument until the addictive properties of nicotine and the extent of children's tobacco use became known. The case for smoking as simply another autonomous value choice became difficult to make for an addictive substance whose use often began in childhood or adolescence.

Ethics and the Public's Health: Protecting Children and Nonsmokers

Although a moral argument based on the freedom to exercise individual autonomy could be made for not restricting competent adults from engaging in tobacco-related behaviors that are detrimental to their health, that argument fails because of the propensity of adult smokers to begin smoking in childhood or adolescence and the known effects of active and passive smoke on nonsmokers, children, and fetuses. According to a 1994 surgeon general's report, most first-time smoking occurs before graduation from high school, and the younger a child is when he or she begins smoking, the greater are the negative health effects (U.S. Department of Health and Human Services, 1994). Smoking and ETS are associated with decreased fetal growth during pregnancy and respiratory problems in school-age children who were exposed to smoke during early development (American Academy of Pediatrics). Children exposed to passive smoke are more likely to develop respiratory and middle-ear problems (Cook and Strachan).

Maternal smoking has been associated with sudden infant death syndrome, and passive smoke has been associated with an increase in hospital admissions among children with cystic fibrosis (Cook and Strachan). Because of these and other significant health risks to children and adolescents, the American Academy of Pediatrics has identified the reduction of children's exposure to both active and passive smoke as a primary goal of preventive health (American Academy of Pediatrics Committee on Substance Abuse).

The moral obligation to protect a vulnerable population is heightened by the dangers of tobacco to children in all stages of development and the fact that those risks are preventable. Although children potentially may be harmed by actively smoking or by their parents' smoking, children are also at risk from ETS outside the home.

The harm from ETS in all age groups is well established. The increased risks of respiratory and heart diseases and the role of passive smoke as an irritant were summarized in a 1986 surgeon general's report (U.S. Department of Health and Human Services, 1986). More recent meta-analyses of epidemiological studies have continued to affirm ETS as a cause of lung cancer (Hackshaw et al.) and have provided further evidence of the negative cardiac effects associated with ETS (He et al.). The continuing confirmation through scientific evidence of the detrimental health effects of passive smoking and the recognition of nicotine as addicting have moved smoking from the realm of personal value choice to the realm of public health.

The ethics involved in public health issues may differ in some respects from those involved in clinical medicine in that obligations to society as a whole may be different from or conflict with obligations to an individual patient. Although some conflicts between the rights of society and the rights of individuals may entail controversy, the overwhelming scientific evidence for the detrimental effects of tobacco has effectively eliminated controversy and promoted consensus among health professionals. The evidence justifies the imposition of restrictions such as workplace bans and restrictions on smoking in public places, whereas the lack of a total ban allows adult individuals to make the choice to smoke. Rather than being viewed as restrictions on personal liberty or intolerance of diverse values, those restrictions can be seen as analogous to the imposition of speed limits to protect the public's safety on highways. Occasional challenges to the scientific evidence still appear, but it is recognized increasingly that one reason for the public's (and some health professionals') delay in accepting the scientific evidence regarding the negative effects of smoking was an active campaign by the tobacco industry to market tobacco use aggressively and discredit scientific evidence about its negative health effects (Ong and Glantz).

Scientific Integrity and Corporate Morality

Since the 1990s confidential tobacco industry documents have become public as a result of litigation and increased public knowledge about the health effects of active tobacco use and ETS. Those documents demonstrate the efforts of the tobacco industry to publicly deny its own research results confirming the dangers of ETS, alter data to support its desired conclusions, and discredit legitimate scientists whose work demonstrated negative effects of ETS (Barnes et al.). Elisa K. Ong and Stanton A. Glantz describe how between 1993 and 1998 lawyers and marketing firms employed by Philip Morris directed a campaign to distort epidemiological standards with contrived concepts of *sound science* in order to attack legitimate scientific evidence on the negative health

effects of tobacco use. Because further regulation of the tobacco industry appeared inevitable, the industry's goal was to raise the standards for scientific proof of harm so that legitimate studies demonstrating harm could never reach those standards and thus could be dismissed as *junk science* (Ong and Glantz).

The campaign was insidious but lost its force when epidemiological organizations refused to agree to some of the statistical standards being pushed by the tobacco industry (Ong and Glantz). This example of the tobacco industry's unethical attempts to manipulate public opinion is only one of many. Policies related to the sale of tobacco to foreign countries also raise difficult issues, including the promotion of cigarettes to children or to people who lack adequate information about the risks of smoking. Vigorous opposition by tobacco companies to efforts to inform Third World consumers about the effects of smoking and attempts to manipulate those efforts have exacerbated the problem (Emri, Bagci, Karakoca, Baris). Corporate morality leading to conflicts of interest and potential harm to individuals remains an unresolved problem.

Legal Regulation of the Tobacco Industry

All defensible theories of just laws recognize the harmfulness of a conduct to others as a good reason for regulating that conduct (Feinberg). In the environment of recognized health risks and the deceptive marketing practices of the tobacco industry lawsuits and regulations have become increasingly common.

Historically, legal decisions and regulations have been decided for and against both the tobacco industry and consumers. For example, the Federal Cigarette Labeling and Advertising Act of 1965 required the warning label that is familiar today but at the same time prohibited warning labels on cigarette advertisements for a period of three years (Center for Disease Control). The Controlled Substance Act of 1970, regulating addictive substances; the Consumer Product Safety Act of 1972, regulating hazardous substances; and the Toxic Substances Control Act of 1976, regulating injurious chemicals, specifically excluded tobacco from their lists of hazardous or addictive substances (Center for Disease Control). Other notable regulations include policies and laws in 1973, 1987, and 1989 to segregate and then ban smoking on domestic airline flights and bans on smoking in government workplaces in 1987, 1994, and 1997 (Center for Disease Control). The CDC website provides a summary of the numerous government regulations pertaining to tobacco since the early twentieth century (Center for Disease Control).

Over the years legal battles by individuals against the tobacco industry were fought with varying degrees of success, but eventually more consumers began to prevail in the courts. Although most disputes were heard in lower courts, two cases involving state laws, cigarette advertising, and injury or potential injury reached the U.S. Supreme Court and resulted in rulings that were partially favorable to each side (*Thomas Cipollone*; *Lorillard Tobacco Company*). In a third case, a victory for the tobacco industry, the U.S. Supreme Court ruled that the U.S. Food and Drug Administration did not have the authority to regulate tobacco products as it did other drugs.

By the mid-1990s four individual states had sued the tobacco industry to obtain reimbursement for healthcare costs related to tobacco use. In an effort to avoid more lawsuits the six major tobacco companies entered into an agreement with the attorney generals and representatives of the remaining forty-six states, along with U.S. territories and the District of Columbia. This so-called Master Settlement provides billions of dollars in payments to states from the tobacco industry beginning in June 2000 and extending over the following twenty-five years (Wilson). In addition to settlement payments, provisions of the Master Settlement include the prevention of industry targeting of children and adolescents in advertising, the regulation of tobacco industry lobbying, and public access to industry records and research (Wilson).

Since the last two decades of the twentieth century the changes in the ways in which the public thinks about and uses tobacco have been sweeping. The moral considerations of individual personal choice and freedom in smoking have become issues of public health, the protection of children, the integrity of science and scientists, and the morality of corporations. On January 27, 2003, Philip Morris changed its name to Altria Group, Inc., to demonstrate, it claimed, "To better clarify its identity as the owner of both food and tobacco companies that manage some of the world's most successful brands" (according to <http://www.philipmorris. com>). However, the moral tensions between the industry and the public continue. What the industry changes will mean in the long term remains to be seen.

MICHAEL LAVIN (1995)
REVISED BY JACQUELYN SLOMKA

SEE ALSO: *Addiction and Dependence; Advertising; Alcohol and Other Drugs in a Public Health Context; Alcoholism; Behavior Modification Therapies; Freedom and Free Will; Genetics and Human Behavior; Harm; Harmful Substances, Legal Control of; Hazardous Wastes and Toxic Substances;* *Human Dignity; Life, Quality of; Maternal-Fetal Relationship; Patients' Responsibilities; Race and Racism; Responsibility*

BIBLIOGRAPHY

American Academy of Pediatrics. 1994. "Tobacco-Free Environment: An Imperative for the Health of Children and Adolescents." *Pediatrics* 93: 866–868.

American Academy of Pediatrics Committee on Substance Abuse. 2001. "Tobacco's Toll: Implications for the Pediatrician." *Pediatrics* 107: 794–798.

Barnes, Deborah E.; Hanauer, Peter; Slade, John; et al. 1995. "Environmental Tobacco Smoke: The Brown and Williamson Documents." *Journal of the American Medical Association* 274: 248–253.

Broders, A. C. 1920. "Squamous-Cell Epithelioma of the Lip: A Study of 537 Cases." *Journal of the American Medical Association* 74(10): 656–664.

Cook, Derek G., and Strachan, David P. 1999. "Health Effects of Passive Smoking: 10. Summary of Effects of Parental Smoking on the Respiratory Health of Children and Implications for Research." *Thorax* 54(4): 357–366.

Emri, Salih; Bagci, Tulay; Karakoca, Yalcin; et al. 1998. "Recognition of Cigarette Brand Names and Logos by Primary Schoolchildren in Ankara, Turkey." *Tobacco Control* 7: 386–392.

Feinberg, Joel. 1986. *Harm to Self: Moral Limits of the Criminal Law*, Vol. 3. Oxford, Eng.: Oxford University Press.

Fichtenberg Caroline M., and Glantz, Stanton A. 2000. "Association of the California Tobacco Control Program with Declines in Cigarette Consumption and Mortality from Heart Disease." *New England Journal of Medicine* 343: 1772–1777.

Food and Drug Administration, et al. v. Brown and Williamson Tobacco Corporation, et al. 98–1152. Supreme Court of the United States. Argued December 1, 1999. Decided March 21, 2000.

Goodin, Robert E. 1989. *No Smoking: The Ethical Issues.* Chicago: University of Chicago Press.

Hackshaw, A. K.; Law, M. R.; and Wald, N. J. 1997. "The Accumulated Evidence on Lung Cancer and Environmental Tobacco Smoke." *British Medical Journal* 315: 980–988.

He, Jiang; Vupputuri, Suma; Allen, Krista; et al. 1999. "Passive Smoking and the Risk of Coronary Heart Disease: A Meta-Analysis of Epidemiologic Studies." *New England Journal of Medicine* 340: 920–926.

Lorillard Tobacco Company, et al. v. Thomas F. Reilly. Attorney General of Massachusetts, et al.; Altadis U.S.A. Inc., etc., et al. v. Thomas F. Reilly, Attorney General of Massachusetts, et al. Nos. 00–596 and 00–597. Supreme Court of the United States. Argued April 25, 2001 Decided June 28, 2001.

Mill, John Stuart. 1975 (1859). *On Liberty.* New York: Norton.

Ong Elisa K., and Glantz, Stanton A. 2001. "Constructing 'Sound Science' and 'Good Epidemiology': Tobacco, Lawyers, and Public Relations Firms." *American Journal of Public Health* 91: 1749–1757.

Thomas Cipollone, Individually and as Executor of the Estate of Rose D. Cipollone, Petitioner v. Liggett Group, Inc., et al. No. 90–1038. Supreme Court of the United States. Argued October 8, 1991. Decided June 24, 1992.

U.S. Department of Health, Education and Welfare. 1964. *Smoking and Health.* Washington, D.C.: U.S. Government Printing Office.

U.S. Department of Health and Human Services. 1986. *The Health Consequences of Involuntary Smoking: A Report of the Surgeon General.* Publication CDC 87–8398. Washington, D.C.: U.S. Government Printing Office.

U.S. Department of Health and Human Services. 1992. *Smoking and Health in the Americas.* Publication CDC 92–8419. Washington, D.C.: U.S. Government Printing Office.

U.S. Department of Health and Human Services. 1994. *Preventing Tobacco Use Among Young People: A Report of the Surgeon General.* Washington, D.C.: U.S. Government Printing Office.

U.S. Department of Health and Human Services. 2000a. *Healthy People 2010,*Vols. 1 and 2. Washington, D.C.: U.S. Government Printing Office.

U.S. Department of Health and Human Services. 2000b. *Reducing Tobacco Use: A Report of the Surgeon General—Executive Summary.* Washington, D.C.: U.S. Government Printing Office.

INTERNET RESOURCES

Agency for Healthcare Research and Quality. 2003. Available from <http://www.ahrq.gov>.

American Cancer Society. Available from <http://www.cancer.org>.

American Lung Association. 2002. "Trends in Tobacco Use." American Lung Association. Best Practices and Program Services Epidemiology and Statistics Unit. Available from <http://www.nicpp.org/files/ALA_Trends_in_Tobacco_Use_2002.pdf>.

Centers for Disease Control and Prevention. Available from <http://www.cdc.gov/tobacco/>.

Chronology of Significant Developments Related to Smoking and Health. Centers for Disease Control (a). Updated April 14, 2003. Available from <http://www.cdc.gov/tobacco/overview/chron96.htm#1992>.

Fact Sheet—Smoking. 2003. New York, NY: American Lung Association. Available from <http://www.lungusa.org/tobacco/smoking_factsheet99.html>.

National Institutes of Health. 2003. Available from <http://www.nih.gov>.

National Library of Medicine. 2003. Availbale from <http://www.nlm.nih.gov>.

Philip Morris. 2003. Available from <http://www.philipmorris.com>.

Selected Actions of the U.S. Government Regarding the Regulation of Tobacco Sales, Marketing and Use. Centers for Disease Control (b). Updated March 31, 2003. Available from <http://www.cdc.gov/tobacco/overview/regulate.htm>.

U.S. Department of Health and Human Services. 2003. Available from <http://www.os.dhhs.gov>.

Wilson, Joy J. 1999. *Summary of the Attorneys General Master Tobacco Settlement.* Washington, D.C.: National Conference of State Legislatures. Available from <www.ncsl.org/statefed/tmsasumm.htm>.

SOCIAL MEDICINE

• • •

Throughout most of medical history the physician's role has been seen predominantly as a personal one in which, for the most part, the one-to-one patient–physician relationship is the one that is considered in medical ethical principles. Although the shocking evidence of physician participation in genocidal activities during World War II led to new ethical statements, such as the Declaration of Geneva, that place physicians' behavior in a social context, such statements nevertheless largely remain codifications of the ethical behavior of a physician toward a particular patient.

Origin and Meaning of Social Medicine

Enlargement of the role of the physician to include social and community aspects of disease prevention, diagnosis, and treatment is of relatively recent development, and is referred to as *social medicine.* Many definitions of social medicine have been attempted, the more generally accepted ones reflecting the relationship of social factors to disease and death. Today there is a general consensus that social medicine represents the study of the medical needs of society and the interaction of medicine and society, along with the practice of inclusion of social factors in public health, preventive medicine, and the clinical examination and treatment of patients.

The concept grew from a variety of experiences over the centuries. In seventeenth-century London, weekly "Bills of Mortality" listing the previous week's deaths began to be published. Incomplete and inaccurate as they were, they inspired John Graunt (1620–1674) and, later, Edwin Chadwick (1800–1890) to relate social and economic circumstances to death rates.

Similarly, in Italy, Bernardino Ramazzini (1633–1714) documented the relationship of disease to a series of occupations. In the nineteenth century, these inchoate efforts came together into social-policy constructs. In Austria, Johann

Peter Frank (1745–1821) published a monumental six-volume work on medical policy as a governmental endeavor—to ensure clean water and sewage disposal, for example, and to promote other regulatory efforts for the benefit of society. Chadwick, in Britain, urged government to take responsibility under the Poor Laws to protect the health of the growing population impoverished by increasing industrialization (Chadwick).

The industrial revolution fostered turmoil throughout Europe and increased the awareness of social causation of disease and death as it brought about far-reaching changes in the lives of working people. Friedrich Engels's study, *The Condition of the Working Class in England in 1844,* described the relationship of diseases such as tuberculosis, typhoid, and typhus to malnutrition, inadequate housing, contaminated water supplies, and overcrowding (Engels; Waitzkin).

The early nineteenth century therefore saw the beginning of a transformation of the physician's role (Rosen, 1974). As physicians increasingly recognized the impact of social factors on their patients' health, they saw that helping individual patients made it necessary to assess and respond to the social aspects of their lives along with everything else that might cause or prolong their patients' illnesses.

The term *social medicine* was first used in 1846 to mean "all those aspects of medicine that affect society" (Guérin, p. 203), but its popularization in Europe is usually attributed to Rudolf Virchow (1821–1902; see Erwin Heinz Ackerknecht's 1953 work, and George A. Silver's 1987 work). Virchow, who later became a highly respected pathologist (known by his colleagues as the "Pope of Medicine"), was an early exponent of the importance of social factors as contributors to disease. In 1847, at the Prussian government's request, Virchow investigated a severe typhus epidemic in rural Upper Silesia. In his report he recommended a series of dramatic economic, political, and social changes that included increased employment, better wages, local autonomy in government, agricultural cooperatives, and a more progressive tax structure. He described disease causation as multifactorial, including the conditions of people's lives. To be effective, he argued, a healthcare system must go beyond treating pathological problems in individual patients, and health professionals therefore must take responsibility for political action. In a radical medical-political newspaper he edited, the masthead read: "The physician is the natural attorney of (advocate for) the poor." Virchow insisted that "medicine is a social science, and politics nothing but medicine on a grand scale" (Silver, 1987, p. 85).

Early on, social medicine was basically an approach to medical practice; proponents recognized the effects of social

conditions and took them into consideration in dealing with illness in patients. During the first half of the twentieth century, when Alfred Grotjahn published his *Soziale Pathologie* (1912) and René Sand his *Vers la Médecine Sociale* (1952), social medicine became more than an aspect of medical practice. These works, among others, established the importance and perhaps even the predominance of social factors in disease causation, maintenance, and remission. A whole new field of scholarly study emerged that understood health, disease, and the role of medicine in these terms. Beyond the traditional ethic of a physician's responsibility to a patient or to other physicians, social medicine, which was concerned with the relationship between health and the conditions of society, imposed an added discipline of responsibility to society (Grotjahn; Sand).

The discipline was further refined by John Ryle, professor of medicine at Cambridge University, who included social factors in the analysis of the varied responses of patients to illness. Since individual responses were influenced by the patient's family, work, and economic circumstances, he regarded the study and clinical application of these factors as part of the practice of social medicine (Galdston; Ryle). Ryle wrote that social medicine

> embodies the idea of medicine applied to the service of man as socius, as fellow or comrade, with a view to a better understanding and more durable assistance of all his main and contributory troubles which are inimical to active health…. It embodies also the idea of medicine applied in the service of societas, or the community of man with a view to lowering the incidence of all the preventable diseases and raising the general level of human fitness.

As it became clear that many of the causative agents of disease were social in nature, social medicine embraced not only what is usually called *preventive medicine*—that is, advice on the prevention of illness provided to individuals and families within medical practice—but also what is usually called *public health*—efforts to prevent disease in whole communities. For health and disease, an interface was seen to exist between society and medicine, not just between the doctor and a patient. The family itself, the home, the workplace, the environment, and various other social conditions played a part in whether or not people became sick, how long they remained sick, whether they recovered, and even whether medical care and other healthcare services were available.

Social medicine ranges from the doctor's use of social factors in making a better diagnosis or offering better treatment (that is, an approach to clinical problems) as well as providing preventive medicine, to helping the medical profession recognize social factors that are *pathological* or *therapeutic* in society (that is, an approach to public health). In its contemporary interpretation, social medicine also means influencing the doctor's frame of mind as a professional, so he or she will recognize the need to modify social factors (in effect, an approach to social reform).

Social medicine therefore includes four components:

1. *medical care*: treatment of the individual patient (or family) to provide comfort and hope, ease symptoms, and, when possible, prolong satisfying and productive life or even "cure" the disease;
2. *preventive medicine*: guidance for the individual patient (or family) in promoting health and preventing disease;
3. *public health*: advocacy and action for health promotion and disease prevention in the community; and
4. *social well-being* (as used in the definition of "health" in the Constitution of the World Health Organization), including amelioration of hunger, homelessness, unemployment, poverty, and hopelessness.

Social medicine in action attempts to

1. ensure equitable access to an effective and efficient medical-care system;
2. encourage preventive medicine by, for example, educating practitioners;
3. support extensive public-health activities; and
4. increase resources and services to improve social well-being.

Social Medicine as an Ethical Model

Physicians engaged in the field of social medicine must concern themselves with a wide variety of problems, disciplines, and factors that encompass what are conventionally understood to be outside the proper concerns of the medical profession. Once the physician recognizes a person as a social creature, the whole range of a patient's needs becomes relevant. Traditionally, physicians have rarely seen themselves as responsible for intervention to correct a social situation outside the family that might be contributing to the patient's illness or obstructing recovery. A socially-oriented medical profession may need to take vigorous action in its patients' interest to promote improved housing, nutrition, and educational opportunities or to combat racism, discriminatory practices, or the inequities and inadequacies of the medical delivery system and its distribution or availability.

Social medicine holds that the physician has an ethical responsibility to take steps to change pathogenic situations to protect society, of which the particular patient for whom he or she bears responsibility is a part. In such circumstances, the practice of social medicine may place a physician in serious opposition to many powerful forces in society, not excluding the majority membership of his or her own profession. A physician may thereby incur social and professional opprobrium. This was the fate of playwright Henrik Ibsen's Dr. Stockmann, described by his community as an "enemy of the people" because he questioned the safety of the town's springs, the source of its prosperity (Ibsen).

Even in milder efforts, physicians who undertake the practice of social medicine may face resistance in utilizing their professional role to ameliorate pathogenic social situations such as inadequate nutrition or malnutrition; accidents and disease that befall those who live in inadequate housing; unsafe working conditions; environmental hazards or decayed neighborhoods; and polluted air and water. Again, since many of these factors are the result of neglect commonly visited upon the poor, the physician who seeks to modify such situations may find it necessary to engage in social movements that attempt to mitigate or eliminate poverty and to encourage poor people to take action on their own. The physician may be forced to take a political position, even initiate political action, in pursuing this end, just as those who do not act or who oppose such actions are taking political positions.

The remainder of this article will cover specific aspects of social medicine. These aspects—environmental and occupational health, medical-care systems, responsibility of the profession, and medical education—illustrate the range of the field and its relevance to current issues.

Environmental and Occupational Health

When a physician, as a responsible practitioner of social medicine, recognizes the potent and often baleful influence of industry on the health not only of its workers but of the community in which it is located, community education and further action may be indicated. There is increasing recognition of the environmental origins of cancer, for example, including the role of carcinogens in the workplace. Some workplaces are hazardous by the nature of the job; in others, accidents—commonly the result of inadequate safety measures or careless disregard for safety standards—result in thousands of deaths and millions of injuries. Further, in an unfortunately large number of instances, the effluent of factories poisons rivers, lakes, and air, contributing to chronic morbidity and increased mortality among the workers and in the community.

The physician with social concern may find both political action and educational efforts unwelcome in a community torn between its need for the jobs provided by the industrial presence and fear of the industry's lethal qualities. In some communities, the answer has been to keep the lethal factory rather than accept unemployment, poverty, and starvation without it. Doctors and communities must begin to deal with a novel ethical conflict: How to modify the paradox of democratic capitalism—the need to restrain the profit motive in order to protect the community from destructive exploitation.

These actions include something more than professional response. The requirements for social change and political action (e.g., nutrition for the children of the poor or occupational safety measures) also demand that the physician act as citizen. In some situations the physician may very well be torn between social concern and his or her livelihood. The physician who works for an industry whose work processes are unsafe or pathogenic may jeopardize his or her job by taking a stand against the employer or the industry of which the employer is a part. Yet failing to take a stand makes him or her complicit and endangers the lives of countless others. A physician cannot be expected ethically to remain silent when the work situation is likely to produce trauma or disease.

Some employed physicians are expected to minimize reports of injury or disease in order to reduce the employer's financial commitment. That is the "job," as the employer sees it, for which the physician was hired. But is the physician's job to put first the interests of the employer who pays his or her salary, or the interests of the patient?

The dilemma of dual responsibility is most vividly apparent in wartime. In addition to the medical oath the physician may have taken at the completion of medical school, on entering military service the physician, like all military officers, must agree to obey military orders. These orders, for example, usually require the military physician to return wounded military personnel to action as quickly as possible. The decision as to which patient to treat first may therefore be determined by which one can be returned to duty most quickly rather than by the urgency of each patient's individual need for medical care. In an extreme case, the military physician would be expected to let a seriously wounded soldier die in order to save the life of one less seriously wounded who was able to return more quickly to battle. And if there were enemy wounded who were more urgently in need of care, when would their turn be?

Medical-Care Systems

In its scholarly manifestation, social medicine initiates studies on a nation's economic and social systems' influence on the structure and function of its healthcare system. Studies and procedures of healthcare in individual countries and cross-national comparisons are an important part of the analytic work of social medicine (Allende; Cochrane; Navarro; Roemer; Sidel and Sidel, 1982, 1983; Waitzkin).

The ethical imperative that arises from this work invites agitation for change and improvement in the structure of the medical-care system to improve its functioning. To that end the results of social medicine studies may generate promotion of the values and methods observed in other national systems, toward better access and improved quality in meeting the needs of the poor and the geographically isolated, and of marginally self-supporting workers. At the turn of the twenty-first century, for example, the inflation of medical costs resulting from disorganization and inequities bankrupted many families and barred adequate access to medical care for many others. What is the physician's role in this situation?

If access to medical care is dependent upon ability to pay, and many people are unable to obtain care for lack of funds, is the physician ethically obliged to oppose ability to pay as a condition for service? Of whom, if anyone, should the physician ethically demand payment? Should physicians demand that medical care be free to everyone at the time of service? When ability to pay interferes with access to medical care, does not the profit motive operate against the best interests of the patient and the ethical principles of the physician?

Newspaper reports and medical journal articles offer accounts of unequal medical treatment by race or gender. Blacks receive fewer advanced technological studies than whites for the same conditions (Kahn, Pearson, Harrison, et al.; Kjellstrand; Wenneker and Epstein); women receive less intensive studies and procedures for heart disease than men (Ayanian and Epstein; Kjellstrand). Ethical principles require reversal of such situations, and social medicine studies and principles guide physicians in taking action (Perkins; Hurowitz).

Evidence accumulates that, with the increase of managed care as a method of cost control in medicine, physicians are urged to limit expenditures by reducing services or narrowing access to expensive studies, hospitalization, or medications. Physicians in medical groups under managed-care controls are offered incentives to conform with such regulations or may be punished financially for not complying.

Official reports as well as media accounts about the scandalous treatment of elderly people confined to nursing homes is another example in point. The profit motive too often leads not only to cutting corners on services and allowing short weights in food or supplies, but to making substitutions of less qualified staff, eliminating necessary services, and waiving safety and protective measures for the helpless inhabitants. Aside from the corrupt financial dealings it encourages in such cases, profit-making often prevents and obstructs both the best care and the provision of alternatives to institutional care. Physicians cannot insulate themselves morally from the mistreatment of elderly people in nursing homes nor from the exploitation of patients through the entrepreneurial mechanics of the pharmaceutical drug industry.

Is it part of the ethics of social medicine to condemn investment in drug industry stocks, in private proprietary hospitals, and in a variety of entrepreneurial enterprises such as laboratories, radiological centers, and other diagnostic and treatment modalities to which they refer their patients? The U.S. Congress and the American Medical Association have strongly condemned "self-dealing" of this nature.

Responsibility of the Profession

In addition to the question of the individual physician's ethics in financial dealings that may compromise patients' best interests, there is the associated question of the physician's responsibility for taking action when he or she observes any unethical or unprofessional behavior on the part of a colleague. If a physician knows first-hand about the poor quality of a particular nursing home, even if his or her particular patient is not affected by it, is the physician required to take steps to correct the situation? Legal steps? Professional steps? Or, more narrowly, if the physician knows of colleagues who do not or cannot adequately carry out their obligations as physicians because of incompetence or because of lack of training, illness, or addiction, what should be done about it? Social medicine holds that there is an ethical responsibility to call attention to these facts even if they do not cause risk to the physician's particular patients.

The physician as social medicine practitioner is asked to make a difficult choice, as a citizen and as a doctor. Social medicine as an ethical model imposes an obligation on the physician to serve his or her individual patient by serving all patients. And, as a member of a profession, the physician must act not only as an individual but as representative of that profession, adopting an advocacy role for the groups in society that require special attention and care. The profession is being asked to act toward society as the individual physician is asked in traditional ethical statements to act toward an individual patient.

Finally, the ethical physician has a responsibility to inform and educate the community on the social nature of health and illness. An educated and knowledgeable constituency is required to provide the necessary support for the political social action. Discussing the dangers of smoking, for example, is hardly enough. Physicians ought also to discuss the economics of the tobacco industry and suggest that steps need be taken to cushion workers from unemployment if the tobacco industry is diminished or eliminated. Moreover, if there is an industrial hazard that needs correction, physicians ought to advise not only on the danger but on means for correcting it.

It is clear, nonetheless, that for physicians to discharge social medical responsibilities in complex areas, they need to see themselves as part of a group larger than the medical profession alone. In 1956, Theodore Fox described the "Greater Medical Profession" and urged "converting the medical empire into a commonwealth" (Fox). To respond ethically to social needs is to recognize the contribution of all health workers and to act in concert with others in the health field and outside it. In doing this the physician may wish to join with others in professionally oriented groups—such as the American Public Health Association, the International Physicians for the Prevention of Nuclear War, Physicians for Human Rights, and Physicians for Social Responsibility.

Social Medicine in Medical Education

Medical education should include not only the technical, laboratory, and clinical models of what a physician can do, must know, and be able to deal with; it should also give the future physician the tools to recognize the social circumstances—industrial, neighborhood, legislative, administrative—that play a part in the production of disease or that influence medical care. Exposure to social medicine as an important component of medical education, along with the example of role models and the fact that faculty members have such interests, will influence students' and later practicing physicians' ideas as to what their responsibilities are and how these responsibilities can be discharged (Silver, 1973).

Although departments of social medicine had long existed in medical schools and hospitals in other countries, it was not until the 1950s that Ephraim Bluestone and Martin Cherkasky organized the first department of social medicine in a U.S. medical institution, Montefiore Medical Center in New York City (Levenson). Other institutions such as Harvard Medical School, the University of North Carolina College of Medicine, and the Albert Einstein College of Medicine later adopted the term in department names or titles of professorships, but the pace of this development in the United States has languished.

Conclusion

Early medical ethics was largely restricted to the concept of a physician–patient dyad. Social relationships of pathogenic factors were unknown or ignored. By the beginning of the twenty-first century, it had become clear that the social aspects of the prevention, causation, maintenance, or cure of disease cannot be adequately dealt with solely in the one-to-one relationship. Expanded notions of the physician's responsibility based on social factors ought to be included in modern medical ethics statements. The physician should learn to recognize and articulate social demands for change in situations that are harmful to patients and to the community, and not simply deal with problems as they arise in his or her patients.

To this end, physicians must know more about the social situations in which disease occurs or which contribute to disease; they must adopt an advocacy role in pursuing change, and join with other health workers in ensuring appropriate social action for correction. In addition to oaths and declarations in which physicians bind themselves to serve individual patients honorably and ethically, service to society must also be required of physicians. Social medicine deserves an integral place within a more traditional medical ethics. Unfortunately, issues of social medicine are often assigned low priority in medical education and in medical practice.

GEORGE A. SILVER
VICTOR W. SIDEL (1995)
REVISED BY VICTOR W. SIDEL

SEE ALSO: *AIDS: Public Health Issues; Conflict of Interest; Epidemics; Eugenics: Historical Aspects; Genetics and Environment in Human Health; Healthcare Resources, Allocation of; Health Screening and Testing in the Public Health Context; Medical Education; Medicine, Anthropology of; Medicine, Sociology of; Occupational Safety and Health; Population Ethics: Elements of Population Ethics; Public Health; Race and Racism; Responsibility; Sexism; Warfare: Medicine and War; Whistleblowing*

BIBLIOGRAPHY

Ackerknecht, Erwin Heinz. 1953. *Rudolf Virchow: Doctor, Statesman, Anthropologist.* Madison: University of Wisconsin Press.

Allende, Gossens Salvador. 1939. *La Realidad Medico-Social Chilena: Sintesis.* Santiago, Chile: Ministerio de Salubridad, Prevision y Asistencia Social.

Ayanian, John Z., and Epstein, Arnold M. 1991. "Differences in the Use of Procedures Between Women and Men for Coronary Heart Disease." *New England Journal of Medicine* 325: 221–225.

Chadwick, Edwin. 1842 (reprint 1965). *Report on the Sanitary Conditions of the Labouring Population of Great Britain,* ed. M. W. Flinn. Edinburgh: Edinburgh University Press.

Cochrane, Archibald Leman. 1972. *Effectiveness and Efficiency: Random Reflections on Health Services.* London: Neuffield Provincial Hospitals Trust.

Engels, Friedrich. 1845 (reprint 1968). *The Condition of the Working Class in England in 1844.* Stanford, CA: Stanford University Press.

Fox, Theodore F. 1956. "The Greater Medical Profession." *Lancet* 2(6946): 779–780.

Galdston, Iago, ed. 1949. *Social Medicine: Its Derivations and Objectives.* New York: Commonwealth Fund.

Grotjahn, Alfred. 1912. *Soziale Pathologie.* Berlin: A. Hirschwald.

Guérin, Jules. 1848. "De l'intervention du corps médical dans le situation actuelle; programme de médecine sociale." *Gazette Médicale de Paris,* series 3, 3(12): 203.

Hurowitz, James C. 1993. "Toward a Social Policy for Health." *New England Journal of Medicine* 329(2): 130–133.

Ibsen, Henrik. 1882 (reprint 1935). "An Enemy of the People." In *Eleven Plays of Henrik Ibsen.* New York: Modern Library.

Kahn, Katherine L.; Pearson, Marjorie L.; Harrison, Ellen R.; et al. 1994. "Health Care for Black and Poor Hospitalized Medicare Patients." *Journal of the American Medical Association* 271: 1169–1174.

Kjellstrand, C. M. 1988. "Age, Sex, and Race Inequality in Renal Transplantation." *Archives of Internal Medicine* 148: 1305–1309.

Levenson, Dorothy. 1984. *Montefiore: The Hospital as Social Instrument: 1884–1984.* New York: Farrar Straus Giroux.

McKeown, Thomas, and Lowe, Charles Ronald. 1974. *An Introduction to Social Medicine,* 2nd edition. Oxford: Blackwell Scientific Publications.

Navarro, Vicente. 1992. "Has Socialism Failed? An Analysis of Health Indicators Under Socialism." *International Journal of Health Services* 22(4): 563–601.

Perkins, Jane. 1993. "Race Discrimination in the American Health Care System." *Clearinghouse Review* (special issue): 371–383.

Roemer, Milton. 1991. *National Health Systems: Comparative Strategies.* New York: Oxford University Press.

Rosen, George. 1947. "What Is Social Medicine? A Genetic Analysis of the Concept." *Bulletin of the History of Medicine* 21(5): 674–733.

Rosen, George. 1974. *From Medical Police to Social Medicine: Essays on the History of Health Care.* New York: Science History Publications.

Ryle, John A. 1943. "Social Medicine: Its Meaning and Its Scope." *British Medical Journal* 2(4324): 633–636.

Sand, René. 1952. "The Advent of Social Medicine." In *The Advance to Social Medicine.* London: Staples Press.

Sidel, Ruth, and Sidel, Victor W. 1982. *The Health of China.* Boston: Beacon Press.

Sidel, Victor W., and Sidel, Ruth. 1983. *A Healthy State: An International Perspective on the Crisis in U.S. Medical Care.* New York: Pantheon.

Silver, George A. 1973. "The Teaching of Social Medicine." *Clinical Research* 21(2): 151–155.

Silver, George A. 1987. "Virchow, the Heroic Model in Medicine: Health Policy by Accolade." *American Journal of Public Health* 77(1): 82–88.

Waitzkin, Howard. 1989. "Marxist Perspective in Social Medicine." *Social Science and Medicine* 28(11): 1099–1101.

Wenneker, Mark B., and Epstein, Arnold M. 1989. "Racial Inequalities in the Use of Procedures for Patients with Ischemic Heart Disease in Massachusetts." *Journal of the American Medical Association* 261: 253–257.

SOCIAL WORK IN HEALTHCARE

• • •

Social workers have played a vital role in healthcare settings since the early twentieth century. Social work was introduced to medical settings in the United States by Dr. Richard C. Cabot in 1905. Cabot, a professor of both clinical medicine and social ethics at Harvard University, was instrumental in adding social workers to his clinic staff at Massachusetts General Hospital. Under the direction of their first department head, Ida Cannon, these social workers helped patients and their families cope with illness, disease, disability, and hospitalization by focusing particularly on their psychosocial needs, including their emotional reaction and adaptation (Rossen).

Over time, social work's function and influence in healthcare settings have expanded significantly (Miller and Rehr). In addition to assisting hospitalized patients and their families, social workers provide genetic counseling, hospice services, psychotherapy and counseling in mental-health agencies, and treatment of people with eating disorders and substance abuse problems. These opportunities exist in hospitals, neighborhood health and family planning clinics, psychiatric institutions, community mental-health centers, nursing homes, rehabilitation centers, and other long-term care facilities. Social workers' specialized role is to help patients and their families cope with illness and disability.

Many social workers in healthcare settings provide patients and their families with counseling, and information about and referral to needed resources (e.g., home healthcare, financial assistance, nursing home placement). Social workers are also skilled in organizing and facilitating support groups for various populations, such as cancer patients, rape victims, and parents of seriously impaired infants. They work to enhance the availability of community-based resources (e.g., healthcare clinics in low-income neighborhoods or residential programs for children with AIDS), advocate on behalf of individual patients who are in need of services, and advocate to ensure that important public policy issues related to healthcare are addressed (e.g., funding for lead screening or guidelines concerning involuntary commitment of mentally ill individuals to psychiatric hospitals).

Social workers typically function as part of an interdisciplinary team, which may include physicians, nurses, nutritionists, rehabilitation staff, clergy, and healthcare administrators. On occasion, they facilitate the process through which healthcare professionals negotiate differences of opinion or conflict among themselves concerning specific ethical issues. Social workers' skilled use of mediation techniques can help to resolve disagreements that sometimes arise in healthcare settings. Their sensitivity to ethnic and cultural diversity can be particularly helpful when there is a clash between patients' and families' ethnically or culturally based values and prevailing ethical norms, policies, and healthcare practices (e.g., concerning the use of mood-altering medication, autopsy, or blood transfusion).

Bioethical issues in healthcare settings present social workers with complex challenges (Reamer, 1985, 1987). Some of these ethical issues pertain to specific medical conditions. Examples include ethical dilemmas related to a family's decision about withdrawal of a patient's life support, abortion following a rape, organ transplantation, the use of restraints with a noncompliant psychiatric patient, or a patient's decision to refuse neuroleptic medication. When such issues arise, social workers often serve as important intermediaries in relationships among patients, their families, and healthcare professionals. In these instances, social workers help patients and their families make difficult personal decisions, facilitate communication among members of the healthcare team, advocate on a patient's or family's behalf, or raise policy issues that need to be addressed by a hospital, nursing home, or rehabilitation center.

Other bioethical issues concern the nature of relationships and transactions between social workers and patients or their families. For example, social workers in healthcare settings must be familiar with privacy and confidentiality norms that govern relationships with patients and families. They must also be sensitive to complex ethical issues involving patients' right to self-determination, informed consent procedures, truth telling, professional paternalism, and whistleblowing (Loewenberg and Dolgoff; Reamer, 1990).

In particular, social workers can clarify differences among the ethical obligations that guide various professions. For example, social workers in a healthcare setting can help clarify the ethical responsibilities of various professionals when staff suspect child abuse or that a patient with AIDS poses a threat to a third party.

Healthcare social workers are also involved in discussion and formulation of the ethical aspects of healthcare policy and administration. This may take several forms. Social workers may participate as members of institutional ethics committees (IECs) that discuss ethically complex cases and policies. They may have a particularly valuable perspective because of their extensive contact with patients and their families and can, therefore, contribute to discussions about, for example, resuscitation guidelines, patients' right to refuse treatment, advance directives, organ transplantation, treatment of severely impaired infants, and the privacy rights of AIDS patients. Similarly, social workers are active participants on institutional review boards (IRBs) that examine a variety of ethical issues in research on human subjects.

In addition, social workers may be involved in discussions about the ethical aspects of healthcare financing mechanisms and cost-containment measures. They may also propose ways to advocate on patients' behalf or to advocate for policy reform that may provide a more just allocation of scarce healthcare resources at the local, national, or international level. An example is social workers' participation on a hospital committee to assess the pressure to limit care provided to, and hasten discharge of, psychiatric patients covered under *managed care* programs operated by private insurers. In these instances, social workers may help identify the psychosocial consequences of various strategies to allocate limited healthcare resources.

As a profession, social work has its formal origins in nineteenth-century concern about the poor, and is an outgrowth of the pioneering work of charity organization societies and settlement houses, primarily in England and the United States (Brieland; Leiby). Thus, social workers are inclined to be attentive to the needs of low-income, culturally diverse, and oppressed patients and families.

Although contemporary social workers provide services to individuals and families at all points on the socioeconomic spectrum, the profession continues to have an abiding concern for the disadvantaged. As a result, social workers in healthcare settings are alert to ethical issues that involve such populations as low-income patients, abused children and elders, women, refugees and immigrants, substance abusers, ethnic minorities, and gay or lesbian individuals. Concern about such vulnerable groups—for example, with respect to their access to healthcare, their privacy rights, or discrimination against them by healthcare providers—is one of social work's principal hallmarks. Social workers may advocate for individual patients and families whose rights are threatened or who are victims of institutional abuse or discrimination. They also may advocate for public policy that will enhance protection of the rights of these populations.

Like all healthcare professionals, in order to participate fully in discussions of bioethical issues and dilemmas, social workers need specialized knowledge and training. First, they need to be familiar with the history, language, concepts, and theories of bioethics, particularly as they have evolved since the early 1970s. Second, social workers should be knowledgeable about formal mechanisms that can help healthcare professionals monitor and address bioethical issues. These include phenomena such as IECs, IRBs, utilization review and quality assurance committees, informed consent procedures, and advance directives. It is also useful for social workers to be acquainted with relevant codes of ethics and legal considerations (statutes and case law) related to patients' rights and healthcare professionals' obligations.

Finally, social workers should be familiar with the various schools of thought that pertain to ethical decision making and ethical theory. This can be particularly useful when social workers are involved in discussion of cases with professional ethicists, for example, when a decision must be made about when and how to tell a fragile, terminally ill patient the truth about his or her diagnosis, or to disclose confidential information, against a patient's wishes, in order to protect a third party. This training may be offered as part of agency-based in-service education, professional conferences, or undergraduate and graduate social work education.

Especially since the early 1970s, social workers have been aware of the diverse and complex bioethical issues involved in healthcare, whether it involves acute or chronic, inpatient or outpatient, or medical, rehabilitative, nursing, or psychiatric care. Social workers' growing awareness of, and enhanced expertise in addressing, bioethical issues helps to ensure the protection of patients' and families' rights and the soundness of ethical decisions made in healthcare settings.

FREDERIC G. REAMER (1995)
BIBLIOGRAPHY REVISED

SEE ALSO: *Bioethics Education: Other Health Professions; Clinical Ethics: Institutional Ethics Committees; Confidentiality; Family and Family Medicine; Informed Consent:*

Meaning and Elements of Informed Consent; Palliative Care and Hospice; Paternalism; Privacy in Healthcare; Teams, Healthcare; Whistleblowing

BIBLIOGRAPHY

Brieland, Donald. 1987. "History and Evolution of Social Work Practice." In *Encyclopedia of Social Work*, vol. 1, 18th ed., ed. Anne Minahan. Silver Spring, MD: National Association of Social Workers.

Bullis, Ronald K. 1995. *Clinical Social Worker Misconduct: Law, Ethics, and Personal Dynamics.* Belmont, CA: Wadsworth Publishing Company.

Kirk, Stuart A., ed. 1998. *Current Controversies in Social Work Ethics: Case Examples.* Washington, D.C.: National Association of Social Workers.

Leiby, James. 1978. *A History of Social Welfare and Social Work in the United States.* New York: Columbia University Press.

Linzer, Norman. 1998. *Resolving Ethical Dilemmas in Social Work Practice.* Boston, MA: Allyn and Bacon.

Loewenberg, Frank, and Dolgoff, Ralph. 1992. *Ethical Decisions for Social Work Practice*, 4th ed. Itasca, IL.: F. E. Peacock.

Miller, Rosalind S., and Rehr, Helen, eds. 1983. *Social Work Issues in Health Care.* Englewood Cliffs, NJ: Prentice-Hall.

National Association of Social Workers. 1979. *Code of Ethics of the National Association of Social Workers.* Silver Spring, MD.: Author.

Pawar, Manohar. 2000. "Australian and Indian Social Work Codes of Ethics." *Australian Journal of Professional and Applied Ethics* 2(2): 72–85.

Reamer, Frederic G. 1985. "The Emergence of Bioethics in Social Work." *Health and Social Work* 10(4): 271–281.

Reamer, Frederic G. 1987. "Values and Ethics." In *Encyclopedia of Social Work*, vol. 2, 18th ed., ed. Anne Minahan. Silver Spring, MD: National Association of Social Workers.

Reamer, Frederic G.. 1990. *Ethical Dilemmas in Social Service*, 2nd edition. New York: Columbia University Press.

Reamer, Frederic G. 1998. *Ethical Standards in Social Work: A Critical Review of the National Association of Social Workers Code of Ethics.* Washington, D.C.: National Association of Social Workers.

Reamer, Frederic G., 1999. *Social Work Values and Ethics.* New York: Columbia University Press.

Reamer, Frederic G. 2001. *Social Work Ethics Audit: A Risk Management Tool.* Washington, D.C.: National Association of Social Workers.

Robison, Wade L. and Reeser, Linda Cherrey. 1999. *Ethical Decision Making in Social Work.* Boston: Allyn and Bacon.

Rossen, Salie. 1987. "Hospital Social Work." In *Encyclopedia of Social Work*, vol. 1, 18th ed., ed. Anne Minahan. Silver Spring, MD.: National Association of Social Workers.

Thyer, Bruce A., and Pruger, Robert. 2002. *Controversial Issues in Social Work Practice.* Boston: Allyn and Bacon.

SPORTS, BIOETHICS OF

• • •

The use of banned substances (doping), genetic enhancement, and gender issues are three topics central to the discussion of bioethics in sports.

Doping in Sport

Prior to the inception of the World Anti-Doping Agency (WADA) in 1999 and the World Anti-Doping Code (2003), banned substances and practices in organized sport were identified by the International Olympic Comittee (IOC). In its *International Olympic Charter against Doping in Sport* (1990), the IOC declared that "the use of doping agents in sport is both unhealthy and contrary to the ethics of sport, and that it is necessary to protect the physical and spiritual health of athletes, the values of fair play and of competition, the integrity and unity of sport, and the rights of those who take part in it at whatever level." This charter contains a list of substances and practices that are banned from the Olympic Games. The use of these banned substances and practices is referred to as *doping*. However, the IOC lacked a clear ethical framework that could justify the banning of these items by showing them to be relevantly different from permitted substances and practices.

Each of the IOC's reasons for banning certain substances and practices can be found in more developed forms in the literature of the philosophy and ethics in sport. These include arguments against cheating, unfair advantage, and harm,as well as the ideas that doping perverts the nature of sport and that doping is dehumanizing. The basis for a potential coherent and enforceable ban on doping in sport derives from a view of the intrinsic goods of sport.

THE INADQUACY OF CURRENT ARGUMENTS TO SUPPORT BANS. There are four arguments that are generally proposed to justify banning drugs in sport. All of them have some merit, though none of them provide a sufficient justification for banning doping.

Cheating and unfairness. The argument that doping amounts to cheating was used by Justice Charles Dubin of the Canadian Royal Commission, which was established by the Canadian Federal Government after the Ben Johnson scandal during the 1988 Seoul Olympics. The *Dubin Report* states that the most vigorous opponents of cheating in sport are those who insist that sports must be conducted in accordance with the rules. The moral disapprobation of doping is thus seen as coming from the fact that doping is cheating.

The major problem with this position is that an activity only becomes cheating once there is a rule prohibiting it. So while the fact that doping is cheating may well provide a reason for enforcing the rules against doping, and while the fact that doping is cheating may give other athletes a reason to have an extremely negative attitude towards those who dope, there is not yet a clearly argued reason for creating the rule banning doping in the first place.

There are alternative interpretations of this argument. One is that there is something in the concept of *cheating* that implies a notion of *unfair advantage* of one competitor over another. The use of certain substances and practices falls into this category. However, for this view to justify banning a substance, the notion of unfair advantage must be independent of the rules of sport (unlike cheating). In other words, if *unfair advantage* turns out to be just rule-breaking, then it cannot do the work that the concept of "cheating as rule-breaking" could not do. This raises a variety of philosophically interesting questions: What is cheating? Why is cheating wrong? And, independent of the answer to these questions, *Why should doping been banned?* From a bioethics perspective, it will not do to say simply that one should not dope because it is banned. What is significant is the justification for banning it in the first place.

The argument that doping is unfair suffers from a similar weakness. The simplest idea of fairness is one connected to adherence to the rules: an action is unfair if it is against the rules. An alternative notion of fairness is independent of the rules of sport. But this notion would have to show how doping was inherently unfair, even if the contestants agreed that all could do it, and even if the rules of the game permitted it. Thus, the concept of unfair advantage is no better justification for banning a substance than cheating is.

The concepts of cheating and unfair advantage would have to exist independently outside of sport in order to be brought to bear to evaluate sport. For example, the concepts of cruelty or brutality, which are moral evaluations, have been used to ban sports such as bare-knuckle boxing. It may well have been the case that bare-knuckle bouts were free of cheating and quite fair, they were, however, brutal and cruel, and on these grounds they were banned. Unless the concepts of cheating and unfair advantage can similarly be grounded outside of sport, they will be unavailable to justify or criticise the rules of sport.

Harm to the athlete. The second most commonly cited argument used to justify the ban on doping is that it is harmful. Doping is viewed as being: (1) harmful to users, (2) harmful to other athletes, (3) harmful to society, and (4) harmful to the sports community. However, these arguments cannot be expected to provide a general justification for prohibiting doping, but must be addressed sport by sport and substance by substance.

The argument that a ban is justified because doping is harmful to the user assumes that a particular substance or pracice is harmful, and that potential users need to be protected from the substance or practice. Anabolic steroids provide a good example of such a substance. The assertion that medically supervised steroid use harms the user is, at the turn of the twenty-first century, scientifically unproven. Much of the evidence concerning harm is derived from anecdotal testimony of athletes using very high doses in uncontrolled conditions, and the medical evidence from controlled low-dose studies tends to show minimal harm. Society's abhorrence of the practice has prevented the gathering of hard scientific evidence, because such research has yet to be approved by ethics committees. Autologous blood-doping has not been shown to have adverse side-effects at all.

There are two elements to the charge of harm to the user of a substance: the bad effects of the substance, and the causal linkage of these effects to doping. It has not been scientifically proven just what the "bad effects" from doping are. For the sake of argument, however, one can grant that steroids do indeed harm their users (not an implausible assumption). It would then be necessary to address each particular steroid on its own merits, rather than formulated a general argument against doping.

It can also be argued that the desire to protect competent adults from the consequences of their own actions is paternalistic. Paternalism has both acceptable and unacceptable forms. For example, some would argue that banning doping for minors is acceptable, but that banning doping for adults is unacceptable. There are, however, instances where certain practices are banned for adults, such as banning driving without seatbelts. The question thus becomes whether banning steroids, and other substances and practices, is acceptable paternalism?

Much of the thrust of modern bioethics has been directed against medical paternalism. It may be argued that to ban steroids solely to protect competent adults is to treat those adults athletes as children who are unable to make choices that directly impact their lives. This position is generally inconsistent with the nature of high-performance sport, in which athletes are constantly pushing their limits.

Some would argue that it is inconsistent, and even hypocritical, for the governing bodies of sports to attempt to justify a ban by appealing to the athlete's well-being. There are many training practices, and indeed many sports, that carry a far greater likelihood of harm to the athlete than does the controlled use of steroids. If the reason for banning doping in sport really were a concern for the health and well-being of athletes, then many other practices (and many sports) should also be banned.

One might argue that the risks incurred by the nature of the sport (e.g., brain damage from having one's head pummelled in boxing) are different from the risks that are incurred from practices that have nothing to do with competition in the sport per se (e.g., liver damage from steroid use). The basis of this argument might be tied to a distinction between the *external good* and the *internal good* that are derived from participation in a sport. Internal goods (skill, strategy, self-fulfillment, etc.) are gained from participation in the activity itself, while external goods (fame, prestige, money, etc.) are gained from societal recognition of success. Some might argue that the only way one can gain these internal goods is to take the risks involved in participation. However, this distinction is invalid if the justification for the ban is that a substance harms the user, because the athlete can be harmed in either case (i.e., both brain damage and liver damage are harmful).

There is little evidence to suggest that banning doping will protect athletes. As long as a subculture exists that believes that doping brings benefits—and that it is an occupational hazard of highlevel competitive sport—athletes will continue to use these substances in clandestine, unsanitary, and uncontrolled ways. Only a change in values will end such use, and this will only happen after a logically consistent position for the ban has been put forward (presumably, a ban would be intended as part of a larger process aimed at producing just such a change in values).

Harm to other athletes. It is also argued that steroids should be banned because of the harm their use causes to other athletes. ("Others" are usually deemed to be "clean," or nondoping, athletes.) This is called the *coercion* argument, and it is more difficult to dismiss quickly. The same liberal tradition that prohibits paternalistic interventions permits interventions designed to prevent harm to others. What must be determined is how great the harm is to other athletes, and how severe the limitation on personal action is.

In order to assess this argument one needs to consider whether or not the potential coercion of clean athletes outweighs the infringement on the liberties of athletes caused when a substance or practice is banned. Clean athletes are harmed, so the argument goes, because the dopers "up the ante." If some competitors are using steroids, then all competitors who wish to compete at their level will need to take steroids or other substances to keep up. This argument has some merits, but it is still incomplete, for elite-level sport is already highly coercive. If full-time training, altitude training, or diet control are shown to produce better results, then everyone is forced to adopt these measures to keep up. The feeling that somehow steroid use is worse than longer or more specialized training just raises the question of *why* it is worse. Why can't an athlete accept two "raises of the ante" but not accept a third, or even an unlimited number?

The answer to this question relies on a demand for consistency. There must be some reason why a particular practice is banned, and that reason cannot be merely that it raises the ante too high. This is a qualitative question, not a quantitative one, that necessarily requires an explanation for banning a substance on its own merits.

On the other hand, the coercion argument has merit if it can be shown that doping is irrelevant to a particular view of what is important to sport. If sports and sporting contests are about testing skills, then it can be argued that the improved performance that comes with doping is irrelevant to that test of skill (especially when one bears in mind that if some athletes dope, others will be forced to dope in order to keep up, thus obviating the original advantage that came with doping). If doping is irrelevant to sport, the athletes can shun it as being unnecessarily coercive.

Harm to society. This position says that doping harms others in society, especially children who see athletes as role models. If children see athletes having no respect for the rules of the games they play, there will be an undermining of respect for rules, and for law in general. This argument only works if doping is against the rules, however, and so cannot function as a justification for banning doping in the first place.

Athletic drug use is also seen as part of a wider social problem of drug use. The argument here is that if children see athletes using drugs to attain sporting success, then other drugs may be seen as a viable means to other ends. The limitation of this argument is that there are many things that are considered appropriate for adults but not for children. Alcohol and cigarettes are obvious examples, as is sex, but, in North America at least, these substances or activities are not banned for adults simply because they would be bad for children.

A further response to the suggestion that athletes should be role models—and, in particular, *moral* role models—is to ask why. People expect widely varying things of their public figures. No one seriously expects musicians or actors and actresses to be moral role models, so why should athletes be singled out for special treatment? Why should more be expected from athletes than from other public figures?

Some philosophers have argued that sport is one of the very first areas young people experience, and one of the first in which they hope to gain excellence. From a societal perspective, if the heros and heroines of young people are morally despicable, then they will exert a negative influence. Young people will not separate the athletic abilities of their heroes or heroines from the quality of their personal lives, especially when fame and glamour surround such persons. The achievement of excellence in athletics comes prior to, and will greatly influence, the achievement of excellence in adult arenas such as business, academia, and politics. Perhaps for these reasons people are more concerned about the moral image of athletes than of other public figures.

What is it about drug use in sport that people find morally repugnant? No one else is prevented from using cold remedies, even if they drive public transportation, or from using caffeine as a stimulant to work harder. So it is not even the case that athletes are asked to meet the standards every one else meets, but rather, at least in regard to substance use, they must meet more rigorous standards.

Harm to the sport community. One other group that is potentially harmed is the sports-watching public. These people will be harmed, the argument goes, if they are being cheated—if they expect to see dope-free athletes battling it out in fair competition and are denied this form of entertainment. This harm can be removed in other ways than through banning steroid use, however. One could, for example, remove the expectation that athletes be dope-free. The feeling of being cheated is dependent on the idea that what was expected was a particular type of competition. However, this means asking people to settle for less than what they really want. They might, therefore, suffer other harms, such as the loss of the chance to watch doping-free competition. Of course, this does not address the question of why people value doping-free competition.

HARM CAUSED BY BANS. Because any bans that are imposed need to be enforced, there are potential harms caused by the bans themselves. Enforcement of bans on substances or practices designed to help one train, rather than improve one's performance on the day of competition, requires year-round, random, unannounced, out-of-competition testing. This is an intrusion into the private lives of athletes. Thus, athletes are harmed by being required to consent to such testing procedures (and to give out constant updated information on their whereabouts) in order to be eligible for competition.

One aspect of the harm caused by bans is abstract. Any time one's choices are restricted, one has been harmed. One could argue that the athlete is harmed when deprived of the chance to dope in order to improve performance. On the other hand, the spectator is harmed when deprived of the chance to watch doping-free sport. There is, however, a more direct harm. If one bans drugs or practices, one must necessarily take steps to enforce that ban. Despite the number of positive tests during a competition, the only effective way to test for banned substances is to introduce random, unannounced, out-of-competition testing. This is because some substances, such as anabolic steroids, can be discontinued before competition, and still retain their effects and also because of the prevalence of masking agents and urine substitution using catheters. The demand that athletes be prepared to submit to urine (or blood) testing at any time is considered by some to be a serious breach of their civil and human rights. It could also be argued, however, that such interference is just part of the price of being in sports—no one is forced to become an athlete, let alone an elite athlete.

Many who discuss this topic suggest that "sport is different," that it is not "real life," but "only a game." They argue that, because of this difference, the limitations imposed by the requirements of consent do not apply. The suggestion is that participation in high-performance sport is a privilege, not a right. Therefore, athletes are not deprived of their rights if they are deemed ineligible because they will not submit to a drug test, because they do not have a right to participate in the first place. The serious consequences of this argument is that it would allow the imposition of any rules, no matter how absurd.

Further, this argument is unclear. It may mean that no person has the right to be selected for a national team or for financial support. This is certainly true, but it is also true that there is some obligation to select the best available people for national teams and, barring income tests, for financial support as well. It could then be argued that the "best available person" means the best person available who abides by the rules of the game. However the rules of sport are not arbitrary, and they are open to moral scrutiny. If the format of the drug test is unacceptable on the moral grounds that it invades privacy, then it is also unacceptable for there to be a rule of eligibility that requires it. Sport may well be different, but nothing is so special or different that it can escape all moral scrutiny.

Perversion of sport. The concepts of cheating and unfairness and of harm are moral concepts. Cheating and unfairness presuppose a set of rules, so logically these concepts cannot be used to justify a rule. The concepts of cheating and unfairness are are thus *inside* sport. The arguments related to harm utilize a principle found outside of sport and applied to it, thus working from the outside in.

In contrast, arguments related to the perversion of sport do not operate from moral principles, but from metaphysical ones. What the arguments seek to show is that there is some feature of sport, which, if properly understood, would be demonstrably incompatible with doping. Thus, doping should be banned because it is somehow antithetical to the true nature of sport.

Part of the problem when dealing with this question is that sport is socially constructed, and there is no obvious reason why it could not be constructed to include doping. A view of sport which places at its center the testing of sporting skills, with sporting skills defined by the nature of the game concerned, suggests that doping is not so much antithetical to sport, but rather irrelevant to it (Schneider and Butcher, 1994). Doping is irrelevant to sport because it does not improve skill, but merely provides a competitive advantage over those who do not dope. But a prerequisite for this justification is that it must come from the athletes themselves, not from sport administrators.

Unnaturalness and dehumanization. It is also argued that doping should be banned because it is either unnatural or dehumanizing. The unnaturalness argument does not get very far for two reasons. The first is that it is not clear what would count as *unnatural*. The second is that it is inconsistent. Some things designated unnatural are permitted (e.g., spiked shoes) while certain natural substances (e.g., testosterone) are banned.

The dehumanization argument is interesting but incomplete. There is no agreed upon conception of what it is to be human. Without this it is difficult to see why some practices should count as dehumanizing. We also have a problem with consistency. Some practices, such as psycho-doping (the mental manipulation of athletes using the techniques of operant conditioning) are not banned, whereas the re-injection of one's own blood is banned.

An Alternative Approach

A two-tiered approach has been proposed that could justifiably prohibit doping in sport. This approach tries to show: (1) why athletes should not want to dope, and (2) why the community should support doping-free sport.

WHY ATHLETES SHOULD NOT WANT TO DOPE. Sports are practices that provide the opportunity for individuals to acquire and demonstrate skills. A well-executed back-hand volley is a demonstration of skill because of the kinds of things that are necessary to win at tennis. The shot is difficult and effective, and it is just this sort of manifestation of skill that makes participating in sport so worthwhile. The joy of sport comes from acquiring the goods that are internal to sport, the goods that come with the mastery and demonstration of skill. If this joy is the primary reason for participation in sport, then doping is irrelevant to the internal goods of sport.

Every sport is a sort of game, a game where obstacles have been artificially created to prevent one from readily achieving the object of the game. Skill is demonstrated in the overcoming of those obstacles, within the limits provided by the rules of the game. What makes sport interesting and worthwhile is the mastery of skill, and its demonstration in a fair contest with equally skilled opponents. Doping does not help one to acquire sporting skills, but simply provides a competitive advantage over those who do not dope.

Further, as long as one's competitors do not dope, there is no reason for any athlete to dope, even if the risks are minimal and the probabilities of harm are small. Because there is no game-productive reason for doping, athletes would be wise to avoid it as an unnecessary risk.

Finally, the coercive effect of doping is such that if athletes believe that a good number of their opponents dope, they will feel compelled to dope in order to keep up. But this has the effect of removing the competitive advantage that those who first doped sought to gain. Doping is only an advantage—in terms of *winning*—if you dope and your opponent does not. That advantage is lost if everyone dopes.

These arguments point the way to a method of avoiding the invasion of privacy caused by the enforcement of bans. If athletes want doping-free sport, they will also want to be assured that the competition is fair. Athletes, then, would be in the position to request the enforcement of the rules of self-limitation that they themselves have rationally and prudently chosen.

WHY THE COMMUNITY SHOULD SUPPORT DOPING-FREE SPORT. The sporting community, both participants and fans, is in a position to defend a view of human excellence that can put limits on the pursuit of performance excellence in sport. Given that in most countries amateur sport is publicly funded, the community can promote a view of sporting excellence that places it within the context of a complete, and excellent, human life. So, despite the fact that excellence in certain sports (i.e. boxing and downhill skiing) requires running dreadful risks, society is in a position to limit those risks because it does not want to promote downhill speed over long and healthy lives. The message from those who support sport should be that an athlete's sporting life is only a part of his or her entire life. While excellence in sport is a worthy pursuit, it should not be pursued at the expense of one's health and well-being. Because amateur sport is publicly funded, the community is in a position to put limits on its support, limits that come from the desire to promote human excellence across a complete lifetime.

Genetic Enhancement in Sport and Bioethics

Gene transfer technology will revolutionize the way people view illness and health, and it will also transform the way we diseases are treated and prevented. While this work is still in the research phase, the most imminent applications of gene transfer research to sport performance include muscle growth factors and oxygen transport and utilization.

CONCEPTUAL ISSUES. The primary challenge in gene transfer technology is in drawing the line between therapy and enhancement. The standard approach in sport has been that therapy (repair to bring one back to *normal*) has been permitted, but enhancement (going beyond *normal*) has been banned. This approach does not fit neatly with current medical practice and thinking. For example, in many forms of prevention, the body's normal responses to disease are enhanced to enable a person to avoid infection or illness. Some muscle-repair therapies may have the effect of making the muscle stronger than it was before the injury, thus enhancing performance.

The wording used in a particular ban or regulatory list needs careful consideration. It is easy to be either too specific (thus missing a significant new development) or too general (thus encompassing a variety of acceptable uses of technology). Because of the relation of sport to society, the language used in the World Anti-Doping Code attempts to deal with the development of genetic technology. This code addresses the use and impact of gene transfer technology in sport, while acknowledging that sport operates in a social context. In regard to genetic enhancement, even if sport organizations decided that enhancements should not be permitted, if it became standard medical and social practice to enhance memory and mental acuity, or to enhance muscle growth and strength in the elderly, it would be extremely difficult for sport to stand apart in opposition. There are many areas where enhancement is not only accepted, but encouraged, valued, and highly rewarded (e.g., cosmetic surgery) and even sport—some drug use is permissible in baseball in North America, for instance. If it is socially acceptable in some settings, why not in sport?

The World Anti-Doping Agency (WADA) attempted to initiate discussion on the development of some core agreements by hosting a conference on genetic enhancement and sport at the Banbury Centre in New York in February 2002. WADA has the opportunity to influence and shape the discussion, and to define and direct policy, before gene transfer technologies become available for general use.

OBJECTIONS TO GENE TRANSFER TECHNOLOGY FOR PERFORMANCE ENHANCEMENT. Despite a lack of clarity in exactly what is meant by *treatment* and *enhancement,* it is generally agreed that enhancement for sport purposes is unacceptable. However, within medicine and science this is a very complicated issue, partly because the technology is in the early stages of development. It is difficult for medical scientists to state, in the abstract, that enhancement for sport is unacceptable. This position is thus far more appropriate as a statement from the sport community. Scientifically, it would certainly be unacceptable when the technology is in this immature state.

There is strong agreement that action is required on this issue, and that this action will be complex and multifaceted. It should include: (1) ongoing cooperation between the research and sport community, (2) communication between the sport community and regulatory bodies for review and regulation of research and biotechnology, (3) inclusion of wording covering gene transfer technology in the World Anti-Doping Code, (4) research into detection mechanisms, (5) ongoing discussions between the sport community and the medical and scientific communities concerning standards of practice, (6) ongoing discussions between the sport community and the biotech and pharmaceutical industries, (7) education of athletes, the professions (especially medicine), industry, governments, and the public.

UNDISCOVERED COUNTRY. A number of themes and issues related to genetic therapy and genetic information have yet to be discussed in the sport context. The first of these is *genetic design,* which involves "designing" babies for specific (athletic) traits. The second of these issues is *germ-line,* or heritable, therapy. Other uses of genetic technology include *in vitro* genetic screening, which, in principle, makes it possible to screen embryos for genetic characteristics, and then implant into the womb only those with the "desirable" genetic makeup. It is not known if it will be possible to do this for genes associated with traits that predispose to greater athletic performance, but such a possibility raises numerous ethical questions.

There is also the possibility of genetic screening *in vivo,* where genetic screening techniques could be used (as a form of potential aptitude testing) to determine which children or young people were most likely to benefit from specialized sport training. There has been no comprehensive discussions of the acceptability of these procedures for sport purposes, nor of the privacy issues associated with this genetic information.

REGULATION AND REVIEW. Research on the human applications of gene transfer technology is highly regulated and reviewed at local and national levels in the United States, and, to some extent, by similar mechanisms in other nations. However, review and regulation vary by jurisdiction and nation. The research is currently highly sophisticated and expensive.

There are gaps in regulation in regard to sport applications. For example, a study would not be likely to be described as having the purpose of exploring the enhancement of sport performance, though it could have that effect. The prospective regulation of gene transfer technology for sport purposes must be multifaceted and include: (1) regulation of research, (2) regulation of professional medical practice, and (3) regulation of athletes and support staff.

TESTING. There is general agreement in the sport community that the possibility of testing requires the development of more efficient methods for detection of genetic modification or of the physiological effects of genetic modification. Testing may well be difficult, and it may raise additional ethical issues, but it involves technical issues that are soluble by improved research and technology development. Testing could be aimed at both the primary genetic modification and at secondary indicators. The incorporation of *markers,* or tags, into foreign therapeutic genes to make them more readily detectable may help in detection programs, though this would be contrary to best principles of drug design, in which only therapeutic efficacy should be relevant.

RESEARCH AND EDUCATION. There needs to be increased research and development in the areas of *in vivo* gene and vector detection and the identification of the physiological effects of genetic modification, along with careful and constant ethical review. General education, as part of social change, is viewed as essential. Education should be values-based and target-specific. Researchers need to be educated on the potential uses of their research for sport enhancement purposes—and why this would be harmful to sport and athletes. Biotech companies need to be educated on the potential uses of their products and processes, and on their role (and self-interest) in avoiding misuse. The professions (particularly medicine) need to be educated on standards of professional practice and distinctions between therapy and enhancement. Finally, athletes need to be educated on the values of sport and the side effects and hazards of gene transfer technology.

Bioethics, Sport, and Gender

Many elite-level sports require pushing human limits, and thus present high risks of injuries. Generally speaking, elite-level training can produce fit, but not necessarily healthy, athletes. The results of the pressure to can be different for men and women, however. Three issues in particular—disordered eating, amenorrhea, and osteoporosis—are commonly referred to as *the female athlete-triad.* These problems surface most often in sports such as gymnastics, where victory is the result of judging. In such cases, the physical requirements and resulting risks are directly caused by decisions about what counts as excellent sport. The judging criteria for these sports need to be tailored so as to minimize the health risks they impose on the athletes.

Women athletes have a much higher prevalence of disordered eating than men. Women athletes have, at various times, faced different body-type ideals, but the greatest tension is that between the traditional ideal athlete and the traditional ideal woman. This reflects the higher level of eating disorders among women in the general population, a result of unattainable ideals among many women regarding their bodies. Thus, this problem is partly cultural, and medical control may not be the best, and is certainly not the only, way of addressing the issue.

Historically, some medical authorities have viewed menstruation, pregnancy, menopause, body size, and some feminine behaviors as diseases. For the female athlete the situation becomes even more complicated, because she can be classified as even more abnormal when reproductive changes are evaluated in the context of the traditional male sports arena. If a normal healthy woman is considered unhealthy because the model of the ideal healthy adult is based on being male, then the female athlete starts out as an unhealthy adult simply because she is a woman. If the female athlete then shows signs of becoming masculine through excellence in sports, this only increases her "abnormality." Following this kind of medical classification, when a woman bleeds, she is ill, yet if she does not bleed she is also ill. Pregnancy, then, theoretically constituting a state of health for the traditional ideal woman, should not be treated as disease.

Serious charges of irresponsibility can occur when the relationship between women athletes and their fetuses are characterised as adversarial. Some countries (e.g., Canada, the United States, Australia) have begun to imprison women for endangering their fetuses (Sherwin). Most pregnant women athletes face, at the very least, moral pressure based on the view that simultaneously being pregnant and participating in sport is socially unacceptable. However, genuine harm to the fetus may occur with participation in sport (e.g., through oxygen deprivation). This is a problem best dealt with through education, however, not through prohibition and criminal penalties.

The classification of the reproductive aspects of women's lives as illnesses has led to wide-scale paternalistic medical management of women under claims of beneficence (Sherwin). In sport, these so-called illnesses have been part of the basis for excluding women. Certainly, serious complications requiring medical interventions can occur with any aspect of a female athlete's reproductive life or life-cycle changes. The physical and emotional pain experienced by older women athletes during menopause has always been a fact. Sport physicians, however, who are predominately male, had to learn to take their female patients seriously before they could recognize that this pain was real, and not just "in their heads." There are instances where the label of illness or disease is appropriate, but it is important that this does not lead to harming women athletes from a policy perspective (e.g., banning them from participation, rather than educating them about coping with their illness and participating in sport).

The Logic of Gender Verification and Transsexualism

Having entirely separate sports for men and women inevitably leads to the question of the logic of gender verification. If there are to be separate sporting events for women, it must be possible to exclude any men that may wish, for whatever reason, to compete in these events. This means that there must be a rule of eligibility that excludes men. (Conversely, if there is such a rule, the question arises of whether there should also be such a rule excluding women from men's events, even if the women believed they would inevitably lose.) This requires a test of gender that can be applied fairly to any potential participant. There are at least three methods of applying any such test. The first would be to test all contestants, the second would be to test random contestants, and the third would be to test targeted individuals.

It is not beyond the realm of imagination, however, that a money-hungry promoter might decide to enter men in a women's event. A male may even, with good intentions, choose to enter a women's event (such as synchronized swimming) as a form of protest against gender discrimination. Without a test to decide just who is eligible, women's events could be forced to accept participants who were quite obviously and unashamedly male, but who professed to be female.

There is a great deal of debate about how sex roles and gender are established. One school of thought takes the position that *sex* refers to biological characteristics and *gender* to socially learned characteristics. The standard practice in the Olympic Games has been to have medical experts verify gender. But, by delegating gender verification to medical experts, the sport community (and society in general) has given great power to medical experts on an issue that is in dispute by researchers.

One famous case that illustrates the conceptual and moral issues of gender verification is that of Renée Richards. Richards was previously a male elite-level tennis player who underwent what is commonly termed a "sex-change operation." The U.S. Women's Tennis Federation wanted to exclude a player who was genetically male, and they therefore introduced the requirement that players take a chromosomal test known as the Barr Test. Richards refused, and went to court to demand the right to participate in women's events. In court she was deemed to be female on the basis of the medical evidence. In the media, this story played as an example of a courageous individual fighting for personal rights against an intransigent and uncaring system, though there are, of course, other ways of viewing the story.

What makes a woman a woman? Is it chromosomes, genitalia, a way of life or set of roles, or a medical record? It is not clear why medical evidence of surgery and psychology should outweigh chromosomal evidence, nor is it clear why any one answer should be taken as categorically overriding any other. Some women argue that any gender or sex test is demeaning (especially visual confirmation of the "correct" genitalia) and discriminatory if it is not also applied to men. Clearly the use of any test, given the complexity of human sex and gender, may lead to anomalies and surprises. Yet many women wish to have sporting competitions that exclude men. One thing that does seem to become clear when faced with the complexity of this issue is that women athletes themselves should be the guardians and decision makers concerning women's sport. The best result will be one that arises through discussion, debate, and consensus.

THOMAS H. MURRAY (1995)
REVISED BY ANGELA J. SCHNEIDER

SEE ALSO: *Addiction and Dependence; Conflict of Interest; Cybernetics; Enhancement Uses of Medical Technology; Harmful Substances, Legal Control of; Human Dignity; Transhumanism and Posthumanism*

BIBLIOGRAPHY

Brown, W. 1980. "Ethics, Drugs, and Sport." *Journal of the Philosophy of Sport* 11: 15–23.

Brown, W. 1984. "Comments on Simon and Fraleigh." *Journal of the Philosophy of Sport* 11: 33–35.

Brown, W. 1984. "Paternalism, Drugs, and the Nature of Sports." *Journal of the Philosophy of Sport* 11: 14–22.

Brown, W. 1990. "Practices and Prudence." *Journal of Philosophy of Sport* 17: 71–84.

Butcher, R. B., and Schneider, A. J. 1993. *The Ethical Rationale for Drug-Free Sport.* Ottawa: Canadian Centre for Drug-Free Sport.

Cohen, G. 1993. *Women in Sport: Issues and Controversies.* Thousand Oaks, CA: Sage.

Creedon, P., ed. 1994. *Women, Media and Sport: Challenging Gender Values.* Thousand Oaks, CA: Sage.

Dubin, C. 1990. *Commission of Inquiry into the Use of Drugs and Banned Practices Intended to Increase Athletic Performance.* Ottawa: Canadian Government Publishing Centre.

Fausto-Sterling, A. 1985. *Myths of Gender: Biological Theories about Women and Men.* New York: Basic Books.

Fost, N. 1986. "Banning Drugs in Sport: A Skeptical View." *Hasting Centre Report* August: 5–10.

Hargreaves, J. 1995. "A Historical Look at the Changing Symbolic Meanings of the Female Body in Western Sport." In *Sport as Symbol, Symbols in Sport,* ed. F. van der Merwe. ISHPES Studies, Vol. 4. Germany: Academia Verlag.

Houlihan, Barrie. 2002. *Dying to Win: Doping in Sport and the Development of Anti-Doping Policy,* 2nd edition. Strasbourg, France: Council of Europe Publishing.

International Olympic Committee. 1987. *The Olympic Movement.* Lausanne, Switzerland: Author.

International Olympic Committee. 1990a. *International Olympic Charter Against Doping in Sport.* Lausanne, Switzerland: Author.

International Olympic Committee. 1990b. *The Olympic Charter.* Lausanne, Switzerland: Author.

Lenskyj, H. 1986. *Out of Bounds: Women, Sport and Sexuality.* Toronto: Women's Press.

Mahowald, M. 1978. *Philosophy of Woman: An Anthology of Classic and Current Concepts.* Indianapolis, IN: Hackett.

Murray, Tom H. 1987. "The Ethics of Drugs in Sport." In *Drugs and Performance In Sports,* ed. Richard M. Strauss. Philadlphia: W. B. Saunders.

Noddings, N. 1984. *Caring: A Feminine Approach to Ethics and Moral Education.* Berkeley: University of California Press.

Okruhlik, K. 1995. "Gender and the Biological Sciences." *Canadian Journal of Philosophy* 20: 21–42.

Schiebinger, L. 1993. *Nature's Body: Gender in the Making of Modern Science.* Boston: Beacon Press.

Schneider, A. J. 1992. "Harm, Athletes' Rights and Doping Control." In *First International Symposium for Olympic Research,* eds. R. K. Barney and K. V. Meier. London, Ontario: University of Western Ontario, Centre for Olympic Studies.

Schneider, A. J. 1993. "Doping in Sport and the Perversion Argument." In *The Relevance of the Philosophy of Sport,* ed. G. Gaebauer. Berlin: Academia Verlag.

Schneider, A. J., and Butcher, R. B. 1993. "For the Love of the Game: A Philosophical Defense of Amateurism." *Quest* 45(4): 460–469.

Schneider, A. J., and Butcher, R. B. 1994. "Why Olympic Athletes Should Avoid the Use and Seek the Elimination of Performance-Enhancing Substances and Practices in the Olympic Games." *Journal of the Philosophy of Sport* 20/21: 64–81.

Sherwin, S. 1992. *No Longer Patient: Feminist Ethics and Health Care.* Philadelphia: Temple University Press.

Simon, R. L. 1984. "Good Competition and Drug-Enhanced Performance." *Journal of the Philosophy of Sport* 11: 6–13.

Spears, B. 1988. "Tryphosa, Melpomene, Nadia, and Joan: The IOC and Women's Sport." In *The Olympic Games in Transition,* ed. J. Segrave and D. Chu. Champaign, IL: Human Kinetics Books.

Suits, B. 1988. "Tricky Triad: Games, Play, and Sport." *Journal of Philosophy of Sport,* 8: 1–9.

Tong, R, 1995. "What's Distinctive About Feminist Bioethics?" In *Health Care Ethics in Canada,* eds. F. Baylis, J. Downie, B Freedman, B. Hoffmaster, and S. Sherwin. Toronto: Harcourt Brace Canada.

Wolfe, Mary L. 1989. "Correlates of Adaptive and Maladaptive Musical Performance Anxiety." *Medical Problems of Performing Artists* March: 49–56.

INTERNET RESOURCE

World Anti-Doping Agency. 2003. "World Anti-Doping Code." Available from <http://www.wada-ama.org>.

STUDENTS AS RESEARCH SUBJECTS

• • •

Why does it matter if research subjects are students? Three answers surface immediately: first, students might be children; second, students might be in school; and third, students might be engaged in learning. None of these answers is always true, but they are true often enough to deserve consideration in research plans involving students as research subjects. Research involving students, be they minors or adults, should be conducted in accord with ethical principles and applicable regulations to protect students from potential coercion and harm. Paradoxically, these regulations and ethical codes send conflicting signals: The regulations carve out certain kinds of education research as being exempt from the umbrella of regulatory protection, while various ethical statements, disciplinary codes, and guidance—most notably from the American Educational Research Association—single out students as deserving careful treatment (Office for Human Research Protections; Strike, Anderson, Curren, et al.; American Psychological Association; American Sociological Association).

Primary and Secondary Education Students

The vast majority of students in primary and secondary schools have yet to reach adult maturity, legally and developmentally. Given the ethical principle of respect for persons, from which arises the practice of informed consent, research involving young students raises the question of students' abilities to make voluntary, competent and informed decisions about whether or not to participate in proposed research. Human development and experience affect the level of student understanding of research participation. Language and literacy skills affect students' ability to receive and interpret relevant information, much less appreciate the implications of what the consequences of participation could be. Children are generally less familiar than adults with key concepts relevant to research participation and risk, such as confidentiality, experimental trials, or the estimated probability of a particular outcome. Such cognitive tools are essential to grasping a specific research activity and the involvement of research subjects. As they develop and learn, students gradually become more like adults in their capacity to truly understand what involvement in research entails (Bruzzese and Fisher). Some education systems set standards regarding what students should know and be able to do in science at various grade levels, as illustrated by the American Association for the Advancement of Science and the National Research Council. Such standards may provide useful guidance regarding what prospective young research subjects should be expected to understand about participation in research.

Young students also vary significantly from adults in their perceptions and assessments of risks and benefits. Their abilities to make practical judgments are less well developed than those of adults. They may attach very different values to specific harms and benefits, and most concern themselves with short-term consequences. A typical sixth grader views the sacrifice involved in giving up math class to participate in research differently from how an adult would understand it. Children and adolescents also have their own views about common forms of research compensation such as money or material goods. Young people's faculties of moral judgment,

including the reasons they use to justify practical decisions, also vary from adults in patterned ways (Bebeau, Rest, and Narvaez).

Students' voluntary decision-making is also shaped by various influences. Very young children are strongly affected by their parents and other significant adults, while adolescents become more susceptible to their friends' and peers' value orientations and pressures as adult influences wane (Steinberg, Brown, and Dornbusch) These influences obviously bear upon how researchers should construct the circumstances in which students are asked to participate in research.

Parents, Guardians, and School Officials

These developmental considerations lead ethicists and some federal agency regulations to view the agreeable young person as providing *assent*, that is, an affirmative expression of willingness to participate voluntarily in research. U. S. federal regulations generally require assent from minors and supplement that requirement with the *permission* of a parent or guardian. Requirements are less rigidly established in other countries, and practices vary widely. Permission is construed according to standard criteria for informed consent with respect to the parent or guardian's decision on behalf of the student.

Permission generally provides an appropriate mechanism for protecting the autonomy, interests and welfare of the young student, but it may also present challenges. If permission comes from the parents, the research team needs twice the number of affirmative responses to its request for participation. Parents often are not as easy to contact as students, and research suggests that some parents do not give permission for their children to participate in research not because they object, but simply because they don't get around to signing and returning a consent form (Singer). Other parents have reservations about a research team's overtures that are unrelated to any concerns about their children's welfare; they may be embarrassed to reveal their lack of literacy skills, or believe that signing a form reflects a legal concession, or even fear that their signature somehow puts them in jeopardy. Some parents have interests contrary to the students whose welfare they are expected to protect; they may worry that their child's responses to a research survey may embarrass or incriminate the parents. On the other side, students' hesitation about participation may stem from apprehensions about what their parents may find out about sensitive survey questions or how they answered them.

Other adults have a role in protecting prospective student research subjects, which may lead to tension over who has authority to permit student participation in research. School officials are responsible for students' welfare and directly supervise students' school day activities. Since proposed research activities may disrupt normal school life, researchers are generally obliged to obtain school officials' permission to carry out research with students as research subjects. Researchers might also view school officials as appropriate sources for permission to involve students in research. This view is contestable, however, as conflicts arise about parents having control over, or at least a say in, what happens to their children in schools. In the United States, federal laws—most notably the *Family Educational Rights and Privacy Act* and the *Protection of Pupil Rights Amendment*—and state and local laws and policies reflect efforts to prescribe when parents must be consulted before researchers may collect data about students through school records, surveys, or other means. Since federal regulations do allow for waiver or alteration of elements of consent or documentation of consent under certain conditions, researchers sometimes request such waivers, particularly for large scale surveys where the researchers point to the low level of risk involved and the difficulties of securing adequate unbiased samples if active parental permission is required. For some parents, however, it is the sensitivity of survey topics and the potential invasion of privacy that concerns them, not the degree of risk involved.

The School Site

The question of who has authority over what happens to students in schools also raises the issue of the convenience of conducting research with students in schools. Most primary and secondary schooling is compulsory in affluent countries; consequently, researchers can expect to find in schools large and fairly representative samples of young people, neatly segregated by age, under adult supervision, engaged in activities not of their own choosing, and legally required to stay. The opportunities for relatively inexpensive and efficient data collection are obvious. Thus some research efforts seek to involve populations of students as research subjects not because the research objective is focused on understanding education or the lives of students per se, but rather because students in schools offer a convenient way to study a wide variety of phenomena concerning youth. This approach may be viewed by some as a form of exploitation that could be unwelcome and disruptive to the educational process. Frequently students are surveyed about their health and development, extracurricular activities, and perceptions of themselves and society, for reasons unrelated to their educations. Research studies focused on areas outside of education may detract from the school's pursuit of its educational mission, and may pose risks for students by asking for sensitive information about criminal, antisocial, or private behavior.

Education Research and Practice

Education research involves students for the specific purpose of studying the formal and informal processes of learning. Such research projects raise their own set of important ethical concerns, particularly when they involve educational practice and practitioners. Some of these concerns resemble those raised in clinical trials of therapeutic medical interventions.

Education research may involve the educational equivalent of the *therapeutic misconception*: the mistaken belief that the nature of the subject's involvement in research in designed to improve that subject's welfare, rather than in developing generalizable knowledge (Appelbaum, Roth, Lidz, et al.). Students, parents, and researchers may all fall prey to the *educational misconception,* especially in the context of educational practice.

Education researchers often involve teachers or other practitioners in data collection or as co-researchers, and the dual roles of researcher and practitioner sometimes conflict (Hammack), as they do in biomedical research (Koski). What should a practitioner/investigator do in a classroom situation where pursuing a research question comes at the expense of delivering an important lesson? What if one uncovers sensitive information about the students that an educator would not otherwise have known? If a practitioner/investigator discovers that a student cheated on a test, should he or she, as an educator, discipline the student and alter the grade, or, as a researcher, protect the research subject from harm? Note that in such circumstances the protective research device of confidentiality is rendered useless, because the person who collects the information is the selfsame person as the one from whom the potentially harmful information is supposed to be kept.

Education research also raises issues of justice or fairness with regard to the selection of research objectives and selected student populations. Should the focus be on research that will benefit the largest possible number of students, with current level of success in the middle range? Or should the focus be on those students who possess the potential to improve the most from better educational interventions, even if they are already doing relatively well? And what of those students who are currently doing relatively poorly in the current educational system, whose level of achievement may be the most difficult to improve? Do students of one ethnic or linguistic minority deserve more attention than students of another, because their numbers in the education system are larger? Such questions of beneficence and justice are reflected in any research project proposing a selective sample of students, and are framed by deeply held cultural beliefs about the importance of education as a vehicle for equality of opportunity and social mobility.

Education research frequently involves the evaluation of interventions delivered at a collective level in classrooms and schools. Reducing class size, changing teacher behavior, altering curricula, attaching high stakes to test performance, and reforming school culture are all educational interventions that can only be accomplished and studied at a group level. In a study where classrooms or schools are randomly assigned to an innovative approach (treatment) or to the standard educational practice (control), by the time the results are available, students may have outgrown the opportunity to benefit from the more effective intervention if they did not receive it during the study. Individual students and their guardians may be able to decline to have the data about them collected or included in research analyses, and sometimes accommodations such as classroom re-assignment can be made to enable students to opt out of a research study. In many cases, though, if a student or guardian wants to avoid the student's participation in a research evaluation of an educational practice at a participating school, the options may be severely constrained or costly. Such collective decisions about the involvement of students as research subjects must face the challenge of striking a reasonable balance between majority will and minority freedoms (Oakes)

The use of qualitative methods and the involvement of practitioners in many education research studies significantly transform the relations and ethical orientations among researchers, practitioners, and students. Qualitative research strategies in education characteristically intertwine the prescriptive and descriptive dimensions, place research activities in specific moral and political frameworks, and recognize the essential contributions of the "insider" subjects' perspectives, abandoning disinterested stances in favor of "advocacy" positions (Howe and Moses). Likewise, practitioner/investigators often find themselves sharing control over the nature, objectives, and credit for research projects with their colleagues and students, making the relationships among the participants more egalitarian, changeable, and complex (Zeni). In such cases the ethical responsibilities shift accordingly.

Tertiary Education Students

Undergraduate and graduate students generally have the background knowledge, literacy skills, and abilities to appreciate potential harms and benefits at a level resembling those of adults. Indeed, nearly all are adults, removing the need for parental permission for the vast majority of tertiary education students. The typical college student also has relatively good health, more flexible schedule commitments, few or no dependents, limited financial resources, considerable disposable time, and openness to new experiences. More than fifteen million students attend degree-granting tertiary education institutions in the United States, where they are easily accessible to academic researchers. Tertiary education students are prime candidates for research involvement.

DEPARTMENTAL SUBJECT POOLS. Academic researchers, most notably psychologists, have capitalized on the ready availability of students, often their own students. The vast majority of findings in human studies by psychologists come from research involving students as research subjects (Chastain and Landrum). In order to avoid the coercive situation of faculty asking their students to participate in their own research, many institutions set up departmental subject pools (DSPs) through which they arrange for students to participate in faculty research projects.

The practical arrangements of DSPs vary. Some are entirely voluntary, while others are attached to course selection—usually introductory psychology or other lower-division social science courses—and are either required of students or award extra credit for the course. Most DSPs allow students other options, such as writing a paper, as an alternative to participation in research. The ethical rationale generally put forward for this practice is that the DSP arrangements for research participation provide an educational benefit to the research subjects while efficiently supplying sufficient numbers of research subjects to enable faculty to carry out a more robust research agenda of valuable studies.

Some DSPs are ethically better than others, depending on specific features of the DSP, including the following:

- Clear, timely information is provided to prospective students.
- Investigators demonstrate respect for research subjects through their conduct.
- Student participation in the system is efficient and non-punitive.
- Students choose from a variety of research studies.
- Research studies are appropriate for a sample population of college students.
- Research studies are generally low in risk.
- Subject participation is structured to provide educational consent and debriefing experiences.
- A variety of alternatives to participation in research are offered, involving comparable

educational value, time commitment, and enjoyment (Sieber).

The 2002 revision of the American Psychological Association's ethical code reaffirms its previous position on students as research subjects, allowing DSPs if students have alternative options: "8.04 Client/Patient, Student, and Subordinate Research Participants (b) when research participation is a course requirement or an opportunity for extra credit, the prospective participant is given the choice of equitable alternative activities" (American Psychological Association).

There are reasons for skepticism about whether DSPs are ethical at all, unless they are entirely voluntary. Given the imbalances in power, authority, and autonomy inherent in the relationship between teacher and student, complete voluntariness may not be possible. Whatever degree of latitude DSPs permit in student choice of research projects or alternatives, required participation still reflects researchers' use of their control over students' educational choices to induce them to participate.

The claim that DSP participation represents a genuinely beneficial and authentic educational experience is open to objection. DSPs present students with consent situations that do not reflect the ideal of voluntary participation: Outside of DSPs, research subjects are either volunteers or are offered compensation in forms they value. Extraordinary briefing or debriefing experiences may provide students with better understanding of the substance of a particular research project, but to the extent that they succeed in this regard they also provide a distorted picture of the educational benefits of the typical non-DSP research subject's experience. It is also difficult to accept the idea that well-designed debriefing exercises will overcome the inherent differences in the educational potential of the research subject's actual experience of participation in a given research study. If the goal throughout is really supposed to be educational, it seems a more effective approach would be for faculty to involve their students in mock research activities specifically designed to demonstrate key features of research subject participation connected to the rest of the course's curricular content. In sum, the rationale for DSPs may be said to represent the institutionalization of the educational misconception. What is especially intriguing in this regard is the fact that the educational value of research subject participation in DSPs is seldom even assessed, and few if any rigorous research studies have been conducted comparing the educational effectiveness of research participation to the frequently utilized alternative educational options. Some educational institutions have taken steps to eliminate DSPs or impose additional oversight procedures to ensure that when

and if they are permitted, they are closely scrutinized. For some, recruitment of students through broad-based appeals to the general public is considered preferable both ethically and scientifically, as a less selected population of subjects may enhance the generalizability of study results.

STUDENTS IN GRADUATE OR PROFESSIONAL TRAINING. Outside of DSPs, students sometimes participate in research studies related to their field of study, some of which focus on their regular education and training. These studies present challenges resembling those discussed above with regard to primary and secondary school practitioner researchers, with respect to the general issues of possible coercion, the educational misconception, and the inherent limits of confidentiality protections. What is different, however, is that the researcher/subject relationship has grown in some ways: The student research subject is now an adult, and the researcher is now someone whose authority over the student has taken on a different shade. For example, graduate or medical students may view the investigator as an important mentor and career influence, in addition to whatever control the investigator might possess over students' grades, recommendations, teaching or research assignments, and opportunities for postdoctoral work or residency programs. Even if the researcher wishes the students to view a decision to participate as a research subject as entirely voluntary, the students may see themselves as having no choice.

At the same time, academic faculty may view participation in research as an obligation students should accept as a function of their having chosen to pursue a profession in which research plays an integral part. Where faculty are doing research to evaluate the effectiveness of their educational practices, they may feel that students have an obligation to contribute to improving those practices, because the students are benefiting from lessons drawn from studying previous students' experiences (Dubois). At the same time, faculty may be conscious of the importance of providing role models of researchers who treat their subjects with the utmost respect, and must therefore solicit their voluntary consent (Henry and Wright). Hans Jonas argued that those persons who are most knowledgeable, committed, and autonomous should be the first to participate as research subjects, which presumably implies that graduate and medical students should be the first to volunteer for such studies, after the faculty themselves. This argument construes the idea of autonomy more broadly, in the sense that while the student may feel pressured to volunteer for a study at the given moment, the student has chosen to pursue a highly-rewarded profession in which research—with its incumbent risks and sacrifices for human subjects such as themselves—plays an important role. To the extent that a student's autonomy is limited by the personal and professional circumstances of their participation, Jonas's presumption may not be true.

Conclusion

Students' decisions to participate in research may be affected by various influences, incentives, rewards, or compensation, and yet the pressure of these factors does not always rise to the level of undue influence or coercion. Students occupy a wide range of locations along the spectrum of opportunities for participation in research, ranging from invitation to attraction to enticement to pressure to force. Some influences may be altered, while others are endemic to the student's natural condition. As long as investigators and institutions are cognizant of and responsive in the design and execution of their studies to the special situations that arise in research involving students, they can reduce the likelihood that additional social and regulatory limits to their work will be imposed. Unless society is willing to forego all research in which students are the research subjects, the challenges of enlisting students as research subjects under circumstances of mixed voluntariness will continue.

IVOR ANTON PRITCHARD
GREG KOSKI

SEE ALSO: *Informed Consent, Consent Issues In Human Research; Research Policy, Subject Selection; Military Personnel as Research Subjects; Minorities as Research Subjects; Prisoners as Research Subjects; Research, Unethical*

BIBLIOGRAPHY

American Association for the Advancement of Science. 1993. *Benchmarks for Science Literacy.* New York: Oxford University Press.

Appelbaum, Paul S.; Roth, Loren H.; Lidz, Charles W.; et al. 1987. "False Hopes and Best Data: Consent to Research and the Therapeutic Misconception." *The Hastings Center Report* 17(2): 20–24.

Bebeau, Muriel J.; Rest, James R.; and Narvaez, Darcia. 1999. "Beyond the Promise: A Perspective on Research in Moral Education." *Educational Researcher* 28(4): 18–26.

Bruzzese, Jean-Marie, and Fisher, Celia B. 2003. "Assessing and Enhancing the Research Consent Capacity of Children and Youth." *Applied Developmental Science* 7(1): 13–26.

Chastain, Garvin, and Landrum, R. Eric, eds. 1999. *Protecting Human Subjects: Departmental Subject Pools and Institutional Review Boards.* Washington, D.C.: American Psychological Association.

DuBois, James. 2002. "When is Informed Consent Appropriate in Educational Research? Regulatory and Ethical Issues." *IRB: Ethics & Human Research* 24(1): 1–8.

Hammack, Floyd M. 1997. "Ethical Issues in Teacher Research." *Teachers College Record* 99(2): 247–265.

Henry, Rebecca C., and Wright, David E. 2001. "When Do Medical Students Become Human Subjects of Research? The Case of Program Evaluation." *Academic Medicine* 76(9): 871–875.

Howe, Kenneth R., and Moses, Michele S. 1999. "Ethics in Educational Research." In *Review of Research in Education,* ed. Ashghar Iran-Nejad and P. David Pearson. Washington, D.C.: American Educational Research Association.

Jonas, Hans. 1969. "Philosophical Reflections on Experimenting with Human Subjects." In *Experimentation with Human Subjects,* ed. Paul Freund. New York: George Braziller.

Koski, G. 1999. "Resolving Beecher's Paradox: Getting Beyond IRB Reform." *Accountability in Research* 7: 213–225.

Oakes, J. Michael. 2002. "Risks and Wrongs in Social Science Research: An Evaluator's Guide to the IRB." *Evaluation Review* 26(5): 443–479.

Sieber, Joan E. 1999. "What Makes a Subject Pool (Un)Ethical?" In *Protecting Human Subjects: Departmental Subject Pools and Institutional Review Boards,* ed. Garvin Chastain and R. Eric Landrum. Washington, D.C.: American Psychological Association.

Singer, Eleanor. 1993. "Informed Consent and Survey Response: A Summary of the Empirical Literature." *Journal of Official Statistics* 9(2): 361–375.

Steinberg, Laurence; Brown, B. Bradford; and Dornbusch, Sanford M. 1996. *Beyond the Classroom: Why School Reform Has Failed and What Parents Need to Do.* New York: Touchstone.

Strike, Kenneth A.; Anderson, Melissa S.; Curren, Randall; et al. 2002. *Ethical Standards of the American Educational Research Association: Cases and Commentary.* Washington, D.C.: American Educational Research Association.

Zeni, Jane, ed. 2001. *Ethical Issues in Practitioner Research.* New York: Teachers College Press.

INTERNET RESOURCES

American Psychological Association. 2002. "Ethical Principles of Psychologists and Code of Conduct." Available from <http://www.apa.org/ethics/>.

American Sociological Association. 1997. "American Sociological Association Code of Ethics." Available from <http://www.asanet.org/members/ecoderev.html>.

Family Policy Compliance Office, Department of Education. *Family Educational Rights and Privacy Act.* Available from <http://www.ed.gov/offices/OII/fpco/ferpa/leg_history.html>.

Family Policy Compliance Office, Department of Education. *Protection of Pupil Rights Amendment.* Available from <http://www.ed.gov/offices/OII/fpco/hot_topics/ht_10–28-02.html>.

National Committee on Science Education Standards and Assessment, National Research Council. 1996. *National Science*

Education Standards. Available from <http://www.nap.edu/books/0309053269/html/index.html>.

Office for Human Research Protections, Department of Health and Human Services. *Federal Policy for the Protection of Human Subjects.* Available from <http://ohrp.osophs.dhhs.gov/humansubjects/guidance/45cfr46.htm>.

SUICIDE

• • •

Philosophical issues concerning suicide arise in a wide range of contemporary end-of-life dilemmas: the withdrawal or withholding of medical treatment; involuntary treatment; high-risk, experimental, and unconventional treatment; euthanasia, assistance, and physician assistance in suicide; requests for maximal treatment; and many others. Although suicide is often popularly understood in a narrower sense of active, pathological self-killing, traditionally abhorred, the underlying issue most broadly conceived concerns the role that individuals may play in bringing about their own deaths.

Two focal issues concerning suicide are evident in these broader dilemmas. First, should suicide be recognized as a right, and if so, under what conditions? On this first question rest the foundations for various applications of the "right to die," as well as a variety of other issues in high-risk and self-sacrificial behavior.

Second, what should the role of other persons be toward those intending suicide? On this second question rest practical, legal, and public-policy issues in suicide prevention and suicide assistance. Both focal issues concerning suicide raise larger questions about the nature of choices to die and the relevance of mental illness, about the role of the state, about conceptual issues in determining what actions are to be counted as suicide, about the role of religious belief concerning suicide, about the possibility of an autonomous choice of suicide, and about the moral status of suicide.

The Incidence of Suicide

The United States exhibits a rate of reported suicide—10.7 per 100,000 year (year 2000 figures)—that falls approximately midway between societies in which reported suicide rates are extremely low, such as the Islamic countries, and those in which reported rates are extremely high, for example, Hungary. In the United States, there are almost 30,000

reported suicides per year and twenty-five times that many reported attempts; it is the eleventh highest cause of death for the U.S. population as a whole, ahead of homicide, the fourteenth highest. This means that, as John L. McIntosh points out, more Americans kill themselves than are killed by others.

Suicide rates are approximately equivalent across socioeconomic groups. Suicide rates are four times higher for males than females, but attempted suicide rates are four times higher for females than males. Attempt rates for whites and blacks are equivalent; rates of death by suicide are twice as high for whites. Suicide is the third leading cause of death for fifteen- to twenty-four-year-olds. For white males, suicide rates increase with age, rising to a peak of 61.7 per 100,000 in the age range eighty-four to eighty-nine; for women, suicide rates peak in midlife and decline thereafter; and elderly black women have the lowest rate of all adult groups, with those eighty-five and above showing the lowest risk (0.04 per 100,000, a rate based on such a low number of deaths that it is considered unreliable). In the United States, suicide rates declined throughout the 1990s and early 2000s—possibly due, among other factors, to the increased availability of antidepressant medications. Nevertheless, the number of deaths remains high. On average, one person commits suicide in the United States every eighteen minutes.

There are no reliable estimates of the number of unreported suicides, particularly those in medical situations involving terminal illness, the very cases that raise the most pressing current ethical issues. Suicide statistics, including those just cited, primarily reflect suicide in the narrower sense of active, pathological self-killing, whereas deaths brought about by refusal of treatment, by self-sacrifice or voluntary martyrdom, by high-risk behavior, or by self-deliverance in terminal illness are rarely described or reported as suicides. Rates of physician-assisted suicide where legal are quite low: In the Netherlands, where both voluntary active euthanasia and physician-assisted suicide are legal, the former comprises approximately 2.4 percent of the total annual mortality and the latter approximately 0.2 percent, figures fairly constant over the sixteen-year period, 1985 to 2001, for which reliable data is available. In Oregon, where physician-assisted suicide has been legal since 1997 under Measure 16, the Oregon Death with Dignity Act, 125 patients used lethal prescriptions provided legally by their physicians during the first five years of the act, representing less than 0.1 percent of the total annual deaths in the state.

Scientific Models of Suicide

Contemporary scientific understandings of the nature of suicide, primarily in the narrower sense, tend to fall into three groups: the "medical" model; the "cry-for-help," "suicidal career," or "strategic" model; and the "sociogenic" model.

THE MEDICAL MODEL. This model, heavily influential throughout most of the twentieth century, has understood suicide in terms of *disease:* If suicide is not itself a disease, then it is the product of disease, usually mental illness. Suicide is understood as largely involuntary and nondeliberative, the outcome of factors over which the individual has little or no control; it is something that "happens" to the victim. Studies of the incidence of mental illness in suicide often tacitly appeal to this model by attempting to show that mental illness—usually depression, less frequently other mental disorders—is always or almost always present in suicide. This invites the inference that the mental illness or depression "caused" the suicide.

More recent work presupposing the medical model has focused on biological factors associated with suicide, exploring among other findings decreases of serotonin in spinal fluid; drug challenges with fenfluramine; twin studies and other avenues of detecting heritable genetic patterns in families with multiple suicides; and environmental and disease exposures during pregnancy. While work to date remains provisional and in any case establishes correlations rather than causes, it nevertheless points to biological factors that may play a role in suicide.

THE CRY-FOR-HELP MODEL. A second model, developed in the pioneering work of Edwin S. Shneidman and Norman L. Farberow in the 1950s, understands suicide as a communicative strategy: It is a cry for help, an attempt to seek aid in altering one's social environment. Thus it is primarily *dyadic,* making reference to some second person (or less frequently, an institution or other entity) central in the suicidal person's life. In this view, it is the suicidal gesture that is clinically central; the completed suicide is an attempt that is (often unintentionally) fatal. While the cry for help is manipulative in character, it is also often quite effective in mobilizing family, community, or medical resources to assist in helping change the circumstances of the attempter's life, at least temporarily. Later theorists have developed related models that also interpret suicide attempts as strategic: The concept of *suicidal careers* interprets an individual's repeated suicide threats and attempts as a method of negotiating the world, though—as for the American poet Sylvia Plath (1932–1963)—an attempt in such a "career" may prove fatal.

THE SOCIOGENIC MODEL. Originally developed by the French sociologist Émile Durkheim (1858–1917) in his landmark work *Suicide* (1897), the sociogenic model sees suicide as the product of social forces varying with the type of social organization within which the individual lives. "It is not mere metaphor," Durkheim wrote, "to say of each human society that it has a greater or lesser aptitude for suicide, … a collective inclination for the act, quite its own, and the source of all individual inclination, rather than their result" (p. 299). In societies in which individuals are very highly integrated into the society and their behavior is rigorously governed by social codes and customs, suicide tends to occur primarily when it is institutionalized and required by the society (as, for example, in the Hindu practice of *sati,* or voluntary widow-burning); this is termed *altruistic* suicide. In societies in which individuals are very loosely integrated into the society, suicide is *egoistic,* almost entirely self-referential. In still other societies, Durkheim claimed, individuals are neither over- nor underintegrated, but the society itself fails to provide adequate regulation of its members; this situation results in *anomic* suicide, typical of modern industrial society. In Western societies of this sort, institutionalized suicide has been extremely rare but not unknown, confining itself to highly structured situations: the sea captain who was expected to "go down with his ship" and the Prussian army officer who was expected to kill himself if he was unable to pay his gambling debts.

Like the medical model, the sociogenic model considers suicide to be "caused," but it identifies the causes as social forces rather than individual psychopathology. Like the cry-for-help model, the sociogenic model sees suicide as a responsive strategy, but the responses are not so much matters of individual communication as conformity to social structures and reaction to the social roles a society creates.

Prediction and Prevention

Two principal strategies are employed to recognize the prospective suicide *before* the attempt: the identification of verbal and behavioral clues and the description of social, psychological, and other variables associated with suicide. Suicide prevention includes alerting families, professionals (especially those likely to have contact with suicidal individuals, such as schoolteachers), and the public generally to the symptoms of an approaching suicide attempt. They are trained to recognize and take seriously both direct warnings (e.g., "I feel like killing myself") and indirect warnings (e.g., "I probably won't be seeing you anymore") and behavior (e.g., giving away one's favorite possessions). They are also encouraged to be especially sensitive to these symptoms in those at highest risk, especially in males, those who are older, live alone, are alcoholic, have negative interactions with important others, are isolated, have poor or rigid coping skills, are less willing to seek professional help, have low religiosity, and have a history of previous suicide attempts—the last of these being a particularly at-risk group. Prevention strategies take a vast range of forms, from the *befriending* techniques developed by the Samaritans in England and the crisis *hot lines* widely used in the United States to involuntary commitment to a mental institution. Prevention strategies also include *postvention,* or post-occurrence intervention, for the survivors—spouse, parents, children, or important others—of a person whose suicide attempt was fatal, because such survivors are themselves at much higher risk of suicide, especially during the first year following the death.

These models of suicide and the associated forms of prediction and prevention are ubiquitous in contemporary medical and psychiatric practice. Yet although suicide has been treated largely as a medical or psychiatric matter, the conceptual, epistemological, and ethical problems it raises have reemerged in two central contexts: that of right-to-die issues in terminal illness and that of political phenomena such as self-sacrifice and suicide terrorism.

Conceptual Issues

The term *suicide* carries extremely negative connotations. There is little agreement, however, on a formal definition. Some authors count all cases of voluntary, intentional self-killing as suicide; others include only cases in which the individual's primary intention is to end his or her life. Still others recognize that much of what is usually termed suicide neither is wholly voluntary nor involves a genuine intention to die, such as suicides associated with depression or other mental illness. Many writers exclude cases of self-inflicted death that, while voluntary and intentional, appear aimed to benefit others or to serve some purpose or principle—for instance, the Greek philosopher Socrates (c. 470–399 B.C.E.), who drank the hemlock; Captain Lawrence Oates (1880–1912), thean English explorer who, after falling ill during the return trip from an expedition to the South Pole, deliberately walked out into a blizzard to allow his fellow explorers to continue without him; or the Buddhist monk Thich Quang Duc, who immolated himself in the streets of Saigon in June 1963 to protest the Diem regime during the Vietnam war. These cases are usually not called suicide, but *self-sacrifice* or *martyrdom,* terms with strongly positive connotations.

However, attempts to differentiate these positive cases from negative ones often seem to reflect moral judgments, not genuine conceptual differences. Conceptual and linguistic framing of a practice plays a substantial role in social policies; for example, supporters of physician-assisted suicide often use the term *aid-in-dying* as well as earlier euphemisms such as *self-deliverance* to avoid the negative connotations of *suicide,* while opponents insist on the more negative term *suicide.* The term suicide is not used in Oregon's Death with Dignity Act to describe the practice it makes legal, and indeed the statute stipulates: "Actions taken in accordance with this Act shall not, for any purpose, constitute suicide, assisted suicide, mercy killing or homicide, under the law" (Section 3.14). In contrast, the U.S. Supreme Court cases *Washington v. Glucksberg* and *Vacco v. Quill* (decided jointly in 1997) expressly considered the issue as one involving "suicide." Similarly, Palestinian militants attacking Israeli civilians have been called *suicide bombers* by their targets and by the Western press, but they are called *martyrs* by their supporters and those who recruit them for this role.

Cases of death from self-caused accident, self-neglect, chronic self-destructive behavior, victim-precipitated homicide, high-risk adventure, refusal of lifesaving medical treatment, and self-administered euthanasia—all of which share many features with suicide but are not usually termed such—cause still further conceptual difficulty. Consequently, some authors claim that it is not possible to reach a rigorous formal definition of suicide, and prefer a *criterial* or operational approach to characterizing the term, noting its varied, shifting, and often inconsistent range of uses. Nevertheless, conceptual issues surrounding the definition of suicide are of considerable practical importance in policy formation, affecting, for instance, coroners' practices in identifying causes of death, insurance disclaimers, psychiatric protocols, religious prohibitions, codes of medical ethics, and laws prohibiting or permitting assistance in suicide.

Suicide in the Western Tradition

Much of the extremely diverse discussion of suicide in the history of Western thought has been directed to ethical issues. The Greek philosopher Plato (c. 428–c. 348 B.C.E.) acknowledged Athenian burial restrictions—the suicide was to be buried apart from other citizens, with the hand severed and buried separately—and in the *Phaedo,* he also reported the Pythagorean view that suicide is categorically wrong. But Plato also accepted suicide under various conditions, including shame, extreme distress, poverty, unavoidable misfortune, and "external compulsions" of the sort that had been imposed on his teacher Socrates by the Athenian court when it condemned him to drink the hemlock. In the *Republic* and the *Laws,* respectively, Plato obliquely insisted that the person suffering from chronic, incapacitating illness or uncontrollable criminal impulses ought to allow his life to end or cause it to do so. Plato's pupil, the Greek philosopher

Aristotle (384–322 B.C.E.) held more generally that suicide is wrong, claiming that it is "cowardly" and "treats the state unjustly." The Greek and Roman Stoics, in contrast, recommended suicide as the responsible, appropriate act of the wise man, not to be undertaken in emotional distress, but as an expression of principle, duty, or responsible control of the end of one's own life, as exemplified by Cato the Younger (95–46 B.C.E.), Lucretia (sixth century B.C.E.), and Seneca (c. 4 B.C.E.–65 C.E.).

Although Old Testament texts describe individual cases of suicide (Abimilech, Samson, Saul and his armor-bearer, Ahithophel, and Zimri), nowhere do they express general disapproval of suicide. The Greek-influenced Jewish general Josephus (c. 37–c. 100 C.E.), however, rejected it as an option for his defeated army, and clear prohibitions of suicide appear in Judaism by the time of the Talmud during the first several centuries C.E., often appealing to Genesis 9:5, "For your lifeblood I will demand satisfaction." The New Testament does not specifically condemn suicide, and mentions only one case: the self-hanging of Judas Iscariot after the betrayal of Jesus. There is evident disagreement among the early church fathers about the permissibility of suicide, especially in one specific circumstance: Eusebius of Caesarea (c. 260–c. 339), Ambrose (339–397), Jerome (c. 347–c. 419), and others all considered whether a virgin may kill herself in order to avoid violation.

While Christian values clearly include patience, endurance, hope, and submission to the sovereignty of God, values that militate against suicide, they also stress willingness to sacrifice one's life, especially in martyrdom, and absence of the fear of death. Some early Christians (e.g., the Circumcellions, a subsect of the rigorist Donatists) apparently practiced suicide as an act of religious zeal. Suicide committed immediately after confession and absolution, they believed, permitted earlier entrance to heaven. Rejecting such reasoning, Augustine (354–430) asserted that suicide violates the commandment "Thou shalt not kill" and is a greater sin than any that could be avoided by suicide. Whether he was simply clarifying earlier elements of Christian faith or articulating a new position remains a matter of contemporary dispute. In any case, it is clear that with this assertion the Christian opposition to suicide became unanimous and absolute.

This view of suicide as morally and religiously wrong intensified during the Christian Middle Ages. Thomas Aquinas (c. 1225–1274) argued that suicide is contrary to the natural law of self-preservation, injures the community, and usurps God's judgment "over the passage from this life to a more blessed one" (*Summa theologiae* 2a 2ae q64 a5). By the High Middle Ages the suicide of Judas, often viewed earlier as appropriate atonement for the betrayal of Jesus, was seen as a sin worse than the betrayal itself. Enlightenment writers began to question these views. The English statesman Thomas More (1478–1535) incorporated euthanatic suicide in his *Utopia* (1516). In his *Biathanatos* (1608, published posthumously in 1647), the English poet John Donne (1572–1631) treated suicide as morally praiseworthy when done for the glory of God—as he claimed was the case for Christ. The Scottish philosopher and historian David Hume (1711–1776) mocked the medieval arguments, justifying suicide on autonomist, consequentialist, and beneficent grounds.

Later thinkers such as the French writer Madame de Staël (Anne-Louise-Germaine, née Necker, the baroness Staël-Holstein, 1766–1817) and the German philosopher Arthur Schopenhauer (1788–1860) construed suicide as a matter of human right—although Mme. De Staë subsequently reversed her position. Throughout this period, other thinkers insisted that suicide was morally, legally, and religiously wrong: Among them, the English evangelist and founder of methodism John Wesley (1703–1791) said that suicide attempters should be hanged, and the English jurist William Blackstone (1723–1780) described suicide as an offense against both God and the King. The German philosopher Immanuel Kant (1724–1804) used the wrongness of suicide as a specimen of the moral conclusions the categorical imperative could demonstrate. In contrast, the Romantics tended to glorify suicide, and the German philosopher Friedrich Nietzsche (1844–1900) insisted that "suicide is man's right and privilege" (Nietzsche, p. 210).

Although religious moralists have continued to assert that divine commandment categorically prohibits suicide, that suicide repudiates God's gift of life, that suicide ruptures covenantal relationships with other persons, and that suicide defeats the believer's obligation to endure suffering in the image of Christ, the volatile discussion of the moral issues in suicide among more secular thinkers ended fairly abruptly at the close of the nineteenth century. This was due in part to Émile Durkheim's insistence (1897) that suicide is a function of social organization, and also to the views of psychological and psychiatric theorists, developing from the French physician Jean Esquirol (1772–1840) to the Austrian neurologist Sigmund Freud (1856–1939), that suicide is a product of mental illness. These new "scientific" views reinterpreted suicide as the product of involuntary conditions for which the individual could not be held morally responsible. The ethical issues, which presuppose choice, reemerged only in the later part of the twentieth century, stimulated primarily by discussions in bioethics of terminal illness and other dilemmas at the end of life.

Suicide and Martyrdom in Religious Traditions

The major monotheisms, Judaism, Christianity, and Islam, all repudiate suicide, though in each martyrdom is recognized and venerated. Judaism rejects suicide but venerates the suicides at Masada, where in May of the year 73 C.E. some 960 Jews trapped in a fortress built on a high rock plateau killed themselves rather than be taken prisoner by the Romans, and accepts *kiddush hashem,* self-destruction to avoid spiritual defilement. At least since the time of Augustine, Christianity has clearly rejected suicide but accepts and venerates martyrdom to avoid apostasy and to testify to one's faith. Islam also categorically prohibits suicide but at the same time defends and expects martyrdom to defend the faith. Yet whether the distinction between suicide and martyrdom falls in the same place for Judaism, Christianity, and Islam is not clear. Judaism appears to accept self-killing to avoid defilement or apostasy; Christianity teaches passive submission to death when the faith is threatened but also celebrates the voluntary embrace of death in such circumstances; some Islamic fundamentalists support the political use of *suicide bombing,* viewing it as consistent with Islam and its teachings of jihad, or *holy war,* though others view this as a corruption of Islamic doctrine. Thus while all three traditions revere those who die for the faith as martyrs and all three traditions formally repudiate suicide, at least by that name, the practices they accept may be quite different: Christians would not accept the mass suicide at Masada; Jews do not use the suicide-bombing techniques of their Islamic neighbors in Palestine; and Muslims do not extol the passive submission to death of the Christian martyrs, appealing on Koranic grounds to a more active self-sacrificial defense of the faith.

Non-Western Religious and Cultural Views of Suicide

Many other world religions hold the view that suicide is prima facie wrong, but that there are certain exceptions. Still others encourage or require suicide in specific circumstances. Known as *institutionalized suicide,* such practices have included the *sati* of a Hindu widow, who was expected to immolate herself on her husband's funeral pyre; the seppuku or hara-kiri (suicide by disembowelment) of traditional Japanese nobility out of loyalty to a leader or because of infractions of honor; and, in traditional cultures from South America to Africa to China, the apparently voluntary submission to sacrifice by a king's retainers at the time of his funeral in order to accompany him into the next world. Eskimo, Native American, and some traditional Japanese cultures have practiced voluntary abandonment of the elderly, a practice closely related to suicide, in which the elderly are left to die, with their consent, on ice floes, on mountaintops, or beside trails.

In addition, some religious cultures have held comparatively positive views of suicide, at least in certain circumstances. The Vikings recognized violent death, including suicide, as guaranteeing entrance to Valhalla (the central hall of the afterlife). Some Pacific Islands cultures regarded suicide as favorably as death in battle and preferable to death by other means. The Jains, and perhaps other groups within traditional Hinduism, honored deliberate self-starvation as the ultimate asceticism and also recognized religiously motivated suicide by throwing oneself off a cliff. On Mangareva, members of a traditional Pacific Islands culture also practiced suicide by throwing themselves from a cliff, but in this culture not only was the practice largely restricted to women, but a special location on the cliff was reserved for noble women and a different location assigned to commoners. The Maya held that a special place in heaven was reserved for those who killed themselves by hanging (though other methods of suicide were considered disgraceful), and they recognized a goddess of suicide, Ixtab. Many other pre-Columbian peoples in the western hemisphere engaged in apparently voluntary ritual self-sacrifice, notably the Aztec practice of heart sacrifice, which was generally characterized at least during some historical periods by enhanced status and social approval. The view that suicide is intrinsically and without exception wrong is associated most strongly with post-Augustinian Christianity of the medieval period, surviving into the present; this absolutist view is not by and large characteristic of other cultures.

Contemporary Ethical Issues

Is suicide *morally* wrong? Both historical and contemporary discussions in the Western tradition exhibit certain central features. Consequentialist arguments tend to focus on the damaging effects a person's suicide can have on family, friends, coworkers, or society as a whole. But, as a few earlier thinkers saw, such consequentialist views would also recommend or require suicide when the interests of the individual or others would be served by suicide. Deontological theorists in the Western tradition have tended to treat suicide as intrinsically wrong, but, except for Kant, are typically unable to produce support for such claims that is independent of religious assumptions. Contemporary ethical argument has focused on such issues as whether hedonic calculus of self-interest—weighing pleasures and pains, or benefits against harms—in which others are not affected, provides an adequate basis for an individual's choice about suicide; whether life has intrinsic value sufficient to preclude choices of suicide; and whether any ethical theory can show that it would be wrong, rather than merely imprudent, for the ordinary, nonsuicidal person, not driven by circumstances or acting on principle, to end her life.

Epistemological Issues

Closely tied to conceptual issues, the central epistemological issues raised by suicide involve the kinds of knowledge available to those who contemplate killing themselves. The issue of what, if anything, can be known to occur after death has, in the West, generally been regarded as a religious issue, answerable only as a matter of faith; few philosophical writers have discussed it directly, despite its clear relation to theory of mind. Some writers have argued that because we cannot have antecedent knowledge of what death involves, we cannot knowingly and voluntarily choose our own deaths; suicide is therefore always irrational. Others, rejecting this argument, instead attempt to establish conditions for the rationality of suicide. Others consider whether death is always an evil for the person involved, and whether death is appropriately conceptualized as the cessation of life. Still other writers examine psychological and situational constraints on decision making concerning suicide. For instance, the depressed, suicidal individual is described as seeing only a narrowed range of possible future outcomes in the current dilemma, the victim of a kind of *tunnel vision* constricted by depression. The possibility of preemptive suicide in the face of deteriorative mental conditions such as Alzheimer's disease is characterized as a problem of having to use the very mind that may already be deteriorating to decide whether to bear deterioration or die to avoid it.

Public-Policy Issues

It is often, though uncritically, assumed that if a person's suicide is *rational,* it ought not to be interfered with or prohibited. This assumption, however, raises policy issues about the role of the state and other institutions in the prevention of suicide.

RIGHTS AND THE PREVENTION OF SUICIDE. In the West, both church and state have historically assumed roles in the control of suicide. In most European countries, ecclesiastical and civil law imposed burial restrictions on the suicide as well as additional penalties, including forfeiture of property, on the suicide's family. European attitudes and legal sanctions concerning suicide were translated into colonial societies as well, for example in India, Africa, and various Pacific Islands. In England, suicide remained a felony until 1961,

and in Canada until 1971. Suicide has been decriminalized in most of the United States and in England, primarily to facilitate psychiatric treatment of suicide attempters and to mitigate the impact on surviving family members; in most U.S. states, however, assisting another person's suicide is a violation of statutory law, case law, or recognized common law. In Germany assisting a suicide is not illegal, provided the person whose death it will be is competent and acting voluntarily; in the Netherlands, physician-assisted suicide is legal under the same guidelines as voluntary active euthanasia: In Switzerland, assisted suicide is legal if it is done without self-interest on the part of the assister; and in Belgium, physician-performed voluntary active euthanasia is legal but physician-assisted suicide is not. Ongoing ferment characterizes the legal status of physician-assisted suicide in many countries.

Building on Shneidman and Farberow's early work, suicide-prevention strategies have been enhanced by considerable advances in the epidemiological study of suicide, in the identification of risk factors, and in forms of clinical treatment. Suicide-prevention professionals welcome increased funding for education and prevention measures targeted at youth and other populations at high risk of suicide. Nevertheless, philosophers are increasingly alert to the more general theoretical issues these strategies raise, for example, the effect of high false-positive rates on the right to avoid unjustified coercion. Restrictions to prevent suicide— such as involuntary incarceration in a mental hospital or suicide precautions in an institutional setting—typically limit liberty, but because the predictive measures of suicide risk that are available are neither perfectly reliable nor perfectly sensitive, they identify some fraction of persons as potential suicides who would not in fact kill themselves and fail to identify others who actually will. There are two distinct issues here. First, how great an infringement of the liberty of those erroneously identified is to be permitted in the interests of preventing suicide by those correctly identified? Second and more generally, can restrictive measures for preventing suicide be justified at all, even for those who will actually go on to commit suicide? Civil rights theorists are generally disturbed by the first of these problems, libertarians by the second.

Although U.S. law does not prohibit suicide, suicide has not been recognized as a right. There has been considerable pressure from right-to-die groups in favor of recognizing a broad right to self-determination in terminal illness not only by refusal of life-prolonging treatment but also by bringing about one's own death. In the *Washington v. Glucksberg* and *Vacco v. Quill* cases, the U.S. Supreme Court ruled unanimously that there was no constitutional right to assisted suicide, though the Court's ruling did not prohibit states from establishing laws that would legalize it. Cases such as these, however, tend to conflate the notion of a negative right to assistance in suicide, which would prohibit interference when a willing physician wished to provide assistance to a patient, with the far more controversial notion of a positive right to assistance in suicide—something that would give patients a claim to be provided with help from physicians when they sought it.

Other rights issues raised by suicide include, for example, freedom of expression. When Hemlock Society president Derek Humphry's *Final Exit*—a book addressed to the terminally ill that provided explicit instructions on how to commit suicide, including lethal drug dosages—was published in the United States in 1991 and sold over half a million copies, its publication was protected on the grounds of freedom of expression; yet in several other countries, including France and Australia, *Final Exit* was banned. More recent controversy surrounds web sites that provide explicit how-to information about suicide, including how to do so using readily available materials, and internet chat rooms that encourage or dare visitors to kill themselves.

PHYSICIAN-ASSISTED SUICIDE. Although issues of the permissibility of suicide generally have been the focus of sustained historical discussion, contemporary public-policy debate tends to focus on a narrower, specific issue: that of physician-assisted suicide, usually coupled with the question of voluntary active euthanasia. There are two principal arguments advanced for the legalization of these practices. First, claims about autonomy appeal to a conception of individuals as entitled to control as much as possible the course of their own dying. To restrict the right to die to the mere right to refuse unwanted medical treatment and so be *allowed* to die, this argument holds, is an indefensible truncation of the more basic right to choose one's death in accordance with one's own values. Thus, advance directives, such as living wills and durable powers of attorney, "do not resuscitate" (DNR) orders, and other mechanisms for withholding or withdrawing treatment, are inadequate to protect fundamental rights. Second, arguments for the legalization of physician-assisted suicide, usually together with arguments for voluntary euthanasia, involve an appeal to what is variously understood as mercy or nonmaleficence. Because not all terminal pain can be controlled and because suffering encompasses an even broader, less controllable range than pain, it is argued, it is defensible for a person who is in irremediable pain or suffering to choose death if there is no other way to avoid it.

Two principal arguments form the basis of the opposition to legalization of these practices. The first is that killing (in both suicide and euthanasia) is simply morally wrong,

and hence wrong for doctors to facilitate or perform. The second argument is that legalization would invite a "slippery slope" leading to involuntary killing. The slippery slope argument contends, among other things, that permitting assistance in suicide or the performance of euthanasia would make killing "too easy," so that doctors would turn to it for reasons of bias, greed, impatience, or frustration with a patient who was not doing well; that it would set a dangerous model for disturbed younger persons who were not terminally ill; and that, in a society marked by prejudice against the elderly, the disabled, racial minorities, and many others, and motivated by cost considerations in a system that does not guarantee equitable care, "choices" of death that were not really voluntary would be imposed on vulnerable persons. Suicide in these circumstances would become a matter of social expectation or imperative. The counterargument for legalization replies that more open attitudes toward suicide would reduce psychopathology by allowing more effective counseling, and that by bringing practices that have always gone on in secrecy out into the open—and hence under adequate control—legalization would provide the most substantial protection for genuine patient choice.

Data from the Netherlands, where physician-assisted suicide and voluntary active euthanasia have been legally tolerated since the mid-1980s and are now legal, and from Oregon, where physician-assisted suicide became legal in 1997, do not support claims about a slippery slope, though full legalization is comparatively recent in both. In both only a very small fraction of patients who die actually die with physician assistance. Most are patients with cancer: 75 percent in the Netherlands, 79 percent in Oregon. Even so, of patients with cancer, the vast majority of those who die in either the Netherlands or Oregon do not die with this form of assistance. There is no evidence of disparate impact on groups of patients understood as vulnerable—the elderly, the poor, people with disabilities or with developmental delays, and others, although prior to the development of the protease inhibitors, was high for people with AIDS. Pain has not been the central issue; rather, most patients who have elected physician assistance in dying have done so, according to family members, physicians, and hospice caregivers, to avoid deterioration and loss of control over their circumstances. In Oregon, for example, the most frequently reported concerns by patients who died in 2001 included loss of autonomy (94%), decreasing ability to participate in activities that make life enjoyable (76%), and loss of control of bodily functions (53%); inadequate pain control and the financial implications of treatment were mentioned by just 6 percent each.

Particularly relevant to public-policy discussions is the contention of some contemporary writers that suicide will become "the preferred way of death" because it allows control over the time, place, and circumstances of dying. Others claim that as pain control in terminal illness improves, interest in physician-assisted euthanatic suicide will disappear. These may seem to be mere predictive claims. But in the technologically developed nations, where the epidemiologic transition in causes of death now means that the majority of the population will not die of parasitic and infectious disease, as was the case in all societies until the middle of the nineteenth century and is still the case in many less developed nations, but will die of late-life degenerative diseases with prolonged downhill courses, these claims may seem to harbor quite different normative visions of the roles people may—and should—play in their own deaths. One now faces a death that is comparatively predictable and prolonged, often perceived as burdensome to oneself and to those one loves.

Several particularly contentious issues have been raised in view of these facts. One concerns the question of whether a person can have a "duty to die." Some theorists have argued that as the burdens and costs of terminal care increase, both to the patient and to the family, a person becomes obligated to end his life; other commentators find this claim repugnant, an example of the kind of thinking that would fuel a slide down the slippery slope. Resolution of this issue rests on whether an individual's preferences and personal sense of concern for and obligation to family or others can be disentangled from social expectations about costs and savings.

Another issue of growing philosophical concern is that of suicide in old age, for reasons of old age alone rather than illness that accompanies old age. Despite extensive discussion among the Stoics of this matter—they held it to be a reasonable choice—and despite the prospects of vastly extended life expectancies of people in advanced industrial societies, such matters as preemptive suicide to avoid the deterioration of old age have been very little discussed.

Nor has the issue of altruistic suicide, not only in order to spare healthcare costs or other burdens for family members or others, but also in situations such as political protest and military strategy, received adequate philosophical analysis. In situations in which individuals committing suicide believe themselves to be acting for the common good, even at extreme personal sacrifice, is suicide—though it might be labeled with such euphemisms as martyrdom or heroism—morally acceptable or even praiseworthy? Such issues will form the basis for some of the many ethical challenges concerning suicide to be faced in future years.

MARGARET PABST BATTIN (1995)
REVISED BY AUTHOR

SEE ALSO: *Aging and the Aged: Old Age; Autonomy; Death; Dementia; Emotions; Human Rights; Life, Quality of; Life Sustaining Treatment and Euthanasia; Medical Codes and Oaths; Medical Ethics, History of Europe; Mental Illness: Conceptions of Mental Illness; Mental Institutions, Commitment to; Natural Law; Pain and Suffering; Pastoral Care and Healthcare Chaplaincy*

BIBLIOGRAPHY

Alvarez, Albert. 1971. *The Savage God: A Study of Suicide.* London: Weidenfeld and Nicolson.

Baechler, Jean. 1979. *Suicides,* tr. Barry Cooper. Oxford: Basil Blackwell.

Barraclough, Brian M. 1992. "The Bible Suicides." *Acta Psychiatrica Scandinavia* 86(1): 64–69.

Battin, Margaret Pabst. 1982. *Ethical Issues in Suicide.* Englewood Cliffs, NJ: Prentice-Hall.

Battin, Margaret Pabst. 1994. *The Least Worst Death: Essays in Bioethics on the End of Life.* New York: Oxford University Press.

Battin, Margaret Pabst, and Maris, Ronald W., eds. 1983. "Suicide and Ethics." Special issue of *Suicide and Life-Threatening Behavior* 13(4).

Battin, Margaret Pabst, and Mayo, David J., eds. 1980. *Suicide: The Philosophical Issues.* New York: St. Martin's Press.

Battin, Margaret P.; Rhodes, Rosamond; and Silvers, Anita, eds. 1998. *Physician-Assisted Suicide: Expanding the Debate.* New York: Oxford University Press.

Beauchamp, Tom L. 1996. *Intending Death: The Ethics of Assisted Suicide and Euthanasia.* Upper Saddle River, NJ: Prentice-Hall.

Brock, Dan W. 1993. *Life and Death: Philosophical Essays in Biomedical Ethics.* Cambridge, Eng.: Cambridge University Press.

Brody, Baruch A., ed. 1989. *Suicide and Euthanasia: Historical and Contemporary Themes.* Dordrecht, Netherlands: Kluwer.

Daube, David. 1972. "The Linguistics of Suicide." *Philosophy and Public Affairs* 1(4): 387–437.

Donne, John. 1982. *Biathanatos,* ed. Michael Rudick and Margaret Pabst Battin. New York: Garland.

Droge, Arthur J., and Tabor, James D. 1992. *A Noble Death: Suicide and Martyrdom among Christians and Jews in Antiquity.* San Francisco: HarperCollins.

Durkheim, Émile. 1951. *Suicide: A Study in Sociology,* tr. John A. Spaulding, ed. George Simpson. New York: Free Press.

Emanuel, Linda L., ed. 1998. *Regulating How We Die: The Ethical, Medical, and Legal Issues Surrounding Physician-Assisted Suicide.* Cambridge, MA: Harvard University Press.

Fedden, Henry Romilly. 1938. *Suicide: A Social and Historical Study.* London: Peter Davies.

Hardwig, John. 1997. "Is There a Duty to Die?" *Hastings Center Report* 27(2): 34–42.

Hume, David. 1777 (reprint 1963). "Of Suicide." In *Essays: Moral, Political, and Literary,* ed. T. H. Green and T. H. Grose. London: Oxford University Press.

Humphry, Derek. 1991, 1996, 2002. *Final Exit: The Practicalities of Self-Deliverance and Assisted Suicide for the Dying.* Eugene, OR: National Hemlock Society. 2nd edition, New York: Dell. 3rd edition, New York: Delta.

Humphry, Derek, with Wickett, Ann. 1978. *Jean's Way.* London: Quartet Books.

Kant, Immanuel. 1980. *Lectures on Ethics,* tr. Louis Infield. Indianapolis, IN: Hackett.

Kant, Immanuel. 1983. *Ethical Philosophy: The Complete Texts of the Grounding for the Metaphysics of Morals, and Metaphysical Principles of Virtue, Part II of the Metaphysics of Morals,* tr. James W. Ellington. Indianapolis, IN: Hackett.

Kant, Immanuel. 1993. *The Critique of Practical Reason,* tr. Lewis White Beck. 3rd edition. New York: Macmillan.

Landsberg, Paul-Louis. 1953. *The Experience of Death; The Moral Problem of Suicide,* tr. Cynthia Rowland. New York: Philosophical Library.

Maris, Ronald W.; Berman, Alan L.; and Silverman, Morton M. 2000. *Comprehensive Textbook of Suicidology.* New York: Guilford Press.

Minois, George. 1999. *History of Suicide: Voluntary Death in Western Culture,* tr. Lydia G. Cochrane. Baltimore: Johns Hopkins University Press.

Murray, Alexander. 1998. *Suicide in the Middle Ages,* vol. 1: *The Violent against Themselves.* Oxford: Oxford University Press.

Nietzsche, Friedrich. 1953 (1881). *The Dawn of Day (Morgenrote),* p. 210. Stuttgart: Kroner Verlag.

Perlin, Seymour, ed. 1975. *A Handbook for the Study of Suicide.* Oxford: Oxford University Press.

Prado, Carlos G. 1990. *The Last Choice: Preemptive Suicide in Advanced Age.* Westport, CT: Greenwood.

Putnam, Constance E. 2002. *Hospice or Hemlock? Searching for Heroic Compassion.* Westport, CT: Praeger.

Quill, Timothy E. 1996. *A Midwife through the Dying Process: Stories of Healing and Hard Choices at the End of Life.* Baltimore, MD: Johns Hopkins University Press.

Seneca, Lucius Annaeus. 1920. "Letter on Suicide" and "On the Proper Time to Slip the Cable." In *Ad Lucilium Epistulae Morales,* tr. Richard M. Gummere. London: W. Heinemann.

Shneidman, Edwin S., ed. 1976. *Suicidology: Contemporary Developments.* New York: Grune and Stratton.

Shneidman, Edwin S., and Farberow, Norman L., eds. 1957. *Clues to Suicide.* New York: McGraw-Hill.

Sprott, Samuel E. 1961. *The English Debate on Suicide: From Donne to Hume.* La Salle, IL: Open Court.

Thomasma, David C.; Kimbrough-Kushner, Thomasine; Kimsma, Gerrit K.; et al., eds. 1998. *Asking to Die: Inside the Dutch Debate about Euthanasia.* Dordrecht, Netherlands: Kluwer.

van der Maas, Paul J.; van der Wal, Gerrit; Haverkate, Ilinka; et al. 1996. "Euthanasia, Physician-Assisted Suicide, and Other Medical Practices Involving the End of Life in the Netherlands, 1990–1995." *New England Journal of Medicine* 335(22): 1699–1705.

INTERNET RESOURCES

McIntosh, John L. 2003. "Recent Suicide Statistics." Available from <http://www.iusb.edu/˜jmcintos/>.

Onwuteaka-Philipsen, Bregje D.; van der Heide, Agnes; Koper, Dirk; et al. 2003. "Euthanasia and Other End-of-Life Decisions in the Netherlands in 1990, 1995, and 2001," *The Lancet* 361. Available from <http:/image.thelancet.com/extras/03art3297webpdf>.

Oregon Department of Health Services. "Death with Dignity Act." Available from <http://www.dhs.state.or.us/publichealth/programs.cfm>.

van der Heide, Agnes; Deliens, Luc; Faisst, Karin; et al., on behalf of the EURELD consortium. 2003. "End-of-life Decision-Making in Six European Countries: Descriptive Study." *The Lancet* Available from <http://image.thelancet.com/extras/03art3298web.pdf>.

SURROGACY

SEE *Reproductive Technologies: VI. Contract Pregnancy*

SURROGATE DECISION-MAKING

• • •

It is well established in medical ethics, practice, and law that the informed consent of competent patients must be secured before treatment. However, patients frequently are unable to participate in decision making about their treatment because of the effects of the illness, treatment, or underlying condition. This is especially common when patients are critically ill or near death, but it can happen at any time in the course of treatment. More specifically, patients who cannot make their own decisions are those who have been found to be incompetent to make a particular treatment choice; the determination of competence sorts patients into those whose treatment choices must be respected even if others disagree with them and those for whom decision-making authority will be transferred to another person.

When someone else must make decisions for a patient, a possible alternative is for their physicians to do that; when decisions are routine and uncontroversial, this is often what happens. However, when decisions have significant consequences for the patient, it is common practice to seek a surrogate or proxy to take the patient's place in decision making with the patient's physician.

The practice of and requirement for informed consent with competent patients are based on two central moral values: self-determination and patient well-being. Self-determination is the interest of ordinary persons in making important decisions about their lives for themselves and according to their own values; informed consent respects patients' self-determination. Patients' well-being is served by informed consent because the consent process allows a patient to decide which alternative treatment, including the alternative of no treatment, will best serve his or her values and life plans; the practice of informed consent usually, though not always, results in decisions that serve the patient's well-being. These two values can support the practice of surrogate decision making when a patient is not able to take part in decision making. The surrogate can be the person the patient authorized or would authorize to decide for him or her and can reflect the patient's values and life plans.

This entry examines in more detail how surrogate decision making can serve a patient's self-determination and well-being by considering two central issues: Who should be selected to be a patient's surrogate? and By what standards should a surrogate make decisions about a patient's care? (Buchanan and Brock). The entry then briefly considers some controversies about surrogate decision-making.

Selection of a Surrogate

Who should be selected to be a patient's surrogate? If the goal is to serve a patient's self-determination when that patient is unable to take part in decision making, it is appropriate to select the person whom the patient wanted or would want to act as a surrogate. If the goal is to serve the patient's well-being, it is appropriate to select a person who will be well positioned to represent the patient's interests and values. Sometimes the patient will have authorized another individual explicitly to act as his or her surrogate through an advance directive. In most states in the United States a durable power of attorney for healthcare (DPAHC) allows a patient to legally designate a surrogate to make healthcare decisions for him or her in the case of the patient's incompetence. Many other countries also have procedures for designating a surrogate. Ethically, there is a strong presumption that the surrogate should be the person whom the patient selected.

Most patients who become incompetent, however, do not have an advance directive to select a surrogate. In that case the surrogate should be the person whom the patient would have wanted to serve as a surrogate. In most cases it will be clear who that is: either a close family member or a friend who cares about the patient and knows the patient's values and wishes (Brock). When it is clear who the patient would have wanted to be the surrogate, there is a strong presumption that that is who should be selected. In the absence of a DPAHC or guardianship, many states in the United States have statutes authorizing a family member to make healthcare decisions for an incompetent patient; these statutes often list the order of the family members in terms of their relationship to the patient who should be selected. This presumption that a close family member should be the surrogate when the patient has not chosen one explicitly is justified by the fact that a close family member is the person whom most patients would want to be the surrogate. A close family member also usually will be most concerned to secure what is best for the patient and usually will know the patient best and thus be in the best position to represent the patient's wishes and values in decision making.

In cases where it is clear that the patient would have wanted someone besides the closest family member to be the surrogate, however—for example, because of conflict with or estrangement from that family member—that other person should be selected. In other cases there may be conflict between family members over who should serve as the surrogate. In either case it often is possible to resolve the question of who should be surrogate informally with the healthcare team or within the family. If those attempts fail, the healthcare team can have the responsibility to utilize the courts to attempt to obtain an appropriate surrogate for the patient.

In some cases there is no appropriate person available and willing to serve as the patient's surrogate. This typically occurs when no family members or friends can be located, or located in time, to make the necessary decisions. Different healthcare institutions have different procedures and practices for these cases. Relatively routine and uncontroversial decisions often are made by the healthcare team. For more consequential or controversial decisions, such as the patient's resuscitation status or the withdrawing or withholding of life-sustaining treatment, practice varies. Some institutions allow such decisions to be made by the healthcare team after consultation with others, such as the chief of service or an ethics committee. Others go to court to have a legally authorized surrogate appointed for the patient. It is important that healthcare institutions have clear procedures to follow when patients lack a natural surrogate so that decision making is not paralyzed but can proceed appropriately.

Standards for Surrogate Decision Making

What standards should surrogates employ in making decisions for incompetent patients? As in the selection of a surrogate, the standards for surrogate decision making should support the values of patient self-determination and well-being that underlie all treatment decision making. Viewed from this perspective, there are three ordered principles to guide surrogate decision-making. They are ordered in the sense that the first should be applied when possible; if that cannot be done, the second should be used, and if the second cannot be applied, the third should be used. This ordering means that the three principles should be understood as applying in different circumstances rather than as competing for application in the same circumstances.

The first principle is the advance directives principle, according to which decisions should be made in accordance with the patient's advance directive when one exists with instructions that relate to the decision at hand. The advance directive might be either a so-called treatment directive such as a living will with specific instructions about treatment the patient does or does not want in specific circumstances (whereas advance directives typically are used to decline treatment, they also can be used to indicate what treatment the patient wants) or a DPAHC that names a surrogate but also includes instructions about the patient's treatment wishes for the surrogate. Despite great efforts at the end of the twentieth century to increase the use of advance directives, most patients do not have one when they are incompetent to make their own decisions. Moreover, the instructions in advance directives are often so vague—for example, "if I am terminally ill no extraordinary measures should be applied"—that it is unclear what their implications are for the specific treatment decision at hand. As a result there usually will not be an advance directive available that clearly and decisively states the patient's wishes regarding the treatment choice in question.

When the advance directives principle cannot be applied for these or other reasons, the substituted judgment principle should be used. This instructs the surrogate to attempt to make the decision the patient would have made if he or she had been competent in the circumstances that obtain. More informally, it tells the surrogate to use his or her knowledge of the patient and the patient's values, wishes, and concerns to try to determine what the patient would have wanted. Even in the absence of explicit instructions from the patient, a surrogate often will know the patient well enough to have considerable evidence about what the patient would have wanted. However, some caution is needed when there has not been a prior explicit discussion between the patient and the surrogate about treatment because a

number of studies have shown that family members frequently are mistaken in their judgments about patients' wishes, and physicians tend to do even less well in predicting patients' wishes in the absence of explicit prior discussions (Seckler et al.).

One of the most important functions of the substituted judgment principle is to emphasize that surrogates' role is not to determine what they would want in the circumstances if they were the patient or what they want for the patient but what the patient would want for himself or herself. An important responsibility of healthcare providers in working with surrogates is to help them understand their appropriate role however much what they might want for themselves differs from what the patient would want.

When there is no surrogate available who knows the patient well or, more specifically, has knowledge of the patient bearing on the treatment choice at hand, the best interests principle should be employed. That principle instructs the surrogate to attempt to make the choice that best serves the patient's interests. In practice this generally entails making the choice that most reasonable persons would make in the circumstances. This standard is justified because in the cases in which it is used the surrogate does not have knowledge about how the patient might differ from most reasonable persons in respects that are relevant to the decision to be made.

In actual practice decision-making circumstances cannot be characterized as neatly as they have been in this discussion of these three principles. For example, sometimes an advance directive may give some, but not decisive, guidance, and so the surrogate must interpret it by using substituted judgment reasoning. In other cases, there may be no advance directive and a surrogate may have only incomplete knowledge of the patient's likely wishes; in this case substituted judgment reasoning must be supplemented by best interests reasoning to arrive at a treatment choice. The relative weight that should be given in these cases to advance directives versus substituted judgment reasoning or to substituted judgment versus best interests depends on the particular circumstances of the case and how decisive or indeterminate the prior principle is for the choice and thus to the extent to which the subordinate principle must be used to supplement it.

Controversies about Surrogate Decision Making

One of the main controversies in surrogate decision making concerns the degree of discretion surrogates should have in making decisions for incompetent patients. It is not possible to be precise about this and there will be disagreement in particular cases, but the standards for surrogate choice make it clear that surrogate discretion should not be unlimited. More specifically, surrogates should make decisions that are reasonably in accordance with the appropriate principle or standard for decision; "reasonable accord," however, does not mean that others, such as the healthcare providers, must always be convinced that a surrogate is making the best choice. The important point is that it is a mistake for healthcare providers to believe that they must do whatever the surrogate wants no matter how unreasonable that choice appears to be. The law reflects such limits as well; for example, DPAHCs typically do not give surrogates the authority to make choices that conflict with the patient's known wishes or fundamental interests.

A second controversy concerns conflicts between advance directives or substituted judgment standards and the best interests standard (Dworkin). Defenders of the best interests standard (Dresser) argue that an incompetent patient's prior wishes, especially when the patient is no longer aware of or identifies with them, should not be followed when they are in conflict with the current interests of the patient. An example would be a patient with pneumonia who needs antibiotics, is demented, and can no longer recognize friends or family members but enjoys his or her existence watching television and previously said that he or she would want no life-sustaining treatment in those circumstances. Here the patient's previous wishes expressed when the patient was competent appear to be in conflict with the patient's current interests. There is no consensus about how these conflicts should be resolved, although they are probably relatively uncommon.

A third controversy concerns whether and to what extent the interests of others justifiably can override the wishes or interests of the patient (Hardwig). Especially when patients are very near death, decisions about treatment may have little impact on their interests but a considerable impact on others, such as family members. Some have argued that in this case the standard patient-centered model for decision making should be set aside to recognize the needs and interests of family members.

DAN W. BROCK

SEE ALSO: *Advance Directives and Advance Care Planning; Autonomy; Beneficence; Cancer, Ethical Issues Related to Diagnosis and Treatment; Care; Clinical Ethics: Clinical Ethics Consultation; Compassionate Love; Competence; Death; Dementia; Ethics: Normative Ethical Theories; Informed Consent; Life Sustaining Treatment and Euthanasia; Medical Futility; Mentally Disabled and Mentally Ill Persons; Palliative Care and Hospice; Pediatrics, Adolescents; Pediatrics, Intensive Care in; Right to Die: Policy and Law*

BIBLIOGRAPHY

Brock, Dan W. 1996. "What Is the Moral Authority of Family Members to Act as Surrogates for Incompetent Patients?" *Milbank Quarterly* 74(4): 599–619.

Buchanan, Allen E., and Brock, Dan W. 1989. *Deciding for Others: The Ethics of Surrogate Decision Making.* Cambridge, Eng., and New York: Cambridge University Press.

Dresser, Rebecca. 1986. "Life, Death, and Incompetent Patients: Conceptual Infirmities and Hidden Values in the Law." *Arizona Law Review* 28: 373–405.

Dworkin, Ronald M. 1993. *Life's Dominion: An Argument about Abortion, Euthanasia and Individual Freedom.* New York: Knopf.

Hardwig, John. 1990. "What about the Family?" *Hastings Center Report* 20(2): 5–10.

Seckler, A.B.; et al. 1991. "Substituted Judgment: How Accurate Are Proxy Predictions?" *Annals of Internal Medicine* 115: 289–294.

SURVEILLANCE

SEE *Confidentiality*

SUSTAINABLE DEVELOPMENT

• • •

The idea of sustainable development dominates late-twentieth-century discussions of environment and development policy. It is a key term in international treaties, covenants, and programs and is being written into the constitutions of nation-states. An immense literature has gathered around it (Marien). Even those who reject the term must define their views in reference to it. In spite of this influence, serious empirical, conceptual, and normative problems must be addressed if the term is to serve as a comprehensive framework for efforts to sustain the biosphere and advance human fulfillment, economic security, and social justice throughout the world.

The Appeal of Sustainable Development

If the peoples of the world are to cooperate in solving their economic, social, and environmental problems, they must share a common understanding of the relationships among these problems and a common vision of a sustainable and just future. The economic expansion that began in the West several centuries ago has spread to embrace the world, transforming all societies in its wake and creating a global economic system and attendant monoculture with powerful human and environmental impacts. Given the dominance of this system, there needs to be a comprehensive policy framework to guide it—even if the framework adopted is critical of the system itself and seeks to redirect or even dismantle it.

Sustainable development is an appealing candidate for this office. "The key element of sustainable development is the recognition that economic and environmental goals are inextricably linked" (National Commission on the Environment, p. 2). This premise, bolstered by empirical claims that poverty and environmental degradation feed one another and that conservation need not constrain development nor development result in environmental degradation, has obvious political advantages. It allows persons with conflicting positions in the environment-development debate to search for common ground without appearing to compromise their positions. New coalitions of nongovernmental organizations (NGOs) concerned for justice, population, environment, and development issues have formed under the flag of sustainable development. Business leaders have come forward to propose new business-to-business and business-to-government partnerships in the name of sustainable development (International Chamber of Commerce; Schmidheiny). In addition, sustainable development has broad moral appeal among those motivated by concern for present as well as future generations, since it purports to be the name for a process and a future state in which everyone and the environment as a whole will benefit.

"Sustainable" qualifies the idea of development. After World War II it was widely assumed that economic development would lead to greater freedom, justice, and security for the world's peoples. When environmental issues first appeared on the international agenda at the Stockholm Conference on the Human Environment in 1972, the debate was whether—and how—concerns for environment and equity could be reconciled with economic development. In succeeding years, as economic development strategies failed to close the gap between rich and poor, within or between nations, and studies showed growth in world population and consumption approaching Earth's biophysical limits, questions were raised about whether the theory of development could serve either human or environmental needs and whether it did not need to be modified to include ecological, political, social, cultural, and spiritual considerations.

By 1992, for most participants at the World Conference on Environment and Development (UNCED) held at Rio de Janeiro, these issues appeared settled. The principal agreement of the conference, *Agenda 21,* affirms that "integration of environment and development ... will lead to the fulfillment of basic needs, improved living standards for all, better protected and managed ecosystems and a safer, more prosperous future. No nation can achieve this on its own; but together we can—in a global partnership for sustainable development" (United Nations, p. 15).

This entry analyzes why the concept of sustainable development occupies the center of thought on development and environment policy, how it is being defined, what criticisms are being raised about it, and what kind of work is needed if the concept truly is to meet the needs of the planet.

Sustainable development nicely expresses the progressive evolutionary worldview that emerged in the West in the late nineteenth century, with all the presumed objective support of the natural sciences, and the positive attitude toward social change often associated with it (Esteva). This progressivist ideology recognizes the problems posed by the interactions of population growth, resource use, and environmental degradation but is guardedly optimistic about the capacities of modern societies to solve those problems, given public understanding, technological and structural improvements in keeping with sound scientific research, and strong political leadership. As the Stockholm Declaration affirmed: "[T]he capability of man to improve the environment increases with each passing day" (Weston et al., p. 344).

The discourse of sustainable development thus occupies a middle-of-the-road position between those perspectives that take an uncritically optimistic attitude toward growth and technological change and those that predict the inevitability of global collapse. It also confirms the liberal insistence that the meaning of the goal of human development, fulfillment, or quality of life be stated in purely formal terms so that individuals and groups have the opportunity to define it for themselves (Kidd).

The Meaning of Sustainable Development

Mainstream thinking on sustainable development views it as a form of societal change that adds the objective or constraint of resource sustainability to the traditional development objective of meeting basic human needs (Lélé). "Mainstream thinking" refers to those ideological frameworks typical of international environmental agencies such as the United Nations Environment Programme (UNEP); international development agencies, including the World Bank; research organizations such as the International Institute for Environment and Development; and NGOs such as the Washington-based Global Tomorrow Coalition.

The concept of resource sustainability originated in the late nineteenth century in the context of renewable resources such as forests or fisheries, where it informed such ideas as *maximum sustainable yield.* When the language of *sustainable development* came into international usage with the publication by the International Union for the Conservation of Nature and Natural Resources (IUCN), UNEP, and the World Wildlife Fund (WWF) of the *World Conservation Strategy* in 1980, this original meaning was retained but broadened to include the maintenance of ecosystem *carrying capacity* and the management and conservation of all living resources as a necessary prerequisite to development. Thus a clear line of intellectual (and often institutional and professional) descent runs from Gifford Pinchot, the first director of the U.S. Forest Service, and other turn-of-the-century advocates of the *resource conservation ethic* in Europe and the United States, to contemporary mainstream thought on sustainable development. Pinchot's utilitarian notion that "conservation … stands for development … the use of natural resources … for the greatest number for the longest time" remains at the root of contemporary thinking on sustainable development (Pinchot, pp. 42–48).

It is possible to interpret *sustainable development* literally to mean sustaining indefinitely the process of economic growth, change, or development. But this viewpoint is not representative of the U.N. World Commission on Environment and Development, chaired by Gro Harlem Brundtland, prime minister of Norway, the group most responsible for marshaling the data, argument, and political influence necessary to put the term on the agenda of international debate. In the commission's view, although a new era of more efficient technological and economic growth is needed in order to break the link of poverty and environmental degradation, "ultimate limits [to usable resources] exist" and indefinite economic expansion is therefore impossible (World Commission on Environment and Development, pp. 8–9).

Nonetheless, like the goal of equity, the prerequisite of ecological sustainability is often either downplayed or presumed, as in the classic definition offered by the World Commission on Environment and Development: "Sustainable development is development that meets the needs of the present without compromising the ability of future generations to meet their own needs" (World Commission on Environment and Development, p. 43). Ecological sustainability is more likely to be mentioned in a list of *requirements* of sustainable development, such as those composed by the organizers of the Ottawa Conference on Conservation and Development in 1986 (Jacobs and Munro):

- integration of conservation and development
- satisfaction of basic human needs
- achievement of equity and social justice
- provision for social self-determination and cultural diversity

- maintenance of ecological integrity

Issues of Sustainable Development

For many critics, sustainable development lacks clarity of definition, including criteria for and examples of successful achievement (Yanarella and Levine). As early as 1984, UNEP Executive Director Mostafa K. Tolba lamented that sustainable development had become "an article of faith, a shibboleth; often used, but little explained" (Lélé, p. 607). A recent survey of the literature on sustainable development found that "case studies are surprisingly few and often hard to come by" (Slocombe et al.). It is notable that the second version of the *World Conservation Strategy, Caring for the Earth,* acknowledges the ambiguity of the term, and places its emphasis on "building a sustainable society" (IUCN, UNEP, WWF, 1991).

For other critics, the concept of sustainable development is all too clear and fundamentally mistaken. Negative critiques of sustainable development cluster around its (1) empirical accuracy; (2) idea of justice; (3) idea of sustainability; (4) economic assumptions; (5) view of science; and (6) metaphorical and spiritual assumptions.

EMPIRICAL ACCURACY. The empirical basis of sustainable development thinking is criticized both for its analysis of the problems of poverty and environmental degradation and for its proposed solutions to them. Thijs de la Court and Richard B. Norgaard (1988a), among others, argue that mainstream thinking typically ignores the two major factors responsible for both of these problems—the shift of local economies to production of exports for the world market and the adoption by traditional societies of the values of Western urban and capitalist society. Thus global free trade, the solution often offered by sustainable development proponents as the way to greater integration of the local community into the world economic system, will only intensify the problems, lending support to massive, hierarchically managed, capital-intensive industrial projects— dams, plantations, factories, urban settlements—that destroy the diversity and integrity of human communities and environments alike (Sachs). Nor will most of the other policies typically promoted in the name of sustainable development be of much help: more scientific data, more efficient technology, improved managerial capabilities, and more effective environmental education. Much more fundamental and difficult actions are necessary, such as community control of the economy, land reform, changes in cultural values, and reductions in the consumption of industrial commodities and in birthrates (Lélé).

SOCIAL JUSTICE. Most pronouncements on sustainable development hold that social justice, especially in the form of equity between wealthy and poor nations, is essential to the process. Critics contend that these ideas are seldom explicated in any detail, however. The issue of population stabilization is generally avoided, conflicting claims of intragenerational versus intergenerational equity are not addressed, and fundamental civil and political rights are seldom mentioned. In keeping with traditional development theory, there is abstract emphasis on meeting *basic human needs* and, in recent years, *participation of all stakeholders,* but it is seldom clear what these needs are, which ones should have priority, what kind of participation is required, or how sustainable development will result in greater justice or environmental protection.

These questions have become especially acute in the sphere of gender. One of the primary challenges to mainstream thinking on sustainable development has come from the international women's movement through organizations such as INSTRAW (United Nations International Research and Training Institute for the Advancement of Women) and ecofeminist theoretical perspectives, such as those of Vandana Shiva and Maria Mies (Braidotti et al.). Within the women's movement there is widespread recognition of the deep-seated patriarchal assumptions in development discourse and the connections between the destruction of nature and the exploitation of women and other marginal groups in the development process. Mainstream sustainable development theory does little to change this. *Agenda 21,* the blueprint for sustainable development adopted by the United Nations Conference on Environment and Development in 1992, retains a patriarchal orientation, evident in its failure to recognize the special role of "subdominants"—women, people of color, children, native and indigenous people—in each of its seven major themes (Warren). In order to address this problem, the Women's Environmental and Development Organization (WEDO) and other organizations have argued for the need for women to gain control over natural resources and the benefits that are derived from them and for recognition of women's special knowledge and skills in environmental care.

IDEA OF SUSTAINABILITY. Environmental ethicists and scientific ecologists are critical of the idea of sustainable development because of its reductionist approach to environmental values. Discussions of sustainable development typically assume that what needs to be sustained is human use, especially human agricultural use and industrial production. Yet instrumental value is only one of the many environmental values that need to be sustained in the complex interplay of human enjoyment, respect, use, and care of nature, and there is empirical evidence that single-minded pursuit of instrumental value through such policies, for example, as "maximum sustainable yield" seldom succeeds (Ludwig et al.). *Agenda 21* is criticized for its exclusive concentration on the need to sustain the environment for human use. Chapter 15, for example, argues that the primary reason for preserving biodiversity is that it provides a potential source of genetic materials for biotechnological development (Sagoff). This emphasis reflects a strong anthropocentric value orientation, explicit in Principle 1 of the Rio Declaration on Environment and Development: "Human beings are at the centre of concerns for sustainable development" (United Nations, p. 9).

In an unprecedented policy decision in 1991, the Ecological Society of America challenged the widely held assumption that what ought to be sustained is human use of the biosphere. It set the goal of a "sustainable biosphere" as its priority for research in ecology in the closing decade of the twentieth century, thus implying that the biosphere has value in and for itself and that above all else this is the value that must be sustained (Risser et al.).

Failure to recognize that nature has value of its own (as well as for the sake of humans) has serious practical consequences. Not only does it inhibit acceptance of the idea of sustainable development by many environmental and religious groups whose traditions embrace a more generous understanding of nature's values, but it eliminates consideration of those meanings of sustainability having to do with the way life nourishes life—with sustenance. Certain methods of subsistence agriculture, for example, built up over many generations, especially by women, simultaneously nourish human communities and the soil, yet fail to receive public recognition and support (Shiva).

ECONOMIC ASSUMPTIONS. Criticisms of the economic analysis and prescriptions of sustainable development thinking have been suggested above and may be summarized under two primary headings. First, and most generally, are those criticisms that find in the idea of sustainable development only another example of the triumph of *homo economicus* in modern society. There is a prevalent assumption that sustainable development is equivalent to sustainable *economic* development. Thus economists at the International Institute for Environment and Development argue in circular fashion that their "sustainability paradigm," a version of the "conventional economic paradigm, illustrated by utilitarian benefit-cost analysis," if modified to allow for the concept of intergenerational equity, is preferable to the "bioethics paradigm" that recognizes intrinsic values in nature, because, among other things, the latter "inhibits [economic] development" (Turner and Pearce, p. 2).

The second sort of criticism concentrates on the failure of sustainable development thinking to challenge the assumption that economic growth can break the link between poverty and environmental degradation. Although the Brundtland commission recognized "ultimate limits," it nonetheless recommended a five- to tenfold increase in global economic productivity to reduce poverty and provide the resources for environmental protection (World Commission on Environment and Development). Ecological economists such as Herman Daly point out the biophysical impossibility of such growth and the need to arrest, or even reduce, the total "throughput" or flow of matter-energy, from natural sources, through the human economy, and back to nature's sinks. They believe that a strict distinction should be made between *growth,* defined as "quantitative expansion in the scale of the physical dimensions of the economic system," which cannot be sustained indefinitely, and *development,* defined as the "qualitative change of a physically nongrowing economic system in dynamic equilibrium with the environment," which can be so sustained (Daly and Cobb, p. 71). In their view, limited progress can be made in arresting economic growth by enforcing accepted maxims of sound economics, for example, increased resource efficiency and environmental accounting to show how income is actually a drawdown of natural capital or stock resources. Such measures alone, however, will be insufficient without redistribution of wealth and income between nations and classes, as well as population stabilization.

VIEW OF SCIENCE. Mainstream sustainable development thinking is dominated by the policy languages of science, economics, and law. Typical of such discourse is the view that science can provide a value-neutral definition of sustainability acceptable to persons with widely differing value perspectives (Brooks). But critics point to hidden norms in scientific methodology that support the status quo and are inconsistent with the personal and political transformations needed for justice and care of Earth. Moreover, only a very narrow range of considerations can be scientifically determined, thereby effectively eliminating challenges to established value judgments. In addition, the use of *risk analysis* focuses on involuntary costs that ecological changes may impose on society rather than on what should be the most important concern: the altering of ecosystems that risk-free business-as-usual will effectuate (Sagoff). Donald Ludwig, Ray Hilborn, and Carl Walters (1993) argue that the history of resource exploitation teaches the necessity of action before scientific consensus is achieved and that while science can help recognize problems, it cannot provide solutions. They caution that spending money on more scientific research is often a way to avoid addressing problems of population growth and excessive use of resources.

METAPHORICAL AND SPIRITUAL ASSUMPTIONS. Some critics consider the concept of *development* a dangerous mystification of history and do not believe adding the adjective *sustainable* appreciably alters the difficulty. Biologically speaking, *development* means progress from earlier to later, or from simpler to more complex, stages in the growth of an organism. In post–World War II development discourse, it was used as a metaphor for the transition of traditional societies into modern industrial societies (leading to distinctions between "underdeveloped," "developing," and "developed" societies). Used in this way, the metaphor implies a step forward in a linear progression, a natural, organic flowering, rather than a deliberate, culturally specific invention. It also implies that the most modern nations, such as the United States, are the most civilized and therefore models to imitate. Adding *sustainable* to *development* only confirms these biological connotations and hence strengthens its potential to obscure differences among cultures and the drawbacks of modernization.

But more than a misplaced analogy is at issue. *Development* is a powerful secular religion, in the words of Peter Berger, "the focus of redemptive hopes and expectations" (Berger, p. 17). Viewed in these terms, *development* means more than an improvement in material living standards. Development as religion means that human fulfillment is to be found in activities that improve material living conditions, for oneself and for others. Development as religion is a messianic mission to bring the fruits of material progress to the world, and it is questionable whether the idea of *sustainable development* substantially changes this. To depart from the religion of development would require defining the ends of development in terms of qualitative, as well as quantitative, goods—goods such as truth, beauty, freedom, friendship, humility, simplicity. Not only are such moral and spiritual goods the most worthy ends of human life; they may be the only way to empower persons to reduce their consumption, limit their procreation, and live sustainable lives (Goulet, 1990).

The Future of Sustainable Development

Given the value placed upon unthrottled economic growth in industrial and nonindustrial societies alike, acceptance of the goal of sustainable development, even in a weak sense, is a remarkable and positive step (Marien). Moreover, acceptance of the idea of sustainable development in international circles and by the government, business, and NGO leadership of many nations, north and south, means that there now exists an opportunity for dialogue and new social compacts between diverse political constituencies. It is possible to argue, therefore, that the idea of sustainable development offers a realistic way of effecting a potentially radical transformation in global environment and development policy. The question is whether (1) these diverse constituencies can be engaged in a process of mutual inquiry, criticism, and discussion that will lead, step by step, toward improvements in the empirical, conceptual, and normative adequacy of the idea and in meaningful attempts to embody it in practice; and (2) an international political constituency, uniting mainstream and marginal groups and actors, can be mobilized to challenge the entrenched powers that will inevitably be threatened by changes in policy. There is also the question of whether these things can happen quickly enough, before disillusionment sets in and a fragile consensus is shattered. There are several ways of advancing this kind of agenda over the next decade. Empirical understanding of sustainable development will improve with a more issue-driven and democratically structured scientific approach that recognizes the uncertainty of facts, conflicts in values, and the urgency of decisions. Such an approach needs to be transdisciplinary and practically focused on the dynamics responsible for poverty, injustice, and environmental degradation and on how these dynamics may be changed without economic growth through resource depletion. It requires analyses of factors such as human motivation and ownership patterns, neglected in most studies to date. Studies of alternative development policies in the Indian state of Kerala present good examples (Franke and Chasin).

Empirical adequacy also will improve through initiatives such as those now underway to design quantitative "indicators" of sustainability (Trzyna), especially those indexes that can challenge, and eventually replace, the Gross National Product (GNP) as the measure of economic and social well-being. For example, Daly and Cobb (1989) propose an Index of Sustainable Economic Welfare that measures not only levels of consumption but also income distribution, natural resource depletion, and environmental damage. Macroeconomic criteria and indicators of sustainability have been proposed in areas such as population stability, greenhouse gases, soil degradation, and preservation of natural ecosystems (Ayres). Specific moral and material incentives to meet these criteria are also being developed (Goulet, 1989).

The conceptual and normative adequacy of the idea of sustainable development will improve as it is expanded to include the full range of moral and public policy criteria necessary to sustain the biosphere and advance human fulfillment, economic security, and social justice throughout

the world (Corson). Such a redefinition of the goals of sustainable development will need to include (1) development conceived primarily as improvement in the quality of human life; (2) sustainability conceived as the sustainability of Earth's biosphere, with protection and restoration of ecosystems and biodiversity and sustainable use of renewable resources contributing to that end; (3) the transition to a steady-state global economy by reducing consumption among affluent classes while at the same time promoting economic growth in poor communities to meet basic human needs and provide the resources necessary for environmental protection; (4) redistribution of wealth and income between rich and poor nations; (5) population stabilization and eventual reduction to more optimal levels; (6) guarantees of basic human rights, including environmental rights, to all persons, with special attention to the empowerment of women and children; (7) new nondominating and nonreductionsitic ways of producing and transmitting knowledge of the environment and sustainable livelihood; and (8) freedom for local cultures, Western and non-Western, to pursue a variety of alternative visions and strategies of sustainable development.

The philosophy of sustainable development will also improve as discussion moves beyond the confines of economics and resource management into larger multidisciplinary and public arenas. Most mainstream thought on sustainable development has taken place without the benefit of philosophy, theology, the arts, or humanities and with only limited benefit from scientific ecology. Yet intellectual leaders in these fields, from diverse cultures and faiths throughout the world, have been trying to understand the meaning of just, participatory, and sustainable ways of life for several decades (Engel and Engel). Citizens also have substantial contributions to make to an enlarged understanding of sustainable development, as the peoples' alternative treaties signed at the NGO-led Global Forum at Rio de Janiero demonstrate (Rome et al.).

Nowhere is the challenge to mainstream sustainable development thinking more difficult—or more fateful—than in the area of comprehensive spiritual values and morals. In 1987 the U.N. Commission on Environment and Development concluded that "human survival and well-being could depend on success in elevating sustainable development to a global ethic" (World Commission on Environment and Development, p. 308). Faced with the prospect that the mainstream interpretation of sustainable development might well become a global ethic, critics argue for what they believe to be more adequate understandings of human nature and destiny, calling instead for "authentic development," "just, participatory ecodevelopment," or simply "good life." Sustainable development need not be anthropocentric or androcentric; it may be theocentric or coevolutionary (Norgaard, 1988b), a human activity that nourishes and perpetuates the historical fulfillment of the whole community of life on Earth.

J. RONALD ENGEL (1995)
BIBLIOGRAPHY REVISED

SEE ALSO: *Endangered Species and Biodiversity; Environmental Ethics; Environmental Health; Environmental Policy and Law; Population Ethics; Population Policies; Technology*

BIBLIOGRAPHY

Ayres, Robert U. 1991. *Eco-Restructuring: The Transition to an Ecologically Sustainable Economy.* Fontainebleau, France: INSEAD.

Berger, Peter. 1976. *Pyramids of Sacrifice: Political Ethics and Social Change.* Garden City, NY: Anchor/Doubleday.

Braidotti, Rosi; Charkiewicz, Ewa; Hausler, Sabine; and Wieringa, Saskia. 1994. *Women, the Environment and Sustainable Development: Towards a Theoretical Synthesis.* London: Zed and INSTRAW.

Bromley, Daniel W. and Paavola, Jouni, eds. 2002. *Economics, Ethics and Environmental Policy: Contested Choice.* Boston, MA: Blackwell.

Brooks, Harvey. 1992. "The Concepts of Sustainable Development and Environmentally Sound Technology." *ATAS Bulletin* 7:19–24.

Boylan, Michael, ed. 2001. *Environmental Ethics: Basic Ethics in Action.* Englewood Cliffs, NJ: Prentice-Hall.

Cobb, John B., Jr. 1992. *Sustainability: Economics, Ecology, and Justice.* Maryknoll, NY: Orbis.

Corson, Walter H. 1994. "Changing Course: An Outline of Strategies for a Sustainable Future." *Futures* 26(2): 206–223.

Daly, Herman E.; Cobb, John B., Jr.; and Cobb, Clifford W. 1989. *For the Common Good: Redirecting the Economy Toward Community, the Environment, and a Sustainable Future.* Boston: Beacon Press.

Davidson, Julie. 2000. "Sustainable Development: Business As Usual or a New Way of Living?" *Environmental Ethics* 22(1): 25–42.

Davison, Aidan. 2001. *Technology and the Contested Meanings of Sustainability.* Albany: State University of New York Press.

De la Court, Thijs. 1990. *Beyond Brundtland: Green Development in the 1990s.* New York: New Horizons.

Engel, J. Ronald, and Engel, Joan Gibb, eds. 1990. *Ethics of Environment and Development: Global Challenge, International Response.* Tucson: University of Arizona Press.

Esteva, Gustavo. 1992. "Development." In *The Development Dictionary: A Guide to Knowledge as Power,* ed. Wolfgang Sachs. London: Zed.

Franke, Richard W., and Chasin, Barbara H. 1992. *Kerala: Development Through Radical Reform.* New Delhi: Promilla.

Goulet, Denis. 1989. *Incentives for Development: The Key to Equity.* New York: New Horizons.

Goulet, Denis. 1990. "Development Ethics and Ecological Wisdom." In *Ethics of Environment and Development: Global Challenge, International Response,* pp. 36–49, eds. J. Ronald Engel and Joan Gibb Engel. Tucson: University of Arizona Press.

Herkert, Joseph R. 1998. "Sustainable Development, Engineering and Multinational Corporations: Ethical and Public Policy Implications." *Science and Engineering Ethics* 4(3): 333–346.

International Chamber of Commerce. 1991. *The Business Charter for Sustainable Development.* Paris: Author.

International Union for the Conservation of Nature and Natural Resources (IUCN); United Nations Environmental Programme (UNEP); and World Wildlife Fund (WWF). 1980. *World Conservation Strategy.* Gland, Switzerland: IUCN.

International Union for the Conservation of Nature and Natural Resources (IUCN); United Nations Environmental Programme (UNEP); and World Wildlife Fund (WWF). 1991. *Caring for the Earth: A Strategy for Sustainable Living.* Gland, Switzerland: IUCN.

Jacobs, Peter, and Munro, David A., eds. 1987. *Conservation with Equity: Strategies for Sustainable Development.* Gland, Switzerland: IUCN.

Kidd, Charles V. 1992. "The Evolution of Sustainability." *Journal of Agricultural and Environmental Ethics* 5(1): 1–26.

Kitamura, Minoru. 2000. "Constructing a Paradigm for Sustainable Development." *Nature, Society, and Thought* 13(2): 253–260.

Langhelle, Oluf. 2000. "Sustainable Development and Social Justice: Expanding the Rawlsian Framework of Global Justice." *Environmental Values* 9(3): 295–323.

Lélé, Sharachchandra M. 1991. "Sustainable Development: A Critical Review." *World Development* 19(6): 607–621.

Ludwig, Donald; Hilborn, Ray; and Walters, Carl. 1993. "Uncertainty, Resource Exploitation, and Conservation: Lessons from History." *Science* 260(5104): 17, 36.

Marien, Michael. 1992. "Environmental Problems and Sustainable Futures." *Futures* 24(8): 731–757.

National Commission on the Environment. 1993. *Choosing a Sustainable Future: The Report of the National Commission on the Environment.* Washington, D.C.: Island Press.

Newton, Lisa H. 2002. *Ethics and Sustainability: Sustainable Development and the Moral Life.* Englewood Cliffs, NJ: Prentice Hall.

Norgaard, Richard B. 1988a. "The Rise of the Global Exchange Economy and the Loss of Biological Diversity." In *Biodiversity,* eds. Edward O. Wilson and Frances H. Peter. Washington, D.C.: National Academy Press.

Norgaard, Richard B. 1988b. "Sustainable Development: A Coevolutionary View." *Futures* 20(6): 606–619.

Payne, Dinah, and Raiborn, Cecily A. 2001. "Sustainable Development: The Ethics Support the Economics." *Journal of Business Ethics* 32(2): 157–168.

Pinchot, Gifford. 1910. *The Fight for Conservation.* New York: Doubleday, Page.

Risser, Paul G.; Lubchenco, Jane; and Levin, Simon A. 1991. "Biological Research Priorities—A Sustainable Biosphere." *BioScience* 41(9):625–627.

Rome, Alexandra; Patton, Sharyle; and Lerner, Michael, eds. 1992. *The Peoples' Treaties from the Earth Summit.* Bolinas, CA: Commonweal Sustainable Futures Group, Common Knowledge Press.

Sachs, Wolfgang, ed. 1993. *Global Ecology: A New Arena of Political Conflict.* London: Zed.

Sagoff, Mark. 1994. "Biodiversity and *Agenda 21*: Ethical Considerations." In *Proceedings from the Conference on the Ethical Dimensions of the United Nations Programme on Environment and Development, January, 1994, at the United Nations, New York,* ed. Donald A. Brown. Harrisburg, PA.: Earth Ethics Research Group Northeast.

Sarre, Philip. 1995. "Towards Global Environmental Values: Lessons from Western and Eastern Experience." *Environmental Values* 4(2): 115–127.

Schmidheiny, Stephan. 1992. "The Business of Sustainable Development." *Finance and Development* 29(4): 24–27.

Shiva, Vandana. 1988. *Staying Alive: Woman, Ecology and Development.* London: Zed.

Slocombe, D. Scott; Roelof, Julia K.; Cheyne, Lirondel C.; et al., eds. 1993. *What Works: An Annotated Bibliography of Case Studies of Sustainable Development.* Sacramento, CA: International Center for the Environment and Public Policy.

Stefanovic, Ingrid Leman. 2000. *Safeguarding Our Common Future: Rethinking Sustainable Development (SUNY Series in Environmental and Architectural Phenomenology).* Albany: State University of New York Press. 2000.

Trzyna, Thaddeus C., ed. 1994. *Indicators of Sustainability.* Sacramento, CA: International Center for the Environment and Public Policy.

Turner, R. Kerry, and Pearce, David W. 1990. *The Ethical Foundations of Sustainable Economic Development.* London: International Institute for Environment and Development.

United Nations. 1993. *Agenda 21: The United Nations Programme of Action from Rio.* New York: U.N. Department of Public Information.

Warren, Karen J. 1994. "Eco-feminism and *Agenda 21*." In *Proceedings from the Conference on the Ethical Dimensions of the United Nations Programme on Environment and Development, January, 1994, at the United Nations, New York,* ed. Donald A. Brown. Harrisburg, PA: Earth Ethics Research Group Northeast.

Weston, Burns H.; Falk, Richard A.; and D'Amato, Anthony A., eds. 1980. *Basic Documents in International Law and World Order.* St. Paul, MN: West.

World Commission on Environment and Development [Brundtland Commission]. 1987. *Our Common Future.* Oxford: Oxford University Press.